THE PHARMACY TECHNICIAN

Foundations and Practices

MIKE JOHNSTON

Publisher: Julie Levin Alexander
Publisher's Assistant: Regina Bruno
Editor-in-Chief: Marlene McHugh Pratt
Executive Editor: Joan Gill
Program Manager: Faye Gemmellaro
Editorial Assistant: Stephanie Kiel
Development Editor: Jill Rembetski, iD8-TripleSSS Media
   Development, LLC
Director of Marketing: David Gesell
Executive Marketing Manager: Katrin Beacom
Senior Marketing Coordinator: Alicia Wozniak
Marketing Specialist: Michael Sirinides
Project Management Team Lead: Cindy Zonneveld
Project Manager: Yagnesh Jani

Full-Service Project Management: Jared Sterzer
Senior Operations Specialist: Nancy Maneri-Miller
Senior Media Editor: Matt Norris
Media Project Manager: Lorena Cerisano
Creative Director: Andrea Nix
Senior Art Director: Maria Guglielmo Walsh
Cover and Interior Designer: Ilze Lemesis
Cover Image: Jezper/Shutterstock; Monkey Business Images/
   Shutterstock; katrinaelena/Fotolia
Composition: PreMediaGlobal Inc.
Printing and Binding: R.R. Donnelley/Willard
Cover Printer: Lehigh-Phoenix Color
Text Font: Times LT Std 10/12

Credits and acknowledgments for material borrowed from other sources and reproduced, with permission, in this textbook appear on the appropriate page within the text.

Notice: Care has been taken to confirm the accuracy of information presented in this book. The authors, editors, and the publisher, however, cannot accept any responsibility for errors or omissions or for consequences from application of the information in this book and make no warranty, express or implied, with respect to its contents.

Library of Congress Cataloging-in-Publication Data
Johnston, Mike (Pharmacy technician), author.
   The pharmacy technician : foundations and practices / Mike Johnston. — 2nd edition.
      p. ; cm.
   Includes bibliographical references and index.
   ISBN-13: 978-0-13-289759-4
   ISBN-10: 0-13-289759-8
 I. Title.
   [DNLM: 1. Pharmacy. 2. Pharmaceutical Preparations. 3. Pharmacists' Aides. 4. Technology, Pharmaceutical. QV 704]
   RS122.95
   615.1023—dc23
                                                                                              2013036302

10 9 8 7 6 5 4 3 2 1

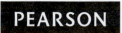

ISBN 10:   0-13-289759-8
ISBN 13: 978-0-13-289759-4

Dedication

This textbook is dedicated to the memory of

Emily

Emily passed away, at the age of 2, as a result of a medication error made by a pharmacy technician. I hope that this textbook, along with more stringent regulations, will help prevent such tragedies in the future.

To Eric

Thank you for your constant support, patience, and understanding. I am a better man for having met you and blessed to have you by my side.

Contents

CHAPTER 3
Communication and Customer Care   28

CHAPTER 4
Pharmacy Law and Ethics   40

CHAPTER 7
Referencing and Drug Information Resources   110

....

II. COMMUNITY AND INSTITUTIONAL PHARMACY 122

....

CHAPTER 10
Technology in the Pharmacy   177

CHAPTER 13

Over-the-Counter (OTC) Products   206

CHAPTER 14

Introduction to Compounding   232

CHAPTER 15
Introduction to Sterile Products 247

III. PHARMACY CALCULATIONS 262

CHAPTER 16
Basic Math Skills 262

Preface

Introduction

The Pharmacy Technician: Foundations and Practices addresses today's comprehensive educational needs for one of the fastest growing jobs in the United States—that of the pharmacy technician. The pharmacy technician career is ranked number 19 among the 100 fastest-growing jobs in the United States. According to the U.S. Bureau of Labor Statistics, the pharmacy technician career is growing at approximately 32%, a much higher rate than other jobs in the health professions. This equates to an anticipated net increase in employment opportunities of 108,300 between 2010 and 2020.

In addition to the tremendous workforce demand for pharmacy technicians, professional regulations and requirements are being established for pharmacy technicians across the United States. With many state boards of pharmacy either considering, or having already enacted, requirements for mandatory registration, certification, and/or formal education, the need for a comprehensive and up-to-date pharmacy technician textbook such as *The Pharmacy Technician: Foundations and Practices, 2nd edition* has never been greater.

Learning Made Easy

The core chapter features include:

- Clearly defined chapter learning objectives inform students of the expected educational outcomes and provide instructors with tools to measure their students' mastery of the material presented.
- Chapter introductions and summaries provide students with a clearer understanding of the scope and rationale for the content being covered.
- Key terms listed at the beginning of each chapter familiarize students with new terminology; key terms are then bolded and defined within the margins of text to reinforce students' learning.
- Numerous full-color illustrations and photographs allow students to visualize content.
- Step-by-step procedures in relevant chapters provide students with clear directions on how to perform the numerous tasks required of pharmacy technicians.
- *Workplace Wisdom* boxes feature tips, comments, and advice from a seasoned pharmacy technician.
- *Profile in Practice* boxes offer practical exercises that simulate real-world pharmacy problems, giving students the opportunity to apply their learning.
- Review exercises at the end of every chapter assess student comprehension. Exercises include multiple-choice questions, Internet-based assignments, and critical thinking questions.

New to This Edition

The second edition of this text contains extensive updates and additions to ensure *The Pharmacy Technician: Foundations and Practices* remains the most relevant and practical textbook for pharmacy technician education. Check out all the updates to this edition:

Updates to Section I

- New chapter on Referencing and Drug Information Resources that identifies and discusses the proper use of the numerous print and electronic drug information resources that are available to pharmacy technicians; includes steps on evaluating the credibility of a reference website.
- Expanded key historic figures/events and added new content on the evolution of the pharmacy technician profession to Chapter 1.
- Added updated and expanded content on the qualifications, educational, and continuing education requirements for becoming a pharmacy technician to Chapter 2.
- Expanded content on nonverbal communication, clarified the differences between internal and external customers, and added terminally ill patients as a type of customer to Chapter 3.
- Updated laws included in Chapter 4, including addition of the Patient's Bill of Rights, USP <797>, and the Medicaid Tamper-Resistant Prescription Pad Law of 2008.
- Added table of symbols commonly used in health care and pharmacy to Chapter 5.
- Moved content on Dosage Formulations and Routes of Administration (formerly Chapter 18) to Unit 1 as Chapter 6 and reorganized content.

Updates to Section II

- New chapter on Over-the-Counter (OTC) Products that explains over-the-counter drugs, presents an overview of the commonly used OTC products by body system, and describes the pharmacy technician's role in relation to OTC products and patients.
- Split Inventory Management and Insurance and Third-Party Billing to become two separate chapters with expanded coverage in each.
- Added direct patient care, drug utilization review, medical information systems, medication use review, productivity and workflow management and ringing up customers, plus expanded coverage of packaging and labeling and pharmacy technician responsibilities to Chapter 8.
- Added content on protocol and formularies, tech-check-tech, and pharmacy technician responsibilities to Chapter 9.

- Added information on health care information technology and electronic prescribing to Chapter 10.
- Added content on evaluating costs and sources, ordering atypical products, and communicating changes in product availability in the new chapter dedicated to Inventory Management (Chapter 11).
- Added formularies, drug utilization reviews, TRICARE, fraud, and information systems to the new chapter dedicated to insurance and third-party billing (Chapter 12).
- Added information on USP <795>, calibrating devices, incompatibilities, PCAB accreditation, and specialized certification to Chapter 14.
- Added new procedures on cleaning a horizontal laminar flow hood, cleaning a vertical laminar flow hood or BSC, dressing/garbing up, proper hand washing, withdrawing from a vial, reconstituting a powder vial, and removing fluid from an ampule to Chapter 15, as well as information on regulations and guidelines.

Updates to Section III

- New chapter on Business Math that includes how to calculate cost, selling price, and markup, understand copayments and average wholesale price, and calculate gross and net profits.
- Revised over 25% of the math practice problems in all Unit 3 chapters.

Updates to Section IV

- Deleted separate chapter on drug classifications and integrated content within other chapters in Unit 4.
- Expanded anatomy and physiology content to Unit 4 chapters as appropriate.
- Added more than 30 new conditions to Unit 4 chapters as appropriate, including prostate cancer, osteoporosis, hyperthyroidism, renal failure, prostatitis, hypotension, and pneumonia, to name a few examples.
- Revised, updated, and reorganized tables and lists of pharmaceutical, OTC, and alternative treatments for the various conditions within all Unit 4 chapters.
- Updated review questions, web challenges, and references/resources as appropriate.

Updates to Section V

- New chapter on Medication Errors that includes statistics, categories of common errors, best practices for avoiding errors, and oversight agencies.
- Added a new chapter on Workplace Safety and Infection Control.
- Added information on poisoning, cognitive impairment, and elder abuse to Chapter 37.

Other Changes

- Updated chapter review questions, web challenges, and references/resources as appropriate.

- Updated and consolidated appendices as appropriate.
- Corrected errors identified by current users as needed.
- Added new photos, illustrations, and tables.

Organization of the Text

The Pharmacy Technician: Foundations and Practices, 2nd edition, contains five sections and 38 chapters. The following is a brief description of each section and its chapters.

Section I—Introduction to Pharmacy

The first section of the book (Chapters 1–7) provides students with an introduction to pharmacy practice and establishes a framework for the student to build upon. This section includes a comprehensive account of the history of medicine and pharmacy (Chapter 1); an examination of the characteristics, traits, and attributes of a professional pharmacy technician (Chapter 2); a discourse on effective communication, customer service, and patient care (Chapter 3); a detailed explanation of pharmacy law and ethics matters (Chapter 4); an exhaustive review of medical terminology and abbreviations used in pharmacy practice (Chapter 5); an overview of the various dosage formulations and routes of administration (Chapter 6); and a guide to referencing and drug information resources (Chapter 7).

Section II—Pharmacy Practice

The second section of the book (Chapters 8–15) provides students with an understanding of contemporary pharmacy practice. This section includes a detailed explanation of community-based pharmacy operations (Chapter 8); a thorough explanation of health-system-based pharmacy operations (Chapter 9); an overview of the use of technology in the pharmacy (Chapter 10); an overview of inventory management (Chapter 11) and insurance and third-party billing (Chapter 12); a detailed review of over-the-counter products (Chapter 13); an introduction to nonsterile, or extemporaneous, compounding (Chapter 14); and an introduction to aseptic technique and preparation of sterile products (Chapter 15).

Section III—Pharmacy Calculations

The third section of the book (Chapters 16–22) provides students with systematic understanding of how to properly perform pharmacy and dosage calculations. This section includes a review of basic math skills necessary to perform advanced pharmacy calculations (Chapter 16); an overview of the various systems of measurement used in pharmacy practice (Chapter 17); a detailed explanation of how to do various dosage calculations (Chapter 18); an introduction on how to perform concentration and dilution calculations (Chapter 19); an overview of how to solve alligations (Chapter 20); an overview of how to do parenteral-based calculations (Chapter 21); and an introduction to business math (Chapter 22).

Section IV—Pharmacology

The fourth section of the book (Chapters 23–34) provides students with a thorough comprehension of pharmacology, including anatomy and physiology. This section includes an introduction to the subject of pharmacology (Chapter 23). It also contains a thorough review of anatomy, physiology, and pharmacology by body system, related to the skin (Chapter 24), the eyes and ears (Chapter 25), the gastrointestinal system (Chapter 26), the musculoskeletal system (Chapter 27), the respiratory system (Chapter 28), the cardiovascular system (Chapter 29), the immune system (Chapter 30), the renal system (Chapter 31), the endocrine system (Chapter 32), the reproductive system (Chapter 33), and the nervous system (Chapter 34).

Section V—Special Topics

The fifth section of the book (Chapters 35–38) gives students an understanding of medication errors (Chapter 35); a thorough comprehension of workplace safety and infection control (Chapter 36); an introduction to special considerations in pharmacy practice for pediatric and geriatric patients (Chapter 37); and an introduction to the use of biopharmaceuticals (Chapter 38).

Appendices

- *Appendix A—Common Over-the-Counter Products* is a current listing of the most commonly used OTC products, organized by drug category.
- *Appendix B—Top 200 Drugs* is a current listing of the most-prescribed medications in the United States, in the order of both total dollars and prescription count.
- *Appendix C—Advanced Career Path Options* offers students a closer look at various advanced practice settings, including long-term care, home infusion service, mail-order pharmacy, nuclear pharmacy, and federal pharmacy.
- *Appendix D—Practice Certification Exams* offers students three unique exams that simulate the national certification exam in both content coverage and question format. Each exam contains 90 questions developed using the content outline of the Pharmacy Technician Certification Board (PTCB) national certification exam. Answers to the exams appear in the Instructor's Resource Manual.

Available Ancillaries

For Students

- Textbook
- *Lab Manual and Workbook*—The Student Workbook contains chapter objectives, critical reivew questions, pharmacy calculation and PTCB review questions, activities, case studies, and lab exercises that test students' knowledge of the key concepts presented in the core textbook.

For Instructors

- *Instructor's Resource Manual*—The Instructor's Resource Manual contains chapter learning objectives, lesson plans for each learning objective (with a customizable section for instructor notes), teaching tips, concepts for lecture, PowerPoint lecture slides that correspond to each concept for lecture, suggestions for classroom activities, and answers to all of the textbook exercises, including the three practice certification exams located in Appendix D.
- *PowerPoint slides*—Includes more than 1600 lecture note slides as well as full image bank.
- *MyTest test bank*—Includes 3800 test questions

MyHealthProfessionsLab for The Pharmacy Technician

The ultimate personalized learning tool is available at www.myhealthprofessionslab.com This online course correlates with the textbook and is available for purchase separately or for a discount when packaged with the book. MyHealthProfessionsLab for the Pharmacy Technician is an immersive study experience that includes pretests and posttests to asses the skills the student learns in each chapter. Videos focused on math and other special topics, games, and anatomy & physiology activities round out the experience. Learners track their own progess through the course and use a personalized study plan to achieve successs.

MyHealthProfessionsLab saves instructors time by providing quality feedback, ongoing individualized assessments for students, and instructor resources all in one place. It offers instructors the flexibility to make technology an integral part of their course or a supplementary resource for students.

Visit www.myhealthprofessionslab.com to log into the course or purchase access. Instructors seeking more information about discount bundle options or for a demonstration should contact their Pearson sales representative.

About the Author

Mike Johnston is one of the most recognized and influential pharmacy technician leaders in the world. In 1999, Mike founded the National Pharmacy Technician Association (NPTA) and led the association from 3 members to more than 20,000 in less than two years, and now more than 60,000 members. Today, as chairman/CEO of NPTA and publisher of *Today's Technician* magazine, he spends the majority of his time meeting with and speaking to employers, manufacturers, industry leaders, and elected officials on issues related to pharmacy technicians, both across the United Sates and internationally.

Mike serves as the sole pharmacy technician delegate to the *United States Pharmacopeia* (USP) and is the only North American representative member of the European Association of Pharmacy Technicians (EAPT). He is also a CPE administrator and field reviewer approved by the Accreditation Council on Pharmacy Education (ACPE).

Mike's background includes experience in community-based pharmacy practice, health-system pharmacy practice, extemporaneous compounding, and as a pharmacy technician instructor. Mike has been nationally certified since 1997 (CPhT) and is also certified in IV/sterile products, chemotherapy, and extemporaneous compounding.

In 2013, Mike opened his own pharmacy—SCRIPTS Compounding Pharmacy—located in the suburbs of Houston, Texas. In addition, he is the author of eight previous textbooks on pharmacy technician education and *Rx for Success—A Career Enhancement Guide for Pharmacy Technicians*.

Mike holds a B.S. with honors in Business Management and Ethics from Dallas Christian College and is currently working on his Masters in Business Administration at Dallas Baptist University.

About NPTA

The NPTA is the world's largest professional organization specifically for pharmacy technicians. The association is dedicated to advancing the value of pharmacy technicians and the vital roles they play in pharmaceutical care. In a society of countless associations, we believe that it takes much more than just a mission statement to meet the professional needs of and provide the necessary leadership for the pharmacy technician profession—it takes action and results.

The organization is composed of pharmacy technicians practicing in a variety of practice settings, such as retail, independent, hospital, mail-order, home care, long-term care, nuclear, military, correctional facilities, formal education, training, management, sales, and many more. NPTA is a reflection of this diverse profession and provides unparalleled support and resources to members.

NPTA is the foundation of the pharmacy technician profession; we have an unprecedented past, a strong presence, and a promising future. We are dedicated to improving our profession while remaining focused on our members.

Pharmacy technician students are welcome to join more than 60,000 practicing pharmacy technicians as members of NPTA.

For more information:
- call 888-247-8706
- visit www.pharmacytechnician.org

Acknowledgments

The author wishes to give special acknowledgment and thanks to the following individuals who represent the greatest contributors to this text.

Joan Gill—for your strong leadership, guidance, and insight on this project as an executive editor. It is an honor and privilege to work with you.

Jill Rembetski—for your persistence, dedication, and amazing talent as a developmental editor. Thank you for keeping me on track with all of the overlapping deadlines and the intense schedule. You are the best in the business, and it is a blessing to work with you.

Stephanie Kiel—for your ability to keep everything organized and on track as an editorial assistant.

Julie Alexander—for your ongoing commitment and support as a publisher.

Mark Cohen—for your initial efforts in signing me with Pearson Education.

Jared Sterzer and the entire team at PreMediaGlobal—for your attention to detail and editing contributions.

Sandy Andrews, Jennifer Susan O'Reilly, Paul Sabatini, and Robin Luke—for being the most amazing team of researchers and assistant writers.

Reviewers

We wish to thank the following individuals for reviewing this textbook for accuracy and providing invaluable suggestions and feedback.

Sheree N. Bryant, MS
Pharmacy Technology Instructor and Program Coordinator
Ashland Community and Technical College
Ashland, KY

Linda Goetz, AA, CPhT
Pharmacy Technician Program Director
CNI College
Orange, CA

Joni Jefferson, CPhT
Pharmacy Technician Instructor
Black Hawk College: PaCE
Davenport, IA

Joshua Kramer, BS, CPhT
Director of Technology
Pharmacy Technician Program Director
Arizona College
Glendale, AZ

Kathryn McGlothlen, MHA, CPhT
Program Director
Brookline College
Phoenix, AZ

Michael C. Melvin, RPh /BS PHR
Pharmacy Technology Director
Southern Crescent Technical College
Griffin, GA

Loretta Montano, CPhT
Program Director
Pharmacy Technician
Brookline College
Albuquerque, NM

Shelby L. Newberry, MCPhT
Pharmacy Technician Program Director
Externship Coordinator
Vatterott College
Kansas City, MO

Carol A Penrosa, MS, RN
Faculty, Associate Degree Nursing
Southeast Community College
Lincoln, NE

Karen Snipe, CPhT, MEd
Department Head
Pharmacy Technician Program Coordinator
Trident Technical College
Charleston, SC

Reviewers from the 1st Edition

Julette Barta, CPhT, BSIT
Pharmacy Technician Instructor
San Joaquin Valley College
Rancho Cucamonga, CA

Kathleen M. Beall, BS, RT (R)
Clinical Instructor
Pima Medical Institute
Mesa, AZ

Amy Elias, CPhT, RPhT
Instructor
Richland College
Dallas, TX

Michelle Goeking, BM, CPhT
Instructor
Black Hawk College
Moline, IL

Jeff Gricar, CPhT, MEd
Faculty, Pharmacy Technician Program
Houston Community College
Houston, TX

Michael M. Hayter, PharmD, MBA
Adjunct Instructor, Pharmacy Technology and Health Information
Virginia Highlands Community College
Abingdon, VA

Anne P. LaVance, BS, CPhT
Director
Pharmacy Technician Program
Delgado Community College
New Orleans, LA

Michele Benjamin Lesmeister, MA
Renton Technical College
Renton, WA

Chris Neer, CPhT
Lead Pharmacy Tech Instructor
Remington College—Memphis Campus
Memphis, TN

Vincent Range
Assistant Professor of Mathematics
ATS Math Chairman
Jefferson College
Hillsboro, MO

DeEtta Ryan, MBA
Basic Studies Instructor
Renton Technical College
Renton, WA

Paula Denise Silver, BS Biology, PharmD
Medical Instructor
Medical Careers Institute
Newport News, VA

Karen Snipe, CPhT Med
Department Head
Diagnostic and Imaging Services
Trident Technical College
Charleston, SC

Bobbi Steelman, CPhT, MEd, Specialist in School Administration
Pharmacy Technician Program Manager
Draughons Junior College
Bowling Green, KY

Benjamin Walker, CPhT
Program Director
ATI Career Center
Dallas, TX

Chapter Features

Learning Objectives

Each chapter opens with a list of learning objectives, which can be used to identify the material and skills the student should know upon successful completion of the chapter.

LEARNING OBJECTIVES

After completing this chapter, you should be able to:

- Describe the origins of pharmacy practice from the Age of Antiquity.

- Discuss changes in pharmacy practice during the Middle Ages.

- Describe changes in pharmacy practice during the Renaissance.

- List significant milestones for pharmacy practice from the 18th, 19th, 20th, and 21st centuries.

- Discuss the role biotechnology and genetic engineering could have on the future of pharmacy practice.

Key Terms

The **Key Terms** section appears at the beginning of each chapter. The terms are listed in alphabetical order, and the terminology appears in boldface on first introduction in the text. A feature in the margin gives the definition of the term so that students have definitions immediately available in the context of the chapter content.

KEY TERMS

apothecary, p. 2
biotechnology, p. 8
compounding, p. 2
pharmacogenomics, p. 9
pharmacopoeia, p. 6
pharmacy, p. 1
prescription, p. 7

Information Boxes

Information Boxes containing additional historical, technical, or interesting content related to the chapter appear throughout each chapter.

info — Working for an Insurance Comapny

Many insurance companies are now recruiting and hiring pharmacy technicians because of their extensive knowledge of medications, insurance benefits, and the billing process.

Profile in Practice

Profile in Practice boxes in each chapter feature short scenarios that depict realistic pharmacy problems. Students use knowledge they have gained from the chapter to answer the critical thinking questions related to the scenario.

PROFILE IN PRACTICE

Dave is a pharmacy technician working in a retail pharmacy. He is processing a prescription for 90 Zoloft 100 mg tablets to be taken one at bedtime. The insurance company has rejected the prescription, citing "Incorrect Days Supply," but the patient insists that her paperwork stated she could get a three-month supply of her medications.

▶ *How should Dave assist his patient?*

Workplace Wisdom

Workplace Wisdom boxes interspersed throughout each chapter offer helpful tips, comments, and additional resources and provide additional information the student might use on the job.

Workplace Wisdom HMOs

Common HMO providers include Aetna, Cigna, Humana, Kaiser, and TRICARE (CHAMPUS).

Chapter Summary

Each **Chapter Summary** is an excellent review of the chapter content.

Summary

Insurance billing requires a comprehensive knowledge of billing terms, codes, and policies, such as DAW codes, authorized days supply, and formularies. Many insurance claim rejections can be prevented by ensuring that all information is correctly entered into the pharmacy's computer system before a claim is submitted.

When properly trained, pharmacy technicians are able to assist the pharmacist by handling these responsibilities and allowing the pharmacist to focus on more clinical aspects of providing pharmaceutical care. These responsibilities vary by facility, but with time and experience, pharmacy technicians can effectively manage these aspects of pharmacy practice.

Chapter Review Questions

Multiple-Choice Questions appear at the end of every chapter to measure the student's understanding and retention of the material presented in the chapter. These tools are available for use by the student or can be used by the instructor as an outcome assessment. Answers appear in the *Instructor's Resource Manual*.

Chapter Review Questions

1. Medicare is the federally funded insurance program for people, including those _____.
   a. aged 60 or older
   b. with disabilities
   c. with cardiac disease
   d. in active duty in the military

2. What is the correct DAW code for a prescription on which the physician does not permit generic substitution?
   a. 0
   b. 1
   c. 2
   d. 3

6. An error code of "Patient Not Covered" means _____.
   a. the insurance coverage has been terminated
   b. the name is entered incorrectly
   c. the date of birth is incorrect
   d. any of the above

7. Aetna is an example of a(n) _____.
   a. HMO
   b. PPO
   c. drug discount card
   d. worker's compensation plan

8. Which of the following actions would *not* affect

Additional Features

Critical Thinking Questions

Thought-provoking **critical thinking questions** appear at the end of chapters to test student's comprehension on the chapter content. Students must rely on the content in the text and their own critical thinking skills to answer the questions.

Critical Thinking Questions

1. What incentive do drug manufacturers have to establish patient-assistance programs?

2. If an individual has a worker's compensation claim, yet requests to use his or her personal insurance plan, what are the potential consequences?

3. Why would January typically be the month with the most insurance rejections? What strategies could a pharmacy implement to reduce rejections?

Web Challenges

Web Challenges at the end of chapters lead students to perform Internet research related to a chapter's content on the Internet, and then either answer questions related to their search, or prepare information about what they have discovered.

Web Challenge

1. Using the Internet, research various prescription insurance plans and write a brief report on an HMO plan, a PPO plan, and a drug discount card program that you find.

2. To learn more about both Medicare prescription drug coverage and formularies, review the CMS Medicare Formulary at http://www.cms.gov Search under the Medicare tab from the home page, and then review the options under Prescription Drug Coverage.

References and Resources

This listing at the end of each chapter provides additional information (organization contact information, websites, etc.) that is related to chapter content, as well as location information for references used in preparation of the text.

References and Resources

"A Primer on Pharmacy Information Systems." *Journal of Healthcare Information Management*. Web. 6 June 2012.

American Society of Health-System Pharmacists. "ASHP Guidelines on Medication-Use Evaluation." *American Journal of Health-System Pharmacy*. 53 (1996): 1953–1955. Print.

"Definition of Pharmacy Benefit Manager." MedicineNet .com. Web. 20 September 2012.

Johnston, Mike. *The Pharmacy Technician: Foundations and Practices*. 1st ed. Upper Saddle River, NJ: Pearson, 2009. Print.

"Retail Pharmacies." *Prodigy Systems*. Web. 13 June 2012.

"The Laws That Govern The Securities Act." *Securities and Exchange Commission*. Web. 30 August 2012.

"What are Drug Utilization Reviews (DUR)?" *The Academy of Managed Care Pharmacy's Concepts in Managed Care Pharmacy*. Web. 6 June 2012.

"What do pharmacy system costs?" *Pharmacy Management Software*. Web. 6 June 2012.

"What is CHAMPVA?" *U.S. Department of Veterans Affairs*. Web. 6 June 2012.

Procedures

Step-by-step **Procedures** appear where relevant throughout the text to help students systematically work through processes and procedures they will perform on the job.

Examples

Numerous **Examples** appear in the Pharmacy Calculations chapters to help students visualize the most effective ways to work through different problem types.

EXAMPLE 16.22 DIVIDING FRACTIONS

$$\frac{2}{8} \div \frac{3}{7} = \underline{\hspace{2cm}}$$

$$\frac{2}{8} \times \frac{7}{3} = \underline{\hspace{2cm}}$$

$$2 \times 7 = 14$$

$$8 \times 3 = 24$$

So, $\frac{2}{8} \div \frac{3}{7} = \frac{14}{24}$, which can be reduced to $\frac{7}{12}$.

Practice Problems

Practice Problems are also interspersed throughout the Pharmacy Calculations chapters to give students ample opportunities to apply the information they have learned in the chapter.

Practice Problems 16-10
Ratios as Percentages

Convert the following ratios to percentages.

1. 6:8 = _____
2. 1:25 = _____
3. 1:250 = _____
4. 1:10 = _____
5. 4:16 = _____

Illustrations and Photos

Numerous **full color illustrations and photos** appear throughout the chapters to provide students with visuals and comparisons to reinforce the lesson.

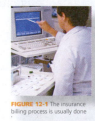
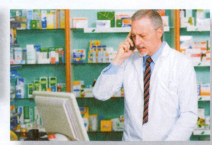

FIGURE 12-1 The insurance billing process is usually done

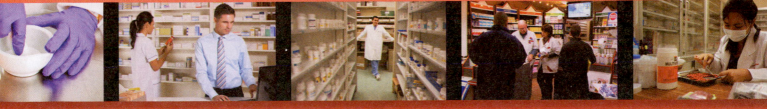

CHAPTER 1

History of Pharmacy Practice

LEARNING OBJECTIVES

After completing this chapter, you should be able to:

- Describe the origins of pharmacy practice from the Age of Antiquity.

- Discuss changes in pharmacy practice during the Middle Ages.

- Describe changes in pharmacy practice during the Renaissance.

- List significant milestones for pharmacy practice from the 18th, 19th, 20th, and 21st centuries.

- Discuss the role biotechnology and genetic engineering could have on the future of pharmacy practice.

KEY TERMS

apothecary, p. 2
biotechnology, p. 8
compounding, p. 2
pharmacogenomics, p. 9
pharmacopoeia, p. 6
pharmacy, p. 1
prescription, p. 7

INTRODUCTION

Pharmacy is an ancient profession. Although the word *pharmacy* comes from the ancient Greek word *pharmakon*, meaning "drug," the actual origin of pharmacy practice has been traced back to ancient times more than 7,000 years ago.

At first glance, learning about the history of pharmacy practice may seem unnecessary for someone who is preparing to become a pharmacy technician. However, if you are to understand many of the concepts, theories, and practices that are covered in the following chapters, you must understand the evolution of the profession. Many of the principles used in pharmacy thousands of years ago are still practiced. Knowing this history will help you appreciate the evolution of this profession and the development of professional guidelines and regulations.

---

pharmacy the art and science of preparing and dispensing medication.

Rx Symbol

Rx is commonly considered an abbreviation for the Latin word *recipere* or *recipe*, which means "Take, thou." Additional medical abbreviations also use *x*: For example, sx = signs and symptoms, tx = treatment, hx = history, and dx = diagnosis. However, the Rx symbol is not really the standard letters "R" and "x," but actually a symbol of an italic R with a leg that hangs down below the line with a line crossing it like an x (Figure 1-1). According to the 1931 book *Devils, Drugs, and Doctors*,

"Rx is not, as is frequently supposed, an abbreviation of a Latin word meaning recipe or compound, but is an invocation to Jupiter, a prayer for his aid to make the treatment effective. . . . [S]ometimes in old medical manuscripts all the R's occurring in the text were crossed."

In other words, the Rx symbol was a corruption of the ancient symbol for the Roman god Jupiter.

FIGURE 1-1 The Rx symbol.

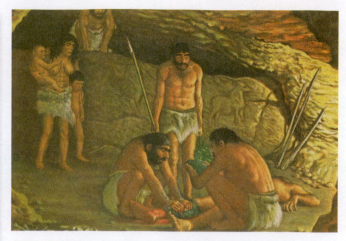

FIGURE 1-2 Ancient humans and medicine. (Images by Robert Thom. Printed with permission of American Pharmacists Association Foundation. Copyright 2009 APhA Foundation.)

symptoms of illness, as well as prescriptions and instructions for **compounding**, or preparing, remedies.

Mithradates VI

Mithradates VI, also known as Mithradates the Great, was king of Pontus and Armenia Minor (modern-day Turkey) from 120 BCE to 63 BCE (Figure 1-3). For seven years after the assassination of his father, Mithradates lived in the wilderness and developed an immunity to poisons by regularly consuming them in small, nonlethal doses. In addition, he used his prisoners as

The Age of Antiquity

The Age of Antiquity refers to the time span of 5000 BCE (BC) up through (AD) 499 CE. This is the time of ancient humans and the great ancient empires.

Ancient Humans

The origin of pharmacy can be traced back to the crude and simple discoveries of ancient humans, who are most commonly referred to as cavemen (Figure 1-2). Ancient humans learned from observing their environment, as well as acting on instinct. They watched as both birds and beasts applied cool water, leaves, dirt, or mud to themselves; consequently, these materials became the first soothing remedies for humans as well. By trial and error, humans learned which plant and mineral remedies worked best, and eventually they began to share this knowledge with others.

Ancient Mesopotamia

Babylon, which is referred to as the cradle of civilization, provides the earliest known record of **apothecary** practice. Around 2600 BCE, healers were priest, pharmacist, and physician all in one. Archaeologists have found clay tablets that record the

---

apothecary Latin term for pharmacist; also used as a general term to refer to the early practice of pharmacy.

compounding producing, mixing, or preparing a drug by combining two or more ingredients.

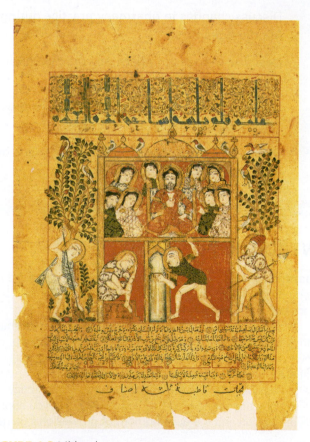

FIGURE 1-3 Mithradates.
Source: DEA/J. E. BULLOZ/Getty Images

subjects for testing poisons and antidotes. Based upon his experiences, studies, and writings, Mithradates developed a "universal antidote" for poisoning, known as Mithradates' antidote. He is regarded as the father of toxicology.

Ancient China

According to legend, in 2000 BCE, Chinese Emperor Shen Nung took interest in and researched the medicinal value of several hundred herbs, testing many of them on himself. Additionally, he wrote the first *Pen T-Sao*, or native herbal, recording 365 drugs. In modern times, Shen Nung is worshipped as the patron god of native Chinese drug guilds.

Ancient Egypt

The practice of pharmacy in ancient Egypt was conducted by two classes of workers: echelons and chiefs of fabrication. Echelons were gatherers and preparers of drugs, similar to the modern-day pharmacy technician, whereas chiefs of fabrication were the head pharmacists.

Although our knowledge of Egyptian medicine comes from records made as early as 2900 BCE, the most important Egyptian pharmaceutical document is the *Papyrus Ebers*, written in 1500 BCE. The *Papyrus Ebers* is a collection of 800 prescriptions that specifically mentions 700 unique drugs.

Ancient India

More than 2,000 drugs are recorded in the *Charaka Samhita*, an ancient Indian manuscript originating from as early as 1000 BCE. The *Charaka Samhita*, which means "compendium of wandering physicians," is the work of multiple authors and was written in Sanskrit, an ancient Indian language.

Ancient Greece and Rome

Terra Sigilata, or "sealed earth," was the first therapeutic agent to bear a trademark. Originating in ancient Greece prior to 500 BCE off the island of Lemnos, Terra Sigilata was a small clay tablet, similar in size to an aspirin. Each year, the people of Lemnos dug clay from a pit on a Lemnian hillside in the presence of political and religious leaders. The clay was washed, refined, shaped into uniform tablets, impressed with an official seal, sun-dried, and then distributed commercially. Thus, it is a precursor to today's branded and marketed drugs.

Hippocrates

Hippocrates of Cos was an ancient Greek physician who lived between 460 BCE and 377 BCE (Figure 1-4). He was a third-generation physician, philosopher, and professor at the Cos School of Medicine. Known as the father of medicine, Hippocrates is commonly regarded as one of the most notable figures of all time in medicine. One of his writings, *Corpus Hippocraticum*, rejected the widely held view that illness was connected to mystical or demonic forces; instead, it positioned medicine as a branch of science.

Hippocrates developed the theory of humors, in which an individual's health was supposed to be connected to the balance, or harmony, of four basic bodily fluids, known as *humors*, which also related to a mood or personality characteristic: blood (joyful/happy), phlegm (lethargic), yellow bile (irritable), and dark or black bile (angry).

In total, Hippocrates published more than 70 writings related to or referencing the practice of medicine and apothecary. Modern physicians still take the Hippocratic Oath, as part of which they pledge to "do no harm."

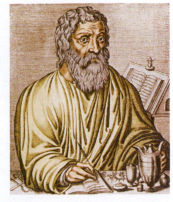

FIGURE 1-4 Hippocrates of Cos. (Stock Montage/Hulton Archive/Getty Images.)

Theophrastus

Theophrastus, one of the greatest early Greek philosophers and natural scientists, observed and wrote extensively on the medicinal qualities of herbs (Figure 1-5). Known as the father of botany, his observations and writings, which date back to about 300 BCE, were surprisingly accurate, as measured by present research and knowledge. Among his work, Theophrastus classified plants according to their methods of growth, locales, sizes, and practical uses.

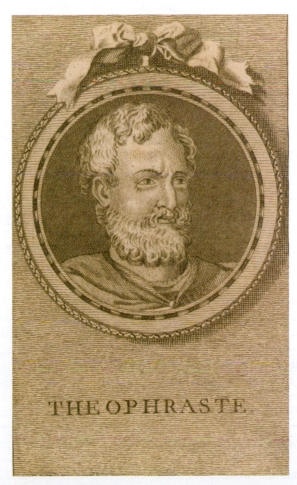

THEOPHRASTE

FIGURE 1-5 Theophrastus.

A Comparison of the Original Hippocratic Oath with the Modern Version

The Original Hippocratic Oath (translated into English)	The Modern Hippocratic Oath
I swear by Apollo, the healer, Asclepius, Hygieia, and Panacea, and I take to witness all the gods, all the goddesses, to keep according to my ability and my judgment, the following Oath and agreement: To consider dear to me, as my parents, him who taught me this art; to live in common with him and, if necessary, to share my goods with him; to look upon his children as my own brothers, to teach them this art, without charging a fee; and that by my teaching, I will impart a knowledge of this art to my own sons, and to my teacher's sons, and to disciples bound by an indenture and oath according to the medical laws, and no others. I will prescribe regimens for the good of my patients according to my ability and my judgment and never do harm to anyone. I will not give a lethal drug to anyone if I am asked, nor will I advise such a plan; and similarly I will not give a woman a pessary to cause an abortion. But I will preserve the purity of my life and my arts. I will not cut for stone, even for patients in whom the disease is manifest; I will leave this operation to be performed by practitioners, specialists in this art. In every house where I come I will enter only for the good of my patients, keeping myself far from all intentional ill-doing and all seduction and especially from the pleasures of love with women or with men, be they free or slaves. All that may come to my knowledge in the exercise of my profession or in daily commerce with men, which ought not to be spread abroad, I will keep secret and will never reveal. If I keep this oath faithfully, may I enjoy my life and practice my art, respected by all men and in all times; but if I swerve from it or violate it, may the reverse be my lot.	I swear to fulfill, to the best of my ability and judgment, this covenant: I will respect the hard-won scientific gains of those physicians in whose steps I walk, and gladly share such knowledge as is mine with those who are to follow. I will apply, for the benefit of the sick, all measures [that] are required, avoiding those twin traps of over-treatment and therapeutic nihilism. I will remember that there is art to medicine as well as science, and that warmth, sympathy, and understanding may outweigh the surgeon's knife or the chemist's drug. I will not be ashamed to say "I know not," nor will I fail to call in my colleagues when the skills of another are needed for a patient's recovery. I will respect the privacy of my patients, for their problems are not disclosed to me that the world may know. Most especially must I tread with care in matters of life and death. If it is given to me to save a life, all thanks. But it may also be within my power to take a life; this awesome responsibility must be faced with great humbleness and awareness of my own frailty. Above all, I must not play at God. I will remember that I do not treat a fever chart, a cancerous growth, but a sick human being, whose illness may affect the person's family and economic stability. My responsibility includes these related problems, if I am to care adequately for the sick. I will prevent disease whenever I can, for prevention is preferable to cure. I will remember that I remain a member of society with special obligations to all my fellow human beings, those sound of mind and body, as well as the infirm. If I do not violate this oath, may I enjoy life and art, respected while I live and remembered with affection thereafter. May I always act so as to preserve the finest traditions of my calling and may I long experience the joy of healing those who seek my help.

Dioscorides

During the 1st century of the common era, another Roman named Pedanios Dioscorides accompanied the Roman armies on their journeys throughout the known world, in order to study medicinal treatments. He recorded his observations and developed precise rules for collecting, storing, and using drugs. His writings, a five-volume book titled *De Materia Medica*, were used by medical professionals as late as the 16th century and contained information on more than 600 plants and minerals (Figure 1-6). *De Materia Medica*, considered the precursor to all modern pharmacopoeias, is the principal historical reference on the medicines used by the Greeks, Romans, and other cultures of antiquity.

Galen

Galen practiced and taught both pharmacy and medicine in Rome during 130–200 CE (Figure 1-7). After attending medical schools in Greece and Egypt, he eventually became the personal physician for the Roman imperial family. Galen contributed to the study of medicine by writing more than 100 books on topics that included physiology, hygiene, pathology, pharmacology, blood-letting, and therapeutics. His principles for preparing and compounding medicines reigned in the Western world for 1,500 years, and his name is still associated with the class of pharmaceuticals compounded by mechanical means—galenicals.

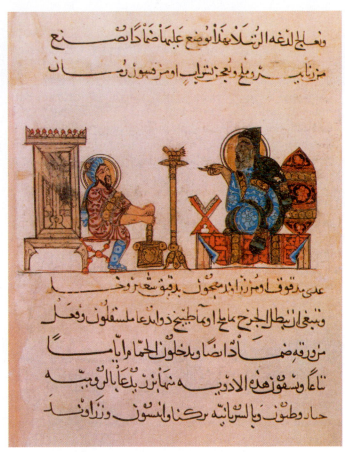

FIGURE 1-6 Dioscorides.

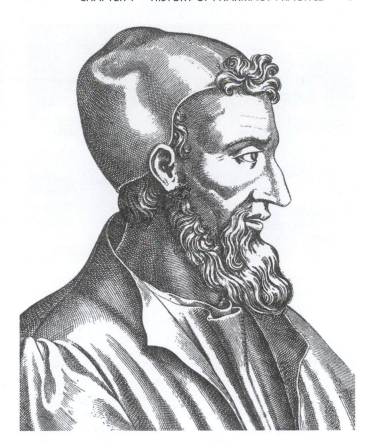

FIGURE 1-7 Galen.
Source: Photo Researchers/Getty

The Middle Ages

The Middle Ages lasted from 500 CE through 1500 CE. Once called the Dark Ages, while this historic period is not noted for cultural or scientific progress, a number of significant developments occurred in the practice of pharmacy.

Monasteries

During the Middle Ages, pharmacy and medicine were practiced and preserved in the monasteries; scientists are known to have been taught in the cloisters as early as the 7th century. The monks gathered herbs in the wild or raised them in their own gardens and then prepared them according to the art of the apothecary to aid the sick and injured. Medicinal herb gardens can still be found at many monasteries in numerous countries.

The First Apothecaries

Late in the 8th century, the Arabs separated the roles of the apothecary and physician, establishing the first apothecaries (privately owned drug stores) in Baghdad (Figure 1-8). In addition to the Greco-Roman knowledge of apothecary, the Arabs used their natural resources to develop syrups, confections, conserves, distilled waters, and alcoholic liquids. As the Muslims traveled across Africa, Spain, and southern France, they brought this new system of pharmacy with them, and it was eventually adopted by Western Europe, where public

pharmacies began to appear. However, it was not until 1240 CE, in Sicily and southern Italy, that pharmacy was separated from medicine. At the palace of Frederick II of Hohenstaufen, who was both Emperor of Germany and King of Sicily, pharmacists were presented with the first European edict completely separating their responsibilities from those of medical practitioners.

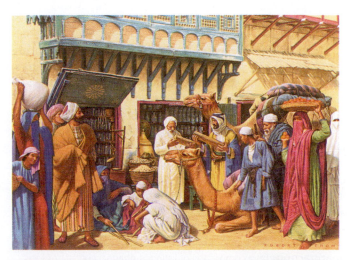

FIGURE 1-8 The first apothecaries. (Images by Robert Thom. Printed with permission of American Pharmacists Association Foundation. Copyright 2009 APhA Foundation.)

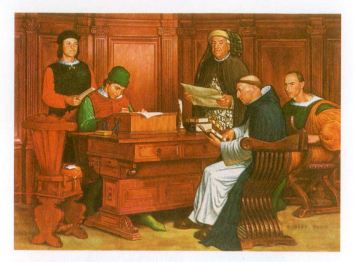

FIGURE 1-9 The first pharmacopoeia. (Images by Robert Thom. Printed with permission of American Pharmacists Association Foundation. Copyright 2009 APhA Foundation.)

The First Pharmacopoeia

It was in Florence, Italy, that the idea of a **pharmacopoeia** with official status, to be followed by all apothecaries, originated (Figure 1-9). The *Nuovo Receptario*, as originally titled in Italian, was published and became the legal standard for the city-state of Florence in 1498. It was the result of collaboration between the Guild of Apothecaries and the Medical Society, marking one of the earliest manifestations of constructive interprofessional relations. The professional groups received advice and guidance from the powerful Dominican monk Savonarola, who at the time was the political leader in Florence.

The Renaissance

The Renaissance period, which includes the 16th and 17th centuries (1500–1600 CE), was filled with scientific advancements, a renewed interest in culture and the arts, and expanded exploration, which included the European exploration of the Americas.

The First Anglo-Saxon Organization for Pharmacists

Trade in drugs and spices had been very lucrative during the Middle Ages. In the British Isles, the Guild of Grocers, which represented shopkeepers, monopolized this trade and maintained jurisdiction over the apothecaries. After years of effort, the apothecaries found allies among court physicians; in 1617 King James I granted them a charter to form a separate company known as the "Master, Wardens and Society of the Art and Mystery of the Apothecaries of the City of London"—despite vigorous protests from the grocers. This marked the first organization of pharmacists in the Anglo-Saxon world.

---

pharmacopoeia a compilation or listing of pharmaceutical products that also contains their formulas and methods of preparation.

prescription an order, by an authorized individual, for the preparation or dispensing of a medication.

The First Apothecary in the American Colonies

Many Europeans, particularly those who had some wealth and those who were religious nonconformists, were attracted to the opportunities presented by the American colonies. John Winthrop, the first governor of the Massachusetts Bay Colony and the founder of Boston, sought advice from English apothecaries and physicians when he was unable to persuade professionals to emigrate from Britain to the colony. In 1640, he began providing apothecary products by selling imported drugs, as well as those derived from plants native to New England.

The 18th Century

During the 18th century, the American colonies united, fought the British Empire to gain their independence, and ultimately formed the United States of America. Notable advancements in the practice of pharmacy and medicine, however, were occurring on both sides of the Atlantic Ocean.

Elizabeth Marshall: America's First Female Pharmacist

In 1729, Christopher Marshall, an Irish immigrant, established an apothecary shop in Philadelphia. Over 96 years, the shop became a leading retail store, one of the first large-scale chemical manufacturers, a training school for pharmacists, and an important supply depot during the American Revolution. Eventually, management of the apothecary shop was taken over by Marshall's granddaughter Elizabeth, America's first female pharmacist.

Benjamin Franklin: America's First Hospital

Founded by Benjamin Franklin, colonial America's first hospital was established in Philadelphia in 1751, with the hospital's pharmacy beginning operations in 1752 (Figure 1-10). Although Jonathan Roberts was the first hospital pharmacist in America, it was his successor, John Morgan, whose influence upon pharmacy and medicine made important changes to the development of professional pharmacy in North America. First as pharmacist, and later as physician, Morgan supported the

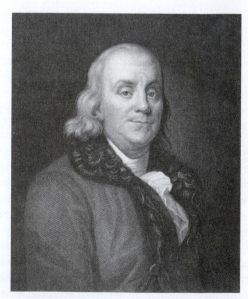

FIGURE 1-10 Benjamin Franklin.

use of written **prescriptions** and advocated for the independent practice of the two professions.

Andrew Craigie: America's First Apothecary General

Andrew Craigie, a Bostonian, was the first man to hold the rank of a commissioned pharmaceutical officer in the American army. Appointed commissary of medical stores by the Massachusetts Committee of Safety, less than two months later Craigie was present at the Battle of Bunker Hill, on June 17, 1775, taking care of the sick and wounded. When Congress reorganized the Medical Department of the army in 1777, Craigie became the first Apothecary General; his duties included procurement, storage, manufacture, and distribution of the army's required drugs. He also developed an early pharmaceutical wholesaling and manufacturing business.

The 19th Century

During the 1800s (the 19th century), America was a young country and the practice of American pharmacy was being established.

America's First College of Pharmacy

In the early 1800s, pharmacists were faced with two major threats: deterioration of the practice of pharmacy as they had known it and a discriminatory classification by the University of Pennsylvania medical faculty. Pharmacists held a protest meeting in Carpenters' Hall on February 23, 1821, in Philadelphia. At a second meeting, on March 13, the pharmacists voted to form the Philadelphia College of Pharmacy, a school of pharmacy with a self-policing board, which became America's first educational institution for pharmacy.

The American Pharmaceutical Association

In October 1852, Daniel B. Smith, William Procter, Jr., and 20 delegates of the Philadelphia College of Pharmacy founded the American Pharmaceutical Association (APhA) to meet the needs for better communication among pharmacists, standards for education and apprenticeship, and quality control over imported drugs. Membership was opened to "[a]ll pharmacists and druggists of good character who subscribed to its Constitution and to its Code of Ethics."

Workplace Wisdom APhA

After more than 150 years, APhA continues to serve the profession, although it was recently renamed the American Pharmacists Association (APhA). For more information, go to www.pharmacist.com

The Father of American Pharmacy

William Procter, Jr., is known as the father of American pharmacy (Figure 1-11). In 1837, he graduated from the Philadelphia College of Pharmacy; Procter operated a retail pharmacy, served the college as professor of pharmacy for 20 years, was a leader in founding the American Pharmaceutical Association, served that organization as its first secretary and later as its president, served 30 years on the USP Revision Committee,

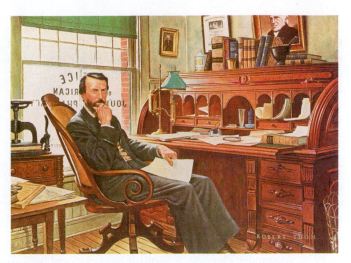

FIGURE 1-11 The father of American pharmacy, William Procter, Jr. (Images by Robert Thom. Printed with permission of American Pharmacists Association Foundation. Copyright 2009 APhA Foundation.)

and was editor of the *American Journal of Pharmacy* for 22 years. In 1869, though retired, Procter continued to edit the journal in a small publication office. He returned to chair the Philadelphia College of Pharmacy in 1872, before passing away in 1874.

The *United States Pharmacopoeia*

Published in 1820, the first *United States Pharmacopoeia* (USP) was the first book of drug standards to achieve acceptance by an entire nation. In 1877, the USP was in danger of discontinuation, because of a lack of interest from the medical profession, but Dr. Edward R. Squibb, a manufacturing pharmacist and physician, took the problem to the APhA, which formed a USP Revision Committee. The publication quickly regained authoritative stature and continues to be published today.

Workplace Wisdom USP

To learn more about USP standards and publications, go to www.usp.org

info The Role of USP in Pharmacy Practice

After more than 150 years, the relevance of the USP to pharmacy practice continues to evolve and grow. Today, the USP is considered the official public standards-setting authority for all prescription and over-the-counter medicines, dietary supplements, and other health care products manufactured and sold in the United States. Currently, the National Pharmacy Technician Association (NPTA) serves as an official delegate member of USP, providing insights and a voice for pharmacy technicians.

The Father of Modern Genetics

Gregor Mendel (1822–1884) is known as the father of modern genetics (Figure 1-12). An Austrian priest and scientist, Mendel showed that the inheritance of traits follows particular laws, through his study of inherited traits in pea plants. The significance of Mendel's work was not recognized until his research was rediscovered at the turn of the 20th century.

The 20th Century

The 20th century (1900s) was a period of impressive scientific discoveries and advancement, including in the field of medicine. In addition, it was in the early 1900s that the federal government began to regulate the practice of pharmacy.

The Discovery of Penicillin

In 1928, Alexander Fleming, a Scottish physician and bacteriologist discovered penicillin by accident. While studying the properties of staphylococci, Fleming stacked all of his cultures on a bench in his unkempt laboratory prior to taking a month long vacation with his family. Upon his return, he noticed that one culture had become contaminated with a fungus. The staphylococci that was directly in contact with the fungus had been destroyed. Afterward, Fleming grew the mold in a pure culture and discovered that it produced a substance, which he initially called "mould juice," which killed a variety of disease-causing bacteria. In 1929, Fleming named the substance penicillin, but mass production of the world's first antibiotic did not begin until World War II.

The American Council on Pharmaceutical Education

In 1932, multiple pharmacy-related associations cofounded the American Council on Pharmaceutical Education (ACPE) as an autonomous agency to establish standards for pharmacy education. ACPE initially established standards for the baccalaureate degree in pharmacy, and then added the doctor of pharmacy standards as an alternative. In the year 2000, it announced a conversion to the doctor of pharmacy (PharmD) as the sole entry-level degree for the profession of pharmacy. In 1975, ACPE developed standards for the approval of continuing pharmacy education providers. In 2003, the agency's name was changed to the Accreditation Council for Pharmacy Education (ACPE).

The Polio Vaccine

In the 1950s, polio was considered the most frightening public health epidemic in the postwar era in America. It was the deadly disease that left President Franklin Roosevelt crippled. In 1952 alone, there were more than 58,000 reported cases, which left over 3,100 dead and 21,000 paralyzed. Jonas Salk developed an injectable vaccine for the disease in the late 1940s, and it was tested on nearly two million school children (Figure 1-13). The successful trial results and the vaccine for polio were released in 1955.

Biotechnology

Biotechnology drugs are produced using living organisms such as yeast, bacteria, or mammalian cells. Although producing drugs from living organisms is not new, modern biotechnology has greatly expanded the number of different drugs that can be produced by using living organisms.

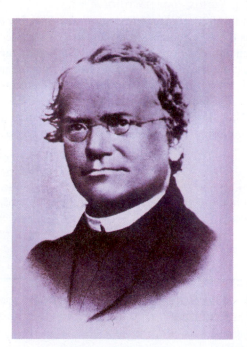

FIGURE 1-12 Gregor Mendel. (Image from the National Library of Medicine.)

biotechnology a technique that uses living organisms to make or modify specific products.

pharmacogenomics the study of individual genetic differences in response to drug therapy.

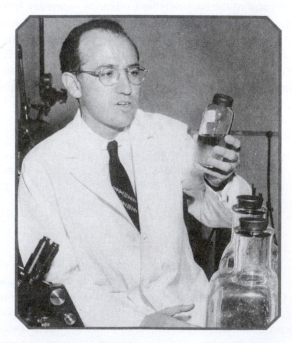

FIGURE 1-13 Jonas Salk.
Source: NYPL/Science Source/Getty Images

The majority of biotechnology drugs are manufactured through a process called *recombinant DNA technology*, in which a human gene that is capable of triggering the production of a specific protein is inserted into a living organism that is then cultured in a laboratory (Figure 1-14). The organism incorporates the gene into its cell structure and begins producing the desired protein (drug).

The proteins (drugs) produced by recombinant DNA technology are very fragile and can be administered only by injection into the vein or under the skin. If taken orally, the proteins will be destroyed by stomach acids and enzymes before they enter the patient's bloodstream.

Some of the drugs now produced by biotechnology were once made by different means. Insulin, for example, was once extracted from the tissue of animals. Most, however, are not producible by other methods.

The majority of biotechnology drugs now under development are being tested for use in the treatment of cancer or cancer-related conditions, which could have a major impact on the future health care of cancer patients. Currently, the Food and Drug Administration (FDA) has approved 254 biotechnology drugs for 385 indications.

Pharmacogenomics

It is not uncommon for patients to be given medications that either do not work effectively for them or that cause unwanted or dangerous side effects. These patients return to their doctors again and again, hoping to find a drug that will work for them. Enter **pharmacogenomics**, a very promising and appealing alternative.

Imagine that you go to your doctor's office. After a simple and rapid test of your DNA, your doctor changes his or her mind about the drug he or she was intending to prescribe for you because the genetic test indicates that you could suffer a severe negative reaction to that particular medication. Upon further examination of your test results, the doctor finds that you would benefit greatly from a new or different drug and

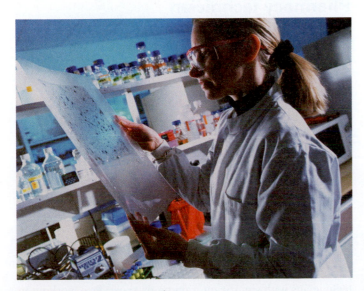

FIGURE 1-14 DNA sequencing.
Source: SPL/Custom Medical Stock Photo

that there would be little likelihood that you would react negatively to it. This is how the promise of pharmacogenomics is portrayed, and it is not as far off in the future as you might expect.

According to the Biotechnology Industry Organization (BIO),

> "the topics of pharmacogenomics, the use of genomic or genetic information to predict [a] drug's efficacy…. and personalized medicine, the tailoring of medical treatment to individuals, have been garnering increasing attention in Washington policy circles. BIO member companies are involved in using innovative pharmacogenomics and personalized medicine approaches across the full spectrum of drug development and commercialization. . . . [C]hanges in the regulatory review process and the healthcare reimbursement system are already underway, and will accelerate in coming months and years."

Evolution of the Pharmacist's Role

The 20th century saw the role of the modern American pharmacist evolve through four unique stages or eras: the traditional era, the scientific era, the clinical era, and the pharmaceutical care era.

The Traditional Era

From the early 1900s through the 1930s, pharmacists continued the traditional, preexisting practice of pharmacy, in which their role consisted primarily of formulating and dispensing drugs derived from natural sources.

The Scientific Era

Beginning in the late 1930s, the practice of pharmacy began to take a significantly more scientific-based approach. This era was marked by the development of new drugs, scientific testing of the effects of drugs on the human body, new regulations pertaining to the efficacy of medications, and the mass production of synthetic drugs and antibiotics. Several factors caused this shift in practice. Both world wars required the production of massive quantities of drugs, both existing and newly developed, for the soldiers. A large number of new drugs were discovered and manufactured. In particular, the discovery and development of penicillin-based drugs saved countless lives during World War II. Unfortunately, the era also saw numerous recorded incidents of fatalities and adverse reactions to non-regulated drugs.

The Clinical Era

In the 1960s, the pharmacy practice shifted again, with the approval of many new medications. Pharmacists were now expected to dispense not only medications but also drug information, warnings, advice, and helpful suggestions to their patients. This era transformed pharmacy into a cognitive-based profession slightly before the United States as a whole entered the ongoing information age.

The Pharmaceutical Care Era

Toward the end of the 20th century, the practice of pharmacy shifted yet again. This time, however, it transformed into a combination of the three prior eras. The practice of pharmacy and the role of the pharmacist became focused on ensuring positive outcomes for drug-related therapies. This overarching philosophy, known as *pharmaceutical care*, is actually a combination of formulation and dispensing of drugs (traditional era), a scientific approach to evidence and outcome-based results (scientific era), and provision of expanded consultations and cognitive-based services (clinical era). Going forward into the 21st century, there are many new and ever-changing trends in the pharmaceutical era. The era continues to evolve with new inventions and changes in technology—all areas of which the pharmacy technician should keep abreast of.

Evolution of the Pharmacy Technician

As previously discussed, the role of pharmacy technician can be traced back to the echelons in ancient Egypt. However, this role did not evolve significantly until the late 20th century. In the early and mid-1900s, pharmacy technicians were referred to as clerks, assistants, aides, or pharmacy support personnel. Most pharmacy assistants were the children of pharmacists who worked at the family-owned pharmacy. Any training they received was informal and acquired on the job.

Military Pharmacy Technicians

In the mid-1940s, the U.S. military pioneered the evolution of the professional pharmacy technician by developing standardized training and competency requirements and delegating more responsibilities to more knowledgeable pharmacy technicians. The original military classification was "pharmacy specialist," but the position evolved into today's pharmacy technician.

Move for Standardization

Although the move for standardizing pharmacy technician requirements, competencies, and job duties first took root during the 1970s, it was not until the 1990s that they began to transform notably. Some of these changes included the development of a national certification examination, formation of a model curriculum for training, and specific mention of technicians in state pharmacy practice acts. While the industry as a whole has adopted various standards for pharmacy technicians, the standards are unfortunately neither equal nor consistent across some state lines. National organizations and stakeholders continue to push for collective standardization among pharmacy technician regulations, competencies, and duties.

National Certification

Since 1995, the Pharmacy Technician Certification Board (PTCB) has certified over 425,000 pharmacy technicians through their certification exam and transfer process. Research indicates that there are approximately 275,000 actively certified pharmacy technicians through PTCB, individuals who

have met the requirements to maintain their certification. Several thousand additional pharmacy technicians have completed the national certification process through the Exam for the Certification of Pharmacy Technicians (ExCPT), administered by the National Healthcareer Association (NHA). The NHA recently acquired the ExCPT from the Institute for the Certification of Pharmacy Technicians (ICPT) to add to its large and diverse portfolio of health career certification programs. Certification requirements vary by state, so it is imperative to check with your State Board of Pharmacy to determine if a specific certification exam is required in your state.

This push for professional certification demonstrates the seriousness of this profession and the need for standardized competencies in the workplace. Prior to the PTCB exam, most technicians had only a high school diploma, although it was not mandatory; also, background checks were not done in every state.

Where We Are Today

As of 2013, all but six states (Colorado, Hawaii, Michigan, New York, Pennsylvania, and Wisconsin) regulate the practice of pharmacy technicians. Although a lack of consistency among state regulations pertaining to pharmacy technicians continues, momentum for standards and regulations have been evidenced over the past decade. Some states require mandatory, accredited formal education and training, while others require certification (either national or state), and many states now require registration, licensure, or a combination of all three. It is critical that you contact your own State Board of Pharmacy and educate yourself about the most current standards, guidelines, and regulations required to practice as a pharmacy technician as these requirements vary state by state and are evolving quickly. Table 1-1 shows some important milestones for pharmacy technicians.

The Future of Pharmacy and the Pharmacy Technician

As we move further into the 21st century, the future of medicine and pharmacy practice appears to be poised for the greatest and most significant advancements to date.

Occupational Outlook for Pharmacy Technicians

According to the Bureau of Labor Statistics (BLS), employment for pharmacy technicians with training and experience is expected to increase much faster than the average job, and opportunities are expected to be good. The BLS anticipates employment of pharmacy technicians to increase by 25% to 31% from 2008 to 2018. They cite that "job opportunities for pharmacy technicians are expected to be good, especially for those with previous experience, formal training, or certification." In addition, advancement opportunities, such as lead tech and supervisory positions, are most readily available for pharmacy technicians with significant training or experience working in large pharmacies and health systems.

TABLE 1-1 Pharmacy Technician Milestones

Mid-1940s	The U.S. Army establishes a training program for "pharmacy specialists."
1968	The U.S. Department of Health, Education, and Welfare recommends "the Bureau of Health Manpower should support … the development of a pharmacist aide curriculum in junior colleges and other educational institutions."
1969	The American Society of Hospital (now Health-System) Pharmacists (ASHP) workshop notes "the establishment of nationally recognized educational standards for pharmacy technicians would be of value." The American Pharmaceutical (now Pharmacists) Association (APhA) task force delineates tasks that pharmacists and technicians may perform.
1970	ASHP releases *Statements on Supportive Personnel in Hospital Pharmacy.*
1971	ASHP establishes a mechanism to accredit hospital-based pharmacy technician training programs.
1973	The National Association of Chain Drug Stores (NACDS) supports greater use of pharmacy technicians and favors on-the-job training.
1975	ASHP releases *Training Guidelines for Hospital Pharmacy Technicians: Supportive Personnel.*
1977	The American College of Apothecaries (ACA) suggests that the education of pharmacy technicians be conducted exclusively by accredited colleges that offered the doctor of pharmacy degree; ASHP publishes *Manual for Hospital Pharmacy Technicians: A Programmed Course in Basic Skills.*
1980	ASHP develops *Minimum Competencies for Institutional Pharmacy Technicians with Training Guidelines.*
1981	The Michigan Pharmacists Association (MPA) creates a certification exam for pharmacy technicians; ASHP creates a technical assistance bulletin on outcome competencies and training guidelines for institutional pharmacy technician training programs; ASHP recommends the establishment of an accreditation standard for pharmacy technician training programs.
1982	ASHP creates standards for accreditation of pharmacy technician training programs.
1983	ASHP accredits the first technician training program; ASHP approves resolution endorsing certification and registration of pharmacy technicians.
1987	The Illinois Council of Hospital Pharmacists (ICHP) creates a certification exam for pharmacy technicians.
1988	APhA advocates training in programs under a pharmacist's guidance; ASHP hosts first conference on pharmacy technicians.
1991	The Pharmacy Technician Educators Council (PTEC) is established.
1995	APhA, ASHP, ICHP, and MPA create the Pharmacy Technician Certification Board (PTCB).
1996	APhA and ASHP release *White Paper on Pharmacy Technicians.*
1999	The National Pharmacy Technician Association (NPTA) is established.
2001	NABP becomes a partner of PTCB; second edition of the *Model Curriculum for Pharmacy Technician Training* is released.
2003	The *White Paper on Pharmacy Technicians 2002* is released.

Medication Therapy Management and Pharmacists

Medication therapy management (MTM) is a service that optimizes therapeutic outcomes for individual patients, and since the mid-2000s it has become an increasingly focused trend for the practice of pharmacists. Through MTM services, pharmacists are able to provide medication therapy review, pharmacotherapy consultations, immunizations, and disease state management and health and wellness programs. As the practice of MTM evolves and pharmacists move more toward a path of providing clinical and consultative services, pharmacy technicians will be relied upon to assist with specific MTM activities and become increasingly involved in the general pharmacy practices traditionally handled by pharmacists.

Summary

The practice of pharmacy has deep, historic roots, in addition to an innovative and promising future. Although it has taken 7,000 years of progress, this profession has evolved from applying dirt and leaves to developing genetically tailored medications that are prepared specifically for each individual's unique DNA structure. The key concepts for this chapter include:

- The need for pharmaceutical products, services, and knowledge has existed since prehistoric times.
- As the profession gains new information and technology, pharmacy continues to evolve to better serve patients.

Chapter Review Questions

1. Which civilization provides the earliest known record of apothecary practice?
   a. Ancient Egypt
   b. Ancient China
   c. Ancient Mesopotamia
   d. Ancient Greece

2. The _____ is an ancient collection of prescriptions, mentioning more than 700 unique drugs.
   a. *Pen T-Sao*
   b. *Papyrus Ebers*
   c. Terra Sigilata
   d. *Charaka Samhita*

3. Echelons, from ancient _____, were similar to the modern-day pharmacy technician.
   a. China
   b. Egypt
   c. India
   a. Mesopotamia

4. Which individual is recognized as the father of American pharmacy?
   a. Christopher Marshall
   b. Benjamin Franklin
   c. William Procter, Jr.
   d. Dr. Edward R. Squibb

5. Which era of pharmacy practice in the 20th century is characterized by new regulations pertaining to medication efficacy?
   a. the traditional era
   b. the scientific era
   c. the clinical era
   d. the pharmaceutical care era

6. Which organization was established to autonomously set standards for pharmacy education?
   a. ACPE
   b. APhA
   c. BIO
   d. USP

7. Who is responsible for separating the practices of pharmacy and medicine?
   a. Savonarola
   b. King James I
   c. Hippocrates
   d. Frederick II

8. The first official pharmacopoeia originated in which country?
   a. England
   b. Greece
   c. Italy
   d. the United States

9. Which individual is recognized for shifting the view of medicine from the mystic to the scientific?
   a. Hippocrates
   b. Galen
   c. Savonarola
   d. Frederick II

10. The U.S. _____ marked a major milestone in the evolution of pharmacy technicians, by establishing a training program for "pharmacy specialists," in the mid-1940s.
    a. Air Force
    b. Army
    c. Marine Corp
    d. Navy

Critical Thinking Questions

1. In what ways has the practice of modern pharmacy remained consistent from the Age of Antiquity to today?

2. Describe the crucial differences in the practice of pharmacy during the Middle Ages and today.

Web Activity

1. Take the University of Arizona's History of Pharmacy Museum Virtual Tour: Go to http://www.pharmacy. arizona. Then select the Visitors menu, and then select Museum.

References and Resources

"ACPE Website." *Accreditation Council for Pharmacy Education.* ACPE. 2012. Web. 3 January 2012.

Bender, George A. *Great Moments in Pharmacy.* Detroit, MI: Northwood Institute Press, Print. 1996.

Cowan, David L. and William H. Helfand. *Pharmacy: An Illustrated History.* New York, NY: Harry N. Abrams, Print. 1990.

"ExCPT Exam." *National Healthcareer Association.* NHA. 2012. Web. 3 January 2012.

Haggard, Howard W. *Devils, Drugs, and Doctors.* New York, NY: Harper & Brothers, Print. 1929.

"MTM Central." *American Pharmacists Association.* APhA. 2012. Web. 3 January 2012.

"NPTA Website." *National Pharmacy Technician Association.* NPTA. 2012. Web. 3 January 2012.

Orum-Alexander, Gail G. and James J. Mizner, Jr. *Pharmacy Technician: Practice and Procedures.* New York, NY: McGraw Hill. Print.

"Pharmacogenomics and Personalized Medicine." *Biotechnology Industry Organization.* BIO. 2012. Web. 3 January 2012.

"Pharmacy Technicians and Aides." *Occupational Outlook Handbook, 2010–2011 Edition.* Bureau of Labor Statistics. 2011. Web. 3 January 2012.

"PTCB Website." *Pharmacy Technician Certification Board.* PTCB. 2012. Web. 3 January 2012.

"Report of the Sesquicentennial Stepping Stone Summits— Summit Two on Pharmacy Technicians." *Accreditation Council for Pharmacy Education.* ACPE. 2002. Web. 3 January 2012.

Rouse, Mike. "White Paper on Pharmacy Technicians 2002: Needed Changes Can No Longer Wait." *American Journal of Health-System Pharmacy.* 60 (2003): 37–51. Print.

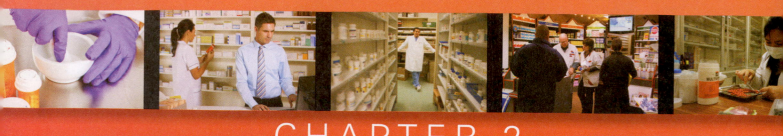

CHAPTER 2

The Professional Pharmacy Technician

LEARNING OBJECTIVES

After completing this chapter, you should be able to:

- Summarize the educational requirements and competencies of both pharmacists and pharmacy technicians.

- Describe the two primary pharmacy practice settings and define the basic roles of pharmacists and pharmacy technicians working in each setting.

- Explain six specific characteristics of a good pharmacy technician.

- Demonstrate the behavior of a professional pharmacy technician.

- Explain the registration/licensure and certification process for becoming a pharmacy technician.

KEY TERMS

ambulatory pharmacy, p. 16

association, p. 24

attire, p. 18

attitude, p. 18

certification, p. 22

community pharmacy, p. 16

compassion, p. 22

direct patient care, p. 15

doctor of pharmacy (PharmD), p. 15

empathy, p. 22

health-system pharmacy, p. 16

institutional pharmacy, p. 16

licensing, p. 22

pharmacist, p. 15

pharmacy, p. 15

pharmacy technician, p. 15

profession, p. 15

registration, p. 22

INTRODUCTION

A pharmacy technician is an integral part of the pharmacy staff and a member of the larger field of health occupations. Pharmacy technicians are professionals, working within the most trusted profession in the United States. It stands to reason, then, that a pharmacy technician must maintain specific competencies, undergo specialized education and training, and exhibit key personal characteristics.

This chapter provides an overview of the pharmacy profession, the traits and characteristics of a good pharmacy technician, and the framework within which one prepares for a future as a professional pharmacy technician.

Overview of the Pharmacy Profession

A **profession** is an occupation that requires advanced education and training; each profession generally has a professional association, code of ethics, and process of certification or licensing. Historically, there were only three recognized professions: medicine, ministry, and law. **Pharmacy**, which evolved from the profession of medicine, is the profession of preparing and dispensing medications, as well as supplying drug-related information to patients and consumers. Today, the practice of pharmacy is based upon delivering **direct patient care**, which can encompass many aspects of the health care of a patient, including providing pharmaceutical care, counseling, patient education, and in some cases even the administration of medication, such as immunizations.

By definition, a *professional* is any individual engaged within a specific profession. Pharmacy includes two classifications of practicing professionals: **pharmacists** and **pharmacy technicians**. Pharmacists are educated, skilled individuals licensed to practice pharmacy and dispense medications, whereas pharmacy technicians are educated, skilled individuals who are trained to work in a pharmacy under the supervision of a pharmacist.

Qualifications and Educational Requirements

Pharmacy professionals are subject to regulations that impose educational and training requirements, so that they will have the knowledge base and competencies necessary to practice pharmacy.

Pharmacists

Pharmacists graduate from pharmacy school with a **doctor of pharmacy (PharmD)** degree, although up until the year 2000, the entry-level degree for pharmacists was the bachelor of science in pharmacy (BS Pharm) degree. A PharmD degree requires a minimum of six years of college, which include at least two years of prepharmacy study and four years of study at a college of pharmacy accredited by the Accreditation Council for Pharmacy Education (ACPE). In addition to the academic requirements, individuals must complete an extensive internship, usually consisting of 1,500 hours, at a local pharmacy under the supervision of a licensed preceptor. Some states require that internship hours must be completed solely after graduation from pharmacy school. To become a licensed pharmacist, an individual must pass the North American Pharmacist Licensure Examination (NAPLEX) and in most states a drug law exam, such as the Multistate Pharmacy Jurisprudence Examination (MPJE). Age requirements vary by state. Pharmacists are required to be licensed with their State Board of Pharmacy (SBOP), as well.

Pharmacy Technicians

In the past, most pharmacy technicians were simply trained on the job, but on-the-job training (OJT), by its very nature, is employer specific and limited to the precise tasks required in the job for which the person was hired. In most cases, OJT does not provide instruction in or guarantee understanding of the theory or background surrounding pharmacy practice. Therefore, formal education requirements, competency exams, and registration with an SBOP are progressively replacing OJT. Most states require, at a minimum, that individuals have a high school diploma or GED equivalent and/or are 18 years of age and have no history of felonies or drug-related misdemeanors, in order to practice as a pharmacy technician, as are the qualifications for the national certification exams. Later in this chapter you will learn more about preparing for your future as a pharmacy technician.

Accredited Pharmacy Technician Training Programs The American Society of Health-System Pharmacists (ASHP) accredits pharmacy technician training programs. Although ASHP accreditation is voluntary in most states, the organization and their accreditation program has set the benchmark for standardized pharmacy technician curriculum and program guidelines. A list of the modules prescribed in ASHP's Model Curriculum for Pharmacy Technician Training is provided in Table 2-1.

Roles of Pharmacy Professionals

Although pharmacy is a collaborative practice, in which pharmacists and pharmacy technicians work as a team, specific—and even regulated—differences between their roles, responsibilities, and authority exist.

Pharmacists

The role of the pharmacist is extensive and varies significantly depending on the practice setting. For example, in a community pharmacy setting the pharmacist might counsel patients about over-the-counter remedies, whereas in a hospital pharmacy setting the pharmacist might advise physicians about the best drugs to prescribe for certain indications. The following discussion explores the basic duties of a pharmacist and should not be considered absolute or exhaustive.

The primary jobs of all pharmacists are to dispense medications prescribed by authorized medical professionals and provide vital information to patients about medications and their use. Pharmacists also monitor the health and progress of

---

profession an occupation that requires advanced education and training.

pharmacy the profession of preparing and dispensing medications, as well as supplying drug-related information to patients and consumers.

direct patient care care provided to a patient that encompasses various aspects, including pharmaceutical care, counseling, patient education, and medication administration.

pharmacist educated, skilled individual licensed to practice pharmacy and dispense medications.

pharmacy technician educated, skilled individual trained to work in a pharmacy, under the supervision of a pharmacist.

doctor of pharmacy (PharmD) a doctoral degree in pharmacy practice.

TABLE 2-1 ASHP's Model Curriculum for Pharmacy Technicians

1. Orientation to Pharmacy Practice	20. Preparation of Nonsterile Compounded Products
2. Therapeutic Agents for the Nervous System	21. Preparation of Sterile Compounded Products
3. Therapeutic Agents for the Skeletal System	22. Preparation of Cytotoxic and Hazardous Medication Products
4. Therapeutic Agents for the Endocrine System	23. Medication Distribution
5. Therapeutic Agents for the Muscular System	24. Identification of Patients for Counseling
6. Therapeutic Agents for the Cardiovascular System	25. Medication Safety
7. Therapeutic Agents for the Respiratory System	26. Collection of Payment (Billing)
8. Therapeutic Agents for the Gastrointestinal System	27. Monitoring Medication Therapy
9. Therapeutic Agents for the Renal System	28. Maintenance of Equipment and Facilities
10. Therapeutic Agents for the Reproductive Systems	29. Investigational Medication Products
11. Therapeutic Agents for the Immune System	30. Personal Qualities of Technicians
12. Therapeutic Agents for Eyes, Ears, Nose, and Throat	31. Certification
13. Therapeutic Agents for the Dermatologic System	32. Pharmacy Organizations
14. Therapeutic Agents for the Hematologic System	33. Management of Change
15. Collecting, Organizing, and Evaluating Information	34. Acute Care Practice (Option Long-Term Care) Experience
16. Purchase of Pharmaceuticals, Devices, and Supplies	35. Home Care Practice Experience
17. Control of Inventory	36. Ambulatory Clinic with Infusion Services Practice Experience
18. Assessment of Medication Orders/Prescriptions	37. Community or Outpatient Pharmacy Practice Experience
19. Preparation of Noncompounded Products	

patients in response to drug therapy to ensure that the medications being used are safe and effective.

Pharmacists in ambulatory (community-based) pharmacies counsel patients about prescription drugs and answer questions pertaining to possible side effects or interactions among various drugs. In addition, they provide information about and make recommendations of over-the-counter drugs and medical devices. Some pharmacists in community pharmacies provide specialized services to help patients manage specific conditions, such as diabetes, and some are trained to administer vaccines.

Pharmacists who work in **health-system pharmacies**, such as in hospitals, nursing homes, and long-term care facilities, prepare and dispense medications for individual patients, and advise the medical staff on the selection and effects of drugs. They also assess, plan, and monitor drug regimens (see Figure 2-1). Pharmacists may also evaluate drug use patterns and outcomes for patients in hospitals or other institutional settings.

health-system pharmacy common name for an institutional pharmacy.

community pharmacy name commonly used for an ambulatory or retail pharmacy.

ambulatory pharmacy community-based pharmacy; includes chain retail drugstores, grocery store pharmacies, home health care, mail-order facilities, and other pharmacies from which patients can obtain medications without living on-site.

institutional pharmacy a pharmacy found in places such as hospitals, long-term care facilities, extended-living facilities, and retirement homes, which require patients to reside on-site.

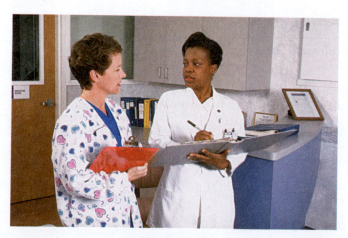

FIGURE 2-1 A pharmacist in a hospital setting often advises other medical personnel or monitors patient drug regimens.
Source: Michal Heron/Pearson Education/PH College

Pharmacy Technicians

As with the pharmacist, the role of a pharmacy technician varies considerably depending on the practice setting and state regulations. The following information explores the basic duties of a pharmacy technician and again should not be considered absolute or exhaustive.

Pharmacy technicians assist pharmacists to provide pharmaceutical care. It is common for technicians to perform routine tasks, such as computer entry, medication preparation, selection, counting, and labeling. The pharmacist is required to review and verify every prescription before it is dispensed to a patient. Technicians are also required to refer any patient questions regarding prescriptions, drug information, or related health matters to the pharmacist. In addition, pharmacy technicians routinely prepare reports, maintain documentation, and order supplies.

In **community pharmacies**, technicians also create and maintain patient profiles, handle insurance (third-party) billing, and manage the inventory.

In health-system pharmacies, technicians may review patient charts; prepare and deliver medications to nursing stations; perform unit-dose packaging; and, if trained and/or certified to do so, prepare sterile products such as intravenous (IV) antibiotics and chemotherapy (see Figure 2-2). Detailed information on the duties and practices of pharmacy technicians working in retail and health-system pharmacies is provided in Chapters 8 and 9, respectively.

Practice Settings

The two general classifications of pharmacy practice settings are ambulatory pharmacies and institutional pharmacies. **Ambulatory pharmacies** are community-based pharmacies, often referred to as retail pharmacies, which include chain retail drugstores, grocery store pharmacies, home health care, mail-order facilities, and other pharmacies from which patients can obtain medications without living on-site (see Figure 2-3). **Institutional pharmacies**, or health-system pharmacies, are found in places such as hospitals, long-term care facilities, extended-living facilities, and retirement homes (see Figure 2-4). Additional practice settings, such as specialty pharmacies, include home infusion, managed care, nuclear pharmacies, and the military.

As a rule of thumb, if patients can travel to the pharmacy or have the pharmacy travel to them, they are using an ambulatory pharmacy. If patients and the pharmacy are housed in the same facility, the pharmacy is called an institutional pharmacy.

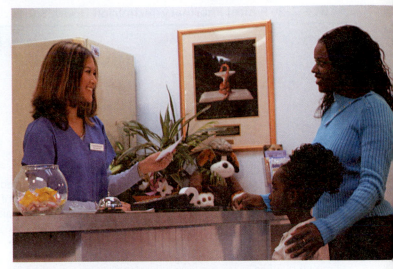

FIGURE 2-3 An ambulatory (community) pharmacy.

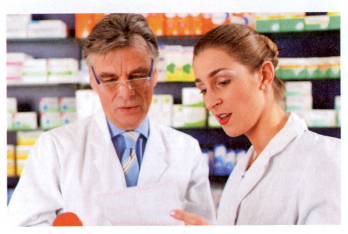

FIGURE 2-4 An institutional (health-system) pharmacy.
Source: Matthew Borkoski/Getty

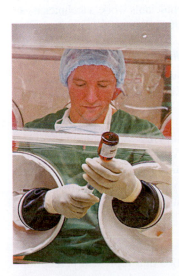

FIGURE 2-2 Trained or certified pharmacy technicians may prepare sterile products.
Source: Edwige/Science Source

Working Hours

Schedules and shifts vary from pharmacy to pharmacy, depending on the practice setting and the hours of operation for each specific pharmacy. Pharmacy technicians routinely work evenings, weekends, and/or holidays; this is particularly true for newer technicians who have less seniority on the job.

The majority of chain retail pharmacies are open seven days a week. Independently owned community pharmacies are typically open on weekdays only, although some may be open on the weekends as well. Most institutional pharmacies operate 24 hours a day, and many chain pharmacies now also operate a number of 24-hour pharmacies, dispersed geographically, within a specific city. Table 2-2 shows an example of the hours and shift schedules for pharmacy technicians at a typical chain retail pharmacy, specialty pharmacy, and 24-hour pharmacy.

TABLE 2-2 Typical Pharmacy Technician Hours/Shifts

	Day	Pharmacy Hours	First Shift	Second Shift	Third Shift
Typical chain pharmacy hours/shifts	Monday–Friday	8:00 a.m.–10:00 p.m.	8:00 a.m.–4:00 p.m.	11:00 a.m.–7:00 p.m.	2:00 p.m.–10:00 p.m.
	Saturday/Sunday	10:00 a.m.–6:00 p.m.	10:00 a.m.–6:00 p.m.	n/a	n/a
Specialty pharmacy hours/shifts	Monday–Friday	9:00 a.m.–5:00 p.m.	9:00 a.m.–5:00 p.m.	n/a	n/a
	Saturday/Sunday	Often closed on both days of the weekend, althoug this varies by pharmacy	n/a	n/a	n/a
24-hour pharmacy hours/shifts	Monday–Friday	12:00 a.m.–12:00 p.m.	8:00 a.m.–4:00 p.m.	4:00 p.m.–12:00 a.m.	12:00 a.m.–8:00 a.m.
	Saturday/Sunday	12:00 a.m.–12:00 p.m.	8:00 a.m.–4:00 p.m.	4:00 p.m.–12:00 a.m.	12:00 a.m.–8:00 a.m.

Staggered 30-minute lunch is included in this time block.

" Workplace Wisdom Work Shifts

First shift is commonly referred to as the "day shift."

Second shift is also known as the "swing shift."

Third shift is often referred to as the "graveyard shift."

Remember, the pharmacy hours and shift schedules outlined in this chapter are only examples. Each pharmacy has its own specific hours of operation and schedules, including breaks and mealtime allowances. The schedules described here refer to full-time positions, but many part-time positions are available for pharmacy technicians. In addition, some pharmacy technicians work seven days on followed by seven days off, or work 10- or 12-hour shifts, similar to nurses.

"

Pharmacy Technician Pay

Pharmacy technician pay and salaries vary from state to state as do certification requirements. Salaries also vary depending on the employment status of the tech, meaning that if they are a lead tech or have been with the hospital or retail pharmacy for a while, then their pay is often more than a tech who just started working. Technicians can also obtain raises and bonuses for a job well done.

Characteristics of a Good Pharmacy Technician

Pharmacy technicians must possess a wide range of knowledge and skills. Successful pharmacy technicians are intimately involved in providing critical health care to all types of people. They operate in strict compliance with written procedures and

guidelines and answer directly to the pharmacist for the quality and accuracy of their work. The pharmacist is ultimately responsible for technicians' activities and performance and is their direct supervisor.

Because pharmacy technicians deal with private medical and insurance information as well as dangerous substances, they must act according to the highest ethical and professional standards. Breaches of this public trust can lead to serious consequences. When a one-hour-photo clerk makes a mistake, you lose your pictures and he or she could lose his or her job. When a pharmacy technician makes an error, the result can be serious health consequences and even death. Although the pharmacist is ultimately responsible for checking each technician's work, a technician can be held liable in court for errors of negligence or omission.

Display a Professional Manner and Image

"If you aren't managing your own professional image, others are," according to Harvard Business School professor Laura Morgan Roberts. She adds,

> "People are constantly observing your behavior and forming theories about your competence, character, and commitment, which are rapidly disseminated throughout your workplace. It is only wise to add your voice in framing others' theories about who you are and what you can accomplish."

As defined by Roberts, "Your professional image is the set of qualities and characteristics that represent perceptions of your competence and character as judged by your key constituents." As a pharmacy technician, your "key constituents" are your patients, customers, coworkers, and managers. Among the many attributes that contribute to a professional image,

---

attitude a way of acting, thinking, or feeling.

attire clothing.

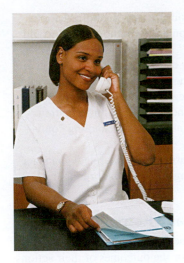

FIGURE 2-5 Displaying a positive attitude, in direct contact with customers, with coworkers, or while on the telephone, demonstrates your professionalism as a pharmacy technician.
Source: Michal Heron/Pearson Education/PH College

attitude, attire, and grooming consistently rank at the top.

Attitude

Attitude is a psychological concept. It can be positive, negative, or ambivalent, and generally it is a result of social learning from one's environment. When pursuing a professional image, however, a positive attitude is the only option. Attitude is technically defined as:

- The posture of the body in connection with an action or mood
- A way of acting, thinking, or feeling
- The position of an aircraft in relation to the horizon line

These definitions provide tremendous insight. Although most individuals recognize that attitude is a way of acting, thinking, or feeling, many forget the connection between attitude and the posture of the body—this is body language. You can say all the right things and take all the proper actions, but your body language cannot hide your true feelings and attitude (see Figure 2-5).

The last definition may at first seem inapplicable or inappropriate, but under the surface there is a great correlation. The attitude reading on a pilot's flight deck provides him or her with critical information regarding the position of the aircraft in relation to the horizon. If the attitude is in check and correctly aligned, the pilot is then able to proceed safely and increase the altitude (height) of the plane. The same can be said about one's professional image and attitude: So long as it is in check and correctly aligned, the individual is positioned to advance and grow within his or her profession.

" Workplace Wisdom Tips on Having a Positive Attitude

- Create and maintain a can-do mindset.
- Approach and respond to others in a pleasant and upbeat manner.
- Maintain enthusiasm despite criticism.
- Express support, loyalty, and appreciation.
- Demonstrate an "I care" policy.   "

Attire

Attire, or clothing, refers to all items used to cover the body, including the hands, feet, and head. Attire has two primary purposes: function and image. Numerous attire elements are required and necessary when working in pharmacy environments;

many (such as gloves, shoe covers, and face masks) are related to specific skills and practice settings (see Figure 2-6).

We discuss personal protective equipment and other items in later chapters. However, there is one common item that both serves as a functional attire element and relates to maintaining a professional image: the lab coat or smock. It is customary for pharmacy personnel to wear a lab coat in all practice settings, and, interestingly, it serves both defined purposes for attire, function, and image. The lab coat is functional in that it is a protective garment that keeps the individual's clothing from coming into contact with liquid medications, ointments, and chemicals. It also provides numerous, spacious pockets for storing reference booklets, notepads, calculators, and pens.

In addition, the lab coat contributes to a pharmacy technician's professional image. It is immediately recognizable by patients and customers, and inspires trust in the person wearing it. The public shares an unspoken expectation that a healthcare professional, such as a pharmacist or pharmacy technician, who is wearing a lab coat is knowledgeable and trustworthy.

Most pharmacies also establish a specific dress code for their employees for the primary purpose of maintaining a professional image. In general, pharmacies use one of two dress codes: business or scrubs.

Business Pharmacy personnel are expected to dress above business-casual standards; however, the traditional definition of business attire is altered to be practical in the pharmacy environment. Men should wear slacks or dress pants, a button-down shirt, and a tie. Women can wear slacks, conservative skirts, blouses, shells, cardigans, or dresses. Most fabrics are appropriate, but denim is usually not acceptable. Business dress codes are most often adopted by retail pharmacies and management at health-system pharmacies.

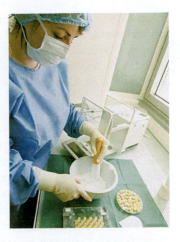

FIGURE 2-6 The attire and protective equipment you use on the job depends on your job function and the practice setting in which you work.
Source: Edwige/Science Source

General Lab Coat Guidelines

- White lab coat (short or long)—pharmacist
- Colored lab coat (short)—pharmacy technician
- White smock—pharmacy technician
- Sleeveless vest—pharmacy technician, pharmacy clerk, cashier

Scrubs Many pharmacies require personnel to wear scrubs, a medical uniform consisting of a pullover shirt and pants. The pharmacy typically predetermines the color of scrubs required and may or may not issue uniform scrubs to the staff. This dress code is most often adopted by health-system pharmacies.

Grooming

People present themselves to the public in a variety of ways. They may cut, dye, and style their hair; grow facial hair; use makeup or perfume and cologne; wear jewelry; mark their skin with tattoos; or have body piercings. All these options contribute to one's image, but do not constitute clothing per se; these elements are collectively classified as *grooming*.

Pharmacy professionals represent both their employer and the profession to patients and customers; therefore, it is important for each employee to use good judgment and good habits in grooming and personal hygiene.

Grooming standards vary, and in some cases are regulated, by practice setting and employer. However, the following are basic grooming standards for professionals:

- Hair should be kept neat, clean, and professional; coloring should appear natural.
- Men should be clean shaven or maintain a neat, trimmed mustache and/or beard.
- Makeup should be used in moderation, and a natural skin color should be maintained.
- Fingernails should be kept trimmed and clean.
- A single pair of appropriate earrings may be worn.
- Additional piercing and tattoos should not be visible when one is in professional attire.
- Perfume/cologne should be used sparingly, or avoided altogether, at the workplace.

Be Trustworthy and Confidential

National surveys consistently show that pharmacy is among the most trusted professions in the United States, more so than doctors and clergy. Patients have an unmatched, inherent trust in their pharmacists and by extension their pharmacy technicians. Trust is a treasured gift and one that should be handled reverently. As a pharmacy technician, it is your responsibility to deserve and maintain your patients' trust. After all, with the potential of fatal errors, patients are essentially putting their lives in your hands each time you type and fill their prescription. One large component of being trustworthy is confidentiality. Aside from explicit and stringent laws, such as the Health Insurance Portability and Accountability Act (HIPAA), confidentiality is a primary responsibility of any health care professional. As a pharmacy technician, you will be given access to very detailed, private information regarding your patients and you are to be responsible and respectful when handling such details. The following are a few tips on how to be trustworthy and maintain confidentiality:

- Always be truthful and honest, especially when you make a mistake.
- Be reliable and accountable; keep your promises.
- Remember that open and honest dialogue is reciprocated.

- Safeguard the privacy of your patients and information.
- Treat others and their personal information as you would desire yours to be treated.
- Study HIPAA privacy laws carefully to make sure you are fully informed of your responsibilities and liabilities.
- Never make assumptions regarding who may or may not have access to privileged and confidential information.
- Always err on the side of caution when handling confidential information.
- When in doubt, ask the pharmacist or pharmacy manager before taking action, sharing information, or making comments.

Demonstrate Initiative and Responsibility

Pharmacy technicians should be proactive in their role in the pharmacy and be accountable for the outcomes of their actions and behavior. In other words, a pharmacy technician should demonstrate initiative and responsibility within professional boundaries. The following are some practical examples of how to express these characteristics:

- Use professional resources and references effectively.
- Anticipate problems and develop solutions in advance.
- Become a valuable resource through personal research, knowledge, and networking.
- Brainstorm and suggest innovative ideas and solutions.
- Follow through on all promises and commitments.
- Take full responsibility for mistakes made and learn from them.

info | Steps to Problem Solving

Be prepared to address and solve problems in your role as a pharmacy technician. Problems will arise, despite everyone's best efforts and intentions; the key is to be able to solve them when they do occur. As a pharmacy technician, you will encounter a wide variety of problems. Some problems will be clinical and practice related, while others will be emotional and individual related. Sometimes the problem will be with a patient or customer; other times it will be with a manager or coworker. Here are four basic steps to problem solving:

1. Understand the problem. Ask yourself: Can you clearly identify and state the problem? What are you trying to accomplish? What information or outcome is needed?
2. Devise a solution. You can develop a solution in a variety of ways, such as looking for a pattern, examining related problems, reviewing best practices or case studies, or establishing subgoals and working backward from the desired result.
3. Carry out the solution. Once you have devised a solution, take action. Implement the solution and check for results along the way.
4. Review the outcomes. After fully implementing the solution, take a look back and ask yourself: Did the solution produce the desired results? Has the problem in fact been solved? Was there a better alternative to solve the problem? Upon review, make any necessary changes and continue to progress.

Work as a Team Member

The efficiency of a pharmacy depends directly on the effectiveness of its team-centered approach to practice. The best teams have strong leaders, committed members, a shared vision, and effective communication. Although the pharmacist-in-charge (PIC) or pharmacy manager is the team leader of the pharmacy, your participation and attitude can greatly shape the work outcomes and stability of your team. Here are some specific examples of how to work as a team member:

- View yourself as an integral part of the team, neither above nor below it.
- Build positive working relationships with all pharmacy staff members.
- Share information, knowledge, and experience openly with your coworkers.
- Cooperate with other staff members to achieve desired outcomes.
- Be open to feedback from your coworkers and provide feedback when appropriate.
- Work to remove any barrier to your team's effectiveness.

Tips on Building Consensus

The pharmacy staff is typically a small group of individuals with inherent small group dynamics, such as the importance of consensus building. Consensus allows a group to achieve goals more efficiently, resolve conflict, and create workable solutions. Here are some tips on how to build consensus:

- Always look for areas of agreement.
- Develop genuine relationships with your coworkers.
- Listen more than you speak.
- Support and reinforce positive actions, behaviors, and mindsets.
- Never make assumptions or judge others.

PROFILES IN PRACTICE

Sydney is the lead pharmacy technician at a local community pharmacy; having worked there for nearly seven years, she makes sure that everyone is mindful of her seniority. Sydney refuses to stock the vials, collect the trash, or check out customers, as she feels that she is above these duties.

- What impact does Sydney's perspective likely have on her coworkers?
- How can Sydney improve her professionalism and serve as a better role model for the other pharmacy technicians?
- With a clear attitude of arrogance, what reason(s) might the pharmacist or manager use for justifying Sydney's status as lead tech?
- How would you handle working in that environment?

Adapt to Change

The practice of pharmacy is in a constant state of evolution and change. As the demand for pharmaceutical services grows, new drugs become approved, and advances in technology are implemented, the scope and standards of pharmacy practice change. As a pharmacy technician, you must anticipate changes with a positive attitude and a readiness to adapt. Here are some practical examples of demonstrating adaptability:

- Be flexible.
- View changes as progress or improvements.
- Adapt your own attitudes and behavior to work effectively with different people and situations.
- Accept and learn to work with changing priorities, strategies, procedures, and methods.
- Maintain work effectiveness in new or changing situations.
- Handle pressure and stress properly.

Be Knowledgeable

Pharmacy technicians are required to master a great deal of knowledge and information. From being able to recognize the brand name and generic name equivalent of drugs to performing pharmaceutical calculations to understanding pharmacology—these are but a few of the many areas in which a pharmacy technician must be knowledgeable. Your pharmacists, patients, and coworkers will all be depending upon you having a mastery of the information you need to perform your job. On top of that, pharmacy information is constantly changing—new drugs, indications, drug recalls, best practices, or regulations are always being introduced—so your journey of learning will never cease. Here are some tips on remaining well informed:

- Learn the Top 200 Drugs, including brand/generic equivalence, classification, therapeutic indication, strengths, and dosage forms, as soon as possible. Until you have mastered this information, be sure to keep a pocket reference guide with you.

Principles of Negotiation

One of the best approaches to conflict resolution is principled negotiation, which goes along with the characteristic of being adaptable. In 1981, Roger Fisher and William Ury published their now classic book on conflict resolution, *Getting to Yes*. According to their book, the following are the four essential principles of negotiation, which are still valid:

1. Separate the people from the problem.
2. Focus on interests, not positions.
3. Develop mutually beneficial options.
4. Insist on objective criteria.

- Subscribe to and read industry trade journals, such as *Today's Technician*, *Drug Topics*, *US Pharmacist*, and *Pharmacy Times* to keep abreast of the latest news, trends, and information.
- Attend pharmacy conferences, local, statewide, or national, to network and learn from both industry leaders and your peers.
- Select and complete continuing education (CE) programs that are relevant to your job and that will improve your knowledge base. Take the time to truly study the information presented, as opposed to simply rushing through the course to obtain the necessary credits.
- Join a professional organization, such as the National Pharmacy Technician Association (NPTA), and become active. One of the primary benefits of membership in a professional organization is receiving timely news and information on industry trends and best practices.

Pharmacy professionals are required to complete CE programs to remain knowledgeable, but continuous professional development is also important. Here are some recommendations regarding CE and professional development:

- Stay informed by reading trade journals and maintaining active membership in professional organizations.
- Attend pharmacy seminars and conferences.
- Take the initiative to learn new skills.
- Learn from and seek others' ideas, perspectives, and experiences.
- Seek feedback on performance.
- Adopt others' appropriate suggestions for improving your performance.
- Look for new ideas to improve personal, team, and pharmacy effectiveness.

Remember Compassion and Empathy

It is a basic principle, but one that is often overlooked: Pharmacy professionals serve patients who may be sick and/or in pain. With few exceptions, the customers or patients with whom a pharmacy technician interacts are seeking relief or treatment for an illness, disease, or other medical condition. It is important to treat all patients with **compassion** and **empathy**. Here are some points to keep in mind:

- Treat all people with dignity and respect.
- Be considerate, caring, and kind.

---

compassion a deep awareness of and sympathy for another's suffering.

empathy a feeling of concern and understanding for another's situation or feelings.

registration the process of listing or being named to a list.

licensing permission granted by a government entity for an individual to perform an activity.

certification recognition granted by a nongovernmental agency, attesting that an individual has met the required levels of competency.

- Focus your efforts on helping the patient.
- Be understanding and forgiving of patients' behaviors and attitudes.
- Assume the best about others.
- Try to imagine yourself in the patient's situation.

Preparing for Your Future as a Pharmacy Technician

Professionals are identified by several means, all of which are useful in the proper settings. Registration, licensing, and certification are some of the most common. It is important to understand these terms, as there has been much confusion in the pharmacy profession over their use.

- **Registration** is simply the process of listing or being named to a list.
- **Licensing** is permission granted by a government entity for an individual to perform an activity. The person has to meet certain standards, which are often set by law and are usually intended to protect the public.
- **Certification** is recognition granted by a nongovernmental agency, attesting that an individual has met the required levels of competency.

Registration/Licensure for the Pharmacy Technician

Most states now require pharmacy technicians to become either registered or licensed with the SBOP. Each state decides whether it will register or license, and the baseline eligibility requirements for either also vary by state. Common eligibility requirements include the following:

- High school graduation or GED equivalent
- Attainment of a certain age, such as 18 years or older
- No felony conviction(s)
- Formal education or training as a pharmacy technician
- Passage of an SBOP competency exam
- Certification

These regulations and requirements vary by state, so you should consult your SBOP for specific information.

Certification for the Pharmacy Technician

When a pharmacy technician becomes certified, the certification agency verifies that the candidate has met the agency's or board's standards for skills and knowledge necessary to practice as a pharmacy technician. This signifies to employers, coworkers, and patients that a certain level of competence has been verified.

National certification for pharmacy technicians became possible in 1995 with the founding of the Pharmacy Technician Certification Board (PTCB). Although the PTCB continues to be the standard in technician certification, other agencies have recently emerged and achieved recognition. Of these newer exams, the Exam for the Certification of Pharmacy Technicians (ExCPT) has received the greatest recognition and acceptance.

Exam for the Certification of Pharmacy Technicians

The ExCPT was developed by the Institute for the Certification of Pharmacy Technicians (ICPT) and is now a part of the National Healthcareer Association (NHA). The ExCPT is accredited by the National Commission for Certifying Agencies (NCCA), nationally recognized and endorsed by the National Community Pharmacists Association and the National Association of Chain Drug Stores (NACDS).

The ExCPT is offered as a computerized exam at over 600 PSI Testing Centers throughout the United States. The exam consists of 110 multiple-choice questions, which must be completed within 2 hours. The exam measures the candidate in three areas of competence:

1. *Regulations and technician duties*, such as the role of pharmacists and pharmacy technicians, functions that a technician may and may not perform, prescription department layout and workflow, pharmacy security, the role of government agencies, inventory control, and pharmacy law (25% of exam).
2. *Drugs and drug products*, such as drug classification, mechanisms of action, dosage forms, and knowledge of the most commonly prescribed drugs (25% of exam).
3. *The dispensing process*, including preparation of prescriptions, dispensing of prescriptions, pharmacy calculations, sterile products, unit dosing, and repackaging (50% of exam).

Complete information on the ExCPT is available at **www.nhanow.com/pharmacy-technician**.

Candidates must meet certain qualifications in order to sit for the exam. For example, the candidate must be at least 18 years old; have a high school diploma or GED; have completed a training program or have one-year work experience in the field; not have been convicted of a felony; and not have any registration or license revoked, suspended, or subject to any disciplinary action by a state health or regulatory board.

The cost of the exam is $105. Individuals who fail to pass the exam must wait 30 days before retaking the exam. After three failed attempts, the individual must wait one year before retaking it again.

Renewal of certification, or *recertification*, is required every two years. To be recertified, individuals must have completed 20 hours of CE, including 1 hour of pharmacy law. The fee for recertification is $50.

Pharmacy Technician Certification Exam

The Pharmacy Technician Certification Exam (PTCE) is offered by the PTCB, based in Washington, D.C. The PTCE is accredited by NCCA and nationally recognized and endorsed by the National Association of Boards of Pharmacy, the American Pharmacists Association, and the ASHP. More than 425,000 individuals have passed the PTCE, which is officially recognized by 44 individual SBOPs.

The PTCE is offered as a computerized exam at over 220 Pearson VUE Testing Centers. The exam consists of 90 multiple-choice questions and must be completed within 110 minutes (1 hour 50 minutes). The content of the exam has been reorganized into nine knowledge areas:

1. Pharmacology for Technicians
2. Pharmacy Law and Regulations
3. Sterile and Nonsterile Compounding
4. Medication Safety
5. Pharmacy Quality Assurance
6. Medication Order Entry and Fill Process
7. Pharmacy Inventory Management
8. Pharmacy Billing and Reimbursement
9. Pharmacy Information Systems Usage and Application

Complete information on the PTCE is available at **www.ptcb.org**.

Candidates must meet certain qualifications in order to sit for the exam. For example, the candidate must have a high school diploma or GED; not have been convicted of a felony or have any drug- or pharmacy-related conviction including misdemeanors; have had no denial, suspension, revocation, or restriction of registration or licensure by any SBOP; and have no admission of misconduct or violation of regulations of any SBOP.

The cost of the exam is $129. Individuals who fail to pass the exam must wait 60 days before retaking the exam. After three failed attempts, the individual must appeal to PTCB to request to take the exam again.

Renewal of certification, or recertification, is required every two years. To be recertified, individuals must have completed 20 hours of CE, including 1 hour of pharmacy law. The fee for recertification is $40 if done online or $65 if done by mail.

The American Council on Pharmacy Education (ACPE) accredits organizations as approved providers of continuing pharmacy education (CPE), which is more commonly referred to as continuing education, or rather CE. ACPE does not develop and accredit individual programs, but rather develops and enforces the standards for CPE as well as accredit and monitor ACPE-approved providers. Each CPE activity, or course, is assigned a unique identification number, known as the Universal Activity Number (UAN), such as 0384-0000-10-008-H04-T. Each component of the UAN represents specific information pertaining to the activity. The first four digits indicate the official ACPE-approved provider number. For example, the NPTA is provider number 0384, so each of its accredited CPE activities will begin with that code; the second four digits represent the provider number of the cosponsor of the program, with 0000 indicating no cosponsor and 9999 indicating a nonaccredited cosponsor; and the next two digits indicate the year of the activity's initial release date. Most CPE activities are approved for three years. Following the two-digit year code, a three-digit unique course identification number is provided. After the course number, a three-digit code, beginning with either an "H" or an "L" followed by a two-digit topic designator of 01, 02, 03, 04, or 05, is provided. "H" indicates that the CPE activity is a home study course, whereas "L" denotes that it is a live course. The topic designators indicate that the activity is based upon disease state management or drug therapy (01), AIDS therapy (02), pharmacy law (03), general pharmacy (04), or patient safety (05). Finally the course ends with either a target audience designator of "P" for pharmacists or "T" for pharmacy technicians. This information can be very valuable when you are looking for CPE activities that meet specific requirements, such as being approved for pharmacy technicians, a live course, and an activity that will meet the pharmacy law credit requirement. For more information on ACPE accreditation, visit www.acpe-accredit.org.

In addition to the CE requirements associated with recertification as a certified pharmacy technician, many states also require pharmacy technicians to complete CE in order to maintain their registration or licensure. In most cases, CE credits completed for recertification can also apply toward state requirements. CE requirements vary by state, so it is important to check with your SBOP for current requirements.

Specialized Certifications

In addition to national certification, several specialized certifications are available for qualified pharmacy technicians. The NPTA offers the following advanced certification programs: sterile products/IV certification, chemotherapy certification, and nonsterile/extemporaneous compounding certification. Each of these specialized certifications consists of a home study module, hands-on training, and skill technique validations. Applicants must be either nationally certified or currently enrolled in an approved pharmacy technician training program. By obtaining advanced training and specialized certifications, such as those offered by the NPTA, pharmacy technicians have greater career opportunities and earning potential. Employers generally prefer to hire qualified individuals with advanced certifications, and several SBOPs actually require

such training and certification in order for pharmacy technicians to be permitted to practice these advanced skills. More information on the NPTA's certificate programs can be found at www.pharmacytechnician.org.

Professional Organizations

In general, an **association**, or professional organization, is a group of individuals united for a specific purpose or cause. Associations are organized for various reasons, but typical recurring benefits they provide to their members include the following:

- Continuing education
- Professional development
- Information, research, and statistics
- Professional standards
- Networking
- Advocacy
- Professional recognition

According to the American Society of Association Executives (ASAE), "Believing in the mission of an organization is a powerful incentive.... Associations have a responsibility to achieve results, not only for their members but for society at large."

There are four national organizations that are primarily focused on the practice of pharmacy and that individual pharmacy technicians are permitted to join. Information on these four associations is outlined in Table 2-3.

In addition to the national pharmacy associations, there are also pharmacy organizations in individual states/cities, relating to specific practice settings, and targeted to race, religion, and other cultural variations. Research the various associations and determine which one(s) would be of greatest benefit to you—then get involved!

Career Opportunities

Being a pharmacy technician is among the best career opportunities that do not require a college degree. The NPTA reports that pharmacy technician ranks 60th in the 100 fastest-growing jobs in the United States and 19th in the 500 best jobs.

The U.S. Bureau of Labor Statistics confirms that pharmacy technician is among the most promising occupations, as the job is forecast at an annual growth rate of 31%, which equates to 99,800 additional positions between 2008 and 2018.

Pharmacy technicians are no longer limited to working in drugstores and hospitals. Numerous unique career-path options are now opening to pharmacy technicians, such as:

- Clinical practice
- Compounding
- Nuclear medicine
- Training/education
- Management
- Sales
- Research and development
- Consulting

association a group of individuals who voluntarily form an organization to accomplish a common purpose.

TABLE 2-3 **National Pharmacy Associations**

Organization	Founded	Memberships	Benefits[1]	Dues	Membership Size[2]	Contact Information
AAPT— American Association of Pharmacy Technicians	1970s	Technicians[3] Pharmacists Students	e-Newsletter with CE (4x) (A hardcopy newsletter is available for an additional $25 per year); annual seminar; regional chapter seminars; member discounts	$40	700	**pharmacytechnician.com** Phone: 877-368-4771 Fax: 336-333-9068
APhA— American Pharmacists Association	1852	Technicians Pharmacists[3]	*Pharmacy Today* magazine (12x); annual meeting; CE—through **pharmacist.com**; member discounts; affinity programs	$67 $249	50,000	**pharmacist.com** Phone: 1-202-628-4410 Fax: 202-783-2351
ASHP— American Society of Health-System Pharmacists	1942	Technicians Pharmacists[3] Students (RPh)	*ASHP Action Line* newsletter (12x); annual meetings; CE—TechTopics (10 hours); member discounts; affinity programs	$69[5] $275[4] $43[6]	30,000	**ashp.org** Phone: 1-866-279-0681
NPTA— National Pharmacy Technician Association	1999	Technicians[3]	*Today's Technician* magazine (6x); annual and regional meetings; CE—unlimited/online; member discounts; affinity programs	$69	60,000	**pharmacytechnician.org** Phone: 888-247-8700 Fax: 888-247-8706

[1]Benefits provided with listed technician membership dues, according to content published on website.
[2]Estimated total membership, including all categories.
[3]Primary membership category.
[4]Pharmacist/associate membership dues per year.
[5]Technician membership dues per year.
[6]Student membership dues per year.

Summary

Pharmacy is an industry that consists of professionals: pharmacists and pharmacy technicians. As with any profession, pharmacy requires an individual to be educated, trained, diligent, and ethical. You will have to study and work hard to attain your goal, but tremendous career opportunities await the professional pharmacy technician. The key concepts for this chapter include:

- The pharmacy profession includes both pharmacists and pharmacy technicians. Both groups have defined educational requirements and specific roles within the pharmacy.

- The professional pharmacy technician maintains a proper image, is responsible and a team player, adapts quickly and appropriately to change, seeks continuing education and development, and demonstrates compassion.

- The process of preparing for your future as a pharmacy technician includes formal education and training, registration/licensure, national certification, and involvement with a professional organization.

Chapter Review Questions

1. Which of the following is classified as a health-system pharmacy?
   a. home health care
   b. chain drugstore
   c. mail-order facility
   d. extended-living facility

2. Pharmacists are required to complete _____ years of college-level education.
   a. two
   b. four
   c. six
   d. eight

3. Which agency provides state-specific regulations for practice?
   a. ACPE
   b. NABP
   c. PTCB
   d. SBOP

4. Attitude refers to a way of _____.
   a. acting
   b. feeling
   c. thinking
   d. all of the above

5. Which two agencies are recognized providers for national pharmacy technician certification?
   a. ICPT and PTCB
   b. APhA and ASHP
   c. NABP and NACDS
   d. ACPE and SBOP

6. Certified pharmacy technicians are required to complete _____ hours of continuing education every two years.
   a. 5
   b. 10
   c. 20
   d. 40

7. _____ refers to permission granted by a government entity for an individual to perform an activity.
   a. Certification
   b. Licensure
   c. Registration
   d. Specialization

8. There are _____ specific content areas that comprise the PTCE.
   a. three
   b. six
   c. seven
   d. nine

9. Certified pharmacy technicians are authorized to _____.
   a. dispense medications
   b. provide drug information
   c. prepare and deliver medications to nursing stations
   d. none of the above

10. Which professional organization publishes *Today's Technician* magazine?
    a. NPTA
    b. AAPT
    c. APhA
    d. ASHP

Critical Thinking Questions

1. Why is it important that pharmacists and pharmacy technicians have specific and distinct competency requirements, roles, and responsibilities?

2. Which of the characteristics of a good pharmacy technician do you currently possess? Of the characteristics described in this chapter, which is your strongest area and which is your weakest area?

3. Why do you think that pharmacy has consistently been rated as the most trusted profession in the United States, even over doctors and clergy?

Web Challenge

1. Find the website for your State Board of Pharmacy and then perform a search for information and requirements for pharmacy technicians in your state. Print out the information you find. (Hint: A list of SBOP contact information is available at www.nabp.net.)

2. Visit the website of each of the national pharmacy organizations listed here. Review the full list of membership benefits offered by each association.

   AAPT—www.pharmacytechnician.com
   APhA—www.pharmacist.com
   ASHP—www.ashp.org
   NPTA—www.pharmacytechnician.org

References and Resources

"AAPT Website." *American Association of Pharmacy Technicians*. AAPT. 2012. Web. 7 January 2012.

"ACPE Website." *Accreditation Council for Pharmacy Education*. ACPE. 2012. Web. 7 January 2012.

"APhA Website." *American Pharmacists Association*. APhA. 2012. Web. 7 January 2012.

"ASAE Website." *American Society of Association Executives*. ASAE. 2008. Web. 21 March 2008.

"ASHP Website." *American Society of Health-System Pharmacists*. ASHp. 2012. Web. 7 January 2012.

"ExCPT Exam." *National Healthcareer Association*. NHA. 2012. Web. 13 January 2012.

Fisher, Roger and William Ury. *Getting to Yes*. New York, NY: Penguin, 1981. Print.

"Human Resources." *Michigan State University*. MSU. 2008. Web. 21 March 2008.

Johnston, Mike. *Certification Exam Review*. Upper Saddle River, NJ: Pearson, 2005. Print.

Johnston, Mike. *Fundamentals of Pharmacy Practice*. Upper Saddle River, NJ: Pearson, 2005. Print.

"Model Curriculum for Pharmacy Technician Training." *American Society of Health-System Pharmacists*. Web. 4 January 2012.

"NPTA Website." *National Pharmacy Technician Association*. NPTA. 2012. Web. 3 January 2012.

"Pharmacy Technician: Occupational Outlook Handbook." *U.S. Bureau of Labor Statistics*. BLS. Web. 29 March 2012.

"Pharmacy Technicians and Aides." *Occupational Outlook Handbook, 2010–2011 Edition*. Bureau of Labor Statistics. 2011. Web. 3 January 2012.

"PTCB Website." *Pharmacy Technician Certification Board*. PTCB. 2012. Web. 13 January 2012.

Roberts, Laura M. et al. "How to Play to Your Strengths." *Harvard Business Review*. January 1, 2005. Web. 21 March 2008.

Stark, Mallory. "*Creating a Professional Image*." Harvard Business School, 2005. Web. 21 March 2008.

"2010 Survey of Pharmacy Law." *National Association of Boards of Pharmacy*. Web. 11 January 2011.

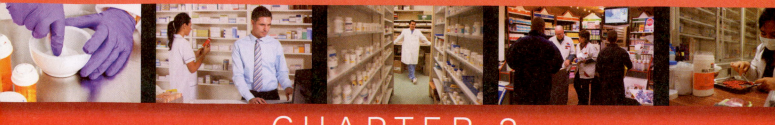

CHAPTER 3

Communication and Customer Care

LEARNING OBJECTIVES

After completing this chapter, you should be able to:

- Describe and illustrate the communication process.
- List and explain three types of communication.
- Summarize various barriers to effective communication.
- List and describe primary defense mechanisms.
- Describe specific strategies for eliminating barriers to communication.
- Summarize the elements of and considerations in caring for patients.
- List the five rights of medication administration.

KEY TERMS

channel, p. 29
context, p. 29
defense mechanisms, p. 34
denial, p. 35
diction, p. 30
displacement, p. 35
feedback, p. 29
inflection, p. 30
intellectualization, p. 35
kinesics, p. 32
message, p. 29
nonverbal communication, p. 31
oculesics, p. 32
pitch, p. 30
projection, p. 35
pronunciation, p. 30
proxemics, p. 32
rationalization, p. 35
reaction formation, p. 35
receiver, p. 29
regression, p. 35
repression, p. 35
sender, p. 29
sublimation, p. 35
verbal communication, p. 29
volume, p. 30
written communication, p. 31

INTRODUCTION

Communication is simply the process of transferring information, but it is not a simple process. The purpose of communication is to get your message across to others clearly. Communicating takes effort from everyone involved. During the process, errors can arise, resulting in confusion, misunderstandings, and sometimes a complete failure of the information transfer system. Customer service and pharmaceutical care both directly relate to the effectiveness of communication in the pharmacy. Thus, this topic is crucially important to the pharmacy technician.

The Communication Process

Communication is a process (Figure 3-1). More specifically, it is a two-way process. Communication is more than just talking, or even just listening; there is an art to communication.

The Communications Process

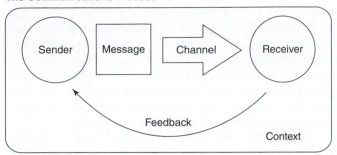

FIGURE 3-1 The communication process.

To better illustrate the communication process, let's use the following scenario: A patient, Mr. Matthews, is at the pharmacy to pick up his son's medicine. After locating the prescription, the pharmacy technician, Rebecca, sees a note on the bag stating, "Insurance denied; must pay cash."

The Sender

The communication process is initiated by the **sender**, the individual who has a statement to make or a question to ask. In our scenario, the pharmacy technician, Rebecca, becomes the sender and initiates the communication process, by explaining, "I am sorry, Mr. Matthews, but apparently the insurance company denied the prescription. Your total is going to be $143.90."

The Message

The **message** is the information that the sender provides, when making a statement, or requests, when asking a question. Although the concept of a message may seem elementary, many factors influence and create the full meaning of the message; these factors are discussed later in this chapter.

Rebecca's message was a statement; she provided information to Mr. Matthews about the insurance company's action. In addition, Rebecca's message informed Mr. Matthews how much money he needed to pay to receive his son's medication.

The Channel

The term **channel** simply refers to the mode by which the sender transmits the message. Communication occurs through written channels, such as letters and e-mails; verbal channels, such as

---

sender the person who originates or imparts a communication message.

message the substance, or information, being transferred in communication.

channel a gesture, action, sound, written or spoken word, or visual image used in transmitting information.

receiver the person to whom a communication message is sent.

feedback the return of information, or a message, in the communication process.

context the setting, or circumstances, in which communication occurs.

verbal communication the imparting or interchanging of thoughts, opinions, or information through the use of spoken words.

---

phone calls; and nonverbal channels, such as the sender's body language. The channel of communication in our scenario is verbal. Both Rebecca and Mr. Matthews are physically present at the pharmacy, and they are speaking face to face.

The Receiver

The **receiver** in the communication process is the individual to whom the sender is transmitting the message. In verbal communication, it is the person to whom the sender is speaking or questioning. In our scenario, Mr. Matthews is the receiver as he hears Rebecca explain her message, "I am sorry, Mr. Matthews, but apparently the insurance company denied the prescription. Your total is going to be $143.90."

Feedback

Feedback is the aspect of communication that makes it a two-way process. The receiver provides the sender with feedback—a reaction, either verbal or nonverbal—to the communicated message. Feedback is critical to ensure that the receiver properly understood the message. Returning to our scenario, Mr. Matthews lets out a loud sigh and shakes his head when he hears Rebecca's message. In a sense, feedback actually reverses the communication process, because the initial receiver becomes the sender and the initial sender becomes the new receiver. In effective communication, the process continues to reverse as it flows back and forth, creating a clear and useful conversation.

Context

Context refers to the situation, or environment, in which the message is delivered. In our scenario, one context is the pharmacy and the attitudes and beliefs related to pharmacy professionals. Pharmacy has for many years been cited as the most trusted and respected profession in the United States, ranking above medical practice, law, and ministry. This honor, however, comes with a responsibility to communicate in a trustworthy and professional manner.

Another context of our scenario is Mr. Matthews's personal situation. It could be that his son is very sick, but he cannot afford the medication; therefore, his family's health and financial resources are also a part of the background to the feedback he is providing.

Communication Types and Methods

The three primary types of communication are verbal, written, and nonverbal. As a pharmacy technician, you will need to communicate effectively in all three modes. Within the pharmacy practice setting (in fact, in any setting), we use a variety of methods for effective communication within any one type. To illustrate the types and methods of communication, we will continue to extend the scenario between Mr. Matthews and Rebecca.

Verbal Communication

The first type of communication is **verbal communication** (Figure 3-2). Although this is an auditory type of communication,

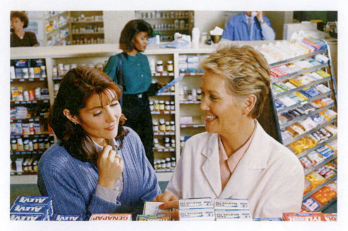

FIGURE 3-2 Verbal communication.
Source: Corbis

it encompasses much more than words alone. Verbal communication includes one's tone of voice, inflection, pitch, volume, and pronunciation and diction, as well as the specific words used.

The first, and most important, point to remember regarding verbal communication—or any type of communication, for that matter—is the accuracy and clarity of the message. Even if you handle every aspect of the communication process professionally, your efforts will not matter if the message you are sending is inaccurate.

The sender's tone of voice greatly influences the message and consequently the feedback received. Consider the message sent by Rebecca: "I am sorry, Mr. Matthews, but apparently the insurance company denied the prescription. Your total is going to be $143.90." As words printed on a page, the message appears clear and professional, but what effect could Rebecca's tone of voice have?

Read Rebecca's statement aloud, using a sympathetic, caring tone of voice: "I am sorry, Mr. Matthews, but apparently the insurance company denied the prescription. Your total is going to be $143.90."

Now read her statement aloud again, using a monotone, impersonal tone of voice: "I am sorry, Mr. Matthews, but apparently the insurance company denied the prescription. Your total is going to be $143.90."

Finally, read her statement aloud once more, using a condescending, annoyed tone of voice: "I am sorry, Mr. Matthews, but apparently the insurance company denied the prescription. Your total is going to be $143.90."

Although not one single word was different, three entirely different messages were sent to Mr. Matthews. It is easy to imagine how Mr. Matthews's feedback would vary depending on the tone of voice Rebecca used.

Inflection is a change in the tone of voice, the emphasis, or word stress used, or the pronunciation of a specific word or phrase. Inflection too can greatly influence a sender's message. To see the differences, repeat Rebecca's statement several times aloud, each time emphasizing a different word or phrase: "I am sorry, Mr. Matthews, but apparently the insurance company denied the prescription. Your total is going to be $143.90."

The sender's voice **pitch** (how high or low the voice is in sound wave frequency) and the **volume** at which the sender speaks can affect the receiver's ability to properly understand the message. If Rebecca speaks to Mr. Matthews too softly, he might not be able to hear what Rebecca said and then become confused or agitated. In contrast, if Rebecca speaks too loudly, Mr. Matthews might become embarrassed, self-conscious, uncomfortable, or defensive. This aspect of verbal communication is particularly important with geriatric patients, who may not hear very well or may have specific ranges of hearing loss.

Finally, the sender's **pronunciation** and **diction** are critical to ensuring that the receiver properly understood the message. Incorrect pronunciation and/or the use of slang will both impair the message and reduce the receiver's perception of your credibility and professionalism.

There are two primary methods of verbal communication: face to face and by telephone.

Face-to-Face Communication

As a pharmacy technician, you will be involved in face-to-face communication nearly all day long, excluding a few specialty practice settings. This face-to-face communication will be with your pharmacists, your coworkers, and your patients and customers. Here are some tips for effective face-to-face communication:

- Smile. Be a pleasant individual to communicate with.
- Speak clearly and at an appropriate volume.
- Use professional and appropriate tones of voice, inflections, and diction.
- Listen actively when someone is speaking to you; acknowledge the speaker by nodding your head.
- Do not interrupt while someone is speaking. Wait until the speaker is finished.
- Ask questions to ensure that you both completely understood the conversation.

Telephone-Based Communication

Pharmacy technicians spend a great deal of time communicating on the telephone. They may use the phone to speak with patients, request refill authorizations from doctors' offices, or get assistance from an insurance company's help desk (see Figure 3-3). In any case, telephone-based communication can be more complicated than face-to-face

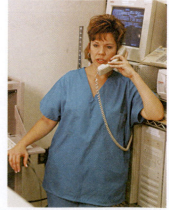

FIGURE 3-3 Telephone communication.

---

inflection alteration in pitch or the tone of voice.

pitch the property of sound that is determined by the frequency of sound wave vibrations reaching the ear.

volume the loudness of a communication.

pronunciation the manner in which someone utters a word.

diction clarity and distinctness of pronunciation in speech.

written communication the imparting or interchanging of thoughts, opinions, or information through the use of written words.

nonverbal communication the imparting or interchanging of thoughts, opinions, or information without the use of spoken words.

communication because of the lack of additional information from nonverbal communication (discussed later in this chapter).

Personal Phone Calls It is not professional to make personal phone calls while on the job. If you do, then you are risking your reputation as a pharmacy technician, plus you are running the risk of getting written up by your supervisor, or you may face more serious consequences such as getting fired from your job.

Written Communication

The second type of communication is **written communication**. Although many of the considerations concerning verbal communication apply to written messages as well, other factors come into play when you communicate in writing.

As a pharmacy technician, you will communicate in writing in a variety of ways, such as notes, messages, lists, reports, and other documentation. The most common written communications that pharmacy technicians receive are prescriptions and medication orders.

Just as with verbal communication, accuracy is fundamental with written messages. Legible handwriting and correct grammar both play a large role in creating accurate written messages. If your handwriting is illegible—that is, difficult or impossible to read—your communication will cause at the least delay and possibly confusion or an outright error.

▣ Procedure 3-1

Receiving a Voicemail

1. Record the date and time the message was left.
2. Record the caller's name and phone number.
3. Indicate the individual for whom the message was left.
4. Clearly document the request made on the voicemail.
5. Sign or initial the documentation.

▣ Procedure 3-2

Leaving a Voicemail

1. State your full name and the pharmacy's name.
2. Provide the pharmacy's phone number and hours of operation.
3. Indicate the purpose of your call, but say you are calling about personal business. If you give out too much health information, then you may be breaking privacy and/or HIPAA laws.
4. Make any specific requests needed.
5. Give your name and the pharmacy's phone number a second time.

Nonverbal Communication

The final type of communication, and the most underestimated, is **nonverbal communication**, which is communication that is neither spoken nor written by an individual. Research indicates that up to 80% of communication is nonverbal. However, most individuals are unaware of their nonverbal cues or, rather, do not realize that they are sending messages this way. Sometimes they inadvertently send nonverbal messages that contradict or oppose their verbal message. Silence, for example, can deliver either positive or negative feedback, depending on the context of the communication.

There are many methods of nonverbal communication, some of which are used subconsciously. However, when you realize that more than three-fourths of human communication is nonverbal, you should also realize that it is imperative for you to take control over these cues if you are to be an effective and accurate communicator. Nonverbal communication consists of kinesics, oculesics, proxemics, work environment, and even distractions.

Voicemails and Patient Confidentiality

Patient confidentiality is a major issue in all pharmacy work, but you must take special care regarding confidentiality when leaving voicemail messages. If you are calling a doctor's office to get a refill authorization, at the patient's request, obviously you will need to provide detailed information, including the patient's name and the medication. If, however, you are leaving a voicemail for the patient, on either a home answering machine or a work voicemail, it is inappropriate to include any detailed or confidential information. A proper message would be "Hello, this is Brad with Main Street Pharmacy calling to speak with Ms. Chan. You can call me back at 281-555-7900. Again, this is Brad at Main Street Pharmacy. The telephone number is 281-555-7900. Thank you."

Kinesics

Kinesics, commonly called body language, refers to communication through body movement and facial expressions.

- Facial expressions—communicate emotions, such as happiness, anger, or surprise.
- Arm positions—crossing one's arms across his or her chest can indicate that the individual is guarded and placing a subconscious barrier up, whereas an open stance with one's arms hanging by his or her sides suggests comfort and ease.
- Gestures—can communicate thoughts, requests, or strong emotions.
- Posture—communicates confidence and energy level; good posture indicates a confident, professional, and alert individual.
- Body movement—fidgeting with one's hands, or rocking back and forth, or swinging one's foot can communicate either disinterest in or agitation with the dialogue. Such movement often indicates a desire to end the communication as soon as possible. Frequent blinking or touching the face while speaking can indicate deceit or the act of withholding information.

Oculesics

Oculesics refers to the study of eye contact, which is a major contributor to nonverbal communication. Although the customs and significance of eye contact varies between cultures, it is recommended to always maintain proper eye contact with your patients and coworkers. Doing so ensures that you are signaling your interest in the communication, and it allows you to observe the other individual's nonverbal communication.

- Eye contact—communicates interest in the dialogue. Looking away, or gazing, indicates disinterest in the communication.

Proxemics

Proxemics refers to the study of measurable distance between individuals as they interact. According to American anthropologist and cross-cultural researcher Edward T. Hall's research, a distance of 6 to 18 inches refers to an intimate zone reserved for close family members; a distance of 1.5 to 4 feet is considered a personal zone and is generally used for friends and associates; a social space of 4 to 12 feet is reserved for coworkers or social environments, and 10 to 25 feet is considered public distance. Socially accepted personal space varies among cultures; however, most interactions in the pharmacy occur within the social space of 4 to 12 feet.

- Personal space—the distance one stands from another person when talking can communicate one's level of comfort and trust with the other individual. However,

personal space can also simply be a cultural norm, as opposed to a nonverbal cue.

Environment

The environment in which communication occurs is also noteworthy. A proper environment is clean, organized, and free from distractions, including loud sounds or music. Consider the nonverbal message that your patient would receive if he or she approached the pharmacy to find it dirty, unorganized, hectic, and noisy.

Active Listening

Have you ever had a conversation in which you were "heard" by the other individual but the individual was not truly "listening?" Active listening is a structured technique used to improve communication. As a pharmacy technician it is critical that you actively listen to your patients, as opposed to simply hearing them. Here are the four primary steps involved in active listening:

1. Hearing—listen attentively to ensure that you understand what the other person is saying.
2. Interpreting—confirm your understanding of what you heard the other person say.
3. Evaluating—ask the other person questions regarding what you heard.
4. Responding—acknowledge to the other person that he or she has been heard and properly understood; nonverbal communication techniques can also be used to express your interest in what the other person has said.

Barriers to Communication

Problems with communication can arise at any stage of the communication process (sender, message, channel, receiver, feedback, or context). Any problems have the potential to create misunderstandings and confusion (see Figure 3-4).

To be an effective communicator, and to get your point across without misunderstanding or confusion, your goal should be to reduce the occurrence of problems at each stage of the process by using clear, precise,

---

kinesics the study of nonlinguistic bodily movements, such as gestures and facial expressions, as a systematic mode of communication.

oculesics direct visual contact with another individual's eyes.

proxemics the study of the cultural, behavioral, and sociological aspects of spatial distances between individuals.

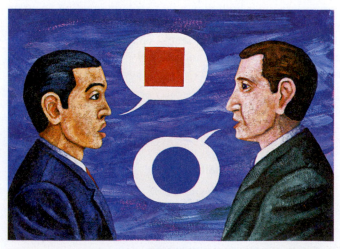

FIGURE 3-4 Language barriers.

well-planned communication. If your message is too long, jumbled, or inaccurate, you can expect it to be misunderstood or misinterpreted. Poor grammar and conflicting body language can also make a message unclear or send additional, unintended meanings. You must commit to breaking down the barriers that exist in each stage of the communication process. This section examines some common barriers to the communication process, their impact, and tips on how to eliminate them.

Language Barriers

One of the leading barriers to communication in the United States is language. This barrier arises when a patient or coworker is unable to speak or understand the English language. This communication barrier affects one out of every five people in the United States:

- Twenty-one million people speak English less than adequately.
- Thirty million people do not speak English as their primary language.

As a pharmacy technician, you must be prepared to deal with patients who speak little or no English. Although it is the role of the pharmacist to counsel patients on their prescriptions and medications, technicians are the frontline employees who communicate with patients directly about many important issues.

> ❝ **Workplace Wisdom** **Bilingual Benefits**
>
> Bilingual pharmacy technicians are a valuable asset to any pharmacy and typically have a greater earning potential. There is a great need for pharmacy professionals who are fluent speakers of languages other than English, particularly Spanish, Vietnamese, Chinese, and French, across the United States. Be sure that you include details on your résumé pertaining to any other language(s) you speak. ❞

Here are some tips on how to overcome a language barrier:

- **Use the client's native language, if possible**—Many pharmacy technicians are bilingual. If you can speak the patient's language, do so.
- **Offer to use a translator**—A translator could be a coworker, a member of the client's family, another health care provider, or even an employee from a different department. In any case, it should be someone that patients feel they can trust.
- **Provide written instructions in the client's native language**—The computer systems in most pharmacies are able to print prescription labels and drug monographs in nearly any language. Offer this service to any patient for whom English is not the primary or native language.

Communication Impairments

Outside of language barriers, there are two primary communication impairments: hearing impairment and illiteracy. Both of these impairments can become significant obstacles in communicating with patients and customers, if you do not know how to properly address them.

Hearing Impairment

Hearing-impaired individuals have a relative insensitivity to sound in the speech frequencies, meaning that conventional speech and language itself become barriers to communication (see Figure 3-5).

Hearing impairment is categorized according to severity. The scale includes deafness, being "hard of hearing," and unilateral hearing loss.

- Deafness—little or no residual hearing capability; the patient is unable to hear.
- Hard of hearing—partially unable to hear; the patient typically requires hearing aids.
- Unilateral hearing loss—hears normally in one ear, but has trouble hearing with the other ear.

Here are some tips for communicating with clients who have hearing impairments:

- **Look directly at the patient when speaking**—Individuals who suffer from impaired hearing rely heavily on lip reading as people speak. To ensure that clients are able to read your lips, look directly at them as you speak. If you can see their lips, you know that they can see yours.
- **Speak louder**—Many people who are hard of hearing, or have unilateral hearing loss, need you to speak at a louder-than-normal volume to communicate effectively. Keep in mind, however, the nature of your comments or questions. You must still protect your patient's confidential information. Be subtle when speaking loudly, because proper tone and inflection are still important.
- **Reduce background noise**—Background noise, which is common at most places of business, can further impair an individual's ability to hear you. When possible, particularly when communicating with those who have unilateral hearing loss, speak in a location with little or no background noise, such as in the patient consultation room.

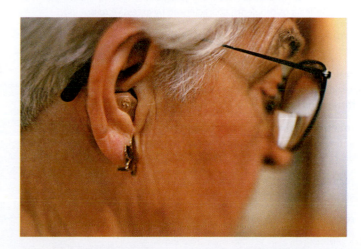

FIGURE 3-5 A hearing-impaired person will often wear a hearing aid.
Source: Keith Brofsky/Getty Images, Inc.

An Internet-based resource for learning ASL online is available at **www.signingonline.com**.

- **Always have the pharmacist provide counseling on new prescriptions**—By ensuring that the pharmacist consults each patient on new prescriptions, you guarantee that, at a minimum, patients receive verbal instructions and warnings related to their medication(s).
- **Always ask patients if they have any questions**—Regardless of whether patients are picking up refills of existing prescriptions, dropping off new prescriptions, or purchasing over-the-counter (OTC) medications, ask if they have any questions. This approach provides an opportunity for those with insufficient reading skills to gain information without feeling embarrassment or shame.
- **Watch for indicators of low-level literacy skills**—Although it is not appropriate to profile individuals according to their literacy skills, certain indicators can be useful. For example, if a patient seems to have difficulty reading or completing a new patient profile, this could indicate low literacy skills. If you suspect that a patient may have literacy complications, ask him or her to write the address, date of birth, or other common profile information on the prescription as he or she drops it off to be filled. This allows you to screen for literacy problems and therefore better understand the patient's communication needs. Compassion and empathy are crucial when dealing with persons who cannot read. They may be embarrassed, but they still need to understand their medicines. It is up to you to help them feel comfortable and receptive to important information.

- **Learn sign language**—The preceding tips probably will not help you communicate with totally or profoundly deaf patients. However, learning American Sign Language (ASL) may allow you to communicate effectively with these patients.

---

defense mechanisms unconscious mental processes used to protect one's ego.

denial a defense mechanism characterized by refusal to acknowledge painful realities, thoughts, or feelings.

displacement a defense mechanism characterized by an unconscious shift of emotions, affect, or desires from the original object to a more acceptable or immediate substitute.

intellectualization a defense mechanism used to protect oneself from the emotional stress and anxiety associated with confronting painful personal fears or problems; characterized by excessive reasoning.

projection a defense mechanism whereby one's own attitudes, feelings, or suppositions are attributed to others.

rationalization a defense mechanism whereby one's true motivation is concealed by explaining one's actions and feelings in a way that is not threatening.

reaction formation a defense mechanism characterized by actions at the opposite extreme of one's true feelings, as overcompensation for unacceptable impulses.

regression a defense mechanism characterized by reverting to an earlier or less mature pattern of feeling or behavior.

repression a defense mechanism characterized by the exclusion of painful impulses, desires, or fears from the conscious mind.

sublimation a defense mechanism in which unacceptable instinctual drives and wishes are modified to take more personally and socially acceptable forms.

PROFILE IN PRACTICE

Toby works as a pharmacy technician at a chain retail pharmacy. A new patient arrived and requested to have a prescription filled, but was unable to complete the patient profile form when asked to do so. Toby's patient is illiterate.

▸ *How can Toby assist without embarrassing the patient?*
▸ *What special considerations, if any, will the patient need when picking up his prescription?*

Defense Mechanisms

Another common barrier to communication is the utilization of **defense mechanisms**, which are unconscious behaviors or reactions that are generally prompted by anxiety. Pharmacy professionals serve individuals who are sick, ill, or fighting a disease, and most of these individuals are simultaneously experiencing anxiety and worry. When anxiety occurs, the mind initially responds with an increase in problem-solving thinking, seeking ways to escape the situation. At that point, a variety of defense mechanisms may be triggered.

All defense mechanisms share two common properties. First, they are often used unconsciously. Second, they tend to distort, transform, or otherwise misrepresent reality. Sigmund Freud, a pioneer of psychotherapy, identified nine primary defense mechanisms: denial, displacement, intellectualization, projection, rationalization, reaction formation, regression, repression, and sublimation. This section includes a brief overview of each one, to help familiarize you with these behaviors that you may see in customers or in yourself.

Denial

Denial is a defense mechanism whereby an individual avoids confronting a problem by denying the very existence of the problem. An example is the patient who is diagnosed with diabetes, but denies that he or she really has the disease and therefore decides not to take the prescribed medications and test his or her blood glucose levels.

Displacement

Displacement occurs when an individual transfers his or her own negative emotions to someone, or something, that is completely unrelated to the individual's feelings. An example of displacement is the patient who has been yelled at by his or her boss all day and then transfers his or her anger and resentment to the pharmacy technician when he or she is at the pharmacy that evening.

Intellectualization

Intellectualization is the defense mechanism whereby an individual deals with conflict or stressors by making generalizations to minimize disturbing feelings. An example is the impatient customer who becomes irate when hearing that it will take an hour to fill his or her prescription—because, after all, "How long does it actually take to pour 30 tablets into a bottle and put a label on it?"

Projection

Projection occurs when an individual attributes his or her own thoughts or impulses to another person. For example, a patient who is prejudiced against minorities complains that both the African-American and Asian-American staff pharmacists treat the patient with disrespect, because they do not like him or her.

Rationalization

Rationalization is a defense mechanism whereby an individual offers a socially acceptable and apparently logical explanation for an act or decision that is actually produced by unconscious impulses. An example is the patient who decides to take twice the prescribed dosage of his or her medication, believing that if 500 mg is good, then 1,000 mg would be even better.

Reaction Formation

Reaction formation occurs when someone goes to the opposite extreme of behavior, overcompensating for unacceptable impulses. Consider the patient who is confronted by his or her physician about requesting an unnecessary number of prescription drugs, and then stops taking any medications at all.

Regression

Regression is a defense mechanism in which an individual suffers a loss of some of the development already attained and reverts to a lower level of adaptation and expression. An example is the adult who suddenly becomes incapable of taking tablets or capsules, and requires all of his or her medication in liquid form.

Repression

Repression involves an involuntary exclusion of a painful thought, impulse, or memory from awareness. For example, a patient immediately changes the subject when asked how the patient is doing after the death of his spouse.

Sublimation

Sublimation is a defense mechanism whereby individuals redirect their socially unacceptable impulses or emotions into a socially acceptable form. An example is the patient who has been diagnosed with a debilitating disease: To divert his or her attention, the patient begins to work excessively long hours at the office.

Conflict

Conflict will certainly arise in the pharmacy setting, just as it does in any workplace. Serious disputes, disagreements, and arguments are all considered conflict, and they may arise with your patients or your coworkers. Strategies on resolving conflict include the following:

- Get assistance from your pharmacy manager.
- Identify attitude shifts to show respect for others' needs.
- Transform problems into creative opportunities.
- Develop communication tools to build rapport. Use listening skills to clarify understanding.
- Apply strategies to attack the problem, not the person.
- Manage your emotions. Express fear, anger, hurt, and frustration wisely to effect change.
- Identify personal issues that may be involved in the situation.
- Evaluate the problem in its broader context.

The best strategy for pharmacy technicians to use in conflict resolution is to request the assistance of the pharmacist or pharmacy manager. It is important to remember your scope of authority and duties. Conflict that arises with a patient will often require the pharmacist to become involved or handle the situation. When conflict develops between coworkers, the matter should be taken to the pharmacy manager or supervisor.

Eliminating Communication Barriers

So far in this section, we have explored various barriers to effective communication, in addition to strategies and tips on how to eliminate them. The universal keys to eliminating communication barriers include:

- Fully understanding the communication process
- Recognizing that numerous barriers to communication exist
- Knowing and effectively using strategies to overcome communication barriers
- Being willing to recognize and eliminate communication barriers as they arise

The final key—willingness to recognize and eliminate communication barriers as they arise—is the most important of the four. Unless you are willing to actively address communication barriers, they will continue to hinder and reduce the effectiveness of your communication.

Caring for Customers and Patients

In addition to dispensing prescription medications, pharmacy professionals provide comfort, care, advice, and instructions. They also guarantee specific rights, such as patient confidentiality. Patients are just one type of customer whom the pharmacy technician serves, however. There are two main types of customers: internal and external.

Internal Customers

Within any pharmacy, or company for that matter, there are a number of internal customers who must be treated with respect and care. Examples of internal customers include the pharmacy manager; pharmacists; fellow pharmacy technicians and clerks; upper management staff; and individuals who work in other departments within the organization, such as information technology (IT), human resources, accounting, and legal. Within health systems, internal customers can extend to physicians, nursing staff, and other health professionals.

External Customers

The patient is the primary external customer, regardless of practice setting; however, pharmacy technicians also serve other external customers such as the patient's family or caregiver, pharmaceutical representatives, and, in the case of community pharmacies, physicians, nurses, and other health professionals.

Patient Rights

In pharmacy practice, patients are guaranteed five specific rights, known as the *Five Patient Rights*. These rights ensure that the *right* patient receives the *right* medication, at the *right* strength, by the *right* route, at the *right* time. By following the Five Rights, medication safety is ensured.

1. Right patient—The prescription must be labeled for, dispensed to, and billed to the right customer.
2. Right medication—The prescription for medication must be accurately interpreted and the correct medication dispensed.
3. Right strength—The dosage, or strength, prescribed must be accurately interpreted and the medication accurately labeled and dispensed.
4. Right route—The intended dosage form or route of administration must be used.
5. Right time—The proper directions for administration must be correctly interpreted from the prescription, included in the medication labeling, and explained to the patient.

> ❝ **Workplace Wisdom** **The Five Rights**
> - Right patient
> - Right medication
> - Right strength
> - Right route
> - Right time ❞

In addition to the long-standing (but unofficial) Five Rights, Congress passed the Patient's Bill of Rights in 2005. In general terms, the Patient's Bill of Rights guarantees that patients have the right to:

- The best care available for their health needs
- Be treated with courtesy and respect

- Know their illness, condition, and treatment
- Give or refuse permission for care, treatment, or research
- Plan and participate in their own care
- Be examined and treated in private
- Receive care in a manner that supports comfort and dignity
- Have communications and records concerning their care treated in a confidential manner
- Have their families and significant others treated respectfully
- Know the names and positions of the persons caring for them
- Make health care decisions by completing a living will, or by appointing a person to make health care decisions on their behalf
- Take part in discussion of ethical issues that arise regarding their care
- Spiritual care and religious support consistent with personal beliefs
- Know how issues, complaints, and grievances about their care will be handled
- Care that respects their growth and development
- Effective assessment and management of pain
- An interpreter or assistive devices when they have a communication impairment or do not speak or understand the language of the health care team
- Family involvement in decisions about organ, tissue, and eye donation
- Leave the hospital or outpatient clinical site even if their physicians advise against it
- Ethical business practices

The Patient's Bill of Rights covers all aspects of medical and pharmaceutical care, so certain guarantees in it may not relate directly to the practice of pharmacy. It is essential, however, that pharmacy technicians familiarize themselves with the Patient's Bill of Rights and abide by its directives.

Greeting Customers

Pharmacy technicians are, most often, the frontline employees in the pharmacy, meaning that a technician is usually the first and last person to speak with a patient. In addition, as much as 75%, or more, of the communication and interaction the customer has at the pharmacy will be with you, the pharmacy technician.

It is important to remember that most patients who come to the pharmacy are sick or feeling badly. Customers may be confused about which OTC medication to purchase or may be emotional because of news just received at the doctor's office. Whatever the situation, it is important to greet your customers in a timely, caring, and positive manner. Here are several keys to greeting your patients and customers effectively:

- Smile.
- Speak and act sincerely.
- Look at your customer attentively.
- Introduce yourself and ask for your customer's name.
- Build trust and establish a personal relationship with your patient over time.
- Refer customers to the pharmacist to address any questions outside of your scope of practice.

Protecting Confidentiality

Confidentiality is essential in pharmacy practice and is required by law. Although Chapter 4 outlines the legal aspects and requirements of patient confidentiality, it is appropriate to address the relationship of confidentiality to patient care here.

Generally speaking, every piece of data or information pertaining to a patient is considered confidential. In addition to their legal rights, patients have certain expectations regarding this information. They trust that any personally identifiable information will be kept safe and secure from personnel who do not need to know the information. They expect that patient profiles and medication histories will be kept private and used only for pharmacy-related issues. They also assume that any information regarding their medical conditions will not be released to anyone without their permission.

Confidentiality is vital because it is the foundation on which the patient's trust in the pharmacy and pharmacy staff is built. As a pharmacy technician, you will constantly work with private and confidential information. It is imperative that you always protect the confidentiality of your patients.

Pharmacist Consultations

Pharmacist consultations are one of the essential elements of providing pharmaceutical care (see Figure 3-6). Providing advice, instructions, and other clinical information falls outside the scope of practice for pharmacy technicians; these responsibilities are to be handled by the pharmacist on duty. It is the responsibility of the pharmacy technician, however, to ensure that patients and customers speak with the pharmacist when appropriate. A pharmacist consultation is required for any:

- New prescription that a patient has not previously taken
- New prescription or refill when changes were made from previous dispensing
- Prescription or refill that flags a drug utilization review (DUR)
- Request by a customer or patient to speak with the pharmacist

There are certain exceptions to the rule that pharmacy technicians do not provide instructions to patients. Upon the authorization of the pharmacist, the technician may read the instructions or directions for a prescription. Also, after being trained and approved by the pharmacist, many pharmacy technicians assist patients with selecting and understanding OTC medical devices, such as blood glucose meters and nebulizers. These exceptions vary by state regulation and individual pharmacist approval. Under no circumstances, however, should a pharmacy technician ever provide verbal advice or clinical information.

Special Considerations

There are a number of special considerations in providing customer service and patient care, such as the patient's culture and age.

Cultural Differences

The United States is known as the melting pot; nowhere else on Earth will you find a greater diversity in ethnicity and cultural background. This becomes a special consideration at the pharmacy, as it is important to provide the highest quality pharmaceutical care while still respecting your patient's cultural differences. For example, different cultures accept different physical boundaries: Persons from certain cultures prefer a greater distance from their conversation partners, whereas persons from other cultures prefer to stand very close to the person they are speaking with. In addition, different cultures have various methods of greeting, salutations, attire, and even medical beliefs. The key is to be attentive to your customers, learn what they find acceptable, and respect their preferences.

Age

Another special consideration for providing pharmaceutical care is the age of the patient (see Figure 3-7). In general, this becomes a factor only when dealing with the extremes of age, for pediatric and geriatric patients. When providing care for pediatric patients (those under the age of 12), the communication process will be directed toward the parent or guardian. Geriatric (older) patients may themselves be the individuals with whom you communicate,

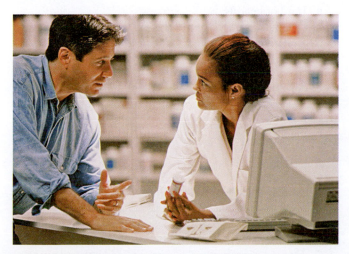

FIGURE 3-6 A pharmacist consults with a patient.
Source: Bruce Ayres/Getty Images, Inc.

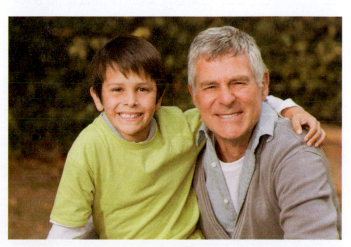

FIGURE 3-7 The age of a patient is a special consideration in pharmaceutical care.
Source: wavebreakmedia/Shutterstock

or they may have a designated caregiver, such as a child, a person designated by a medical power of attorney, or a nurse.

Terminally Ill Patients

When working as a pharmacy technician, you will be providing care for individuals who are terminally ill. Some of your patients will be suffering from acquired immune deficiency syndrome (AIDS), end-stage disease states, cancer, and other deadly conditions. When providing care for terminally ill patients, it is critical that you have empathy, compassion, and an understanding of the emotional stages that occur when an individual knows that he or she is dying. Psychologist Kubler-Ross identified five stages commonly experienced by patients: (1) denial, (2) anger, (3) bargaining, (4) depression, and ultimately (5) acceptance. Depending upon which stage a patient is currently in, you should be prepared to respond appropriately and compassionately, without taking his or her comments, actions, or behaviors personally. Through each individual's grief cycle, we can learn more about the grief process and what that individual goes through when experiencing the emotion of grief.

Summary

As you now know, communication is simply a process, but it is not a simple process. Pharmacy technicians work as front-line employees in the pharmacy, which means that both your management and your patients rely on you to be an effective communicator.

Although barriers to effective communication can and will arise in the pharmacy, it is your responsibility to remain aware and take the initiative to eliminate those barriers or overcome defense mechanisms. This requires a concerted, proactive approach on your part.

In addition, it is important to remember that the practice of pharmacy no longer consists of just dispensing drugs. Rather, it involves dispensing pharmaceutical care, which includes customer service, pharmacist consultations, and other services.

Chapter Review Questions

1. The most important key to eliminating barriers to communication is _____.
   a. fully understanding the communication process
   b. recognizing that numerous barriers to communication exist
   c. knowing strategies on how to overcome communication barriers
   d. being willing to recognize and eliminate communication barriers as they arise

2. A phone call is an example of which element of the communication process?
   a. channel
   b. context
   c. feedback
   d. message

3. How many Americans do not speak English as their primary language?
   a. 30 million
   b. 21 million
   c. 44 million
   d. 46 million

4. An involuntary exclusion of a specific thought or impulse is the defense mechanism referred to as _____.
   a. displacement
   b. reaction formation
   c. repression
   d. sublimation

5. _____ consists of serious disputes, disagreements, or arguments.
   a. Barrier to communication
   b. Conflict
   c. Defense mechanism
   d. None of the above

6. _____ is the condition in which an individual hears normally with one ear, but has trouble hearing with the other.
   a. Hard of hearing
   b. Deafness
   c. Unilateral hearing loss
   d. Selective hearing

7. Verbal communication methods include all of the following, except which one?
   a. diction
   b. pitch
   c. pronunciation
   d. silence

8. Language is the leading communication barrier in the U.S. that affects one out of every _____ people.
   a. 5
   b. 10
   c. 15
   d. 20

9. Offering a socially acceptable, or logical, explanation for an act is the defense mechanism known as _____.
   a. intellectualization
   b. denial
   c. projection
   d. rationalization

10. Pharmacists should be alerted for consultations in the following situations, except for _____.
    a. every new prescription
    b. every refill
    c. DUR prescriptions
    d. OTC advice

Critical Thinking Questions

1. List the Five Rights and discuss the potential consequences of not adhering to each.

2. In what ways are defense mechanisms and conflict connected?

3. Why are pharmacist consultations important, and why are they considered outside the scope of practice for pharmacy technicians?

Web Challenge

1. Go to http://thomas.loc.gov/ and search for the 2005 Patient's Bill of Rights. Print a copy of the complete act to read.

2. Go to http://www.funquizcards.com/quiz/personality/what-is-your-communication-style.php and take the online "What is Your Communication Style?" quiz. Print your assessment.

References and Resources

Conflict Resolution Network. 2008. Web. 20 January 2008.

"Data Centre Summary." *UNESCO Institute for Statistics.* 2005. Web. 20 January 2008.

Gandhi, J.K., et al. "Drug Complications in Outpatients." *Journal of General Internal Medicine.* 15 (1998): 149–154. Print.

Hu, D.J. and R.M. Covell. "Health Care Usage by Hispanic Outpatients as a Function of Primary Language." *Western Journal of Medicine.* 144 (1998): 490–493. Print.

Jacobs, Elizabeth, et al. "Impact of Language Barriers on Patient Satisfaction in an Emergency Department." *Journal of General Internal Medicine.* 4 (1999): 82–87. Print.

Johnston, Mike. *Certification Exam Review.* Upper Saddle River, NJ: Pearson, 2005. Print.

Johnston, Mike. *Fundamentals of Pharmacy Practice.* Upper Saddle River, NJ: Pearson, 2005. Print.

Kirkman-Liff, B. and D. Mondragon. "Language of Interview: Relevance for Research of Southwest Hispanics." *American Journal of Public Health.* 81 (1991): 1399–1404. Print.

Morales, L.S., et al. "Are Latinos Less Satisfied with Communication by Health Care Providers?" *Journal of General Internal Medicine.* 14 (1999): 400–407. Print.

"National Assessment of Adult Literacy (NAAL)." *U.S. National Center for Education Statistics.* 2005. Web. 20 January 2008.

Orum-Alexander, Gail G. and "Overcoming the Language Barrier." *Healthcare Providers Service Organization.* 2008. Web. 20 January 2008.

"Profile of Selected Social Characteristics: 2000." *U.S. Census Bureau, DP-2.* 2008. Web. 20 January 2008.

Weinick, R.M. and N.A. Krauss. "Racial and Ethnic Differences in Children's Access to Care." *American Journal of Public Health.* 90 (2001): 1771–1774. Print.

Woloshin, S., et al. "Is Language a Barrier to the Use of Preventive Services?" *Journal of General Internal Medicine.* 12 (1997): 472–477. Print.

Workman, T.E. and N.T. Lombardo. *Overcoming Language Barriers.* Binghamton, NY: Haworth Press, 2003. Print.

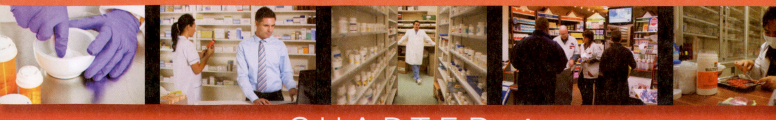

CHAPTER 4

Pharmacy Law and Ethics

LEARNING OBJECTIVES

After completing this chapter, you should be able to:

- Classify the various categories of U.S. law.
- List the regulatory agencies that oversee the practice of pharmacy and describe their function(s).
- Summarize the significant laws and amendments that affect the practice of pharmacy.
- Recognize and use a drug monograph.
- Define *ethics* and *moral philosophy*.
- List and explain the nine ethical theories.
- Summarize the Pharmacy Technician code of ethics.

KEY TERMS

adulterated, p. 43
autonomy, p. 54
beneficence, p. 54
civil law, p. 41
consequentialism, p. 54
criminal laws, p. 41
defendant, p. 41
ethics, p. 51
felony, p. 42
fidelity, p. 54
justice, p. 54
medical device, p. 51
medical ethics, p. 52
medical malpractice, p. 41
misbranded drug, p. 51
misdemeanor, p. 42
monograph, p. 51
nonconsequentialism, p. 54
plaintiff, p. 41
social contract, p. 54
statute, p. 41
veracity, p. 54

INTRODUCTION

Federal and state laws, as well as professional ethics, regulate the practice of pharmacy. The regulations on pharmacy practice in the United States have evolved and increased over the past 100 years, as legislators have responded to outcries from citizens to serve and protect the public interest. The government began to take the initiative in the regulation of pharmacy at the end of the 18th century. Over time, the profession of pharmacy has become subject to more regulations than were, back in the 1800s, ever thought possible. In the United States, a professional degree is a requirement for any individual who wishes to practice pharmacy. This requirement was established to protect the public and set minimum standards, so that citizens could rely on pharmacists having at least a standard level of education and competence.

This chapter focuses primarily on the major federal regulations pertaining to pharmacy practice. However, it does not list all federal laws pertaining to pharmacy, all the regulations included in or promulgated under the laws discussed, or all state regulations. To learn more about these topics, contact your State Board of Pharmacy (SBOP).

Overview of Law

There are four types of law in the United States: constitutional, statutes and regulations, administrative rules and regulations, and legislative intent.

Constitutional Law

The U.S. Constitution outlines the organization of the federal government. All laws passed must conform to the principles and rights set forth in the Constitution. The first 10 amendments to the Constitution are called the Bill of Rights; this is the source of the most fundamental rights, such as freedom of speech and religion, right to a jury trial, and protection against unreasonable searches and seizures.

Statutes and Regulations

Statutes are laws that are passed by federal, state, or local legislatures. Federal statutes are passed by the U.S. Congress and signed into law by the president. Regulations clarify and explain statutes, but they must also be consistent with the enacted statute because they have the same legal effect and power as the statute under which they were promulgated. Statutes often assign the power to create regulations, and delegate the responsibility for doing so, to a regulatory agency.

State Law and Regulations

State constitutions establish the organization of state government. Any laws passed by a state must meet the standards of both the federal and state constitutions, and state statutes must also remain consistent with the United States Code (USC) and the *Code of Federal Regulations* (CFR), which are federal statutes and regulations. State statutes and regulations may provide additional rights to corresponding federal law, but states may not take away rights that are established by or guaranteed under federal law.

Legislative Intent

Statutory and regulatory laws are based on legislative intent. In many cases, the legal interpretation of a law, the meaning of a particular section, or the meaning of a specific word is studied to determine what the legislators wanted the law to do or to cover. Interpretations are influenced by the use of *may* instead of *shall*, or even the location of a semicolon. Justices and judges are often called upon to determine legislative intent. The opinions and decisions they issue are commonly referred to as *case law*.

Criminal, Civil, and Administrative Law

Law can also be categorized as criminal, civil, or administrative.

Criminal Law

Criminal laws are those dealing with homicide, illegal drugs, theft, and other antisocial behavior. These laws are enforced by state agents against specific persons or corporations. The victim cannot prosecute the criminal case and does not have the right to determine if the state will prosecute the alleged criminal, because criminal law is designed to protect society as a whole rather than to compensate individuals who have been victims of criminal activity. This explains why criminal cases are titled *State v. John Smith* and *People v. Doe*.

Civil Law

Civil lawsuits involve personal injuries, business disputes, land deals, libel and slander, and various other commercial interests and noncriminal matters. **Civil law** actions must be brought by an attorney hired by the injured party, known as the **plaintiff**, against the alleged wrongdoer, referred to as the **defendant**. The parties in a civil case may be individuals, corporations, or the state itself.

Tort Law

Tort law is in essence a type of civil law, although it can also overlap into criminal law, in which a private wrong is committed against an individual or his or her property; this wrongdoing is known as a tort. Under tort law, an individual may seek compensation for suffering harm as the result of a wrongful act of an individual. **Medical malpractice** falls under tort law; therefore, pharmacies and pharmacy professionals are most often named in civil lawsuits, brought by plaintiffs claiming that professional errors or omissions were committed. Torts can be either intentional or unintentional, which is referred to as negligence.

Administrative Law

With the exception of the Defense Department and law enforcement agencies, the federal government conducts its activities through administrative agencies that enforce the laws. Examples of administrative agencies include the Internal Revenue Service (IRS), the Centers for Medicare and Medicaid Services (CMS), the Social Security Administration (SSA), and many others. States also operate through administrative agencies. Many of these agencies, such as state equal employment opportunity (EEO) commissions, correspond to federal agencies, whereas others, such as SBOPs, have no federal counterpart.

In addition to enforcing laws passed by the legislatures, administrative agencies refine these laws with regulations.

---

statute a law, decree, or edict.

criminal law any law dealing with crime or punishment.

civil law any law dealing with the rights of private citizens.

plaintiff the party that initiates a legal action.

defendant the party against which a legal action is brought.

medical malpractice the negligent treatment of a patient by a health care professional.

Some laws, such as the Americans with Disabilities Act, leave agencies little room for interpretation. With other laws, such as those creating SBOPs, the enabling legislation is vague, giving the agency the authority to determine the scope and detail of any regulations. Agencies must satisfy specific procedural requirements when promulgating regulations, but once the regulations are established, they have the force of law.

Violations of the Law

Any violation of the law is referred to as a *crime*, whether the law is criminal, civil, or administrative in nature. Crimes are further classified as either a **misdemeanor** or a **felony**.

Misdemeanors

Misdemeanor crimes are considered less serious than felonies and, depending on state law, are punishable by community service, parole, a fine, or imprisonment for 12 months or less. Infractions, such as traffic violations, are lesser misdemeanors, which are generally punishable by fines only.

Felonies

A felony, in contrast, is a serious crime, conviction of which typically results in imprisonment for more than a year. Felonies include murder; rape; aggravated assault; arson; robbery; and the manufacturing, sale, distribution, or possession of illegal drugs, among other crimes.

> ## ❝ Workplace Wisdom   Professional Liability
>
> As pharmacy technicians assume more responsibility, take on larger roles, and receive greater recognition in the pharmacy, they also become more subject to legal liability. Professional liability insurance coverage is now offered by a number of providers, including Healthcare Providers Service Organization (HPSO) and Pharmacists Mutual. ❞

PROFILE IN PRACTICE

Jim is a pharmacy technician who works at a local hospital, preparing IVs and chemotherapy. One of the patients at the hospital dies from a medication error because Jim added the wrong medication to an IV bag. The hospital pharmacist is responsible for verifying the technician's work, including IV preparations.

▸ *Who is responsible for the patient's death?*

▸ *What consequences can be expected for both the pharmacist and the pharmacy technician?*

misdemeanor an offense or infraction less serious than a felony.

felony a serious crime, such as rape or murder.

adulterated altered and causing an undesirable effect.

Regulatory Agencies

A number of regulatory agencies, on both the federal and state levels, oversee the practice of pharmacy.

Centers for Disease Control and Prevention

The Centers for Disease Control and Prevention (CDC) is the federal agency that is charged with protecting public health and safety through the investigation, identification, prevention, and control of diseases. Various institutes and centers are operated under the oversight of the CDC, including the National Institute of Occupational Safety and Health (NIOSH).

Centers for Medicare and Medicaid Services

The CMS, formerly known as the Health Care Financing Administration is the agency that regulates the administration of Medicare, Medicaid, the State Children's Health Insurance Program, the Health Insurance Portability and Accountability Act (HIPAA), the Clinical Laboratory Improvement Amendments, and several other health-related programs. The CMS conducts inspections to ensure compliance with its guidelines.

Drug Enforcement Administration

The Drug Enforcement Administration (DEA) regulates the legal trade in narcotic and dangerous drugs, manages a national narcotics intelligence system, and works with other agencies to prevent illegal drug trafficking. In 1982, coordinated joint jurisdiction over drug offenses was given to the Federal Bureau of Investigation (FBI) and the DEA. Agents of the two organizations work together on drug law enforcement, and the administrator of the DEA reports to the director of the FBI. The DEA has offices nationwide and in more than 40 foreign countries.

Food and Drug Administration

The Food and Drug Administration (FDA) is responsible for protecting the public health by ensuring the safety, efficacy, and security of drugs, biological products, medical devices, food, and cosmetics. The FDA is also responsible for reviewing and approving new drug applications (NDAs), new generic equivalents, and new therapeutic indications for existing medications.

The Joint Commission

The Joint Commission evaluates and accredits nearly 15,000 health care organizations and programs in the United States. Since 1951, the Joint Commission has established and enforced standards that focus on improving the quality and safety of care provided by health care organizations. It evaluates and accredits hospitals, hospice facilities, nursing homes, long-term care facilities, rehabilitation centers, and other health care organizations.

Occupational Safety and Health Administration

The Occupational Safety and Health Administration (OSHA) is a division of the U.S. Department of Labor that oversees the administration of the Occupational Safety and Health Act and enforces standards in all 50 states. The mission of OSHA is to ensure the safety and health of U.S. workers by setting and enforcing standards; OSHA establishes protective standards, enforces those standards, and reaches out to employers and employees through technical assistance and consultation programs.

State Boards of Pharmacy

The SBOP is the state agency that registers and regulates pharmacy facilities, pharmacists, and pharmacy technicians. Each state's Board of Pharmacy is responsible for establishing and maintaining a state pharmacy practice act that regulates the actual practice of pharmacy. The SBOP is granted the authority to monitor the activities of and, if necessary, reprimand licensed pharmacy professionals; it may also revoke the licenses of both pharmacy facilities and pharmacy professionals.

Overview of Pharmacy Law

Now that we have reviewed the various types of U.S. law and regulatory agencies, we can discuss legislation that specifically addresses the practice of pharmacy.

State and Federal Functions

Law and medicine are based on different, and sometimes opposing, professional paradigms. Medicine is a science-based profession; law is not based on a scientific paradigm. Nevertheless, the practice of pharmacy and medicine must conform to law.

The United States operates on a federalist system, in which there is a central government that has certain powers, but the state is the basic unit of political power. The distribution of power between the state and the federal government has always been a point of debate.

Historically, the states maintained power over their domestic matters. The federal government was given power over trade between the states and foreign policy issues. The federal government took greater power over domestic affairs during the Civil War and has continued to expand its authority. The 1980s saw the federal government assume even more power through its mandate of entitlement programs such as Medicare and Medicaid, even while it reduced federal financial support for these programs.

State Pharmacy Law

State law, generally, pertains to the actual practice of pharmacy. For example, state laws and regulations determine which activities related to immunization administration may be delegated by a pharmacist to a technician. States license pharmacies and pharmacy professionals, determine the standards under which pharmacists practice, and may add restrictions to federal laws, such as the food and drug laws.

Federal Pharmacy Law

It is the role of the federal government to determine the extent to which medical practice regulations are uniform among the 50 states, but, in most areas of medical practice, the states maintain the central regulatory role. In general, federal law pertains to the manufacturing, marketing, and distribution of pharmaceutical drugs. However, the federal government has enacted numerous pharmacy-related laws, which are outlined next. If federal and state laws ever conflict, the more stringent of the two laws is to be applied.

The Pure Food and Drug Act of 1906

On June 30, 1906, Congress passed a law that provided for federal inspection of meat products and forbade the manufacture, sale, or transport of **adulterated** food products or poisonous patent medicines. This law was called the Pure Food and Drug Act of 1906.

The Coca-Cola Company advocated for the 1906 Act, so it could advertise that its soft drink was "Guaranteed under the Pure Food and Drug Act." In 1909, however, the federal government attempted to ban the soft drink, citing the Pure Food and Drug Act and Coca-Cola's caffeine and cocaine content. Coca-Cola ultimately settled the case out of court and altered the product ingredients.

Over time, the Pure Food and Drug Act proved to be inadequate, because it did not:

- Cover cosmetics
- Grant the federal government authority to ban unsafe drugs
- Prohibit manufacturers from making false statements about their drugs
- Require labeling to identify the contents of a product

The Sherley Amendment of 1912

In an effort to overcome the ruling of *the United States v. Johnson*, in which the Supreme Court ruled the Pure Food and Drugs Act of 1906 did not prohibit false therapeutic claims but rather only false or misleading statements regarding the ingredients or identity of a drug, the Sherley Amendment of 1912 was enacted. It was designed to prohibit labeling medicines with false therapeutic claims intended to defraud consumers.

The Food, Drug, and Cosmetic Act of 1938

In 1938, U.S. legislators passed the Food, Drug, and Cosmetic Act, commonly referred to as the FDCA. The purpose of the FDCA was to limit interstate commerce in drugs to those that

---

info

Disasters Lead to Regulations

Disasters prompted the U.S. government to establish many of the original laws pertaining to pharmacy practice and the efficacy of medications. In 1937, a manufacturer decided to market a mixture of sulfanilamide and diethylene glycol as a remedy for sore throats. Diethylene glycol, known today as antifreeze, made the mixture into a deadly poison. This product caused 107 reported deaths, which became known as the sulfanilamide disaster of 1937 and prompted passage of the Food, Drug, and Cosmetic Act of 1938.

are safe and effective. Among the many major provisions of this legislation were the following:

- Manufacturers were required to submit evidence that new drugs were safe before they could market the drugs.
- All drugs had to have warnings and adequate directions for use.
- New drugs were required to be tested clinically before being marketed to the public.
- Drugs used as diagnostic agents, therapeutic devices, and cosmetics were required to be regulated for the first time.

The FDCA established an agency within the U.S. Department of Health and Human Services to oversee the new policies: the FDA.

Many of the provisions of the FDCA pertain to requirements for the label of a drug. It is important to understand and recognize the difference between the *label* of a drug and the *labeling* of a drug. Although both sound the same, they are actually two uniquely different components regulated under the FDCA. The label of a drug is "a display of written, printed, or graphic matter upon the immediate container of any article;" it is the information on the outer portion of the package or container. The labeling of a drug refers to "all labels and other written, printed, or graphic[al matter] either upon or accompanying the drug." Thus, labeling is broader in scope than the label; the labeling of a drug includes the package and package inserts, as well as the label.

The FDCA also regulated who could prescribe *legend drugs,* those available only by prescription. The FDCA does not require that the prescriber be licensed in the state where the prescription is actually filled, as long as the prescription is valid in the state in which it was written. A prescriber is permitted to delegate an authorized individual to transmit a prescription; however, the prescriber cannot delegate the authority to prescribe or authorize a refill.

Legend Drugs

According to the FDCA, only a practitioner licensed to administer and prescribe legend drugs may do so. Such practitioners include physicians, surgeons, veterinarians, dentists, physician assistants, nurse practitioners, and even pharmacists in certain states and according to specific regulations.

These laws and regulations govern drugs dispensed for human use. Be aware that additional or modified requirements are in place for drugs dispensed for animal use.

Labeling requirements for dispensed prescriptions include the following (see Figure 4-1):

- Pharmacy name and address
- Serial number (Rx number)
- Date of fill
- Expiration date
- Prescriber's name
- Patient's name
- Directions for use
- Cautionary statements

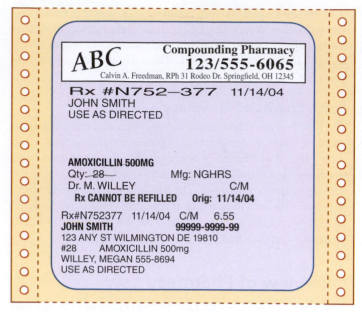

FIGURE 4-1 Sample prescription label.

The FDCA requires that legend drugs include the following information on the label of a drug (see Figure 4-2):

- Established name and quantity of each active ingredient
- Statement of new quantity
- Statement of usual dosage
- Federal legend
- Route of administration
- In the case of habit-forming drug—a federal warning
- Name of all inactive ingredients, if intended for route of administration other than the oral
- Unique lot or control number
- Statement specifying the type of container to be used for dispensing
- The name and place of business of the manufacturer, packer, or distributor
- Expiration date, if applicable

Although the label is considered a component of the labeling of a drug, the FDA also requires additional information in

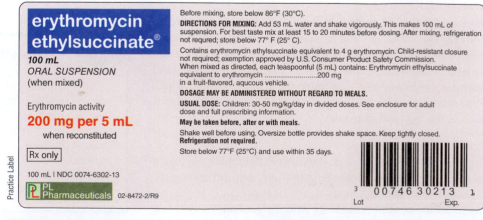

FIGURE 4-2 Sample legend drug label.

the labeling that accompanies a legend drug. The following information is required by the FDA and is usually provided in the package insert:

1. Description, which is usually a chemical structure
2. Clinical pharmacology
3. Indications and usage
4. Contraindications—situations in which the drug should not be used
5. Warnings of side effects and potential safety hazards
6. Precautions—details as to special care that must be taken
7. Adverse side effects
8. Drug abuse and dependence
9. Dosage
10. Statement as to how the drug is supplied
11. Date of the most recent revision to the labeling

Over-the-Counter Drugs

The FDCA requires that drugs approved for over-the-counter (OTC) distribution include the following information on the label of a drug (see Figure 4-3):

1. Product name
2. Name and address of the manufacturer and distributor and name of the person or place that repackages the product and others in the chain of commerce
3. Established name of all inactive or active ingredients and the quantities of certain other ingredients
4. Net contents
5. Required cautions and warnings
6. Name of any potentially habit-forming drug contained in the formula
7. Adequate directions for use or consumption

Drug Facts

Active ingredient (in each caplet)	Purpose
Acetaminophen 650 mg.....	Pain reliever/ fever reducer

Uses
- temporarily relieves minor aches and pains due to:
  - muscular aches
  - backache
  - headache
  - toothache
  - the common cold
  - menstrual cramps
  - minor pain of arthritis
- temporarily reduces fever

Warnings
Liver warning: product contains acetaminophen. Severe liver damage may occur if you take
- more than 6 caplets in 24 hours, which is the maximum daily amount
- with other drugs containing acetaminophen
- 3 or more alcoholic drinks every day while using this product

Overdose warning: Taking more than the recommended dose (overdose) may cause liver damage. In case of overdose, get medical help or contact a Poison Control Center right away. (1-800-222-1222) Quick medical attention is critical for adults as well as for children even if you do not notice any signs or symptoms.

Do not use
- if you are allergic to acetaminophen
- with any other drug containing acetaminophen (prescription or nonprescription).
  If you are not sure whether a drug contains acetaminophen, ask a doctor or pharmacist.

Ask a doctor before use if you have liver disease.

Ask a doctor or pharmacist before use if you are taking the blood thinning drug warfarin

Stop use and ask a doctor if
- pain gets worse or lasts for more than 10 days
- fever gets worse or lasts for more than 3 days
- new symptoms occur
- redness or swelling is present
These could be signs of a serious condition. ▶

Drug Facts (continued)

If pregnant or breast-feeding, ask a health professional before use.

Keep out of reach of children.

Directions
- do not take more than directed (see overdose warning)
- adults and children 12 years and over: take 2 caplets every 8 hours with water
- swallow whole – do not crush, chew or dissolve
- do not take more than 6 caplets in 24 hours
- do not use for more than 10 days unless directed by a doctor
- children under 12 years: do not use

Inactive ingredients
carnauba wax, colloidal silicon dioxide, croscarmellose sodium, FD&C red #40 aluminum lake, hypromellose, magnesium stearate, maltodextrin, microcrystalline cellulose, polyethylene glycol 400, polysorbate 80, povidone, pregelatinized starch, stearic acid, titanium dioxide

Store at room temperature (68°–77°F).
Questions or comments? 1-888-777-6666

FIGURE 4-3 Sample OTC drug label.

There have been numerous amendments to the original FDCA of 1938 as well as related legislative acts. This text cannot cover all of these amendments and acts, but the following subsections describe several of the most prominent ones.

The Durham–Humphrey Amendment of 1951

Also known as the Prescription Drug Amendment, the Durham–Humphrey Amendment of 1951 required that prescription drugs bear the legend, "Caution: Federal law prohibits dispensing without a prescription." This required legend is the reason why prescription drugs are referred to as *legend drugs*. Later amendments approved a substitute legend that simply reads "Rx only."

The Federal Hazardous Substance Labeling Act of 1960

The Federal Hazardous Substance Labeling Act of 1960 authorized the FDA to regulate hazardous substances, including those that are toxic, corrosive, irritants, strong sensitizers, flammable, or pressure generating. Specifically, this act required hazardous substances to bear labels, cautioning consumers of the potential hazards.

The Kefauver–Harris Amendment of 1962

Also known as the Drug Efficacy Amendment, the Kefauver–Harris Amendment of 1962 focused on drug manufacturers' accountability for the efficacy, or effectiveness, of drugs. Several provisions of this amendment are important to pharmacy practice:

- Good manufacturing practices (GMPs) were established for manufacturers.
- Prior to marketing any new drug, manufacturers were required to supply proof of the effectiveness and safety of the drug.
- Advertising of prescription drugs was placed under the supervision of the FDA.
- Procedures for NDAs and investigational drugs were established.

The Comprehensive Drug Abuse Prevention and Control Act of 1970

In 1970, the Comprehensive Drug Abuse Prevention and Control Act essentially combined all of the federal laws dealing with narcotics, stimulants, depressants, and abused designer drugs.

More commonly referred to as the Controlled Substances Act (CSA) of 1970, the Comprehensive Drug Abuse Prevention

The Thalidomide Disaster

The Kefauver–Harris Amendment was a legislative response to the thalidomide disaster of 1962, caused by a sedative thalidomide, which had been developed and was widely available abroad, and began to be used for antinausea treatment in early pregnancy. Children of women who had taken the medication during their first trimester of pregnancy were often born with severe deformities, especially of the extremities.

TABLE 4-1 Controlled Drug Schedules

Schedule	Symbol	Examples
Schedule I	C-I	Heroin, LSD, marijuana
Schedule II	C-II	Cocaine, morphine, Ritalin
Schedule III	C-III	Vicodin, Lortab, Tylenol #3, anabolic steroids
Schedule IV	C-IV	Valium, Librium
Schedule V	C-V	Lomotil

and Control Act established the DEA, which is an agency within the U.S. Department of Justice. It establishes a closed system in which the distribution of controlled substances is permitted only between entities registered with the DEA.

The CSA established five classes, referred to as *schedules*, of controlled substances. These schedules represent the potential for abuse of each drug. This legislation was enacted to help ensure public safety. The schedules range from I to V, with Schedule I having the highest potential for abuse and Schedule V having the lowest (see Table 4-1).

Schedule I

Schedule I drugs have a high potential for abuse. They have no currently accepted medical use in the United States, or there is no accepted safety standard for the use of these drugs. Examples of drugs in Schedule I include heroin, LSD, and marijuana. C-I is the symbol for this class of drugs.

Schedule II

Schedule II drugs have a currently accepted medical use in the United States, but they also have a high potential for abuse, or the abuse of these drugs or other substances may lead to severe dependence. Examples of drugs in Schedule II include cocaine, morphine, and Ritalin. C-II is the symbol for this class of drugs.

Schedule III

Schedule III drugs have less potential for abuse than those in Schedules I and II and have a currently accepted medical use in the United States. Abuse of Schedule III drugs may lead to moderate physical dependence or high psychological dependence. Examples of drugs in Schedule III include Vicodin, Lortab, Tylenol #3, and anabolic steroids. C-III is the symbol for this class of drugs. Schedule III substances may be refilled if authorized by the prescriber; however, refills are limited to five and all refills must be within six months from the date the original prescription was issued.

Schedule IV

Schedule IV drugs have a low potential for abuse and have a currently accepted medical use in the United States, or the abuse of these drugs may lead to limited dependence. Examples include Valium and Librium. C-IV is the symbol for this class of drugs. Schedule IV substances may be refilled if authorized by the prescriber; however, refills are limited to five and all refills must be within six months from the date the original prescription was issued.

Schedule V

Schedule V drugs have a low potential for abuse and have a currently accepted medical use in the United States, or the abuse of these drugs may lead to limited dependence in relation to all other controlled substances. An example of a Schedule V drug is Lomotil. C-V is the symbol for this class of drugs. There are no additional requirements on refills of Schedule V substances, and a prescription can be refilled for up to one year according to the prescriber's directions.

Registration

Participation in any of the following activities requires registration with the DEA:

- Manufacturing controlled substances
- Distributing controlled substances
- Dispensing controlled substances
- Conducting research with controlled substances
- Conducting instructional activities with controlled substances
- Conducting a narcotic treatment program
- Conducting chemical analysis with controlled substances
- Importing or exporting controlled substances
- Compounding controlled substances

Those who engage in any of these activities must register with the DEA, using either Form 225 (to manufacture or distribute), Form 224 (to dispense), or Form 363 (to compound or conduct a narcotic treatment program). Initial registration is granted for a period of 28 to 39 months, after which the registration period is every 36 months.

Registrants (those who are approved by the DEA) receive a unique identification number, referred to as their DEA number, to be used within the closed system.

Prescribing

According to the CSA, prescriptions for controlled substances must include the following:

- Full name and address of the patient
- Name, address, and registry number of the prescriber
- Date issued
- Manual signature of the prescriber

Prescriptions for C-III and C-IV medications may be authorized for up to five refills; however, C-II prescriptions are not permitted to have refills authorized. In addition, prescriptions for controlled substances are required to be written in ink, or with a typewriter or an indelible pencil. There are additional requirements for prescribing a Schedule II substance, such as many states that require that these prescriptions be completed on a triplicate prescription form.

Dispensing

The dispensing of controlled substances is similar to the dispensing of legend drugs under the FDCA; however, there are several exceptions and additional regulations. Although federal law states that C-II prescriptions are valid for sixty days, many states permit C-II prescriptions to be valid for only seven days. In this case, the seven-day limitation is enforced, as it is the more stringent of the opposing laws. Prescriptions for C-III and C-IV medications are valid for six months, including refills. If necessary, C-II prescriptions may be partially filled; however, the remaining quantity must be supplied within 72 hours. Prescriptions for C-III, C-IV, and C-V medications may be transferred to a different pharmacy one time only, whereas C-II prescriptions are prohibited from being transferred. In addition to the information required on the label for a noncontrolled legend prescription, controlled substances require a federal transfer warning.

Refilling

Prescriptions for C-III and C-IV medications may be refilled, if authorized, up to five times within six months from the original written date. Labels for refills of C-III or C-IV substances are required to include the date of initial filling, in addition to the date of the refill. C-II prescriptions are prohibited from being refilled.

Ordering

To order Schedule I or II substances, a registrant must complete a triplicate form (DEA Form 222) or use the DEA Controlled Substance Ordering System (CSOS), which is electronic. However, registrants are not required to use the federal order form to obtain controlled substances in Schedules III, IV, or V, because of the lower potential for abuse of these substances (at least in comparison to the other schedule substances).

Recordkeeping

The CSA dictates that registrants keep records of the following items:

- On-hand inventory of controlled substances
- Biennial inventory, after the initial inventory of controlled substances

Additional records may be required depending on the activity of the registrant.

The DEA requires reporting of exact quantities of Schedules I and II substances; however, registrants are permitted to estimate quantity for Schedules III through V substances.

There are three approved filing methods for prescriptions of controlled substances:

1. Three-drawer—there is one file for C-II; one file for C-III, C-IV, and C-V; and one file for all other prescriptions.
2. Two-drawer—there is one file for all controlled substances and a different one for all other prescriptions. All prescriptions for substances in Schedules III through V must have a red "C" stamped in the lower-right corner.
3. One-drawer—there is one drawer for C-II and one drawer for all other prescriptions, including those for Schedules III through V substances. Again, prescriptions for substances in Schedules III through V must have a red "C" stamped in the lower-right corner.

Reporting

If theft of controlled substances is discovered, the registrant must report the theft to both the DEA and the local police. The disposal of controlled substances must be reported to the DEA on DEA Form 41.

Inspections

The DEA may inspect any location registered for controlled substances. It may inspect all records, reports, forms, physical inventories, prescriptions, containers, labels, and equipment pertaining to controlled substances. The DEA may also inspect security systems and/or take a physical inventory of all controlled substances.

The Poison Prevention Packaging Act of 1970

According to the Poison Prevention Packaging Act (PPPA) of 1970, all legend and controlled drugs, with some exceptions, must be dispensed in a childproof container. For patients such as the older people, who do not wish to have their medications dispensed in such containers, a signed, written request to that effect should be kept on file at the pharmacy. Exceptions to the PPPA include sublingual doses of nitroglycerin, contraceptives, drugs dispensed to inpatients in hospitals, and certain emergency medications.

> ## ❝ Workplace Wisdom PPPA Exceptions
> - Sublingual nitroglycerin
> - Sublingual/chewable isosorbide dinitrate (10 mg or less)
> - Erythromycin granules for oral suspension
> - Cholestyramine in powder form
> - Unit-dosed potassium supplements
> - Sodium fluoride (264 mg or less)
> - Betamethasone tablets (12.6 mg or less)
> - Pancrelipase preparations
> - Prednisone tablets (105 mg or less)
> - Mebendazole tablets (600 mg or less)
> - Methylprednisolone tablets (84 mg or less)
> - Colestipol in powder form (5 g or less)
> - Erythromycin in tablet form (16 g or less)
> - Drugs dispensed to inpatients in hospitals
> - Upon request of the prescriber or patient ❞

The Occupational Safety and Health Act of 1970

Congress passed the Occupational Safety and Health Act to ensure worker and workplace safety. The goal was to make sure that employers provide their workers with a place of employment free from recognized hazards to safety and health, such as exposure to toxic chemicals, excessive noise levels, mechanical dangers, heat or cold stress, or unsanitary conditions.

To establish standards for workplace health and safety, the Occupational Safety and Health Act also created the NIOSH, a research institution.

The Drug Listing Act of 1972

The Drug Listing Act of 1972 amended the Federal FDCA to require drug establishments (manufacturers, repackagers, and distributors) to register their products and list all of their commercially marketed drug products with the FDA. This requirement includes establishments that repackage or otherwise change the container, wrapper, or labeling of any drug package in the course of distribution of the drug from the original place of manufacture to the person who makes final delivery or sale to the ultimate customer. The Drug Listing Act applies to all drug firms that manufacture or process human drugs, veterinary drugs, and medicated animal feed premixes.

Each drug is assigned a unique and permanent product code, known as the National Drug Code (NDC), which identifies the drug establishment, the formulation, and the size/type of product packaging.

The Medical Device Amendment of 1976

The Medical Device Amendment of 1976 required, for the first time, that the safety and effectiveness of life-sustaining and life-supporting devices have premarket approval from the FDA.

The Orphan Drug Act of 1983

Congress passed the Orphan Drug Act of 1983 to stimulate the development of drugs for rare diseases (those that affect 200,000 people or fewer). Before passage of this legislation, private industry had little incentive to invest money in the development of drugs for treating small patient populations, because the drugs were expected to be unprofitable. The law provides three primary incentives:

1. Seven-year market exclusivity to sponsors of approved orphan products
2. A tax credit of 50% of the cost of conducting human clinical trials
3. Federal research grants for clinical testing of new therapies to treat and/or diagnose rare diseases

In 1997, Congress created an additional incentive when it granted companies developing orphan products an exemption from the usual drug application or user fees charged by the FDA.

The Drug Price Competition and Patent Term Restoration Act of 1984

Commonly known as the Hatch–Waxman Act, the Drug Price Competition and Patent Term Restoration Act of 1984 established the modern system of generic drugs. Manufacturers can file Abbreviated New Drug Applications (ANDAs) to seek FDA approval for generic versions of drugs, for which patent protection is set to expire.

The Prescription Drug Marketing Act of 1987

The Prescription Drug Marketing Act was enacted to address certain prescription drug marketing practices that have contributed to the diversion of large quantities of drugs into a secondary "gray" market.

These marketing practices, including the distribution of free samples, the use of coupons redeemable for drugs at no cost or low cost, and the sale of deeply discounted drugs to hospitals and health care entities, helped create a multimillion-dollar drug diversion market that provided a portal through which mislabeled, subpotent, adulterated, expired, and counterfeit drugs were able to enter the nation's drug distribution system.

The Anabolic Steroid Control Act of 1990

The Anabolic Steroid Control Act of 1990 placed anabolic steroids in Schedule III of the CSA. The CSA defines *anabolic steroids* as any drug or hormonal substance chemically and pharmacologically related to testosterone (other than estrogens, progestins, and corticosteroids) that promotes muscle growth.

The Omnibus Budget Reconciliation Act of 1990

Known as OBRA '90, the Omnibus Budget Reconciliation Act of 1990 focused on federal funding of the Medicare and Medicaid programs. This was the act that created an increased need for pharmacy technicians. While determining that funding, OBRA also mandated that the pharmacist perform drug utilization reviews (DURs) and offer counseling to patients, and even provided funding and set reimbursement fees for such activities. In addition to elevating the profession of pharmacist in the United States, OBRA, by its nature, created a real need for pharmacy technicians to assist pharmacists.

The Dietary Supplement Health and Education Act of 1994

The provisions of the Dietary Supplement Health and Education Act define dietary supplements and dietary ingredients, establish a framework for assuring safety, outline guidelines for literature displayed where supplements are sold, provide for use of claims and nutritional support statements, require ingredient and nutrition labeling, and grant the FDA the authority to establish GMP regulations. The law also established an executive-level Commission on Dietary Supplement Labels and an Office of Dietary Supplements within the National Institutes of Health.

> **❝ Workplace Wisdom** The FDA's Role in Regulating Herbal Products and Dietary Supplements
>
> Most individuals are unaware that herbal products and dietary supplements are not regulated by the same standards and guidelines as drugs—whether prescription or OTC. Dietary supplements, which include most herbal products, fall under a general umbrella of "foods," not drugs, and although still regulated under the FDA, through the Center for Food Safety and Applied Nutrition they fall under different guidelines from drugs. All supplements are required to be labeled as a dietary supplement. ❞

The Health Insurance Portability and Accountability Act of 1996

The Health Insurance Portability and Accountability Act of 1996, also known as HIPAA, was enacted to ensure patient confidentiality and privacy. Initially, HIPAA gave patients the right

to review their medical records and established the requirement of patient consent for the transfer of medical records and for oral, written, and electronic communications regarding medical records. Today, patient consent is required for a pharmacist or pharmacy technician to fill a prescription.

HIPAA considers the following to be protected health information (PHI):

- Any information created or received by the pharmacy
- Information relating to a patient's health—mental or physical, past, present, or future
- Information that may identify a patient

Privacy standards, however, were only one of four major components of the act. In addition, HIPAA regulated electronic health transaction standards, unique identifiers, and security and electronic signature standards. The electronic health transaction standards require that all health organizations adopt a standard set of codes to be used in health records and transactions, such as for diseases, injuries, causes, symptoms, and actions taken. Unique identifiers were addressed to simplify and standardize the multiple identification numbers that health organizations previously used to identify themselves in various communications. The security standard established a mandate for safeguarding the storage, maintenance, and transmission of individual's health information and applied standards for acceptance of electronic signatures.

The Food and Drug Administration Modernization Act of 1997

This act was designed to simplify various FDA regulations and procedures. Specifically, the Food and Drug Administration Modernization Act allowed greater ease and speed with which the FDA can approve new drugs and grant access to investigational medications. The required federal legend was also abbreviated to simply "Rx only."

The Drug Addiction Treatment Act of 2000

This act was established to permit physicians, who complete a training course and register with the DEA, to prescribe pre-approved C-III, C-IV, and C-V medications, as a means of maintenance or detoxification, to individuals with an opioid addiction. Specific restrictions are placed upon the number of patients an approved physician may treat.

The Medicare Modernization Act of 2003

This act marked a significant change to Medicare, the government-managed insurance program for seniors. As a result of this act, Medicare beneficiaries were provided with the opportunity to enroll in Medicare Advantage, or Medicare Part D, which is a voluntary prescription drug benefit plan for seniors. Prior to this act, Medicare patients were provided prescription drug benefits only when hospitalized (Medicare Part A) or through nursing homes and physician offices (Medicare Part B).

USP Chapter <797>

In 2004, the *U.S. Pharmacopoeia* established the first enforceable standards for sterile compounding with the release of USP Chapter <797>. This chapter outlines procedures and practices required for the safe and proper compounding of sterile preparations. The standards established in USP <797> are applicable to all settings in which sterile preparations are compounded, including pharmaceutical manufacturers. Revisions to USP <797> went into effect in 2007.

The Combat Methamphetamine Epidemic Act of 2005

Known as the CMEA, the Combat Methamphetamine Epidemic Act of 2005 regulates, among other things, retail OTC sales of ephedrine, pseudoephedrine, and phenylpropanolamine products. Retail provisions of the CMEA include daily sales limits and 30-day purchase limits, placement of product out of direct customer access, sales logbooks, customer identification verification, and employee training.

The Medicaid Tamper-Resistant Prescription Pad Law of 2008

This law required that all written prescriptions for covered outpatient drugs are required to be written on a tamper-resistant prescription pad. In order to be considered tamper resistant, a prescription must contain at least one of the following characteristics:

1. One or more industry-recognized features designed to prevent unauthorized copying of a completed or blank prescription form

---

■ Procedure 4-1

Selling Methamphetamine-Related Products

1. Ensure that the request does not exceed daily or monthly limits.
2. Verify the customer's photo identification (e.g., driver's license).
3. Complete necessary paperwork and documentation of sale, including:
   - customer's name
   - customer's address and telephone number
   - customer's identification number (e.g., driver's license number)
   - product name
   - product strength
   - product quantity
   - date
   - customer's signature
   - your name and signature.
4. Process the sales transaction at the pharmacy.

---

2. One or more industry-recognized features designed to prevent erasure or modification of information written on the prescription pad by the prescriber
3. One or more industry-recognized features designed to prevent the use of counterfeit prescription forms

Prescriptions transmitted from the prescriber to the pharmacy verbally, by fax, or electronically are not subject to these requirements.

The Affordable Care Act of 2010

Sometimes referred to as "Obamacare," the purpose of the Affordable Care Act (ACA) was to ensure Americans access to insurance coverage. Americans will have the ability to choose insurance coverage through an open-market insurance exchange, which will pool buying power and give Americans new affordable choices of private insurance plans.

Under the ACA, all individuals are required to have healthcare insurance or face the penalty of a fee administered as a "shared responsibility payment." The IRS is responsible for assessing and collecting the penalty as reported on federal tax returns. The penalty, which is to begin in 2014, would initially be either $95.00 or one percent of income, whichever number is greater. In 2015 it increases to $325.00 or two percent of income and in 2016, $695.00 or 2.5 percent of income. After 2016, the penalty amount would be appraised to fall into conjunction with the cost-of-living. There are, however, those who are not subject to the individual mandate or the shared responsibility payment.

Persons who are not subject to the individual mandate of ACA:

- Undocumented immigrants
- Religious objectors
- Those who are serving jail time

Persons who are not subject to the shared responsibility payment:

- Those who pay insurance premiums, which are more than eight percent of their adjusted household income
- Any person who is a member of an American Indian tribe
- Those who apply for a financial hardship waiver
- Any person who was without insurance for less than three months of the year
- Any person whose income falls below the federal tax filing threshold

Adulteration Versus Misbranding

According to the FDA, an *adulterated* drug is a drug that is in a condition contrary to the intentions of the manufacturer. Adulteration focuses on the physical condition of the drug or device. In contrast, *misbranding* focuses on the representations made by the manufacturer. Following are some criteria, of which any one is sufficient to constitute adulteration or misbranding.

---

misbranded drug a drug that has been misleadingly or fraudulently labeled.

medical device any instrument or apparatus used in the diagnosis, prevention, monitoring, treatment, or alleviation of disease.

monograph a detailed document pertaining to a specific drug.

Adulterated drugs

- Are prepared, packaged, packed, or held under unsanitary conditions
- Are manufactured in a way that does not conform to established GMPs
- Have a container composed of a poisonous or deleterious substance
- Contain an unsafe color additive
- Vary from an official compendium standard
- Are new, unsafe, animal drugs or animal feeds containing such drugs
- Are a Class III device without premarket approval (a banned device)
- Are OTC drugs that are not packaged in tamper-resistant packaging

Misbranded drugs

- Have false or misleading labels
- Have labels that fail to state the name and place of business of the manufacturer, packager, packer, or distributor and that lack an accurate statement of quantity
- Have labels with required information not prominently placed on them
- Have labels that do not state "Warning: May Be Habit Forming" in the case of habit-forming substances
- Have labels that, in the case of legend drugs, do not include the generic name or the names of ingredients, or have type on the label that is not less than one-half the size of the trade/brand name
- Are not listed in an official compendium (unless they are labeled and packaged by compendium standards)
- Are in packages that are misleading
- Are subject to deterioration, and have the label that does not bear corresponding precautionary statements
- Endanger one's health if used in the manner suggested by the labeling
- Are composed of either insulin or an antibiotic drug and are not batch certified
- Contain a color additive and are not labeled accordingly
- Are produced by manufacturers who are not registered with the FDA and who do not list the drug as one they manufacture
- Are subject to the PPPA of 1970 and are not packaged accordingly
- Are touted in advertisements that fail to mention the generic or established names (if they are prescription drugs) and that omit the side effects, warnings, contraindications, effectiveness, and quantitative formulas of the drugs
- Have labels with inadequate directions for use and inadequate warnings about the effects of the drugs
- Have labels that fail to bear the statement "Caution: Federal law restricts this drug to use by or on the order of a licensed veterinarian," in the case of veterinary drugs

New Drugs

According to the FDCA, there are in essence only two ways in which drugs can be lawfully sold in the United States. The drug must either be exempted through the 1962 amendments or be approved by the FDA under the procedures for an NDA.

The process by which the FDA approves new drugs includes the approval of an investigational new drug through the filing of an NDA. It can take years before approval is gained through this process, not counting the many years of research and development—and approval is never guaranteed.

Samples

The following is considered a drug sample by the FDA: any drug that is habit forming; bears the federal legend or is restricted to investigational use; or is not intended to be sold, but rather is purveyed to promote the sale of the drug. The FDA permits manufacturers and distributors to distribute drug samples upon written request of a prescriber, under a system that requires the recipient to execute a written receipt for the sample and return the receipt to the manufacturer.

Medical Devices

A **medical device** is an instrument or machine that is recognized in either the National Formulary or *U.S. Pharmacopoeia*. It is intended for the diagnosis, cure, mitigation, treatment, or prevention of disease, or it is intended to affect the structure or any function of the body of a human or animal.

The FDCA categorizes medical devices into three classes. Class I devices are those that have relatively low potential to cause harm, such as scissors or needles. Class II devices are subject to specific performance standards established by a panel of experts. Examples of Class II devices are thermometers, hearing aids, and catheters. Class III medical devices are life-supporting systems whose failure could cause death or serious injury, such as a pacemaker or a heart valve.

Monographs

Drug **monographs**, commonly known as *package inserts*, are a necessary component of a drug's labeling (see Figure 4-4). The monograph provides all the clinical information required by the FDA. Most monographs are similar in layout and style, and contain the following sections.

Description—provides a written description of the visual elements of the drug and packaging, as well as the basic chemical structure of the drug.

Clinical pharmacology—includes information on the drug's mechanism of action, absorption, distribution, metabolism, elimination, and administration. It also includes any notes relevant to specific patient populations, such as pediatric patients.

Indications and usage—describes the specific conditions or symptoms that the drug has been approved by the FDA to prevent or treat.

DESCRIPTION

Methylprednisolone is a glucocorticoid. Glucocorticoids are adrenocortical steroids, both naturally occurring and synthetic, which are readily absorbed from the gastrointestinal tract. Methylprednisolone occurs as a white to practically white, odorless, crystalline powder. It is sparingly soluble in alcohol, in dioxane, and in methanol, slightly soluble in acetone, and in chloroform, and very slightly soluble in ether. It is practically insoluble in water.

The chemical name for methylprednisolone is preng-1, 4-diene-3,20-dione, 11, 17, 21-trihydroxy-60methyl-(6α, 11β)-, and the molecular weight is 374.48. The structural formula is represented below:

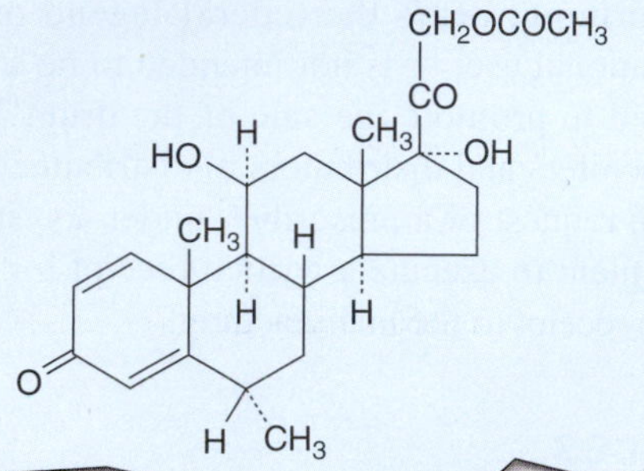

Each MethylPREDNISolone Tablet for oral administration contains 4 mg methylprednisolone. Inactive ingredients: magnesium stearate, microcrystalline cellulose and sodium starch glycolate.

CLINICAL PHARMACOLOGY

Naturally occurring glucocorticoids (hydrocortisone and cortisone), which also have salt-retaining properties, are used as a replacement therapy in adrenocortical deficiency states. Their synthetic analogs are primarily used for their potent anti-inflammatory effects in disorders of many organ systems.

Glucocorticoids cause profound and varied metabolic effects. In addition, they modify the body's immune responses to diverse stimuli.

INDICATIONS AND USAGE

MethylPREDNISolone Tablets are indicated in the following conditions:

1. Endocrine Disorders
Primary or secondary adrenocortical insufficiency (hydrocortisone or cortisone is the first

FIGURE 4-4 Drug monograph.

Contraindications—lists the types of patients who should not use the medication, whether that is a class of patients (such as diabetics) or individuals taking another specific class of drug.

Warnings—details the serious side effects that can be caused by the medication and instructions on what the patient should do if these effects are experienced.

Precautions—lists all of the remaining possible, or potential, side effects that the patient should be aware of.

Drug abuse and dependence—provides notification if the medication has shown signs of a potential for abuse or dependence.

Adverse reactions—covers reactions that are unexpected and potentially life threatening.

Dosage—includes the recommended dosage of medication; dosages are typically categorized by patient age and/or weight.

How supplied—describes how the medication is supplied, including strengths, dosage formats, and storage requirements.

---

ethics a system of principles and duties; often associated with a profession.

medical ethics principles and moral values of proper medical care.

Patient's Bill of Rights

All states establish what is known as Patient's Bill of Rights, which outlines the patients' proper expectations regarding their quality of care, privacy, and individual health care provider's responsibilities. Health care providers and facilities, such as physician offices and hospitals, are obligated to provide all patients with access to a written copy of the Patient's Bill of Rights. Figure 4-5 shows an example of Patient's Bill of Rights for a major Texas medical facility:

Ethics and the Pharmacy Technician

As in many professions, **ethics** is a factor in decision making for pharmacy professionals, including pharmacy technicians. Many situations can and will arise in which you or your colleagues will be required to make ethical decisions. Ethical decisions are required in those gray areas where there is no clear-cut, black-or-white, correct, or incorrect response or choice. These decisions require an understanding of a professional code of ethics, as well as an understanding of moral principles and their application to your own life.

Ethics is not law, religion, or morals, but all of these can affect your ethical decisions. Ethics is as personal as your individual faith and influences much of your behavior. In a profession, members of that profession often adopt an ethical code. This code can serve as a guidepost or parameter to aid your reasoning process when a decision is required. Keeping your ethical decisions within the limits of an ethical code can also help protect you, if you are called upon to defend your actions.

Defining Ethics

The term *ethics* derives from the Greek word *éthos*, referring to character. Ethics is commonly defined as the considered reflection and systematic analysis of the morality of certain behavior when required actions are unclear. An ethical decision is not an emotional, knee-jerk reaction, but something that has been weighed and measured carefully. **Medical ethics** is the discipline of evaluating the merits, risks, and social concerns of activities in the field of medicine.

Moral Philosophy

A *moral*, or *principle-based*, *philosophy* is an individualized set of values or value system. It is the moral reasoning process that guides you as you decide the rightness or wrongness of conduct. Such a philosophy will guide you in reaching ethical decisions that align with professional standards of conduct.

Sample Patient Bill of Rights

You have the right to:

Be Treated with Respect

It is our privilege to serve every patient that comes through our door. We pledge to serve patients with consideration and without discrimination at all times.

Participate in Your Healthcare

You have the right to all the information you need to make the best possible decisions, including treatment options, test results, and an explanation of costs involved. You have the right to accept or reject a treatment plan. Your care will be improved if you participate in the decisions regarding your health.

Access Your Medical Record

Your medical record is kept in the facility, but it is your medical information and you have the right to access it. You may order a copy of your record at any time for a small administrative fee.

A Second Opinion

Do not hesitate to ask your doctor if you want a second opinion. Many times, when a disease is serious, complex or demands a surgical intervention, patients seek a second opinion.

Confidentiality

You have the right to talk in confidence with your healthcare providers and, within legal limits, to have your privacy protected at all times.

Have a Family Member with You

You may have a family member accompany you during your discussion with the doctor.

Know the Names and the Titles/Roles of Our Staff

We expect our staff to wear identification badges. If you do not see a badge, please feel free to ask any of us for our name and our role (doctor, nurse, receptionist, etc.).

Have Your Advance Directive on File

Many patients develop "advance directives," or living wills. You can give this to your doctor and it will be filed in your medical record.

Be Examined in Private

Your provider may be working with a healthcare student. You have the right to request that your examination be completed without anyone else in the room (unless a chaperone is required for sensitive exams).

Questions/Concerns

If you have any concerns about your visit, you may:
- Contact the department you visited
- Contact our patient care representatives at 713-555-0101
- Contact the facility's Chief Medical Officer Dr. John Smith, 713-555-1212
- Contact the Texas Board of Medical Examiners at 1.800.201.9353

FIGURE 4-5 Sample Patient's Bill of Rights.

PROFILE IN PRACTICE

To better illustrate this topic, as well as later discussions on ethical theories, consider the following scenarios, which are commonplace situations in pharmacy practice.

▶ *Mrs. Montgomery, a regular customer, arrives at your pharmacy and needs a refill for her Synthroid, a prescription drug. While processing her order, you discover that she has no refills left on her prescription. It is 9:00 p.m. on Friday night, and Monday is the Fourth of July. You notify the pharmacist of the situation and await further instructions.*

▶ *A distribution problem arises when there is a vaccine or medication shortage. What factors must be considered when determining to whom those items will be dispensed or administered?*

Practicing Ethics

Several moral principles concern pharmacy professionals. These principles are the basis for the theories of ethical practice discussed next. While reviewing the principles, keep in mind that there may be conflicts between them. For instance, beneficence may help the most people, but require you to abandon veracity. Here are the five principles:

- **Beneficence**—bringing about good. Your role as a pharmacy technician places you in a position to benefit others (e.g., your patients).
- **Fidelity**—keeping a promise. This is illustrated by a pharmacy technician who strictly fills prescriptions in the order in which they were dropped off, thereby keeping a promise to have patients' prescriptions ready by a certain time.
- **Veracity**—telling the truth. Pharmacy technicians demonstrate veracity when they report any inappropriate actions or behaviors occurring within the pharmacy, such as drug diversion or unreported medication errors.
- **Justice**—acting with fairness or equity within the law. An example of this occurred years ago, when a new OTC product was introduced: Cold Eze. The product received extensive media coverage, and word-of-mouth testimonials caused the demand to quickly outgrow the supply. Pharmacy technicians acted justly by limiting the quantities sold per individual and setting up waiting lists for new shipments.
- **Autonomy**—acting with self-reliance. Pharmacy technicians demonstrate autonomy by working interdependently within the pharmacy; in other words, the technicians work by supporting the pharmacist, but also are reliable, dependable, and show appropriate initiative.

Ethical Theories

The following nine theories can help you measure possible ethical decisions. To better illustrate these theories, we will return to the ethical scenarios presented earlier.

---

beneficence the quality of being kind or charitable.

fidelity faithfulness to obligations and duties.

veracity truthfulness; the quality of conforming with the truth.

justice the principle of moral rightness and equity.

autonomy the condition or quality of being independent.

consequentialism the theory that the value of an action derives solely from the value of its consequences.

nonconsequentialism the theory that certain actions, in and of themselves, are wrong.

social contract an understood agreement between individual members of a society.

Consequentialism

Consequentialism is the theory that the value of an action derives solely from the value of its consequences. Returning to Mrs. Montgomery's situation (as mentioned previously), how does the theory of consequentialism treat her problem? What about restricting the use of flu vaccine in the case of a medication shortage? How could that decision be guided under this theory?

Nonconsequentialism

Nonconsequentialism is the study of actions themselves without regard to outcome. In other words, it is the argument that the ends justify the means. Could the pharmacist argue that Mrs. Montgomery having her medication is more important than the law that says legend drugs cannot be dispensed without a valid prescription? In the case of a shortage, could we say that first come–first served is the fairest way to distribute vaccine?

Social Contracts

Pharmacists, technicians, and patients recognize certain expectations of each other and act accordingly. Such expectations are called **social contracts**. Can Mrs. Montgomery argue that she entrusts the pharmacist with the responsibility to provide for her medication needs? Could the pharmacist, in turn, argue that Mrs. Montgomery's situation is not her problem, because Mrs. Montgomery has a responsibility to keep her prescriptions current and the pharmacist, in turn, should expect such behavior? How would this theory apply to the vaccine situation?

The Ethics of Care

The *ethics of care* is a "principle [that] requires the decision-maker to more clearly focus on such basic moral skills as kindness, sensitivity, attentiveness, tact, patience, and reliability." In the situation with Mrs. Montgomery, should the pharmacist ask herself what the kind and reliable action would be? Could she argue that "teaching" Mrs. Montgomery to be more conscientious by refusing to fill her expired prescription would be the better path? What is the most humane action in the face of a vaccine shortage?

Rights-Based Ethics

Rights-based ethics is a theory based on an understanding of human rights—the belief that an individual in a democratic society should be shielded from undue forces and allowed to enjoy and pursue personal projects; in short, the theory that each individual has certain moral rights as well as legal rights. Does Mrs. Montgomery have a right to receive her medication despite any rules or regulations? Could the pharmacist argue that she should fill Mrs. Montgomery's prescription because it is the patient's right? How would rights-based ethics apply to the vaccine shortage?

Principle-Based Ethics

Principle-based ethics states that moral principles are general, universal guides to action. This is a more personal approach. The pharmacist could say that going against a law is immoral for her. However, it could also be argued that refusing medication to anyone who needs it is also immoral. You could ask, "Is it ever moral to deny medication to someone in need?" How does that question, and your answer, change in a shortage situation?

Virtues-Based Ethics

Virtues-based ethics is the use of virtues, or the idealization of specific morals, establishing right reason in action. In Mrs. Montgomery's case, what would the most virtuous action be? What about in the vaccine shortage case?

Law

Law is closely related to the system of ethics and sometimes overlaps it, creating confusion and tension about the "right thing to do" in a given situation. Mrs. Montgomery's case is a good example. The laws governing prescriptions are very clear. They do not allow exceptions. The pharmacist could definitely quote the law to Mrs. Montgomery and refuse to fill her prescription, arguing that the law is the law and the pharmacist's hands are tied. Are there any laws governing the distribution of drugs? Would they apply to the vaccine case? Should there be new laws for just such a case?

Professional Code of Ethics

Pharmacy technicians are health care professionals who assist pharmacists in providing the best possible care to patients. The principles of this code, which apply to pharmacy technicians working in any and all settings, are based on the application and support of the moral obligations that guide the pharmacy profession in relationships with patients, health care professionals, and society.

An identifying benchmark for all professions is their sincere acceptance of the responsibility to maintain a standard of conduct beyond either an unthinking conformity to the law or the routine performance of technical skills. The code of ethics that follows is an example of the ninth ethical theory, virtues-based ethics. It was written by technicians for technicians and adopted by both the American Association of Pharmacy Technicians and the National Pharmacy Technician Association. Can you find an answer here that works for you to the dilemma in Mrs. Montgomery's case?

The Pharmacy Technician Code of Ethics

Preamble

I. A pharmacy technician's first considerations are to ensure the health and safety of the patient and to use knowledge and skills to the best of his or her ability in serving others.

II. A pharmacy technician supports and promotes honesty and integrity in the profession, which includes a duty to observe the law, maintain the highest moral and ethical conduct at all times, and uphold the ethical principles of the profession.

III. A pharmacy technician assists and supports the pharmacist in the safe, efficacious, and cost-effective distribution of health services and health care resources.

IV. A pharmacy technician respects and values the abilities of pharmacists, colleagues, and other health care professionals.

V. A pharmacy technician maintains competency in his or her practice and continually enhances his or her professional knowledge and expertise.

VI. A pharmacy technician respects and supports the patient's individuality, dignity, and confidentiality.

VII. A pharmacy technician respects the confidentiality of the patient's records and discloses pertinent information only with proper authorization.

VIII. A pharmacy technician never assists in the dispensing or distributing of medications or medical devices that are not of good quality or do not meet the standards required by law.

IX. A pharmacy technician does not engage in any activity that will discredit the profession, and he or she will expose, without fear or favor, illegal or unethical conduct in the profession.

X. A pharmacy technician associates with and engages in the support of organizations that promote the profession of pharmacy through the use and enhancement of pharmacy technicians.

Liability

Now that you have a thorough understanding of the various laws, regulations, and ethical framework that pharmacy technicians practice within, it is time to discuss liability. As a health care professional, you will be liable for your work, actions, behaviors, and even comments. If, for some reason, a patient suffers damages as a result of negligence or tort, in which you were responsible or contributed, you can be held professionally liable. Charges resulting from negligence or unintended tort, can result in punitive, or monetary, damages as well as potentially having your ability to practice as a pharmacy technician suspended or revoked. Charges from criminal activities, such as insurance fraud, theft, or drug diversion, is considered intentional tort and could result in imprisonment.

As a health care professional, who is subject to professional liability, it is vital that you ensure that you protect yourself. The primary and preferred method of protecting oneself from liability claims is to avoid errors or actions that can result in civil or criminal charges. In addition, however, it is highly recommended that you maintain professional liability insurance to protect yourself financially from punitive damages. Civil cases will almost always focus on seeking punitive damages from the pharmacy (corporation) and the pharmacist, as they will have greater financial assets to make claims against, but as a pharmacy technician you are not immune from similar claims. A professional liability insurance policy should always be maintained. Many employers provide, at least a minimal amount of coverage, for their employees, but it is your responsibility to research if you will be covered and to what limit.

Individual professional liability policies are quite affordable, averaging around $100 per year for sufficient coverage for a pharmacy technician, and thus it is recommended to always maintain an individual policy in addition to any employer-provided coverage.

For more information on professional liability insurance policies, check out:

HPSO—www.hpso.com

Pharmacists Mutual—www.phmic.com

Summary

Many of the regulations pertaining to practice as a pharmacy technician are established and overseen by your specific state's board of pharmacy. In general, federal laws pertain to the manufacturing of pharmaceutical products, and state laws pertain to the actual dispensing of those products. It is imperative that you familiarize yourself with both the federal laws and the laws of your particular state pertaining to pharmacy practice. In addition, you should fully understand the basic ethical theories and the code of ethics for pharmacy technicians, in preparation for the ethical dilemmas and questions that will inevitably arise in the pharmacy setting.

Chapter Review Questions

1. The _____ requires that prescription drugs bear the legend, "Caution: Federal law prohibits dispensing without a prescription."
   a. Drug Listing Act
   b. Kefauver–Harris Amendment
   c. Food, Drug, and Cosmetic Act
   d. Durham–Humphrey Amendment

2. _____ law cases may be initiated only by the state, not by victims.
   a. Administrative
   b. Case
   c. Civil
   d. Criminal

3. Which of the following is an example of a C-IV medication?
   a. Valium
   b. Ritalin
   c. Vicodin
   d. Lomotil

4. The chemical structure of a drug is listed within the _____ section of a drug's official monograph.
   a. adverse reaction
   b. clinical pharmacology
   c. description
   d. dosage

5. Which of the following moral principles refers to telling the truth?
   a. fidelity
   b. veracity
   c. beneficence
   d. autonomy

6. Which agency is responsible for registering and regulating pharmacy facilities and pharmacy professionals?
   a. CMS
   b. FDA
   c. OSHA
   d. SBOP

7. A hearing aid is classified as a Class _____ medical device.
   a. I
   b. II
   c. III
   d. IV

8. Which of the following is commonly referred to as the Drug Efficacy Amendment?
   a. Kefauver–Harris Amendment
   b. Durham–Humphrey Amendment
   c. Medical Device Amendment
   d. none of the above

9. Which of the following ethical theories states that pharmacists, technicians, and patients recognize certain expectations of each other and act accordingly?
   a. nonconsequentialism
   b. principle-based ethics
   c. social contracts
   d. virtues-based ethics

10. Which pharmacy-related law was determined to be inadequate because it did not require labeling to identify a product's contents?
   a. Controlled Substances Act
   b. Food, Drug, and Cosmetic Act
   c. Poison Prevention Packaging Act
   d. Pure Food and Drug Act

Critical Thinking Questions

1. Contrast the role the federal government plays in the regulation of pharmacy practice with that of the state government.

2. An individual, who clearly abuses illegal drugs, asks to purchase a box of syringes at the pharmacy. On the one hand, if the pharmacy staff sell the syringes to the individual, they are in some way aiding in his addiction; on the other hand, they are ensuring that he does not feel obligated to share or reuse needles. What do you believe is the ethical thing to do? Why?

3. Why is it important that pharmacy technicians have a professional code of ethics?

Web Challenge

1. Pharmacy technicians can be, and have been, held liable in civil lawsuits related to medication errors. Several companies offer professional liability insurance designed for pharmacy technicians. Visit www.phmic.com and www.hpso.com and compare the policies they offer to technicians.

2. Using a search engine, search for "pharmacy technician sued" or "pharmacy technician lawsuit." While researching, print out information on three civil lawsuits in which a technician has been sued.

References and Resources

Andrews, Sandra. *The Affordable Care Act*. Houston, TX: *Today's Technician*, 2012. Print.

Buerki, Robert A. and Louis D. Voterro. *Ethical Practices in Pharmacy: A Guidebook for Pharmacy Technicians*. Madison, WI: American Institute of the History of Pharmacy, 1997. Print.

"CDC Website." *Centers for Disease Control and Prevention*. CDC. 2012. Web. 6 January 2012.

"DEA Website." *Drug Enforcement Administration*. DEA. 2012. Web. 6 January 2012.

"FDA Website." *Food and Drug Administration*. FDA. 2012. Web. 6 January 2012.

"Healthcare.gov Website." *U.S. Department of Health and Human Services*. HHS. 2013. Web. 21 May 2013.

Johnston, Mike. *Certification Exam Review*. Upper Saddle River, NJ: Pearson, 2005. Print.

Johnston, Mike. *Fundamentals of Pharmacy Practice*. Upper Saddle River, NJ: Pearson, 2005. Print.

Mugler, Mark W. "A Brief History of the FDA." *Lynch*. 2006. Web. 6 January 2012.

Nielsen, James R. *Handbook of Federal Drug Law*. 2nd ed. Philadelphia, PA: Williams & Wilkins, 1992. Print.

Orum-Alexander, Gail G. and James J. Mizner, Jr. *Pharmacy Technician: Practice and Procedures*. New York, NY: McGraw Hill, 2010. Print.

Richards, Edward P. and Katharine C. Rathbun. *Law & the Physician: A Practical Guide*. Boston, MA: Little Brown, 1993. Print.

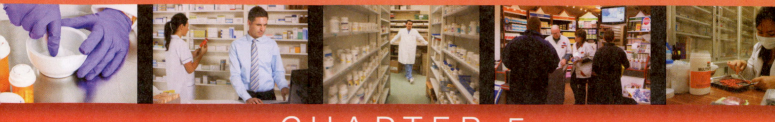

CHAPTER 5

Terminology and Abbreviations

LEARNING OBJECTIVES

After completing this chapter, you should be able to:

- Identify selected root words used in pharmacy practice.

- Identify and correctly use selected prefixes and suffixes in conjunction with root words.

- Recognize and interpret common abbreviations used in the pharmacy and medicine.

- List abbreviations that are considered dangerous and explain why.

- Recognize and interpret symbols commonly used in pharmacy and medical practice.

- Recognize and list common drug names and their generic equivalents.

- Recall and define common pharmacy and medical terminology used in the pharmacy field.

INTRODUCTION

To understand the pharmacy industry and profession, you must learn the appropriate language, which consists of terminology and abbreviations. Most medical terms are derived from Greek and Latin words and consist of a root word, prefix, and/or suffix. By learning selected roots, prefixes, and suffixes, you will be able to understand words you may have never seen or heard before.

This chapter covers the most common words and phrases as well as prefixes and suffixes used for communication in the practice of pharmacy. This chapter gives you an overview of the standard terminology that you will need to know, if you are to succeed. The information is arranged by topic and then alphabetically for easier reference in the future. This chapter is not all-inclusive, and you should continue to learn as much terminology as possible to increase your knowledge base.

Understanding Selected Roots

Root words are words or parts of a word that identify the major meaning of a term. Root words are the essential part of the whole word. More specifically, root words can identify the part of the body or condition to which a term relates. Table 5-1 lists some of the common root words used in various pharmacy settings.

TABLE 5-1 Selected Roots

Root	Meaning	Example
arter	artery	arterial
arthr	joint	arthritis
bronch	bronchus	bronchitis
carcin	cancer	carcinoma
cardi	heart	cardiac
cyst	bladder	cystoscopy
derma	skin	dermatology
enter	abdomen/intestine	enteral
gastr	stomach	gastric
gluco	sugar	glucose
hemo	blood	hematology
hepat	liver	hepatoma
my	muscle	myalgia
nasa	nose	nasal
nephr	kidney	nephrology
neur	nerve	neurology
oste	bone	osteoporosis
patho	disease	pathologist
phleb	vein	phlebotomy
pneum	lung	pneumonia
psych	mind	psychosis
procto	rectum	proctology
pulmo	lung	pulmonary
ren	kidney	renal
rhin	nose	rhinoplasty
thromb	blood clot	thrombosis
vas	(blood) vessel	vascular

root words words or parts of a word that identify the major meaning of a term.

prefix a part of a word attached to the beginning of a root word that gives a specific meaning to the root.

suffix a part of a word attached to the end of a root word that gives a specific meaning to the root.

Understanding Selected Prefixes

A **prefix** is a part of a word attached to the beginning of a root word that gives a specific meaning to the root. For example, *bio-* means living organisms. If you recognize this prefix in a medical term, you will know that the term pertains in some way to living organisms. Prefixes are commonly used in the medical field to signify the meaning of a bigger word. Table 5-2 presents some of the common prefixes you will encounter as a pharmacy technician.

Understanding Selected Suffixes

A **suffix** is a part of a word attached to the end of a root word that gives a specific, new meaning to the root. For example, *-logy* is a suffix that means "the study of." If you add *-logy* to

TABLE 5-2 Common Prefixes

Prefix	Meaning	Example
a-, an-	without	anesthesia
ante-	before	anterior
anti-	inhibit, oppose	antibiotic
bio-	living organisms	biology
brady-	slow	bradycardia
con-	together	conception
contra-	against	contraindication
dia-	complete	diagnosis
dys-	abnormal, difficult	dyslipidemia
en-	in	enteral
ex-	out	external
hyper-	too much	hyperglycemia
hypo-	too little	hypoglycemia
inter-	between, among	interstitial
intra-	within	intradermal
macro-	large	macronutrients
mal-	abnormal	malabsorption
micro-	small	microscope
neo-	new	neonatal
para-	around	parasite
poly-	many, much	polydipsia
post-	after, behind	postmenopausal
pre-	before, in front	prenatal
sub-	below, underlying	sublingual
tachy-	fast	tachycardia

the prefix *bio-*, you end up with *biology*, or the study of living organisms. Table 5-3 includes the common suffixes a pharmacy technician should be familiar with and understand.

Understanding Combining Forms

A **combining form** is a root word with an added vowel. The vowel does not give a new meaning to the root word; its sole purpose is to make it easier to combine the root word with a suffix or another root. The combining form simply makes the new term easier to say and does not change the meaning of the other word parts.

For example, *cardi-* is a root word meaning "heart." When the suffix *-ac* is added to the root, it becomes *cardiac*, which means pertaining to the heart. When the suffix *-logy* is added to the root, we add an extra "o" to connect the root and suffix, producing *cardiology*, which means the study of the heart.

Pharmacy Abbreviations

As in the medical field, you will encounter numerous abbreviations, acronyms, and codes in the pharmacy setting. To completely understand the language of pharmacy, you must be able to understand and interpret these abbreviations. Although the abbreviations are not federally recognized, they are favored as substitutes, with a standard meaning, for a whole word or phrase. It is much easier to read a couple of symbols than to interpret several lines in a physician's poor handwriting. Symbols and abbreviations are also used as a time-saving measure for the physician and pharmacy staff. To prepare a prescription for dispensing correctly, you must be able to interpret the medication order as written by the physician. Tables 5-4 through 5-8 present the common abbreviations used in writing prescriptions, as well as those used in standard pharmacy practice. These include abbreviations related to pharmacy in general, directions and SIG codes, routes of administration, dosages and measurements, and medicines.

Dangerous Abbreviations

Effective January 1, 2004, the Joint Commission issued a list of dangerous abbreviations, acronyms, and symbols that are not to be used, known as the "Do Not Use" list. One of the major problems with certain abbreviations is that they may have more than one meaning. For example, "DC" could mean *discharge* in one instance and *discontinue* in another. Also, these abbreviations are prone to misinterpretation: Poorly written, *QD* could look like *QID* to someone other than the writer.

With communication and use of medical records and documentation spanning various health care venues, abbreviations increase the risk of misinterpretation and error. In addition, some health care staff may be unfamiliar with certain abbreviations, which can delay getting appropriate health care to the patient. The primary objective of excluding dangerous abbreviations is patient safety.

TABLE 5-3 Common Suffixes

Suffix	Meaning	Example
-ac	pertaining to	cardiac
-al	pertaining to	renal
-algia	pain	fibromyalgia
-ase	enzyme	protease
-cide	kill, killer	suicide
-cyte	cell	leukocyte
-dipsia	thirst	polydipsia
-ectomy	surgical removal	hysterectomy
-emia	blood condition	anemia
-ic	pertaining to	toxic
-itis	inflammation	rhinitis
-logist	specialist	oncologist
-logy	study of	biology
-oid	resembling	steroid
-oma	tumor	carcinoma
-osis	condition	histoplasmosis
-pathy	disease	neuropathy
-plasty	surgical repair	rhinoplasty
-rrhage	bursting of blood	hemorrhage
-rrhea	flowing discharge	diarrhea
-sclerosis	hardening	arteriosclerosis
-scope	instrument	microscope
-scopy	viewing of	colonoscopy
-stasis	control	homeostasis
-uria	urine	polyuria

By permission. From Merriam-Webster's Collegiate® Dictionary, 11th Edition © 2013 by Merriam-Webster, Inc.

The following items are affected by this Joint Commission initiative:

- Medication orders
- Clinical documentation
- Progress notes
- Consultation reports
- Operative reports
- Educational materials
- Protocols
- Other related

---

combining form a root word with an added vowel.

TABLE 5-4 General Pharmacy Abbreviations

Meaning	Abbreviation
adverse drug effect	ADE
adverse drug reaction	ADR
amount	amt
average wholesale price	AWP
compound	cmpd; cpd
concentration	conc
dextrose 5% in 0.45% sodium chloride	D5/1/2NS
dextrose 5% in 0.9% sodium chloride	D5NS
dextrose 5% in water	D5W
diagnosis-related group	DRG
diluent	dil
discontinue	D/C; DC
dispense	disp.
dispense as written	DAW
Drug Enforcement Administration	DEA
drug utilization review	DUR
elixir	elix
enteric coated	EC
extended release	XL
fluid	fl.
Food and Drug Administration	FDA
lactated ringer's solution	LR
liquid	liq
lotion	lot
maximum allowable cost	MAC
metered dose inhaler	MDI
national formulary	NF
no known allergies	NKA
no known drug allergies	NKDA
normal saline (sodium chloride 0.9%)	NS
nothing by mouth	NPO
ointment	oint; ung
over-the-counter	OTC
patient	pt

TABLE 5-4 General Pharmacy Abbreviations *(Continued)*

Meaning	Abbreviation
pediatric	ped
powder	pwdr
prescription	Rx
Schedule I	C-I
Schedule II	C-II
Schedule III	C-III
Schedule IV	C-IV
Schedule V	C-V
solution	soln
suppository	supp
suspension	susp
syrup	syr
vitamin	vit
water	aq; aqua
wholesale acquisition cost	WAC

TABLE 5-5 Pharmacy Abbreviations—Directions/ SIG Codes

Meaning	Abbreviation
after	p
after meals	pc
after meals and at bedtime	pc & hs
afternoon	pm
as desired	ad lib
as directed	u.d.
as needed	prn
as much as needed	ad lib
as soon as possible	ASAP
at bedtime	hs
before meals	ac
before meals and at bedtime	ac & hs
both ears	AU
both eyes	OU
by mouth (orally)	po; PO

(Continued)

TABLE 5-5 Pharmacy Abbreviations—Directions/SIG Codes *(Continued)*

Meaning	Abbreviation
daily	qd; QD
dispense as written	DAW
double strength	DS
every	q; Q
every day	qd; QD
every day at bedtime	qhs; QHS
every afternoon/evening	qpm; QPM
every hour	qh; QH
every morning	qam; QAM
every other day	qod; QOD
every week	qw
four times daily	qid; QID
hour	hr; h
immediately	STAT
left ear	AS
left eye	OS
may repeat	MR
of equal parts	aa
quantity sufficient	qs
right ear	AD
right eye	OD
three times daily	tid; TID
two times daily	bid; BID
weekly	w; wk
with	ć,
without	ś
while awake	W/A; WA
24 hours	24H

TABLE 5-6 Pharmacy Abbreviations—Routes of Administration

Meaning	Abbreviation
buccal	BU
by mouth	PO

TABLE 5-6 Pharmacy Abbreviations—Routes of Administration *(Continued)*

Meaning	Abbreviation
external	EX
inhalation	IN
injection	Inj
intradermal	ID
intramuscular	IM
intrathecal	IT
intravenous	IV
intravenous piggyback	IVPB
intravenous push	IVP
intrauterine	IU
metered dose inhaler	MDI
mouth/throat	MT
nasal	NA
ophthalmic	oph; opth
oral	OR
otic	OT
rectally	PR; RE
subcutaneous	SC
sublingual	SL
tincture	tinct.
topical	TOP
transdermal	TD
urethral	UR
vaginally	PV; VA

TABLE 5-7 Pharmacy Abbreviations—Dosages and Measurements

Meaning	Abbreviation
ampule	amp
capsule	cap
centimeter	cm
cubic centimeter	cc
drop	gtt

(Continued)

TABLE 5-7 Pharmacy Abbreviations—Dosages and Measurements *(Continued)*

Meaning	Abbreviation
drops	gtts
each	aa; ea
fluid ounce	fl. oz.
grain	gr.
gram	g; gm
hour	h; hr
kilogram	kg
liter	L
microgram	mcg
milligram	mg
milliequivalent	mEq
milliliter	ml; mL
millimeter	mm
millimole	mmol
ounce	oz
pound	lb; #
tablespoon	tbsp; TBS
tablet	tab
teaspoon	tsp
units	U
½	ss

TABLE 5-8 General Medical Abbreviations

Meaning	Abbreviation
acetaminophen	apap; APAP
acquired immune deficiency syndrome	AIDS
albumin	alb
aspirin	asa; ASA
attention deficit disorder	ADD
attention deficit hyperactivity disorder	ADHD
autonomic nervous system	ANS
basal metabolic rate	BMR
beats per minute	BPM

TABLE 5-8 General Medical Abbreviations *(Continued)*

Meaning	Abbreviation
before surgery	pre op
birth control pills	BC; BCP
blood pressure	BP
blood sugar	BS
body weight	BW
bowel movement	BM
calcium	Ca
carbohydrate	carb
catheter	cath
central nervous system	CNS
chest X-ray	CXR
chronic obstructive pulmonary disease	COPD
complete blood count	CBC
congestive heart failure	CHF
coronary artery disease	CAD
cystic fibrosis	CF
dextrose 5% in water	D5W
diabetes mellitus	DM
diagnosis	diag, dx
discontinue	D/C; DC
do not resuscitate	DNR
doctor of dental surgery	DDS
doctor of osteopathy	D.O.
ear, nose, and throat	ENT
electrocardiogram	ECG; EKG
electroencephalogram	EEG
fasting blood sugar	FBS
gastrointestinal	GI
genitourinary	GU
headache	HA
health maintenance organization	HMO
heart rate	HR
hemoglobin	HgB

(Continued)

TABLE 5-8 General Medical Abbreviations (Continued)

Meaning	Abbreviation
herpes simplex virus	HSV
high blood pressure	HBP
history	Hx
human immunodeficiency virus	HIV
hydrochlorothiazide	HCTZ
hydrogen peroxide	H_2O_2
hypertension	HTN
intensive care unit	ICU
iron	Fe
licensed practical nurse	LPN
magnesium	Mg
magnesium oxide	MgO; MagOx
magnetic resonance imaging	MRI
managed care organization	MCO
measles, mumps, rubella vaccine	MMR
medication administration record	MAR
methicillin-resistant *Staphyloccus aureus*	MRSA
milk of magnesia	MOM
multiple sclerosis	MS
multiple vitamin (injection)	MV; (MVI)
myocardial infarction (heart attack)	MI
nausea and vomiting	N/V; N&V
nitroglycerine	NTG
nonsedating antihistamines	NSAs
nonsteroidal anti-inflammatory drugs	NSAIDs
normal saline	NS
oxygen	O_2
penicillin	PCN
physician assistant	PA
potassium	K
potassium chloride	KCl
preferred provider organization	PPO
quality assurance	QA

TABLE 5-8 General Medical Abbreviations (Continued)

Meaning	Abbreviation
recommended daily allowance	RDA
red blood cell	RBC
rheumatoid arthritis	RA
sexually transmitted disease	STD
shortness of breath	SOB
sodium	Na
sodium chloride	NaCl
symptoms	Sx
tetracycline	TCN
total parenteral nutrition	TPN
treatment	Tx, Rx
tuberculosis	TB
urinary tract infection	UTI
zinc	Zn
zinc oxide	ZnO

In 1999, the Institute of Medicine issued a report stating that between 44,000 and 96,000 deaths each year may be attributed to medical errors. In light of this information, numerous health care entities are continuously evaluating and developing strategies for reducing these occurrences. One result has been the development of the "Do Not Use" list, which is based on the most commonly mistaken and misunderstood written abbreviations used in all forms of medical communication. As of January 1, 2004, a "minimum" list of dangerous abbreviations, acronyms, and symbols was approved by the Joint Commission (see Table 5-9). From January 1, 2004, the items listed in Table 5-9 *must* be included on each accredited organization's "Do not use" list.

In addition to this basic list of items that must not be used, as of April 1, 2004, each organization had to identify at least three additional "Do not use" abbreviations, acronyms, or symbols (of its own choosing) to go on to its mandatory "Do not use" list. Table 5-10 offers suggestions for items that should be considered for each facility's "Do not use" list.

In addition, the Institute for Safe Medical Practices (ISMP) has suggested other abbreviations, acronyms, and symbols that should be considered suspect. Optimally, all these terms should be prohibited as well (see Table 5-11).

TABLE 5-9 The Joint Commission's "Minimum" Do Not Use List

Abbreviation	Potential Problem	Preferred Term
IU (for international unit)	Mistaken as IV (intravenous) or 10 (ten).	Write "international unit."
MS, MSO$_4$, MgSO$_4$	Confused for one another; can mean morphine sulfate or magnesium sulfate.	Write "morphine sulfate" or "magnesium sulfate."
Q.D., Q.O.D. (Latin abbreviation "for once daily and once every other day)	Mistaken for each other. The period after the Q can be mistaken for an "I" and the "O" can be mistaken for "I."	Write "daily" and "every other day."
Trailing zero (X.0 mg), lack of leading zero (.X mg)	Decimal point is missed.	Never write a zero by itself after a decimal point (X mg), and always use a zero before a decimal point (0.X mg).
U (for unit)	Mistaken as zero, four, or cc.	Write "unit."

Source: © The Joint Commission, 2013. Reprinted with permission.

TABLE 5-10 The Joint Commission's "Recommended" Do Not Use List

Abbreviation	Potential Problem	Preferred Term
μg (for microgram)	Mistaken for mg (milligrams), resulting in a 1,000-fold overdose.	Write "mcg."
A.S., A.D., A.U. (Latin abbreviations for left, right, or both ears); O.S., O.D., O.U. (Latin abbreviations for left, right, or both eyes)	Mistaken for each other (e.g., AS for OS, AD for OD, and AU for OU).	Write "left ear," "right ear," or "both ears"; "left eye," "right eye," or "both eyes."
c.c. or cc (for cubic centimeter)	Mistaken for U (units) when poorly written.	Write "mL" for milliliter.
D/C (for discharge)	Interpreted as discontinue whatever medications follow (typically discharge meds).	Write "discharge."
H.S. (for half-strength or bedtime)	Mistaken for either half-strength or hour of sleep (at bedtime). q.H.S. mistaken for every hour. All can result in a dosing error.	Write out "half-strength" or "at bedtime."
S.C. or S.Q. (for subcutaneous)	Mistaken as SL for sublingual, or "5 every."	Write "Sub-Q," "subQ," or "subcutaneously."
T.I.W. (for three times a week)	Mistaken for three times a day or twice weekly, resulting in an overdose.	Write "3 times weekly" or "three times weekly."

Source: © The Joint Commission, 2013. Reprinted with permission.

TABLE 5-11 ISMP's "Recommended" Do Not Use List

Abbreviation/ Dose Expression	Intended Meaning	Misinterpretation	Correction
3	dram	Misunderstood or misread (symbol for dram misread as "3" and minim misread as "mL").	Use the metric system.
> and <	greater than and less than	Mistakenly used for the opposite of intended meaning.	Use "greater than" or "less than."
/ (slash mark)	separates two doses or indicates "per"	Misunderstood as the number 1 ("25 unit/10 units" read as "110" units).	Do not use a slash mark to separate elements in doses. Use "per."
x3d	for three days	Mistaken for "three doses."	Use "for three days."
ARA°A ara-V	vidarabine	cytarabine ARA°C (ara-C)	Write out drug name.
AU	aurio uterque (each ear)	Mistaken for OU (oculo uterque—each eye).	Do not use this abbreviation.
AZT	zidovudine (Retrovir)	Azathioprine	Write out drug name.
BT	bedtime	Mistaken as "BID" (twice daily).	Use "hs."
cc	cubic centimeters	Misread as "U" (units).	Use "mL."
CPZ	Compazine (prochlorperazine)	Chlorpromazine	Write out drug name.
D/C	discharge, discontinue	Premature discontinuation of medications when D/C (intended to mean "discharge") is misinterpreted as "discontinued" when followed by a list of drugs.	Use "discharge" and "discontinue."
DPT	Demerol–Phenergan–Thorazine	diphtheria–pertussis–tetanus (vaccine)	
HCl	hydrochloric acid	potassium chloride (the "H" is misinterpreted as "K")	
HCT	hydrocortisone	hydrochlorothiazide	
HCTZ	hydrochlorothiazide	hydrocortisone (seen in misinterpretation of HCT250 mg)	
IU	international unit	Misread as IV (intravenous).	Use "units."
mg	microgram	Mistaken for "mg" when handwritten.	Use "mcg."
$MgSO_4$	magnesium sulfate	morphine sulfate	
MSO_4	morphine sulfate	magnesium sulfate	
MTX	methotrexate	Mitoxantrone	
"Nitro" drip	nitroglycerin infusion	sodium nitroprusside infusion	
"Norflox"	norfloxacin	Norflex	
o.d. or OD	once daily	Misinterpreted as "right eye" (OD—oculus dexter), causing administration of oral medications in the eye.	Use "daily."

TABLE 5-11 ISMP's "Recommended" Do Not Use List *(Continued)*

Abbreviation/ Dose Expression	Intended Meaning	Misinterpretation	Correction
per os	orally	The "os" can be mistaken for "left eye."	Use "PO," "by mouth," or "orally."
q6PM, etc.	every evening at 6 P.M.	Misread as every six hours.	Use 6 p.m. "nightly."
q.d. or QD	every day	Mistaken for q.i.d., especially if the period after the "q" or the tail of the "q" is read as an "i."	Use "daily" or "every day."
qhs	nightly at bedtime	Misread as every hour.	Use "nightly."
qn	nightly or at bedtime	Misinterpreted as "qh" (every hour).	Use "nightly."
q.o.d. or QOD	every other day	Misinterpreted as "q.d." (daily) or "q.i.d." (four times daily) if the "o" is poorly written.	Use "every other day."
SC	subcutaneous	Mistaken for SL (sublingual).	Use "subcut." or write "subcutaneous."
ss	sliding scale (insulin) or 1/2 (apothecary)	Mistaken for "55."	Spell out "sliding scale." Use "one-half" or 1/2.
sub q	subcutaneous	The "q" has been mistaken for "every" (e.g., one heparin dose ordered "sub q 2 hours before surgery" misinterpreted as every two hours before surgery)	Use "subcut." or write "subcutaneous."
TAC	triamcinolone	tetracaine, Adrenalin, cocaine	
TIW or tiw	three times a week	Mistaken as "three times a day."	Do not use this abbreviation.
U or u	unit	Read as zero (0) or four (4), causing a 10-fold overdose or greater (4U seen as "40" or 4u seen as "44").	"Unit" has no acceptable abbreviation. Use "unit."
$ZnSO_4$	zinc sulfate	morphine sulfate	
Name letters and dose numbers run together (e.g., Inderal40 mg)	Inderal40 mg	Misread as Inderal 140 mg.	Always use space between drug name, dose, and unit of measure.
Zero after decimal point (1.0)	1 mg	Misread as 10 mg if the decimal point is not seen.	Do not use terminal zeros for doses expressed in whole numbers.
No zero before decimal dose (.5 mg)	0.5 mg	Misread as 5 mg.	Always use zero before a decimal when the dose is less than a whole unit.

Reproduced by permission of Institute for Safe Medication Practices.

Further details are available on the following Joint Commission and ISMP websites:

- www.jointcommission.org
- www.ISMP.org

Commonly Used Symbols

Table 5-12 provides a list of symbols commonly used in pharmacy and medical practice.

Drug Names

Table 5-13 provides a comprehensive list of often-used brand names of drugs and their generic equivalents.

Terminology

Terminology is the set of technical or special terms used in a business, art, science, or specific profession. Like many professions, pharmacy and medical professionals use a unique language and terminology. The following lists are not complete, but are a good reference when working in a pharmacy.

TABLE 5-12 Common Symbols

Symbol	Meaning
Δ	change
↑	increase
↓	decrease
>	greater than
<	less than
=	equals
✠	none
°	degree
'	minutes
"	seconds
↕	minim

TABLE 5-13 Common Brand Names and Generic Names of Drugs

Brand/Trade Name	Generic Name	Brand/Trade Name	Generic Name
Abbokinase	urokinase	Advil, Motrin, Nuprin	ibuprofen
Accolate	zafirlukast	AeroBid, Nasalide	flunisolide
Accupril	quinapril HCl	Aerosporin	polymyxin B sulfate
Accutane	isotretinoin	Afrin, Allerest, Dristan Long Lasting, Duration, Sinex Long Acting	oxymetazoline HCl (nasal)
Achromycin, Sumycin	tetracycline HCl		
Aciphex	rabeprazole sodium		
Aclovate	alclometasone dipropionate	Aftate, Tinactin	tolnaftate
Acthar, ACTH	corticotropin	Aggrastat	tirofiban
Acticin	permethrin	Agoral Plain, Kondremul	mineral oil emulsion
Actifed, Triafed	triprolidine HCl & pseudoephedrine HCl	Akineton	biperiden
		Alamast	pemirolast potassium
Actigall	ursodiol	Albalon, Privine, Vasocon	naphazoline HCl
Activase	alteplase	Albamycin	novobiocin
Actonel	risedronate sodium	Albenza	albendazole
Adenocard	adenosine	Aldactazide	hydrochlorothiazide & spironolactone
Adrenalin Chloride, Sus-Phrine	epinephrine HCl		
		Aldactazide	spironolactone & hydrochlorothiazide
Adrucil	fluorouracil		

TABLE 5-13 Common Brand Names and Generic Names of Drugs *(Continued)*

Brand/Trade Name	Generic Name	Brand/Trade Name	Generic Name
Aldactone	spironolactone	Antilirium	physostigmine salicylate
Aldomet	methyldopa	Antivert, Bonine	meclizine HCl
Aldoril	methyldopa & hydrochlorothiazide	Anturane	sulfinpyrazone
Aleve, Anaprox	naproxen sodium	Anzemet	dolasetron mesylate
Alfenta	alfentanil HCl	Aphthasol	amlexanox
Alkeran	melphalan	Apresazide	hydralazine & hydrochlorothiazide
Allbee w/C, Stresscaps, Surbex-T	vitamin B complex with C	Apresoline	hydralazine HCl
Allegra	fexofenadine HCl	Aquasol A	vitamin A
Alomide	lodoxamide tromethamine	Aquasol E	vitamin E
Alphagan	brimonidine tartrate	Aquatensen, Enduron	methyclothiazide
Altace	ramipril	Aralen HCl	chloroquine HCl
Alupent	metaproterenol sulfate	Aramine	metaraminol
Amaryl	glimepiride	Arava	leflunomide
Ambien	zolpidem tartrate	Aredia	pamidronate disodium
Amerge	naratriptan	Aricept	donepezil HCl
Americaine	benzocaine	Arimidex	anastrozole
A-Methapred, Solu-Medrol	methylprednisolone sodium succinate	Artane	trihexyphenidyl HCl
Amicar	aminocaproic acid	Arthrotec	diclofenac sodium & misoprostol
Amidate	etomidate	Asacol, Pentasa, Rowasa	mesalamine
Amikin	amikacin sulfate	Ascorbic acid	vitamin C
Amoxil	amoxicillin	Ascriptin, Bufferin	aspirin, buffered
Amphojel	aluminum hydroxide gel	Asendin	amoxapine
Amytal	amobarbital sodium	Aspirin	a.s.a (acetylsalicylic acid)
Anadrol-50	oxymetholone	Astelin	azelastine HCl
Anafranil	clomipramine HCl	Astramorph PF, Duramorph, MS Contin, Roxanol	morphine sulfate
Ancef, Kefzol	cefazolin sodium		
Ancobon	flucytosine		
Androlone-D, Deca-Durabolin	nandrolone decanoate	Atacand	candesartan cilexetil
		Atarax	hydroxyzine HCl
Ansaid	flurbiprofen	Ativan	lorazepam
Antabuse	disulfiram	Atromid-S	clofibrate
Antagon	ganirelix acetate	Atrovent	ipratropium bromide

(Continued)

TABLE 5-13 Common Brand Names and Generic Names of Drugs *(Continued)*

Brand/Trade Name	Generic Name	Brand/Trade Name	Generic Name
Attenuvax	measles (rubeola) virus vaccine, live	Bleph-10, Sulamyd Sodium	sulfacetamide sodium
Augmentin	amoxicillin & potassium clavulanate	Blocadren, Timoptic	ticlopidine HCl
Auralgan	antipyrine & benzocaine	Brethine, Bricanyl	terbutaline sulfate
Avapro	irbesartan	Bretylol	bretylium tosylate
Aventyl, Pamelor	nortriptyline HCl	Brevibloc	esmolol HCl
Avita, Renova	tretinoin	Brevital sodium	methohexital sodium
Axid	nizatidine	Bumex	bumetanide
Aygestin	norethindrone acetate	Buphenyl	sodium phenylbutyrate
Azactam	aztreonam	Buprenex	buprenorphine HCl
Azmacort, Kenalog, Nasacort	triamcinolone acetonide	BuSpar	buspirone HCl
		Butisol sodium	butabarbital sodium
Azo-Gantrisin	phenazopyridine HCl & sulfisoxazole	Cafergot	ergotamine tartrate & caffeine
Azopt	brinzolamide	Calan, Isoptin, Verelan	verapamil HCl
Azulfidine	sulfasalazine	Calciferol	vitamin D
Bacid, Lactinex	lactobacillus	Calciferol, Drisdol	ergocalciferol
Bactrim, Septra	sulfamethoxazole & trimethoprim	Calcijex, Rocaltrol	calcitriol
		Calcium Pantothenate, Pantothenic Acid	vitamin B_5
Bactroban	mupirocin	Camptosar	irinotecan HCl
Beepen-VK, Pen-Vee K, Veetids	penicillin V potassium	Cantil	mepenzolate bromide
Bemote, Bentyl, Antispas	dicyclomine HCl	Capastat sulfate	capreomycin
Benadryl	diphenhydramine HCl	Capitrol	chloroxine
Benemid	probenecid	Capoten	captopril
Benylin	dextromethorphan HBr	Capozide	captopril & hydrochlorothiazide
Benzedrex	propylhexedrine		
Betadine	povidone-iodine	Carafate	sucralfate
Betapace	sotalol HCl	Carbatrol, Tegretol	carbamazepine
Betoptic, Kerlone	betaxolol HCl	Carbocaine, Polocaine	mepivacaine HCl
Biaxin	clarithromycin	Cardene	nicardipine HCl
Bicillin C-R	penicillin G benzathine & procaine	Cardioquin	quinidine polygalacturonate
		Cardizem, Dilacor XR	diltiazem HCl
Bicitra	sodium citrate & citric acid	Cardura	doxazosin mesylate
BICNU	carmustine (BCNU)	Carnitor	levocarnitine
Blenoxane	bleomycin sulfate	Cartrol	carteolol HCl

TABLE 5-13 **Common Brand Names and Generic Names of Drugs** *(Continued)*

Brand/Trade Name	Generic Name	Brand/Trade Name	Generic Name
Cataflam	diclofenac potassium	Cogentin	benztropine mesylate
Catapres	clonidine HCl	Cognex	tacrine HCl
Caverject	alprostadil	Colace, Diocto	docusate sodium (dss)
Ceclor	cefaclor	Colestid	colestipol HCl
Cedax	ceftibuten	Coly-Mycin M	colistimethate sodium
CeeNU	lomustine	Coly-Mycin S	colistin sulfate (polymixin E)
Cefadyl	cephapirin sodium	Combivent	ipratropium bromide & albuterol sulfate
Cefizox	ceftizoxime sodium		
Cefobid	cefoperazone sodium	Combivir	lamivudine & zidovudine
Cefotan	cefotetan disodium	Compazine	prochlorperazine
Ceftin, Kefurox, Zinacef	cefuroxime	Copaxone	glatiramer acetate
Cefzil	cefprozil	Cordarone	amiodarone HCl
Celebrex	celecoxib	Corgard	nadolol
Celestone	betamethasone	Corlopam	fenoldopam mesylate
Celexa	citalopram hydrobromide	Cortef, Hydrocortone	hydrocortisone
Celontin Kapseals	methsuximide	Cortisporin	neomycin, polymyxin B, hydrocortisone
Cerebyx	fosphenytoin sodium		
Chirocaine	levobupivacaine	Cortone	cortisone acetate
Chloroptic, Chloromycetin	chloramphenicol	Cortrosyn	cosyntropin
		Corvert	ibutilide fumarate
Chlor-Trimeton	chlorpheniramine maleate	Corzide	bendroflumethiazide & nadolol
Choledyl	oxtriphylline		
Chronulac, Cephulac	lactulose syrup	Cosmegen	actinomycin D
Cinobac	cinoxacin	Cosmegen	dactinomycin
Cipro	ciprofloxacin	Cotazym, Viokase, Creon, Ilozyme, Pancrease	pancrelipase
Claforan	cefotaxime sodium		
Claritin	loratadine		
Cleocin	clindamycin	Coumadin	warfarin sodium
Climara, Estraderm	estradiol transdermal	Crixivan	indinavir mesylate
Clinoril	sulindac	Cuprimine, Depen	penicillamine
Clomid, Serophene	clomiphene citrate	Cutivate, Flonase	fluticasone propionate
Clorpres, Combipres	clonidine HCl & chlorthalidone	Cyanocobalamin	vitamin B_{12}
		Cyclocort	amcinonide
		Cyclospasmol	cyclandelate
Cloxapen	cloxacillin sodium	Cycrin, Depo-Provera, Provera	medroxyprogesterone acetate
Clozaril	clozapine		

(Continued)

TABLE 5-13 Common Brand Names and Generic Names of Drugs *(Continued)*

Brand/Trade Name	Generic Name	Brand/Trade Name	Generic Name
Cylert	pemoline	Depakene	valproic acid
Cystadane	betaine anhydrous	Depakote	divalproex sodium
Cystagon	cysteamine bitartrate	Depo-Medrol	methylprednisolone acetate
Cytadren	aminoglutethimide	Depo-Testosterone	testosterone cypionate
Cytomel, Triostat	liothyronine sodium	Desenex	undecylenic acid
Cytosar-U	cytarabine	Desferal	deferoxamine mesylate
Cytotec	misoprostol	Desoxyn	methamphetamine HCl
Cytovene	ganciclovir sodium	Desquam, Persa-Gel	benzoyl peroxide
Cytoxan, Neosar	cyclophosphamide	Desyril	trazodone HCl
D.H.E. 45, Migranal	dihydroergotamine mesylate	Detrol	tolterodine tartrate
		Dexedrine	dextroamphetamine sulfate
Dalgan	dezocine	DiaBeta, Glynase, Micronase	glyburide
Dalmane	flurazepam HCl		
Danocrine	danazol	Diabinese	chlorpropamide
Dantrium	dantrolene sodium	Diamox	acetazolamide
Daranide	dichlorphenamide	Dibenzyline	phenoxybenzamine HCl
Daraprim	pyrimethamine	Didrex	benzphetamine HCl
Daricon	oxyphencyclimine HCl	Didronel	etidronate disodium
Darvocet-N	propoxyphene napsylate & acetaminophen	Differin	adapalene
		Diflucan	fluconazole
Darvon	propoxyphene HCl	Digibind	digoxin immune FAB
Darvon compound-65	propoxyphene HCl, aspirin, caffeine	Digitek, Lanoxin	digoxin
Darvon-N	propoxyphene napsylate	Dilantin	phenytoin
DaunoXome	daunorubicin citrate liposomal	Dilaudid	hydromorphone HCl
		Dilaudid cough syrup	hydromorphone HCl & guaifenesin
Daypro	oxaprozin		
Decadron, Hexadrol	dexamethasone	Dimetane	brompheniramine maleate
Decholin	dehydrocholic acid	Dimetapp	brompheniramine maleate & phenylpropanolamine HCl
Declomycin	demeclocycline HCl		
Delestrogen, Valergen	estradiol valerate	Diovan	valsartan
Delta Cortef, Prelone	prednisolone	Dipentum	olsalazine sodium
Demadex	torsemide	Diprivan	propofol
Demerol HCl	meperidine HCl	Diprosone	betamethasone dipropionate
Demser	metyrosine	Disalcid	salsalate
Denavir	penciclovir	Ditropan	oxybutynin chloride

(Continued)

TABLE 5-13 Common Brand Names and Generic Names of Drugs *(Continued)*

Brand/Trade Name	Generic Name	Brand/Trade Name	Generic Name
Diuril	chlorothiazide	Emete-Con	benzquinamide HCl
Dobutrex	dobutamine HCl	Emetrol	phosphated carbohydrate solution
Dolobid	diflunisal	Eminase	anistreplase, anisoylated PSAC
Dolophine HCl	methadone HCl		
Dolorac	capsaicin	Empirin with Codeine	aspirin with codeine
Donnatal	belladonna alkaloids & phenobarbital	E-Mycin, Eryc, Ery-Tab, Ilotycin, PCE	erythromycin base
Dopar, Larodopa	levodopa	Enbrel	etanercept
Dopram	doxapram	Enduronyl	methyclothiazide & deserpidine
Doral	quazepam		
Dostinex	cabergoline	Engerix-B, Recombivax HB	hepatitis B vaccine
Dramamine	dimenhydrinate	Enlon, Reversol, Tensilon	edrophonium chloride
Drixoral	dexbrompheniramine maleate & pseudoephedrine sulfate	Entex LA	phenylpropanolamine HCl & guaifenesin
DTIC-Dome	dacarbazine	Epogen	epoetin alfa
Dulcolax	bisacodyl	Epsom salt	magnesium sulfate
Durabolin, Hybolin	nandrolone phenpropionate	Equagesic	meprobamate & aspirin
		Ergamisol	levamisole HCl
Duragesic	fentanyl transdermal	Ergocalciferol	vitamin D_2
Duranest HCl	etidocaine HCl	Ergomar, Ergostat	ergotamine tartrate
Duricef	cefadroxil	Ergotrate	ergonovine maleate
Dycill, Dynapen, Pathocil	dicloxacillin sodium	Erythrocin Stearate	erythromycin stearate
Dymelor	acetohexamide	Estinyl	ethinyl estradiol
DynaCirc	isradipine	Estrace	estradiol
Dyrenium	triamterene	Ethmozine	moricizine HCl
E.E.S., EryPed	erythromycin ethylsuccinate	Ethyol	amifostine
Ecotrin	enteric-coated aspirin	Eurax	crotamiton
Edecrin	ethacrynic acid	Euthroid, Thyrolar	liotrix
Effexor	venlafaxine	Evista	raloxifene
Elavil	amitriptyline HCl	Exosurf	colfosceril palmitate
Eldepryl	selegiline HCl		
Ellence	epirubicin HCl	Famvir	famciclovir
Elmiron	pentosan polysulfate sodium	Fareston	toremifene citrate
		Fastin, Zantryl	phentermine HCl
Elspar	asparaginase	Felbatol	felbamate

(Continued)

TABLE 5-13 Common Brand Names and Generic Names of Drugs *(Continued)*

Brand/Trade Name	Generic Name	Brand/Trade Name	Generic Name
Feldene	piroxicam	Gastrocrom, Intal, Nasalcrom	cromolyn sodium
Femcare, Gyne-Lotrimin, Lotrimin, Mycelex	clotrimazole	Gas-X, Mylicon, Phazyme	simethicone
Femiron	ferrous fumarate	Gemzar	gemcitabine
Feosol, Fer-In-Sol	ferrous sulfate	Geocillin	carbenicillin indanyl sodium
Fergon	ferrous gluconate	Geref	sermorelin
Fioricet	butalbital, caffeine, & acetaminophen	Glucophage	metformin HCl
		Glucotrol	glipizide
Fiorinal	butalbital, caffeine, & aspirin	Glyset	miglitol
Flagyl, Metrogel, Protostat	metronidazole	Gonal-F	follitropin alfa
Fleet Enema	sodium phosphate enema	Grifulvin V, Grisactin, Fulvicin PG	griseofulvin
Flexeril	cyclobenzaprine HCl	Habitrol, Nicoderm, Prostep	nicotine transdermal
Florinef acetate	fludrocortisone acetate		
Floxin, Ocuflox	ofloxacin	Halcion	triazolam
Fludara	fludarabine phosphate	Haldol	haloperidol
Flumadine	rimantadine HCl	Halotestin	fluoxymesterone
Fluothane	halothane	Herplex	idoxuridine
Folex, Rheumatrex	methotrexate	Hespan	hetastarch
Folvite	folic acid	Hibiclens	chlorhexidine gluconate
Fortaz, Tazidime	ceftazidime	Hiprex, Urex	methenamine hippurate
Fortovase, Invirase	saquinavir	Hismanal	astemizole
Fosamax	alendronate sodium	Hivid	zalcitabine
FUDR	floxuridine	Humalog	insulin lispro
Fungizone	amphotericin B	Humatin	paromomycin
Furadantin	nitrofurantoin	Humibid, Robitussin	guaifenesin (glycerol guaiacolate)
Gabitril	tiagabine HCl		
Galzin	zinc acetate	Humorsol	demecarium bromide
Gamastan, Gammar	gamma globulin IM	Hyalgan, Vitrax, Synvisc	sodium hyaluronate
Gamastan, Gammar	immune globulin IM	Hycamtin	topotecan HCl
Gamimune N, Gammagard, Gammar-IV, Sandoglobulin	immune globulin IV (IGIV)	Hycodan	hydrocodone bitartrate & homatropine methylbromide
Gantanol	sulfamethoxazole	Hydeltra—T.B.A.	prednisolone tebutate
Gantrisin	sulfisoxazole	Hydeltrasol, Pediapred	prednisolone sodium phosphate
Gan-Xene, Tranxene	clorazepate dipotassium		
Garamycin, Genoptic	gentamicin	Hydergine	ergoloid mesylates

(Continued)

TABLE 5-13 **Common Brand Names and Generic Names of Drugs** *(Continued)*

Brand/Trade Name	Generic Name	Brand/Trade Name	Generic Name
Hydrea	hydroxyurea	Isordil, Sorbitrate	isosorbide dinitrate
HydroDIURIL, Esidrix, Oretic, Microzide	hydrochlorothiazide	Isuprel	isoproterenol
		Kantrex	kanamycin sulfate
Hydromox	quinethazone	Kaon	potassium gluconate
Hydropres	hydrochlorothiazide & reserpine	Kaon-Cl, K-Dur, K-Lor, Klorvess, K-Lyte/Cl, K-Tab, Micro-K, Slow-K, Ten-K, Klor-Con, Klotrix	potassium chloride
Hygroton	chlorthalidone		
Hylorel	guanadrel sulfate		
Hyperstat, Proglycem	diazoxide	Kaopectate	kaolin & pectin
Hyper-Tet	tetanus immune globulin	Karidium, Luride, Pediaflor	sodium fluoride
Hy-Phen, Vicodin	hydrocodone bitartrate & acetaminophen	Kayexalate	sodium polystyrene sulfonate
Hytrin	terazosin	Keflex	cephalexin
Idamycin	idarubicin HCl	Keflin	cephalothin sodium
Ifex	ifosfamide	Keftab	cephalexin monohydrate
Ilopan	dexpanthenol	Kemadrin	procyclidine HCl
Ilosone	erythromycin estolate	Kenacort, Aristocort	triamcinolone
Imdur, ISMO	isosorbide mononitrate	Ketalar	ketamine HCl
Imitrex	sumatriptan succinate	Kinevac	sincalide
Imodium	loperamide HCl	Klonopin	clonazepam
Imuran	azathioprine	Kristalose	lactulose (crystallized)
Inapsine	droperidol	Kwell	lindane
Inderal	propranolol HCl	Kytril	granisetron HCl
Inderide	propranolol HCl & hydrochlorothiazide	Lacril, Isopto Plain	methylcellulose drops
		Lamisil	terbinafine HCl
Indocin	indomethacin	Lamprene	clofazimine
Infasurf	calfactant	Lariam	mefloquine HCl
InfeD	iron dextran	Lasix	furosemide
Innovar	fentanyl citrate & droperidol	Lescol	fluvastatin sodium
Inocor	amrinone lactate	Leukeran	chlorambucil
Integrillin	eptifibatide	Leukine	sargramostim
Intropin	dopamine HCl	Leustatin	cladribine
Inversine	mecamylamine HCl	Levatol	penbutolol sulfate
Ismelin	guanethidine monosulfate	Levo-Dromoran	levorphanol tartrate
Isopto Carpine, Pilocar, Pilostat	pilocarpine HCl	Levophed	norepinephrine (levarterenol)

(Continued)

TABLE 5-13 Common Brand Names and Generic Names of Drugs (Continued)

Brand/Trade Name	Generic Name	Brand/Trade Name	Generic Name
Levsin, Cystospaz, Anaspaz	l-hyoscyamine sulfate	Luvox	fluvoxamine maleate
Lexxel extended release	enalapril maleate/felodipine	Lysodren	mitotane
Librax	chlordiazepoxide HCl & clidinium bromide	Maalox	aluminum hydroxide, magnesium hydroxide suspension
Librium, Libritab	chlordiazepoxide HCl	Macrobid, Macrodantin	nitrofuratoin macrocrystals
Lidex	fluocinonide	Magan	magnesium salicylate
Limbitrol	chlordiazepoxide HCl & amitriptyline HCl	Mandelamine	methenamine mandelate
Lincocin	lincomycin	Mandol	cefamandole naftate
Lioresal	baclofen	Maolate	chlorphenesin carbamate
Lipitor	atorvastatin	Marcain, Sensorcaine	bupivacaine HCl
Lithane, Lithobid, Eskalith	lithium carbonate	Marezine	cyclizine
		Marinol	dronabinol
Lithostat	acetohydroxamic acid (AHA)	Matulane	procarbazine HCl
Livostin	levocabastine HCl	Mavik	trandolapril
Lodine	etodolac	Maxair	pirbuterol acetate
Lodosyn	carbidopa	Maxalt	rizatriptan benzoate
Lomotil	diphenoxylate HCl with atropine sulfate	Maxaquin	lomefloxacin HCl
		Maxipime	cefepime HCl
Loniten, Rogaine	minoxidil	Maxzide, Dyazide	triamterene & hydrochlorothiazide
Lopid	gemfibrozil		
Lopressor	metoprolol	Mazanor, Sanorex	mazindol
Loprox	ciclopirox olamine	Mebaral	mephobarbital
Lorabid	loracarbef	Meclan	meclocycline sulfosalicylate
Lotemax	loteprednol etobonate	Meclomen	meclofenamate sodium
Lotensin	benazepril HCl	Medrol	methylprednisolone
Lotrel	amlodipine/benazepril HCl	Mefoxin	cefoxitin sodium
Lotrisone	clotrimazole & betamethasone dipropionate	Megace	megestrol acetate
		Mellaril	thioridazine HCl
Lovenox	enoxaparin sodium	Mentax	butenafine HCl
Loxitane	loxapine succinate	Mepergan	meperidine HCl & promethazine
Lozol	indapamide		
Ludiomil	maprotiline HCl	Mephyton, Aquamephyton, Phytonadione	phytonadione (vitamin K_1)
Lufyllin	dyphylline		
Luminal, Solfoton	phenobarbital	Mepron	atovaquone
Lupron	leuprolide acetate	Meridia	sibutramine

(Continued)

TABLE 5-13 Common Brand Names and Generic Names of Drugs *(Continued)*

Brand/Trade Name	Generic Name	Brand/Trade Name	Generic Name
Merrem IV	meropenem	Mustargen, HN_2	nitrogen mustard (mechlorethamine)
Meruvax II	rubella virus vaccine, live	Mutamycin	mitomycin
Mesantoin	mephenytoin	Myambutol	ethambutol HCl
Mesnex	mesna	Mycifradin	neomycin sulfate
Mestinon, Regonol	pyridostigmine bromide	Mycobutin	rifabutin
Methergine	methylergonovine maleate	Mycogen II, Mycolog II	nystatin & triamcinolone
Meticorten, Orasone, Deltasone	prednisone	Mycostatin, Nilstat	nystatin
Mevacor	lovastatin	Mylanta	aluminum hydroxide, magnesium hydroxide with simethicone suspension
Mexitil	mexiletine HCl	Myleran	busulfan
Mezlin	mezlocillin sodium	Myochrysine	gold sodium thiomalate
Miacalcin, Calcimar	calcitonin-salmon	Mysoline	primidone
Micardis	telmisartan	Mytelase	ambenonium chloride
Micatin, Monistat-Derm	miconazole nitrate	Nalfon	fenoprofen calcium
Midamor	amiloride HCl	Nallpen, Unipen	nafcillin sodium
Milk of magnesia (MOM)	magnesium hydroxide	Naprosyn	naproxen
Miltown, Equanil	meprobamate	Naqua, Metahydrin	trichlormethiazide
Minipress	prazosin HCl	Narcan	naloxone HCl
Minitran, Nitro-Bid, Nitrostat, Tridil	nitroglycerin	Nardil	phenelzine sulfate
Minizide	prazosin HCl & polythiazide	Naropin	ropivacaine HCl
Minocin	minocycline HCl	Natacyn	natamycin
Miradon	anisindione	Navane	thiothixene
Mirapex	pramipexole	Nebcin, Tobrex	tobramycin sulfate
Mithracin	mithramycin	NegGram	nalidixic acid
Mithracin	plicamycin	Nembuta	pentobarbital sodium
Mivacron	mivacurium chloride	Neo-Synephrine	phenylephrine HCl
Moban	molindone HCl	Neptazane	methazolamide
Moduretic	amiloride HCl & hydrochlorothiazide	Nesacaine	chloroprocaine HCl
Monocid	cefonicid sodium	Neumega	oprelvekin
Monopril	fosinopril sodium	Neupogen	filgrastim
Monurol	fosfomycin tromethamine	Neurontin	gabapentin
Mucomyst	acetylcysteine	Niacin, Nicotinic acid	vitamin B_3
Murine Plus, Tyzine, Visine	tetrahydrozoline HCl	Nicobid, Nicolar, Nicotinex	niacin (nicotinic acid)

(Continued)

TABLE 5-13 Common Brand Names and Generic Names of Drugs *(Continued)*

Brand/Trade Name	Generic Name	Brand/Trade Name	Generic Name
Nilandron	nilutamide	Orgaran	danaparoid sodium
Nimbex	cisatracurium besylate	Orinase	tolbutamide
Nimotop	nimodipine	Orudis, Oruvail	ketoprofen
Nitrek, Nitro-Dur, Transderm-Nitro	nitroglycerine (transdermal)	Oxsoralen	methoxsalen
		OxyContin	oxycodone HCl
Nitropress	nitroprusside sodium	Pamine	methscopolamine bromide
Nizoral	ketoconazole	Paradione	paramethadione
Noctec	chloral hydrate	Parafon Forte DSC, Paraflex	chlorzoxazone
Nolvadex	tamoxifen citrate		
Norcuron	vecuronium bromide	Paral	paraldehyde
Norflex	orphenadrine citrate	Paraplatin	carboplatin
Norgesic	orphenadrine citrate, ASA, & caffeine	Paregoric	camphorated tincture of opium
Normodyne, Trandate	labetalol HCl	Parlodel	bromocriptine mesylate
Noroxin, Chibroxin	norfloxacin	Parnate	tranylcypromine suflate
Norpace	disopyramide phosphate	Patanol	olopatadine HCl
Norpramin	desipramine HCl	Pavabid	papaverine HCl
Norvasc	amlodipine	Pavulon	pancuronium bromide
Norvir	ritonavir	Paxil	paroxetine HCl
Novafed, Sudafed	pseudoephedrine HCl	Paxipam	halazepam
Novantrone	mitoxantrone HCl	PBZ	tripelennamine HCl
Novocain	procaine HCl	Pediazole	erythromycin ethylsuccinate/sufisoxazole
Nubain	nalbuphine HCl		
Numorphan	oxymorphone HCl	Peganone	ethotoin
Nuromax	doxacurium chloride	Penetrex	enoxacin
Nutropin	somatropin	Pentam 300, Nebupent	pentamidine isethionate
Nydrazid, Laniazid	isoniazid	Penthrane	methoxyflurane
Ogen, Ortho-Est	estropipate	Pentothal	thiopental sodium
Omnicef	cefdinir	Pepatavlon	pentagastrin
Omnipen, Principen, Totacillin, Polycillin	ampicillin	Pepcid	famotidine
		Percocet, Roxicet	oxycodone HCl & acetaminophen
Oncovin, Vincasar	vincristine sulfate	Percodan	oxycodone HCl & aspirin
Optimine	azatadine maleate	Periactin	cyproheptadine HCl
Oreton methyl, Android, Testred	methyltestosterone	Peri-Colace	docusate sodium with casanthranol (dss+)
Organidin	iodinated glycerol	Permax	pergolide mesylate

(Continued)

TABLE 5-13 Common Brand Names and Generic Names of Drugs *(Continued)*

Brand/Trade Name	Generic Name	Brand/Trade Name	Generic Name
Permitil, Prolixin	fluphenazine HCl	Procardia, Adalat	nifedipine
Persantine	dipyridamole	Proleukin	aldesleukin
Pfizerpen	penicillin G potassium	Proloprim, Trimpex	trimethoprim
Phenergan	promethazine HCl	Pronestyl, Procan-SR	procainamide HCl
Pipracil	piperacillin sodium	Propacet, Wygesic	propoxyphene HCl & acetaminophen
Pitocin, Syntocinon	oxytocin	Propecia, Proscar	finasteride
Pitressin	vasopressin	Propine	dipivefrin HCl
Placidyl	ethchlorvynol	Propulsid	cisapride
Plaquenil sulfate	hydroxychloroquine sulfate	ProSom	estazolam
Plasma-Plex, Plasmanate	plasma protein fraction	Prostaphlin, Bactocill	oxacillin sodium
Platinol	cisplatin	Prostigmin	neostigmine
Plavix	clopidogrel	Prostin E2	dinoprostone
Plendil	felodipine	Proventil, Ventolin	albuterol
Polaramine	dexchlorpheniramine maleate	Provigil	modafinil
Ponstel	mefenamic acid	Prozac	fluoxetine HCl
Pontocaine HCl	tetracaine HCl	Pulmicort, Rhinocort	budesonide
Prandin	repaglinide	Pulmozyme	dornase alfa
Pravachol	pravastatin sodium	Purinethol	mercaptopurine (6-MP)
Precose	acarbose	Pyridium, Urodine	phenazopyridine HCl
Pregnyl	chorionic gonadotropin	Pyridoxine HCl	vitamin B_6
Premarin	conjugated estrogens	Quarzan	clidinium bromide
Prempro	conjugated estrogens & medroxyprogesterone acetate	Quelicin, Anectine	succinylcholine chloride
		Questran	cholestyramine
Prevacid	lansoprazole	Quinaglute Dura-Tabs	quinidine gluconate
Priftin	rifapentine	Quinora, Quinidex Extentabs	quinidine sulfate
Prilosec	omeprazole		
Primacor	milrinone lactate	Rapamune	sirolimus
Primaxin	imipenem–cilastatin	Raplon	rapacuronium bromide
Prinivil, Zestril	lisinopril	Raxar	grepafloxacin
Prinzide, Zestoretic	lisinopril & hydrochlorothiazide	Refludan	lepirudin (rDNA)
		Regitine	phentolamine mesylate
Priscoline HCl	tolazoline HCl	Reglan	metoclopramide HCl
ProAmatine	midodrine HCl	Regranex	becaplermin
Pro-Banthine	propantheline bromide	Regroton	chlorthalidone & reserpine

(Continued)

TABLE 5-13 **Common Brand Names and Generic Names of Drugs** (Continued)

Brand/Trade Name	Generic Name	Brand/Trade Name	Generic Name
Relafen	nabumetone	Ser-Ap-Es	hydralazine, hydrochloro-thiazide, & reserpine
Relenza	zanamivir	Serax	oxazepam
Remeron	mirtazapine	Serentil	mesoridazine
Remicade	infliximab	Serevent	salmeterol
Renagel	sevelamer	Seromycin	cycloserine
Renese	polythiazide	Serzone	nefazodone
Requip	ropinirole HCl	Silvadene	silver sulfadiazine
Rescriptor	delavirdine mesylate	Sinemet	carbidopa & levodopa
Restoril	temazepam	Sinequan	doxepin HCl
Retavase	reteplase	Singulair	montelukast sodium
Retrovir	zidovudine (AZT)	Solganal	aurothioglucose
Riboflavin	vitamin B_2	Solu-Cortef	hydrocortisone sodium succinate
Ridaura	auranofin	Soma	carisoprodol
Rimactane, Rifadin	rifampin	Sonata	zaleplon
Riopan	magaldrate	Sparine	promazine HCl
Risperdal	risperidone	Spectrobid	bacampicillin HCl
Ritalin	methylphenidate HCl	Sporanox	itraconazole
Rituxan	rituximab	Stadol	butorphanol tartrate
Robaxin	methocarbamol	Stelazine	trifluoperazine HCl
Robaxisal	methocarbamol & aspirin	Stilphostrol	diethylstilbestrol diphosphate
Robinul	glycopyrrolate	Streptase	streptokinase
Rocephin	ceftriaxone sodium	Stromectol	ivermectin
Romazicon	flumazenil	Sublimaze	fentanyl
Rubex, Adriamycin	doxorubicin HCl	Sucraid	sacrosidase
Rythmol	propafenone HCl	Sufenta	sufentanil citrate
Salutensin	hydroflumethiazide & reserpine	Sular	nisoldipine
Sandostatin	octreotide acetate	Sulfamylon	mafenide acetate
Sansert	methysergide maleate	Suprane	desflurane
Seconal sodium	secobarbital sodium	Suprax	cefixime
Sectral	acebutolol HCl	Surfak	docusate calcium
Seldane D	terfenadine & pseudo-ephedrine HCl	Survanta	beractant
Selsun Blue, Selsun	selenium sulfide	Sustiva	efavirenz
Senokot, Senolax	senna	Symmetrel	amantadine HCl

(Continued)

TABLE 5-13 Common Brand Names and Generic Names of Drugs *(Continued)*

Brand/Trade Name	Generic Name	Brand/Trade Name	Generic Name
Synalar	fluocinolone acetonide	Timolide	hydrochlorothiazide & timolol maleate
Synercid	quinupristin/dalfopristin	TobraDex	tobramycin & dexamethasone
Synthroid, Levothroid	levothyroxine sodium	Tofranil	imipramine HCl
Tagamet	cimetidine	Tolectin	tolmetin sodium
Talacen	pentazocine & acetaminophen	Tolinase	tolazamide
Talwin	pentazocine	Tonocard	tocainide HCl
Tambocor	flecainide acetate	Topamax	topiramate
Tao	troleandomycin	Topicort	desoximetasone
Tapazole	methimazole	Toprol XL	metoprolol tartrate
Tasmar	tolcapone	Toradol	ketorolac tromethamine
Tavist	clemastine fumarate	Torecan	thiethylperazine maleate
Taxol	paclitaxel	Tracrium	atracurium besylate
Taxotere	docetaxel	Transderm-scop	scopolamine HBr
Temodar	temozolomide	Trecator-SC	ethionamide
Temovate	clobetasol propionate	Trental	pentoxifylline
Tenex	guanfacine HCl	Triavil	perphenazine & amitriptyline HCl
Tenoretic	atenolol & chlorthalidone		
Tenormin	atenolol	Tridione	trimethadione
Tenuate	diethylpropion HCl	Trilafon	perphenazine
Terazol	terconazole	Tritec	ranitidine bismuth citrate
Terramycin, Uri-Tet	oxytetracycline HCl	Trobicin	spectinomycin
Teslac	testolactone	Tronolane, Tronothane HCl, Prax	pramoxine HCl
Tessalon	benzonatate		
Thalomid	thalidomide	Trovan	trovafloxacin mesylate
Theo-Dur, Slo-Phyllin, Gyrocaps	theophylline	Tums	calcium carbonate
		Tussionex	chlorpheniramine polistirex & hydrocodone polistirex
Thiamine HCl	vitamin B$_1$		
Thorazine	chlorpromazine HCl	Tuss-Ornade	caramiphen edisylate & phenylpropanolamine HCl
Thypinone	protirelin		
Ticar	ticarcillin disodium	Tylenol, Tempra	acetaminophen
Tigan	trimethobenzamide HCl	Tylenol #3	acetaminophen & codeine
Tikosyn	dofetilide	Tylox	oxycodone HCl, acetaminophen, & sodium metabisulfite
Tilade	nedocromil sodium		
Timentin	ticarcillin & clavulanate potassium	Ultiva	remifentanil HCl
		Ultram	tramadol HCl

(Continued)

TABLE 5-13 Common Brand Names and Generic Names of Drugs *(Continued)*

Brand/Trade Name	Generic Name	Brand/Trade Name	Generic Name
Ultravate	halobetasol propionate	Vioform	clioquinol (iodochlorhydroxyquin)
Unasyn	ampicillin sodium & sulbactam sodium	Vira-A	vidarabine
Uni-Cap hexavitamin, Theragran	multivitamin	Viracept	nelfinavir mesylate
		Viramune	nevirapine
Unicap-T, Theragran-M	multivitamin with minerals	Virazole	ribavirin
Uniretic	moexipril HCl & hydrochlorothiazide	Visken	pindolol
Urecholine, Duviod	bethanechol chloride	Vistaril	hydroxyzine pamoate
Urispas	flavoxate HCl	Vistide	cidofovir
Urolene Blue	methylene blue	Vitamin B$_{12}$	cyanocobalamin
Valisone	betamethasone valerate	Vitamin C	ascorbic acid
Valium	diazepam	Vitravene	fomivirsen sodium
Valstar	valrubicin	Vivactil	protriptyline HCl
Valtrex	valacyclovir HCl	Voltaren	diclofenac sodium
Vanceril, Beclovent, Beconase, Vancenase	beclomethasone dipropionate	Vontrol	diphenidol
		Wellbutrin, Zyban	bupropion HCl
Vancocin, Vancoled	vancomycin	Wellcovorin	leucovorin calcium
Vansil	oxamniquine	Wycillin	penicillin G procaine
Vantin	cefpodoxime proxetil	Wydase	hyaluronidase
Vascor	bepridil HCl	Wytensin	guanabenz acetate
Vaseretic	enalapril maleate & hydrochlorothiazide	Xalatan	latanoprost
Vasodilan, Voxsuprine	isoxsuprine HCl	Xanax	alprazolam
Vasotec	enalapril maleate	Xeloda	capecitabine
Vasoxyl	methoxamine HCl	Xylocaine, Nervocaine	lidocaine HCl
Velban	vinblastine sulfate	Yutopar	ritodrine HCl
Velosef	cephradine	Zaditor	ketotifen fumarate
VePesid	etoposide	Zagam	sparfloxacin
Vermox	mebendazole	Zanaflex	tizanidine HCl
Versed	midazolam HCl	Zanosar	streptozocin
Viagra	sildenafil citrate	Zantac	ranitidine HCl
Vibramycin, Doxychel, Doxy, Doryx, Monodox	doxycycline hyclate	Zarontin	ethosuximide
		Zaroxolyn	metolazone
Vicoprofen	hydrocodone bitartrate & ibuprofen	Zebeta	bisoprolol fumarate
		Zefazone	cefmetazole sodium
Videx	didanosine	Zemplar	paricalcitol

(Continued)

TABLE 5-13 Common Brand Names and Generic Names of Drugs *(Continued)*

Brand/Trade Name	Generic Name	Brand/Trade Name	Generic Name
Zenapax	daclizumab	Zomig	zolmitriptan
Ziac	bisoprolol fumarate & hydrochlorothiazide	Zosyn	piperacillin sodium & tazobactam sodium
Ziagen	abacavir sulfate	Zovirax	acyclovir
Zithromax	azithromycin	Zyflo	zileuton
Zocor	simvastatin	Zyloprim	allopurinol sodium
Zofran	ondansetron HCl	Zyprexa	olanzapine
Zoloft	sertraline HCl	Zyrtec	cetirizine HCl

Pharmaceutical Terminology

A

Absorption is the time it takes for a drug to work after it has been administered; the rate at which the drug passes from the intestines into the bloodstream.

Active ingredient is the chemical in a medication that is known or believed to have a therapeutic effect.

Acute refers to a disease or illness with a sudden onset and a short duration.

Additive is a substance added to a liquid solution that is intended for IV use.

Admixture is a substance produced by mixing two or more substances.

Adverse reaction denotes an unwanted or unexpected side effect or a reaction to a medication; it may also result from an interaction among two or more medications.

Aerosol is a medication dosage form that uses a gaseous substance consisting of fine liquid or solid particles.

Alcoholic solution is a solution that contains only alcohol as the dissolving agent.

Allergen is a substance, like pollen, that causes an allergy.

Allergic reaction denotes a sensitivity to a specific substance that is absorbed through the skin, inhaled into the lungs, swallowed, or injected.

Allergy is a sensitivity of the immune system to a chemical or drug; an allergy causes symptoms ranging from rashes to more severe symptoms such as irregular breathing.

Amphetamines are substances that are frequently abused as stimulant medications; they can be used to treat the medical conditions of narcolepsy and eating disorders.

Analeptic refers to a substance that stimulates the central nervous system.

Analgesic refers to a substance used to relieve acute or chronic pain.

Anaphylactic shock is a hypersensitivity reaction to a substance.

Anesthetic refers to relief of pain by the process of interfering with the nerve transmission alerting the brain of pain.

Angiotensin-converting enzyme (ACE) inhibitors are used to treat hypertension (high blood pressure) and heart failure by blocking the enzyme that activates angiotensin—a natural substance that narrows the blood vessels and thereby raises blood pressure.

Anorectic refers to a substance that suppresses the appetite.

Antacid is a substance that relieves high acid levels in the gastric (stomach) area.

Antagonist refers to a substance that opposes the action of another drug or substance.

Antianxiety describes substances that reduce or relieve anxiety.

Antibiotic is a substance used to kill or stop the growth of bacteria in the body.

Antibody is a protein produced by the immune system to respond to foreign substances in the body.

Anticholinergic refers to a substance that inhibits hypersecretion and gastrointestinal motility.

Anticoagulant refers to a substance that stops blood clotting (also known as a blood thinner).

Anticonvulsant refers to a substance that stops brain nerve firing to suppress convulsive seizures.

Antidepressant is a substance that helps to maintain proper hormone balance levels to decrease depressive moods.

Antidiarrheal relieves and decreases gastrointestinal activity that produces diarrhea.

Antidote is a substance or remedy that counteracts the effects of a poisoning agent.

Antiemetic is a substance that relieves nausea and vomiting.

Antiflatulent refers to a substance that relieves the pressure of excess intestinal gas.

Antifungal refers to a substance that kills fungi growing in or on the body.

Antigen is a substance that stimulates the body to produce antibodies.

Antihistamine refers to a substance that stops the effects of histamine release, which causes sneezing, watery eyes, and congestion.

Antihypertensive refers to a substance that works to lower blood pressure.

Anti-inflammatory is a substance that reduces and relieves inflammation.

Antineoplastic refers to a substance that is used to kill cancer cells.

Antioxidants are chemical substances that reduce or prevent oxidation (chemical binding of oxygen with other chemicals or molecules).

Antiplatelets   are substances that reduce the ability of platelets to stick together and form a clot.

Antipruritic   denotes a substance that relieves itching.

Antipsychotics   are substances that block and inhibit the stimulatory actions of dopamine.

Antipyretic   refers to a substance that relieves and lowers high fever.

Antiseptic   is an agent that is capable of preventing infection by inhibiting the growth of microorganisms.

Antispasmodics   relieve stomach muscle spasms.

Antitussives   relieve severe cough.

Antiviral   refers to drugs that fight viral infections in the body.

Aqueous   means "containing water."

Aseptic techniques   are used to get rid of bacteria and other microorganisms and thus protect against infection.

Astringent   refers to a substance that stops secretions or controls bleeding.

Auxiliary labels   are placed on the medication package to provide information and instructions for use.

B

Bacteriocide   is an agent that kills bacteria.

Bacteriostat   is an agent that inhibits bacterial growth.

Beta-blockers   are substances used in the treatment of hypertension, angina, arrhythmia, and cardiomyopathy; they may also be used to minimize the possibility of sudden death after a heart attack.

Binding agent   is a substance that holds all the ingredients in a tablet together.

Bioequivalence   describes a substance acting on the body with the same strength and similar bioavailability as the same dosage of another substance.

Blood sugar level   is the measure of glucose (sugar) level in the bloodstream.

Brand name   is the proprietary name of a drug exclusive to a manufacturer for selling and distributing purposes.

Bronchodilator   is a substance that relaxes the bronchial smooth muscles in the respiratory system.

Buccal tablet   is a tablet that is dissolved in the lining of the cheek instead of being swallowed whole.

Bulk compounding   is the process of compounding large quantities of a substance for dispensing or distributing.

Bulk manufacturing   is the process of manufacturing large quantities of a substance for sale and distribution.

Bulking agent   is a chemical substance required to produce a certain desired result.

C

Calcium-channel blockers   are substances used to treat and reduce hypertension (high blood pressure) and disorders that affect the blood supply to the heart; also used in the treatment of irregular heartbeat.

Capsule   is a solid dosage form of a medication; usually made of gelatin, which surrounds and holds fine particles of a solid or liquid.

Chemotherapy   is the treatment of cancer using specific chemical agents or drugs.

Chewable tablets   are meant to be chewed instead of swallowed whole.

Chronic   refers to a disease or illness that has a long duration (e.g., lifetime).

Clinical trials   are scientific experiments that test the effect of a drug on human test patients; required by the FDA for approval of a new medication.

Communicable   refers to a disease or illness that can be transmitted to another person.

Compound   refers to a substance made from a combination of two or more substances.

Contagious   refers to the time period when an infectious person can transmit a disease to another person through direct or indirect contact.

Contraception   is the process of preventing conception or impregnation.

Contraceptive   refers to any device, drug, or chemical agent that prevents contraception.

Contraindication   is an aspect of a patient's condition that does not fit with the proposed treatment.

Controlled release medications   are released and metabolized over a period of time in the body.

Controlled substance   refers to a drug with a high potential for abuse; manufacturing and distribution of these substances are regulated by the federal government to limit abuse and harm.

Corticosteroids   are substances used to prevent minor asthma attacks or to treat severe attacks.

Cream   is a semisolid dosage form of a medication, usually applied externally to soothe, lubricate, or protect.

Cure   is the effective treatment of a disease or illness, leading to elimination of all symptoms.

D

Decongestant   refers to a substance that shrinks the mucous membranes that produce congestion.

Defecation   refers to the voiding of feces from the bowels.

Dehydration   refers to the excessive loss of water from the body.

Diagnosis   is a process by which a health care professional (doctor, nurse, or technician) determines the patient's condition or disease, after tests and examinations.

Disease   is a physical process in which the body or specific organs are being attacked or destroyed, causing harm and characteristic symptoms to the patient.

Distribution   is the process following absorption by which a drug is passed to the cells of various organs.

Diuretic   is a substance that increases the water output in the kidneys; reduces water retention in the body.

Dopamine   is a neurotransmitter associated with the regulation of movement, emotions, pain, and pleasure.

Drops   are a liquid dosage form of medication; they usually are placed in the eyes or ears.

Drug   is a chemical compound intended for use in the diagnosis, treatment, or prevention of a disease in human or animals; any substance that is intended to produce an alteration of the chemistry and/or functioning of the body.

E

Effervescent tablet   is a tablet that is dissolved into a liquid before administration.

Electrolytes   are salts that the body requires in its fluids; they are essential for nerve, muscle, and heart functions.

Elimination   is the process following distribution by which a drug is broken down and the excess is excreted.

Elixir   is a liquid dosage form that contains a flavored water and alcohol mixture.

Emesis refers to vomiting.

Emulsion is a liquid dosage form of a mixture of two products that normally do not mix together.

Enema is the process by which a medicated fluid is injected into the rectum.

Esophagitis is a condition characterized by inflammation, swelling, and irritation of the esophagus.

Estrogens are hormones produced in the ovaries; they are responsible for the development and maintenance of female secondary sex characteristics.

Excretion is the process by which the body eliminates waste after metabolism and distribution.

Expectorants are substances that remove mucus from the upper respiratory system.

F

Food and Drug Administration (FDA) is the federal agency responsible for the approval, review, and regulation of drugs and dietary supplements.

Formulary refers to a list of preferred medications that insurance plans allow their members to get at a lower out-of-pocket expense.

Fungicide refers to a substance that kills fungi.

G

Generic name is the nonproprietary name of a drug.

Genetically engineered drugs are substances produced by organisms that have had foreign genes artificially inserted into their genetic codes.

Globulin is a plasma protein.

Glucagon is a hormone produced in the pancreas that causes the automatic release of glucose.

Glucose is the sugar found in the bloodstream; it is the primary energy source for bodily functions.

Glycogen is the principal substance the body uses for storing carbohydrates; stored in the liver, glycogen turns into glucose and is released into the bloodstream when the blood sugar level gets low.

H

Half-life defines the amount of time it takes for half of a substance to be broken down in the body and excreted.

Hazardous waste is any substance that is potentially dangerous and toxic to living organisms; these wastes must be disposed of properly.

Health is the physical, emotional, or mental well-being of a person.

Health care is the procedures, techniques, tests, and examinations that are used to prevent, treat, and maintain a patient's health and well-being.

Hematemesis refers to the vomiting of blood.

Histamine (H2) blockers reduce acid secretion by preventing histamine from reaching the H2 receptors.

Hydroalcoholic solutions contain water and alcohol.

Hyperemesis refers to excessive vomiting.

Hypersensitivity is an exaggerated response to a given stimulus.

Hypnotic refers to a substance that relaxes the central nervous system to produce sleep.

I

Immediate-release medications are available to the body and metabolized immediately following administration.

Immunosuppressant refers to substances that are used to prevent the body from rejecting an organ transplant (also known as antirejection drugs).

Inactive ingredients are the ingredients found in a drug, other than the active ingredient; used to flavor, digest, color, and bind the whole substance.

Infection is an invasion and multiplication of pathogenic microorganisms in body parts or tissues.

Infusion is the process of slowly injecting a solution or emulsion into a vein or subcutaneous tissue.

Inhalation is the administration of a medication directly into the lungs via the mouth or nose.

Inhaler is a device that uses a gaseous substance to force fine solid or liquid particles into the respiratory system through the nose or mouth.

Insulin is a hormone secreted by the pancreas that helps the body digest sugars and starches; manufactured insulin is used when the patient's pancreas does not produce enough on its own.

Intolerance is an extreme sensitivity to a drug or other substance.

Intracardiac denotes the administration of a medication by injection directly into the heart.

Intradermal denotes the administration of a medication by injection into the skin.

Intramuscular refers to the administration of a medication within or into a muscle.

Intravenous refers to the administration of a medication within or into a vein.

Inventory refers to the supplies of medications that the pharmacy stocks for dispensing.

L

Labeling is the process of identifying a particular medication with the patient's and physician's information for dispensing.

Laxative is a substance that increases defecation.

Legend drug is a medication that requires a prescription written by a physician before it can be dispensed to the patient.

Local refers to a small area or single part of the body (e.g., local anesthetic).

Lotion is a liquid dosage form that contains a powdered substance in a suspension; used externally to soothe, cool, dry, and protect.

M

Medical devices are devices or products used for medical procedures or diagnostic tests.

Medication order is a prescription written in a hospital or other institutional setting.

Migraines are severe headaches caused by extreme changes in the blood vessels in the brain.

Muscle relaxants are used to treat involuntary, painful contraction of muscles by slowing the passage of nerve signals that cause pain to the muscles.

N

Narcotic is a drug for pain relief that has a high potential for abuse; can cause dependency and tolerance.

Narrow therapeutic range is the bioequivalence range of a brand-name drug and its generic counterpart where very small changes in dosage level could result in toxicity.

Nausea is a feeling of sickness to the stomach, usually accompanied by the urge to vomit.

Nonaqueous means "contains no water."

Nonlegend drugs are medications that do not require a prescription before dispensing; more commonly referred to as over-the-counter medications.

Nonsteroidal anti-inflammatory agents are substances that inhibit the production of the enzymes necessary for the synthesis of prostaglandins, thereby reducing pain and inflammation.

O

Ointment is a semisolid (mixture of a liquid and solid) dosage form that is applied externally to deliver medication, lubricate, and protect.

Ophthalmic refers to the administration of a medication through the eye.

Opiate is a drug derived from the opium poppy, such as morphine or codeine.

Opioid is a drug, hormone, or other substance that has sedative or narcotic effects similar to substances containing opium or its derivatives.

Oral refers to the administration of a medication into the mouth.

OSHA is the Occupational Health and Safety Association; responsible for developing safety guidelines for the workplace.

Otic denotes the administration of a medication into the ear.

Overdose is the action of, and condition resulting from, ingesting too much of a substance or drug; may result from one dose or multiple doses over the course of time.

P

Package insert is a supplement, provided by the manufacturer, containing specific details, instructions, and warnings about the medication.

Parenteral denotes the administration of medication by any route other than oral; administration by injection.

Patch is a dosage form in which the medication is delivered through a solid application applied to the skin and absorbed into the bloodstream.

Patent is a federally granted, exclusive right to a product for a specific period of time (before other manufacturers can create and sell an identical product).

Pharmacist is a licensed, skilled health care professional who has been trained to dispense medications as ordered by physicians and to counsel patients on drug therapies.

Pharmacokinetics is the study of the rates at which drugs are metabolized, distributed, and excreted from the body after consumption.

Pharmacology is the study of drugs and their effects on the body.

Placebo is a pill-like preparation that contains no active chemical ingredients; usually given for its psychological effects (commonly referred to as a sugar pill).

Prescription includes a direction given by a physician for the preparation and use of a medication for a specific patient, to be dispensed by a pharmacist.

Progestins are female reproductive hormones; they cause menstruation as they trigger the shedding of the uterine lining.

Proton pump inhibitors are substances that reduce gastric acid build-up by blocking the release of protons in the stomach.

Psychotherapeutic drugs are substances used to relieve the symptoms of mental and psychiatric illnesses, such as depression, psychosis, and anxiety.

Psychotropic denotes a substance that affects a person's ability to distinguish the real from the imaginary.

R

Recreational drugs (usually illegal) are often used in a social setting for their pleasurable effects instead of their medicinal value.

Rectally refers to the administration of a solid or liquid medication through the rectum.

S

Schedule I drugs are classified by the Drug Enforcement Administration as having a high potential for abuse and have no FDA approval for medicinal use (illegal drugs).

Schedule II drugs are classified by the Drug Enforcement Administration as having a high potential for abuse, with severe dependence liability (e.g., narcotics, amphetamines, stimulants).

Schedule III drugs are classified by the Drug Enforcement Administration as having less abuse potential than Schedule II drugs and moderate dependence liability (e.g., nonnarcotic stimulants, nonbarbituate sedatives, anabolic steroids).

Schedule IV drugs are classified by the Drug Enforcement Administration as having less abuse potential than Schedule III drugs and limited dependence liability (e.g., sedatives, antianxiety agents, nonnarcotic analgesics).

Schedule V drugs have limited abuse potential; they are available as prescription or over-the-counter drugs (e.g., cough syrups with small amounts of codeine, antitussives, antidiarrheals).

Sedatives relieve anxiety and tension; calm and relax the patient.

Side effects are predicted, unwanted reactions to a substance or combination of substances.

Slow-release medications are released and metabolized over a period of time in the body.

Solution is a liquid dosage form in which the medication is completely dissolved in a liquid.

Sterilize means to cleanse (objects, wounds, burns, etc.) of microorganisms such as bacteria.

Steroids are a group of chemical substances that include hormones, vitamins, sterols, and various drugs.

Stimulants are a class of medications that are intended to increase alertness and physical activity.

Subcutaneous refers to the administration of a medication under the skin.

Sublingual tablet is a tablet that is dissolved under the tongue instead of being swallowed whole.

Suppository denotes the administration of a solid medication through the vagina or rectum.

Suspension is a liquid dosage form in which the solid particles are not completely dissolved.

Symptom is a condition that usually occurs before the onset of a disease or illness; an abnormality that provides evidence of the existence of a disease or illness.

Syrup is a liquid dosage form that consists of water and sugar mixed with the medication.

T

Tablet is a solid dosage form in which the ingredients are compacted into a small, formed shape.

Tolerance is the condition in which the body has become unresponsive to a substance after prolonged exposure.

Topical refers to a substance used externally for relief from swelling, itching, or infection.

Toxin refers to a poisonous substance.

Transdermal refers to the administration of a medication through the skin (e.g., patches).

U

U.S. Pharmacopoeia (USP) is a nonprofit organization, recognized by the FDA, that publishes standards on prescription drugs, over-the-counter medications, dietary supplements, and health care products.

V

Vaginal tablet is a tablet that is dissolved in the mucous lining of the vagina.

Vaginally denotes the administration of a solid or liquid medication through the vagina.

Vasodilator is a substance that causes the blood vessels to widen.

Vomit refers to ejecting all or part of the stomach contents through the mouth.

W

Withdrawal symptom is an effect that can occur as the result of suddenly stopping the use of a substance after prolonged use.

Medical Terminology

A

Acidosis is an abnormal increase in the acidity of body fluids.

Acne vulgaris is a skin condition that occurs due to the overproduction of oil by the oil glands of the skin; results in pimples, blackheads, and whiteheads on the surface of the skin.

Addiction is physical or psychological dependence on a chemical substance, such as alcohol; any habit that cannot easily be given up.

Alkalosis is an abnormally high alkalinity of the blood.

Allergists are physicians who finalize in the diagnosis and treatment of allergies.

Amebiasis is an infection caused by an amoeba.

Amnesia is a loss of memory (may be short- or long-term).

Anatomy is the study of the structures in living things.

Androgen is a steroid, or hormone, that conroles the development of masculine characteristics.

Anemia is a condition in which the bloodstream has very few red blood cells that can carry oxygen to the tissues.

Anesthesiologists are physicians who specialize in administering drugs to anesthetize or sedate patients before surgical procedures; they monitor a patient's vital signs while the patient is under anesthesia.

Aneurism is a localized blood clot.

Angina pectoris is a condition characterized by attacks of chest pain caused by an insufficient supply of oxygen to the heart.

Angioplasty refers to the surgical repair of blood vessels.

Anorexia is an eating disorder characterized by a refusal to maintain body weight at a healthy range, low self-esteem, and an intense fear of gaining weight.

Apnea is a temporary cessation in breathing.

Arrhythmia is an irregular heartbeat.

Arteriosclerosis is a condition characterized by thickening and hardening of the arteries.

Arthritis is a condition characterized by inflammation of the joints.

Ascites is the accumulation of fluid in the abdominal cavity.

Asthma is a condition that affects a patient's breathing by restricting the airways and oxygen supply due to inflammation, swelling, and irritation.

Attention deficit disorder (ADD) is a mental disorder characterized by developmentally inappropriate levels of attention, concentration, activity, distractibility, and impulsivity.

Attention deficit hyperactivity disorder (ADHD) is a mental disorder characterized by constant impulsive behavior; difficulty in concentration; and hyperactivity that decreases social, academic, or occupational functioning.

Autoimmune disorders are characterized by an immune response against the body's own tissues.

B

Bacteria are single-celled microorganisms that are abundant in most living things; may be beneficial or harmful to a person.

Benign refers to a condition or abnormal growth that is not cancerous (e.g., tumor, cyst).

Biopsy is the removal and examination of a sample tissue.

Blood pressure measures the force exerted by blood against the walls of the arteries; measured when the heart contracts and relaxes.

Bloodstream is a general term for the area in which the blood flows; includes capillaries, veins, and arteries.

Body mass index (BMI) is the measurement of body fat relative to the patient's height and weight.

Bradycardia is a slower than normal heart rate.

Bronchitis is a medical condition characterized by an acute inflammation of the bronchial tubes in the lungs.

C

Carcinogen is any agent capable of causing cancer.

Carcinoma is an invasive malignant tumor from the epithlial tissue that tends to infiltrate other areas of the body.

Cardiac arrest refers to the absence of a productive heart beat.

Cardiologists are physicians who specialize in the treatment of heart disorders and illnesses.

Cardiovascular disease refers to conditions of the heart and circulation system.

Catalyst is a substance that speeds up a chemical reaction.

Cataract is an opacity of the lens or capsule of the eye, causing vision impairment or blindness.

Cavity is a hollow space in a structure.

Cerebral refers to the brain.

Cerumen is the medical term for earwax.

Chemotherapy is the prevention or treatment of cancerous disease by the use of toxic chemical agents.

Cholesterol is a substance produced in the liver and used for normal body functions, including production of hormones, bile, and vitamin D.

Clinical refers to diagnostic tests, lab work, and procedures that require close observation of patients.

Coagulation refers to the blood-clotting process.

Colostomy is a surgical construction of an artificial opening from the colon for excretion.

Congestive heart failure is a potentially fatal condition of the cardiovascular system wherein the heart has lost its ability to pump blood.

Contraceptives are drugs or devices used for the prevention of pregnancy; can also be used for hormone regulation.

Cortisone is a naturally occuring corticosteroid.

Cranial refers to the skull or head.

Cystitis is a condition of inflammation of the urinary bladder.

D

Dementia is a disease characterized by progressive memory loss as well as learning and thinking disorders; it is often a symptom of Alzheimer's disease, though it may have other causes as well.

Dependency is physical and/or psychological reliance on a habit or chemical substance.

Depression is a mental disorder wherein the person feels sad and helpless; characterized by personality changes and a loss of socialization, communication, and energy.

Dermatologists are physicians who specialize in the treatment of skin disorders and illnesses.

Detoxification is the process by which the patient is medically supervised for withdrawal from alcohol or drug dependency.

Diabetes is a condition characterized by failure of the pancreas to produce insulin, which is essential for digestion and for retrieving energy from food.

Dieresis refers to the increased formation of urine.

Diplopia is the medical term for double vision.

Distal refers to the part that is farthest from the point of attachment.

Dysparenunia refers to difficult or painful sexual intercourse.

Dyspepsia is difficulty in digestion.

Dysphasia is difficulty in swallowing.

Dyspnea is difficulty in breathing.

Dysuria is difficult or painful urination.

E

Ecezema refers to an inflammatory skin condition.

Edema refers to abnormal swelling of the body or a body part caused by an increased buildup of fluids in tissues and organs.

Ejaculation is the process of ejecting or discharging semen.

Embolism is a sudden blocking of a blood vessel.

Emergency medicine specialists are physicians who specialize in the treatment of emergency situations and trauma.

Emphysema is an irreversible disease (often caused by long-term smoking) in which there has been severe damage to the alveoli (tiny air sacs) in the lungs; results in a decrease in the ability of the lungs to exchange gases; symptoms are wheezing, coughing, shortness of breath, and difficulty in breathing.

Endorphin is a chemical or ingredient produced by the body that relieves pain and stress.

Epididymitis is the inflammation of the epididymis.

Epinephrine is a hormone produced by the adrenal medulla; the most potent stimulant of the sympathetic nervous system.

Epistxis is the medical term for a nose bleed.

Erythrocyte is a red blood cell.

Esophagitis is an inflammation of the esophagus due to acid buildup.

Estrogen is a hormone, produced by the ovaries, which stimulates the female secondary sex characteristics.

Etiology is the study of diseases.

Euphoria is a feeling of great happiness and well-being.

Excretion is the process by which waste is eliminated from the body.

External refers to the outer or outside part of a structure.

F

Febrile refers to an above normal body temperature; fever.

Fibrilation is the rapid twitching of individual muscle fiber with little or no movement of the muscle as a whole; an ineffectual heartbeat.

Flatus refers to the gas generated in or expelled from the digestive tract.

G

Gastric ulcer is a tear in the normal tissue lining of the stomach wall.

Gastritis is an inflammation of the normal tissue lining of the stomach wall.

Gastroenterologists are physicians who specialize in the treatment of digestive disorders and illnesses.

Gastroesophageal reflux disease (GERD) is a condition that occurs when food that has not been completely digested is forced back up the esophagus; the food is very acidic and irritates the esophagus, causing heartburn and other symptoms.

Gastrointestinal tract is the part of the digestive system that includes the mouth, esophagus, stomach, and intestines; aids in digesting and processing food in the body.

Genitalia refers to the human reproductive organs.

Geriatrics is the treatment of older patients.

Gingivitis is an inflammation of the gums.

Glaucoma is an eye condition in which pressure builds up in the eye because of reduced drainage of fluid from the eye; can result in the loss of vision in the affected eye.

Glycosuria refers to the presence of glucose in the urine.

Gynecologists are physicians who specialize in the treatment of disorders of women's reproductive organs.

H

Heartburn is a painful burning sensation in the throat (esophagus) just below the breastbone.

Hematuria refers to the presence of blood in the urine.

Hemoptysis refers to spitting up blood.

Hemorrhage refers to severe, uncontrollable bleeding (can be external or internal).

Hemostasis refers to the stoppage of bleeding or hemorrhage.

Heparin is an organic acid that prevents platelet agglutination and blood clotting.

Hepatitis is a condition associated with inflammation of the liver.

Herpes simplex is an acute viral disease characterized by watery blisters on the skin and mucous membranes; commonly known as cold sores.

Hives is a condition associated with skin eruptions and whelps.

Hormone is a chemical substance that stimulates and regulates certain bodily functions.

Hormone replacement therapy (HRT) is a therapy developed for women to help increase estrogen levels that are declining during menopause.

Hyperglycemia is the condition of high blood glucose (sugar).

Hyperkalemia is the condition of excessive amounts of potassium in the blood.

Hyperlipidemia refers to high cholesterol.

Hypertension refers to long-term high blood pressure.

Hypoglycemia is the condition of low blood glucose (sugar).

Hypotension refers to long-term low blood pressure.

Hypoxia refers to a low concentration of oxygen in the tissues.

Hysterectomy refers to the surgical removal of the uterus.

I

Immunity is the body's ability to fight off infections from bacteria and viruses.

Impotence is the inability to achieve and maintain penile erection.

Incontinence refers to the inability to hold or control urination or defecation.

Inflammation is any redness, swelling, pain, or heat in a body tissue or tissues caused by physical injury, infection, or irritation.

Influenza is a contagious viral infection of the nose, throat, and lungs, which often occurs in the winter season; also called flu.

Inpatient   refers to a person who has been admitted to a hospital or other medical facility to receive treatment for a disease or injury.

Internal   denotes the inner or inside part of a structure.

J

Jaundice   is a condition associated with a yellow appearance of the skin and is associated with problems with the liver.

K

Ketonuria   refers to the presence of ketones in the urine.

L

Laryngitis   is the inflammation of the larynx.

Lavage   refers to washing out a hollow organ, such as the stomach, with repeated injections of water.

Leukemia   is a condition characterized by elevated white blood cell counts.

Leukocyte   is a white blood cell.

Lipids   are organic compounds consisting of fats and other substances; used to measure cholesterol.

Lymph   is the clear, watery fluid derived from body tissues that contains white blood cells.

Lymphoma   refers to a tumor of the tissue in the lymph glands.

M

Malignant   refers to an abnormal condition or growth in which a group of cells (e.g., cancerous cells) cause harm and destruction to other cells and tissues.

Mamoplasty   refers to the surgical removal of a breast.

Melanoma   is a skin cancer.

Meningitis   is the inflammation of the meninges of the brain and spinal cord.

Menopause   refers to the cessation of the menstrual cycle.

Metabolism   consists of the physical and chemical processes of the body that convert consumed food into energy for use by the tissues and organs.

Metastasis   is the spreading of a disease from one organ or part of the body to another organ or part of the body.

Myocarditis   is the inflammation of the heart muscle.

N

Narcolepsy   is a rare, chronic sleep disorder characterized by constant daytime fatigue and sudden attacks of sleep.

Nephritis   is the inflammation of the kidney.

Neurologists   are physicians who specialize in the treatment of disorders and illnesses within the brain and central nervous system.

Neuropathic   relates to a disease of the nerves.

Neurotransmitter   is a chemical substance released by one nerve cell that activates or inhibits a neighboring nerve cell.

Nocturia   refers to excessive urination during the night.

O

Obstetricians   are physicians who specialize in the care of pregnant women before and during childbirth.

Occlusion   is a blockage of a blood vessel.

Oncologists   are physicians who specialize in the treatment of cancer; they are usually expert in radiation therapy, chemotherapy, and other cancer treatments.

Ophthalmologists   are physicians who specialize in the treatment of poor vision and eye disorders, using medication, corrective lenses, and surgery.

Organ   is a part of the body made up of specialized tissues that performs a specialized function or functions; part of an organ system.

Orthopedists   are physicians who specialize in the treatment of injuries and structural disorders of the bones and joints.

Osteoporosis   is a medical disease characterized by a loss in total bone density; it can be the result of calcium deficiency, menopause, certain endocrine diseases, advanced age, medications, or other risk factors.

Otolaryngologists   are physicians who specialize in the treatment of disorders and illnesses of the ear, nose, and throat.

Outpatient   refers to a patient who receives treatment from a hospital or other medical facility on a scheduled basis without being admitted for overnight or continuous stay.

P

Pain   is a feeling of slight or severe discomfort caused by an injury or illness.

Palpitation   refers to a forceful heartbeat felt by the patient.

Panic attack   is a sudden, repeated episode of extreme fear, panic, and anxiety.

Parietal   refers to the wall of a structure or cavity.

Pathogen   is a microorganism (bacteria or virus) that causes disease.

Pathologists   are clinicians who study the history, causes, and progress of diseases by examining specimens of body tissues, blood, body fluids, and body secretions.

Pathology   is the study of the nature of disease(s).

Peripheral   denotes a location at or toward the surface of the body or a body part.

Pertussis   refers to whooping cough.

Pharyngitis   is the inflammation of the pharynx.

Phlebitis   is the inflammation of a vein.

Physiology   is the study of the function of living things.

Plasma   refers to the fluid portion of the blood.

Pneumonia   is the inflammation of the lung.

Polydipsia   refers to an excessive thirst.

Polyuria   refers to excessive urine formation.

Prevention   is the process of taking steps to keep a health condition or other abnormality from occurring or worsening.

Primary care   is the medical care a person receives from a general practitioner or family physician.

Primary care physician   is usually the internal medicine or family physician, who treats a variety of illnesses; this physician may refer a patient to a specialist if further specialized care or treatment is necessary.

Prognosis   refers to the medical assessment of the expected outcome and course of a particular disease.

Proximal   denotes the location of the part that is nearest to the point of attachment.

Pruritic   is the sensation of intense itching of the skin.

Psychiatrists   are physicians who specialize in the treatment of mental, emotional, and behavioral disorders by the use of medications and psychotherapy.

Psychotherapy   is the nondrug treatment of psychological disorders; usually performed as behavioral or cognitive therapy.

Pulmonary   refers to the lungs and respiratory system.

R

Radiologists   are technicians who use technologies such as X-rays, radiation methods, and ultrasound machines to view and assess medical problems.

Receptor   is the part of the nerve cell that recognizes the neurotransmitter and communicates with other nerve cells.

Respiration   is the process by which gases are passed through the lungs and distributed throughout the body.

S

Seasonal affective disorder (SAD)   is a type of depression that occurs during the fall and winter months, or during other times of the year or in parts of the world where exposure to natural sunlight is limited.

Secondary care   is medical care that a person receives from a specialist after being referred by the primary care physician.

Serotonin   is a neurotransmitter in the brain that regulates moods, appetite, sensory perception, and other central nervous system functions.

Sinusitis   is the inflammation of the sinuses.

Spasm   is an involuntary muscle contraction.

Specialists   are physicians who are experienced in a certain area of medicine or the study for treatment and prevention.

Surgeons   are physicians who specialize in and are trained to perform surgical procedures and operations on patients to provide treatment or cure for an illness or injury.

Syndrome   refers to a set of symptoms that are characteristic of a particular disease.

Systemic   refers to the whole body.

T

Tachycardia   is a rapid heart beat.

Tachypnea   refers to rapid or fast breathing.

Terminally ill   refers to the condition of having an illness or disease for which no treatment or cure is available; the expected outcome is death.

Testosterone   is a hormone produced in high amounts in males and that regulates certain characteristics of muscle building, sexual organs, hair growth, and deepening of the voice during puberty.

Thrombosis   is a condition associated with a blood clot in the vascular system.

Tinnitus   refers to a ringing sound in the ear.

Toxic   refers to a poisonous substance.

Tumor   is an uncontrollable and progressive new growth of tissue.

U

Urinary incontinence   is the inability to control the passage of urine from the bladder.

Urologists   are physicians who specialize in the treatment of disorders in the urinary tract, as well as problems in the male reproductive organs.

V

Vaccine   is a preparation that contains weakened or killed viruses, or bacteria, and is administered to a person to activate immunity to the disease caused by that virus.

Vascular   refers to the blood vessels and circulatory system.

Vasodilation   refers to the contraction of smooth muscles that surround the blood vessels.

Vasodilator   is a nerve or drug that causes vasodilation.

Venereal   refers to that which is associated with, or transmitted via, sexual intercourse.

Vertigo   is a condition characterized by dizziness.

Virus   is a very small infectious organism that requires a living host cell for reproduction.

Visceral   refers to the structures inside the body.

Void   refers to emptying the bladder.

Summary

The ability to recognize and understand the language of pharmacy and medicine is necessary to practice as a pharmacy technician. This language includes terminology, abbreviations, and drug names. It is unlikely that you will immediately retain all the information presented within this chapter, but over time and with experience, you should gain a strong working knowledge of the information presented. This chapter will serve as a valuable reference as you continue your studies and begin practicing as a pharmacy technician.

Chapter Review Questions

1. The root word *rhin* refers to which of the following?
   a. intestines
   b. kidney
   c. mind
   d. nose

2. Which of the following is the generic equivalent for Dalmane?
   a. loratadine
   b. flurazepam
   c. digoxin
   d. clindamycin

3. The prefix *hypo-* refers to which of the following?
   a. against
   b. large
   c. too little
   d. too much

4. The suffix *-algia* refers to which of the following?
   a. tumor
   b. pain
   c. inflammation
   d. control

5. Which of the following is the brand-name equivalent for furosemide?
   a. Lasix
   b. Medrol
   c. Paxil
   d. Toprol XL

6. The root word *oste* refers to which of the following?
   a. bone
   b. heart
   c. lung
   d. vein

7. What is the abbreviation for "after meals"? _____

8. What does the abbreviation "ADR" stand for? _____

9. What is the abbreviation for "four times daily"? _____

10. What does the abbreviation "DUR" stand for? _____

Critical Thinking Questions

1. Why are some abbreviations, such as "d/c," considered dangerous and need to be avoided?

2. How can recognizing root words, prefixes, and suffixes assist you in becoming and working as a pharmacy technician?

3. Why are abbreviations used on prescriptions?

Web Challenge

1. Go to www.jointcommission.org and print out the Joint Commission's Official Abbreviation "Do Not Use List," as well as tips on implementing the list in the pharmacy.

2. Visit Medic8's Online Medical Dictionary at http://www.medic8.com/MedicalDictionary.htm. Find three medical terms that are not listed in this chapter and define them by using the root, prefix, and/or suffix.

References and Resources

Dorland's Illustrated Medical Dictionary. 32nd ed. Philadelphia, PA: Elsevier, 2012. Print.

Drug Facts and Comparisons. 2011 ed. Sr. Clinical Ed. Andrea L. Williams. St. Louis, MO: Wolters Kluwer, 2011. Print.

Fremgen, Bonnie F. and Suzanne S. Frucht. *Medical Terminology: A Living Language*. 5th ed. Upper Saddle River, NJ: Pearson, 2012. Print.

"ISMP's List of Error-Prone Abbreviations, Symbols, and Dose Designations." *Institute for Safe Medication Practices*. 2011. Web. 13 January 2012.

Johnston, Mike. *Certification Exam Review*. Upper Saddle River, NJ: Pearson, 2005. Print.

Johnston, Mike. *Fundamentals of Pharmacy Practice*. Upper Saddle River, NJ: Pearson, 2005. Print.

"Official Do Not Use List." *The Joint Commission*. June 2010. Web. 13 January 2012.

Rice, Jane. *Medical Terminology: A Word Building Approach*. 7th ed. Upper Saddle River, NJ: Pearson, 2011. Print.

Stedman's Medical Dictionary. 2nd ed. Boston, MA: Houghton Mifflin, 2004. Print.

Turley, Susan M. *Medical Language*. 2nd ed. Upper Saddle River, NJ: Pearson, 2010. Print.

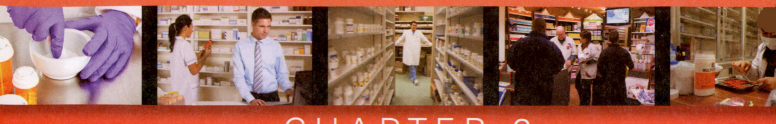

CHAPTER 6

Dosage Formulations and Routes of Administration

LEARNING OBJECTIVES

After completing this chapter, you should be able to:

- Explain drug nomenclature.

- Identify various dosage formulations.

- Identify the advantages and disadvantages of solid and liquid medication dosage formulations.

- Explain the differences between solutions, emulsions, and suspensions.

- Explain the difference between ointments and creams.

- Identify the various routes of administration and give examples of each.

- Give examples of common medications for various routes of administration.

- Identify the advantages and disadvantages of each route of administration.

- Identify the parenteral routes of administration.

- Explain the difference between transdermal and topical routes of administration.

- Explain the difference between sublingual and buccal routes of administration.

- Identify the abbreviations for the common routes of administration and dosage formulations.

KEY TERMS

anhydrous, p. 98

aqueous, p. 98

aromatic, p. 99

dosage form, p. 95

emollient, p. 98

emulsion, p. 98

formulary, p. 94

health maintenance organizations (HMOs), p. 94

homogenous, p. 99

hydrophobic, p. 98

nomenclature, p. 94

occlusive, p. 98

oleaginous, p. 98

route of administration (ROA), p. 102

semisynthetic, p. 94

synthesized, p. 94

synthetic, p. 94

viscous, p. 99

volatile, p. 100

INTRODUCTION

Technological advances over the last century have vastly changed the way the world lives and have given us a wider variety of choices in our daily lives. Pharmacy is no longer restricted to using plants and animals as the basis for new medications, and advances have enabled the pharmaceutical industry to produce even more new medications in a greater variety of forms than ever before. This chapter discusses the different sources from which medications are derived, how medications are named, various dosage formulations, and routes of administration, and introduces common medications in each of the categories.

Sources of Drugs

Although most people are familiar with the trade or brand names of the medications they take, they may be unfamiliar with the various names used to identify the same drug products or the fact that their medications are derived from many different sources, including plants and animals. Drugs are derived from a variety of sources that can be put into three categories: natural, synthetic, and genetically engineered. This section briefly discusses each category.

Natural Drug Sources

Natural drugs are substances that occur in nature and are naturally occurring. These include substances that are derived or extracted from plants, animals, and minerals.

Plant Sources

The plant kingdom provides a rich and varied source of natural products that can be used as drugs, either as the active ingredient or as a precursor for the synthesis of a drug. Examples of natural drugs derived from plant sources include:

- Acetylsalicylic acid (aspirin)—analgesic derived from white willow bark.
- Cocaine—local anesthetic derived from the coca plant (see Figure 6-1).
- Codeine, morphine—analgesics derived from the opium poppy plant (see Figure 6-2).
- Digoxin—cardiac glycoside derived from the foxglove plant (see Figure 6-3).
- Vincristine, vinblastine—anticancer drugs derived from the periwinkle plant (see Figure 6-4).

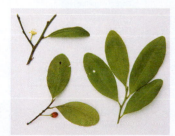

FIGURE 6-1 Coca plant (*Erythroxylum coca*).
Source: Matthew Ward, Dorling Kindersley

Animal Sources

In addition to plants, animals are another primary source for natural drugs. Examples of natural drugs derived from animal sources include:

- Bovine insulin—derived from the pancreas of a cow.
- Porcine insulin—derived from the pancreas of a pig.
- Pepsin—derived from the stomach of a cow.
- Thyroid hormones—derived from thyroid glands of a pig.

Mineral Sources

Minerals, which are naturally occurring solid chemical substances found in the earth and soil, are another natural source for drugs. Examples of natural drugs from mineral sources include:

- Ferrous sulfate (iron)—used to treat iron deficiencies.
- Gold—used to treat arthritis.
- Magnesium—used in milk of magnesia, a laxative and antacid.
- Potassium—used to treat low blood levels of potassium.
- Sodium chloride—a common base solution for IV therapies.
- Zinc—used in skin protectants and sunscreen.

Synthetic Drug Sources

Synthetic drugs are produced in the laboratory and are not naturally occurring. A drug is **semisynthetic** if it is a naturally occurring substance that has been chemically altered. A drug is considered to be **synthesized** if it is made in a laboratory to imitate a drug that is naturally occurring. In the pharmacy practice, it is common for any drug that does not occur in nature and is produced in the laboratory to be called *synthetic*. Examples of synthetic drugs include:

- Adrenalin—synthesized epinephrine for the treatment of hypersensitivity and asthmatic attacks.
- Amoxicillin, ampicillin, piperacillin—semisynthetic penicillins used to treat various infections.
- Barbiturates—synthetic central nervous system depressants.
- OxyContin—synthetic opiate used for pain management.

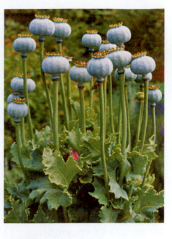

FIGURE 6-2 Opium poppy (*Papaver somniferum*).
Source: Roger Smith, Dorling Kindersley

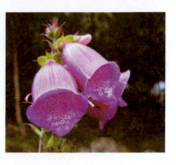

FIGURE 6-3 Foxglove (*Digitalis purpurea*).

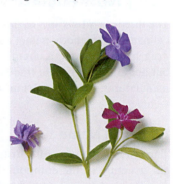

FIGURE 6-4 Periwinkle (*Vinca minor*).
Source: Matthew Ward, Dorling Kindersley

TABLE 6-1 Drug Nomenclature Examples

Chemical Name	Generic Name	Trade Name(s)
(±)-2-(p-isobutylphenyl) propionic acid	ibuprofen	Motrin, Advil
4'-hydroxyacetanilide	acetaminophen	Tylenol
4-thia-1-azabicyclo[3.2.0]-heptane-2-carboxylic acid, 3,3-dimethyl-7-oxo-6-[(phenoxyacetyl)amino]-, monopotassium salt, [2S-(2a,5a,6b)]-	penicillin VK	Veetids

Genetically Engineered Drug Sources

Genetically engineered drugs are synthetic drugs produced by means of recombinant DNA (rDNA) or monoclonal antibodies (MAbs). When manufacturers use *recombinant DNA*, they combine two different DNA strands to produce a new strand of DNA (deoxyribonucleic acid) or rDNA. MAbs are hybrid cells created in the laboratory from animals. These new cells can be used to treat tumors and diagnose various conditions. Examples of rDNA and MAb drugs include:

- Human insulin—created by rDNA to treat diabetes.
- Recombinant hepatitis B vaccine—created by rDNA to vaccinate against hepatitis B.
- Rituxan, Zevalin, Erbitux, Avastin—MAbs used in the treatment of various cancers.

Drug Nomenclature

The three classifications of drug **nomenclature** are the chemical name, the generic name, and the brand or trade name. All drug products have a chemical name and a generic name, but not all drugs have a trade name. Understanding drug nomenclature is very important and necessary for a pharmacy technician.

Chemical Name

The *chemical name* of a drug product reflects the chemical structure of the compound. The chemical name is often complicated, extremely lengthy, and difficult to remember and pronounce (see Table 6-1). Each drug is named according to the strict nomenclature guidelines of the International Union of Pure and Applied Chemistry, an organization whose main purpose is to advance worldwide aspects of the chemical sciences. The chemical names of drugs are used primarily in chemistry and pharmaceutical research; they are not commonly used in daily pharmacy practice.

Generic Name

The *generic name* of a drug is a convenient and concise name used by the public to identify the active ingredient in the drug. The generic name is assigned to the drug by the manufacturer in collaboration with the Food and Drug Administration (FDA). A generic drug name is usually not capitalized and may be used by anyone because it is not restricted by copyright or trademark. It is also the name used in the *United States Pharmacopoeia* (USP) and the *United States Pharmacopoeia National Formulary* (USP-NF). The USP is the official standards-setting authority for prescription and over-the-counter (OTC) drugs; the USP-NF is the publication containing the official standards. Identical substances always use the same generic name; that is, a substance never has more than one generic drug name assigned to it. The generic name is also known as the *nonproprietary name* (see Figure 6-5).

In efforts to contain escalating drug costs, many insurance companies and **health maintenance organizations (HMOs)** pay the pharmacy only for generic medications, according to their **formularies**. In addition, many pharmacies stock their shelves alphabetically by generic name.

---

synthetic drugs that are not naturally occurring; produced in a laboratory.

semisynthetic a naturally occurring compound that has been chemically altered.

synthesized produced in a laboratory to imitate a naturally occurring compound.

nomenclature set of names; way of naming.

health maintenance organization (HMO) a type of health care/insurance plan.

Formulary a listing of drugs approved for use or reimbursement.

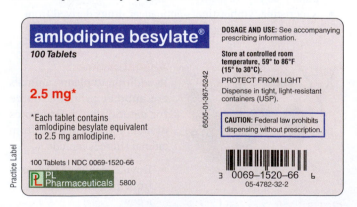

FIGURE 6-5 Generic name: amlodipine besylate.

Trade or Brand Name

The *trade* or *brand name* of a drug is registered or trademarked by a specific producer or manufacturer to identify its particular drug. Because a trade name is trademarked, it cannot be used by other manufacturers. Trade names are normally capitalized, and a single generic drug, such as ibuprofen, may be produced, marketed, and sold under more than one trade name. The trade or brand name may also be referred to as the *proprietary name*. Table 6-1 lists some examples of drug nomenclature.

Classification of Drugs

A drug may be placed into a specific category based on any one or more of the following considerations:

- Chemical ingredients
- Method by which the drug is used (e.g., by mouth, by injection, topical application)
- Area of the body that is treated (e.g., stomach, head, heart)

These categories are also called *classifications*, and any drug fitting the designated criteria belongs to that class of drugs. Many drugs fit into more than one category because they may be indicated and used for entirely different conditions.

Although there are numerous ways to classify drugs, they are often classified into groups according to two methods. The first method is according to therapeutic classification as determined by a drug's therapeutic use. For example, *diuretic* (an agent that promotes the excretion of urine) is an example of a pharmacological classification, as it describes the drug's effect on the body. The second method is determined by a drug's mechanism of action. A therapeutic classification, such as *antinausea* drug (a drug to combat vomiting), more straightforwardly describes the clinical action of the drug.

Dosage Formulations

Medications are available in various **dosage forms**; the term refers to how the medication is prepared for administration to the patient. The two primary dosage preparations are liquid and solid. Common dosage forms include tablets, solutions, suspensions, inhalants, creams, and ointments. A single medication may be available in multiple dosage forms to allow use for various disease states, patient age ranges, and desired results.

Solid Dosage Forms

Medications are most widely available as solid dosage forms (see Figure 6-6). They may be administered via different routes,

---

dosage form the actual form of the drug (tablet, capsule, suppository, solution, etc.); also called dosage formulation.

---

such as orally, rectally, vaginally, or topically.

A physician must review many factors when deciding if a solid dosage form is an appropriate choice for the patient. Solid medications have several advantages over other forms of medication, including:

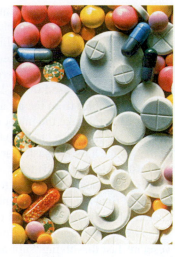

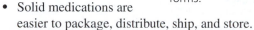
FIGURE 6-6 Solid dosage forms.

- Patients are able to self-administer solid medications more easily.
- Solid medications usually have a longer shelf life before reaching the expiration date.
- Solid medications are easier to package, distribute, ship, and store.
- Dosing is more accurate with solid dosage forms because the medication is already in a distinctive unit/measure.
- Solid medications usually have little or no taste, whereas liquid medications often have a bad taste.
- Solid dosage forms have been created to release the medication over a longer period of time in the patient's body, as in extended-release medications. This allows the patient to take fewer doses while still getting the desired effects.

Solid medications also have several disadvantages:

- Some patients may have difficulty swallowing large tablets or capsules.
- Solid medications are not an appropriate choice for patients who are unconscious or are using nasal/mouth breathing tubes for ventilation.
- Solid medications take longer to be absorbed, broken down, and distributed in the body. The stomach has to metabolize the medication before it can take effect.
- Solid medications are not fast enough for immediate-action treatments. When immediate-action treatments are required, liquids or injectable medications are more appropriate.

Tablets

Tablets are solid medications that are compacted into small, formed shapes. They are usually taken by mouth (oral administration). Tablets consist of several components that work together to ensure that the tablet is easy to swallow, has flavorings or sweeteners for improved taste, is properly digested in the body, and releases the drug at the proper time to produce the desired effect. All of the ingredients in a medication except the active drug(s) are called *inactive*, or *inert*, *ingredients*.

Tablets are classified by the way they are made. The two most common tablet classifications are molded and compressed. *Molded* tablets are made by using a mold and wet materials. *Compressed* tablets are formed by die-punching compressed, powdered, crystalline, or granular substances into a uniform shape. One characteristic of a compressed tablet is the film, sugar coating, or enteric coating on the outside of the tablet, commonly used to mask a bad taste or foul smell and protect the tablet from the air and humidity. The film coating is also used to make the tablet smooth and easier to swallow. Enteric coating is used to keep the tablet from being dissolved in the stomach by the gastric acids and to protect the lining of the gastrointestinal (GI) tract and stomach from irritation by the drug. Medications that are to be released in the body over a period of time are made with enteric coatings. *Caplets* are film-coated tablets in the shape of a capsule.

The six common types of tablets are chewable, effervescent, fast dissolving, sublingual, buccal, and vaginal. The following text briefly describes each type and its unique characteristics and uses.

Chewable Tablets Chewable tablets are tablets that should be chewed instead of being swallowed whole to achieve the desired results. Chewable tablets are most commonly used for pediatric medications because small children have a difficult time swallowing tablets. Most chewable tablets include sweeteners and flavorings to mask bad tastes and make the medication easier to take. Some adult medications are also chewable, such as antacids and aspirin.

Effervescent Tablets Effervescent tablets are dissolved into a liquid before administration. These tablets contain special ingredients that release the active chemical ingredient by reacting with the liquid; this is what causes the bubbling and fizzing when an effervescent tablet is placed in a liquid. Effervescent tablets have the advantage of being completely dissolved in the liquid before the patient takes the medication. This allows for quicker absorption in the body than a solid tablet.

Fast-Dissolving Tablets Fast-dissolving, or rapidly disintegrating, tablets are a rather new dosage formulation, in which a tablet can be taken orally, with or without water. These tablets begin disintegrating immediately upon entry into the mouth. This dosage formulation is particularly beneficial for medications used to treat nausea/vomiting, seizures, and migraines. Various OTC medications are also now available in this formulation, to provide convenience since water is not required to take the tablet. This formulation differs from effervescent tablets, in that it is not intended to be dissolved in a liquid prior to administration but rather eliminates the need for liquid altogether.

> ### 💬 Workplace Wisdom Effervescent Preparations
>
> Effervescent tablets or granules *must* be dissolved in a liquid before they are administered. Effervescent tablets or granules should *never* be chewed, swallowed whole, or dissolved on the tongue. Effervescent preparations release carbon dioxide when they come in contact with liquid, and this release of gas into the GI system could cause serious harm to the patient.

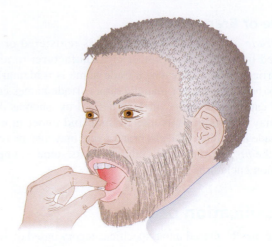

FIGURE 6-7 Sublingual tablet and route.

Sublingual Tablets Sublingual tablets are disintegrated and absorbed when the tablet is placed sublingually—under the tongue (see Figure 6-7). The ingredients in these tablets are absorbed through the lining of the mouth into the bloodstream; thus, sublingual tablets are useful for medications that are destroyed by stomach acids or poorly absorbed through the GI tract.

Buccal Tablets Buccal tablets are similar to sublingual, except that they are disintegrated in the buccal pouch of the mouth, located between the gums and the cheek, and absorbed into the bloodstream through the lining of the cheek.

Vaginal Tablets Vaginal tablets are solid dosage forms that are administered into the vagina and are dissolved and absorbed through the mucous lining of the vagina. Vaginal tablets are useful if immediate treatment and medication are needed within the walls of the vagina.

Capsules

Capsules are solid medication forms in which the active and inactive ingredients of a drug are contained in a shell. The most common shell is composed of gelatin, which is made of protein from animals. The smooth surface of the gelatin shells allows easier swallowing. Gelatin shells may be either soft or hard.

Soft Gelatin Shells Soft gelatin shells have had ingredients added to the shell to give it a soft and elastic consistency. This consistency allows the capsule to be flexible during administration. The two halves of a soft capsule are sealed together and cannot be broken apart. The shape of soft capsules can vary from round to oblong (see Figure 6-8). They

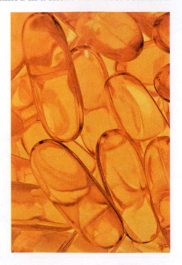

FIGURE 6-8 Soft gelatin shell capsules.
Source: Colin Cuthbert/Science Source

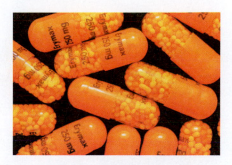

FIGURE 6-9 Hard gelatin shell capsules.
Source: Sinclair Stammers/Science Source

are filled with powdered, pasty, or liquid medications. The soft gelatin capsule dissolves once in the body, allowing the medication to be absorbed and distributed to the body tissues. *Gel caps* are soft gelatin capsules that contain an oil-based medication.

Hard Gelatin Shells Hard gelatin capsules are characterized by two oblong halves joined together (see Figure 6-9). These capsules are filled only with powdered medications, never liquid, as liquid would dissolve the capsule shells. Hard gelatin capsules are most often intended for oral administration, and such capsules should be swallowed whole. However, an advantage of a hard gelatin capsule is that it can be opened and its contents can be sprinkled over a food substance or into water before administration. This is helpful for patients who are not able to swallow a whole capsule. The ingredients will be dissolved more quickly outside the gelatin shell.

Lozenges

Also called *pastilles* or *troches*, *lozenges* are a hard, disk-shaped solid dosage form that contains a sugar base. Lozenges are used to deliver a variety of local therapeutic effects to the patient's mouth and throat, including antiseptic, analgesic, anesthetic, antibiotic, decongestant, astringent, and antitussive effects. The lozenge remains in the patient's mouth until it has completely dissolved and all the medication has been released.

Powders

Powders are a solid preparation in which fine, uniform particles of active and inactive ingredients are ground up. Powders are usually manufactured and packaged as large supplies for bulk compounding. They may be applied internally or externally. Internal administration is done after the powder mixture has been dissolved in a liquid. External powders can be applied directly to the skin to be absorbed into the bloodstream. External powders are also referred to as *dusting powders*. Commonly used internal powders are potassium supplements, which must be dissolved in water or juice for administration. Mycostatin powder is an external powder used to treat fungal infections on the skin.

Powders packaged in bulk supply are difficult to measure accurately. This accuracy is achieved at the individual dose level by packaging the powder in a *powder paper*, a small piece of paper that measures out exactly one dose. BC Powder comes packaged in powder papers, each one equivalent to one dose.

Granules

Granules are made from powders that are wetted and then dried. Once completely dried, the powder is ground into coarse, nonuniform particles. Granules are commonly used in pediatric antibiotic suspensions. Distilled water is added to the package of granules, and the suspension is shaken until the solid particles dissolve completely in the liquid.

Medicated Sticks

Medicated sticks are a unique solid dosage form used in topical application of local anesthetics, sunscreens, antivirals, antibiotics, and, of course, cosmetics. For example, a lip balm, which moisturizes the lips, may contain both an antiviral and a sunscreen for use in the treatment and prevention of a herpes simplex outbreak.

Semisolid Dosage Forms

Certain medications are only partly solid, as they have a viscosity and rigidity between that of a solid and a liquid. Examples of semisolid dosage forms include suppositories, creams, ointments, and pastes.

Suppositories

Suppositories are a semisolid dosage form used to administer medication by way of the rectum, the vagina, or the urethral tract. They are meant to melt or undergo dissolution at body temperature, delivering the needed drug either locally or systemically. The route of delivery and the intended patient determine the size and shape of the suppository. Suppositories are often used to deliver medication to babies, since oral ingestion is not a practical option. In addition, suppositories can be very useful to deliver antivomiting medications, such as Phenergan, since oral dosage forms may not be a practical option.

Creams

Creams are semisolid preparations that may or may not contain medication and are composed of an oil-in-water base or a water-in-oil base. They are lighter than ointments and can be applied to the skin more easily. Creams function to soothe, cool, dry, and protect the skin. Creams are usually preferred over ointments because they are easier to apply and wash off the skin.

Ointments

Ointments are semisolid dosage forms composed of solid and liquid medications. Ointments are applied externally to the skin or mucous membrane and are used to deliver medication to the skin, lubricate the skin, or protect the skin. Ointments may or may not contain medication. They are categorized into the following types: oleaginous, water-soluble, anhydrous, and emulsions. The choice of an ointment depends on the specific characteristics and desired results. Certain medications are more effective in a water-based ointment than in a heavy, greasy base.

Oleaginous Ointments Oleaginous ointments are **emollients** used to soothe and cool the skin or mucous membrane. Their primary function is to protect the surface from the air. An advantage of an oleaginous ointment is that it is **hydrophobic** and not easily washed off. These ointments keep moisture from leaving the skin and, therefore, are commonly used as lubricants. They can remain on the skin for a long period of time. One disadvantage of oleaginous ointments is their greasy feel.

Water-Soluble Ointments Water-soluble ointments have characteristics that are the opposite to those of oleaginous ointments. They are nongreasy to the touch and easily wash off with water. These types of ointments usually do not contain fats or water. Water-soluble ointment bases can be mixed with a nonaqueous or solid medication.

Anhydrous Ointments Anhydrous ointments are emollients similar to oleaginous ointments. The major difference between the two is that anhydrous ointments absorb water instead of repelling it, because anhydrous ointments contain no water. A main function of these ointments is to soften and moisturize the skin, but not to the same degree as ointments with an oleaginous base. As it absorbs water, the anhydrous ointment turns into a water-in-oil emulsion.

Emulsions Emulsions are emollient bases that are comprised of water and oil. The two types of emulsions are oil-in-water and water-in-oil. The water-in-oil bases are heavy, greasy, emollient, and **occlusive**. The oil-in-water bases are the opposite: water-washable, nongreasy, and nonocclusive.

Pastes Pastes are stiff or very viscous ointments that do not melt or soften at body temperature. They are intended to be used as protectant coverings over the area(s) where applied. Pastes usually contain at least 20% solids.

Liquid Dosage Forms

The most common liquid dosage forms are syrups, solutions, emulsions, and suspensions (see Figure 6-10). The fluid medium is also called the *vehicle* or *delivery system* and is considered to

---

oleaginous containing oil; having oil-like properties.

emollient softening and soothing to the skin.

hydrophobic repels water.

anhydrous without water.

emulsion liquid mixture of water and oil.

occlusive closing or blocking; refers to a substance that closes or covers a wound and keeps the air from reaching the wound.

aqueous containing water.

homogenous having all the same qualities within a group.

viscous thick; almost jelly-like.

aromatic having a strong or fragrant smell (aroma).

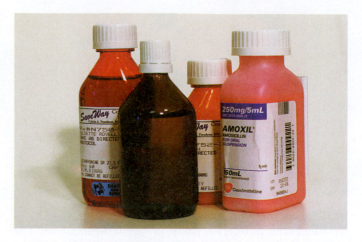

FIGURE 6-10 Liquid dosage forms.

carry the active ingredient or medication. The vehicle may be **aqueous** (water), or the liquid used may be oil or alcohol. The medication may be dissolved in the vehicle or may remain as a fine solid particle suspended in the fluid. The consistency of the liquid can be as thin as water or as thick as syrup.

Liquids have several advantages over other dosage forms, including:

- Patients who have difficulty swallowing solid dosage forms, such as tablets, can better tolerate liquid dosage forms.
- Liquid medications are absorbed faster in the body than solid dosage forms, because the active ingredient has already begun to break down and can readily be absorbed in the bloodstream. Solid dosage forms must be dissolved and broken down in the body before absorption of the active medication can take place.
- Liquid forms provide much more flexibility for achieving the proper dosage of the medication.

Liquids also have several disadvantages compared to other dosage forms, including:

- Liquids often have a shorter life before expiration than other dosage forms.
- Liquids may have a bad taste, as the medication is already dissolved, and, like a tablet or capsule, this dosage form cannot have a protective coating. This may make compliance especially difficult for children who do not like the taste of the medication. Sweeteners and flavorings are often used to make liquid medications tolerable for the patient. (Solid medications such as tablets and capsules are often coated to diminish contact with the taste receptors before they are swallowed.)
- Liquids may be more difficult to administer for some patients; thick liquids can be hard to pour, and patients often spill liquids.
- Liquids may promote dosage errors, as some patients may not measure a liquid correctly.
- Liquids usually have special storage requirements that must be maintained for the medication to work properly. For example, if refrigeration is needed, patient travel and compliance may be difficult.

Solutions

Solutions are a dosage form in which the medication is completely dissolved and evenly distributed in a **homogenous** mixture. The molecules of the solid, liquid, or gas medications are equally distributed among the molecules of the liquid vehicle. Solutions are usually absorbed quickly, because the medication is already completely dissolved; this allows the medication to take effect faster. This may be the greatest advantage of solution dosage forms. There are several subcategories of solutions, based on the characteristics of the vehicle in which the medication is dissolved.

Aqueous Solutions

Aqueous solutions are liquid mixtures that use purified or sterile water as the vehicle. They are available for oral, topical, or parenteral administration. Aqueous solutions are available as douches, irrigating solutions, enemas, gargles, washes, and sprays.

Douches are directed into a body cavity or against a part of the body to clean and disinfect. These can be used to remove debris from the eyes, nose, throat, or vagina.

Irrigating solutions are also used to cleanse parts of the body, such as the eyes, urinary bladder, abraded skin, or open wounds. These types of solutions contain antibiotics and antimicrobial medications to rid the site of infection. Irrigating solutions are often used over a larger part of the body and, in surgical procedures, to clear blood and debris.

Enemas are aqueous solutions administered rectally to empty the bowel or treat infections and diseases of the lower GI tract. Enemas are also often used to relieve constipation and to cleanse the bowel before a surgical procedure.

Gargles and *washes* are used to cleanse and treat diseases of the mouth and throat. Gargles are swished in the patient's mouth and then spit out. Washes are used more often for cosmetic and disinfecting purposes in the mouth. Like gargles, washes are used in the mouth and not swallowed.

Viscous Aqueous Solutions

Viscous aqueous solutions also use purified or sterile water as the liquid vehicle. These liquid preparations are thick, sticky, sweet solutions that may be either liquid or semisolid preparations. Viscous aqueous solutions include syrups, jellies, and mucilages.

Syrups are concentrated mixtures of sugar and water, and may be medicated or nonmedicated. Syrups are distinguished from other solutions by the high concentration of sugar contained in the mixture. In addition to the active ingredient, syrups may also contain flavorings or sweeteners that have no medicinal value. Nonmedicated syrups may be used as a vehicle for unpleasant-tasting medications. The biggest advantage of syrup is its ability to cover up the bad taste of a medication; because it is so thick, only a small portion of the medication comes in contact with the taste receptors in the mouth. The thicker consistency of syrup can also have a soothing effect on irritated or infected tissues of the mouth and throat. The most common use of syrups is in pediatric and adult cough and cold syrups.

Jellies are semisolid preparations that contain water. They are most often used as lubricants for surgical gloves, vaginal contraceptive agents, and rectal thermometers. Jellies can be used as lubricants to aid in the insertion and removal of diagnostic probes into orifices or to reduce friction during an ultrasound procedure.

Mucilages are much thicker, viscous, adhesive liquids that contain water and the thick components of vegetable matter. They are useful to prevent insoluble, solid medication particles from settling at the bottom of the liquid.

Nonaqueous Solutions

Nonaqueous solutions use dissolving agents other than water, although the vehicle may be combined with water. Vehicles commonly used in nonaqueous solutions include alcohol, glycerin, and propylene glycol. The solutions that use only alcohol as the dissolving agent are called *alcoholic* solutions.

Hydroalcoholic Solutions

Hydroalcoholic solutions are nonaqueous solutions, but differ from pure aqueous solutions in that they contain alcohol in addition to water to act as the vehicle or dissolving agent. The most common example of a hydroalcoholic solution is an elixir.

Elixirs are liquid preparations that contain flavored water and alcohol mixtures intended for oral administration. They are clear, sweet solutions that may or may not contain medication. The amount of alcohol in the mixture varies, depending on the ability of the other ingredients to dissolve easily in pure water. Many drugs dissolve more easily in a water-and-alcohol mixture than in water alone. The range of alcohol contents in one solution may vary from 2% to 30%.

Alcohol, the greatest advantage of an elixir, may also be its greatest disadvantage. Many patients are not able to consume alcohol, and it may have undesired side effects or interactions with other medications currently being taken. Patients, especially pediatric and older adults, should pay attention to the ingredient contents in elixirs. These populations can be extrasensitive to even the smallest alcohol content. Medicated elixirs are often given to patients who have a difficult time swallowing tablets or capsules.

Two examples of commonly prescribed medicated elixirs are phenobarbital and digoxin. Elixirs can also be used as sweeteners or flavoring agents. **Aromatic** elixirs are nonmedicated and are used as vehicles to mask the unpleasant taste of a medication.

Alcoholic Solutions

Alcoholic solutions contain only alcohol as the dissolving agent and have no water. The most common alcohols used in preparing alcoholic solutions are ethyl alcohols (ethanol). Examples of alcoholic solutions include collodions, spirits, and glycerite solutions.

Collodions are alcoholic solutions that contain pyroxylin (which is found in cotton fibers) dissolved in ethanol. When this liquid preparation is applied to the skin, the alcohol evaporates, leaving only a thin film covering of the pyroxylin. An added advantage of a collodion is that it can carry an added medication. These preparations are used to treat and dissolve corns or warts. A more common example of a collodion is the Band-Aid liquid bandage, which applies a medication and a thin covering to prevent infection.

Spirits are liquid solutions that may be either alcoholic or hydroalcoholic. Spirits contain **volatile** and aromatic substances. Alcohol dissolves these substances more easily than water, allowing a greater concentration of these materials. Spirits may be administered internally or inhaled. Spirits are also known for their flavoring ability, such as peppermint spirits. Other spirits, known as aromatic ammonia spirits or smelling salts, may be inhaled through the nose. If spirits contain water in addition to alcohol, they are identified as hydroalcoholic solutions.

Glycerite solutions are nonaqueous solutions that contain a medication dissolved in glycerin. Glycerin is a sweet, oily fluid made from fat and oils. Glycerin is considered a flexible vehicle. It can be used alone or in any combination with water or alcohol. Glycerin is often used as a solvent for medications that do not easily dissolve in water or alcohol alone. Usually, a medication is dissolved in glycerin, which is then further mixed into a water or alcohol vehicle. Glycerite solutions are often viscous and have the thick consistency of a jelly. Glycerite solutions are rarely used today.

Suspensions

Suspensions contain very fine solid particles mixed with a gas, liquid, or solid preparation. Most suspensions are solid particles dispersed in a liquid. A suspension is often used when a solid medication form is not appropriate for a particular patient. Because the solid particles in the suspension are very small, the breakdown and absorption process is much quicker than that with tablets or capsules. The medication reaches the bloodstream much sooner than it would if a solid medication form were used.

The key difference between a solution and a suspension is that a suspension must be shaken well before use, to redistribute any of the solid particles that have settled in the liquid mixture. Suspensions are usually intended for oral ingestion in cases where a large amount of medication is needed. Suspensions are also available for administration by other routes, including ophthalmic, parenteral, otic, and rectal. Suspensions for oral use are combined with water, although other suspensions may use oil as the vehicle or dissolving agent.

Magmas and Milks

Magmas and *milks* are suspensions of undissolved medications in water. They are very thick, viscous liquids. These suspensions are intended only for oral use and must be shaken thoroughly before use. Milk of Magnesia is the most common example of a magma suspension.

Lotions

Lotions are suspensions for external use only. They are made up of a powdered medication in a liquid mixture. Lotions are used to soothe, cool, dry, and protect irritated skin and wounds. Lotions can function as disinfectants, protectants, moisturizers, and anti-inflammatories. Lotions have an advantage over other external medications in that they can easily be applied over large areas of the skin. They do not leave an oily or greasy feel on the skin after application. The most common OTC example of a lotion is Calamine lotion.

Gels

Gels are suspensions similar to magmas and milks, but the solid particles in gels are much smaller. Gels can be used for oral or topical administration. OTC antacids are common examples of gel suspensions.

Extractives

Extractives are liquid mixtures made from concentrated active ingredients that are derived from plants or animals. The drug is withdrawn by soaking the dried tissue in a solvent. After the liquid is evaporated, the only thing remaining is the active, or crude, drug ingredient. Some examples of extractives are tinctures, extracts, and fluidextracts. The various types of extractives are distinguished by the potency of their active ingredient.

Tinctures are extractive alcoholic or hydroalcoholic solutions. The potency of each mixture is adjusted so that each milliliter of tincture contains the exact potency of 100 mg of crude ingredient. Iodine and paregoric tinctures are two common examples of this type of extractive.

Fluidextracts are more potent than tinctures, as each milliliter of fluidextract contains 1,000 mg of the crude drug.

Extracts are very similar to tinctures and fluidextracts, except for potency. The potency of the crude drug in extracts is two to six times stronger than that in the others. Common examples of extracts are vanilla, peppermint, and almond extracts used for cooking.

Emulsions

Emulsions are liquid mixtures of water and oil, which normally do not mix. One liquid is broken down into smaller elements and evenly distributed throughout the other liquid. The liquid that was broken down into small elements is called the *internal phase*; the other liquid is the *external phase*. The external phase may also be referred to as the *continuous phase*, because it remains a liquid substance.

Emulsions are named for the emulsifying agent that is used with the two phases. The emulsifying agent is added to the liquid mixture to prevent the internal phase from fusing together and separating from the external phase. If an emulsifying agent is not used, the two liquids will eventually separate and create two distinct layers. This is commonly seen in a bottle of oil and vinegar salad dressing. Before you shake the bottle, you can see the individual layers of oil and vinegar that have settled and separated. Once shaken, the two layers are mixed together again. This is an example of what happens when an emulsifying agent is not added to a liquid mixture.

volatile evaporates rapidly.

Water-in-oil emulsions are liquid mixtures of water droplets distributed throughout an oil substance. These mixtures are commonly used on unbroken skin wounds. Water-in-oil emulsions spread out more evenly than oil-in-water emulsions, because the skin's natural oils mix well with the external oil phase in the emulsion. The oils also soften the skin better by adding moisture and remaining on the skin when washed with water. These emulsions are often avoided, though, because they easily stain clothing and have a greasy texture.

Oil-in-water emulsions contain small oil globules dispersed throughout water. These mixtures are commonly used as oral medications. The undesirable oily medications are broken down into small particles and dispersed in a sweetened, flavored aqueous vehicle. These small particles can then be swallowed without coming into contact with the taste buds. The small size of the particles increases absorption in the stomach and bloodstream. Oil-in-water emulsions are lighter and nongreasy. For these reasons, they are the first choice for application to a hairy part of the body. The two common types of oil-in-water emulsions are mineral oil and castor oil.

Comparison of Water-in-Oil and Oil-in-Water Emulsions

Each type of emulsion has several advantages and disadvantages. Several factors drive the choice of the proper emulsion; the rule of thumb is:

- Medications that dissolve more easily in water are applied as water-in-oil emulsions.
- Medications that dissolve more easily in oil are applied as oil-in-water emulsions.

Liniments

Liniments are medications that are applied to the skin with friction and rubbing. They can be solutions, suspensions, or emulsions and are used to relieve minor cuts, scrapes, burns, aches, and pains. Most contain a medication that produces a mild irritation or reddening of the skin when applied. This irritation then produces a counterirritation, or mild inflammation, of the skin. This counterirritation relieves the inflammation of a deeper structure, such as tissues or muscles. Ben-Gay is the most commonly used OTC liniment today.

Transdermal Patches

Transdermal patches are medicated adhesives that deliver medication directly into the bloodstream after being applied to the skin. This dosage formulation is beneficial for administering medication on a controlled release through the skin. Patches are available for OTC products, such as nicotine patches, as well as for various prescription medications, such as those used for motion sickness, pain, hormones, angina/chronic heart disease, and even depression.

" Workplace Wisdom Transdermal Patches

In most cases, patients should rotate the spots where transdermal patches are applied, to avoid skin irritation. In addition, to avoid pulling hair out during removal, patches should not be applied to hairy skin areas.

Sprays

Medicated sprays are available in pump-type dispensers and used to deliver various types of medications. The most common medicated sprays are administered nasally, which provides quick absorption and onset of action; however, nitroglycerin is available in a translingual spray, which is administered under the tongue.

Inhalants

Inhalants are medications that contain a fine powder or solution delivered through a mist into the mouth or nose. The medication immediately enters the respiratory tract for absorption. The most common inhalant medications are inhalers used to treat asthma. Allergy nasal sprays may also be delivered as an inhalant through the nose.

Aerosols

Aerosols are very fine liquid or solid particles mixed in a vehicle. The aerosol mixture is packed with gas and pressure to be administered via the respiratory tract or applied topically. When used properly, the gaseous pressure forces the liquid or solid particles out of the inhaler. Internal aerosols are contained in inhalers and can be used in the nose or mouth. The inhaler forces the medication directly into the lungs and respiratory system so that the medication can immediately provide relief. External aerosols are usually applied topically. Common external aerosols are Tinactin and Bactine sprays. One advantage of external aerosols is that they can be used in hard-to-reach areas or on severely irritated areas of the skin. Aerosols do not cause as much irritation to the wound as other topical treatments, such as ointments or creams.

Delayed and Extended Releases

Some medications are made to be released in the body over a period of time, rather than all at once. Referred to as extended release (ER), long acting (LA), sustained release (SR), time release (TR), or controlled release (CR), these medications dissolve in the body, but allow only a portion of the active ingredient to be absorbed into the bloodstream at a time. ER medications are most commonly available in tablets and capsules. There are also a few liquid preparations that are made to slowly release over a period of time. ER medications are available for many common illnesses, such as hypertension,

info

Caution with Liniments

Liniments are prepared with alcohol or acetone; contain other irritants such as capsaicin; and should not be applied to bruised or broken skin, as pain and irritation would occur.

Dosage Form Variety for Animals

The need for a variety of alternative dosage forms is not exclusive to humans. Animals need variety, too! Think of trying to give a cat a capsule by mouth—depending on the cat's mood, it is probably not going to happen. Specialty pharmacies can, however, compound the prescribed medication into a transdermal gel that the owner can simply rub onto the back of the feline's ear. There are also other alternative dosage forms, not discussed in this chapter that may be used for animals. For example, sometimes it is necessary to use a fish or a mouse as the dosage form or vehicle for patients such as dolphins and snakes.

Synonymous for Delayed or Extended Release

Other names commonly used to indicate delayed or extended release include:

- Constant release
- Continuous action
- Continuous release
- Controlled action
- Controlled release
- Delayed absorption
- Delayed action
- Extended action
- Gradual release
- Long acting
- Long lasting

- Long-term release
- Programmed release
- Prolonged action
- Prolonged release
- Slow acting
- Slow release
- Sustained action
- Sustained release
- Time coated
- Time released

diabetes, depression, and bacterial infections, and pain. The following characteristics are considered when selecting an ER medication:

- The same amount of medication is released into the bloodstream over a slow, consistent period.
- There is added convenience for patients, as they will take fewer doses per day to achieve the same (or better) results than they would have to take of an immediate-action medication. Most ER medications are taken q12h or q24h.
- Patient compliance increases when there are fewer doses and pills to take per day.
- Costs are often lower, as the patient does not need as many pills or doses. Lower prescription costs also help increase patient compliance.
- Adverse reactions and side effects are reduced, because the medication is introduced into the body slowly.

ER medications are made possible by advanced technologies. Gelatin capsules can be made to contain very small beads of medication. The stomach immediately dissolves the gelatin capsule, exposing the beads for absorption. The beads of medication are then dissolved and absorbed over a period of time. Many cold and allergy medications are made in this fashion to provide relief for 6 to 12 hours after taking one dose. Some ER medications are made with two layers. One layer is dissolved and absorbed immediately, while the other one dissolves gradually over time.

Another method of making ER medications is to embed the medication in a plastic or wax matrix. As the medication is released from the matrix, it is dissolved and absorbed in the body. The matrix itself does not dissolve, but is excreted from the body as waste. A more advanced technology uses an osmotic pump to deliver the medication over a period of time. The system consists of a membrane surrounding the medication. Through the process of osmosis, and depending on the concentration, medication is diffused out to the body. Medication is pushed from the membrane to the body with the entrance

PROFILES IN PRACTICE

Adam is a pharmacy technician who works in central pharmacy. An intensive care unit (ICU) nurse calls stating that a patient received her morning dose of Razadyne, but needs an evening dose of the medication, because the patient is taking the drug BID.

▶ What actions should Adam take at this point?
▶ What is the generic name of Razadyne, and what is it used for?

and exit of water. Examples of ER medication are Procardia XL and Cardizem CD.

Routes of Administration

Medications are delivered to a patient by a variety of routes of administration. The **route of administration (ROA)** is simply the method by which a medication is introduced into the body for absorption and distribution (see Figure 6-11). The ROA can vary from patient to patient and depends on the effect desired from the administered medication. Several factors are considered when determining the ROA, including:

- Patient's age—Younger and older patients may have difficulty swallowing medications.
- Patient's physical state—The state of consciousness may determine the best route.
- Patient's medical condition—Oral medications may not be appropriate for patients with stomach or GI complications.

---

route of administration (ROA) how a drug is introduced into or on the body.

ROUTES

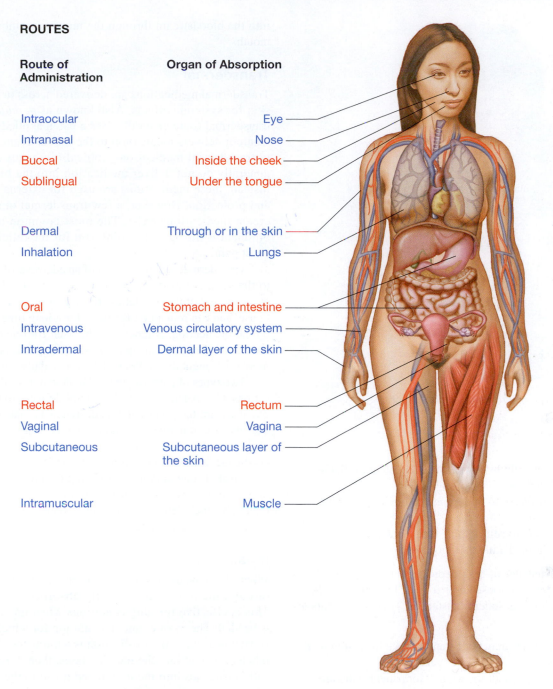

Route of Administration	Organ of Absorption
Intraocular	Eye
Intranasal	Nose
Buccal	Inside the cheek
Sublingual	Under the tongue
Dermal	Through or in the skin
Inhalation	Lungs
Oral	Stomach and intestine
Intravenous	Venous circulatory system
Intradermal	Dermal layer of the skin
Rectal	Rectum
Vaginal	Vagina
Subcutaneous	Subcutaneous layer of the skin
Intramuscular	Muscle

FIGURE 6-11 Various routes of administration.

- Time to achieve results—Injections or IV routes achieve results much faster than other routes.
- Side effects—Possible side effects should be considered when choosing an ROA.

Oral

The most common and uncomplicated ROA is by mouth (see Figure 6-12). The abbreviation for the oral route of administration, PO, is derived from the Latin *per os* (by mouth). Capsules, tablets, caplets, liquids, and emulsions are some of the medication dosage formulations that may be taken orally. Most medications are available for both oral and another route

of administration. For example, one patient may be treated with an oral tablet or suspension, whereas another patient needs an injection of the same medication for immediate treatment. Most tablets, capsules, and liquids are given via the oral ROA.

Advantages of oral medications over other routes of administration include:

- Oral medications are safer, more convenient, and easier to store.
- They may be more readily available in pharmacies. Injections may have to be special-ordered by the physician or pharmacy.

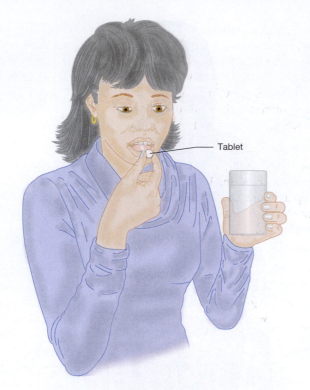

Tablet

FIGURE 6-12 The oral route of administration.

- They are generally less expensive than other available route medications.
- Many are available in both immediate-release and ER dosage forms.
- They are easier to self-administer and generally do not require additional administration supplies.

The disadvantages of oral medications usually lead physicians and patients to choose another route by which to administer the medication in specific instances. These disadvantages include:

- Oral medications may not be appropriate for children or older adults.
- They may be difficult to swallow for patients who are unconscious, ventilated, or having digestion problems.
- They must be broken down and absorbed before they can be distributed throughout the body. For this reason, oral medications take longer to provide effects and relief.

Sublingual

Sublingual medications, specifically tablets, are administered under the tongue. When the medication comes in contact with the mucous membrane underneath the tongue, it is able to bypass the digestive system and is diffused directly into the blood supply through the veins beneath the tongue.

Buccal

Buccal tablets and lozenges/troches are administered by being placed in the mouth between the gum and the cheek. Similar to the sublingual ROA, buccal medications are quickly absorbed

into the bloodstream through the mucous membranes of the mouth.

Transdermal

Transdermal medications are delivered across or through the skin for systemic effects. Also known as *percutaneous*, the transdermal route generally uses a patch applied to the skin, where it delivers medication to the bloodstream. In contrast to transdermal medications, topical ointments and creams generally do not deliver medication into the bloodstream; instead, these medications are used for external treatments and protection. However, a few transdermal ointments and cream medications exist. The most common transdermal ointment is nitroglycerin ointment for the relief of cardiac chest pain.

Transdermal patches consist of an adhesive vehicle applied to the skin; the medication is released into the bloodstream over a period of time. Patches are easy to store, are convenient to use, and can remain on the body for a long time. Depending on the medication, patches may be used for one day or up to a week at a time. Wearing a transdermal patch is considered more convenient than taking a tablet on a daily basis.

Two types of patches are used to deliver transdermal medications. One patch controls the rate of delivery to the skin and bloodstream; the other patch is designed so that the skin controls the rate of delivery. In the patch that controls the delivery, a special membrane that is in direct contact with the skin delivers the medication from a drug reservoir. When the skin is used to control the rate of delivery, the drug is moved from the patch into the blood. The difference between these two routes is the relatively quick delivery of a large amount of medication all at once via the second route.

Inhalation

When the inhalation ROA is used, the medication is inhaled through the mouth and directly absorbed into the lungs. This is effective for lung conditions when immediate relief is needed. The most common condition for which inhalation is used is asthma; the medication is administered through an inhaler inserted into the mouth. Gases, then, force the medication particles into the mouth and down to the lungs. With other respiratory conditions, such as infections and congestion, inhalers may be used to help open the lungs and bronchioles if the airways are temporarily constricted. Common examples of medications administered through inhalation include albuterol (Proventil/Ventolin), Advair Diskus, and OTC Primatene Mist.

Nasal

Medications can be inhaled through the nose and absorbed into the bloodstream or sprayed into the nose for local effects. Like inhalation by mouth, the nasal ROA provides immediate relief for conditions such as nasal allergies and congestion. A nasal inhaler is used by holding it to the nostrils and inhaling through the nose; liquid medications are more commonly sprayed into the nose.

There may be additional conditions for which a nasally administered medication is more effective. One example is a narcotic analgesic, Stadol. When administered nasally, this medication reaches the bloodstream more quickly than through the traditional oral ROA. Common medications available for nasal administration include Flonase, Rhinocort, and Stadol.

Parenteral

The second most commonly used ROA is injection (see Figure 6-13).

Parenteral is the route by which medication does not pass through the GI system for absorption and distribution. The most common parenteral routes are:

1. Intradermal (ID)
2. Subcutaneous (SC)
3. Intramuscular (IM)
4. Intravenous (IV)

Medications that are delivered by the parenteral routes have several advantages over the oral ROA:

- Quicker absorption and distribution
- Convenience for those who cannot take oral medications
- Varied rate of delivery (from a couple of seconds to several hours)

Care must be taken to ascertain that the dosages given parenterally are correct, because the action is usually immediate, and there is no way to reverse the amount of drug administered. For many medications, there are also few or no ways to reverse any adverse effects. Adverse effects can occur when a dose given is too high, or when a dose given is too low.

Parenteral administration of medications is also very invasive. For this reason, some patients are uneasy with these routes and prefer oral medications. Injections can be very painful for children and older people. They also create an opportunity for bacteria and infection to enter the body. The common dosage forms of medications given by the parenteral route include suspensions, solutions, and emulsions.

Intradermal

The intradermal (ID) route injects medications into the top layers of the skin. These injections are not as invasive or as deep as those done by the SC route. The ID route is used to complete skin testing for allergies and some diseases, such as tuberculosis.

Subcutaneous

The subcutaneous (SC) ROA is one of the most utilized of parenteral routes. The medication is injected into the tissue immediately under the skin and is then absorbed in the bloodstream and distributed to the body as needed. The SC route delivers the medication at a slower rate than IM or IV routes. The ability for patients to self-administer SC injections is a great advantage. In addition, because the medication is not being delivered too far into the body, a smaller needle can be used, which is less painful and invasive than IM or IV. One disadvantage is a limitation on the volume of the drug that can be injected under the skin: The volume limit for the SC route is 3 mL.

Intramuscular

With the intramuscular (IM) ROA, medications are injected directly into large muscle masses, such as upper arms, thighs, or buttocks, and then absorbed from the muscle into the

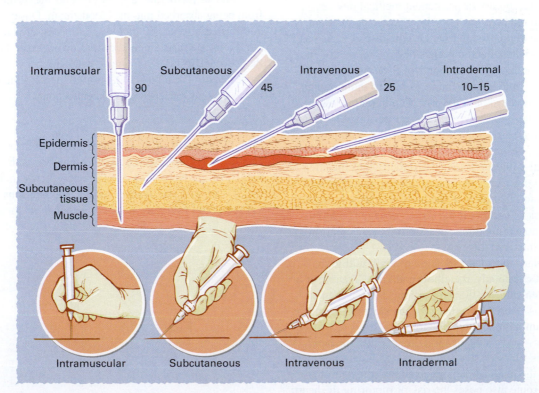

FIGURE 6-13 IM, SC, IV, and ID routes of administration.

bloodstream. Dosage forms administered intramuscularly include solutions and suspensions. IM medications are not as quick to work as medications delivered intravenously.

As with the IV route of administration, the IM rate of delivery can vary from seconds to minutes, and there is little chance for reversal of a medication injected directly into the muscle. Another disadvantage of this route is that the injection is usually painful and can cause irritation.

Intravenous

The most common parenteral route is the IV route. A medication administered IV is injected or administered directly into a vein. The medication can be a solution or suspension.

IV medications can be administered at different rates of delivery. A *bolus* is a larger volume of solution administered at one time for immediate effect. A *continuous infusion* is the administration of a solution over a continued or long period of time. For an *intravenous push* (IVP), a medication is administered directly into the vein with a syringe.

❝ Workplace Wisdom **Needles**

Determining the gauge and length of a needle is important when preparing medications for injection. Here are some industry guidelines. For IV injections, use a 1-inch or 1.5-inch needle with a gauge of 16 to 20. For IM injections, again use a 1-inch or 1.5-inch needle, but with a gauge of 19 to 22. SC injections are usually given with a 1-inch needle with a gauge of 24 to 27. ❞

Other Parenteral Routes

There are several other parenteral routes of administration. These include:

- Implant—a temporary or permanent medical device inserted into the body that slowly releases medication. Implants are often used to treat chronic diseases such as cancer or diabetes. Insulin pumps may be implanted in the body to deliver small amounts of insulin as needed. Norplant, a hormone medication, is placed in an implant inserted under the skin in the arm. The implant slowly releases the hormones over a five-year period. At the end of the five years, the implant is removed, and another one is inserted, if desired.
- Intra-arterial—injects medication directly into the arteries. This route reduces the risk of adverse reactions and side effects to other parts of the body. There is, however, a greater risk of toxicity if the wrong dosage is administered. Chemotherapy drugs, used to fight cancer, are commonly administered this way.
- Intra-articular—injects medication directly within the joints, most commonly, the elbow and knee. Treatment of arthritis often calls for the intra-articular ROA. Medications such as Enbrel and other steroids are used to relieve severe inflammation around the joint.
- Intracardiac—injects medication directly into the heart. This route is very invasive and used only in cardiac emergencies, as the medication is injected into the heart muscle itself. This route also poses the risk of rupturing the heart; therefore, it is not recommended except as a last resort.

- Intraperitoneal—injects medication directly into the abdominal or peritoneal cavity. The common use for this route is to administer antibiotics to treat infections inside the peritoneal cavity.
- Intrapleural—injects medication into the sac (pleura) surrounding the lungs to reduce inflammation and scarring of the tissues lining the sacs and to prevent excessive fluid buildup in the pleura.
- Intrathecal—injects medications into the cerebrospinal fluid surrounding the spinal cord. This too is a very invasive and possibly dangerous procedure. It is used to treat infections or cancers of the central nervous system.
- Intraventricular—one of the most invasive parenteral routes; injects antibiotics or chemotherapy agents into the brain cavities, or *ventricles*.
- Intravesicular—injects medications directly into the urinary bladder; used to treat urinary bladder infections as well as bladder cancer.
- Intravitreal—injects medication directly into the vitreous body of the eye. Most medications do not reach the eye from the bloodstream, so for severe infections of the eye, this route is preferred because the antibiotic goes directly into the eye. Because this route is highly invasive, it is usually used only for severe diseases that are significantly reducing a patient's sight.

Topical

Medications that are administered externally to the skin are referred to as *topicals*. Topical medications are applied to the surface of the skin and absorbed into the mucous membrane (see Figure 6-14). The mucous membrane usually prevents the medication particles from being absorbed into the bloodstream. Dosage forms that are administered topically include ointments, creams, lotions, and emulsions. Because the medications do not enter the bloodstream, these dosage forms can be made with a higher concentration than those that do. The topical ROA is used to treat simple external skin rashes or slightly deeper-layer skin infections.

Rectal

With the *rectal* ROA, medication is applied through the rectum. Medications administered rectally may be solids, liquids, semisolids, or aerosols. Common dosage forms include suppositories, enemas, and aerosol foams. Medications administered via the rectal route are used for either their local or systemic

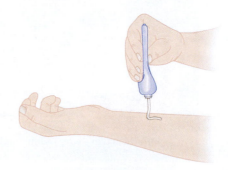

FIGURE 6-14 Topical route: applying an ointment.

effects. For local effects, such as constipation or pain/itching, the medication is not absorbed into the bloodstream. However, for systemic effects, the medication is absorbed into the lower GI tract or the bloodstream, for treatment of conditions such as nausea and vomiting or fever. Rectally administered medications are often used for children when an oral medication is not appropriate. Patients may also prefer a rectally administered medication when they cannot tolerate or swallow an oral form of the medication. For example, rectal suppositories are commonly used to treat severe nausea and vomiting when the patient is not able to keep the solid medication down. Older adult patients who have difficulty swallowing tablets may also prefer rectally administered medications. Some common examples of medications administered rectally include Phenergan suppositories, Fleet enemas, and Proctofoam.

Vaginal

With the *vaginal* ROA, medications are inserted into the vagina for absorption and distribution. Types of dosage forms that can be administered vaginally include solutions, suppositories, tablets, and topical creams or ointments. The most common use for these medications is to treat vaginal infections. However, some medications can be administered through the vagina to deliver medication to the bloodstream to treat systemic conditions. Common examples of vaginally administered

medications are Terazol, Mycostatin tablets, AVC vaginal suppositories, and Massengill douches.

Ophthalmic

Medications that are administered through the eye use the *ophthalmic* route. These medications can be solutions, ointments, suspensions, or gels. Ophthalmic medications are used to directly treat conditions of the eye such as allergies, infections, conjunctivitis, inflammation, or glaucoma. This direct route has the advantage of providing quicker relief than an oral medication that has to be absorbed and distributed throughout the entire body. Medications such as Visine eyedrops immediately relieve the itchiness, redness, and swelling caused by allergies. Ophthalmic medications are also generally very easy to self-administer and are convenient and easy to store. Common examples of medications delivered through the ophthalmic route include Visine, Xalatan, and antibiotic drops.

Otic

Medications that are administered in the ear are said to use the *otic* ROA. These medications are delivered into the ear canal to treat infections, inflammation, and severe wax buildup. Common dosage forms administered through the otic route are solutions and suspensions. These medications are directly absorbed in the ear canal to provide immediate relief.

Information Dosage Forms and Routes of Administration Availability

	Nasal	Ophthalmic	Oral	Otic	Parenteral	Pulmonary	Rectal	Sublingual/Buccal	Topical	Vaginal
Aerosol						X			X	
Capsule			X							
Cream							X		X	X
Elixir			X							
Emulsion									X	
Gel			X						X	
Lotion									X	
Ointment	X	X					X		X	
Paste									X	
Powder			X			X			X	
Spray	X		X			X		X	X	
Solution	X	X	X	X	X	X	X		X	X
Suppository							X			X
Suspension		X	X	X	X					
Syrup			X							
Tablet			X					X		
Troche/Lozenge			X							

Summary

This chapter reviewed the variety of sources from which drugs can be derived, drug nomenclature, common dosage forms, and routes of administration. Most medications are available in multiple dosage forms and can be delivered by multiple routes. It is important to dispense the proper dosage form of medication; otherwise, a patient may not be able to take the medication as the physician instructed. This is a medication error.

Diligence regarding the parenteral routes of administration can be crucial to a patient. If the wrong injection route is used, toxicity can result, and usually very little can be done to reverse the effects of the injection. It is also very important to administer the correct dose of the medication. Too much or too little can be harmful to the patient.

One responsibility of a pharmacy technician is to work with the pharmacist to prepare and dispense medications to patients. The technician must understand drug names as well as the meaning and use of each dosage form and route. Although most dosage forms are commonly administered by one particular route, you cannot make assumptions about the route that is to be used. Many dosage forms may be administered via several different routes. For example, a tablet is commonly administered orally, but it could be administered vaginally as well. Liquid medications can also be administered in a variety of ways. If the prescription order is not clear as to the dosage form and route, the pharmacy staff and medical staff must work together to determine what is best for the patient and to avoid medication errors.

Chapter Review Questions

1. It is possible for a drug to have more than one
   _____ name.
   a. generic
   b. chemical
   c. nonproprietary
   d. brand

2. A drug that is made in a laboratory to mimic a naturally occurring drug is considered _____.
   a. synthetic
   b. semisynthetic
   c. natural
   d. synthesized

3. Which of the following is *not* a liquid dosage form?
   a. suspension
   b. emulsion
   c. cream
   d. enema

4. All of the following are common routes of administration for tablets *except* _____.
   a. buccal
   b. vaginal
   c. sublingual
   d. rectal

5. Which of the following statements is *true*?
   a. Ointments are a semisolid dosage form that are composed of a solid and a liquid medication.
   b. Creams are a semisolid dosage form that may or may not contain medication.
   c. Ointments are usually greasier and oilier than creams.
   d. All of the preceding statements are true.

6. Which of the following is a *false* statement?
   a. An IVP is injected directly into the vein.
   b. A drug administered IM is injected directly into the muscle.
   c. A drug administered ID is injected into the subcutaneous tissue.
   d. All of the preceding statements are false.

7. A medication given by the parenteral route of administration _____.
   a. passes through the skin to aid absorption
   b. requires several hours to be absorbed
   c. can be easily removed from the body after administration
   d. bypasses the GI system for absorption

8. Which of the following drug names is *not* commonly used in daily pharmacy practice?
   a. generic
   b. trade
   c. chemical
   d. nonproprietary

9. Another term for a generic drug is _____.
   a. trade drug
   b. proprietary drug
   c. chemical drug
   d. nonproprietary drug

10. Which of the following is a suspension?
   a. magma
   b. collodion
   c. spirit
   d. emulsion

Critical Thinking Questions

1. Explain why a prescriber might choose an extended-release dosage form over a traditional dosage form and what impact that choice has on the patient.

2. Why is the oral route of administration safer, less complicated, and more convenient than the parenteral route? Why might the parenteral route be a better choice than the oral route?

Web Challenge

1. Go online to research other parenteral routes of administration not discussed in this chapter. List at least five of them and how they are administered.

2. Go online to research one example *each*, of either a prescription or OTC medication, containing the following description in the product's name:

- Extended release (ER)
- Long acting (LA)
- Sustained release (SR)
- Controlled release (CR)

References and Resources

Adams, Michael P. and Leland N. Holland. *Pharmacology for Nurses—A Pathophysiologic Approach.* 4th ed. Upper Saddle River, NJ: Pearson Education, 2013. Print.

American Medical Association. *Know Your Drugs and Medications.* New York, NY: Reader's Digest Association, 1991. Print.

Andreoli, Thomas, et al. *Essentials of Medicine.* 4th ed. Philadelphia, PA: Saunders, 1997. Print.

Ansel, Howard C. *Introduction to Pharmaceutical Dosage Forms.* Philadelphia, PA: Lea & Febiger, 1995. Print.

Berkow, Robert. *The Merck Manual.* 16th ed. Rahway, NJ: Merck Research Laboratories, 1992. Print.

"Drug Nomenclature." *University of Wisconsin.* 2007. Web. 7 July 2007.

Hillery, Anya M., et al. *Drug Delivery and Targeting: For Pharmacists and Pharmaceutical Scientists.* New York, NY: Taylor & Francis, 2001. Print.

Holland, Leland N. and Michael P. Adams. *Core Concepts in Pharmacology.* 3rd ed. Upper Saddle River, NJ: Pearson, 2010. Print.

Johnston, Mike. *Compounding.* Upper Saddle River, NJ: Pearson, 2005. Print.

Lambert, Anita A. *Advanced Pharmacy Practice for Technicians.* 3rd ed. Clifton Park, NY: Thomson Delmar Learning, 2007. Print.

Martelli, Mary Elizabeth. "Sublingual and Buccal Medication Administration." *Healthline.* 2011. Web. 11 January 2012.

"Medication Errors." *Food and Drug Administration.* 2007. Web. 3 July 2007.

Merck Index: An Encyclopedia of Chemicals, Drugs, & Biologicals. 13th ed. Ed. M. O' Neil. New York, NY: John Wiley & Sons, 2001. Print.

Perspective Press. *The Pharmacy Technician.* 5th ed. Englewood, CO: Morton Publishing, 2013. Print.

"Sources of Drugs." *Pharmaceutical Manufacturers and Drug Association.* 2011. Web. 11 January 2012.

"Synthetic Drugs." *Central Connecticut State University.* 2007. Web. 5 July 2007.

Taylor, Leslie. "Plant Based Drugs and Medicines." *Raintree Nutrition.* 2000. Web. 31 March 2008.

"The Basics of Recombinant DNA." *Renssealear.* 2007. Web. 5 July 2007.

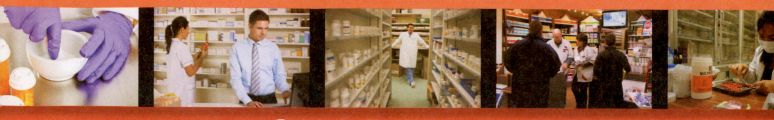

CHAPTER 7

Referencing and Drug Information Resources

LEARNING OBJECTIVES

After completing this chapter, you should be able to:

- Explain the need for referencing and drug information resources.

- Outline and describe the proper steps for referencing drug information resources.

- Explain how package insert monographs are used for referencing.

- List and describe the most commonly used printed drug reference books in pharmacies.

- List and describe the most commonly used electronic and web-based references in pharmacies.

- Outline and describe the proper steps for evaluating the credibility of a website for use as a reference.

- List and describe the most commonly used journals and magazines in pharmacies.

KEY TERMS

apps, p. 117
drug classification, p. 111
drug information resources, p. 111
index, p. 111
off-label usage, p. 111
referencing, p. 111
therapeutic indication, p. 111

INTRODUCTION

Pharmacy practice relies on accurate and timely information, and new, revised, and updated information occurs at a frequent pace within health care sciences. Physicians, nurses, pharmacists, pharmacy technicians, and other health care professionals must stay constantly informed on the latest drugs, therapeutic indications, dosing standards, and clinical evidence. Pharmacy professionals, in particular, must stay well informed as both patients and health care professionals, such as doctors and nurses, often turn to the pharmacist for answers to their medication-related questions. The pharmacist commonly handles these inquiries through the process of **referencing**. As a pharmacy technician, therefore, mastering the ability to reference **drug information resources** is critical. Although in many cases the information will be able to be communicated only by the pharmacist, a pharmacy technician can play a vital role in helping the pharmacist look up the needed information. In other cases, pharmacy technicians will rely on the ability to reference drug information resources for their roles in pharmacy practice.

How to Use Reference Sources

Before taking a detailed look at the most common drug information resources used in pharmacies, you must first understand how reference sources are properly used. In order to access the necessary information in a timely and accurate manner, the pharmacy technician must be familiar with the various reference sources and proper method of referencing (see Procedure 7-1).

The first step is to determine the appropriate reference source. You may need to look up information on a specific medication, such as available strengths, dosage form, information on drug interactions, side effects, compatibility for parenteral medications, formulas for extemporaneous compounds, pricing information, **off-label usage**, or even contact information of a manufacturer. Because each reference source is unique, selecting the correct reference source is important. Although many of the drug information sources contain similar information, meaning that more than one reference source could be selected, you should select the source that you know will have the information needed and that you are most comfortable with using it.

The second step, after selecting the proper reference source, is to look up the drug. Although this seems both easy and obvious, the reality is that each drug information resource organizes information in various ways. There are two primary methods used by drug information resources to organize and

---

referencing the practice of using drug information resources to find evidence-based information.

drug information resources any source providing credible, evidence-based, and evaluated drug information.

off-label usage the practice, regulated by the FDA, of physicians prescribing approved medications for use other than their intended indication.

drug classification a method of grouping drugs together based on similar chemical structures, mechanisms of action, or pharmacologic effects.

therapeutic indication the specific disease or condition a drug is intended to treat.

index an alphabetical listing of names or subjects with page references for ease of use.

Procedure 7-1

How to Use Reference Sources

Step 1. Determine and select the appropriate reference source.
Step 2. Look up the drug by using the reference source's organization system, index, or table of contents.
Step 3. Locate the desired information and read it carefully.

---

arrange information—by drug name or by drug classification/therapeutic usage. References that are organized by drug name may utilize both trade and generic names, using cross-referencing, or they may solely use generic names. This arrangement makes it imperative for you to be familiar with brand–generic equivalents. References that are organized by **drug classification** or **therapeutic indication** can be slightly more challenging and intimidating for new pharmacy technicians. Rather than listing all medications together, these references categorize drug information into sections, or chapters, which focus on specific groupings, such as cardiovascular drugs, respiratory drugs, and gastrointestinal drugs. You should be familiar with how to use the **index**, or table of contents, as a way of expeditiously finding the needed information.

The third and final step is to actually locate the desired information in the selected drug information resource. Once again, this sounds easier than it may be at first. The specific information being researched will likely be contained within a large amount of additional information, and when first learning how to use drug information resources, it can feel like the needed information is buried. Most resources categorize drug information into numerous subcategories, similar to a package insert, which will allow you to go to the appropriate section and locate your information. Other times, however, the information may be presented in tables or charts, which you need to learn how to read and interpret. Be sure to read the information carefully, as inaccurate information can result in serious and even deadly consequences.

Although it may feel a bit overwhelming at the beginning, with time and practice you will develop the ability to quickly and accurately use reference drug information resources. When you do, you will realize the great treasure of information and data that is readily accessible to you.

Resources Used in Pharmacy

There is no shortage of drug information resources available for use in pharmacies. Pharmacy professionals can easily access drug information with package insert monographs, a wide variety of drug reference books, CD-ROMs, online databases, smartphone applications, websites, journals, and magazines. The selection and format of drug information resources will vary by pharmacy. For the purpose of this chapter, we will review the most common and widely used resources for pharmacy (see Figure 7-1).

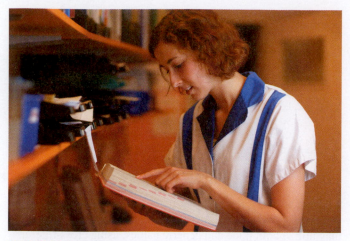

FIGURE 7-1 Pharmacy technician referencing drug information resources.
Source: Robert Kneschke/Shutterstock

Monographs and Package Inserts

One of the most common sources used for drug information and referencing are drug monographs, or package inserts, as discussed in Chapter 4. As an FDA-required element for the labeling of a drug, this resource should always be available for any drug in stock. As a reminder, monographs contain the following sections of information:

Description—provides a written description of the visual elements of the drug and packaging, as well as the basic chemical structure of the drug.

Clinical pharmacology—includes information on the drug's mechanism of action, absorption, distribution, metabolism, elimination, and administration. It also includes any notes relevant to specific patient populations, such as pediatric patients.

Indications and usage—describes the specific conditions or symptoms that the drug has been approved by the FDA to prevent or treat certain conditions or diseases.

Contraindications—lists the types of patients who should not use the medication, whether that is a class of patients (such as diabetics) or individuals taking another specific class of drug.

Warnings—details the serious side effects that can be caused by the medication and instructions on what the patient should do, if these effects are experienced.

Precautions—lists all of the remaining possible or potential side effects that the patient should be conscious of.

Drug abuse and dependence—provides notification, if the medication has shown signs of a potential for abuse or dependence.

Adverse reactions—covers reactions that are unexpected and potentially life threatening.

Dosage—includes the recommended dosage of medication; dosages are typically categorized by patient age and/or weight.

How supplied—describes how the medication is supplied, including strengths, dosage formats, and storage requirements.

Reference Books

Virtually every pharmacy in the United States maintains a collection of reference books, some of which are used daily and others only as needed. As a pharmacy technician, you must be familiar with the most common reference books used in pharmacies, so that you will be able to determine which book to turn to when you are looking for information, either for yourself or at the request of the pharmacist. The collection and number of reference books maintained varies at each pharmacy. Although countless books are available for referencing in pharmacy practice, this chapter outlines the key features of the most commonly used. Each of these books can be ordered online, either directly from the publisher or through online bookstores.

Drug Facts and Comparisons

The most commonly used drug information reference, particularly in community pharmacies, is a book called *Drug Facts and Comparisons*. This reference book provides monographs on more than 22,000 prescription drugs and 6,000 over-the-counter (OTC) products. Monographs are arranged by therapeutic or pharmacological group. In addition, *Drug Facts and Comparisons* contains more than 3,000 unique charts and tables, an appendix of treatment guidelines, a list of manufacturers and distributors, and a Canadian trade-name index. *Drug Facts and Comparisons* is organized into five primary sections:

1. Index (including generic and trade names)
2. Keeping Up (covers orphan, investigational, and temporary listings)
3. Drug Monographs
4. Drug Identification
5. Appendix

The drug monographs are categorized into 14 chapters:

1. Nutrients and Nutritional Agents
2. Hematological Agents
3. Endocrine and Metabolic Agents
4. Cardiovascular Agents
5. Rental and Genitourinary Agents
6. Respiratory Agents
7. Central Nervous System Agents
8. Gastrointestinal Agents
9. Systemic Anti-Infectives
10. Biological and Immunologic Agents
11. Dermatological Agents
12. Ophthalmic and Otic Agents
13. Antineoplastic Agents
14. Diagnostic Aids

A detailed table of contents is provided on the first page of each chapter.

Published by Wolters Kluwer and updated monthly (for the loose leaf edition), the *Drug Facts and Comparisons* is available in hardback print, loose leaf print, pocket-sized print, CD-ROM, and online editions.

Physician's Desk Reference

Another commonly used drug information reference is the *Physician's Desk Reference* (*PDR*). Although many pharmacies maintain a copy of the *PDR*, it is primarily designed for physician office use. The *PDR* contains detailed information on more than 1,000 of the most commonly prescribed drugs and is indexed in four comprehensive sections:

- Manufacturer index
- Product index (trade names)
- Product category index
- Generic/chemical index

The *PDR* provides detailed product information, consistent with FDA labeling, including:

- Chemical information
- Function/therapeutic action
- Indications and contraindications
- Side effects, warnings, and trial research

Published by the PDR Network and updated annually, the *PDR* is available in hardback print, CD-ROM, and online editions.

AHFS Drug Information

Primarily used in health systems, *the American Hospital Formulary Service (AHFS) Drug Information*, or *AHFS DI*, is a collection of drug monographs for virtually every drug available in the United States. The monographs are arranged by pharmacologic–therapeutic classifications and are indexed by trade name, generic name, synonym, abbreviation, pharmacy equivalent name, and former names.

The monographs include:

- Drug interactions
- Adverse reactions
- Cautions and toxicity
- Therapeutic perspective
- Specific dosage and administration information
- Preparations
- Chemistry and stability
- Pharmacology and pharmacokinetics
- Contraindications

The monographs are developed using an independent, evidence-based evaluation process. *AHFS DI* is published by the ASHP and is kept current through ongoing electronic updates and an annual revised print edition. *AHFS DI* is available in printed softback, electronic database, and mobile application editions.

Martindale: The Complete Drug Reference

With nearly 6,000 drug monographs, *Martindale: The Complete Drug Reference* provides detailed monographs and preparation information on drugs and medicines used throughout the world. Monographs are arranged into 49 chapters based on clinical usage. In addition to standard prescription drugs, monographs are included for the following:

- Investigational and veterinary drugs
- Herbal medicines
- Pharmaceutical excipients
- Vitamins
- Vaccines
- Radiopharmaceuticals
- Contrast and diagnostic agents
- Recreational and abused drugs
- Toxic substances
- Disinfectants and pesticides

In addition, *Martindale: The Complete Drug Reference* includes a directory of nearly 16,000 manufacturers; a multilingual pharmaceutical term index, which lists more than 5,000 pharmaceutical terms and routes of administration in 13 major European languages; and a general index prepared from 172,000 entries. One of the key advantages of this reference book is its international scope and usefulness. Published by Pharmaceutical Press, *Martindale: The Complete Drug Reference* is available in a hardback print edition and CD-ROM.

USP–NF

The *USP–NF* is a combination of two official compendia, the *United States Pharmacopeia* (*USP*) and the *National Formulary* (*NF*). This reference set contains standards, which are enforceable by the FDA, for:

- Medicines
- Dosage forms
- Drug substances
- Excipients
- Biologics
- Compounded preparations
- Medical devices
- Dietary supplements

The *USP–NF* features more than 4,500 monographs with detailed information on identity, strength, quality, purity, packaging, and labeling for substances and dosage forms. In addition, the *USP–NF* contains over 230 general chapters, which provide step-by-step instructions for assays, tests, and procedures. The *USP–NF*, which is published by the USP, is updated annually and available in print, CD-ROM, online editions, and USB flash drive editions.

Handbook on Injectable Drugs

Edited by Lawrence A. Trissel, the *Handbook on Injectable Drugs* is the most widely used reference of its kind. Primarily used in health-system pharmacies, this book provides drug monographs for 349 parenteral, or injectable, drugs. Each monograph provides detailed information on compatibility, stability, storage, and preparation. The monographs are arranged alphabetically by its nonproprietary, or generic, name.

Each monograph is divided into the following subheadings:

- Products—lists the sizes, strengths, volumes, and forms in which the drug is commercially available.

- Administration—lists the route(s) by which the drug may be given, rates of administration, and other administration details.
- Stability—describes the stability and storage requirements of the drug.
- Compatibility Information—tabulates the results of primary research on the compatibility of the drug in various infusion solutions, as two or more drugs in intravenous solutions, as two or more drugs in syringes, and injection into Y-sites or administration sets.
- Additional Compatibility Information—provides a narrative account of secondary research.
- Other Information—provides any relevant auxiliary information.

The *Handbook on Injectable Drugs* is available in print, interactive CD-ROM, online editions, and mobile application editions.

Handbook of Nonprescription Drugs

Prescription drugs represent only a fraction of the medication taken by Americans each year; nonprescription, or OTC, drugs, as well as herbal and homeopathic products are taken into consideration. Primarily used in community pharmacy settings, the *Handbook of Nonprescription Drugs* provides detailed information on nonprescription drug pharmacotherapy, nutritional supplements, and complementary and alternative therapies.

Organized by disease-oriented chapters, the *Handbook of Nonprescription Drugs* provides case studies, treatment protocols, comparisons of self-treatment options, patient education boxes, product selection guidelines, and dosage and administration guidelines. An extensive list of chapters covers OTC treatments for conditions ranging from acne to warts, and everything in between. The *Handbook of Nonprescription Drugs*, which is published by the APhA, is available in a printed and online edition.

Approved Drug Products with Therapeutic Equivalence Evaluations "FDA Orange Book"

Commonly referred to as the "*Orange Book*" or "*FDA Orange Book*," *Approved Drug Products with Therapeutic Equivalence Evaluations* identifies drug products approved on the basis of safety and effectiveness by the FDA. This publication is organized into four parts:

1. Approved prescription drug products with therapeutic equivalence evaluations
2. Approved OTC drug products for those drugs that may not be marketed without new drug applications or abbreviated new drug applications because they are not covered under existing OTC monographs
3. Drug products with approval under Section 505 of the Act administered by the Center for Biologics Evaluation and Research

4. A cumulative list of approved products that have never been marketed, are for exportation, are for military use, have been discontinued from marketing, or have had their approvals withdrawn for other than safety or efficacy reasons subsequent to being discontinued from marketing.

The *FDA Orange Book* also includes indices of prescription and OTC drug products by trade or established name and by applicant name. The *FDA Orange Book* is published by the U.S. government and is updated annually. An online version can be accessed free of charge and is updated frequently.

Red Book

For over a century, *RED BOOK* has been a valuable reference guide for pharmacists and pharmacies, providing product information on more than 200,000 prescription and OTC items. One specific distinction of *RED BOOK* is its focus on the latest information on average and wholesale drug costs and pricing, covering:

- Nationally recognized average wholesale prices (AWPs), direct prices, and federal upper-limit prices for prescription drugs
- Direct prices, and federal upper-limit prices for prescription drugs
- Suggested retail prices for OTC products

In addition, *RED BOOK* provides:

- National drug code (NDC) numbers for all FDA-approved drugs
- Complete package information, including dosage form, route of administration, strength, and size
- "Orange Book" codes—FDA-approved drug products with therapeutic equivalent evaluations
- Summaries of drug/food, drug/alcohol, and drug/tobacco
- Sugar-free, alcohol-free, lactose- and galactose-free, and sulfite-containing product listings for customers with special needs
- A complete list of new molecular entities and generics approved by the FDA
- Comprehensive manufacturer, pharmaceutical wholesaler, and third-party administrator directories
- Full-color photographs
- Vitamin comparison table—amounts of vitamins and minerals in over 50 popular multivitamin products
- Common laboratory values—answers to the most common patient questions about urine sugar level, cholesterol, blood pressure, and more
- Guide to leading alternative medicines
- NCPDP billing standards
- Controlled substance inventory sheet

In 2011, *RED BOOK* discontinued being published in print editions and is now exclusively offered as a CD-ROM edition, which is updated four times per year. *RED BOOK* is published by Medical Economics.

American Drug Index

The *American Drug Index* provides a dictionary-style reference of approximately 22,000 brand-name and official USP generic drugs. This reference book provides a thorough explanation and correlation of both prescription and nonprescription drugs. Specifically, each drug listing details:

- Composition
- Strength
- Dosage forms
- Packaging
- Schedule
- Usage
- Name pronunciations

In addition, the *American Drug Index* includes official drug container and storage requirements, a trademark glossary, laboratory values, vaccine and immunologic information, and a listing of manufacturers and distributors. Published by Wolters Kluwer, the *American Drug Index* is available in both printed and CD-ROM editions.

The Merck Index

Referred to as "chemistry's constant companion," *the Merck Index* is among the most established and respected indices of chemicals, drugs, and biologicals. An encyclopedic-style reference book, *the Merck Index,* contains more than 10,000 monographs on:

- Human and veterinary drugs
- Biotech drugs and monoclonal antibodies
- Substances used for medical imaging
- Biologicals and natural products
- Plant and herbal medicines
- Nutraceuticals and cosmeceuticals
- Laboratory reagents and catalysts
- Dyes, colors, and indicators
- Environmentally significant substances
- Food additives and nutritional supplements
- Flavors and fragrances
- Agricultural chemicals, pesticides, and herbicides
- Industrial and specialty chemicals

The Merck Index focuses more on the chemical nature and structure of compounds, making it equally valuable for labs and chemists as it is for pharmacies. Published by Merck, *the Merck Index* is available in printed, CD-ROM, and online editions.

Pediatric & Neonatal Dosage Handbook

The dosing regimens, pharmacokinetics, and pharmacodynamics for pediatric patients, including those from infancy through childhood, require special evaluation and updates. The *Pediatric & Neonatal Dosage Handbook* provides 944 drug monographs and resources designed and evaluated specifically for this patient population. Monographs, which are arranged alphabetically, provide up to 40 fields of information. In addition, more than 100 formulas for extemporaneous pediatric

compounds and 290 pages of appendix information are provided. The *Pediatric & Neonatal Dosage Handbook*, which is published by Lexi-Comp, is available in a printed edition.

Geriatric Dosage Handbook

Just as the pharmaceutical needs of pediatric patients require special attention, so too do geriatric patients. The *Geriatric Dosage Handbook* consists of monographs providing drug information and recommended dosing guidelines for the use of medications for older adult patients. Monographs are arranged in alphabetical order and provide extensive information on drug interactions and drug dosing in older adult patients. The *Geriatric Dosage Handbook*, which is published by Lexi-Comp, is available in a printed edition.

Goodman & Gilman's: The Pharmacological Basis of Therapeutics

Considered the leading text in medical pharmacology, *Goodman & Gilman's: The Pharmacological Basis of Therapeutics* is a trusted reference for pharmacists. Unlike other reference books that consist of drug monographs or indices, this book focuses on pharmacokinetics and pharmacodynamics, drug transport, metabolism, pharmacogenomics, and therapeutics. *Goodman & Gilman's: The Pharmacological Basis of Therapeutics* is categorized into the following sections:

- General Principles
- Neuropharmacology
- Modulation of Cardiovascular Function
- Inflammation, Immunomodulation, and Hematopoiesis
- Hormones and Hormone Antagonists
- Drugs Affecting Gastrointestinal Function
- Chemotherapy of Microbial Diseases
- Chemotherapy of Neoplastic Devices
- Special Systems of Pharmacology
- Appendices

Published by McGraw Hill, *Goodman & Gilman's: The Pharmacological Basis of Therapeutics* is available in a hardback print edition, which includes a DVD image bank, or online.

Remington: The Science and Practice of Pharmacy

For over a century, *Remington: The Science and Practice of Pharmacy* has been one of the most trusted and recognized textbooks and references on the science and practice of pharmacy. Organized in 133 chapters, this reference book covers the full spectrum of pharmacy practice, including:

- Orientation to Pharmacy Practice
- Pharmaceutics
- Pharmaceutical Chemistry
- Pharmaceutical Testing, Analysis, and Control
- Pharmaceutical Manufacturing
- Pharmacodynamics

PROFILE IN PRACTICE

Jared works at the inpatient hospital pharmacy in his hometown. A nurse calls the pharmacy, and speaks with Jared, inquiring about drug interactions and contraindications for a newly approved medication. The staff pharmacists are not available to take the phone call, so Jared writes down all of the information requested.

▶ *To what extent can Jared assist with this request? Should he look up the requested information? Can he provide the answers to the nurse? Can the pharmacist authorize Jared to handle the request independently?*

▶ *Which reference books or sources would be the most beneficial to look up the requested information as quickly as possible? Which reference sources would not be useful for this request?*

- Pharmaceutical and Medicinal Agents
- Fundamentals of Pharmacy Administration
- Social, Behavioral, Economic, and Administrative Sciences
- Patient Care

Published by Lippincott Williams & Wilkins, *Remington: The Science and Practice of Pharmacy* is available in a hardback print edition, which includes a CD-ROM.

Electronic/Web-based References

With the recent advances in technology and connectivity, the number of electronic and web-based references is growing rapidly. It is no longer necessary to maintain a vast physical library of reference books, as many of the titles previously listed, as well as the resources mentioned later, are now available at the click of mouse or even on the tap of one's phone. The following are examples of some of the most widely recognized and used electronic and web-based references.

Micromedex

Micromedex offers many of the leading online and mobile applications that are used by physicians, nurses, and pharmacists. There are a variety of products in the Micromedex product line. The following are examples of products in the Micromedex suite that are particularly useful for pharmacy professionals:

- AltCareDex System—patient education materials on the use of complementary and alternative medicines and practices for various health conditions
- AltMed-REAX for the Patient—evidence-based information on the potential for interactions between alternative

medicines and other drugs, dietary supplements, food, alcohol, and tobacco
- AltMedDex System—evidence-based answers on herbals, dietary supplements, vitamins, and minerals for proper usage and dosing, efficacy, adverse reactions, and interactions; includes complete monographs and summary-level information
- Detailed Drug Information for the Consumer—easy-to-understand materials to help educate your patients about medications and their proper use
- DRUG-REAX System—way to check interacting drug ingredients, their effects, and the clinical significance
- DRUGDEX System—drug resource with fully referenced, unbiased content covering dosage, pharmacokinetics, cautions, interactions, comparative efficacy, labeled and off-label indications, and clinical applications
- IDENTIDEX—accurate identification of unknown drugs by imprint code or slang term
- IV Index—utilizes Trissel's 2 to verify IV compatibility
- KINETIDEX—monitoring drug dosages and serum concentration; pharmacokinetic calculators
- Martindale—access to *Martindale: The Complete Drug Reference*
- P&T QUIK Reports—a series of condensed drug reports to be considered for inclusion in hospital formularies
- Pediatrics—an evidence-based drug dosing tool for pediatric patients
- Thomson Reuters Pharmacy Xpert—a one-of-a-kind clinical intelligence dashboard that combines real-time surveillance with Micromedex evidence to help pharmacists improve outcomes, reduce costs, and manage risk

Medline

Part of the U.S. National Library of Medicine (NLM), Medline is a bibliographic database containing more than 19 million references to journal articles in life sciences, with a concentration on biomedicine. Medline contains references to approximately 5,600 worldwide journals in 39 languages. It is the primary component of PubMed.gov, a website that is used to search the extensive Medline bibliographic database.

MEDMARX

An adverse drug event reporting database, MEDMARX is the largest registry of adverse drug events in the United States, with more than 400 health care facilities registered. MEDMARX allows facilities to anonymously and voluntarily report adverse drug events, enabling participating, subscribing facilities to collect, analyze, and anonymously compare and disseminate their data.

Skyscape

A comprehensive online resource that provides access up to 600 medical resources, including drug guides, medical alerts,

---

apps abbreviation for applications, can refer to use on computers, smartphones, tablets, and so on.

journal summaries, and medical references. In addition, Skyscape features robust search functionality, flowcharts, calculators, and cross-indexing. Skyscape is available for Windows desktop PCs, as well as on all major mobile platforms.

Websites

The Internet has revolutionized the way individuals disseminate and collect information. For the purposes of drug information resources and referencing, the Internet can be both a blessing and a curse. While there are numerous websites on the Internet that provide reliable and useful information for purposes of referencing, there are an even larger number of websites that post drug and health information without any clinical evidence, research, or support. It is critical that the

info **.gov, .edu and .org Websites**

As a general rule of thumb, websites that end with a .gov (government agency), .edu (accredited educational institution) or .org (organization or nonprofit) are considered to provide more reliable and objective information for referencing purposes; however, even these websites should be analyzed for credibility.

TABLE 7-1 Government Websites

Name/Organization	Website
CDC—Centers for Disease Control and Prevention	www.cdc.gov
CMS—Centers for Medicare & Medicaid Services	www.cms.gov
FDA—Food and Drug Administration	www.fda.gov
NIH—National Institutes of Health	www.health.nih.gov
NLM—National Library of Medicine	www.medlineplus.gov
U.S. Department of Health and Human Services (HHS)	www.medicare.gov

credibility of any website is determined prior to using the information it publishes. Steps for evaluating a website are provided in Procedure 7-2.

Tables 7-1 and 7-2 include lists of websites you can use when researching drug information or resources.

The following is a list of additional websites that offer valuable drug information and resources for referencing:

- www.drugs.com
- www.medscape.com
- www.rxlist.com
- www.webmd.com

Smartphone Apps

With the recent technological advances in cell phones, "smartphones," such as the iPhone and Android, have become new avenues for drug information and medical news **apps** (Figure 7-2). The smartphone and apps have essentially antiquated the former personal digital assistants (PDAs), which had become useful mobile tools for health care professionals. Many of the references and resources previously described offer apps or online versions that are configured for mobile phones. Remember to use caution in assessing the credibility of apps, however, just as you do with websites, since virtually

■ Procedure 7-2

Evaluating a Website

Step 1. Determine the website's authority and accuracy by asking the following questions:

Who is the author of the content?

Is the information provided reliable?

What are the qualifications, credentials, or expertise of the content authors/editors?

Step 2. Analyze the website's purpose and content by asking the following questions:

What is the purpose of the website?

Does the website provide clinical, educational, or factual information?

Is the website balanced, objective, and informational, or is it subjective and biased?

Is the website owned or sponsored by a commercial interest, which could impact the accuracy of the information presented? The presence of advertisements, or sponsored content, does not always indicate inaccurate or unbiased information; however, it should serve as a warning to carefully examine the objectivity and accuracy.

Step 3. Review the currentness of the website by asking the following questions:

When was the website last revised or updated?

How current is the information provided?

Step 4. Consider the website's design, organization, and ease of use by asking the following questions:

Is the website clearly organized and easy to navigate and read?

Does the website have an appropriate search capability?

Does the website provide a help section for or instructions on use?

anyone can create an app, publishing information that may or may not be based on clinical evidence.

The following are just a few of the countless drug information resource apps:

- BlackBag—basically a medical mobile newswire, offering the FDA MedWatch Safety wire and recall notices.
- Epocrates Rx—similar to Skyscape, provides a robust collection of medical resources through a single app. It also features drug reference charts, including pictures, and the ability to identify drugs based on their shape, color, or other identifying characteristics.
- MDirectory—an electronic phone book with contact listings of hospitals, physicians, pharmacies, and other medical listings in your area.
- MedAbbreviations—a comprehensive collection and index of more than 13,000 medical abbreviations, medical terms, common shorthand, and professional organizations.
- MedCalc—a calculator with access to a wide array of medical formulas, scores, and classifications.
- Medical Drug Pronunciations—a great resource while trying to learn the proper pronunciation of medications. This app provides pronunciations for over 200 common drugs at the click of a button.
- NPTA—the official app of the National Pharmacy Technician Association, offering access to the latest news articles, continuing education programs, and more.
- Practice Rx—medical safety alert newswire, which also features career and practice tips and advice.
- RxGuide—also similar to Skyscape and Epocrates Rx; however, RxGuide offers electronic copies of actual FDA package inserts.
- Skyscape Rx—collection of four separate information resources, including MedAlert, a mobile medical journal, and RxDrugs, an alphabetical index of every drug currently available on the market.

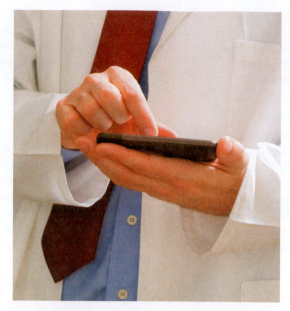

FIGURE 7-2 Smartphones used for drug referencing.
Source: igor.stevanovic/Shutterstock

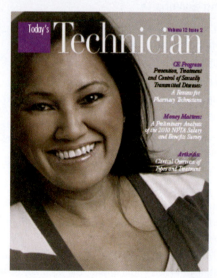

FIGURE 7-3 An example of a pharmacy technician magazine.
(Courtesy of NPTA and Today's Technician)

TABLE 7-2 Drug Information and Reference Guide Websites

Name/Organization	Website
AHFS Drug Information	www.ahfsdruginformation.com
Facts and Comparisons E Answers	online.factsandcomparisons.com
FDA Orange Book	www.accessdata.fda.gov/scripts/cder/ob/default.cfm
MEDMARX	www.medmarx.com
MICROMEDEX	www.micromedex.com
PDR	www.pdrhealth.com
The Merck Index Online	www.cambridgesoft.com/databases/themerckindex/default.aspx

Journals and Magazines

Another excellent source for drug information and resources are industry-related journals and magazines (Table 7-3). As a general rule, journals are considered to be more reliable sources for referencing, as they are scholarly, peer-reviewed publications focusing on clinical data and evidence. Magazines, on the other hand, can provide valuable information and resources, but often contain subjective articles and editorials, which present opinions in addition to facts. Table 7-3 provides a list of pharmacy-related journals and magazines.

TABLE 7-3 Pharmacy-Related Journals and Magazines

Periodical Name	Published	Journal/Magazine	Website
AJHP—American Journal of Health-System Pharmacy	26x/yr	Journal	www.ajhp.org
ComputerTalk	6x/yr	Magazine	www.computertalk.com
DrugStoreNews	16x/yr	Magazine	www.drugstorenews.com
Hospital Pharmacy	12x/yr	Journal	www.hospitalpharmacyjournal.com
JAPhA—Journal of the American Pharmacist Association	12x/yr	Journal	www.pharmacist.com
JPT—Journal of Pharmacy Technology	6x/yr	Journal	www.jpharmtechnol.com
Drug Topics	12x/yr	Magazine	www.drugtopics.com
Pharmacy Times	12x/yr	Magazine	www.pharmacytimes.com
Pharmacy Today	12x/yr	Magazine	www.pharmacytoday.org
U.S. Pharmacist	12x/yr	Magazine	www.uspharmacist.com
Today's Technician	6x/yr	Magazine	www.pharmacytechnician.org

Summary

Current and accurate information is critical to pharmacy practice and pharmaceutical care. As a pharmacy technician, you will be able to use a wide variety of drug information resources and references to look up information for your own needs and to assist the pharmacist in collecting information requested for review or that is requested by patients or health care professionals.

Chapter Review Questions

1. Which reference contains standards that are enforceable by the FDA?
   a. *AHFS DI*
   b. *American Drug Index*
   c. *Drug Facts and Comparisons*
   d. *USP–NF*

2. Which of the following references is a bibliographic database from the U.S. National Library of Medicine?
   a. Micromedex
   b. Medline
   c. MEDMARX
   d. Skyscape

3. Which of the following is an important criterion used to evaluate the credibility of a website?
   a. currentness
   b. organization
   c. purpose
   d. all of the above

4. Which reference covers the full spectrum of pharmacy practice?
   a. *Remington's*
   b. *Martindale*
   c. *Goodman & Gilman's*
   d. *AHFS DI*

5. Which of the following smartphone apps does *not* provide detailed drug product information?
   a. Epocrates Rx
   b. Practice Rx
   c. RxGuide
   d. Skyscape Rx

6. Which reference is noted for providing information on average and wholesale acquisition pricing?
   a. *Orange Book*
   b. *RED BOOK*
   c. *American Drug Index*
   d. *The Merck Index*

7. Which of the following pharmacy journals and magazines is only published bimonthly?
   a. *Computer Talk*
   b. *JPT*
   c. *Today's Technician*
   d. all of the above

8. Which of the following reference books is primarily used in community pharmacies?
   a. *AHFS DI*
   b. *Handbook of Injectable Drugs*
   c. *Handbook of Nonprescription Drugs*
   d. all of the above

9. Which of the following references is *not* arranged by classification or therapeutic usage?
   a. *AHFS DI*
   b. *Drug Facts and Comparisons*
   c. *Handbook on Injectable Drugs*
   d. *USP–NF*

10. Which of the following references would be best used in looking for solubility compatibility information for a parenteral medication?
    a. *AHFS DI*
    b. *Handbook on Injectable Drugs*
    c. *RED BOOK*
    d. *Goodman & Gilman's*

Critical Thinking Questions

1. What are the advantages and disadvantages of arranging reference books by drug classification or therapeutic usage, as opposed to arranging them by trade or generic name?

2. Based upon the resources and references covered in the chapter, list the three references that you feel would be most useful for a health-system pharmacy and the three references that you feel would be most useful for a community pharmacy. Explain your reasoning.

Web Challenge

1. Go online and research a website, not listed in this chapter, that provides drug information. Evaluate the website for credibility and explain why or why not the website would be appropriate for referencing purposes.

2. Choose a prescription drug and then select three of the drug information websites discussed in this chapter. Go to each of the three websites and research the prescription drug you chose. Describe the similarities and differences in the information provided by each website.

3. Go online to research medical or drug information–related smartphone apps not covered in this chapter. List five apps, including their primary features and information provided, and provide an evaluation for each regarding its credibility as a possible reference source.

References and Resources

"AHFS Drug Information." *AHFS Drug Information*. ASHP. 2012. Web. 14 January 2012.

"APhA Website." *American Pharmacists Association*. APhA. 2012. Web. 14 January 2012.

"ASHP Website." *American Society of Health-System Pharmacists*. ASHP. 2012. Web. 14 January 2012.

"Evaluating Web Sites." *Guides to Information Resources*. University of Maryland. 2012. Web. 14 January 2012.

"Facts and Comparisons." *Facts and Comparisons*. Wolters Kluwer. 2012. Web. 14 January 2012.

Hopper, Teresa. *Mosby's Pharmacy Technician: Principles and Practice*. 3rd ed. St. Louis, MO: Elsevier. 2011. Print.

Johnston, Mike. "A Guide to Referencing and Drug Information Resources." *Today's Technician*. 13 (1) (2012). Print.

"Lexicomp." *Lexicomp*. 2012. Web. 14 January 2012.

"The Merck Index." *Merck Publishing*. Merck. 2012. Web. 14 January 2012.

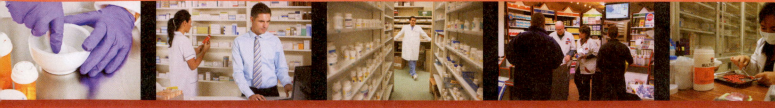

CHAPTER 8

Retail Pharmacy

LEARNING OBJECTIVES

After completing this chapter, you should be able to:

- Explain the ambulatory pharmacy practice setting.

- Describe the two main types of retail pharmacies.

- List the various staff positions in retail pharmacies.

- Describe the typical work environment of a retail pharmacy.

- Discuss the two agencies that regulate retail pharmacy practice.

- List the legal requirements of a prescription medication order.

- Describe the different ways prescriptions arrive at a retail pharmacy.

- List the steps required for a prescription to be filled.

- Discuss the various job duties of technicians in retail pharmacies.

- Discuss the importance of confidentiality for personal health information.

KEY TERMS

adjudication, p. 131

certified pharmacy technician (CPhT), p. 125

chain pharmacy, p. 123

counseling, p. 123

dispense-as-written (DAW), p. 130

doctor of pharmacy (PharmD), p. 126

franchise pharmacy, p. 124

front end, p. 127

household system, p. 132

neighborhood pharmacy, p. 124

over-the-counter (OTC) products, p. 123

patient profile, p. 128

pharmacist in charge (PIC), p. 126

pharmacy clerk/cashier, p. 125

pharmacy manager, p. 125

registered pharmacist (RPh), p. 126

SIG, p. 128

store manager, p. 126

transfer, p. 137

INTRODUCTION

The two main types of pharmacy practice are ambulatory and institutional. Examples of these are hospitals, nursing homes, hospices, and long-term care facilities. Most other pharmacies fall into the category of ambulatory. Ambulatory settings, which are most commonly referred to as *community-based pharmacies*, are privately owned, chain or franchise pharmacies, as well as clinics. These types of pharmacies are also known as *community* or *retail pharmacies* because they serve the local community in which they are located. It is well known that the retail pharmacy is one of the most accessible patient health care settings.

A vast number of career opportunities exist within ambulatory pharmacies. One such opportunity is a position in a retail setting, which is the focus of this chapter.

Direct Patient Care

The definition of direct patient care as it relates to pharmacy is the act of providing knowledgeable and reliable information concerning medication therapy and possible medication-related issues directly to the patient. In 1990, the U.S. Congress passed the Omnibus Budget Reconciliation Act (OBRA). The purpose of this bill required the pharmacist to provide patient medication counseling to Medicaid recipients. State Boards of Pharmacy were required to enact this legislation, and most states broadened the scope of practice to all patient bases, not just Medicaid recipients.

In a retail pharmacy setting, pharmacy technicians are often the first point of contact for the patient. While **counseling** duties are mandated to the pharmacist by law, pharmacy technicians can also share in the development of direct patient care. For example, a technician can recognize those patients who need medication consultation. Being able to provide this significant part of direct patient care requires the pharmacy technician to have explicit knowledge of his or her state's laws and regulations as put forth by the State Boards of Pharmacy. A pharmacy technician armed with this knowledge is able to provide the patient with a better quality of care and safety.

Another aspect of direct patient care in a retail setting centers on the technician's ability to communicate with the patient. A technician who develops informed and logical communication skills can better organize the patient information needed by the pharmacist to perform medication counseling. The diversity of today's world makes it essential for the pharmacy technician to take the steps integral to communicating with those who cannot communicate due to a physical disability, such as patients who are hearing or visually impaired, or do not speak English as a primary language. A technician who learns to communicate effectively portrays the pharmacy in a positive light, not only to the patient, but to other health care professionals as well.

Pharmacy technicians can expand their scope of direct patient care with the proper education and training, along with credentialing and licensing at both the state and national levels. Future duties for a technician related to direct patient care include:

- Gathering and documenting medication information
- Taking new prescriptions from physicians' offices
- Filling patient prescriptions with pharmacist verification

When pharmacy technicians assume these patient care duties, pharmacists are able to provide more clinical duties, such as patient medication consultation. Together, these equate to more favorable and safer outcomes for patients.

Retail Pharmacy

The best-known attribute of retail, or community, pharmacy is the face-to-face interactions among the pharmacist, technicians, and patients. Many people rely on the pharmacy team's knowledge of **over-the-counter (OTC) products**, as well as prescription drugs. Also, when it comes to advice and information related to drugs, the retail pharmacy staff is usually more accessible to the general public than the staff in a doctor's office or clinic.

Within the retail or community setting, ownership of the business can dictate the types of opportunities or tasks a pharmacy technician may have.

Chain Pharmacies

Chain pharmacies are probably what come to mind for most people when they hear the word *pharmacy*. A chain pharmacy by FDA's definition is *"a company that operates four or more pharmacies."* Some of the more familiar chain pharmacies include CVS, Walgreens, Wal-Mart, Target, Rite Aid (Figure 8-1), and Kroger. Chain or franchise pharmacies are further categorized by the key services they provide. For example, Wal-Mart

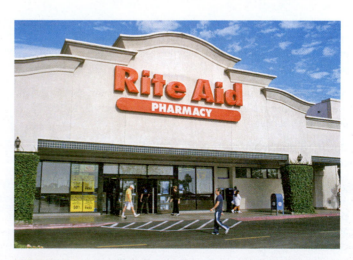

FIGURE 8-1 A retail pharmacy.
Source: A.Ramey/PhotoEdit, Inc.

---

counseling the process of providing patients and customers with pharmaceutical and general health-related advice; provided only by registered pharmacists or doctors of pharmacy.

over-the-counter (OTC) products medications and devices that do not require a prescription for purchase and use.

chain pharmacy a retail, or ambulatory, pharmacy that is owned by a corporation operating multiple pharmacy facilities at various locations.

sells large amounts of merchandise at discounted prices and is considered a mass-merchandiser. A pharmacy such as CVS or Walgreens is considered a chain drugstore because medications are central to its business. Kroger's would be considered a grocery store chain pharmacy because its primary service is selling groceries. Generally, these pharmacies operate at a higher volume than an independent pharmacy might, which can sometimes make for a more strenuous working environment. However, such settings are ideal for technicians who prefer a more vigorous pace.

Career advancement in chain pharmacies is often more readily available than advancement within an independent pharmacy, sometimes locally owned. Advancing to management or developing training for staff can be satisfying for a technician on both a professional, personal, and monetary level. Chain pharmacies can also offer reimbursement for further training, education, national certification, and, where state law requires, licensure. Independent pharmacies often do not have the financial resources available to offer these benefits.

Differences exist between independent and chain pharmacies in hours of operation as well. It is not unusual for some chain pharmacies, particularly those in larger cities, to be open 24 hours a day. Because most chain pharmacies are open longer hours, employees are often scheduled at various shifts, including morning, noon, and night hours. Chain pharmacies are also available to their customers on weekends and most holidays. By contrast, independent pharmacies generally have minimized hours, making it necessary for only one or two shifts. Independent pharmacies are typically closed for most major holidays and have limited hours on the weekend.

Chain pharmacies may also see a spike in prescription volume during a particular time of day or day of the week. The morning hours before noon, and the afternoon, usually from 2:00 PM until 6:00 PM, tend to be the busiest hours. An increase in volume can also be predicted the day prior to a major holiday and the day after a major holiday.

---

franchise pharmacy a retail, or ambulatory, pharmacy that consists of facilities at multiple locations, although each pharmacy may be separately owned.

neighborhood pharmacy an independent pharmacy that is privately owned and small in size, and usually fills an average of 100 to 300 prescriptions per day.

Certified pharmacy technician (CPhT) an individual who is certified to assist pharmacists in providing pharmaceutical care, but is not permitted to dispense medication or counsel patients; certification is achieved by passing a national certification exam.

pharmacy clerk/cashier a noncertified/unlicensed individual who is authorized to do only nonpharmacy-related tasks, such as operating the cash register.

pharmacy manager an individual, almost always a pharmacist, who is appointed to supervise all aspects of the daily pharmacy operations.

Franchise Pharmacies

Franchise pharmacies operate in primarily the same way as chain pharmacies, with one big exception. Franchise pharmacies are owned by an individual, although several different owner–operated locations may exist across the country. In essence, the owner buys the name of the pharmacy, but operates it independently. Chain pharmacies are corporate owned (they have stockholders) and cannot be owned by one individual. Pharmacies such as The Medicine Shoppe, Sav-Mor, and Care are all franchise pharmacies.

There is not much noticeable difference in the day-to-day operations of a franchise and a chain pharmacy. As with the chain pharmacy, the pharmacy technician is usually the first point of contact for the patient. Knowledge, courtesy, and professionalism are still central to the success of the pharmacy technician. State and federal laws governing the scope of pharmacy technicians do not change, regardless of employment setting, and should always be carried out to the letter of the law.

One attractive aspect of working for a franchise pharmacy is the potential for compounding specialized medications. Franchise pharmacies will sometimes move into this area of pharmacy to make them more available to a larger patient base and to be more competitive with the larger chain pharmacies. Learning how to compound specialized medications such as creams, ointments, suppositories, and solutions gives pharmacy technicians a wider range of skills. This makes them a stronger candidate for future advancement.

The hours associated with working for a franchise can vary as they are normally set by the individual owner and not the corporation as with a chain pharmacy. Typically hours of operation will be more like those of the independent.

Independent Pharmacies

Most independent pharmacies are privately owned and relatively small in size, filling, on average, 100 to 300 prescriptions per day. This type of pharmacy is thought of as a **neighborhood pharmacy** (see Figure 8-2). Because of its smaller size and customer base, a neighborhood pharmacy can generally provide

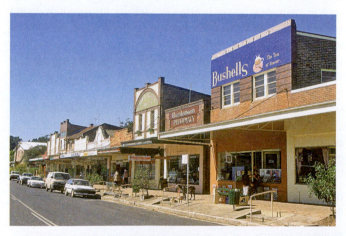

FIGURE 8-2 An independent pharmacy.
Source: Claver Carroll/Getty Images, Inc.

more personalized services to its customers, and pharmacy staff can become better acquainted with their patients.

In addition, some of the independents can provide a wider range of care than the larger chain pharmacies. These expanded services may include offering compounded medications, home health care products, surgical supplies, delivery service, and even patient charge accounts.

Most technicians choose to practice retail pharmacy first because more job opportunities are available in that part of the field as compared to hospital pharmacies. Retail pharmacy also allows a more hands-on approach to pharmacy practice. It involves reviewing, preparing, and recording prescription orders accurately, as well as compounding some special medications. In carrying out these tasks, the pharmacy team efficiently serves and cares for patients.

Outpatient Pharmacies

Outpatient pharmacies are another extension of retail pharmacies, but they are not associated with chain, franchise, or independent pharmacies. Instead, they are normally affiliated with some form of health care system, such as a hospital, clinic, or other ambulatory care facility. The sole purpose of outpatient pharmacies is to provide pharmacy services to patients who are able to leave the health care facility of their own accord from within the health care system. Most health care facilities see outpatient pharmacies as an expansion of direct patient care.

One of the central differences between a chain, franchise, or independent pharmacy and an outpatient pharmacy is the customer base they serve. In the former settings, the customers are primarily people from within the community. Anyone can walk into one of these pharmacies to have his or her prescriptions filled. In an outpatient pharmacy, the customer base is limited to those who have been discharged from the facility to which the pharmacy is associated. Outpatient pharmacies do not fill prescriptions from outside the health care system base. However, as an employee benefit, health care systems will often offer their employees pharmacy services that the outpatient pharmacy provides.

With the rising cost of health care, outpatient pharmacies have become an important part of the health care system. Outpatient pharmacies offer services in a variety of settings: hospitals, clinics, emergency departments, ambulatory care, and long-term care facilities, just to name a few. Outpatient pharmacies can also provide specialty services for their customers, such as compounding of special medications, creams, or ointments. Outpatient pharmacies do not provide IV compounding services as they are usually the job of home health care–based pharmacies.

Outpatient pharmacies are often one of the busiest centers of operation in a health care system. The biggest difference between an inpatient pharmacy and an outpatient pharmacy is that the pharmacist is providing services directly to patients, rather than consulting with a physician about their care. Billing, insurance, and collecting co-pays associated with insurance are also a noticeable difference between outpatient pharmacies and inpatient pharmacies, a job that normally falls on the pharmacy technician. Being versed in prescription billing gives the pharmacy technician a noticeable advantage.

Retail Pharmacy Staff

The operations and management of a retail pharmacy require numerous staff members, each accountable and responsible for various job duties.

Certified Pharmacy Technician

A **certified pharmacy technician (CPhT)** is an individual who is certified to assist pharmacists in providing pharmaceutical care, but is not permitted to dispense medication, or counsel patients (Figure 8-3). Certification is achieved by passing a national certification examination.

Pharmacy Clerk/Cashier

A **pharmacy clerk/cashier** is a noncertified, unlicensed individual who is authorized to assist with only nonpharmacy-related tasks, such as operating the cash register.

Pharmacy Manager

A **pharmacy manager** is an individual, almost always a pharmacist, who is appointed to supervise all aspects of the daily pharmacy operations. The manager's duties may include inventory, scheduling, budgets and financial reports, human resources, customer service, and additional management tasks.

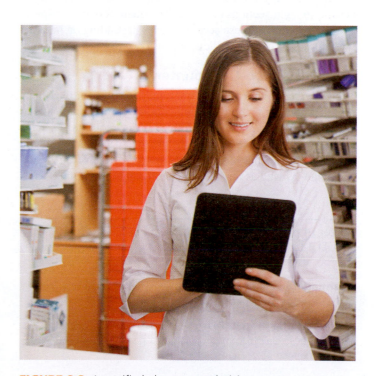

FIGURE 8-3 A certified pharmacy technician.
Source: Tyler Olson/Shutterstock

Doctor of Pharmacy

A **doctor of pharmacy (PharmD)** is an individual who has completed a doctoral degree in pharmacy and is licensed to practice pharmacy in a specific state.

> **❝ Workplace Wisdom** RPh Versus PharmD
>
> Both registered pharmacists (RPh) and doctors of pharmacy (PharmD) are commonly referred to as *pharmacists*. ❞

Pharmacist in Charge

A **pharmacist in charge (PIC)** is an individual designated on the records of the State Board of Pharmacy (SBOP) as the primary, on-site pharmacist. The pharmacist in charge is responsible for ensuring that the pharmacy operates in accordance with state laws and regulations.

Registered Pharmacist

A **registered pharmacist (RPh)** is an individual who has completed a bachelor's degree in pharmacy and is licensed to practice pharmacy in a specific state.

Store Manager

A **store manager** is an individual who has been appointed to supervise all aspects of the daily store operations, including the pharmacy department.

Organization of Retail Pharmacies

The majority of retail pharmacies, regardless of type, are organized into eight sections or areas. The square footage, or space, allotted for each of these sections varies depending on both the size of the pharmacy and the scope or focus of services offered.

Pharmacy Drop-Off Counter

Typically be managed by the pharmacy technician, pharmacy drop-off counter is the first contact point with the patient and where new prescriptions are dropped off or requests are made for refills. It is at this point that the pharmacy technician should verify such information as name, address, date of birth, and physician, as well as any insurance information (Figure 8-4).

---

doctor of pharmacy (PharmD) an individual who has completed a doctoral degree in pharmacy and is licensed to practice pharmacy in a specific state.

pharmacist in charge (PIC) an individual designated on the records of the State Board of Pharmacy as the primary, on-site pharmacist.

registered pharmacist (RPh) an individual who has completed a bachelor's degree in pharmacy and is licensed to practice pharmacy in a specific state.

store manager an individual appointed to supervise all aspects of the daily store operations, including the pharmacy department.

front end the OTC section of a retail pharmacy.

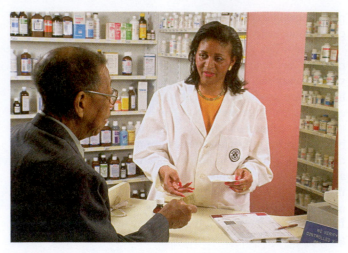

FIGURE 8-4 A customer dropping off a prescription at the pharmacy prescription drop-off area.
Source: Blair Seitz/Science Source

Computer Workstations

Computer workstation should be designated for billing and insurance issues. It may include several computers because it may also be utilized for prescription order entry.

Prescription-Filling Area

Prescription-filling area is supported primarily by the pharmacist. In order for prescriptions to be filled in a safe and timely manner, workflow should be organized and prioritized. An efficient pharmacy technician recognizes these needs and does what is necessary to limit backlog, working in tandem with the pharmacist. Pharmacist and pharmacy technician licenses, registrations, and certifications should be clearly posted in the pharmacy area as mandated by the SBOP.

Patient Consultation Area

Patient consultation area should be away from the center of workflow and traffic to provide the patient with privacy during consultation. HIPAA requires the protection of the privacy of the patient's health information. Pharmacy is not excused from this law and should take every effort necessary to see that it is carried out. Patient consultation is only for a licensed pharmacist; it is unlawful for pharmacy technicians to counsel patients, regardless of their degree of experience.

Prescription Pickup Area

Having separate, clearly marked areas for prescription pickup and drop-off helps to create a better workflow and a safer system of care for the patient.

Medication Storage

Retail pharmacies have multiple storage areas to support the pharmacy operations (see Figure 8-5). Common storage areas are:

- Medication storage, including shelves, cabinets, and a refrigerator/freezer
- Filled prescriptions

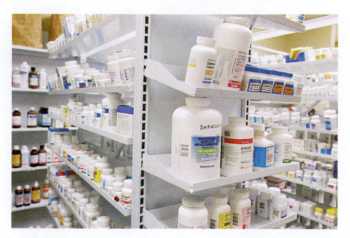

FIGURE 8-5 Typical storage area in the retail pharmacy.
Source: AP Photo/Nati Harnik

- Dispensing supplies, such as vials, bottles, labels, and bags
- Prescription records

Medications should be stored on shelves, alphabetically by generic names, or in a refrigerated system when necessary. These areas should be kept free of clutter to make retrieving an item easy. C-I and C-II drugs must be in locked storage at all times, per DEA regulations. Some medications require refrigeration. Refrigerators should be monitored for any changes in temperature, which could alter the medication. Pharmacist and pharmacy technician licenses, registrations, and certifications should be clearly posted in the pharmacy area as mandated by the SBOP.

OTC/Front End

The over-the-counter (OTC) section, which is referred to as the **front end** in retail terminology, provides customers with various medications, devices, and aids that do not require a prescription to purchase (see Figure 8-6). A comprehensive review of OTC products and devices is covered in Chapter 13.

Regulatory Agencies

Retail pharmacies are regulated, primarily, by three agencies: the SBOP, the DEA, and the Centers for Medicare and Medicaid Services.

State Board of Pharmacy

As you learned in Chapter 4, each state has a state board of pharmacy (SBOP) that registers and regulates retail pharmacy facilities, pharmacists, and pharmacy technicians.

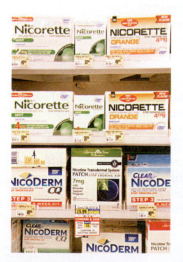

FIGURE 8-6 Examples of medications that are kept behind the counter.
Source: Bill Aron/PhotoEdit, Inc.

The practice of pharmacy is governed at the state level, whereas the pharmaceutical industry is governed at the national level.

The SBOP oversees compliance with the state's pharmacy practice act, and it is for this reason that the SBOP administers unannounced site inspections. The state's enabling legislation gives the state board the authority to require operational changes and to suspend or revoke the license of a pharmacy, pharmacist, or pharmacy technician.

Drug Enforcement Administration

The Drug Enforcement Administration (DEA) is a regulatory department, which is part of the U.S. Department of Justice, set up to regulate the control of narcotics, legal and illegal. Formed in 1972 by an executive order from the Nixon administration, the DEA's primary purpose is to regulate the sale and usage of narcotics. The DEA, an arm of the U.S. Department of Justice, which often works in cooperation with the Federal Bureau of Investigation (FBI), started from 1,470 agents and a budget of 75 million in 1972 to 5,000 agents and a budget of 2.02 billion in 2012.

Centers for Medicare and Medicaid Services

The Centers for Medicare and Medicaid Services (CMS), formerly known as the Health Care Financing Administration (HCFA), is the federal agency that regulates the administration of Medicare, Medicaid, the State Children's Health Insurance Program (SCHIP), the Health Insurance Portability and Accountability Act (HIPAA), the Clinical Laboratory Improvement Amendments,, and several other health-related programs. Approval from the CMS is necessary to receive reimbursement from Medicare or Medicaid, and the CMS conducts inspections to ensure compliance with its guidelines.

The Prescription

Prescriptions are, in essence, orders, either written or verbal, for the dispensing of a medication made by authorized prescribers, such as medical doctors (MDs), physician assistants (PAs), nurse practitioners (CNPs), and dentists (DDS). Prescriptions are the main focus of retail pharmacy practice.

Elements of the Prescription

Every prescription has 10 basic elements (see Figure 8-7). It is the duty of the pharmacy technician to verify that the prescription is complete when it is dropped off or called in to be filled. Each element of the prescription is used in the computer entry, processing, and billing of the order. The 10 basic elements are:

1. *Prescriber information*—the name, address, telephone number, license number, and DEA number of the prescriber. (Note: DEA numbers are not required by law for noncontrolled medications.)

   DEA numbers are license numbers provided by the DEA for registrants who are authorized to prescribe controlled substances. DEA numbers contain two letters followed by seven numbers (e.g., AB1234563). The first letter is typically an A or B; the second letter is typically

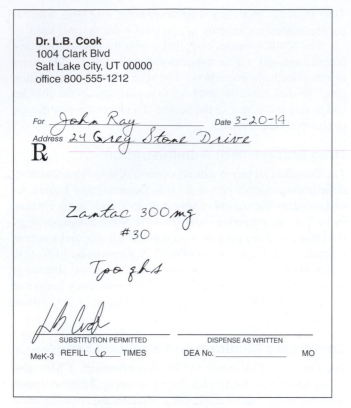

Dr. L.B. Cook
1004 Clark Blvd
Salt Lake City, UT 00000
office 800-555-1212

For _John Ray_ Date _3-20-14_
Address _24 Grey Stone Drive_
R

Zantac 300mg
#30

T po qhs

_____ _____
SUBSTITUTION PERMITTED   DISPENSE AS WRITTEN

MeK-3 REFILL _6_ TIMES   DEA No. _____ MO

FIGURE 8-7 An illustration of a prescription.

■ Procedure 8-1

Verifying a DEA Number

1. Verify that the second letter corresponds to the first letter of the provider's last name.
2. Add the first, third, and fifth digits of the DEA number.
3. Add the second, fourth, and sixth digits.
4. Double the sum of the second, fourth, and sixth digits.
5. Add the sum of steps 2 and 4.
6. Verify that the last digit from step 5 matches the last digit of the DEA number.

the first letter of the registrant's last name. The numbers are designed so that the sum of the first, third, and fifth digits added to twice the sum of the second, fourth, and sixth digits will produce a number that contains the same last digit as the last (seventh) digit of the DEA number. If this formula does not work, the DEA number is fraudulent. Example: Dr. Sarah Byer, DEA AB1234563

1. The B corresponds with "Byer."
2. The sum of the first, third, and fifth digits is 9.
3. The sum of the second, fourth, and sixth digits is 12; 12 doubled is 24.
4. 9 + 24 = 33. The last digit of 33 is 3, which matches the last digit of the DEA number.

2. *Patient name and address*—the name and address of the individual for whom the prescription was written.

❝ Workplace Wisdom **Patient's Address**

Most prescribers do not complete the patient's address, but this should be added when the prescription is dropped off to be filled. ❞

SIG specific directions provided on a prescription for the patient to follow, such as dosages, schedule and frequency of administration, and additional instructions.

patient profile an electronic record, stored in the pharmacy computer system, that details the patient's personal and billing information, prescription records, and medical conditions.

3. *Date prescribed*—the month, day, and year the prescription was written. This will determine the expiration date of the prescription and refills.
4. *Drug name and strength*—the name of the medication being prescribed and its strength, or the amount of active ingredient contained in manufactured prescription products.
5. *Dose and quantity*—the specific dose, or measured amount, of medication being prescribed and a total quantity to be dispensed.
6. *Route of administration*—the route by which the medication should be administered to the patient, such as PO (by mouth).
7. *Signa/directions*—commonly referred to as the **SIG** or SIG code, these are specific directions for the patient to follow, such as dosage, schedule and frequency of dosage, and additional instructions.
8. *Number of refills*—the number of refills authorized by the prescriber, including zero.
9. *Product selection permitted*—the prescriber's authorization for the patient to select a less expensive generic equivalent (if available), or the prescriber's directive to dispense as written (no substitution permitted).
10. *Prescriber's signature*—a prescription is not considered valid unless it is signed by the prescriber.

The Patient Profile

The **patient profile** is an electronic record, stored in the pharmacy computer system, that details the patient's personal and billing information, prescription records, and medical conditions (see Figure 8-8).

To generate a new patient profile, the pharmacy technician must first ask the patient to complete a patient profile form and provide the pharmacy with an insurance card. The patient profile form is used to collect the following critical information:

- Patient's full name
- Patient's address
- Patient's telephone number(s)
- Patient's Social Security number
- Patient's date of birth
- Patient's gender

PATIENT PROFILE

Patient Name

_____ _____ _____
Last   **First**   **Middle Initial**

_____
Street or PO Box

_____
City   State   Zip

Phone   Date of Birth   Social Security No.
( )   _____ ☐ Male ☐ Female _ _ _ _ _ _ _ _ _
             Month   Day   Year

☐ Yes, I would like medication dispensed in a child-resistant container.
☐ No, I do not want medication dispensed in a child-resistant container.

Medication Insurance   Card Holder Name _____
☐ Yes ☐ No   ☐ Card Holder   ☐ Child   ☐ Disabled Dependent
                   ☐ Spouse   ☐ Dependent Parent ☐ Full Time Student

MEDICAL HISTORY

HEALTH   ALLERGIES AND DRUG REACTIONS
☐ Angina   ☐ Epilepsy   ☐ No known drug allergies or
☐ Anemia   ☐ Glaucoma   reactions
☐ Arthritis   ☐ Heart Condition   ☐ Aspirin
☐ Asthma   ☐ Kidney Disease   ☐ Cephalosporins
☐ Blood Clotting Disorders ☐ Liver Disease ☐ Codeine
☐ High Blood Pressure ☐ Lung Disease   ☐ Erythromycin
☐ Breast Feeding ☐ Parkinson's Disease ☐ Penicillin
☐ Cancer   ☐ Pregnancy   ☐ Sulfa Drugs
☐ Diabetes   ☐ Ulcers   ☐ Tetracyclines
Other Conditions _____   ☐ Xanthines
_____   Other Allergies/Reactions_____
_____   _____

Prescription Medication Being Taken   OTC Medication Currently Being Taken
_____   _____
_____   _____
_____   _____

Would You Like Generic Medication Where Possible? ☐ Yes ☐ No

Comments
_____

Health information changes periodically. Please notify the pharmacy of any new medications, allergies, drug reactions, or health conditions.
_____ Signature _____ Date ☐ I do not wish to provide this information

FIGURE 8-8 An illustration of a patient profile.

- Known drug allergies
- Drug sensitivities/reactions
- Medical and health conditions
- Preference on generic drug substitution
- Preference on child-resistant lids

The following details from the patient's insurance card are also added to the patient profile (see Figure 8-9):

- Name of insurance carrier
- Identification (ID) number
- Group code
- Patient code—such as primary, spouse, or dependent

Pearson Community Care

NAME OF BENEFICIARY
MARILOU DOE

MEMBER ID   SEX
ABC112233445 66   **FEMALE**

Rx GROUP   PCC PLAN
123456789   **5678**

Customer Service: 800-111-2222

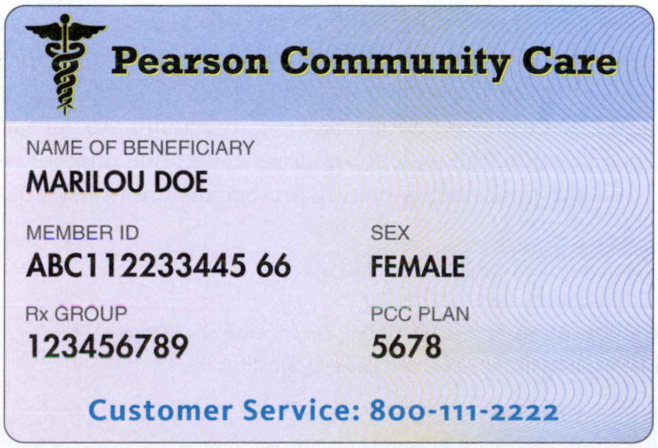

FIGURE 8-9 An example of a patient insurance card.

Processing Prescriptions

Multiple steps are required to process a prescription.

Receiving

Although most prescriptions are brought to the pharmacy in person, this is not the only way a prescription arrives at the pharmacy for processing (see Figure 8-10). For example, in many states faxes are considered legal documents, and it may be more convenient for a prescriber to fax a prescription directly to the pharmacy. A technician may remove a fax from the machine and fill the order because the pharmacist will be reviewing and checking the order. Most pharmacies do not give out their business fax numbers except to prescribers. If a technician is unsure of the source of a fax, he should immediately consult the pharmacist. C-II orders, which are prescriptions for Schedule II drugs (discussed in Chapter 4), are the exception because they must be handwritten original orders and, therefore, cannot be faxed, e-mailed, or phoned into the pharmacy.

Phoned-in prescriptions are also very common in ambulatory pharmacies. In most states, however, pharmacy technicians cannot accept a prescription over the phone. As we get closer to licensing and certification as federal requirements for pharmacy technicians, this may change; for now, though, when the prescriber calls in a prescription, the technician must refer the call to

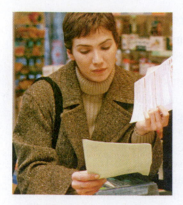

FIGURE 8-10 A patient brings a prescription to a pharmacy.
Source: Veronique Burger/Science Source

a pharmacist, depending on state law. If a patient calls in a refill of an existing order, the technician may take the refill order.

Computers are great communication tools, and ambulatory pharmacies are no strangers to technology. Internet and mail-order pharmacies, among others, may accept prescriptions via e-mail or other Internet transmissions. Some pharmacies are switching to using only electronic prescribing. Because of this technology change, many doctors are required to send their prescriptions through electronic prescribing programs. This practice updates the outdated doctors and health care providers and brings them more into today's technological world.

Reviewing

One of the first steps in providing medication for a patient is receiving and reviewing the order. Remember, legend drugs may not be dispensed without a legal prescription because the government has decided the drug has the potential for addiction or abuse or is dangerous enough to require medical supervision during use. Pharmacy technicians are the front line in the prescription process. By reviewing an incoming prescription for legality and correctness, the technician is not just aiding the pharmacist and serving the patient, but also protecting the public from danger.

Several pieces of information are required before the filling process can begin. It is up to the technician to screen orders to save time (both the pharmacist's and the patient's), and to avoid waste.

The first piece of this puzzle is the patient's name. It is important to get the whole name, not just a nickname. Match the patient's name to the names in your patient profiles, as well as to any possible insurance company records. It is the technician's responsibility to maintain current patient profiles, and this includes making name changes due to divorce or marriage.

Next, verify the date on which the prescription was written. Remember, most prescriptions are good for up to one year.

Current addresses and telephone numbers are also, for the reasons given earlier, important components of a valid prescription. While this information is not legally required to appear on the prescription, the patient's address and phone number need to be in the pharmacy's possession because not only does it confirm the patient's identity, it could also save his life in the event of a problem or recall.

Once the technician verifies the patient for whom the order was written, the next step is to verify the medication being ordered. This includes verifying the correct dosage form, strength, and quantity. If any of these components is missing, the technician should alert the pharmacist immediately and await further instructions.

Next, review the directions for clarity and precision. Does the prescriber allow generic substitution, or is it a **dispense-as-written (DAW)** prescription?

Are any refills available? Remember, according to federal law, a prescription for a C-II drug cannot allow refills; a C-III drug order can be refilled for six months, and prescriptions for C-IV and C-V medications may be refilled for up to a year.

Last, but certainly no less important, is the prescriber's signature. The doctor's signature can also be electronically submitted given the new popularity of electronic prescribing. In some states, a prescriber's assistant can sign for the physician.

Special circumstances apply to certain medications. For instance, prescriptions for C-II drugs must be original, bear no corrections or changes, and contain the prescriber's DEA number.

Errors common to ambulatory pharmacies can be avoided if the technician is knowledgeable and vigilant about accepting prescriptions. Some of the more common problems include:

- Improper patient identification
- Duplicate profiles for the same patient
- Therapeutic discrepancies due to time lapse between time of prescribing and time of dispensing
- Patients who waste time waiting only to find that their prescriptions cannot be filled without further instructions from the prescriber
- Inaccurate or missed insurance billing due to a lack of or incorrect information

One of the most basic services a pharmacy technician provides to a patient, a pharmacist, and society in general is the proper screening of prescriptions. Time, money, and even lives can be saved when this task is performed efficiently and correctly. What transpires in a few moments can affect the lives of many for a lifetime.

Translating

Verifying a prescription order is just the beginning of the pharmacy process. Remember, we have to get the right medication in the right strength and dose to the right patient at the right time! When reduced to a system of clearly defined and meticulously followed steps, the process should run efficiently and without errors.

Computer Entry

After a prescription has been reviewed and properly translated, the information on the prescription must be entered into the pharmacy computer system and the prescription label printed (see Figure 8-11). Nearly every retail pharmacy uses a different, or modified version of, a pharmacy software program. The good news, however, is that the essential elements of computerized prescription processing remain constant.

---

dispense-as-written (DAW) instructions from the prescriber to "dispense as written," without generic substitution.

adjudication the process of transmitting a prescription electronically to the proper insurance company or third-party biller for approval and billing.

PROFILE IN PRACTICE

Mary is a pharmacy technician working at a retail pharmacy. A patient comes in with her sick child and drops off three prescriptions, asking how soon the medications will be ready. Mary indicates that the prescriptions will be ready within 10 to 20 minutes. After entering the prescriptions, printing the labels, and placing them in order to be filled, Mary realizes that the pharmacy is out of stock of one of the medications. The patient is due to return, expecting to pick up the prescriptions, in five minutes.

▸ *What mistake did Mary make?*
▸ *What actions can Mary take to offset her mistake?*

Adjudicating

Online **adjudication** is the process of transmitting a prescription electronically to the proper insurance company or third-party biller for approval and billing. Chapter 9 discusses insurance billing in detail.

Alerting the Pharmacist of Nonformularies

Every prescription plan has a list of medications that are proprietary to the patient's co-pay. Formulary medication lists are generally updated at least once a year, and many times more frequently, by the prescription plan's Pharmacy and Therapeutic Committee (P&T). The P&T committee reviews FDA-approved medications based on their usage, safety, and effectiveness. Once a list has been compiled, it becomes the plan's formulary. Any medications not on this list are considered nonformulary. For example, if the patient's physician prescribes Zocor (simvastatin) and it is on the formulary or preferred medications list, then the patient would be responsible

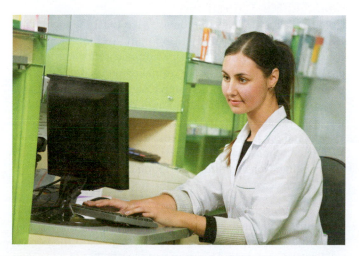

FIGURE 8-11 A pharmacy technician entering a prescription into the pharmacy computer system.
Source: Dmitry Kalinovsky/Shutterstock

Procedure 8-2

Entering a Prescription

The following is a general process for entering a prescription into the pharmacy computer system:

1. Perform a search for the patient, by last name, then first name, and date of birth.
   a. If the patient is already in the system and verified, go to step 2.
   b. If the patient is a new patient, cannot be found in the system, or has changes to the profile, have the patient complete a patient profile form and then create/edit the patient profile, including insurance information.
2. Select the correct patient profile and then select Fill/New Rx, which will prompt the prescription entry screen.
3. Perform a search for the prescriber by last name, then by first name, and DEA number.
   a. If the prescriber is already in the system and verified, go to step 4.
   b. If the prescriber is new or cannot be found in the system, create a new prescriber profile using the information provided on the prescription.
4. Select the correct prescriber.
5. Enter the original date of the prescription.
6. Enter/select the drug prescribed and indicate if generic substitution should be used—based first on availability, then the prescriber's preference, and then the patient's choice. Verify that the correct NDC number is selected for the prescription.
7. Enter the quantity prescribed.
8. Select/enter the directions for the prescription.
9. Enter the number of refills authorized.
10. Select/enter the correct DAW code.
    a. 0—product selection permitted
    b. 1—dispense as written
    c. 2—product selection permitted, but declined by patient
11. Verify/edit the day's supply quantity.
12. Notify the pharmacist of any drug utilization review (DUR) messages, for approval.
13. Transmit/submit for online adjudication by the insurance provider.
14. Approve the adjudication and print paperwork and labels.

only for the amount of the co-pay designated on their prescription card. It is however, important to note that some prescription plans will pay only for the generic formulary medication and not the brand name.

In contrast, nonformulary medications are medications not on the formulary or approved by the prescription plan's P&T committee. Prescription plans will generally pay a percentage of these medications, making the patient's co-pay much higher. For example, the patient's physician specifically orders Crestor (rosuvastatin), but when the technician runs the prescription plan transaction, Crestor is not a medication on the patient's prescription plan formulary. At this point the technician would need to notify the pharmacist. The pharmacist would then speak with the patient to explain the reasons why the co-pay will be significantly higher. The patient might either agree to pay the higher amount or have the pharmacist call the physician to find a substitution drug from the plan's formulary medication list. In some cases the patient requires the specific, prescribed medication. In such cases the pharmacist will phone the physician to request further documentation supporting the need for that specific medication. It then becomes the responsibility of the physician office to provide that information to the patient's prescription plan. Once all information is received and approved, the pharmacist can then fill the medication at the formulary pricing.

Such interruptions can impede workflow and create backlog, making it important for pharmacy technicians to recognize potential issues with nonformulary medications. Each prescription plan has its own specific formulary, and rarely are any two plans the same. However, through careful observation and some experience, the pharmacy technician can learn to recognize where potential formulary issues may arise. Patients rely on the pharmacy to correct issues related to their prescription plans. Knowing how to resolve the issue before it becomes an explosive problem places the pharmacy in the best light, and the patient walks away with a positive experience.

Drug Utilization Evaluation

Drug utilization evaluation (DUE) or drug utilization review is defined by the Academy of Managed Care Pharmacy as "an authorized, structured, ongoing, review of prescribing, dispensing, and use of medication." DUE is an invaluable measurement and patient safety tool used by pharmacists to work with prescribers concerning patient medication therapy and appropriateness. This system of evaluation was set up to alert prescribers to inappropriate or unapproved medication usage. When using DUE, a pharmacist can suggest medication therapies that may be more advantageous to the patient based on FDA-approved medications, prescribed medication usage, appropriate dosing, managed drug therapy, and drug cost.

As pharmacists assume more consulting and counseling duties, pharmacy technicians with a strong knowledge base can assist pharmacists with DUE by collecting essential patient data, including:

- Patient's name and date of birth
- Patient's physician or physicians and their office phone numbers
- Patient's condition, if available
- Patient's current medication, including any new medications or OTC medications they may also be taking
- Patient's current medical and prescription plan
- Patient allergies and reactions

Gathering this information upon the pharmacist's request assists the pharmacist to form a DUE, which will result in the greatest patient outcome both therapeutically and financially.

---

household system the measurement system commonly used by Americans for general measuring and cooking.

NDC Numbers

National Drug Code, or NDC, numbers are identification numbers assigned to each unique drug product, similar to UPC codes for consumer goods. Each NDC number consists of three sets of numbers: The first set indicates the manufacturer; the second set indicates the drug, its strength, and its dosage form; the third and final set of numbers indicates the package size.

Example: NDC 51285-601-05

Preparing

Inventory is a critical responsibility in pharmacy. When the exact medication prescribed is not on the pharmacy's shelves, patients are subjected to unnecessary delays and annoyance. Assuming that the right medication is available, performing a few extra checks can save valuable time and trouble later. The technician should check the lot number and/or the NDC numbers to ensure that the medication selected is the exact medication listed on the patient's label.

It is also important to check the expiration date. The drug must not only be current on the day it is dispensed, but current throughout the entire course of therapy; that is, the expiration date must be far enough away to allow the patient to use all the drug as directed.

When selecting C-II drugs, the technician may be required to enter the medications into a log to aid in inventory control. Make sure you are aware of any state or employer policies before attempting to process a prescription for a C-II drug.

❝ Workplace Wisdom Avoiding Contamination

It is important that medications not be touched directly with the hands, because of the potential for contamination of the medicine and the person touching it. ❞

Counting/Measuring/Pouring

Counting should always be done twice until the technician feels confident in her ability (see Figure 8-12). Prescriptions for C-II drugs should always be counted twice before they are given to the pharmacist for a final recount. Measuring and pouring can be a little more complicated because calculations may be involved. Technicians should not attempt to measure medications until they are comfortable with both the metric system and the **household system**, which is the measurement system commonly used by Americans for general measuring and cooking. Consider the prescription described in the Profile in Practice scenario.

Packaging and Labeling

As simple as it sounds, labeling still requires attention to detail (see Figure 8-13). First, the label must go onto the correct medication container. This may sound silly, but in an assembly-line type of pharmacy, many errors occur over just this detail! For technicians, this is the last chance to check their

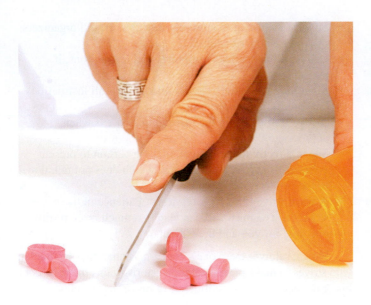

FIGURE 8-12 Counting pills.
Source: Jami Garrison/Shutterstock

PROFILE IN PRACTICE

Dr. Rizzoli has prescribed Amoxil 250 mg suspension TID x10D, but the pharmacy has Amoxil 125 mg/5 mL in stock. Mark, the pharmacy technician, has to know not only mg and mL but also TID and 10D, to calculate the appropriate quantity to dispense. Mark determines that the pharmacy will need to dispense 300 mL of the Amoxil 125 mg/5 mL, by using the following formula: 10 mL (dose) × 3 (frequency) × 10 (duration) = 300 mL.

▶ *What directions must be included on the label to ensure that the patient takes the correct dosage?*

work before submitting it to the pharmacist for a final check. Double-check the directions and drug strength, and affix any auxiliary labels that may be appropriate (see Figure 8-14). The drug label is usually generated by computer and will contain all the information required by law: the name and telephone number of the dispensing pharmacy, the patient's name, the prescription number, the date the prescription was filled and the expiration date of the medication, the medication name and strength, directions, and the prescriber's name. The label also shows the quantity of medication inside, as well as the number of refills.

Container Types and Sizes Today's prescription containers come in various shapes, sizes, and colors. They are made from glass, plastic, and even paper and have advanced quite a bit from the days when they were known as medicinal bottles. Innovations in prescription packaging are being studied as a way to improve patient safety and adherence. Some retail chains, such as Target, have their own proprietary prescription packaging system. Using the appropriate packaging for a prescription is oftentimes as important as choosing the correct medication.

When choosing packaging for medications, there are several factors to take into consideration:

- The medication dosage form—is it a capsule, tablet, liquid, or solid?
- Size, shape or form, and amount—is the chosen container appropriate for the size, the shape or form, and the amount of the medication being placed in the container?
- Restrictions—are there any restrictions with the type of packaging the drug requires, such as protection from heat or light; perhaps does it need refrigeration or even need to be kept frozen?

Once you know these factors, it is much easier to choose the appropriate vessel for the medication.

Prescription vials are typically used to package tablets and capsules. They come in sizes ranging from 6 drams to 60 drams (dram = 1/16 oz). Although prescription vials can be blue or green, the most recognizable and commonly used color is amber.

Prescription bottles are used to package solutions and liquids and come in sizes ranging from 1 ounce to 16 ounces. They can be glass or plastic, although plastic is more common. Bottles are most recognizably amber in color.

Ointment jars are typically used for ointments, creams, or suppositories, which are not commercially available or are special compounds prescribed by the patient's physician. Sizes for ointment jars can range from 1 ounce to 16 ounces.

Prescription dropper bottles are also used to package solutions and liquids, but in a smaller quantity. Medications for eyes, ears, or infants are typically packaged in these bottles.

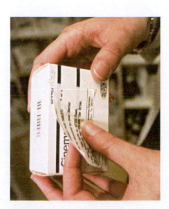

FIGURE 8-13 Labeling a prescription requires attention to detail.
Source: Josh Sher/Science Source

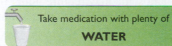
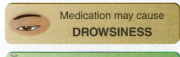
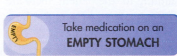
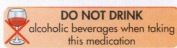
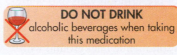
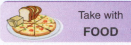

FIGURE 8-14 Examples of auxiliary labels.

Dropper bottles are made from glass and plastic. Dropper bottle sizes are much smaller than regular prescription bottles and can range from 0.5 ounces to 2 ounces.

Blister packing is another available form of medication packaging. It uses a medication card, which includes individual compartments for each tablet. The package is then heat-sealed for safety and security. Blister packs are typically packaged as a 30-day supply and are more readily seen in a long-term care facility setting.

Whatever product you are filling, patient safety and product integrity are two of the most important factors, and neither should ever be compromised.

Packaging for the Physically Impaired, Aged, and Children

In 1970 the U.S. Congress passed the Poisoning Prevention Packaging Act, legislation aimed at reducing the incidence of accidental poisoning and deaths of children under the age of five due to the ingestion of oral medications and common products found in the home. The use of required childproof caps is the cornerstone of this legislation's success.

While keeping children safe is a major goal of parents everywhere, at least 30 children in the United States die annually from accidental poisoning due to drug ingestion or household toxins. The American Association of Poison Control Centers estimates it receives one million phone calls each year concerning accidental poisoning in children under the age of five. So how can this be prevented and what role does the pharmacy technician play in prevention?

- Childproof cap—All oral prescriptions must have a childproof cap unless the patient requests otherwise. If the patient makes such a request, an auxiliary label stating the medication cap is not child proof must clearly be visible on the prescription.
- Auxiliary labels—Auxiliary labels help to warn the patient of medication dangers that may be harmful to children.
- Keeping the medications out of reach—Educating the patient for the need to keep medication from small fingers can help to prevent a disastrous outcome later.

While childproof caps are required by law, they can cause issues for those who are physically impaired or of advanced age. Prescription labels can seem faint or difficult to read for the vision impaired. Being able to open a bottle can be defeating for someone with a physical illness such as arthritis. Medication consultations can seem like whispers to those who struggle to hear. Understanding labels and instructions can be confusing, causing frustration for those who battle with cognitive disabilities including Alzheimer's disease or dementia.

While these issues seem daunting for the patient, there are some steps pharmacy technicians can take to help make these situations more manageable.

- Use non-childproof caps for prescription vials and bottles; make certain to use an auxiliary label stating a non-child-proof cap was used.
- Print pharmacy labels on a solid white background with sharp black letters.

- Suggest the use of magnifying instruments, pill organizers, or dose reminder systems.
- Use braille on patient pamphlets and instructions, if available.
- Make sure the patient clearly understands all instructions before leaving the pharmacy.
- Involve caregivers in the instruction process when appropriate.
- Speak directly to the patient, making certain to present yourself in a clear, audible tone, which does not talk down to the patient.
- Always strive to be a professional. Patience in these situations is a must and can lead to a much more positive outcome for you and the patient.

Patient safety is everyone's concern. A pharmacy technician who strives to make patient safety a priority gains the respect of his or her peers and the confidence of his or her patients.

Categories of Medications Requiring Auxiliary Labels Auxiliary labels are another safeguard pharmacy uses to educate patients about their medication. In addition to the prescription label, auxiliary labels, which are usually brightly colored, are placed on the prescription to draw patients' attention to a particular warning or storage issue regarding their medications. Some of the auxiliary label categories include:

- Administration and route of administration
- Dosing
- Storage
- Dietary restriction
- Expiration
- Warning and caution

Auxiliary labels, an extension of patient education and safety, are used for various categories of medication. Never place auxiliary labels across vital prescription instructions and information; rather they should be placed next to the prescription label or where space clearly allows the patient to read the prescription label instructions.

The following are some of the most common medication categories where auxiliary labels may be necessary:

- Narcotics
- Antibiotics
- Chemotherapy agents
- Ace inhibitors
- Cholesterol medications
- NSAIDS
- Steroids
- Nitrates
- Vitamin K antagonist
- Diuretics

Some medications may require multiple auxiliary labels, and some may require none. If you are unsure, verify the use of auxiliary labels with the pharmacist. Remember, auxiliary labels are a safety measure for the patient; if proper auxiliary labels are not attached to the prescription, patient safety may be compromised.

Visibility Clear instructions that are printed neatly and unhampered by font type, numeric confusion, thin margins, line spaces, unnecessary information, or scattered text—this is the label everyone should have on their prescription. Medication labels can be confusing enough without the addition of mistyped, haphazard label making. Producing a prescription label with optimum visibility is essential for patient medication compliance and safety.

Recommendations from the Institutes for Safe Medication Practices (ISMP) include:

- Making certain text is typed; using an Arial or Verdana font is the most legible.
- Always use numbers instead of letters when describing dosing instructions. For example: 1 tablet 3 times a day.
- Text should never be vertical on prescription labels.
- Barcodes should always be in black.
- Auxiliary labels should not hide any medication instructions, but still be easily visible by the patient.
- Labels should be centered on medication containers, so patients can easily focus on instructions.
- Labels should be white with black lettering. A font size of 12 or 14 is optimal, particularly for older patients with vision impairments.
- Labels should clearly provide pharmacy information—name, address, and phone number—without running over into patient medication instructions. Label should also provide prescriber's name, prescriber's DEA number, patient's name, date prescription was filled, prescription number, and refill information, where applicable.
- Label instructions concerning the medications should include drug name, strength, form, amount being dispensed, and drug manufacture. Medication dosing instructions should be clear and precise.

Patient prescription labels that lack accurate information or visibly hamper a patient's ability to comply with medication instructions not only put the patient at risk, but also can lead the pharmacy into issues of liability. A pharmacy technician who is relentless in their processing of prescription labeling will most likely avoid such issues. If at any time a process or instructions becomes unclear, always consult a pharmacist.

Final Check

The final check is the sole domain of the pharmacist. No medications may be dispensed without the pharmacist's final approval. In an ambulatory setting, this is a relatively simple process. The pharmacist will need the original prescription, the stock bottle used in filling the order, and the labeled container filled with the prescribed medication. Once the pharmacist approves it, the medication may be given to the patient.

State Laws Regarding the RPh Review Prior to Distribution

While today's pharmacy technician is a significant part of the pharmacy team and roles for the technician are expanding, it is never within the scope of the pharmacy technician to dispense medication without a final check from a licensed pharmacist. The law is very clear on this matter. A pharmacist must have the final check before any medication can be received by the patient. While laws regarding pharmacy technicians may vary from state to state, this law remains constant. Essential information a pharmacist requires to perform a final check includes:

- Original medication order or prescription
- Printed and completed medication label
- Bottle used to fill the prescription, which will give the pharmacist the medication's lot number, expiration date, and NDC number
- Signature of the technician who filled the prescription

Once the pharmacist reviews the prescription and signs off on the final check, the medication is ready for distribution to the patient. A new prescription may require a patient consultation; always check with patients before giving them the medication to see if they desire a pharmacist consultation. If it is a refill, chances are the patient will not need consultation, but it is best practice to ask patients if they have any questions regarding their medications.

Storing

After the pharmacist performs the final check, the prescription is ready for storing and dispensing. The prescription is packaged in an appropriately sized prescription bag or box and labeled with a patient prescription receipt and important drug information reports.

For prescriptions that are scheduled for patient pickup, most retail pharmacies store them alphabetically by the patient's last name in a system of bins, drawers, or shelves. Depending on the size of the pharmacy, and the volume it handles, the prescriptions may be alphabetized in groups of letters (e.g., bins labeled "A–C" and "D–F") or by multiple bins per letter (e.g., bins labeled "Aa–Am," "An–Az," "Ba–Bo," and "Br–Ce"). Clearly, the more prescriptions an individual pharmacy fills, the more organized the storage has to be. Properly organized storage of prescriptions ensures that the prescriptions do not become lost and that they can be located quickly when the patient arrives for pickup.

Independent and specialty community pharmacies sometimes offer delivery of prescriptions to the patient's home or office by courier or mail. Regardless of the mode of delivery, these prescriptions are stored in a separate area to be scheduled and prepared for delivery.

Dispensing

Technically speaking, the dispensing of a prescription is the process and time when the medication is released from the pharmacy and given to the patient. For in-store pickups, a prescription is *dispensed* as soon as the pharmacy staff gives the medication to the patient. A delivered prescription is considered dispensed as soon as it leaves the pharmacy.

In other words, once the medication is no longer under the security and control of the pharmacy, it is considered dispensed, and once a medication has been dispensed it cannot be returned to the pharmacy. This is because the pharmacy is no longer able to guarantee the quality and integrity of the medication. Even if, for example, a patient picks up a prescription, walks out to his car, and then immediately comes back inside, the prescription has been dispensed and cannot be returned to stock.

Medication Distribution Systems One type of medication distribution system commonly used in the retail pharmacy setting is an automated counting mechanism. These user-friendly machines are often used to facilitate the medication filling process because they save time, can be more accurate than manual counting, and help improve accuracy and workflow.

Medication distribution systems can be as simple as an automated counting device or as complex as a fully automated robotic system. As the number of prescriptions filled increases, more pharmacies are looking toward the use of some form of medication distribution system. While these machines can save time and improve counting accuracy, there is still an element of possible human error. Use caution when loading medications into the machine, which means remembering the right dose and drug. Also remember to use expiration dates and lot numbers, which are alike when dispensing from two different medication containers.

Automated dispensing cabinets are another type of medication distribution systems. Automated dispensing cabinets, such as Pyxis or Omnicell, are uncommon in a retail setting, but do provide another secure and accurate way of distributing patient medications. Automated dispensing cabinets are often used in ambulatory, long-term care, or hospital settings. The system allows a patient's medication to be securely locked within the cabinet until time of administration. This system works in conjunction with the facility's computer system and continually updates patient medication orders as they are put into the computer system.

As pharmacists move more toward patient counseling duties, the use of medication distribution systems is expected to become more prevalent. A pharmacy technician who familiarizes himself or herself with the workings of these systems has a wider range of abilities and a greater potential for advancement in their pharmacy career.

Supplying Written Patient Information Federal law, P.L. 104–180, written under the direction of the FDA, requires all new medication prescriptions contain Consumer Medication Information (CMI). This law was enacted in order to protect consumers, alerting them to the benefits and dangers of their medications. CMI is usually written by companies outside of the drug manufacture, but all information must be approved by the FDA before it can be distributed to the consumer.

Set forth by FDA regulations, CMI pamphlets must provide the consumer with the following information:

- The name of the medication, both brand and generic
- For what the medication is used
- Do not take medication if you are …
- How to take the medication

- Medication side effects
- General information

Written patient information is an important part of ensuring patient safety and compliance.

It is imperative this information accompany any new prescriptions as it is an extension of patient consultation. The CMI pamphlet often becomes a point of reference if the patient has forgotten the information the pharmacist gave to him or her in consultation. A pharmacy technician who is diligent in helping to ensure that CMI pamphlets accompany new prescriptions gives the patient the information necessary to understand his or her medications. Written patient information should also be given to patients who have questions regarding medication refills. Keeping the patient informed helps to ensure medication safety and compliance.

Counseling is beyond the authorized scope of practice for pharmacy technicians (Figure 8-15). It is reserved only for pharmacists—without exception. Pharmacy technicians do, however, play an important role in the counseling process, in that they alert the pharmacist to the need to counsel patients on new medications, and by always asking patients—even if they are just picking up refills—if they have any questions for the pharmacist.

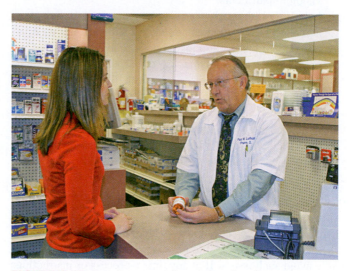

FIGURE 8-15 A customer receives counseling from the pharmacist about a new prescription.
Source: Bonnie Kamin/PhotoEdit Inc.

■ Procedure 8-3

Dispensing a Prescription

1. The pharmacist must complete a final check of the prescription.
2. Verify whether the order is a new prescription or refill.
   a. If a new prescription, have the pharmacist come over to offer counseling.
   b. If a refill, ask the patient if he or she has any questions for the pharmacist.
3. Ring up the customer's order at the cash register.
4. Have the patient sign and date the prescription pickup log.

Transfer situation in which the patient would like to have the prescription refilled at a pharmacy other than where it was originally delivered or filled.

Filing

The final step in processing a prescription is filing the actual hard copy of the prescription. Throughout the entire process, the hard-copy prescription will have been written upon, marked, initialed, and labeled. The label, which is generally placed on the back side of the prescription, contains information generated by the pharmacy computer, including the information labeled on the patient's medication, insurance billing information, and a computer-generated serial number—commonly referred to as the prescription, or Rx number.

The hard-copy prescriptions will be stacked throughout the workday, after the final check. At appropriate times and intervals, the pharmacy technician will organize, verify, and file the hard copies.

The filing process will be determined by the individual pharmacy, but typically is set up as one series for legend prescriptions, one series for controlled prescriptions, and one series for Schedule II drug prescriptions.

Prescriptions are divided by type, or series, and then organized in numerical order of the unique serial number generated by the pharmacy computer. Once the prescriptions have been placed in order, the pharmacy technician will verify that no prescriptions are missing and then file the hard copies—typically in batches of a hundred in specially made prescription file folders.

Refills

Standard prescriptions can usually be refilled as many times as the prescriber orders within one year from the date the prescription was written; in other words, a prescription is good for one year. Exceptions to this rule, in most states, include controlled drugs, which are limited to a maximum of five refills, and C-II medications, which require a new, handwritten prescription for each fill.

In most pharmacies, pharmacy technicians are responsible for handling prescription refill requests. This task includes documenting patient refill orders, verifying prescription refills, processing orders with refills available, and contacting the prescriber to seek approval for additional refills past the number allotted on the original prescription.

Most pharmacies and insurance providers require that a prescription be 75% used before it may be refilled. For example, a patient with a prescription lasting 30 days cannot get a refill until after three weeks. There are exceptions to this rule, however. At her discretion, a pharmacist can provide up to a 72-hour supply of medication, until refills can be approved. Also, many insurance companies will override their refill policy for patients who are traveling overseas or taking extended trips, or in similar situations.

Transfers

Transfers are instances when the patient would like to have the prescription refilled at a pharmacy other than where it was originally delivered or filled (see Figure 8-16).

The laws governing the transfer of prescriptions between pharmacies differ from state to state and depend on the class of drug prescribed. When permitted, a prescription may be

---

■ Procedure 8-4

Requesting a Refill Authorization

1. Ensure that there are no refills remaining on the prescription and that there are no prescriptions on hold, or logged, in the patient's profile for the medication.
2. Print out a copy of the patient's last refill.
3. Call the prescriber and request a refill by providing the following information, either on voicemail or to a nurse:
   a. Patient's name
   b. Patient's date of birth
   c. Drug name
   d. Drug strength
   e. Drug quantity
   f. Date of last fill
   g. Pharmacy's name and phone number
4. Write the date, time, "WCB" (will call back), and your initials on the form.
5. File the form, alphabetically by last name, with the other pending refills.

Note: This process can also be done electronically if the physician's office and pharmacy use an automated refill system.

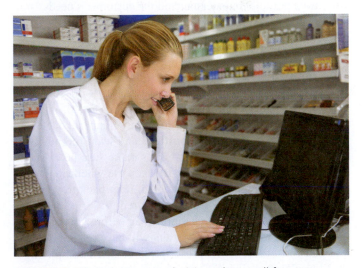

FIGURE 8-16 A pharmacy technician takes a call from a customer who is requesting a prescription transfer.
Source: mangostock/Shuttertstock

---

transferred for only one fill, or the entire prescription may be transferred. The critical factor is that there must be a paper trail for the DEA and SBOP.

The pharmacy's records must track that the prescription was indeed transferred, on a specific date and along with any available refills. If the prescription has already been filled and is being stored, the insurance claim must be reversed and the medication must be returned to stock. The new pharmacy will create a record showing that the prescription was a transfer; the new pharmacy is then responsible for any additional refills or transfers pertaining to that prescription.

In most states, a pharmacist is required to handle the process of transferring a prescription, either in or out. It is standard practice in the industry that the pharmacy that is to receive the transferred prescription should initiate the transfer request and phone call. In addition, most states restrict controlled medications with refills to a maximum of one transfer.

Ringing Up Transactions

Providing customer services is one of the central elements of pharmacy technicians' responsibilities. As with those greeting patients at the pharmacy counter, pharmacy technicians who ring up patient transactions become the identifiable face of the pharmacy. While patients may not remember what the pharmacist has told them, they will always remember a bad experience or an unfriendly encounter, and most of the time the pharmacy technician is the one standing in the center of it all.

Apple has made it their mission to provide customers with the best possible retail experience. They provide their employees with a universal guideline when it comes to customer service, one that is also beneficial to pharmacy customer service. Representatives for Apple are supposed to approach customers in the following manner:

- Approach customers with a personalized warm welcome.
- Probe politely to understand all the customer's needs.
- Present solutions for the customer to take home.
- Listen for and resolve any issues or concerns.
- End with a fond farewell and an invitation to return.

Completing a transaction in retail pharmacy should be handled very much the same way. Always do your best to greet the patient in a friendly, yet professional, manner. Remember, a smile makes you much more approachable. Be patient; patients often have questions and want to know you are listening. If the patient has issues make sure he or she is addressed with the proper tone. Be accurate when ringing up transactions. If you become distracted, refer back to your last item transaction. Make sure any required prescription information is in the patient's prescription bag before you hand it to the patient. In most cases the patient will have to sign a signature pad for receipt of the prescription or when completing a credit card transaction. Be sure to give the patient any change that may due to him or her as well as any credit or insurance cards he or she may have given you. Before the transaction ends, make sure to ask the patient if there is anything else you can help him or her with. If everything is satisfactory to the patient, thank the patient for his or her patronage and wish him or her well.

While it is unrealistic to believe you can satisfy all of the people all the time, keeping a "cool" head goes a long way in defusing situations where the customer is not so happy. There are instances where you may need to call for a manager or pharmacist: If this becomes the case, step away from the situation.

Providing exceptional customer service evokes trust between the pharmacy and the patient, creating security for the patient and longevity for the pharmacy.

Types of Payments

Retail pharmacies accept various forms of payment for prescription medications, OTCs and prescription plan co-payments. The majority are made using a credit card such as Visa, MasterCard, or American Express, or with a credit/debit card linked to the patient's bank account. Credit card transactions are more convenient for most people, and the need to count back change is eliminated. Credit/debit cards work the same way credit cards do. A patient can choose to run a transaction as a credit or a debit, but must input his or her card's pin number to complete a debit transaction. Regardless of which transaction the patient chooses he or she must always sign a receipt of transaction; one copy is for the customer and one copy is for the pharmacy.

While cash and check transactions are less common, they are still a huge part of a pharmacy's payment transactions. When a patient pays with cash, it is important not only to count back any change the patient may be owed, but also to make certain to hand him or her a receipt for the transaction. When accepting a check as payment, remember to ask the patient for proper identification, usually a driver's license, or other form of government-issued ID. Retail pharmacies often use the services of a check verification system such as ChexSystems or TeleCheck, which decrease the chances of a patron's check being returned from the bank unpaid.

Health spending accounts (HSAs) are also a common form of payment for prescriptions, co-pays, and some OTC products. HSAs are a result of the *Medicare Prescription Drug Improvement and Modernization Act* of 2003. These nontaxable savings accounts allow participants to cover health care costs associated with high insurance deductibles or costs not covered by insurance. Each calendar year the participant sets aside a designated dollar amount, which is nontaxable, and puts it into an HSA. The participant can then use this account to pay for co-payments, prescriptions, and other medical services that they are not eligible for payment through their insurance plan. HSAs are used in the same method as credit cards and will have either a Visa or MasterCard logo embedded on the card. It is important to remember, not all pharmacies accept all of the payment types mentioned. The type of payments your pharmacy accepts will be determined by the corporation or the independent owner.

The Cash Register

Cash registers are an important part of a retail pharmacy and over the years have evolved into sophisticated pieces of equipment. The most basic cash registers are electronic with digital displays and numeric buttons. All cash registers will produce a two-part paper receipt: one for the pharmacy and one for the customer.

The advancement of computers has allowed cash registers to do much more than just ring up a patient's medications. Computer-based cash systems can keep track of patient profiles, stock inventory, and medication availability. Point-of-sale (POS) systems are currently the most recognized computer-based cash systems. POS systems work off of a Windows platform and are capable of allowing the operator to perform various types of sales transactions and payments from one machine. The typical setup for a POS system would include:

- Monitor
- Cash drawer
- Bar code scanner
- Printer for receipts
- Keyboard
- Credit card scanner (either integrated into the system or separate equipment)
- Pin pad for debit transactions
- Signature pad

POS systems were designed for the ease of operator use. They allow the operator to simply scan the bar code of an item rather than ringing in the individual price or looking the item up on the keyboard, creating a faster and more accurate transaction. However, for times when a bar code is unavailable, use the keyboard to punch in the bar code and the price will most likely become available on the screen. Or, in those cases where it does not generate a price list, manually enter the price into the machine using the system's keyboard. When this issue occurs, it is best to alert a manager or inventory control person, so the item can be updated within the system, alleviating the problem from happening again.

Software integrated into the POS system can produce reports for inventory control, sales analysis, product trends, and payment types. POS systems can also "talk" with other computer system, automatically generating the patient's co-pay amount when his or her prescription is scanned during checkout. Patient profiles and medication information can also be stored within the POS system, allowing the pharmacy technician to print out any information regarding the patient's medication that the patient may request.

Department Codes

In most retail pharmacy settings, the sale of prescription and OTC drugs is not the only source of revenue. Large retail pharmacies like Walgreens and CVS provide their patrons with products ranging from beauty supplies to candy bars and sometimes, everything in between. Department codes are a way for the pharmacy to track inventory and costs. Department codes will vary from retailer to retailer, but it is important for the pharmacy technician to understand his or her pharmacy's codes in order to produce accurate and seamless transactions for the store's patrons.

Several issues can be tied to using incorrect department codes: Insurance payments can be declined, inventory levels can be incorrectly computed, or taxes can be incorrectly added or dropped from an item. One incorrectly used department code by itself may not seem like a big issue, but the same code or codes entered incorrectly several times can cause headaches, which no one wants.

Voiding Transactions

Voiding transactions is not something anyone likes doing. It can be time consuming and test the patience of those waiting in the checkout line. Transaction voids can happen for a variety of reasons: An item's price is coded incorrectly, the patient changes his or her mind about buying a product, or operator error. Whatever the reason for the void, you most likely will need the assistance of a manager or supervisor to complete the transaction. A receipt for the voided transaction will print out from the system once it is corrected; make certain to place the receipt in the cash register drawer, so it can be reconciled at the end of your shift.

If the void involves a payment transaction, you may need a few additional steps to complete the transaction. If the transaction was paid with cash or a check, you will need to process the void as either cash or a check. If it is a credit card or debit transaction, you will need to swipe the patron's card in order to refund the monies to his or her credit or bank account. If there is a refund due because of the voided transaction, then the patron must receive the refund in the same payment form he or she used to pay for the item. Again, these transactions will mostly likely require assistance from a manager or supervisor.

Taxable Versus Nontaxable Items

Sales tax is a state's way of producing funds for various projects, agencies, and school systems within that state. Determination of what is considered taxable and nontaxable varies from state to state. Prescription medications are not taxable; however, OTC products such as aspirin, cough medicine, or acetaminophen are subject to taxing. In most states items such as hearing aids and hearing aid batteries are not taxable, but items such as an Ace wrap or bandages are taxable. Most states require nontaxable items to be labeled as essentials and taxable items to be labeled as nonessentials. Again, these vary depending upon what state you live in.

Most cash registers will already have a specific state's item taxability requirements integrated into their computer's software. If a question of taxability does arise, it is always best to consult the store's manager or a supervisor. If items are not taxed correctly, it can lead to a store to being audited or having fines imposed from the state.

Pharmacy Technician Job Responsibilities

The daily duties of a pharmacy technician cover a vast number of tasks. One of the main responsibilities of the pharmacy technician in retail pharmacy is to assist the pharmacist in serving patients. Thus, the pharmacy technicians execute a variety of tasks under the supervision of the pharmacist. However, pharmacy technicians cannot counsel or give medical information or advice to patients. It is also the pharmacist's responsibility to perform the final check before a prescription is dispensed to a patient.

Other job responsibilities of the retail pharmacy technician include verifying drug deliveries, storing drugs, rotating stock, ordering drugs, and maintaining inventory records—and this is just the beginning. Pharmacy technicians also verify and accept new prescription and refill orders, as well as create and maintain patient profiles. Filling, compounding, and filing of medication orders are also within the scope of the pharmacy technician's practice. Technicians may also assist the pharmacist in the administration of the retail pharmacy, with duties that can include policy and procedure review, scheduling, and formulary issues. In short, a technician may perform any task that will assist the pharmacist in serving patients or pharmacy operations, with the exception of providing advice or drug-related information or dispensing legend drugs without a pharmacist's approval.

Becoming a pharmacy technician in a retail pharmacy setting is a very good career opportunity. Retail pharmacy is a great way to establish a position of status. Customers trust retail pharmacy technicians and value the services they provide. Most people who come into a local community pharmacy think of the staff almost as members of their families and trust the pharmacy team to provide the highest possible quality of service.

Tasks Requiring Quality Assurance

Quality assurance in pharmacy should really go without saying. Providing quality assurance to your patients in every area of pharmacy is essential not only from a safety aspect, but also to the future of your career. So, how do you make certain quality assurance is taken into consideration in every aspect of what you do as a pharmacy technician? What skills are mandatory for providing quality assurance, and what are the potential effects of not providing quality assurance?

Starting from the time a patient walks into your pharmacy, customer service is the first step in providing quality assurance. As oftentimes the initial point of reference, the pharmacy technician who provides a manner of quality assurance when communicating with patients takes the first step in providing superior patient care; effective and knowledgeable communication when speaking to patients means being able to not only ask the right questions but also look for the ones that go unsaid.

When a pharmacy technician first receives a prescription from a patient, there are some primary elements the pharmacy technician should be looking for:

- Patient name, address, and date of birth
- Name of prescriber and his or her DEA number, office number, and address
- Prescriber's signature on the prescription
- Name of the medication as well as the medication's form, route, directions, and amount to be dispensed
- Details of refills, if any

There are also some questions that the technician must remember to ask the patient:

- Does the patient have any allergies?
- Does the patient have a prescription plan?
- Does the older patient need non-child-resistant caps? If the patient does request non-child-resistant caps, remember to use an auxiliary label stating so.
- If allowable, would the patient like a generic substitution?
- Does the patient have any questions before starting the order entry process?

- Check to see if the patient is already in the computer base. If the patient is in the computer base, verify whether all information is correct, updating any information which is not. If the patient is not in the computer base, add him or her to the system: name, address, date of birth, and any insurance information the patient may have given to you.
- Read the prescription thoroughly before beginning the order entry process. Does it contain all the information necessary to fill the prescription: prescriber's name as well as prescriber's address, DEA number, office number, and signature?
- Does the prescription contain the medication name as well as medication form, strength, amount to be dispensed, and clear directions? If directions are not clear, consult the pharmacist.
- Does the prescription have refills and is a generic substitution allowable?

If all of these questions have been answered, then proceed with computer entry.

Most computer software will have a space where the operator can input the medication's lot number and expiration so this information also prints on the patient's label. Once all information has been entered into the computer, take a moment to double-check your work; if necessary ask for a second set of eyes. Sometimes another person's perspective can pick up the smallest mistake, which could have the potential for becoming a much larger one. Print out the label only after you are certain the information is correct. Read over your label before handing it off to be filled; if you do find a mistake, correct the information before the filling process begins.

Filling the patient's prescription is perhaps an area where quality assurance speaks louder than others. An incorrect medication or dose could cause harm or possibly even death to a patient. Quality assurance when filling a patient's prescription should be at the top of every pharmacy technician's list. There are some precautions the pharmacy technician can take when filling patient medications:

- Read the patient medication label carefully and compare it to the original prescription. Is all the information correct: patient information, prescriber information, medication, and directions?
- Read the medication label before you begin to count. Is it the correct medication and dosage? Do the expiration date and lot numbers match those on the label? What is the amount to be dispensed?
- Count out and package the medication. Did you count correctly? Is the packaging appropriate for the medication? What auxiliary labels might be needed for the medication? Did the patient request non-childproof caps?
- Ask the patient if he or she needs a consultation with the pharmacist. Most of the time this will be for new prescriptions, but a pharmacy technician who recognizes a patient who needs education, even on refills, protects the patient's safety. Under no circumstance should a pharmacy technician give patient medication information. This is a job for the pharmacist only and cannot be re-enforced enough.

- Make sure all consumer medication information is attached to the prescription. This information can sometimes be a reference point for the patient, especially if the patient forgotten what the pharmacist has told him or her.
- Respect the patient's privacy. If a patient has a question concerning the patient's medication or has issues with his or her prescription plan, try to solve the issue in a manner that gives the patient privacy. No one likes to have his or her problems shouted across a busy pharmacy. Remember, the HIPAA provides for the patient's right to privacy concerning the patient's medical information.
- Thank the patient. Everyone likes to know you appreciate his or her patronage, and it may very well be the one thing that keeps the patient returning to your pharmacy in the future.

Many companies succeed or fail because of their quality assurance. Pharmacy is no different. The Merriam-Webster dictionary defines *quality assurance* in this way:

a program for the systematic monitoring and evaluation of the various aspects of a project, service, or facility to ensure that standards of quality are being met.

In pharmacy quality assurance must be a continuous process in order to assure patient safety and satisfaction. The pharmacy technician who evaluates processes in order to improve outcome has quality assurance as a motto and a long, satisfying career in pharmacy.

Providing Requested Information to the Pharmacist

Pharmacists and pharmacy technicians are the backbone of the pharmacy profession. The ability of the two professional disciplines to work in tandem requires trust, knowledge, and integrity. While it is true that pharmacy technicians will never replace pharmacists for duties such as patient medication counseling, it does not mean the pharmacist does not rely on the technician to supply him or her with the information necessary to carry out patient medication counseling.

A pharmacy technician becomes an extension of the pharmacist. On any given day, the pharmacist may ask the technician to supply various types of information necessary for the filling of prescriptions. A pharmacist might request a patient's medication profile when speaking to a prescriber or ask you to call a prescriber's office. A pharmacist may ask the technician to verify information with the patient such as current medications, prescription and OTC, patient allergies and drug reactions, or perhaps even insurance information. It would not be unusual for the pharmacist to request the pharmacy technician check with the wholesaler for the availability and price of a particular medication. When compounding special medications pharmacists will ask the technician to provide them with the steps they will use to complete the compound.

Providing the pharmacist with requested information in an expedient, professional manner builds trust between the technician and the pharmacist. Knowing what information the pharmacist needs to effectively speak with a prescriber or a patient shows the pharmacist that the technician has a sound knowledge base. A technician whose goal is to work with the pharmacist for the betterment of the patient shows they have integrity.

Situations to Alert the Pharmacist

A pharmacy technician is often the right arm of a pharmacist. Still, there are several situations that need the attention of a pharmacist. The pharmacy technician who learns to recognize these situations may sidestep even greater issues later on.

In general taking refill requests can be handled by the pharmacy technician. As long as the prescription has refills available (no more than five in a six-month period), the refill is within the patient's prescription plan refill policy (typically a 30-day window), and the refill request is not for a C-II drug, then most likely the refill can be done. There are, however, times when a pharmacist should be alerted during a refill request.

If a patient who has had an existing prescription refilled several times requests to speak with a pharmacist concerning this medication, alert the pharmacist. A pharmacy technician should never consult or give advice concerning medications. This is a pharmacist's responsibility only and should always be handled as such, no matter how many times the patient has refilled the medication.

Another situation that would call for a pharmacist is refilling C-II narcotics, which cannot be refilled, but instead by law require a new prescription from the prescriber each time the drug is ordered. This is the law and cannot be altered under any circumstances. The pharmacist may call the prescriber requesting a facsimile of the written prescription, but will need the original paper prescription on file before the medication can be dispensed to the patient. Pharmacists may take C-II prescriptions from prescribers over the phone only in an extreme emergency. In such cases, the pharmacist may dispense only a few days' medication and the prescriber must give the original written prescription to the pharmacy within seven days.

Forged and altered prescriptions are a monstrous business, which can be very lucrative for the abuser. A pharmacy technician who recognizes the signs of a forged or altered prescription should always alert the pharmacist if the technician has suspicions. If while taking a refill request from a patient, the pharmacy technician realizes the prescription is stolen, the technician should alert the pharmacist who can then refuse to fill the prescription and alert the proper authorities. The pharmacist can then contact the necessary authorities, helping to curtail the success of the abusers.

If at any time a pharmacy technician has concerns or question regarding a refill request such as a possible drug interaction or allergy, then the technician should notify the pharmacist; being alert to these situations helps to avoid even bigger issues later on.

When if entering a patient's prescription a drug interaction alert pops up on the computer screen, a pharmacy technician should always make the pharmacist aware of the potential interaction. A pharmacy technician should never override an alert because he or she believes it to be harmless or because the pharmacist is too busy. Bypassing such alerts could have irreversible effects for the patient as well as the pharmacy.

The pharmacy technician who alerts the pharmacist to a patient medication counseling need is proactive in preventing unintentional harm to the patient. Since the technician knows patient counseling is a pharmacist duty, alerting the pharmacist when the technician sees a need arise is the only available choice.

A pharmacy technician must also alert a pharmacist when a prescriber needs to give a prescription over the phone. A technician may take refill request, but never new medication prescriptions. If a prescriber has questions concerning a drug, a pharmacist must provide this information. There is never a circumstance where it is OK for a pharmacy technician to provide medication information.

Finally, if a pharmacy technician believes there is a situation that may cause potential harm to a patient such as drug-to-drug interaction, patient allergies, or incorrect dosing, it is well within in the scope of the pharmacy technician to alert the pharmacist to his or her concerns. Presenting the technician's concerns in a professional manner shows the pharmacist that the technician has patient safety as his or her primary goal.

Types of Questions a Technician Can Answer

The Pharmacy Technician Certification Board (PTCB) estimates that as of March 2012 there are 446,872 certified pharmacy technicians in the United States. All but a handful of states, Colorado, Hawaii, Indiana, Michigan, New York, Pennsylvania, and Wisconsin, regulate pharmacy technicians. In some states the regulation is as simple as requiring certification, and in other states educational requirements, licensure, and registration with the SBOP are mandated.

As the role of pharmacy technicians continues to expand, so will the educational needs and state regulations concerning their scope of practice. Still, there are limitations not only on the type of task a pharmacy technician can perform, but also the type of information he or she is allowed to relay to patients.

There is, however, some information that pharmacy technicians may relay to patients. An appropriate circumstance might be if patients request to find out the number of refills available on their prescription, or if they need to know the last time they had the medication filled. Insurance and billing questions are also appropriate for the pharmacy technician to answer. A technician can also answer questions pertaining to the cost of a medication. If a prescriber calls requesting a list of his or her patient's medication, a technician may answer, but only after verifying the prescriber's information. A patient may have a question concerning where the patient might find a particular OTC item; a technician may give him or her directions to the item, but should not give advice on the medication itself such as interactions or usage. A pharmacy technician may also relay information concerning medication form or strength, but again should never relay usage or administration information.

If pharmacy technicians are uncertain whether or not they may answer a question a patient or prescriber has asked them, then they should always check with the pharmacist for verification. In any pharmacy setting the pharmacist has the last word.

A pharmacy technician, who seeks to be a professional, not only respects this, but works to maintain it as well.

Medical Information Systems

A medical information system is the computer hardware and medical base software a pharmacy uses to store information. Advancements in technology have created software for computers, which can process more efficient and more accurate information. Today's medical information systems can not only store patient information, but also connect to a network of other computer systems such as insurance companies, government agencies, and drug wholesalers.

Each individual pharmacy will have a proprietary system for storing medical information. The software associated with the pharmacy's medical information may also be proprietary and requires training from qualified personnel in order to master it. A technician who learns the idiosyncrasies of his or her pharmacy's medical information system places himself or herself at an advantage.

Computer systems that are meant to process and store large amounts of information can sometimes feel daunting to the user, but with training, patience, and time can be a needed ally when processing patient medication prescriptions.

Uses

Medical information systems can be used for any number of situations that might call for secure storage of information. In a retail pharmacy, medical information systems are used as a way to store patient profiles, input patient prescriptions, verify insurance information, alert the pharmacy personnel to possible medication interactions, provide critical patient medication information, store copies of patient prescriptions, check inventory levels, and receive patient payments and insurance co-pays.

Automated dispensing cabinets (Pyxis, Omnicell) also store medical information and are an extension of an institution's computer system. Automated dispensing cabinets have a computer monitor and software integrated into the cabinet. Information is input into the institution's main computer system and connected with the software of the automated dispensing cabinet, automatically updating a patient's information or medication profile.

Pharmacy relies on medical information systems not only as a way to protect the privacy of its patients, but also as a source of information. Drug information sources like Lexicomp and Micromedix can easily be found through an Internet search engine, becoming a useful tool when a pharmacist requests a technician to search for medication information.

The use of medical information systems continues to expand and has become an important link between patient care and prescription medication information. Safeguards encoded in software and bar-coding help to prevent errors during the order entry and filling process. The ability to obtain extensive amounts of information from Internet drug information sites helps to keep prescribers and patients informed.

Career advancement for the pharmacy technician who understands medical information systems increases as the technician becomes more involved with the process of medical information systems.

Impact on Quality Decision Making

Decision making in pharmacy cannot be a haphazard event. Pharmacy technicians must be able to make clear knowledge-based decisions daily. The process of decision making occurs in almost every aspect of a pharmacy technician's responsibilities, from deciding how workflow should progress to what information needs the attention of a pharmacist.

Medical information systems have helped and complicated the decision-making process. Medical information systems have made it easier to compile a patient's medical information in one place; personal, financial, and medication information all live together on the same little microchip. It is a time-saving mechanism, which contains sensitive information essential to the privacy of the patient. A pharmacy technician must make a conscious decision to protect the patient's information. The HIPAA has very stringent rules regarding patient's medical information, and violation of these regulations can lead to substantial fines or, in extreme cases of privacy violation, incarceration.

Medical software is able to put together bits and pieces of a patient's profile, alerting pharmacy personnel to the patient's drug allergies and potential drug interactions. A pharmacy technician should always take these warnings for what that are: a safeguard. A technician who possesses mature decision-making skills knows that these warnings should be brought to the attention of the pharmacist. A licensed pharmacist is the only one capable of deciding the validity of a medication alert.

Medical information systems have also made it easier for pharmacy technicians to obtain medication information. The ability to search a database for needed medication information is much easier than sifting through hundreds of pages of information in a reference book. Still, this information is intended for the use of the pharmacist; bypassing the pharmacist and giving this information directly to the patient constitutes consultation, which is unlawful for the pharmacy technician to do.

Medical information systems can challenge the decision making of the pharmacy technician, but it is the pharmacy technician who thinks clearly through the decision-making process who gains the most benefit.

Characteristics of Typical Database

Medical information databases contain large amounts of information, which are useful for filling patient medication prescriptions and/or providing patient medication information. Patient profiles contain information pertaining to a particular patient: name, address, date of birth, allergies, prescribers, insurance payers, and current medications.

Medical databases also contain information to assist the pharmacist with patient consultation. Pharmacy technicians may also take advantage of this database by printing out consumer medication information for patient medication prescriptions.

Patient insurance information from the pharmacy's medical database can be transported to another medical database, authorizing payment and verifying insurance eligibility.

Databases can help in the management of potential medication interactions, decreasing the chance of an adverse reaction affecting the patient. Databases can alert staff to high-risk medication indicators or medications that may be contraindicated with another.

Inventory control is also a large part of medical databases. Inventory databases store information pertaining to a pharmacy's stock, pricing, and wholesaler. Inventory databases typically have a direct connection to the pharmacy's wholesaler database, giving the pharmacy the ability to know immediately the availability, price, and generic equivalent of any medication.

Finally, for pharmacy technicians or pharmacists who have management responsibilities, medical databases may store information relevant to their pharmacy and its employees. Employee names, Social Security numbers, rates of pay, and hours worked are a few possibilities.

The information within a medical database is sensitive information and should be protected at all times. Pharmacies must abide by the HIPAA regulations in regards to patient information. Employee information should not be shared with anyone who does not have authority to have such information. Protecting this information can be as simple as signing off a computer when leaving a station for any length of time or not sharing your password with coworkers, simple steps that can make a big difference.

Medication Use Review

Medication use review is an extension of the Omnibus Budget Reconciliation Act of 1990. Medication use review is used by state and federal agencies as a way to improve the cost-effectiveness and quality of medication therapies as well as evaluate safety issues, which might exist during the dispensing phase of therapy.

Each state is required to set up its own guidelines concerning medication use review, and committees consist of both pharmacists and physicians. Medication use reviews were initially aimed at Medicaid recipients in order to gain a greater understanding of their medications and provide them with cost-effective and therapy-appropriate medication, but most states have expanded the requirements to include all patients who might receive medication therapies.

Pharmacists have become the most involved members of medication use review. Greater patient counseling duties have increased the need for pharmacy technicians, with job estimates predicting a continued need.

Purpose

The purpose behind patient medication reviews is simple: Provide the patient with the best care possible, in the safest, most cost-effective manner available—a simple concept, with a great potential for improved patient care and safety.

Medication use review committees collect data, which evaluates the cost-effectiveness of a drug, the usefulness of the drug within a therapy, if the drug is being prescribed for its indicated use, and any safety issues. Once these key points are complied, recommendations can be made to continue a patient drug therapy or develop a new plan of therapy.

Medication use reviews were also intended as a way to catch prescription fraud or overuse of prescription writing from a particular prescriber.

Structure

Medication use review involves pharmacists and physicians specifically chosen by the state to conduct regular committee meeting. Physicians and pharmacists discuss specific patient therapies and make recommendations based upon safety, cost-effectiveness, and current prescribing and filling issues.

Once the medication use review collects the necessary data and complies its finding, it will be brought before the Medicaid board for further recommendation. Further recommendation could include discontinuation of a drug or prior authorization measures.

The Pharmacy Technician's Role

The pharmacy technician's role in medication use review involves the need for more technicians. As pharmacists are relegated to more consulting duties, the technician's job responsibilities will change. Regulations regarding technician education, licensure, and certification will be necessary on not only a state but a federal level as well.

Technicians will need to become more versed in the laws affecting patient counseling, learning to detect which patients are in need of consulting with the pharmacist. It is unlawful for technicians to consult patients on any level, but understanding who needs consultation will aid the pharmacist in mandatory patient counseling duties.

Productivity and Workflow Management

Productivity and workflow are two terms that live simultaneously together; you cannot have one without the other. Management of these two terms is essential to the success of any pharmacy. Pharmacy technicians who have a strong conviction for understanding the true depth of the definition of these terms help to provide not only a friendlier workplace environment, but also patient care, which encourages repeated patronage.

No one likes to feel as if he or she is running in circles during his or her workday. Patients do not enjoy standing in long lines. Frustrations can build quickly when these two factors go head to head. A technician who understands his or her productivity is directly related to workflow also understands productivity and workflow are also responsible for patient satisfaction (or dissatisfaction), as well as his or her own personal job satisfaction. If your patients do not return because they are less than satisfied with how long it takes for you to fill their prescription, then chances are the product (patient prescriptions) you have to produce will decrease. However, if your workflow (how you go about production) works as one smooth operation, then you

can produce more (fill more prescriptions) and your patrons will return because of the quality and efficiency of both.

The added benefit to the attention a pharmacy technician takes with production and workflow is the potential for career advancement. Managers and pharmacist recognize when operations run poorly, but they also recognize operations that operate smoothly. Productivity and workflow will be seen not only in the pharmacy's financials, but in the production of the pharmacy as a whole.

Productivity

Productivity—ask any economist or business person, and you will probably get the standard textbook answer—*the rate at which goods or services are produced, especially output per unit of labor*. A much simpler definition might be: Is the value of what you are producing greater than the time it takes to produce? If the answer to this question is *no*, then chances are profits are low, as well as patient and employee satisfaction.

As much as we may not want to believe it, pharmacy is a business and there are several factors that affect its profits; productivity is one of those things. Productivity can be harmed by several factors: cost of drugs from the wholesaler, cost involved with employees (payroll and benefits), standard cost of operation (licensure, insurance, and utilities), cost of equipment (computer systems, software, and medication storage systems), marketing cost (advertisement and sale circulars), cost of medications packaging, and the list can go on and on.

Keeping a tight rein on the cost associated with production will have a much more favorable effect on the bottom line of pharmacy's productivity. A pharmacy technician, who works to control cost when it is possible, without sacrificing patient care, can help to produce a safe, cost-efficient product, which can then be passed onto the patient, gaining satisfaction for all involved.

Use of Productivity Data

What is productivity data? How can it be used to improve productivity? How do you collect productivity data? These are all questions that should be asked when evaluating productivity data. Understanding the effects the data has will do a long way in making the changes necessary to improve productivity.

Productivity data is the measurements used to evaluate if the cost involved with producing a product is greater than the profits gained from production of the product. In pharmacy the product is patient medication prescriptions and the cost of production is the cost necessary for the day-to-day operation of the pharmacy.

Some obvious productivity data that can be collected is the cost associated with purchasing medication from the drug wholesaler. Comparing fluctuation of drug pricing can allow you to adjust pricing, causing less of issue with profit margins. Computer software allows pharmacies to track not only available inventory but also inventory pricing history, making it easier to see where pricing needs to be adjusted.

When it comes to productivity, data computer software is a needed friend. Pharmacy-based computer software can compile daily, weekly, or monthly data on prescription production.

This information coupled with the cost of operation can help a pharmacy see where it might need to cut costs in order for productivity to improve. But productivity is not always simply about cutting cost.

Productivity data can also point to processes that need to be re-evaluated so they run more efficiently and in turn increase the rate of productivity. Evaluating a process for efficiency may involve observation, collecting data, or perhaps even comparing your processes with those of another pharmacy. Bringing all this information together allows the process to be examined and then make the necessary changes.

Productivity data is valuable, but only if it is used from an unbiased perspective, meaning the information should not be used to favor strictly one aspect. In pharmacy productivity in not solely about the amount of profit, but rather how your patient's safety and satisfaction with your production affects your profits. Patients who have to wait in long prescription lines or who feel their question has not been adequately answered will not return. Patient surveys can help produce the data needed to see where improvements need to be made. Surveys that include questions concerning ease of process, customer service, cost, wait times, and medication consultation will help provide a much clearer picture.

Use of productivity data is a must for a positive outcome when evaluating productivity. Pharmacy technicians who have a knowledgeable understanding of how to apply this data elevate productivity and increase chances for future career advancement.

Productivity Measurement Systems

One of the best productivity measurement systems a pharmacy has is its employees. Pharmacist and pharmacy technicians who complete the same tasks and procedures on a daily basis have a keen sense for evaluating a process that they believe may be hampering productivity. Being able to have a physical measurement of issues that need improvement can streamline process and increase productivity.

Computer software is also a valuable system for the measurement of productivity. Computer systems are able to store large amounts of data over any given period of time, making it easier when it comes to comparison of data. A computer-generated report, which gives the user a side-by-side comparison of data, allows the user to not only track production cost and productivity, but also evaluate where changes are necessary for production to improve.

Performance evaluations may not be an immediate thought when it comes to productivity measurement systems, but they are a much more useful tool than one thing. Productivity relies on two things: cost of the product and the time it takes to produce the product. In a pharmacy setting, the time of production is largely dependent upon the efficiency and knowledge of its staff. Yearly performance evaluations separate out areas where employees may need further education or training. Performance evaluation can also suggest what an employee's greatest strengths might be, allowing the employer to use these strengths to its advantage and improving productivity.

Finally, the use of patient surveys cannot be undervalued. Patient-generated surveys can help seal gaps in productivity, which pharmacies do not realize are issues. Suggestions from patients can be a much needed view from outside the pharmacy. Gathering this type of information can cut cost and wait time as well as improve patient medication consultation and the overall safety and satisfaction of the patient.

The Pharmacy Technician's Role

What role can the pharmacy technician play in productivity? A pharmacy's life blood is its employees. No matter how cost-effective a pharmacy might be, if its pharmacists and pharmacy technicians are unable to provide their patrons with quality customer service and trusted, knowledge-based medication information, the patrons will seek the services of another pharmacy.

A pharmacy technician can take a proactive role in the productivity of a pharmacy. Observation is the technician's most valuable asset in the evaluation of productivity. A pharmacy technician who observes a cost or process that is detrimental to productivity should bring his or her concerns to the proper individuals, typically the pharmacy manager or head pharmacist. Simply making those in charge aware of a situation is half the battle.

A pharmacy technician can also help to increase productivity if the technician feels he or she is lacking skills that could improve productivity. If a technician feels he or she needs additional training or further education, the technician should again speak with the pharmacy manager or head pharmacist who will be able to direct the technician through the steps necessary in meeting his or her needs.

Listening to patient's complaints can be an unpleasant task, but a pharmacy technician who realizes he or she is hearing the same complaint multiple times from patients will recognize a need to correct the problem. Correcting issues that are troublesome to a large number of patients may just be the one thing needed to increase productivity.

Finally, a technician who helps to retain pharmacy cost, such as seeking larger discounts from wholesalers, taking full advantage of wholesale specials, seeking discounts for packaging and supplies, conservation of utility cost, or cost associated with wasted and expired medication, proves the technician is in tune with the value of productivity. Technicians who keep this as part of their daily routine will be able to leverage their pharmacy career and have greater job satisfaction, knowing they are an essential part of the pharmacy's productivity.

Workflow Management

Workflow management is an intricate part of the prescription filling process. Workflow is the steps or process taken to complete a task. Workflow management is how the steps or process is controlled. Workflow if left unmanaged will soon become uncontrolled and counterproductive to productivity. In a pharmacy setting unmanaged workflow can have irreversible, negative consequences.

The goal of workflow management is to be able to produce a safe quality product in an efficient, cost-contained method, which returns the highest rate of productivity. In a pharmacy setting, workflow hampered by interruptions, distractions, or processes that are in need of improvement can be costly.

Improperly managed workflow can cause medication errors, waste valuable time, and see tempers flare. Processes are important, and improvement of those processes is a continuous job. Pharmacy technicians who are aware of issues with workflow management can help to minimize problems and suggest solutions, creating a much friendlier atmosphere for workflow management.

Managing Your Own Workflow

Being able to manage one's own workflow is perhaps one of the central solutions for continuous, unhampered workflow and productivity. Feeling overwhelmed or not understanding a process will make a situation worse before it makes it better. But there are several ways a pharmacy technician goes about managing his or her own workflow:

- Be on time. A technician who is chronically late for his or her shift not only starts out at a disadvantage but also puts undue stress on his or her coworkers.
- Come to work ready to work. Unnecessary chatter and interruptions from personnel phone calls can be distracting and lead to a greater chance for mistakes.
- Organize. It is difficult for you to manage workflow if you are constantly searching for the tools you need to complete the task.
- Prioritize. Being able to prioritize tasks or prescriptions will head off potential problems. Recognizing a mom with a sick and crying infant takes priority over a refill request will be well worth the extra effort.
- Clearly understand pharmacy policies and procedures. If you have a clear understanding of the reasons behind a policy or procedure, then chances are you will be able to carry it out more efficiently, making it a sustained part of your workflow.
- Get involved with workflow issues. If you are not part of the solution, then perhaps you are part of the problem. Keeping workflow issues to yourself does nothing to solve them; speaking with the pharmacy manager or pharmacist in charge may just be the answer.
- Actively seek training and educational opportunities. The process of improvement is an unending circle; widening your knowledge base can improve current workflow and create new ideas for workflow where they are needed.

Managing one's workflow is not just case of personal preference, but rather a systematic process constantly open to changes and improvement, which helps increase productivity and makes workflow a seamless process.

Delegation

The act of delegation involves entrusting a person to perform a specific task, which you feel the person is best suited to perform. Everyone has his or her own special talent or skill set; delegating the best person for the task keeps workflow moving and produces the best results for productivity.

Sometimes recognizing what task should be delegated to whom needs to be done by trial and error; after some observation it will become clear who the best candidate is for the job. Productivity and workflow are a team effort; delegating task based upon a person's specialized skill is good business practice and in the aspect of pharmacy sometimes lawfully necessary. A technician cannot be delegated to perform patient medication counseling or make a judgment call concerning a medication alert; by law these duties can be performed only by a licensed pharmacist. Conversely, if a technician has a greater skill set when it comes to inventory, it may be appropriate to make him or her responsible for inventory ordering and control.

Delegation is meant to help improve productivity and workflow; if those who have been delegated a particular task are not helping to improve or, at the very least, keep the process consistent, then it may be time to rethink delegation of duties.

Patient Confidentiality and HIPAA

Patient confidentiality is an important concept for the pharmacy technician, who has access to large amounts of information that patients trust will not be exposed or released unless they grant permission. Electronic health information on a pharmacy's computer system, electronic prescribing data from physicians, transferred patient profiles from outside providers, prescription drug information, and payment records are all examples of information that pharmacy employees are required to maintain as confidential information.

Protected Health Information

A patient's confidential information is commonly referred to as *protected health information* (*PHI*). PHI includes past, present, and future records or information pertaining to treatment or care received for physical or mental health, the rendering of that care, and payment for such services.

The question most commonly asked regarding PHI is, "When are you allowed to disclose or use a patient's confidential information in a pharmacy?" The short answer is that it is acceptable to do so when providing treatment to the patient or the patient's caregiver, when providing information to other health care providers who are caring for the patient, or while processing most payment and operational activities.

The Health Insurance Portability and Accountability Act

A more complex answer to the question requires background knowledge of the primary law governing pharmacies and their disclosure of PHI. The Health Insurance Portability and Accountability Act (HIPAA) of 1996 is a complex law that has greatly affected the entire health care system; it notably affects pharmacy practice because the privacy rules regulate the use of patients' health information.

On April 14, 2003, the HIPAA privacy regulations took effect. On and after that date, pharmacies were required to comply with all requirements relating to protection of patient confidentiality. You may have noticed significant changes in the way pharmacy technicians and pharmacists are now able to transfer and communicate a patient's PHI. New patients at any pharmacy will continue to be required to sign an acknowledgement of receipt of such privacy practices.

Your employer is also required to train all personnel on HIPAA requirements. In addition to the requirements set forth in HIPAA, any pharmacy may create its own systems to further protect and ensure patient confidentiality, as long as the requirements are equivalent to or stricter than those mandated by HIPAA. At the minimum, HIPAA set a standard for protecting patient information to prevent abuse of the privilege of having access to PHI.

Another common question relating to confidentiality of PHI is, "How much of a patient's confidential information can you disclose?" The standard of practice is known as the *minimum necessary standard.* This is interpreted to mean that you use or release the minimum amount of information needed to complete the task that requires you to use or disclose information. It can occasionally be difficult to judge when and where you can use a patient's PHI. Always ask for a second opinion if you feel uncomfortable releasing or revealing PHI.

There are certain circumstances in pharmacy practice in which these requirements do not apply. This includes when you are communicating directly with the patient, there is no need to withhold the patient's personal information from the actual patient. Also, patients may waive their right to confidentiality or authorize you directly to use the information more freely. The most common situation in pharmacy practice in which the minimum necessary standard does not apply is when communicating with other health care providers who are involved in providing care for the patient. In this circumstance, the information is needed to provide congruent care. Finally, if you are ever required by court order or subpoena or government agency regulation to disclose information, you are authorized to do so.

An interesting feature of the HIPAA regulation is that patients were granted explicit rights relating to their PHI. For example, patients have the right to request additional restrictions on disclosure of PHI, obtain copies of their PHI, request changes to their PHI, or request information about to whom the pharmacy has disclosed their PHI outside of the normal pharmacy communications. These are all examples of the affirmative rights provided to patients under the privacy rules enacted with HIPAA.

If you are ever uncertain about whether you are permitted to utilize confidential information, it is best to request permission, or at a minimum discuss the situation with a pharmacist or pharmacy manager. It is always best to be cautious when handling confidential information. It is also acceptable to request written patient authorization to ensure that disclosure or use of information is acceptable to the patient. Note that trash containing any privileged information (e.g. name and Social Security number) must be disposed of properly, such as by shredding or incineration. In addition, PHI should not be discussed around "the water cooler" or within earshot of bystanders, as this is also a violation of HIPAA.

Discretion is also pertinent now that specified consequences can result from improper use of PHI by a pharmacist, pharmacy technician, or other employee. In general, an investigation will occur if any allegations are made relating to violations of the HIPAA privacy rules. Penalties can range from $100 for a single violation to $250,000 and 10 years in jail for aggregate violations within a calendar year.

The HIPAA rules have certainly changed the practice of pharmacy. They have provided enhanced structure and guidance as to the manner in which, and the extent to which, pharmacy personnel can handle PHI. Pharmacy personnel will continue to improve their understanding of the privacy rules of HIPAA as more time elapses and further clarifications are issued concerning various practice settings. Until then, continue to use discretion when handling a patient's PHI and respect the fact that it certainly is a privilege for pharmacy personnel to use such information.

Proprietary Business Information

Proprietary business information is defined as sensitive information owned by a company and that gives the company certain competitive advantages. In other words, it is the company's business secrets. Pharmacies are a business and therefore have proprietary business information that should be protected. Some examples of proprietary business information for a retail pharmacy setting are:

- Monetary information—cost which may be related to a company's overhead, sales contracts, profit margins, or losses
- Merchandising—company-planned advertising, planned or potential merchandise, or a company's position within a certain market
- Production—a company's wholesaler, inventories, prescription record, or future expansion

Proprietary business information is often the key to a business's success and should be protected by its employees. Pharmacy technicians should learn to recognize the information their pharmacy defines as proprietary. Keeping this information confidential portrays the pharmacy technician as trusted professional.

Forged or Altered Prescriptions

The forging or altering of prescription medications has been an issue since the inception of the first known pharmacy, but in recent years the Drug Enforcement Agency has seen a sharp upturn in the number of forged or altered prescriptions. C-II and C-III prescriptions are the most frequently forged or altered prescriptions, but illegal prescriptions for benzodiazepines such as Valium (diazepam), Xanax (alprazolam), and Ativan (lorazapam) as well as stimulants like Ritalin (methylphenidate) and Adderall (amphetamine/dextroamphetamine) are also victimized.

There seems to be no limit of imagination with the criminal mindset of those trying to gain illegal access to prescription medications. Prescription pads are often stolen from physicians' offices, printed illegally and used with a fake physician name, or printed with a real physician's name, but with a different office number, which leads to an accomplish who pretends to be the physician.

Forgery and alterations of prescription medications have gotten so bad, that in April 2008, the Centers for Medicare and Medicaid Services (CMS) passed a law that required prescribers to use tamper-resistant prescription pads any time they wrote a prescription for a patient who used Medicare or Medicaid services. A CMS tamper-resistant prescription pad needed to meet at least one of three allowable requirements: not able to be copied, modified, or counterfeited. In October 2008 CMS expanded its requirement to include all three characteristics. In order for prescribers to receive payment, per CMS, states must ensure all three markers are used in qualifying prescription pads, allowing them to be labeled as tamper-resistant.

Forging and altering prescription medications is a very profitable business for abusers and a very costly business for pharmacies, as well as federal and state agencies. Knowing how to detect a forged or altered prescription helps to attack this issue head on.

Detection

So how do you know if you have a forged or altered prescription? This answer might not be as simple as it seems. Forgers are constantly improving their craft, making it more difficult for authorities to apprehend them. There are, however, some telltale signs pharmacy technicians can use to recognize an illegitimate prescription.

- The handwriting is too neat; prescribers' handwriting is notoriously illegible, and forgery is one of the reasons why.
- Directions are written out with no acceptable abbreviations; 1 tablet q6 h is written out as one tablet every six hours.
- Prescription is not written out in the standard black ink; a prescription written in red, green, or blue ink should be an alert.
- The prescription looks like it has been copied—today's photocopiers can produce copies that look very much like the original; make sure to look closely if you have any suspicions.
- Amount written is an unusually large quantity, or dosing is beyond recommendations.

Even with these alerts illegal prescription passes by pharmacy technicians and pharmacist every day, but there are some simply steps you can take to protect yourself from being taken in by forgers.

- Become familiar with the prescribers in your area; learn to recognize their signatures, most are very distinct.
- Remember your patients; if you have a prescription from someone who has never used your pharmacy before or you do not recognize the person from your community, there may be cause for concern.
- Look at the date on the prescription; if the date is more than a few days from when the prescription was written by the prescriber, then there may be reason to question the prescription's validity.

Detecting a prescription that has been stolen, forged, or altered is not always easy, but having the knowledge needed to alert the pharmacist can be an invaluable tool for the pharmacy technician.

PROFILES IN PRACTICE

Jamie, a certified pharmacy technician, works at an independent pharmacy in her local community. Jamie knows most of her patients and greets them by name as they come into the pharmacy. One day Jamie sees a face she does not recognize, but she continues with her technician responsibilities. The new patron comes to the pharmacy counter and hands Jamie a prescription. Right away there are a few things Jamie sees on the prescription, which are not correct. The prescription is written for 100 Percocet tablets. The instructions are written out as one tablet four times a day and not 1 tablet qid. She does recognize the prescriber, but knows it is not Dr. Franklin's signature.

▶ What should Jamie do?

The first thing Jamie should do if she has any suspicions concerning a prescription is to speak with her pharmacist about why she has suspicions. The pharmacist will then call the prescriber to find out if the prescription was indeed written by him or her, while also verifying the patient name, medication, and directions. If the pharmacist still feels this may be an illegitimate prescription he or she may tell Jamie to ask the patient for identification. If the patient refuses or the identification does not match the patient, then the pharmacist can refuse to fill the prescription. Local authorities should be alerted, as the thief will most likely move on to the next pharmacy.

Strangers are not the only alarm of suspicious prescription activity. Other alerts include:

- A prescriber who writes an unusually large number of prescriptions in a short period of time, particularly if they are C-II or C-III prescriptions.
- A patient who returns to the pharmacy more than normal, several times a month or, sometimes, a week.
- Several patrons who are unrecognizable from the community or who have never used your pharmacy services begin to filter in with several prescriptions, all written by the same prescriber.

As a pharmacy technician, the most important thing to remember is that is OK to alert the pharmacist if the technician suspects the prescription is stolen, forged, or altered. Alerting local authorities, State Boards of Pharmacy, and the DEA helps to combat this growing issue.

Immunizations

The question of whether or not pharmacies should provide immunization services to their patrons is widely contested, yet large chains such as Walgreens, CVS, and Rite Aid and even smaller independent pharmacies have offered flu injections to their patrons for several years. Some of these pharmacies have now expanded their services to include immunizations, the most common being hepatitis A and B, pertussis, and pneumococcal.

Pharmacists are permitted to give immunizations in all 50 states, but the type of immunization, the pharmacist training requirements, and whom they may give immunizations to are determined by individual State Boards of Pharmacy. The increase of immunization services has more than tripled in recent years, expanding the roles of pharmacists and pharmacy technicians alike.

While the process of giving immunizations is strictly a duty for a pharmacist who has been trained and certified to do so, pharmacy technicians also play a valuable part in this process. A few of the variables that might require the attention of a pharmacy technician include ordering of immunization stock, proper storage of immunization stock (most need refrigeration), billing and payment of immunizations, as well as gathering patient information prior to immunizations (particularly allergies or possible allergic reactions).

As the commonality of pharmacies providing immunization services increases, so will the need for pharmacy technicians' knowledge regarding immunizations. Most immunizations have specific storage guidelines, most noticeably the need for refrigeration or freezing. Monitoring of the freezers and refrigerators used to store immunizations will be a daily task. Ordering immunization and collecting daily stock levels of immunizations will also be essential. Payment from patient insurance and prescription plans may require the technician to learn new billing codes. Organizing patient profiles and information concerning allergies, medication reactions, and next dose will be a noteworthy service, which may be added to the pharmacy technicians' responsibilities. No matter what role the pharmacy technician plays, helping the process to be a smooth, safe, and positive transaction for the patient is the most important.

Summary

Retail pharmacy is the largest category of pharmacy in the United States and encompasses chain pharmacies, independent/franchise pharmacies, and clinic pharmacies. Retail pharmacies are staffed by a pharmacist in charge, pharmacy manager, staff pharmacists, pharmacy technicians, and possibly pharmacy clerks. It is a fast-paced work environment, in which pharmacy professionals interact with and directly serve patients face to face.

Chapter Review Questions

1. Which of the following is *not* an example of an ambulatory or a retail pharmacy?
   a. franchise or chain pharmacy
   b. nursing home pharmacy
   c. privately owned pharmacy
   d. hospital outpatient pharmacy

2. The _____ is the agency that registers and regulates retail pharmacy facilities, pharmacists, and pharmacy technicians.
   a. CMS
   b. DEA
   c. FDA
   d. SBOP

3. The third set of numbers in an NDC Number represents the _____.
   a. manufacturer
   b. cost
   c. drug strength
   d. package size

4. A prescription must contain which of the following drug information?
   a. name of the medication
   b. strength
   c. dosage form
   d. all of the above

5. Which of the following is *not* the responsibility of a pharmacy technician?
   a. verifying the patient's name, address, and telephone number
   b. checking for drug name, quantity, strength, dose, and route
   c. verifying the final prescription
   d. entering and billing insurance

6. Which of the following tasks may a pharmacy technician not perform?
   a. fill a prescription from a fax
   b. accept a refill order from a patient
   c. counsel patients about their prescriptions
   d. call an insurer on behalf of a patient

7. Before selecting the medication to fill an order, a pharmacy technician should do which of the following?
   a. check the brand name
   b. check the NDC and/or UPC code
   c. check the contraindications
   d. check with the pharmacist

8. Which of the following does *not* appear on the patient's bottle?
   a. name of the medication being dispensed
   b. quantity of the medication being dispensed
   c. phone number of the prescriber
   d. phone number of the pharmacy

9. Which DAW code indicates that generics were permitted by the prescriber, but denied by the patient?
   a. DAW 0
   b. DAW 1
   c. DAW 2
   d. DAW 3

10. The individual on record with the State Board of Pharmacy as the primary, on-site pharmacist is referred to as the _____.
   a. RPh
   b. PharmD
   c. PIC
   d. POD

Critical Thinking Questions

1. Why do some pharmacies employ pharmacy clerks in addition to pharmacy technicians?

2. Why would retail pharmacies restrict access to certain OTC products, such as glucose meters and insulin syringes, by keeping them behind the pharmacy counter?

3. Describe two situations that would negatively impact a pharmacy's workflow and productivity, and then provide a recommended solution for each situation.

Web Challenge

1. Search the National Association for Chain Drug Stores (NACDS) website to find the current number of community pharmacies in the United States and the volume of prescriptions filled at retail pharmacies last year: http://www.nacds.org

2. Go to the National Community Pharmacists Association (NCPA) website and find the average number of prescriptions filled annually and per day at independent pharmacies: http://www.ncpanet.org

References and Resources

Abood, R. *Pharmacy Practice and the Law*. 7th ed. Boston, MA: Bartlett Publishers, 2012. Print.

"Academy of Manage Care Pharmacy." *Drug Utilization Review*. November 2009. Web. 22 May 2012.

"Adultmeducation." *Dimension 5 Patient-Related Factors*. 2006. Web. 23 May 2012.

"American Medical Association." *Know Your Drugs and Medications*. New York: Reader's Digest Association, 1991. Print.

"American Pharmacist Association." *Pharmacy Based Immunization Delivery*. 2012. Web. 25 May 2012.

"American Society of Healthcare System." *Pharmacist Tech Training Module, Model Curriculum for Pharmacy Technician Training*. n.p. Web. 19 May 2012.

"American Society of Health-System Pharmacist." *Quality Assurance Pharmacist*. n.p. Web. 28 May 2012.

American Society of Hospital Pharmacist. "Innovative Technician Practices Debating in Hospitals. Tech-Check-Tech, Med Rec Show What Technicians Can Do." *ASHP Intersections*. December 2011. Web. 29 May 2012.

Ansel, HC. *Introduction to Pharmaceutical Dosage Forms*. Philadelphia: Lea & Febiger, 1995. Print.

Askew, G. and Stoner-Smith, M. *Assisting in the Pharmacy*. Thomson Delmar. n.p. Print.

Bachenheimer, B.S. *Manual for Pharmacy Technicians*. 4th ed. Bethesda, MD: ASHP. 2010. Print.

Barnett, C., Ellington, A., and Nykamp, D. "Effectiveness of Auxiliary Labeling in Community Pharmacies." *US Pharmacist*. April 2003. Print.

Bernstein, WN. *Clean Spaces—A Look at the Revised, Reissued USP 797 Pharmacy Design Regulation*. 2009. Web. 21 May 2012.

"Blue Shield of California." *Drug Formulary*. 2012. Web. 22 May 2012.

Boyce, A. Allied Health World. *Pharmacy Technician Salary*, January 7, 2010. Web. 18 May 2012.

Bullman, R. "Written Drug Information: Now and the Future." *CMS*. April 2007. Web. 24 May 2012.

"Center for Medicare and Medicaid Services." *Required Use of Tamper-Resistant Prescription Pads for Outpatient Drugs Prescribed for Medicaid Recipients on or after April, 1 2008*. 2008. Web. 24 May 2012.

"ChexSystems." *Consumer Assistance*. 2012 Web. 29 May 2012.

"Commonwealth of Pennsylvania." *Standards of Practice*. 2012. Web. 23 May 2012.

"Consumer Product Safety Commission." *Poison Prevention Packaging Act: A Guide for Healthcare Professions*. 2005. Web. 23 May 2012.

Cooperman, S.H. *Professional Office Procedures*. Upper Saddle River, NJ: Pearson Education, 2006. Print.

Cowen, D. and Helfand, W. *Pharmacy: An Illustrated History*. New York: Harry N. Abrams, 1990. Print.

Crane, A. "An Overview of Pharmacy Automation." *Today's Technician*. 5(4) (2004): 26–37. Print.

Davis, K. *Pharmacy Management Software for Pharmacy Technicians*. 2nd ed. Brookline, MA: DAA Enterprises, Inc. 2012. Print.

Diebold, J. "The Significance of Productivity Data." *Harvard Business News*. May 2009. Web. 30 May 2012.

"Drug Enforcement Administration." *Drug Diversion*. 2012. Web. 25 May 2012.

"Drug Enforcement Administration." *History of the DEA*. 2012. Web. 19 May 2012.

"Drug Enforcement Administration." *Valid Prescription Requirements*. 2012. Web. 24 May 2012.

Drug Information Handbook. 21st ed. Hudson, OH: Lexicomp. 2011. Print.

"Drug Topics." *New Compact Tablet Counter is Fast and Accurate*. October 2010. Web. 24 May 2012.

"EurekAlert." *Tech-Check-Tech*. January 2007. Web. 29 May 2012.

Flaherty, J. "Matters of Privacy—Patient confidentiality." *Today's Technician*. 6(2) (2005): 8, 12. Print.

"Food and Drug Administration." *Pharmaceutical Packing Designed to Reduce Medication Error*. June 2010. Web. 22 May 2012.

"Food and Drug Administration." *Providing Effective Information to Consumers About Prescription Drug Risk Benefits: The Issues Paper*. June 2010. Web. 24 May 2012.

"Food and Drug Administration." *Regulatory Information and Glossary*. 2011. Web. 18 May 2012.

"Formulary and Non-Formulary Medications." *Express Scripts*. 2012. Web. 22 May 2012.

Gable, L. *Centers for Law and Public's Health at Georgetown and John Hopkin's Universities*. February 2003. Web. 25 May 2012.

Garry, M. "Robots on Call." *SuperMarket News*. August 2011. Web. 24 May 2012.

Gebhart, F. "Pharmacy Franchises: Should You Join One?" *Drug Topics*. September 4, 2006. Web. 21 May 2012.

Glatter, R. "How Should We Define Productivity in Healthcare?" *Forbes*. May 2012. Web. 21 May 2012.

Hannabarger, C., Buchman, F., and Economy, P. *Balanced Scorecard Strategy for Dummies*. Hoboken, NJ: Wiley, 2007. Print.

"Health and Human Services." *State Pharmacy Boards Oversight of Patient Counseling Laws*. August 1997. Web. 19 May 2012.

Hanselman, A. "Apple's Customer Service Secrets Revealed: A.P.P.L.E." *The Social Customer*. June 2011. Web. 23 May 2012.

"Health and Human Services." *Medicaid Drug Use Review Programs*. Lessons Learned by States. *HHS*. 1995. Web. 1 June 2012.

"Hewlett Packard." *HP Point of Sales (POS)—Retail Solutions*. 2012. Web. 26 May 2012.

Higby, GJ. and Stroud, EC. *American Pharmacy 1852–2002: A Collection of Historical Essays*. Madison, WI: American Institute of the History of Pharmacy. 2005. Print.

"Idaho Society of Hospital Pharmacist." *Tech-Check-Tech Program*. 2006. Web. 29 May 2012.

"Institutes for Safe Medication Practices." *Principles of Designing a Medication Label for Community and Mail Order Pharmacy Prescription Packages*. 2010. Web. 23 May 2012.

"IQTELL Productivity." *Productivity and Organizations—What Makes Them Important to Us?* December 2011. Web. 30 May 2012.

Johnsen, M. "Walgreens Immunization Studies: Pharmacy Instrumental in Helping States Combat Disease." *Drug Store News*. April 2012. Web. 25 May 2012.

Keefer, A. "How to Buy a Pharmacy." *eHow*. n.p. Web. 21 May 2012.

Kelly, C. and Redman, M. "Rx for Pharmacy Design: A Centered Approach." *Healthcare Design*. November 1, 2009. Web. 21 May 2012.

Kirby Lester. *KL2—Next Generation Counting and Verification System with Workflow Software*. Web. 24 May 2012.

Lambert, A. *Advanced Practices for Pharmacy Technicians*. Clifton Park, NY: Delmar Learning, 2009. Print.

Lankard, K. "What is the meaning of Non-Formulary Drugs?" *eHow*. n.p. Web. 19 May 2012.

Merck. "How Health Care Is Paid For." *Merck Manuel Home Health Handbook for Patients and Caregivers*. 2011. Web. 25 May 2012.

Merriam-Webster Dictionary. Web. 28 May 2012.

"National Association of Chain Drug Stores." *MMA Study on Making Prescription Pharmaceutical Information Accessible for Blind and Visually Impaired Individuals*. June 2004. Web. 23 May 2012.

National Association of Chain Drug Stores, Inc., & Mintz, Levin, Cohn, Ferris, Glovsky, and Popeo, P.C. *HIPAA Privacy Standards: A Compliance Manual for Pharmacies*. Alexandria, VA: NACDS, 2002. Print.

Neighmond, P. "Many Pharmacists Now Administer Vaccines." *National Public Radio*. October 2007. Web. 25 May 2012.

"Organisations for Economic Co-operation and Development." *Defining and Measurement Productivity*. *OECD*. n.p. Web. 30 May 2012.

"Perspective Press." *Pharmacy Technician Workbook and Certification Review*. 5th ed. Englewood, CO: Morton Publishing, 2013. Print.

Pharmacy Technician Certification Board. Web. 29 May 2012.

Plaqakis, J. "Change Is the Air Pharmacist Will Breathe." *Drug Topics*. June 2011. Web. 29 May 2012.

"POS Nation." *POS Cash Registers*. 2011. Web. 26 May 2012.

Radice, C. "Scripting a Change." *Grocery HeadQuarters*. April 2011. Web. 24 May 2012.

"Research Data Assistance Center." *Pharmacy Characteristics Data Dictionary*. 2008 Web. 18 May 2012.

"Rite-Aid Pharmacy." *Immunizations at Rite-Aid*. 2012. Web. 25 May 2012.

Shedd, D. "Tech-Check-Tech Programs." *Pharmacy Tech Resources: The Tech Letter*, Issue 1. August 2011. Web. 29 May 2012.

Sherman, M. "Prescription Containers." *Pharmacy Times*. September 2005. Web. 22 May 2012.

Teeters, J. "Gazing into the Crystal Ball; Health-System Pharmacy 2011 and Beyond." *ASHP InterSections*. March 28, 2011. Web. 19 May 2012.

TeleCheck Services. 2012. Web. 29 May 2012.

Terrie, Y.C. "Vaccinations: The Expanding Role of Pharmacist." *Pharmacy Times*. January 2010. Web. 25 May 2012.

Texas Tech University School of Pharmacy. "A Technician's Role. Optimizing Patient Safety and Minimizing Medication Errors. A Knowledge Base Course for Technicians." *JD Education*. n.p. Web. 28 May 2012.

Thomas, B. and Baron, J. "Evaluating Knowledge Worker Productivity: Literature Review." *Unites States Army*. June 2009. Web. 30 May 2012.

Train Flash. March 2005. Web. 24 May 2012.

United States Department of Health and Human Service. Medicare Prescription Drug, Improvement and Modernization Act. Implementation Tracking System (MTI). 2003.

United States Department of Health and Human Service. "Summary of the HIPAA Privacy Act." *HHS*. n.p. Web. 21 May 2012.

United States Department of the Treasury. "Health Savings Accounts (HSAs)." *US Treasury*. 2012. Web. 25 May 2012.

University of Texas at Austin. "Proprietary Information and Competitive Intelligence." *UT*. November 2011. Web. 25 May 2012.

University of Toledo. "Outpatient Pharmacy." *University of Toledo*. Web. 19 May 2012.

US Legal Definitions. *Proprietary Information Law and Legal Definition*. 2012. Web. 25 May 2012.

US Legal Definitions. *Retail Community Pharmacy Law and Legal Definition*. 2012. Web. 18 May 2012.

Wartell, J. and La Vigne, NG. "The Problem of Prescription Fraud." *Centers for Problem-Oriented Policy*. 2004. Web. 24 May 2012.

Winterstein, AG, Linden, S, Lee, AE, Fernandez, EM, Kimberlin, CL. "Evaluation of Consumer Information Dispensed in Retail Pharmacies." *National Institutes of Health*. August 2010. Web. 24 May 2012.

World Health Organization. "Drug and Therapeutics Committees—A Practical Guide." *Drug Use Evaluation (DUE) (drug utilization review)*. 2003. Web. 22 May 2012.

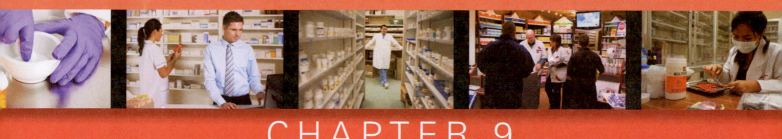

CHAPTER 9

Health-System Pharmacy

LEARNING OBJECTIVES

After completing this chapter, you should be able to:

- Describe the health-system pharmacy practice setting.
- Describe the advantages of a unit-dose system.
- List the necessary components of a medication order.
- Compare the duties of a technician with those of a pharmacist in accepting a medication order in a health-system setting.
- Compare centralized and decentralized unit-dose systems.
- Compare the duties of a technician with those of a pharmacist in filling a medication order in a health-system setting.
- Define the tasks pharmacy technicians perform in health-system settings.

KEY TERMS

blister packs, p. 154

centralized pharmacy system, p. 156

certified nursing assistant (CNA), p. 156

correctional facilities, p. 154

decentralized pharmacy system, p. 156

doctor of medicine (MD), p. 154

doctor of osteopathy (DO), p. 154

emergency medication orders, p. 160

floor stock, p. 158

health-system pharmacy, p. 154

hospice, p. 154

hospital pharmacies, p. 154

inpatient pharmacy (IP), p. 156

institutional pharmacy, p. 153

investigational medication orders, p. 160

licensed nursing assistant (LNA), p. 156

licensed practical nurse (LPN), p. 156

long-term care (LTC) facility, p. 154

medication order, p. 160

nurse practitioner (NP), p. 156

INTRODUCTION

Health-system pharmacy, or **institutional pharmacy**, includes the range of services provided to residents of long-term care facilities (nursing homes), hospitals, hospices, and other residential facilities (see Figure 9-1). In a health-system setting, the pharmacy department is responsible for all patients' medications. The pharmacists must ensure that drug therapies are appropriate, effective, safe, and used correctly. The health-system pharmacist also identifies, resolves, and prevents medication-related problems. The pharmacy technician working in an institutional setting must be familiar with the policies and procedures of the particular institution as well as with state and federal laws.

---

institutional pharmacy a pharmacy found in places such as hospitals, long-term-care facilities, extended-living facilities, and retirement homes, which require patients to reside onsite.

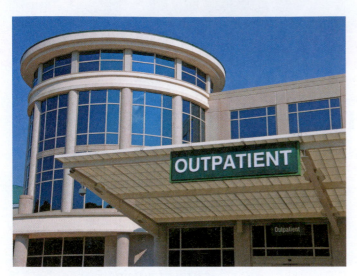

FIGURE 9-1 A health-system pharmacy is often located within a hospital.

Source: Mark Winfrey/Shutterstock

health-system pharmacy a classification of pharmacy setting in which patients reside on-site at the facility where the pharmacy is located (such as hospitals, nursing homes, and long-term care facilities).

blister packs unit-dose packages.

hospital pharmacy the most common type of health-system pharmacy; a pharmacy located within a hospital facility serving patients who have been admitted or are being discharged.

long-term care (LTC) facility facility that provides rehabilitative, restorative, or ongoing skilled nursing care to individuals who need assistance with activities of daily living.

hospice provides palliative care (care designed to help ease suffering) and supportive services to individuals at the end of their lives.

nursing home facility that provides skilled and custodial care to older Americans who do not need the intensive, acute care of a hospital but who can no longer manage independent living.

correctional facilities more commonly referred to as prisons; places in which individuals are physically confined and usually deprived of a range of personal freedoms.

doctor of osteopathy (DO) a licensed individual, trained to examine patients, diagnose illnesses, and prescribe medication and administer treatments using manipulative techniques on the musculoskeletal system in conjunction with conventional treatments.

doctor of medicine (MD) a licensed individual, trained to examine patients, diagnose illnesses, and prescribe and administer medication.

physician assistant (PA) a licensed individual who is trained to coordinate patient care under the supervision of a medical or osteopathic doctor.

Health-System Pharmacies

The **health-system pharmacy** provides around-the-clock delivery service. Health-system pharmacists review patients' drug profiles to avoid possible duplications of treatment and adverse reactions. They are the principal defense against medication errors in the hospital.

Health-system pharmacists often counsel patients on proper medication use, but they also provide drug information and recommendations to doctors and other caregivers. They review patients' drug regimens and oversee medication distribution throughout the institution. In long-term care settings, pharmacists perform a drug therapy review for each patient on a monthly basis or more frequently for special protocols. Health-system pharmacists often discuss the drug therapy of patients with nurses, respiratory therapists, dietitians, laboratory personnel, physicians, and other health care professionals—all with the aim of providing optimal pharmaceutical care.

Health-system pharmacy teams typically provide drug-related products and services 24 hours a day, 365 days a year. Health-system pharmacies also provide medications for emergency departments. Smaller hospitals may be open only for first and second shifts, with an on-call pharmacist after hours. Automated dispensing units are also frequently used to provide safe drug storage for medications required in emergency situations and/or after hours.

Health-system pharmacists and technicians use controlled dispensing systems to ensure that patients have the right drugs at the right time and in the proper dosage and form. They may also provide prescription drugs in individually packaged **blister packs** (unit-dose packages) so that the drugs are dispensed in a convenient and safe manner. You may have also seen blister packs when purchasing medication as a customer.

Health-system pharmacies allow unused, unopened products to be returned for credit (where permitted by state law). When unused, unopened drugs can be returned, medication changes do not result in unused products going to waste. This is very cost-effective.

Health-system pharmacy services are comprehensive in scope and intensity. Older, seriously ill, and chronically ill patients who are often frail and have multiple conditions need more attention than healthier ambulatory patients who are suffering from just one condition. Because the condition of an institutionalized patient constantly changes, frequent updating of drug regimens is required.

This section provides an overview of settings where health-system pharmacy services are typically found.

Hospital Pharmacies

Hospital pharmacies are, by far, the most prevalent type of health-system pharmacy, with more than 5,750 registered hospitals operating in the United States.

Hospitals began as charitable institutions for the needy, aged, sick, or very young. Today, though, they are institutions where sick or injured people receive many levels of medical or surgical care, ranging from outpatient services to long-term intensive care.

Hospital Classifications

The American Hospital Association (AHA) categorizes hospitals as community-based, federal government, psychiatric, long-term care, or institutional hospital units. Community-based hospitals, which include nonprofit, for-profit, and state/local government facilities, represent approximately 85% of the total number of registered hospitals. This chapter focuses primarily on the practices and standards of community-based hospital pharmacies, collectively.

Hospitals are also categorized by their location and size. Depending on their location, hospitals are referred to as either rural or urban. Based on bed capacity, or size, hospitals are categorized as small (25–50 beds), medium-sized (50–100 beds), or large (more than 100 beds).

Long-Term Care Facilities

Long-term care (LTC) facilities provide rehabilitative, restorative, or ongoing skilled nursing care to individuals, referred to as *patients* or *residents*, who need assistance with activities of daily living. The federal government acknowledged the distinctive features of the LTC pharmacy when it passed laws and promulgated regulations to protect the health and well-being of institutional residents (OBRA 1987, OBRA 1990, HCFA'S 1990 nursing home regulations). These laws and rules recognize that drug therapy services for institutional patients are best delivered by LTC pharmacists.

Hospices

Hospices provide palliative care (care designed to help ease suffering) and supportive services to individuals at the end of their lives. Hospices also serve patients' family members and significant others. They operate 24 hours a day, 7 days a week, both in patients' homes and in facility-based settings. Hospices provide pharmaceutical, physical, social, spiritual, and emotional care to patients and their families during the last stages of an illness, the dying process, and the bereavement period.

Nursing Homes

Nursing homes offer skilled and custodial care to older Americans who do not need the intensive, acute care of a hospital but who can no longer manage independent living. Nursing homes are capable of caring for individuals with a wide range of medical conditions.

Nursing homes have different sizes and different names, such as health centers, havens, manors, homes for the aged, nursing centers, care centers, continuing care centers, living centers, or convalescent centers. The number of beds in a particular nursing home can range from approximately 25 to 500; the average number of beds per facility across the United States is 102.

Correctional Facilities

Correctional facilities, more commonly known as *prisons*, are places in which individuals are physically confined and usually deprived of a range of personal freedoms. Usually, these institutions are part of the criminal justice system. Correctional facility pharmacies oversee the provision of pharmaceutical services to those confined to the facility by the operation of law (*inmates*).

Hospital Staff

The operation and management of hospitals require numerous staff members, each accountable and responsible for various job duties.

Doctor of Osteopathy

A **doctor of osteopathy (DO)** is a licensed individual, trained to examine patients, diagnose illnesses, and prescribe medications and administer treatments using manipulative techniques on the musculoskeletal system in conjunction with conventional treatments.

Doctor of Medicine

A **doctor of medicine (MD)** is a licensed individual, trained to examine patients, diagnose illnesses, and prescribe and administer medication. In the hospital setting, the majority of medical doctors specialize in one particular field. For example, a cardiologist specializes in disorders of the heart and circulatory system; an oncologist specializes in diagnosing and treating patients with cancer, and an obstetrician/gynecologist (OB/YN) specializes in both obstetrics and gynecology. Surgeons are trained in the treatment of injury or disease by manual or instrumental procedures.

Physician Assistant

A **physician assistant (PA)** is a licensed individual who is trained to coordinate patient care under the supervision of a medical or osteopathic doctor. Although PAs are authorized to prescribe medications, there are certain restrictions on their ability to prescribe controlled substances. PAs can also be found at drug store clinics and may act as the only type of physician on staff at the drug store clinic. The types of illnesses they treat as well as their ability to prescribe certain medications and controlled substances are limited, as mentioned earlier.

Certified Nursing Assistant

A **certified nursing assistant (CNA)** is an individual who is certified to assist RNs and LPNs in providing patient care, but is not permitted to administer medication.

Licensed Nursing Assistant

A **licensed nursing assistant (LNA)** is an individual who is licensed to assist RNs and LPNs in providing patient care, but is not permitted to administer medication.

Licensed Practical Nurse

A **licensed practical nurse (LPN)** is an individual who is licensed to provide basic care, such as administering medication, under the supervision of a registered nurse. In some states, these individuals are called licensed vocational nurses (LVNs).

---

certified nursing assistant (CNA) an individual who is certified to assist RNs and LPNs in providing patient care, but is not permitted to administer medication.

licensed nursing assistant (LNA) an individual who is licensed to assist RNs and LPNs in providing patient care, but is not permitted to administer medication.

licensed practical nurse (LPN) an individual who is licensed to provide basic care, such as administering medication, under the supervision of a registered nurse.

nurse practitioner (NP) an individual who is licensed to work closely with a physician in providing patient care and typically may prescribe medications under the supervision of a physician.

registered nurse (RN) an individual who is registered to assist physicians with specific procedures, administer medications, and provide patient care.

centralized pharmacy system system in which all pharmacy-related activities are performed from one location and medications are delivered to various patient care units throughout the facility.

decentralized pharmacy system pharmacy service system consisting of a central, or inpatient, pharmacy and multiple satellite pharmacies, as well as an outpatient pharmacy.

inpatient pharmacy (IP) portion of a facility that is responsible for medication packaging, centralized inventory, sterile product preparation, and the preparation and delivery of medication carts. It provides pharmaceutical services to patients admitted to a facility.

outpatient pharmacy a pharmacy that is available to patients who are being discharged from the hospital, or who are being treated by a physician without requiring overnight admission.

satellite pharmacies subunits of a central pharmacy, located near specific patient care areas in a facility, such as cardiology, operating rooms, and chemotherapy treatment centers.

Nurse Practitioner

A **nurse practitioner (NP)** is an individual who is licensed to work closely with a physician in providing patient care. In most states, nurse practitioners are authorized to prescribe medications under the supervision of a physician.

Registered Nurse

A **registered nurse (RN)** is an individual who is registered to assist physicians with specific procedures, administer medications, and provide patient care.

Organization of Hospital Pharmacies

Hospital pharmacies are structured and managed very differently than community-based pharmacies. A hospital pharmacy is organized either on the centralized pharmacy model or on the decentralized pharmacy model, with few exceptions (see Figure 9-2).

Centralized Pharmacy

A **centralized pharmacy system** is operated out of one primary location, the inpatient pharmacy (IP). In this organizational model, all pharmacy-related activities are performed at this one location and medications are delivered to various patient care units throughout the facility.

Decentralized Pharmacies

A **decentralized pharmacy system** can consist of a central, or inpatient, pharmacy with multiple satellite pharmacies, as well as an outpatient pharmacy. The disadvantage of this system is the necessary duplication of staff, inventory, and equipment; however, medium-size and large facilities often have to use this type of system.

Inpatient Pharmacy

The **inpatient pharmacy** is generally responsible for medication packaging, centralized inventory, sterile product preparation, and the preparation and delivery of medication carts. It provides pharmaceutical services to patients admitted to a facility.

Outpatient Pharmacy

The **outpatient pharmacy** is available to patients who are being discharged from the hospital, or who are being treated by a physician in the hospital but do not require overnight admission. It is, in a sense, a retail-style pharmacy located within the hospital facility.

Satellite Pharmacies

Satellite pharmacies are responsible for receiving, processing, and dispensing medication orders for individual patients. Generally, satellite pharmacies provide initial doses and emergency medications, after which medications may be dispensed from floor stock. The number of satellite pharmacies varies by facility, as does their scope of service. In some hospitals, satellite pharmacies are established for specific patient care areas, such as operating rooms, oncology, or pediatrics. Other hospitals have satellite pharmacies spread throughout the facility based on location and access, as opposed to scope of services.

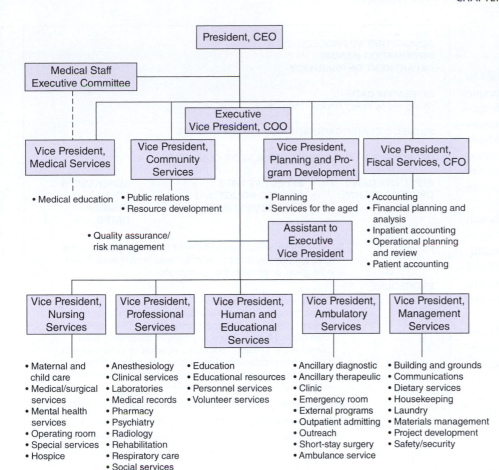

FIGURE 9-2 Typical hospital organization chart.

Regulatory Agencies

Hospital pharmacies are regulated by a variety of agencies, including the Joint Commission, State Boards of Pharmacy, the Centers for Medicare and Medicaid Services, and state Departments of Public Health.

State Board of Pharmacy

The State Board of Pharmacy (SBOP) is the agency that registers and regulates pharmacists and pharmacy technicians; the practice of pharmacy is governed at the state level, whereas the pharmaceutical industry is governed at the national level. Although boards of pharmacy regulate community pharmacy facilities, they do not govern hospital pharmacy departments—just the individuals who work within them. SBOP regulations vary from state to state.

Drug Enforcement Agency

Any institution, manufacturer, or wholesaler who deals with the use, manufacturing, or selling of controlled substances must be registered with the DEA. It is no different with health system pharmacies. The process for a health-system pharmacy to apply for a registered DEA number is the same as any prescriber or retail pharmacy. A number unique to the

health-system pharmacy must be used in all transactions, which involves the selling, transferring, purchasing, or destruction of controlled substances. In a health-system pharmacy the letters that precede their DEA number are used to identify the type of institution: hospital, long-term care, retail.

All pharmacists, technicians, prescribers, wholesalers, and institutions must follow the regulation laid out by the DEA. The role of the DEA in a health-system pharmacy is not much different from its role in a retail pharmacy. The most noticeable difference is the lack of receiving a paper prescription. Prescribers are identified by a DEA number, which is a unique number assigned to them from the DEA. A prescriber's DEA number must be on every outpatient prescription he or she writes. In a health-system setting, the prescriber's DEA number is kept on file in the pharmacy, making it unnecessary to be written on every inpatient order the prescriber writes.

The Joint Commission

The Joint Commission surveys, inspects, and accredits health systems, such as hospitals, every three years. Site inspections, which include the pharmacy department(s), evaluate a facility's compliance with the Joint Commission standards and criteria. These intensive site surveys used to be scheduled in advance, but in 2006 the Joint Commission decided that inspections will now be unannounced. The Joint Commission accreditation is necessary for organizations to receive reimbursement from Medicare and many third-party insurance companies.

Centers for Medicare and Medicaid Services

The Centers for Medicare and Medicaid Services (CMS) is the agency that regulates and administers Medicare, Medicaid, the State Children's Health Insurance Program (SCHIP), the Health Insurance Portability and Accountability Act (HIPAA), the Clinical Laboratory Improvement Amendments, and several other health-related programs. The CMS conducts inspections to ensure compliance with its guidelines; approval from the CMS is necessary for a facility to receive reimbursement from Medicare and/or Medicaid.

State Department of Public Health

A state's Department of Public Health (DPH) is the agency that regulates hospitals, including the hospital pharmacy department(s). The DPH conducts inspections to ensure that the facility is in compliance with the DPH regulations and criteria.

The Policy and Procedure Manual

As do many other well-run organizations, a health-system pharmacy may develop a unique policy and procedure manual to establish specific guidelines and systems for the operations of the facility. *Policies* are definitive methods or courses of action, determined by an organization or a department; *procedures* are the step-by-step directions provided to achieve an organization's policies.

The pharmacy department in a large health system generally has multiple levels of management and supervision, whereas rural health-system pharmacies tend to have fewer staff and managerial layers. The policy and procedure manual provides much-needed structure for the health-system pharmacy.

The policy and procedure manual (Figure 9-3) provides numerous benefits to a health-system pharmacy department. Primarily, it is being used as a resource to:

- Ensure quality assurance throughout the department
- Implement quality control measures, which can reduce medication errors
- Reduce the time required to train employees
- Communicate job responsibilities and scope of authority
- Document compliance for regulatory agencies and accreditation organizations

The organization and contents of policy and procedure manuals vary by facility, but there are several common methods that health-system pharmacies use.

- **Alphabetical**—policies and procedures are listed alphabetically according to their official titles.
- **Categorized**—policies and procedures are divided into topical categories, such as organization, personnel policies, administrative policies, professional policies, and facilities/equipment.

ADMINISTRATIVE PROCEDURES &
INFORMATION MANUAL
DEPARTMENT OF PHARMACY

RE-REVIEW DATE:
(Assigned by Policy Review Committee)

SUBJECT: CLARIFICATION OF MEDICATION ORDERS

RESPONSIBLE DEPARTMENT, DIVISION OR COMMITTEE

EFFECTIVE DATE ORIGINAL POLICY: 8/29/xx	EFFECTIVE DATE REVISED POLICY: 1/12 LAST REVIEW DATE: 10/13.	SUPERSEDES POLICY NUMBER: DATED:

POLICY: No prescription or order is to be filled if there is any doubt in the mind of the pharmacist as to what is called for: the dose, how it is to be given, or whether it is appropriate.

PROCEDURE:

1. Orders being questioned are to be entered on the patient profile as "pending" with documentation of the problem in the clinical notes and a statement in the Special Direction field "See Clinical Notes." The yellow copy of the order is to be placed in the "problem" box with a notation as to the problem. Orders with problems that could pose risk to the patient must contain the phrase "Do not dispense until clarified" on the yellow copy and in the Special Directions Field.
2. No medication is to be dispensed until the order is clarified.
3. It is the responsibility of the pharmacist to contact the prescriber.
4. In the event that the name of the prescriber cannot be determined from the signature or I.D. number, the nurse may be asked for the name of the prescriber.
5. The pharmacist will page the prescriber. If the prescriber is an intern and there is no response in 15 minutes, then page the resident. Repeat this procedure, if necessary. If still no response, contact the attending physician. This last step should be done when, in the pharmacist's professional judgment, the patient could be harmed by further delay.
6. If the matter has not been resolved by the end of the shift, the information must be communicated to a pharmacist on the next shift for follow-up and resolution.
7. Upon receipt of clarification, the pending order is cancelled and the corrected order is entered. Problem resolution is to be documented on the clinical notes.
8. If authorization to change an order has been obtained, a message is to be sent to the unit notifying the nurse of the change. (See "Change in Medication Order").
9. Documentation of a clarification/change will be made in the medical record by the authorized prescriber or the pharmacist.

J. Smith

Director of Pharmacy Services

FIGURE 9-3 Sample policy and procedures manual.

---

floor stock a system in which medications are kept on each floor for distribution to patients.

patient prescription stock system a system in which medication orders are reviewed, prepared, and verified, and then the medications are taken to the floor and dispensed to the patient.

Protocol

Protocols are written agreements, usually created from a formed committee of clinical caregivers such as physicians, nurses, and pharmacists, who agree on a specific plan of action concerning a patient's care. For example, if Mrs. Smith was seen in the emergency department and then admitted to the floor with a diagnosis of pneumonia, a carefully laid out plan of patient care exists for her physician to follow. A standard set of orders would be placed in her chart, and the physician would order her medications and diagnostic tests accordingly. Protocol for a patient diagnosed with pneumonia might include a chest X-ray, IV antibiotic therapy, and respiratory treatment. This set of standard patient orders has been determined by clinical staff to be the best planned treatment for pneumonia.

The pharmacy's involvement in protocol development involves the proper use of medications. When developing a protocol for patient care, it is important to use the medication that will do the most good for the patient's condition, have the least amount of possible interactions, and be cost-effective. Medications that are part of protocols are also determined by a pharmacy's formulary. In this way protocols are also cost savings to the patient. If a prescriber decides to order medications outside of the protocol, the pharmacist will consult with the prescriber, explaining why the medications on the protocol are indicated. Some prescribers are receptive to this; others are not.

In most cases, if the pharmacist consults with the prescriber concerning medications outside of the protocol, and the prescriber decides to continue with the therapy he or she initially ordered, the pharmacist must document this decision in the patient's chart. The prescriber must also have written documentation for going off of protocol. The reason for documentation is more than just liability; most insurance payers recognize protocols for specific diagnosis and may not pay for treatments that are outside of the protocols without documentation stating why the medication protocols were not followed.

Pharmacy technicians can familiarize themselves with their health system's protocols and alert the pharmacist to any issues they may find during the order entry process. If the pharmacist is able to consult the physician prior to the order being completed and filled, then the patient will not only receive the proper protocol, but also have potential cost savings.

Formulary

Medication formularies are a very important part of a health-system pharmacy. Formularies can affect everything from patient care plan protocols to patient medication cost. Because purchasing medications and maintaining formularies is such a large expense, the pharmacy is often one of the most costly departments operating within the health system. So it is extremely important that the health system chooses not only a medication formulary that provides the most benefit for the patient's care needs, but also one that is cost-effective.

Health-system pharmacies are ultimately responsible for maintaining the medication formulary, inventory control, ordering of medications, and contracts with wholesalers, but the medications for a formulary are chosen by the health system's Pharmacy and Therapy (P&T) committee.

P&T committees are comprised of physicians (from various specialties), pharmacists, and other health care workers who have experience in clinical decision making. P&T is responsible for determining which medications will be on a health system's formulary. The committee general meets several times a year

and reviews the medications on the current formulary. The committee evaluates the medications based on their therapeutic usage, safety, cost, and availability. If the P&T feels a medication should be added to the formulary, it will then be added and the pharmacy will be responsible for obtaining the medication into its inventory. If the P&T feels a medication should be deleted from the formulary, then it is deleted and the pharmacy will remove the medication from its current stock and return it to its wholesaler.

Dispensing Systems

Within a single health-system setting, many types of medication distribution systems may exist. This is especially true of a hospital setting, which may even contain multiple pharmacies. The common medication distribution systems are floor stock, patient prescription, and unit dose.

Floor Stock

In the **floor stock** distribution system, medications are kept on each floor for distribution to patients (see Figure 9-4). This system is prone to errors, diversion, and employee theft. However, in recent times, computers have made this system much easier to monitor and fill. The technician stocks the floor unit with a predetermined bulk supply after the pharmacist checks the order. The computerized system tracks the inventory, records who has accessed the unit, and even bills the patient. This system can generate refill orders to the technician, whereupon the process begins again. The floor stock dispensing system requires a great deal of floor space and imposes higher inventory requirements.

Patient Prescription

The **patient prescription stock system** is considered the most inefficient because of waste and the inability of the pharmacy department to properly monitor it. In this system, after reviewing medication orders for a floor, the technician takes the medications to the pharmacist for verification, and then

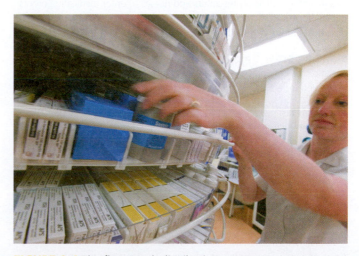

FIGURE 9-4 The floor stock distribution system.
Source: Gusto/Science Source

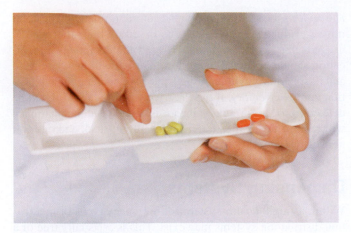

FIGURE 9-5 Filling a patient prescription.
Source: Jochen Tack/Das Fotoarchiv/Getty Images, Inc.

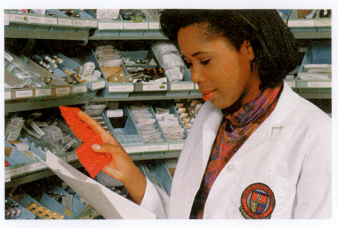

FIGURE 9-6 The unit-dose system makes it very easy to track a patient's medications.
Source: Doug Martin/Science Source

takes the medications to the floor (see Figure 9-5). The orders are usually for several days' supply of the medication (typically three). Once opened, the medication cannot be returned to the pharmacy, since it is considered to have been dispensed and therefore to have left the control and closed system of the health-system pharmacy.

Unit Dose

In contrast to the prescription system, the **unit-dose** system is the most efficient distribution system, and makes it very easy to track a patient's medications (see Figure 9-6). In this system, each medication order is filled in the pharmacy in as close to

---

unit dose a distribution system in which each medication order is filled in the pharmacy in a way that provides each dose in a package ready to administer to the patient. Usually, not more than a 24-hour supply is dispensed at one time.

medication order a term for a patient prescription in a health system.

POE system a point-of-entry computer system networked within the health system to allow prescribers and nurses to enter medication orders directly for the pharmacy; sometimes referred to as a computerized physician order entry (CPOE) system.

standing order a medication order used when a patient is to receive a specific medication at specific intervals throughout the day; also called a scheduled order.

PRN order a medication order used when a patient is to receive a medication only as necessary, as with pain medication.

STAT order a medication order used when a patient requires a medication immediately; this is an urgent order and thus takes priority over other orders and requests.

emergency medication order a specific type of STAT order for a medication that is required for a physician to be able to respond to a medical emergency.

investigational medication order an order for medication used in facilities that participate in research programs.

---

administration form as possible, meaning that not more than a 24-hour supply is dispensed at one time. Scanners may be used to track and bill for the medications when they are dispensed. Unit-dose systems centralize medication preparation in the pharmacy itself, cut the amount of time the nursing staff spend preparing medications, and greatly reduces waste.

Clearly, a unit-dose system requires more technician involvement. In a centralized pharmacy, technicians may have workstations for unit-dose medications (tablets, capsules, and liquids), IVs, sterile preparations, chemotherapy drugs, injections, and compounding. Unit-dose systems can be centralized, decentralized, or a combination of both.

The Medication Order

In health-system pharmacies, prescribers order medications for patients on a **medication order** form, as opposed to the prescription pad used for retail pharmacies. The medication order form is a multipurpose tool for communication among various members of the health care team working within a health system. In addition to prescribed medications, this form can be used by the physician to order lab work, special diets, and X-rays or other medical procedures, so it is imperative that pharmacy personnel be able to properly distinguish and interpret medication orders.

Hospitals can choose to use physical, hard-copy medication order forms, a physician order entry system (**POE system**), or a computerized physician order entry (CPOE) system. The latter is a fully computerized system in which orders are entered electronically into the hospital's networked system.

Medication Order Components

There are some differences between the requirements for a medication order (see Figure 9-7) and those for a prescription. The reasons for the variations are pretty much self-evident. A medication order includes the following:

- Patient information
  - Name
  - Room/bed number

```
16285
CH-7239
(FEB. 13)
```

PHYSICIAN'S ORDER WORKSHEET

NOTE: *Person initiating entry should write legibly, date the form using (Mo./Day/Yr.), enter time, sign, and indicate their title.*

USE BALL POINT PEN (PRESS FIRMLY)

Date	Time	Treatment
		③

PHYSICIAN'S ORDER WORKSHEET	Distribution: (Original) Medical Record Copy (Plies 3, 2, & 1) Pharmacy	**T-5**

FIGURE 9-7 A sample medication order.

- Hospital ID number
- Birth date/age
- Medication information
  - Name
  - Dose
  - Frequency of administration
  - Route
- Signature of the prescriber
- Date and hour the order was written

Types of Medication Orders

The three main types of medication orders are **standing orders**, PRN orders, and STAT orders. A standing, or scheduled, order is used when a patient is to receive a specific medication at specific intervals throughout the day. A **PRN order**, which means an as-needed order, is used when a patient is to receive a medication only as necessary, as with pain medication. A **STAT order**, which stands for immediate order, is used when a patient requires a medication immediately. This is an urgent order that takes priority over other orders and requests.

In addition to these common types of medication orders, there are also emergency medication orders and investigational medication orders. An **emergency medication order** is a specific type of a STAT order for a medication that is required for a physician to be able to respond to a medical emergency. An **investigational medication order** is used in facilities that participate in research programs. Investigational drugs are ordered, prepared, and administered according to stringent protocols specific to the research program.

Point of Entry

Most health-system computers will have software, which allows nursing staff to scan the original order to the pharmacy. The order will then appear in a queue or order-holding area on the computer monitor. The technician can then click on the order in queue, which will bring up the scanned copy of the order. Typically the technician will input the orders into the system in order of time stamp (the time the order was scanned to the pharmacy), but occasionally a medication is needed immediately and the order will have to be placed ahead of all other orders. Medications needed as STATs (emergent) will be highlighted in red in the queue. The technician should make the pharmacist aware of the STAT medication and proceed with getting it to the patient in a timely manner.

Paper Orders

Other health systems do not use a system that allows for orders to be scanned, but instead use a hard copy of the original order. In such cases, one technician is usually assigned to pick up the

info **Order Classifications**

Standing order—to be dispensed routinely

PRN order—to be dispensed as needed

STAT order—to be dispensed immediately

orders from the patient floors on a scheduled basis; an hourly time schedule is typical. Each nursing unit will have a bin, which is specifically for pharmacy medication orders; the technician will then return the orders to the pharmacy, where they will be transcribed into the system by the technician assigned to order entry. Again, it is extremely important that all information is verified before the order entry process begins.

Computerized Physician Order Entry

Computerized physician order entry or CPOE is becoming more prevalent in health-system settings. CPOE allows the physician to electronically order a patient's medication directly into the computer system. The order will then be transmitted to the pharmacy's computer system, where a pharmacist will verify the order and consult the physician on any needed changes or potential medication interactions. The popularity of using CPOE in health systems is increasing, mostly because it provides substantial benefits in regards to management of patient care. Health systems that use CPOE have found a decrease in the time they take to complete an order, virtual elimination of errors related to handwriting and transcription, and reduction of duplicated orders.

CPOE is the last step prior to printing of the medication label and filling of the patient medication order; steps that are missed or not followed correctly can end in errors that may be missed. Systems software like CPOE can help to eliminate these errors, providing a better standard of care for the patient.

Bar Code Point of Entry

Bar code scanning is another method used in health-system pharmacies. Bar code scanning enables pharmacies to implement patient medication safety, decreasing errors and assuring the correct drug is filled for the correct order and associated medication label. Every drug has a National Drug Code (NDC) number that is unique to that particular drug. The NDC number relays information about the drug to a computer system, when the bar code (located directly beneath the NCD number) is scanned. This transmits the drug's information, such as name, dose, form, manufacturer, and cost, into the health-system pharmacy's computer, where it can be viewed on the computer monitor. It is vital in the use of bar coding that the drug's NDC number be entered into the corresponding computer system correctly. Any information that is not entered correctly could cause an order to be filled incorrectly or the pricing of a drug to be incorrect.

Bar coding is also used in health-system pharmacies to verify that the correct drug was used both for order entry and in the filling process. During order entry, the technician will search for the ordered drug in the pharmacy database and then choose the correct drug for the order. This generates a patient medication label that prints with a bar code associated to the drug the technician chose. The technician will then retrieve the drug from stock, scan the bar code on the label, and then scan the drug, and if both of the scans match on the computer monitor, the technician will continue filling the order. This is a verification system that works well, but only if the NDC number has been correctly entered into the computer's system. If a bar code will not scan, most likely the wrong drug has been chosen, or the bar code was entered into the system incorrectly.

Use of bar code systems will continue to increase as the call for better patient medication safety measures becomes a reality. Pharmacy technicians should become aware of the advantages and pitfalls of bar code scanning. A bar code that does not scan properly should never be ignored. If a technician comes across a bar code that does not scan, the technician should first check to see if the correct drug was scanned; if this is not the case and the drug will still not scan, the technician should bring it to the attention of the pharmacy's inventory control person.

Processing Medication Orders

Health-system pharmacy settings are, basically, pharmacies that are located in the "homes" of the patients they serve. The parent facility may be a hospital, nursing home, or hospice. Several differences distinguish a health-system pharmacy practice from an ambulatory pharmacy. The differences in institutional policies and procedures regarding the processing of medication orders can be challenging for technicians unless the technicians receive adequate training beforehand. This section briefly discusses the processing of medication orders and highlights these differences.

Receiving Medication Orders

Just as in an ambulatory setting, no medications are dispensed in a health-system setting without a prescription. In a health system, the medication order is not given to the patient to be filled; rather, it is entered, submitted, filled, billed, and delivered to the patient by the facility staff.

The medication order may arrive in the pharmacy in several different ways:

- The order may be submitted electronically to the pharmacy, utilizing a point-of-entry (POE), or computerized point of entry (CPOE) system.
- The order may be sent by way of a pneumatic tube device (see Figure 9-8).
- The order may be handed directly to the pharmacist.
- The order may be faxed to the pharmacy.
- Orders may be sent through the institutional computer system.
- A technician may be assigned to collect medication orders from many areas throughout the institution.

In addition, medication orders may be submitted directly to the nursing floors, in which case the orders are verified electronically by the pharmacist, and then administered by nurses using floor stock.

Order Entry

Hard-copy medication order forms may be entered into the computer system by pharmacy

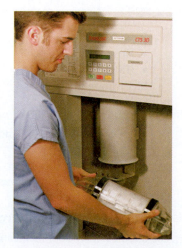

FIGURE 9-8 Receiving a medication order.

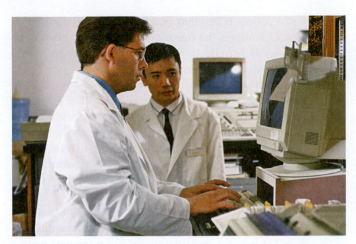

FIGURE 9-9 Entering a medication order.
Source: Keith Brofsky /Getty Images, Inc.

technicians, pharmacists, nursing clerks, nurses, or even physicians (see Figure 9-9). Regardless of who enters the order, the following items must be included:

- Patient's name
- Patient's hospital ID number
- Room number/bed number/location
- Drug name
- Drug strength
- Drug quantity (if a STAT order)
- Route of administration
- Frequency of administration
- Ordering physician
- Date and time of order

Order Verification

Technicians practicing in health-system settings may be assigned to collect and accept medication orders. Technicians may even review the orders for completeness. These orders are called *unverified* and cannot be processed until they have been verified by a pharmacist. Each order must be screened by the pharmacist for correct order entry, potential drug interactions, allergies, drug utilization review, and formulary utilization.

Order Preparation

Just as in an ambulatory setting, medications may be counted out in a health-system setting. The same care must be taken to match lot and UPC numbers, as well as to check expiration dates (see Figure 9-10). The technician performing this task needs to keep the spatula and counting tray clean at all times. Special care should be taken when counting cytotoxic or chemotherapy drugs.

info
Compounded Preparations
Some medications, such as parenteral nutrition, sterile products, and chemotherapy drugs, must be compounded prior to dispensing/administration.

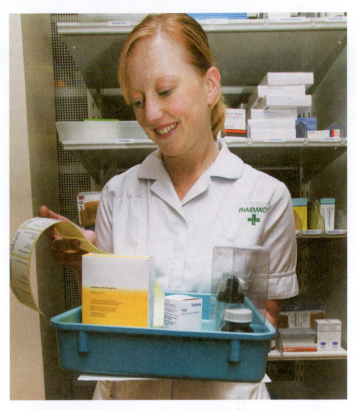

FIGURE 9-10 Preparing an order.
Source: Gusto/Science Source

❝ Workplace Wisdom Counting Medications

A thorough technician will count twice, especially when counting C-II medications.

These facilities may also use automated counting machines that technicians are required to operate and maintain on a daily basis. These machines are popular because they are efficient, reduce errors, and can also reduce drug diversion. An important point to remember is that these machines are only as accurate as the technicians who operate them. At no time should a technician override a machine's built-in checking system. Technicians must also pay close attention to any policies or procedures pertaining to the operation of automated dispensing equipment. ❞

Dispensing Medication Orders

Filling prescriptions or medication orders is one of the most basic duties of a pharmacy technician in any health-system setting. However, filling consists of much more than just counting and basic measuring.

The final check is the sole domain of the pharmacist. No medications may be dispensed without the pharmacist's final approval. In a health-system setting, this is a relatively simple process. The pharmacist will need the original medication order and the labeled container filled with the prescribed medication. Once the pharmacist approves it, the medication may be sent to the proper ward or floor and dispensed to the patient.

State Laws Regarding the RPh Review Prior to Distribution

While there is variation in some of the responsibilities of a pharmacy technician who works in a health-system setting versus a pharmacy technician who works in a retail setting, most of the same set of regulations and standards apply. Pharmacy technicians in a health-system setting are a vital part of the pharmacy team, but just as their retail counterparts, they are not allowed to supersede regulations set forth by their SBOP.

Regulations regarding pharmacy technicians differ from state to state, but protocols regarding pharmacist review of medication orders prior to distribution usually remain consistent. Both health-system technicians and retail technicians must follow the following regulations:

- The pharmacist must have a medication order for comparison; either a copy or the original order must be compared to the medication label.
- The pharmacist must have a completed patient medication label listing: patient's name, medical record number, patient's ID number, date, dosing instructions, pharmacy's name and address, prescriber's name and DEA number, and any another associated medication information such as a bar code.
- The bottle used to fill the medication must accompany the filled medication order so the pharmacist can verify all medication information including expiration date, lot numbers, and NDC number.
- Signature of the pharmacy technician who filled the order; if questions arise the pharmacist will know whom to speak to.
- Signature of a registered pharmacist; this ensures the pharmacist has not only seen the order, but has also verified all information associated with the patient medication order.

Only after the pharmacist signs off on all aspects of the medication order should the medication be brought to the nursing unit for administration. Technicians who ignore these regulations could not only put a patient's safety at risk, but open the health system up for issues of liability and find themselves without a position and with a spotty reputation.

Expediting Emergency Orders

Emergency orders or STAT (emergent) orders are a daily if not hourly (depending upon the decline of the patient's condition) occurrence in a health-system setting. Just as with any medication order, the pharmacy is responsible for making sure the order is filled and sent to the nursing unit for administration. While every medication order should be completed in a timely manner, emergency orders take precedence above all other orders.

Emergency medication orders are for medications that need to be administered to the patient due to situation that is or has become emergent. Situations where emergency orders would be valid might be when a patient's condition suddenly declines or a patient is brought into the emergency room with chest pains. Oftentimes the need for emergency orders will be associated with a life or death issue and should never be pushed aside for orders that are not emergent.

Every health system will have its own protocol in place for handling medication that has been labeled as STAT or emergent. Most health systems will indicate that a emergency medication order must have a turnaround time (the time it takes for the medication to get to the patient from the time it is sent to the pharmacy to the time the nurse administers the medication) of 15 minutes and times greater than this would be subject to being reported as a delay in patient care.

The nursing unit or emergency room will most often alert the pharmacy of an emergency medication order, but if this does not happen most computer software will have a built-in system, which alerts the pharmacy when the order is scanned. There are still some health systems that will fax or use a pneumatic tube system to send orders to the pharmacy. Faxing and the use of pneumatic tube systems can sometimes be unreliable and are not always the best route for emergency orders.

Once the pharmacy receives the order, the technician follows the same protocol for filling regular medication order, making sure to check all patient information. After the label is printed, the order is filled, and the pharmacist has verified the information, the technician will take the medication to the unit where it is needed. Sometimes a nurse or a staff member from the unit where the medication is needed will bring the order to the pharmacy and wait for it to be filled, so the time it takes for the pharmacy to get the order to the unit can be decreased. If the technician has to transport the medication to the unit or emergency room, if possible, it is best practice to hand the medication directly to the nurse or physician who ordered the medication. Handing the medication to the nurse or physician eliminates questions of delay later on.

Pharmacy technicians who are quick to recognize and react to emergency orders help to showcase the efficiency of the pharmacy and understand the pharmacy's importance in patient care.

❝ Workplace Wisdom Tech-Check-Tech

Historically, any task performed by a pharmacy technician related to dispensing a prescription had to be verified and documented in writing by a pharmacist, but certain states have now approved Tech-Check-Tech, a policy that enables hospital pharmacists to spend more time on activities designed to reduce errors and to provide clinical support to physicians and nurses.

In general, hospitals that utilize Tech-Check-Tech employ specially trained pharmacy technicians to check medication cassettes and the work of other technicians. Tech-Check-Tech regulations vary by state, and specific policies vary by institution. Because regulations change frequently, current information on Tech-Check-Tech regulations should be obtained from the SBOP.

Pharmacy Technician Job Responsibilities

To allow pharmacists to focus on the medication-related problems of their patients and provide the best pharmaceutical care, many tasks in the health-system care facility that were once performed by the pharmacist are now delegated to qualified support staff, including pharmacy technicians. The pharmacy technician, under the supervision of a pharmacist and according to the laws of the state in which the technician works, is permitted to perform a wide range of tasks. These tasks may involve a variety of the components of pharmacy practice, including, but not limited to:

- Data collection and reporting (patient satisfaction assessments, compilation of continuous quality improvement data, drug inventory management, formulary maintenance, preparation of billing statements)
- Surveys and inspections (conduct medication room inspections, conduct narcotic audits, check emergency boxes and replace outdated medications, check orders for completeness, inspect and service crash carts)
- Education (assist in facility meetings, help organize and maintain the medical library, and provide in-service training and continuing education for facility personnel)
- Maintenance (assist in the maintenance of devices such as fax machines and automated dispensing systems)
- Dispensing/inventory management (order medication stock, package medications, prepare intravenous solutions, fill and label prescriptions)

No task delegated to a pharmacy technician may involve performing a final check of a medication before it goes to the patient, nor may the technician perform any task that requires the professional judgment of a pharmacist.

To make sure that technicians are properly trained and their performance evaluated, the supervising pharmacist will provide a written job description of the functions performed by the pharmacy technicians, according to the regulations of the state where the facility is located. The initial orientation and training for pharmacy technicians should include information about properly performing their assigned functions, the unique needs of institutionalized patients, and relevant regulations.

The pharmacy technician also needs to receive ongoing training and education. Technicians should be given periodic evaluations of their job performance.

Tasks Requiring Quality Assurance

Quality assurance is the guarantee that a product will have, or process will be carried out with, the highest quality at a consistent rate. In other words, it will be of the same quality all of the time. You are, in a sense, guaranteeing your work. Quality assurance should be the pharmacy's thumbprint. In both retail and health systems, quality assurance should be an expectation.

Quality assurance should be apparent in all aspects of health-system pharmacy, but when it comes to the compounding of IV and chemotherapy agents it should be strictly enforced. There is no room for error in these types of tasks, and

the technician who compounds IV or chemotherapy agents will generally need to have advanced training. IV and chemotherapy compounding requires the use of protocols in order to avoid bringing harm to the patient. There are several ways pharmacy technicians can assure quality when compounding IV or chemotherapy agents:

- Use bar codes. The use of a bar code verification system in an IV room setting greatly reduces the chance of error. But it must be consistent and accurate. It also benefits the technician to do a visual check. Relying solely on bar code scanning can result in missed bar code input errors and a medication associated with the wrong drug.
- Do not inject the medication in the IV bag before it is verified by the pharmacist. Verification from the pharmacist assures the right drug is being used, the right amount of drug is being injected, and it is being injected into the right fluid.
- Double-check your work. Rereading an order before pulling a medication or requesting pharmacist verification can eliminate errors and potential waste of product.
- Make sure your label is correct—right patient, right drug, right instructions, right prescriber.
- Make sure all warning labels, expiration labels, and tamper-resistant materials have been applied to the compound before it is sent to the nursing unit. Chemotherapy agents always need to have a warning, as well as tamper-resistant materials, and some will need light-sensitive packaging. Some IV compounds need refrigeration or are stable only for short periods of time.
- Do a daily nursing unit inventory of all IV and chemotherapy compounds. Return to the pharmacy any compounds that have expired or are past the administration date; doing this will eliminate administration errors and protect the safety of the patient.

Other tasks within the health-system pharmacy that should be subject to quality assurance include:

- Medication order entry
- Filling of medication orders as well as patient medication carts and cassettes
- Service to other health-system professionals
- Timely manner of medication delivery
- Turnaround times for emergency medication orders
- Supplementing floor stock and automated dispensing cabinets (Pyxis and Omnicell)
- Pharmacy nursing unit and emergency code cart inspections, including emergency boxes used for air or ambulance patient transport or operating room emergency kits

Quality assurance should be a health-system pharmacy's only standard for its seal of approval. Health-system pharmacies provide medication therapies and direct patient care needed to support other health-system professionals as well as contribute to the medical needs of the patient. Pharmacy technicians should seek to provide quality assurance in all aspects of their responsibilities, helping to foster a trusting relationship between patients, other health-system professionals, and the pharmacy.

Providing Requested Information to the Pharmacist

In health-system pharmacies, pharmacists and technicians work closely with each other. Some health systems utilize a decentralized pharmacy, which is assigned to specific individual areas of the health system. In a decentralized pharmacy, a pharmacist or pharmacists work together with technicians assigned to the decentralized unit. Many times decentralized pharmacists will specialize in the type of care their decentralized floor provides such as pediatrics or orthopedics. As part of a cohesive team, decentralized pharmacists may rely on technicians to provide them with information necessary for the direct care of the patient.

A pharmacist who works in the centralized pharmacy or main pharmacy also works closely with technicians. There are also times when the centralized pharmacist will rely on the technician to provide him or her with information, which is pertinent to a patient's care.

A pharmacy technician should provide the centralized or decentralized pharmacist with information that is both professional and expedient. This information may include such things as specific information from a patient's medical chart; drug information from Micromedix, Lexicomp, or other reference material; steps taken in compounding a medication; prescriber's phone numbers; pricing and availability of a drug from the wholesaler; or reports concerning daily pharmacy operations.

The need for pharmacists and pharmacy technicians to work together as one team is no less evident in a health-system setting. Technicians who seek to be professional will gain the respect of the pharmacist, other health care professionals, and their peers.

Record Maintenance and Management

Pharmacy technicians are responsible for maintaining accurate, complete, and updated records on patients, procedures, inventory, training, and regulatory compliance.

Cassettes

Medication cassettes in a health-system pharmacy setting allow the pharmacy to fill a 24-hour supply of patient medications to be used on a specific nursing unit for a specific patient. A medication cassette fits into an associated case or cart, and each cassette is dedicated to an individual patient on a specific nursing unit. The cassette is labeled in the pharmacy with the patient information, and then the technician fills the cassette with a 24-hour supply of the patient's medications: both scheduled and PRN.

Each day the technician will run a report from the computer, which lists each patient and his or her medications; the pharmacy technician will then fill the cassette with the medications listed in the report, being sure to take out medications that have been discontinued as well as the medications from patients who have been discharged. Once the cassettes have been filled by the technician and checked by the pharmacist, the technician will exchange the newly filled cassettes with the cassettes currently on the nursing unit. Most health-system pharmacies will have a specific time of day during which this task needs to be done, so that all administration times are covered. Filling medication cassettes is not the same at every health-system pharmacy, but there are some things that apply to filling any medication cassette.

A pharmacy technician needs to remember a few things when filling medication cassettes: Thoroughly and carefully read through the patient's list of medication before you begin filling the cassette. Check to make certain the patient listed at the top of the report is the same patient whose name is on the medication cassette. If there are medications left in the cassette, check to make sure they are on the patient's medication profile. When you exchange medication cassettes, make certain to exchange it with the correct patient; patients are discharged and transferred hourly, oftentimes the patient cassettes are not labeled properly or updated with the correct patient name; it is always best to double-check the name on the patient cassette you are exchanging.

Pharmacy technicians should be aware of their health-system pharmacy's procedure for medication cassettes; it is unlikely any two health-system pharmacies will have the same procedure. If a pharmacy technician does have a question or concern about medication cassettes, he or she should speak with a pharmacist or the technician supervisor.

Unit-Dose Preparation

Pharmacy technicians are in charge of maintaining the unit-dose systems in an institution (see Figure 9-11). They are required to select and prepare medications for dispensing, much as they would in an ambulatory setting.

Medication carts are filled with the medications for each patient in his or her individual drawers. Because many medications do not come in unit-dose form, it is the pharmacy

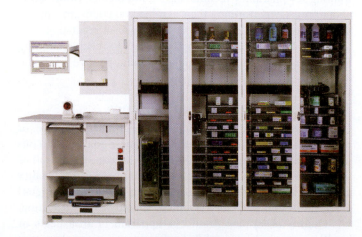

FIGURE 9-11 A view of a unit-dose system (the SP unit dispenser [SPUD]).
Source: Courtesy of ScriptPro

technician's responsibility to prepare all medications. The goal is to prepare each medication in a form as close to its dispensing form as possible. These doses are not labeled for a particular patient, but must be clearly labeled with the drug name and strength. As with any repackaging, strict attention to detail is essential. Each dose must be identifiable up to the time it is administered. All medications must remain sanitary, and in some cases, such as for IV injection, sterile.

- Patient's name
- Location (floor, room, and bed number)
- Drug (name and strength)
- Date

Documentation

Documentation for unit-dose preparations is an essential part of the unit-dose process. Without proper documentation, unit-dose preparations are unsafe to administer to the patient. Documentation procedures for unit-dose preparations vary slightly for each health system, but they all should have the following information:

- Drug name—brand and generic, if applicable
- Form—tablet, capsule, liquid
- Drug strength—liquid or concentration
- Drug's NDC number
- Lot number and expiration date
- Pharmacy expiration date (typically one year from the date of unit dosing; unless the expiration date on the drug bottle is less than one year, then the expiration date would be the bottle's expiration date.)
- Date the drug was packaged
- How many were packaged
- The class number if the drug is a controlled substance
- Initials and signature of the technician who packaged the drug
- Initials and signature of the pharmacist who verified packaging.

Each drug packaged for unit dose should have a separate sheet for documentation. The documentation sheet should then be cataloged in a notebook or other file system, alphabetically by generic name. Unit-dose documentation sheets should be examined periodically to make certain all drug information is being transferred correctly and that there are no changes that need to be made to the documentation procedure.

It is also important to remember that proper labeling of unit-dose products is considered documentation. Each item's unit-dose product will need to be labeled with the proper and correct information. Drug name (brand name where applicable), strength, dose, amount, lot number and expiration date, technician's initials are all vital information, which need to be on a unit-dose product. A unit-dose label should look very much like a manufacturer label and should be placed on the product in a manner that allows staff to read the label with ease and does not cover up any units of measure, which may be on the product, such as milliliters on an oral syringe. On oral syringes, the words "for oral use only" should be visible; be careful not to place the label over this warning.

Bulk Repackaging

The use of unit-dose medications in health-system pharmacies has made processes much easier when it comes to filling patient medication orders or patient medication cassettes, particularly if the order is written for only one dose. A great number of medications are available from the manufacturer as unit dose, but on occasion some are not and need to be repackaged by the pharmacy.

Bulk repackaging is usually a pharmacy technician's responsibility, and depending upon the number of patient beds a pharmacy supports, it can be a very busy job. Bulk repackaging can be done in a number of ways. Automated packagers (Talyst, Med-Pac) can produce from 60 to 120 tablets or capsules per minute. Automated packagers are usually integrated into the pharmacy's computer system. Information from the bulk drug package is entered into the computer system by the technician; once the machine begins to package the product, an imprint of the drug's information appears on one side of the packaging along with a clear side for viewing the drug on the other. The drug will drop down from a bin, which the pharmacy technician fills with the drug prior to starting the packager. Once the drug drops down between the imprinted side and the clear side of the package, it will be heat-sealed, coming out of the packager in one long unit, with perforations at each individual drug package for the ease of separation. After the drug is verified against the proper documentation and checked by the pharmacist, it is ready to be used to fill patient orders.

This process works for most, but not all drugs. There are some drugs that cannot be packaged using an automated packager, due to the size of the product, sensitivity to light, drug class, or cost. Drugs that fall into any of these categories need to be packaged by hand. The quantities packaged for these drugs are usually much smaller than those packaged with an automated packager.

Automated packagers can be a time-saving device, but only if procedures are followed. Verifying the correct drug to be packaged, as well as the drug's lot number and expiration date, can save from having to repeat the process because of an error during input. It is always a best practice to have another technician check your information before you begin the packaging process.

Documentation is also an important part of the repackaging process. Poorly done documentation can lead to patient medication error and other mistakes, which waste time and money. Information verification is always a pharmacy technician's friend and will always pay off in the end.

Documentation with Bulk Repackaging

Documentation with bulk repackaging, whether done manually or with automation, should follow the same documentation process as all other repacked medications. Documentation should include medication name (brand and generic), form, strength, lot number and expiration date, manufacturer's name, NDC number, pharmacy lot number and expiration date, date of packaging, and the technician's and pharmacist's initials and signature.

Improper documentation can lead to patient's medication errors, and in bulk packaging, the error is repeated at a much higher rate, giving a greater chance for the error to be administered to a patient.

Labeling is also a part of documentation. When using an automated bulk packaging process, the label will automatically be imprinted on the package and heat-sealed, but it is still a good idea to check these labels for imprint errors or packages that have not been sealed properly. In addition, occasionally a tablet or capsule may not drop correctly from the machine and you will have an empty package, among ones that are filled with the drug; take time to remove empty packages, so that they are not inadvertently placed in the drug storage bin.

Label making for bulk drugs, which is done manually, will need to be completed in a computer, using the pharmacy's label-making software. This type of label is made specifically for bulk packaging, generally available in a sheet of 30 labels. Proceed with the label-making process as you would with automated bulk packaging; be sure to include all necessary information. Once the item is verified, it can then be labeled and checked by the pharmacist.

All unit-dose packaging needs to be documented in the same manner; each drug should have a filled sheet documenting all information pertaining to the drug, as well as the technician's and pharmacist's initials and signature. Labeling should contain the same information as the documentation sheet and be placed properly on the item for the ease of reading. These steps are important in all types of unit-dose packaging, but most important with bulk repackaging; one error in bulk packaging can quickly turn into several.

🦉 Workplace Wisdom　Repackaging

Capsules and tablets are usually repackaged into blister packs or vials. Liquid medications are usually repackaged into cups or vials.

When repackaging medications, expiration dates must be determined and assigned. In general, expiration dates are established as either six months from the date of repackaging or one-quarter of the manufacturer's remaining expiration date, whichever is less. 🙶

Packaging Special Doses

Special dose packaging involves packaging doses of medication for a very specific dosage. This might be anything from a half tablet to a syringe for an infant in a neonatal unit. Special

---

▮ Procedure 9-1

Determining Expiration Dates

1. Locate the expiration date assigned by the manufacturer.
2. Calculate the total number of months remaining between today's date and the expiration date.
3. Divide the total number of months remaining by 4.
4. Add the result of step 3 to the current date.
5. Compare six months from today's date with the result of step 4 and select the lesser of the two.

PROFILE IN PRACTICE

Joe is a pharmacy technician who works in the centralized pharmacy. He is mainly responsible for repackaging medications into unit dosages. Currently, Joe is repackaging docusate sodium, which bears a manufacturer's expiration date of 10/2015

▶ *What expiration date should Joe assign to this medication?*

---

dose packaging needs to be precise; paying careful attention to the specified dose will remove the chance of medication error later.

Half tablets are one form of special dose packaging. Half-tablet packaging is usually done when a physician prescribes a dose, which may be available commercially, but is not kept in the pharmacy stock. Drug shortages and availability may be other reasons for using half-tablet packaging.

When packaging half tablets, there are a few things the technician must keep in mind. Tablets that are time released, delayed, or enteric coated cannot be cut in half; these are mechanisms of the drug and can directly affect the way the drug is released in the body. These types of drug mechanisms are usually taken on a once-a-day schedule; cutting one of these tablets in half will alter the effect of the drug, giving the patient too much or too little of the drug. Capsules, for obvious reasons, also cannot be cut in half. When cutting tablets in half for packaging, be sure to use a pill cutter that has been thoroughly cleaned; cut slowly and carefully, so as not to crush the tablet.

When printing the label for half tablets make certain that it indicates the packaging contains a half tablet and not a whole tablet; incorrect labeling of half tablets can very quickly lead to patient drug errors.

Finally, when you are packaging half tablets, it is best practice to package only the amount your patient will need for a 24 to 48-hour period; packaging more than this can be a waste of time and money, especially if it is a drug not commonly used in your pharmacy.

Special dose packaging also commonly involves the compounding of specific dosing for oral medications; this is most often used on a neonatal or pediatric unit. Oral dosing can be done when a patient cannot swallow a tablet or capsule or when the commercial strength of a drug is much larger than the dose that was ordered.

When compounding special-dose oral syringes or unit-dose bottles, the technician must take care to draw the exact dose into the oral syringe or bottle; too much or too little could affect patient dosing and, over a period of time, patient care and recovery. Always double-verify your drug before drawing it into the oral syringe or unit-dose bottle. Once the drug has been verified, it can be drawn into the oral syringe or unit-dose bottle. Check for any air bubbles in oral syringes, make certain the oral syringe has "for oral use only" imprinted on the syringe, and then cap the tip of the oral syringe and place tamper-resistant tape over the top of the cap. When using a unit bottle, place the drug in the bottle, cap, and place tamper-resistant tape across the top of the bottle and down along the sides.

When doing any form of special-dose packaging, it is always best to have another technician or pharmacist verify all drug information: drug, packaging, calculations, and dose. Not only could this save your time later, but, if a mistake is discovered, protect a patient.

Documentation with Special-Dose Packaging

There should be no variation in documentation with special-dose packaging; any drug that is packaged by a technician or pharmacist should have the same standard for packaging. In special-dose packaging, documenting the specific dose ordered is extremely important. If the packaging of a special dose comes into question, this documentation becomes a reference point later on. Drug name, strength, dose, manufacturer, lot number and expiration date, as well as the technician's and pharmacist's initials are all standards for package documentation—both for the file copy and the drug label.

Pharmacy technicians should also take care when placing labels on special-dose packaging, particularly when labeling oral syringes. The label should be placed on the oral syringe securely; the label is the only identification of the drug and if it detaches from the oral syringe, the product becomes useless. "Flagging" the label on the oral syringe usually works best. The label should not cover up any lines of measurement on the oral syringe, and, most important, the label should never cover the words "for oral use only."

Remember to place any auxiliary labels the special-dose drug might need: keep in refrigerator, protect from light, or expires on. Taking a few extra steps in the documentation process initially can eliminate questions and confusion later on.

Floor Stock Inspections

Most health systems utilize pharmacy technicians to inspect and maintain the floor stock. The technician inspects the inventory levels, expiration dates, stock condition, and storage conditions. *Floor stock* refers to medications that are located on the patient floors to be administered by nurses. These medications should be inspected daily.

Expired, Discontinued, and Recalled Medications

Floor stock inspections are a common responsibility for the health-system pharmacy technician. Floor stock inspections need to be done on a monthly basis in order to remove any drugs that may be expired, discontinued, and/or recalled. A technician who is diligent with this task saves himself or herself from potential issues later on.

State regulatory bodies as well as the Joint Commission regularly inspect health systems for code violations. They inspect each unit and department of the health system for such things as standards of patient care; fire code; and expired, discontinued, and recalled medications. If an expired, discontinued, or recalled medication is found, it is marked as a violation and the health system has 30 days to correct the issue.

It is for this reason that removing any expired, discontinued, or recalled medication is so important when completing a floor stock inspection. It is very easy to miss the medication of a patient who has been discharged or an expired vial or tablet in an automated dispensing cabinet, but the health-system pharmacy technician should have a plan in place for making certain that these types of medications are removed and returned to the pharmacy. Inventory personnel normally receive the first warnings concerning recalled medications and should alert all pharmacists and technicians. If a technician is alerted to a recall, the technician should make time to remove the drug from his or her assigned floor stock.

Each health-system pharmacy will have its own procedure for expired, discontinued, and recalled medications, which have been returned to the pharmacy from floor stock, but documentation must always be part of the process. Separation of expired, discontinued, and recalled medication is also a common practice in health-system pharmacies. Typically these drugs will be cataloged by the pharmacy's inventory person, so they can be accounted for in the pharmacy inventory and then they will be destroyed by either the health system or an outside company approved by the DEA to destroy medications.

If a technician finds he or she is removing too many expired medications from the automated dispensing cabinet, it may be prudent to decrease the amount of drug level allowed in the dispensing cabinet.

If a technician finds he or she is discovering too many discontinued patient medications in the nursing units, then it may be wise to speak with the technician supervisor so that a solution can be sought for the issue. It may simply be an issue of one person or another not knowing how to handle discontinued medications.

If recalled medications become a problem, then the pharmacy technician should speak with the technician supervisor who may be able to offer a solution.

Removal of expired, discontinued, and recalled medications from floor stock is an essential part of a pharmacy technician's responsibilities and if left undone could cause potential harm or fines imposed upon the health system.

Crash Carts

Pharmacy technicians are often responsible for stocking crash carts, which are sets of trays on a wheeled cart that are used in critical situations or for emergency medical care.

A crash cart typically contains a defibrillator and intravenous medications, plus a variety of medical supplies such as latex gloves and alcohol swabs. While the specific inventory of an institution's crash cart varies, the following are examples of the standard minimum equipment and medication requirements:

Equipment

Airways, all sizes
Forceps, large and small
Nasal canulas, infant, pedi, adult
100% non-rebreather oxygen face masks, infant, pedi, adult
Ambu Bags, infant, pedi, adult

IV Start Paks
1000 cc bag normal saline solution
IV tubing (burotrol for pedi patients)
Angiocatheters
1 cc syringes
3 cc syringes
5 cc syringes
10 cc syringes
20 cc syringes
Gauze
Alcohol preps
Flashlight

Drugs

Aspirin 325 mg tabs
Nitroglycerin 0.4 mg sublingual tabs
Dextrose 50%
Narcan 1 mg amps
Epinephrine 1 mg (1:10,000 conc)
Atropine sulfate 0.1 mg/mL
Lidocaine 100 mg
EpiPen
EpiPen Jr.
SoluMedrol 125 mg vial
Benadryl 50 mg vial
Tagamet 300 mg vial

Compounding

Compounding in health-system pharmacies refers to preparing custom-ordered medications, such as IVs, total parenteral nutrition (TPN), and nonsterile compounds. Technicians preparing orders for IV medications or TPN need specialized training. There are a plethora of machines and measuring systems available, but the equipment is only as good as the operator. Technicians filling these kinds of medication work with less supervision and do more calculations; therefore, they must be well trained. Several accreditations and certifications are available for technicians who wish to specialize in compounding. Technicians who want to perform this type of work should take advantage of those opportunities.

> ❝ **Workplace Wisdom** **USP**
>
> The *US Pharmacopoeia's* (*USP*) revised general chapter "Pharmaceutical Compounding—Sterile Preparations" sets practice standards to ensure that compounded sterile preparations are of high quality. For more information on *USP* go to www.usp.org. ❞

Tech-Check-Tech

As pharmacist roles in health systems continue to move toward more clinical and direct patient care duties, pharmacy technician roles also continue to expand. One of the programs that is gaining popularity in health-system pharmacies is the use of a Tech-Check-Tech system.

Tech-Check-Tech is a system of medication verification where one technician checks the work of another technician. This program employs the use of technicians who are certified

and have passed the health system's required testing to check items such as medication cassettes, floor stock, and refills for automated dispensing cabinets (ADCs).

Tech-Check-Tech is not used in every state; currently only nine states have laws regarding Tech-Check-Tech, which include Texas, California, and Minnesota. Allowance of Tech-Check-Tech is approved by the individual SBOP. Once a state approves Tech-Check-Tech, then the health system must apply for licensure from the SBOP in order to use Tech-Check-Tech in its facility. If the state approves the application, then the health system may institute Tech-Check-Tech, but only if it has a plan in place for stringent technician testing.

Tech-Check-Tech has proven to be a safe and effective verification system, which can free pharmacists to perform much-needed clinical duties within the health system. One study showed a 99.8% accuracy rate with technicians who were part of a Tech-Check-Tech program, having error rates similar to or better than their pharmacist's counterparts.

Technicians who want to be part of a health system's Tech-Check-Tech program will need to pass regulations and testing prior to becoming eligible for the program. Each state and institution sets standards applicable to Tech-Check-Tech, with the following standards being the most common:

- Pharmacy technician certification
- At least one year of work experience as a certified pharmacy technician
- One–on-one training with a pharmacist
- A written test to prove accuracy as well as a didactic component

While Tech-Check-Tech may be useful in some areas of pharmacy, it cannot be used in all aspects. A technician may not check the work of another technician when it comes to matters concerning compounding of IVs or chemotherapy drugs, specialized medication formulations, and first or new drug doses. When using a Tech-Check-Tech program, the pharmacy and the pharmacy technician must operate within the confines of the SBOP; any violation of these regulations results in the discontinuation of the program.

Tech-Check-Tech continues to grow as an institutional practice and is a career opportunity for those technicians who wish to expand their careers; still its continued growth depends upon the success of those who have already employed it. SBOP and institution guidelines for Tech-Check-Tech should never be circumvented because of a backlogged workflow or the busy schedule of a pharmacist. Using Tech-Check-Tech under these circumstances puts patients at risk and will soon eliminate the program from the facility.

If technicians have questions concerning Tech-Check-Tech, they should speak with their pharmacy manager or technical supervisor. Technicians may also find information regarding Tech-Check-Tech on their SBOP website.

Regulations

Regulations for Tech-Check-Tech are established by the SBOP. Institutions must follow these regulations to the letter of the law in order to apply for a Tech-Check-Tech program. If an institution is approved for Tech-Check-Tech, then they may proceed with the program.

An institution may also create its own additional set of standards for technicians wishing to be part of a Tech-Check-Tech. Certification, testing, and accuracy are industry standards. Some institutions may require technicians who want to be part of Tech-Check-Tech to be employed with the institution for a specified period of time. Institutions may require periodic testing of the technician once he or she becomes part of the Tech-Check-Tech program. Continuing education or in-services may become a requirement for Tech-Check-Tech programs.

Regulations are put in place as a form of protection. Regulations should never be tossed aside, regardless of the technician's experience or the trust the pharmacist has for a particular technician. Not respecting regulations defeat the purpose of Tech-Check-Tech programs, forcing the pharmacy to take steps backward rather than forward.

Institutional Policies

Institutional policies for Tech-Check-Tech are built based on the needs of the institution, while incorporating the regulations set forth by the SBOP. If at any time an institution feels as if Tech-Check-Tech is not in the best interest of its patients, it may discontinue the program.

Institutions will generally first form a committee to see if Tech-Check-Tech is an applicable program for their facility. This will be done over an extended length of time: gathering information regarding fill times, time spent on clinical consultation, the pharmacist's and technician's error rates, as well as any issues of safety. Evaluation of the potentials of the program will be done; if a decision is reached to proceed with the program, the pharmacy will apply for licensure from the SBOP to use Tech-Check-Tech.

Once an institution is approved for Tech-Check-Tech, it will begin to single out those technicians whom it feels are good candidates for Tech-Check-Tech. Certification, years of experience as a technician, and accuracy rates are key factors in decision making. Technicians who are chosen must complete an institution-implemented training program, pass written and didactic testing, and have one-on-one informational time with a selected pharmacist.

Institutions may also have additional requirements such as continuing education credits and in-services, yearly testing, and accuracy inspections. Institutions may remove a technician any time they feel the technician does not meet the standards of the program. Quality and success of a Tech-Check-Tech depends not only on the ability of the technician, but also on the dedication of the institution to the needs program.

Methodical Approach

Methodical approach is the way we set about completing a task; in this way it is much like protocol, a specific number of steps in a specific order, which are needed to complete a task accurately and efficiently. In the process of Tech-Check-Tech, methodical approach is not only important, but essential.

In Tech-Check-Tech, a carefully written set of guidelines has been established in order to ensure the safety of the patient; going outside of these guidelines discredits the program and the technician. Technicians chosen for a Tech-Check-Tech program have gained the trust of their institution, trust in their abilities as a technician, and trust showing their desire to follow established guidelines and methods.

No two technicians will ever have the same approach to a method; some may organize themselves before they begin a process; others will just jump right in, regardless of how to go about the method, making certain to use established guidelines when completing the method is the most important.

Methodical approaches such as always verifying "right drug, right patient," bringing concerns and questions regarding medication dosages and possible interactions to the attention of the pharmacist, filling ADCs with the correct drug in the correct drawer, removing discontinued drugs from medication cassettes or a patient's profile, and consistently being accurate are all part of a methodical approach to Tech-Check-Tech.

Using a methodical approach when using Tech-Check-Tech can decrease if not eliminate issues, ease frustrations, and provide excellent standards of care for patients. Methodical approach can also keep productivity and workflow at their highest, providing all involved a much more satisfying experience. Technicians who use a methodical approach gain trust and respect as well as validate the importance of Tech-Check-Tech when it comes to the need for more pharmacist involvement in direct patient care.

Medical Information Systems

Medical information systems in health-system pharmacy are standard equipment; few if any can run effectively without them. As health systems and technology continue to grow, the gap between them seems to become smaller and smaller. Advances in medical software allow the health-system pharmacy to be alerted to potential patient drug allergies or drug interactions, as well as dosing calculations, drug information, and inventory stock and control.

The use of medical information systems has become so extensive that it has allowed pharmacists and technicians to carve out new and expanding career options. Pharmacy informatics is a career field that focuses on medication information data and how it relates to the needs of health systems.

Health system will usually have a proprietary system for storing medical information. Medical software is rarely the same for all health systems and often will require several days of training to learn, depending upon the user's extent and skill level. It may take some time to learn the ins and outs of health-system software, but eventually it becomes second nature.

Health-system medical information systems are sophisticated pieces of technology, which link each of their departments together and with computers outside of the health system. Pharmacy medical information systems are commonly linked with drug wholesalers, SBOPs, DEA, and drug information sites. Pharmacy medical information systems also supply pharmacy personnel with information concerning patient medication profiles, prescribers, insurance, ordered diagnostic testing and results, prescriber's dictation notes, and previous admission information—all information necessary for providing the patient with a well thought-out plan for direct patient care.

Because so much patient information is so readily available, it is important to remember to follow the regulations set forth by HIPAA. Pharmacy is just as responsible as any other department of the health system for seeing that privacy regulations are not compromised. Technicians should remember it is never appropriate to look up patient information they are not authorized to see, including information pertaining to family members or themselves. While it may be tempting to look up your spouse's cholesterol test, it is unlawful and can be grounds for immediate dismissal.

Another type of medical information system used in health-system pharmacies are ADCs such as Pyxis or Omnicell. ADCs can range greatly in size and are used in any areas where medication might be needed urgently or where floor stock may be located.

ADCs have a computer monitor and a computer hard drive integrated into the dispensing cabinet. The ADC is linked to the main frame of the health system as well as the ADC manufacturer, helping to detect any software issues and correcting them before they become a much greater issue. Patient profiles and medication list are updated on the pharmacy computer system and then uploaded to the ADC hard drive, allowing authorized personnel to pull emergency medications, controlled substances, and PRN medications from the cabinet during a scheduled time of administration.

ADC systems are an excellent tool for fighting drug diversion, as every dose taken from the cabinet leaves an imprint of the user's name, patient it was administered to, the medication that was removed, and the amount removed. Inventory of controlled substances stocked in ADCs is typically done by nursing staff prior to shift change; any discrepancies found between the inventoried amount and the ADC-stated amount may require pharmacy to run a report to find the error. Oftentimes it is something as simple as an incorrect count during restock or inventory; either way, all controlled substances stocked in ADCs need to be accounted for.

Medical information systems can make processes much easier to complete, provide pharmacy staff with a greater picture of a patient's needs, bring departments and systems together, illicit tighter inventory controls for controlled substances, and provide patients and health-system staff with safer and better care.

Characteristics of Typical Database

Medical information systems are virtually useless without a well thought-out and comprehensive database. First and foremost, medical databases must be able to store large amounts of sensitive patient information securely. This also means those who operate medical information systems should respect the regulations regarding this information.

A health-system pharmacy database should include not only the basic information concerning a patient, but all aspects related to his or her care. Laboratory testing and results are important for medication therapy consultation. Many

medication orders cannot be written without the results of specific lab tests; TPN, aminoglycoside monitoring, and testing for bacterial strains are all important in deciding the next step in a patient's medication therapy.

Health-system pharmacy databases should also include information useful in patient medication consultations. Reference material is an invaluable tool for pharmacy staff and sometimes needs to be relayed to physicians quickly; databases that contain this information make this a much smoother transaction.

Medical information databases should also contain information regarding a pharmacy's inventory and formulary. Pharmacy databases can easily be connected to wholesalers, giving the pharmacy an up-to-date view of medication availability and cost.

Finally, pharmacy health system databases may contain sensitive departmental information such as employee information, pay rates, and employee evaluations. This information is for authorized users only and should never be shared with those who should not have access to these records.

Uses of medical information databases can be limitless. The pharmacy technician who learns how to use this information raises his or her career to the next level, gaining a career advantage with promising potential.

Medication Use Review

Medication use review (MUR) is a process that was developed as a direct result of the 1990 Omnibus Budget Reconciliation Act (OBRA). OBRA provides mandatory patient medication counseling for new prescriptions as well as the use of MURs.

MURs are a way of looking at a patient's medication therapy in such a way that it allows for the best clinical therapy option while also being cost-effective. Medication therapies also analyze medication safety issues and if the medication is being used for its approved indication.

Medication use reviews also compile information regarding issues that might be seen prior to the filing process such as prescription abuse or fraudulent insurance practices.

MUR is an intended educational tool for prescribers and pharmacists. State's regulatory agencies, such as the SBOP and the State Medical Boards, are required to produce a stand of policy and procedure for their state's MUR. Pharmacists and prescribers who are part of MUR committees help to create a protocol for patient safety and medication therapy, cementing the need for further clinical involvement in patient medication therapy.

The Pharmacy Technician's Role

Pharmacy technicians have always been valuable members of the pharmacy team, but with the creation of OBRA, technicians have become a needed resource. Pharmacist must help fulfill the clinical therapy obligations of OBRA, leaving pharmacy technicians to complete tasks that have traditionally been done by pharmacists.

One current example is the move toward better regulations and education for pharmacy technician. Tech-Check-Tech programs show how technician resources can be used to help decrease medication errors and give additional time to pharmacists in order to complete clinical duties involving direct patient care. Some health systems are even experimenting with Technician Medication Reconciliation.

As pharmacist's careers morph into clinical-based duties, the pharmacy technician's responsibilities will become greater and more involved, ever expanding the realm of career possibilities.

Productivity and Workflow Management

Productivity and workflow management—you cannot have one without the other. In health-system pharmacy productivity is how quickly or efficiently the pharmacy is able to produce its services for the patient and other health-system professionals. Patient medication orders, compounded IV medications, special drug preparations, and patient consultations are all part of a health system's productivity.

Workflow involves the steps the health-system pharmacy takes to produce a product. The more steps it takes to produce a product, the less efficient it is and the more it costs to produce; money, time, and safety become victims of poor workflow management.

Productivity and workflow are oftentimes the hallmark of a health-system pharmacy. Prescribers, nursing staff, and other health-system workers learn to judge the pharmacy department by its performance in these two areas. Pharmacy technicians who understand the necessary connection between productivity and workflow provide outstanding service not only to patients, but to other health-system departments as well; knowing the services these departments provide can oftentimes depend on the service the pharmacy provides to them.

Productivity and workflow can be hampered by any number of issues: improperly trained staff, unclear procedures and protocols or none at all, lack of staff, chronic sick calls, drug and inventory shortages, miscommunication among staff members, or poor management involvement. A technician who recognizes these, or any other problem that hampers productivity and workflow, should speak with his or her pharmacy manager or direct supervisor. A problem that goes unrecognized cannot be fixed, and sometimes management may not be close enough to the problem to understand it is a problem.

Making workflow more efficient increases productivity and increased productivity provides better patient care, which in turn eases strain between departments. Pharmacy technicians should realize their importance in this process and feel free to discuss suggestions that have the potential for improving the process. Well-managed productivity and workflow creates a safe, efficient care for the patient and job satisfaction for the pharmacy technician.

Collaborating with Other Departments

Health systems are made up of various departments, and each one of those departments works together as a team. Health systems need to function as coordinated teams in order to provide safe continuous care for patients. Pharmacy is a very centrally located player in the makeup of the health-system team.

Many departments count on the pharmacy department to provide them with the medications necessary to control their patient's pain, perform surgery, administer medications, or provide them with knowledgeable medication information and therapeutic medication plans. Pharmacy technicians have a large part in producing positive results when collaborating with other departments.

Collaboration between pharmacy departments can be as simple as agreeing on the procedure for emergency medication orders to deciding pharmacy's role in the development of patient care plans. Oftentimes collaboration will involve a pharmacy representative meeting with a representative staff member from another department and asking how pharmacy can help to fill gaps in processes. Pharmacy technicians can be valid representatives for the pharmacy department, using professionalism as a way to collaborate processes and needs with other department.

A health system cannot function with just one department. Collaboration among all departments is necessary for the health system to function as one team, recognizing patient care and safety as their highest priority.

Investigational Drug Products

New drugs are introduced into the U.S. drug market every day, but for those drugs to be approved for use in the United States they must pass strict guidelines set in place by the Food and Drug Administration (FDA).

Any drug manufacturer who wishes to apply for FDA approval must first prove the drug is safe for human consumptions; this is a long, rigorous process, which may take several years. Once the drug is approved by the FDA, it will not receive complete approval until it has completed three clinical phases.

- **Phase I**—a handful of volunteers will be selected for drug testing and levels of toxicity.
- **Phase II**—several doses are used in order to determine which dosage works best with the least amount of side effects.
- **Phase III**—double-blind and controlled placebo studies are done to see how well the drug works

If at the end of phase III the drug manufacture proves the safety and worthiness of the drug, the FDA will approve the manufacturing of the drug, conditional to any changes or restrictions the FDA requires from the drug manufacturer concerning manufacturing, labeling, or distribution.

Investigational drug trials can cost the manufacturer hundreds of thousands of dollars; however, participants in the drug trials can often reap the benefits of the drug's potential.

Development

Development of investigational drug trials in health-system pharmacies is usually taken on by the pharmacy's clinical team. However, there are health-system pharmacies that have specific teams within the department dedicated to the development of investigational drugs.

Typically the pharmacy department is responsible for investigational drug development and will assign a pharmacist or pharmacists, as well as technicians, to be part of the investigational development team. They will work closely with the drug manufacturer, FDA, prescribers, nursing personnel, and any outside state or federal agencies involved in development.

The investigational drug team will meet on a periodic basis to discuss how the drug should be dosed, stored, handled, and disposed of. They will also decide the patient's criteria necessary for drug trial participation. Only volunteers who meet all criteria may participate in the trial. Only prescribers who are recognized as participating in the trail may prescribe the investigational drug. Once all investigation protocols have been developed, the drug manufacturer will supply the pharmacy with the drug and the investigational process can begin.

Record Keeping

Accurate record keeping during an investigational drug process is critical for the approval of the drug. Drug reactions and benefits need to be recorded for investigators to understand all aspects of the drug. The FDA requires the following documentation be kept regarding investigational drug trials:

- Name of those involved in the investigation as well as their titles
- Date the drug was shipped
- Amount of drug shipped
- Code or batch number for shipped drug
- Records of any and all financial reimbursements or payments made to the investigative team or facility by the rug manufacturer

The FDA states these records must be kept for at least two years following the end of the drug trial, as well as a viable sample of the investigational drug.

The investigational team will work closely with the manufacturer to ensure that all required information is documented and released to the FDA. Pharmacy technicians may be called upon to help compile this information by inputting data into the computer base or printing off investigation reports. Pharmacy technicians may also be required to monitor storage, distribution, and disposal of the investigational drug.

Standard Policies and Procedures

Standard policies and procedures for investigational drugs will be determined by the investigational drug team, health-system management, drug manufacturer, and the FDA. The investigational drug team will oversee all aspects of the investigational drug and will determine standards for:

- Labeling
- Storage
- Distribution
- Disposal
- Documentation

Standards for policy and procedures will be based upon FDA regulations as well as health-system policies and required drug manufacturer's information. Any deviation from the standards set forth by the investigational team can be the reason for the investigational drug trial to be terminated.

Pharmacy technicians who are part of an investigational drug trial are under obligation to see all standards for policy and procedure are maintained throughout the investigation. The use of pharmacy technician resources in investigational trial can be useful to all members of the investigational drug team and a move forward in the pharmacy technician's career.

Summary

Health-system pharmacies are designed to serve patients who reside on-site, at the same facility where the pharmacy is located. Health-system pharmacies, also known as institutional pharmacies, include hospital pharmacies and pharmacies in LTC facilities, nursing homes, correctional facilities, and other institutions. Hospital pharmacies are the most common.

Although filling a prescription and filling a medication order are basically the same, health-system pharmacy practice is more varied than community pharmacy practice. Health-system pharmacy technicians work with several distribution systems, repackage medications for specific patients, and also do bulk repackaging for floors and patient care areas. Health-system pharmacies commonly use unit-dose dispensing,

in which patients receive no more than a 24-hour supply of the medications ordered. In hospitals, these medications are dispensed via a centralized pharmacy or a series of satellite pharmacies dispersed throughout the facility. Institutional technicians also deal with sterile and aseptic techniques, cytotoxins, and chemotherapy drugs, as well as a variety of automatic dispensing systems.

The practice of pharmacy in an institutional setting is evolving just as fast, if not faster, as the practice in ambulatory settings. Innovations in medications, drug delivery systems, information systems, and patient care provide technicians' opportunities for more training, education, and responsibility in the health care system.

Chapter Review Questions

1. How often do pharmacists generally perform drug therapy review for each patient?
   a. weekly
   b. monthly
   c. semimonthly
   d. quarterly

2. Which of the following is permitted to administer medication to patients?
   a. CNA
   b. LNA
   c. LPN
   d. CPhT

3. What is the name for an adult care home that is licensed and governed by state and federal regulations?
   a. nursing home
   b. adult day care
   c. homeless shelter
   d. senior center

4. _____ provide rehabilitative, restorative, or ongoing skilled nursing care to individuals who need assistance with the activities of daily living.
   a. Hospices
   b. Hospitals
   c. Correctional facilities
   d. LTC facilities

5. Once a medication order is packaged in a unit-dose container, it must be _____.
   a. rushed to the patient
   b. taken to the attending nurse
   c. properly stored until called for
   d. checked by a pharmacist before being dispensed

6. _____ orders are used for specific medications to be administered at specific intervals throughout the day.
   a. PRN
   b. standing
   c. STAT
   d. CPOE

7. The most efficient medication delivery system in a health-system pharmacy is _____.
   a. individual
   b. floor stock
   c. unit dose
   d. bulk

8. The benefit of an automated dispensing system is that it _____.
   a. is cost-effective
   b. reduces errors when operated properly
   c. helps reduce diversion
   d. all of the above

9. Which regulatory agency administers the State Children's Health Insurance Program?
   a. Joint Commission
   b. SBOP
   c. CMS
   d. DPS

10. Which of the following cannot be repackaged as a unit dose?
    a. C-II medications
    b. liquid medications
    c. eye drops
    d. reconstituted powders

Critical Thinking Questions

1. In what ways is health-system pharmacy practice different from community pharmacy practice?

2. What are the benefits of establishing satellite pharmacies within a health system?

3. Why do health-system pharmacies repackage unit-dose medications?

Web Challenge

1. Go to the National Association for Public Hospitals and Health Systems (NAPH) website and research the definition and characteristics of a *safety net hospital*: http://www.naph.org

2. Visit the American Hospital Association (AHA) website and print out the "Fast Facts on US Hospitals" report: http://www.aha.org

References and Resources

American Hospital Association. *2004 Hospital Statistic Report.* Chicago: AHA, 2004. Print.

American Medical Association. *Know Your Drugs and Medications.* New York: Reader's Digest Association, 1991. Print.

American Pharmacist Association. *Pharmacy Technician Workbook and Certification Review.* Englewood, CO: Morton Publishing, 2001. Print.

American Society of Hospital Pharmacist. "ASHP Statement on the Pharmacy and Therapeutics Committee and the Formulary System."*ASHP.* 2008. Web. 30 May 2012.

American Society of Hospital Pharmacist. "ASHP Technical Assistance Bulletin on Repackaging Oral Solids and Liquids in Single Unit and Unit Dose Packaging." *ASHP.* December 2012. Web. 31 May 2012.

American Society of Hospital Pharmacist. "Guidelines on Preventing Medication Errors in Hospitals." *ASHP.* December 2011. Web. 29 May 2012.

American Society of Hospital Pharmacist. "Innovative Technician Practices Debating in Hospitals. Tech-Check-Tech, Med Rec Show What Technicians Can Do." *ASHP Intersections.* December 2011. Web. 29 May 2012.

American Society of Health-System Pharmacist. *Manual for Pharmacy Technicians.* 2nd ed. Bethesda, MD: ASHP. 1998. Print.

American Society of Health-System Pharmacist. *Quality Assurance Pharmacist.* n.p. Web. 28 May 2012.

Askew, G. and Stoner-Smith, M. *Assisting in the Pharmacy.* Thomson Delmar. n.p. Print.

"CareScout." *Nursing-Home* 2006. Web. 4 March 2006.

Commonwealth of Pennsylvania. *Standards of Practice.* 2012. Web. 23 May 2012.

Davis, K. *Pharmacy Management Software for Pharmacy Technicians.* 2nd ed. Brookline, MA: DAA Enterprises, Inc. 2012. Print.

Diebold, J. "The Significance of Productivity Data." *Harvard Business News.* May 2009. Web. 30 May 2012.

Dixon, B and Zafar, A. "Inpatient Computerized Provider Order Entry (CPOE)." *HHS.* January 2009. Web. 31 May 2012.

"Drug Enforcement Administration." *Drug Diversion.* Web. 25 May 2012.

"Drug Enforcement Administration." *History of the DEA.* Web. 25 May 2012.

"EurekAlert." *Tech-Check-Tech.* January 2007. Web. 29 May 2012.

Food and Drug Administration. *Code of Federal Regulation.* June 2010. Web. 1 June 2012.

Gaunt, M. "Maximizing the Effectiveness of Bar Code Scanning." *Pharmacy Times.* September 2010. Web. 31 May 2012.

Glatter, R. "How Should We Define Productivity in Healthcare?" *Forbes.* May 2012. Web. 21 May 2012.

Health and Human Services. "Medicaid Drug Use Review Programs. Lessons Learned by States." *HHS.* 1995. Web. 1 June 2012.

Idaho Society of Hospital Pharmacist. *Tech-Check-Tech Program.* 2006. Web. 29 May 2012.

IDE Approval Process. June 2010. Web. 1 June 2012.

Institutes for Safe Medication Practices. *Oops, Sorry! Wrong Patient. A Verification System in Needed Everywhere, Not Just at the Bedside.* 2010. Web. 31 May 2012.

IQTELL Productivity. *Productivity and Organizations— What Makes Them Important to Us?* December 2011. Web. 30 May 2012.

Johnston, Mike. *The Pharmacy Technician: Foundations and Practices.* 1st ed. Upper Saddle River, NJ: Pearson, 2009. Print.

Merriam-Webster Dictionary. Web. 28 May 2012.

National Hospice and Palliative Care Organization. *Hospice Standards of Practice.* Alexandria, VA: NHPCO, 2000. Print.

Naylor, H., Woloshuck, D., Fitch, P., and Miller, S., "Retrospective Audit of Medication Order Turn Around Times after Implementation of Standard Definition." *National Institutes of Health.* September–October 2011. Web. 31 May 2012.

Organisations for Economic Co-operation and Development. "Defining and Measurement Productivity." *OECD.* n.p. Web. 30 May 2012.

Pharmacy Technician Certification Board. Web. 29 May 2012.

Plaqakis, J. "Change is the Air Pharmacist Will Breathe." *Drug Topics.* June 2011. Web. 29 May 2012.

Shedd, D. "Tech-Check-Tech Programs." *Pharmacy Tech Resources: The Tech Letter*, Issue 1. August 2011. Web. 29 May 2012.

Teeters, J. "Gazing into the Crystal Ball; Health-System Pharmacy 2011 and Beyond." *ASHP InterSections.* 28 March 2011. Web. 19 May 2012.

Texas Tech University Health Sciences Center. "Minimum Crash Cart Supplies and Drugs." *Texas Tech.* 2008. Web. 12 April 2008.

Texas Tech University School of Pharmacy. "A Technician's Role. Optimizing Patient Safety and Minimizing Medication Errors. A Knowledge Base Course for Technicians." *JD Education.* n.p. Web. 28 May 2012.

The Joint Commission. Web. 31 May 2012.

United States Pharmacopeia. Web. 12 April 2008.

Van Dusen, V. and Sipes, A. "An Overview and Update of the Controlled Substance Act of 1970." *Pharmacy Times.* February 2007. Web. 20 May 2012.

Vanderbilt University Pharmacy Department. "Procedure for the Storage, Handling, and Dispensing of Investigational Drugs, Agents, and/or Biologics in Clinical Trials." *Vanderbilt University.* 2009. Web. 1 June 2012.

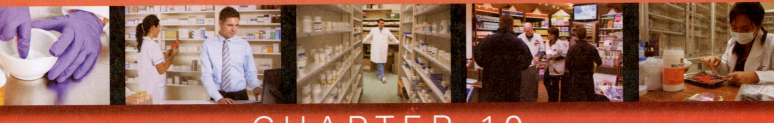

CHAPTER 10

Technology in the Pharmacy

LEARNING OBJECTIVES

After completing this chapter, you should be able to:

- List the hardware and software components used in pharmacy computers and summarize their purpose.

- Describe and discuss the use of automation and robotics in community pharmacies.

- Describe and discuss the use of automation and robotics in health-system pharmacies.

- Define and explain telepharmacy practice.

- Summarize the impact of patient confidentiality regulations on the use of technology in the pharmacy.

KEY TERMS

applications, p. 178

biometrics, p. 182

cassette systems, p. 180

central processing unit (CPU), p. 178

counting machines, p. 180

databases, p. 180

hard drives, p. 178

hardware, p. 178

input devices, p. 178

keyboard, p. 178

modem, p. 178

monitor, p. 178

mouse, p. 178

National Drug Code (NDC) number, p. 184

operating system, p. 178

output devices, p. 178

printer, p. 178

processing components p. 178

random-access memory (RAM), p. 178

read-only memory (ROM), p. 178

scanner, p. 178

software, p. 178

telepharmacy, p. 184

INTRODUCTION

Technology has revolutionized the practice of pharmacy, as it has so many other industries. Gone are the days of writing prescription instructions and labels by hand or with a typewriter, as had been done as recently as the 1970s. Today, virtually every pharmacy uses computers, automated systems, and other technology platforms for its operations and management of pharmaceutical care. This is why a basic understanding of technology is necessary for a pharmacy technician.

Computers

A computer is, in essence, an electronic device used for inputting, storing, processing, and outputting information (see Figure 10-1). A computer system is comprised of both **hardware** and **software** components. This section describes some of the more common hardware and software components used in pharmacy.

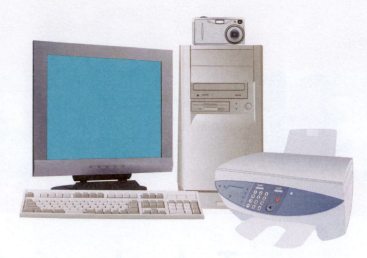

FIGURE 10-1 An example of a computer system and printer.
Source: Risteski goce/Shutterstock

hardware the mechanical and electrical components that make up a computer system.

software the programs and applications that control the functioning of computer hardware and direct the operation of the computer.

input devices hardware that allows information, or data, to be entered into a computer system.

processing components hardware devices used to organize, manage, and store data.

output devices hardware devices that produce and release data in a visual or tangible, printed form.

keyboard the primary input device of a computer system; used to enter information (both alphabetic and numeric) into the computer.

mouse a device that rolls on a hard, flat surface and controls the movement of the cursor, or pointer, on the screen.

scanner a hardware device used to input a photographic image into a computer system.

central processing unit (CPU) the brain of a computer system; it interprets commands, connects the various hardware components, runs software applications, and controls speed and use of memory space.

random-access memory (RAM) temporary memory used while information is being input into the computer.

read-only memory (ROM) permanent memory used for essential operating instructions for the computer system.

hard drive the main storage device of a computer; can be either external or internal.

modem hardware device used for connecting computer systems that are remotely located, via a telephone line or cable; can be installed either internally or externally.

monitor the visual display screen of a computer system.

printer the primary output device of a computer system; used to produce paper documents.

operating system the primary software program that connects the various hardware components of a computer and allows them to perform their essential functions.

applications software programs designed to perform specific functions, such as creating databases, spreadsheets, e-mails, or graphics, or performing word processing.

Hardware

Three types of hardware are required for computers to operate effectively: input devices, processing components, and output devices. **Input devices** allow information, or data, to be entered into the computer system. Then, the **processing components** organize, manage, and store the data. Finally, the **output devices** produce and release the data in a visual or tangible, printed form.

Input Devices

Some familiar examples of computer input devices include:

- **Keyboard**—the primary input device of a computer system; used to enter information (both alphabetic and numeric) into the computer.
- **Mouse**—a device that rolls on a hard, flat surface and controls the movement of the cursor, or pointer, on the screen. Clicking the mouse buttons gives the user control of the computer; each mouse includes one to three buttons, with each one performing different functions.
- **Scanner**—a device used to input a photographic image into a computer system. Some pharmacies are now using scanners to input and store images of each hard-copy, or physical, prescription (see Figure 10-2).

info Scanners

There are two main types of scanners. One works like a copy machine: You place a hard copy face down on the glass plate, close the lid, and press a button. The other type works more like a fax machine: You place a hard copy face down into a machine that feeds the document through after you push a button. The end result, which is the same with both types of scanning devices, is an electronic copy or image of the hard copy that can be stored in, viewed on, and retrieved from within the computer system.

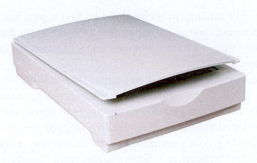

FIGURE 10-2 A computer scanner.
Source: Siede Preis/Getty Images, Inc.

Processing Components

Some of the various computer processing components include:

- **Central processing unit (CPU)**—the brain of the computer system. The CPU is responsible for interpreting commands, connecting the various hardware components, running software applications, and controlling the speed and use of memory space.
- **Memory and storage**—all the information and data being entered, or input, into a computer must be able to be stored. A computer's memory capacity is measured in kilobytes (Kb or K); 1 Kb equals 1,000 characters (bytes) of information. Storage is available through many different options, such as:
  - **Memory chips/cards**—CPUs contain two different types of memory chips: **random-access memory (RAM)** and **read-only memory (ROM)**. RAM is a temporary memory used while information is being input into the computer, whereas ROM is a permanent memory used for essential operating instructions of the system. RAM influences the speed of a computer system; the more RAM a computer has, the faster it will operate. In addition, memory chips and cards are now available in removable formats, such as cards, sticks, and "thumb" drives, all of which can store vast amounts of data on devices as small as keychains.
  - **Hard drives**—the main storage device of a computer; can be either external or internal. Hard drives are magnetic storage devices, usually referred to as the C drive. Many health-system pharmacies have multiple hard drives for their computers.
  - **Tape, disk, CD-ROM, and DVD drives**—in addition to memory chips and hard drives, computers may be equipped with various additional storage devices, including magnetic tapes, floppy disks, CD-ROMs, DVDs, and large-capacity disks, such as Zip or Jaz disks.
- **Modem**—a device used for connecting computer systems that are remotely located, via a telephone line or cable; can be installed either internally or externally. Modems are also used to connect computers to the Internet and company intranets.

Output Devices

Some of the various computer output devices available include:

- **Monitor**—the visual display component of a computer system (see Figure 10-1). The monitor is considered an output device; however, a touch screen—a monitor that allows you to use your finger or a stylus as a mouse—is considered both an input and an output device. The monitor is often referred to as the *screen*.
- **Printer**—the primary output device of a computer system; used to produce paper documents (see Figure 10-1). Within the pharmacy, printers are used for preparing prescription labels, patient information sheets, reports, and receipts.

Software

In general, software can be thought of as the set or sets of instructions the computer follows to perform various functions. For example, a word-processing program is software that allows the user to type words into the computer to create letters, memos, and other types of documents. Examples of software include:

- **Operating system**—the primary software (program) that connect the various hardware components of a computer and allows them to perform their essential functions. The most common operating systems are Microsoft Windows, Linux, and Macintosh OS.
- **Applications**—software programs other than the operating system are referred to as *applications*; these are programs designed to perform specific functions, such as creating databases, spreadsheets, e-mails, or graphics, or performing word processing. There are also numerous apps, such as drug refill reminder programs and medical advice apps, that can be used on mobile devices such as cell phones and other technological mobile devices, like the iPad.

PROFILE IN PRACTICE

Pat is a pharmacy technician and works at an independent, community-based pharmacy. The pharmacy has a very small staff—one pharmacist and two pharmacy technicians. Pat is entering prescriptions into the computer system when she hears a loud boom of thunder during a storm. The entire system shuts down, and the monitor goes blank.

▶ *What should Pat do?*

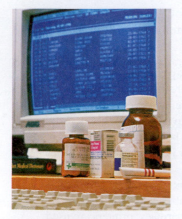

FIGURE 10-3 Within the pharmacy setting, computer systems generate prescription labels, serial numbers, warning labels, and patient's information.
Source: Jerry Mason/Science Source

Computers in the Pharmacy

Within the pharmacy setting, computer systems are used to generate prescription labels, serial numbers, warning labels, and patient information (see Figure 10-3). They also store massive collections of **data-bases** (simply lists of information, ordered in specific ways). With a few keystrokes, a pharmacy technician can pull up a specific prescription or a patient's whole profile of medications from a year ago. Technicians can even retrieve every prescription that has been written for a specific drug in a given period of time.

These systems also offer patient safety mechanisms. The software can alert the technician to potential drug interactions between the drug being filled and a drug or drugs on the patient's current profile. It can also alert the technician if the dose is too high or too low, based on the patient's age, and check new prescriptions against patient allergies.

Chain pharmacies or health-system pharmacies can use their computer systems to electronically link their locations, offering customers greater flexibility when filling and refilling prescriptions, as many community pharmacies are able to access the patient's medication profile, insurance information, and personal details.

Automation and Robotics in Community Pharmacies

Prescription volume in community pharmacies is on the rise and is expected to continue to increase. Thus, the nation's retailers are facing a shortage of licensed pharmacists to fill these prescriptions. These facts present a formidable challenge to already overworked community pharmacies. Not only do these numbers indicate a substantial increase in the pharmacy workload, but, because of the lack of personnel in relation to the number of prescriptions filled, the potential risks to patient safety are alarming. Pharmacy staff members employed in community pharmacies are working as quickly as they can to keep up with current prescription demands. Pharmacies are

increasingly turning to technology to assist pharmacy staff with managing day-to-day operations. Nowhere is the use of technology making a more obvious impact than in the community pharmacy.

One obvious solution is to increase the number of trained pharmacy technician employees in the pharmacy. Most states, in anticipation of the pharmacist shortages to come, are revisiting prior legislation that set a very low ratio of pharmacists to technicians (e.g., one pharmacist to one technician, or one pharmacist to two technicians). Several states have already adjusted this ratio. The other obvious solution, in today's age of computers and data management capabilities, is to add technology.

Pharmacists are no longer as involved with the actual mechanics of prescription filling as they were in the past; rather, they are becoming more involved in patient counseling and disease-state management. Pharmacy technicians are picking up the added responsibilities of prescription filling (although pharmacists are still required to check every prescription before it reaches the patient) and undertaking many of the day-to-day operations required to keep the pharmacy running.

In addition to hiring more technicians, community pharmacies are also employing technology to help ease the burden of ever-increasing prescription volume. The following subsections discuss some examples of the types of technology commonly seen in community pharmacies.

Counting Machines

Many pharmacies use **counting machines** to cut down on the time they take to manually count out oral solids like tablets and capsules. Medications that are poured in bulk into the counting machine fall past an electronic "eye" that counts the tablets. A digital display indicates how many have fallen into the receptacle. Some counters use even more complex technology. Based on the weight of a single tablet of a specific medication, and the number of tablets/capsules desired, the machine will determine how much the final number of tablets/capsules should weigh. This improves the accuracy of counting equipment to around 99.9%.

It is important to note that most pharmacies that use counting machines still require Schedule II (and sometimes Schedules III, IV, and V) narcotics to be counted out by hand because of the stricter inventory and regulatory policies covering controlled substances. In addition, because of the potential for allergic reactions due to cross-contamination, penicillin- and sulfur-containing compounds should not be used in automated counters. Examples of counting machines include the Baker Universal 2010 (McKesson) and the KL15df (Kirby Lester) (see Figure 10-4).

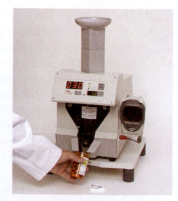

FIGURE 10-4 Example of a counting machine. (Courtesy of McKesson Automation.)
Source: McKesson Corporation

---

databases lists of information, ordered in specific ways.

counting machines electronic devices that automatically and precisely count capsules and tablets, based on weight.

cassette systems drug containers that can hold hundreds or thousands of tablets and are affixed to a counting machine.

Bar-Coding Equipment

Many community pharmacies are using bar coding to increase accuracy and patient safety (see Figure 10-5). These pharmacies scan the bar codes on medication bottles to make sure that the drug therein matches the drug called for on the prescription order. Each bar code contains embedded information that identifies the drug, dosage form, and strength. If the pharmacist or technician has pulled the wrong drug container from the shelf, the bar-code-reading machine will immediately alert the user to the error. Although this technology is somewhat expensive, when you consider what a company must pay to defend it against a lawsuit, the cost–benefit analysis comes down squarely on the side of using this technology.

❝ Workplace Wisdom Bar Codes

The FDA mandates that all prescription medications contain a bar code.

Prescription-Filling Robots

Community and outpatient pharmacies can also use robots and automation technology to fill prescriptions. Perhaps

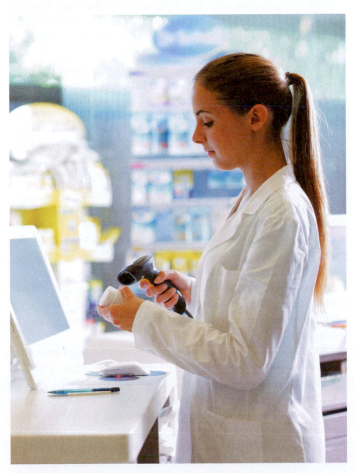

FIGURE 10-5 Bar code technology is now used in many pharmacy applications.
Source: Stokkete/Shutterstock

the most common form of this type of technology is the **cassette system**. These cassettes are essentially drug containers that can hold hundreds, and sometimes thousands, of tablets. The cassette that contains the correct drug is selected by the pharmacy technician and affixed to a counting machine. The user tells the machine how many tablets or capsules are needed, and the machine drops the correct number of tablets or capsules into a prescription vial. In some systems, each individual drug cassette includes its own counting mechanism. This system saves the time of shuttling the cassettes to the counter and placing them back in their original position when finished. Both systems are time savers in the pharmacy and take up a minimum amount of space, but both require human intervention.

There are also true *robots* that are available to fill prescriptions, although these are much more prevalent in institutional pharmacies. Several companies make dispensing robots, like ScriptPro, Parata, and Innovation. These robots work in much the same fashion as a cassette system, except that they do not need a staff member to intervene. A robotic arm and bar code scanning are used within the system to select a vial, dispense medication from a cell, and deliver it for inspection. Some robots will automatically apply the prescription label and auxiliary warnings to the vial. These systems are very accurate and range in size, typically holding 50 to 225 different medications, and most fill up to 150 prescriptions per hour. The drawbacks to this type of robotic automation are the cost and size of the equipment. The cost of these machines is often prohibitive for pharmacies that fill a low (100 or less) to medium (100 to 300) number of prescriptions daily. Another drawback is that the size—the "footprint"—of the equipment is rather large. Even larger community pharmacies often do not have nearly enough floor space to accommodate a large prescription-filling robot. Examples of prescription-filling robots are the Parata Max (Parata) and the ScriptPro SP 200 (ScriptPro) (see Figure 10-6).

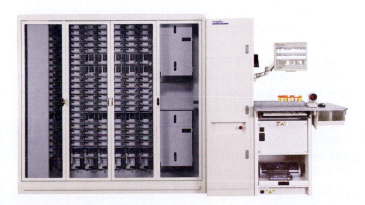

FIGURE 10-6 An example of a prescription-filling robot: the SP 200 Robotic Prescription Dispensing System from ScriptPro.
Source: Courtesy of ScriptPro

Automation and Robotics in Health-System Pharmacies

Health-system pharmacies are increasing their use of automation and robotics. Some automated systems operate completely free of staff intervention, whereas others require daily staff interaction and input. In fact, one company has developed a robot for use in hospitals. These robots have a map of the hospital or facility stored in their memory and are able to navigate to all areas of the hospital using sensors to avoid humans and obstacles. These robots make deliveries between hospital units, the pharmacy, and nursing stations. Some are even able to communicate with hospital staff via voice output. The robots use elevators to move between floors in the hospital, following an assigned route that can be programmed into the memory by the pharmacy.

Currently, it would be cost-prohibitive to install a whole fleet of robots to perform courier duties in a hospital. However, this is just one example of the types of automated systems that are available for institutional use.

There are so many types of automated systems available for health-system pharmacies that they cannot all be mentioned in this chapter. In the sections that follow, though, you will find descriptions of some of the types of technology most commonly used in health-system settings. Most of the focus is on automated medication delivery systems, because this is by far the most prevalent technology in hospitals.

Automated Medication Delivery Systems

Automated medication delivery systems are found in hospitals and some long-term care facilities across the country. These systems allow much faster order turnaround time (the time it takes to fill an order from the time the order was written). They also allow meticulous inventory management of medications, hospital supplies, and narcotics. These systems can save hospitals tens and sometimes hundreds of thousands of dollars every year, simply by recouping lost charges and keeping track of medications and supplies.

Automated medication delivery systems are comprised of cabinets of various sizes that contain drawers and compartments for different medications. The compartments and drawers maintain varying degrees of security, such as password protection or physical locks, based on the requirements of the institution or security needs dictated by the nature of the medication, such as controlled substances. The cabinet hardware also features a computer screen and keyboard that are physically attached to the cabinet. A nurse or other health care practitioner can access medications or other medical supplies by logging on to the computer at the cabinet. The items the individual can retrieve depend on that individual's preprogrammed level of access to the various items stored in the cabinet. For instance, in most health care facilities, respiratory therapists do not have access to any medications other than respiratory supplies. In this instance, the cabinet will deny this individual access to any medications or supplies other than respiratory supplies.

Medication Order—From Physician to Patient

Orders for patient medication are written by a physician in the hospital. A nurse then sends a copy of the order to the pharmacy department for computer order entry (usually done by a technician) and clinical review by a pharmacist. Then, someone from the pharmacy sends the medication back to the nursing unit for administration. Traditionally, with this system, it can take quite a while to get the medication to the patient. However, with the advent of automated delivery systems, the turnaround time for medication orders can be decreased dramatically.

The most time-consuming step in the process is usually the physical delivery of the medication to the nursing unit. With automated medication delivery systems in place, several actions speed up this process. The software that runs the automated cabinet is interfaced to the pharmacy/hospital computer system; consequently, information regarding the patient passes freely between the two systems within minutes of order entry. In addition, a store of the most commonly used medications physically resides in the nursing unit, making it unnecessary for the pharmacy to take the medication to the unit. Instead, the nurse simply goes to the medication cabinet and selects the needed medication from the patient's available medication profile.

Additional benefits provided by automated medication delivery systems are discussed in the following subsections.

Security

Many security issues surround the dispensing and handling of medication. Both controlled substances and other medications must be properly secured. Automated systems provide an extremely high level of security for hospitals and health care facilities via several components.

Every item within an automated cabinet can be password protected. This means that every individual who gains access to any particular medication or supply item is tracked by the computer system, based on that individual's personal password. There are also systems that use **biometrics**, such as fingerprints, to identify and track individual users on the system. Only licensed staff members within the facility are issued user identifications and passwords; thus, only they have access to medications and supplies.

An additional level of security is available for controlled substances and/or items that have a high rate of theft or abuse. Some systems dispense medications one at a time. This is usually referred to as *unit-dose* or *unit-of-use dispensing technology*. This type of system allows user's access only to the exact number of units of medication the user asked for, instead of access to the whole inventory. As an example, think of the difference between a soda vending machine, which dispenses only the item that is paid for and selected by the user, and a newspaper vending machine, where the user pays for a paper but then has access to the machine's entire stock of papers.

---

biometrics technology that measures and analyzes human body characteristics, such as fingerprints, for authentication purposes.

Inventory Control

Automated systems can save health care facilities thousands of dollars a year by recouping lost charges and providing inventory usage reports. These systems can track and bill for hospital supplies and medications used by nursing units and patients. A completely integrated, interfaced system can tell a pharmacy director or materials manager exactly how much of each inventory item is in the hospital at any given point in time. The system can also pull historical data to determine usage rates at any given historical point or for any selected period of time. These reports, which can be generated within minutes, are invaluable tools for managing hospital inventory.

Automated systems also cut down on the number of unexplainable inventory losses. Everyone using the automated supply and medication cabinets is required to log on to the system, via a username and password. This means that everyone who has access to any item in the inventory is tracked and can be identified easily by usage reports.

These systems are also capable of automatic ordering from hospital suppliers and wholesalers. When the inventory of an item reaches a preset point, the system automatically reorders a preset amount of the item. No human intervention is required.

Patient Safety

The most important advantage of automated systems is increased patient safety, which is achieved through a variety of mechanisms.

- *Patient profiles*—because of regulation changes by accrediting bodies, most hospitals using automated systems are either currently using patient medication profiling or converting to it as quickly as they can. Profiling allows a nurse or other user to access only those medications that have been ordered for a particular patient. The user does not select a medication for the patient from the entire drug inventory in the cabinet; rather, he or she selects the desired medication from a list of patient-specific medications. This decreases the possibility of errors due to look-alike or sound-alike drugs. These patient's medication profiles also display the details of the medication order and tell the nurse exactly how much of each drug needs to be given to the patient. Note, however, that there are certain nursing units within a hospital (such as emergency rooms and surgical units) where profiling is not and never will be used, because the patients are not there for long periods of time and usually need to receive medication on an emergency basis.
- *Drug information*—some automated systems are connected to drug information Internet sites. These sites allow users to look up clinical information about a particular drug while at the automated cabinet. Users can look up cautions, interactions, and side effects, and even print out patient information for any medication.
- *Pharmacist review*—because the automated medication dispensing machine is interfaced to the hospital/ pharmacy computer system, a pharmacist has reviewed every order on a patient's medication profile for safety.
- *Administration times*—some systems allow nurse users to access a medication from the patient's profile only when that medication is due to be administered. This ensures that patients receive their medications at the proper times. This also ensures that a patient will not receive double doses of a medication. The system can track and alert users to missed doses.
- *Emergency override*—systems in place within the automated machines allow emergency removal of medication in an acute, critical situation.

Several companies make this type of equipment. Examples of automated medication delivery systems include:

- OmniRx Color Touch (Omnicell, Inc.)
- Omnicell (unit-of-use dispensing) (Omnicell, Inc.)
- Pyxis MedStation (Cardinal Health)
- AcuDose-Rx (McKesson)

Automated Storage and Retrieval Systems

Just as the name indicates, automated storage and retrieval systems are used to store and retrieve inventories of medication kept in the pharmacy. Essentially, the companies that make this type of machinery have automated the pick list. Traditionally, pharmacists and technicians would walk through the pharmacy, manually selecting the items they needed to replenish medication inventories throughout the hospital. However, with the advent of medication carousel systems, the picking process is completely automated, thereby cutting down on pick errors. Because of computer interfaces, the storage and retrieval system knows exactly what items must be restocked on all the hospital units. Users simply tell the carousel system which unit they want to restock; the machine then physically locates all the medications that are needed and gives users access to each location on the carousel, item by item. The carousel system can also automatically generate and send orders to the pharmacy's wholesale distributor to replenish pharmacy supplies. Examples of automated storage and retrieval systems include (see Figure 10-7):

- PharmacyCentral (Omnicell, Inc.)
- Pyxis Carousel System (Cardinal Health)
- MedCarousel (McKesson)
- MedSide (S&S MedCart)

Bar Coding

As mentioned previously, bar-coding technology is being used in all aspects of medication delivery and patient care. Once a medication order is received by the pharmacy, the order is input into the pharmacy's computer system and that item is added to the patient's profile of ordered medications. The technician may then retrieve the medication. To ensure that the proper medication has been selected, the technician may use a handheld bar-code scanner on the item. If the medication is correct, the item is then labeled and sent to the nursing unit. The nurse receives the medication and takes it to the patient's bedside. The nurse then uses another scanner to scan the nurse's own bar-coded badge, the patient's armband, and the medication. This transaction is then logged in the computer system and given a time stamp. This process ensures that the Five Patient Rights are all

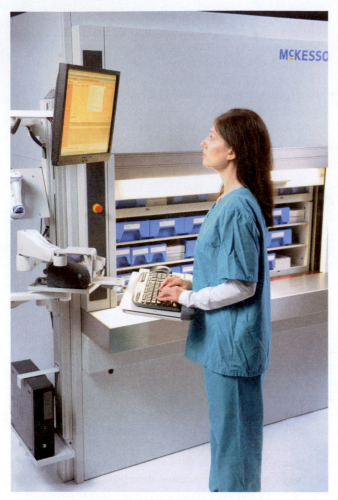

FIGURE 10-7 Example of an automated storage and retrieval system.
Source: McKesson Corporation

electronically checked: The right patient receives the right drug in the right amount at the right time via the right route.

With continuous growth in the use of automation and the number of drugs, in order to reduce the number of medication errors in hospitals and other health care settings, the FDA deemed it necessary to create a method to reduce medication problems using state-of-the-art technology. Therefore, the FDA established a rule that bar coding is mandatory on medications. This mandate applies to all prescription drug products, including biological products and vaccines (except for physician samples), and OTC drugs that are commonly used in hospitals and dispensed in a hospital. Standardized bar codes are also required on prescription drug products used in other settings, such as retail pharmacies.

The required bar code must contain the **National Drug Code (NDC) number** (unique identifying information about

---

National Drug Code (NDC) number a unique identifying number assigned to each drug by the manufacturer.

telepharmacy the practice of using advanced telecommunications technology to provide pharmaceutical care to patients in rural and medically underserved areas at a distance (see Figure 10-8).

---

the drug that is to be dispensed) in a linear bar code as part of the drug label. Bar coding will also allow for the addition of even more information as technology progresses.

Health Care Information Technology and Electronic Prescribing

In 2009, the American Recovery and Reinvestment Act was passed, with the goal of integrating technology into health care delivery nationwide. Part of this bill provides incentives for Medicare and Medicaid providers to use certified electronic health records (EHRs), with the implementation of a nationwide EHR system by 2014. The aim of EHRs is to reduce costs, reduce paperwork, improve safety, reduce duplicated testing, and improve overall the nation's health care system by maintaining a patient's entire health information in one centralized location. Electronic prescribing, or e-prescribing, plays a dominant role in integrating pharmacy professionals in this health care information technology initiative. E-prescribing allows for prescribers to automatically and electronically transmit new prescription orders and refill authorizations directly to the patient's pharmacy of choice. The vision is that, in the near future, patients will no longer be leaving the doctor's office with hand-written prescriptions, but will be able to go directly to their pharmacy and have their prescription(s) ready and waiting for them. Although not perfect, e-prescribing greatly reduces the risk of medication errors resulting from transcribing, the often illegible, handwritten prescriptions.

Telepharmacy

Using advanced telecommunications technology, pharmacists can now provide pharmaceutical care to patients in rural and medically underserved areas at a distance. This is known as **telepharmacy**.

Pharmacy Technology and Patient Confidentiality

Patient confidentiality regulations, such as HIPAA regulations, apply to electronic data just as they do to written information. For this reason, pharmacy computer systems and technology applications must be configured to meet HIPAA privacy guidelines. Only authorized individuals should ever have access to confidential information, including information that is displayed on a computer monitor. Although technology has enabled numerous advances in the practice of pharmacy, it is imperative to keep patient confidentiality in mind, and use technology accordingly.

info **Telepharmacy**

In North Dakota, for example, licensed pharmacists at a central pharmacy site can supervise a registered pharmacy technician at a remote telepharmacy site via teleconferencing. The technician prepares the prescription for dispensing, while the pharmacist communicates face-to-face in real time with both the technician and the patient. All states, however, do not currently permit telepharmacies.

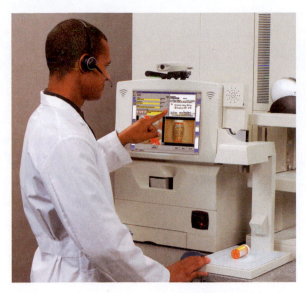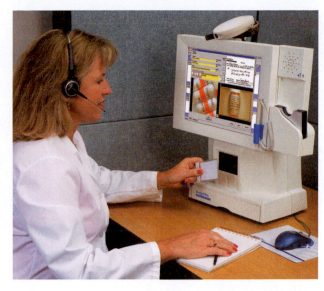

FIGURE 10-8 In an example of telepharmacy, the technician at a remote pharmacy receives and fills the prescription, which is then verified by the support pharmacy.
Source: Courtesy of ScriptPro

Summary

Virtually every pharmacy today relies on computer systems. Computer hardware (e.g., the CPU, memory, monitor, keyboard, mouse, printer, modem, and scanner) and computer software (e.g., the operating system, pharmacy software program, and other applications) allow pharmacies to operate with increased accuracy and efficiency.

In addition to computer systems, both community pharmacies and health-system pharmacies are integrating automation and technology to improve their operations. Such automation and technology include automatic counters, dispensing systems, bar -coding, and even robots.

The advances in pharmacy practice are being driven by the development and use of computers, automation, robotics, and other technologies. The benefits of technology use are recognized in both community and health-system pharmacies. Pharmacy technicians must be computer literate and comfortable with using technology to practice modern pharmacy.

Chapter Review Questions

1. Which of the following is an example of a prescription-filling robot used in community pharmacies?
   a. Baker Cassettes
   b. Kirby Lester KL15df
   c. Baker Universal 2010
   d. SureMed

2. _____ is responsible for interpreting commands and running software applications in a computer.
   a. JAZ
   b. RAM
   c. CPU
   d. ROM

3. The most common type of prescription-filling robots is the _____.
   a. cassette system
   b. counting machine
   c. dispensing robots
   d. automated medication delivery system

4. Microsoft Windows and Linux are both examples of _____.
   a. databases
   b. operating systems
   c. spreadsheets
   d. word processors

5. Pharmacies managed by a registered pharmacy technician, but supervised by a pharmacist at a central, off-site location, are known as _____.
   a. automated dispensing facilities
   b. telepharmacies
   c. satellite pharmacies
   d. automated medication delivery systems

6. Which of the following is a counting machine?
   a. Acu-Dose Rx
   b. Baker Universal 2010
   c. Pyxis MedStat
   d. SureMed

7. Medication bar codes are embedded with all of the following drug information, *except* _____.
   a. dosage form
   b. drug's name
   c. strength
   d. therapeutic indication

8. Which of the following is an automated medication dispensing system?
   a. Acu-Dose Rx
   b. MedCarousel
   c. MedSide
   d. Pharmacy Central

9. According to the American Recovery and Reinvestment Act, a nationwide EHR system is to be implemented by _____.
   a. 2013
   b. 2014
   c. 2015
   d. 2016

10. Which of the following is an automated storage and retrieval system?
    a. Acu-Dose Rx
    b. Pyxis Carousel
    c. Pyxis MedStat
    d. SureMed

Critical Thinking Questions

1. What are some potential disadvantages or dangers of electronic prescribing?

2. In what ways could automation and robotics be a hindrance to the operation of a pharmacy?

3. What precautions can be taken to protect patient confidentiality and secure protected health information (PHI) against hackers and technology-driven identity theft?

Web Challenge

1. Go to www.computertalk.com and click on the link for Vendor Listings. Select any three vendors, visit their websites, and write a brief summary about the technology-based products/services they offer for pharmacies.

2. Go to www.asapnet.org, the website for the American Society for Automation in Pharmacy. Click on the News Archive tab, select an article of interest to you, and write a brief summary of it.

References and Resources

American Society of Health-System Pharmacist. *Manual for Pharmacy Technicians.* 2nd ed. Bethesda, MD: ASHp. 1998. Print.

Crane, A. "An overview of pharmacy automation." *Today's Technician.* 5 (4) (2012): 26–37.

Felton, Jeff, David Nace, and Roger Pinsonneault. "Accountable Care—Concepts and Roles for Pharmacists." *Relay Health.* 2011. Web. 17 June 2012.

Flaherty, J. "Matters of privacy—Patient confidentiality." *Today's Technician.* 6 (2) (2012): 8, 12.

Kolpack, Dave. "Telepharmacies Change the Way Rural America Gets Meds." *Houston Chronicle.* Web. 6 September 2008.

National Association of Chain Drug Stores, Inc. and Mintz, Levin, Cohn, Ferris, Glovsky and Popeo, P.C. *HIPAA Privacy Standards: A Compliance Manual for Pharmacies.* Alexandria, VA: NACDS, 2002.

Pharmacy e-Health Information Technology Collaborative. 2012. Web. 17 June 2012.

Spiro, Rachelle. "The Impact of Electronic Health Records on Pharmacy Practice." *Drug Topics.* April 2012. Web. 17 June 2012.

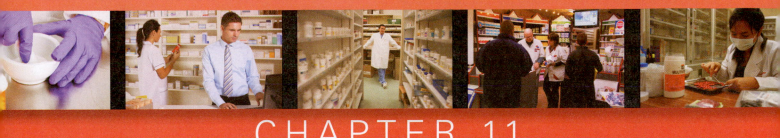

Inventory Management

LEARNING OBJECTIVES

After completing this chapter, you should be able to:

- List and describe the various purchasing systems used in pharmacies.

- List and describe the various methods of purchasing available in pharmacies.

- Define and describe prescription formularies.

- Describe and perform the steps necessary for placing orders.

- Describe and perform the steps necessary for receiving orders.

- List the atypical products to consider with inventory management.

- List the reasons for back-ordered products and outline appropriate methods to communicate changes in product availability.

- Classify the reasons for product returns and describe the process of making returns.

- List and explain the three classifications of drug recalls.

- Describe the process of handling expired drugs.

- Identify the problems with having excessive inventory.

- Describe the issue of drug theft and diversion.

KEY TERMS

contracts, p. 188

expired drugs, p. 192

formularies, p. 188

group purchasing system, p. 188

independent purchasing system, p. 188

purchasing system, p. 188

recall, p. 192

INTRODUCTION

Pharmacy technicians have many duties and responsibilities within a pharmacy practice setting; one of the most common duties is inventory management. The importance of this task is quite clear; the pharmacy cannot dispense prescriptions if proper medications are not in stock.

Purchasing Systems

Pharmacies must determine the most appropriate and advantageous **purchasing system**—the method for obtaining medications, devices, and products—for their organization. In general, there are two types of pharmacy purchasing systems: independent purchasing and group purchasing.

Independent Purchasing

In an **independent purchasing system**, the pharmacy, most often the pharmacy's director or buyer, is responsible for establishing **contracts**, or written agreements, directly with each pharmaceutical manufacturer. Individual contracts set pricing and delivery terms, return policy, and dollar-volume requirements.

Group Purchasing

With a **group purchasing system**, the pharmacy joins a group purchasing organization (GPO), which contracts with pharmaceutical manufacturers collectively for all members of that GPO. In most circumstances, GPOs are able to obtain more competitive pricing and better terms than a pharmacy can get through independent purchasing.

Methods of Purchasing

In addition to the system of purchasing, each pharmacy must determine the method by which it will purchase pharmaceutical products. The three primary methods of purchasing are direct, through wholesaler, and through prime vendor.

Purchasing Direct

When purchasing direct, the pharmacy buyer places separate orders with each pharmaceutical company and receives separate shipments. Purchasing direct requires more time and resources, but can reduce expenses by eliminating markup percentages and fees charged by wholesalers and prime vendors.

Wholesalers

Wholesalers, such as Cardinal Health or Anda Generics, enable the pharmacy to purchase a large number of products, from either various manufacturers or a single source. It is common for wholesalers to offer next-day delivery service; however, their prices are almost always higher.

---

purchasing system an organization's strategy or procedure for obtaining medications, devices, and products.

independent purchasing system a purchasing system in which a pharmacy establishes contracts directly with each pharmaceutical manufacturer.

contracts written agreements.

group purchasing system a purchasing system in which a pharmacy joins a group purchasing organization (GPO), which contracts with pharmaceutical manufacturers collectively for all members of that GPO.

formularies a listing of drugs approved for a specific purpose.

Primary Vendors

Contracting with a prime vendor, such as Amerisource Bergen, Cardinal, or McKesson, has all the benefits of using a wholesaler, as well as better pricing and service terms. Prime vendors, however, require a dollar-volume commitment from the pharmacy and often contractually restrict the pharmacy's ability to enter into additional purchasing agreements.

Formularies

Formularies are, in essence, a listing of drugs approved for a specific purpose. Formularies can be used as a reference manual, as recommendations for prescribing, or even as strict parameters for the medications that are stocked and approved for reimbursement. Formularies are commonly used in health systems, and the listing of selected pharmaceutical drugs reflects the clinical judgment of the medical staff. Health-system formularies are established by the facility's Pharmacy and Therapeutics (P&T) committee, which is composed of physicians, pharmacists, nurses, administrators, and quality-assurance coordinators. Formularies are also discussed in Chapter 9.

Evaluating Costs

Evaluating costs in inventory management can mean completing much research on medications, costs of different drugs on the market, and how each pharmacy differs in its price. Sometimes pharmacies vary greatly in the amount they charge for their Rx's. Chain pharmacies and grocery store pharmacies will generally be cheaper on drug prices, while independent pharmacies may or may not be higher on their prices. There are some major terms to keep in mind when considering ordering and costs of medications. The first term is cost analysis, which refers to all information about financial disbursements of a certain activity, agency, department, or program. Cost control is another important term that refers to the implementation of efforts by the pharmacist and pharmacy technician to realize cost objectives. The costs of medications will vary greatly, depending on the following factors:

- Whether the prescription is a name brand or generic drug
- Drug strength
- Drug manufacturer
- Output or volume of the type of drug sold
- How long the medication has been available on the market
- The range of services the pharmacy offers
- Efficiency, for treating indications, based as a relative factor

Evaluating Sources

As a pharmacy technician, you need to be familiar with ordering practices and where to order medications. Being knowledgeable and familiar with different manufacturers and their products is essential for becoming a quality pharmacy employee. Your research requires utilizing manufacturers' websites and press releases and your contacts with medication representatives to learn about resources and new prescriptions as they become available. In addition, researching the competition and prices of other pharmacies will assist the pharmacy technician in ordering and stocking in both a hospital and retail pharmacy. The procedures for purchasing often involve the following types of buying and purchasing: independent purchasing, group purchasing, and prime vendors. What exactly do these terms mean, and how do they pertain to ordering of drugs and supplies? Those individuals who do the purchasing of drugs and supplies can practice independent purchasing. Independent purchasing is when a pharmacy works solely with pharmaceutical reps to determine delivery, prices, and general quantity. The pharmacy may also choose to participate in group purchasing to order its stock. Group purchasing is when buyers pool their buying power to obtain lower prices. Using prime suppliers is another option that involves the use of a single supplier to meet the pharmacy's drug ordering needs. The advantages of using a prime supplier include lower prices, extended price negotiation, and less paperwork and hassle for the pharmacy staff. To keep track of the drugs they wish to order, pharmacies use a "want book." The want book helps health care professionals to keep track of the many drugs available on the market and also items they wish to order for the pharmacy.

The Ordering Process

The process of ordering medications will vary slightly based on the purchasing system and supplier(s) selected by the pharmacy, but the key steps of ordering are the same.

Generate Order

The first step of the ordering process is to generate an order. This can be done through an automated system, manually, or using a combination of both methods (see Figure 11-1).

Automated

With an automated order, the computer system automatically generates a report (order) based on current inventory levels and preprogrammed reorder points. For example, if the system is programmed to keep a minimum of 200 Lasix 20 mg, and the pharmacy inventory drops to 180 Lasix 20 mg, the system will automatically add one bottle of Lasix 20 mg to the next order.

Role of Judgment with Automated Ordering Systems
Automated ordering systems and perpetual inventory have made the jobs of the pharmacist and the pharmacy technician easier, because they consider drug use on a monthly basis and provide monthly monitoring of information and supply.

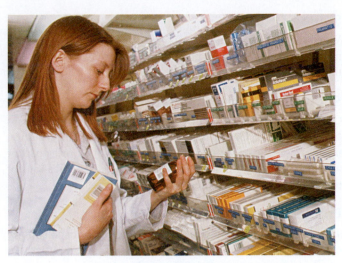

FIGURE 11-1 The first step in the ordering process is generating an order.
Source: Ben Edwards/Getty Images, Inc.

This enables the pharmacy staff to make good judgments when placing orders based on the *call* for a specific drug. Staff can use these systems to manage the budget and monitor the pharmacy's financial gains and losses. Getting stuck with lots of stock can mean great financial losses for the pharmacy, which will have a negative impact on the pharmacy, its employees, and salaries as well.

Manual

In a manual ordering system, the pharmacy buyer reviews the inventory levels and creates an order based on current and forecasted stock needs. The manual method is not commonly used as the primary method of generating orders, as it has been almost entirely supplanted by technology and automated methods. In the manual system of ordering, it is common to use a "want book," which is simply a notebook in which pharmacy staff write down the inventory they need ordered.

Combination of Automated and Manual

The method of ordering most commonly used in modern pharmacy is a combination of the automated and manual methods. The computer system will generate an automated order, which is considered the primary order; additional items are then added manually by the buyer. This is the most efficient method, because it responds easily to changes. For example, restock levels may become outdated within the system, or physicians may suddenly be ordering a new drug in large volume. A combination method can easily handle such variations.

Confirm Order

Once an order has been generated, it must be reviewed and confirmed. It is not uncommon for the automated system to generate orders based on incorrect inventory levels or reorder points, so the buyer should review each order item to determine if it is really needed and that the appropriate quantity is being ordered. Any additions, deletions, or other changes must be entered into the system and then confirmed.

▌Procedure 11-1

Ordering Medications

1. Generate an order.
2. Review the order.
3. Confirm the order.
4. Submit the order.

Submit Order

When the order is finalized and ready, it is electronically submitted to the supplier via phone or the Internet, depending on the vendor.

Supplier's Receipt of Order

Once the supplier has received the order, it will provide confirmation. Order confirmation can consist of a confirmation number given over the phone, sent via an e-mail, or as part of a confirmation report, again depending on the specifications of the vendor and the agreement with the purchaser.

Processing/Shipping of Order

The final step of the ordering process is the full responsibility of the supplier. After receiving and confirming the order, the supplier must process, package, and ship the order to the pharmacy department. Depending on the supplier, shipping of order can require anywhere from 12 hours to 2 weeks.

The Receiving Process

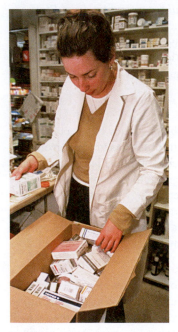

Just as with the ordering process, the procedures for receiving orders will vary by facility. However, the key steps remain the same.

Order Delivery

The first step of the receiving process is the delivery of the order. Orders are most frequently delivered by a supplier-employed courier, most often using secured plastic totes. Deliveries may also be made by FedEx, United Parcel Service (UPS), or the United States Postal Service (USPS).

Order Verification

FIGURE 11-2 Verifying an order.
Source: Josh Sher/Science Source

After the order has been delivered, it must be verified (see Figure 11-2). Accuracy

is an essential element of any inventory management and control system. It is important that the purchase order, the packaging list, the invoice, and the actual order be reconciled against one another. Any errors or discrepancies should be addressed immediately.

Inventory Adjustment

Like the generation of an order, the adjustment of inventory based on a delivered shipment can be handled electronically or manually (see Figure 11-3).

Automated

In an automated system, the computer system automatically updates the inventory levels based on the shipment delivered, not on the order placed. This is the most efficient and accurate method, since some items ordered may not have been shipped because of back-ordering or shortages, for example.

Manual

In a manual system, the pharmacy buyer reviews the shipment and updates the inventory on hand, manually, into the computer system. Manual inventory methods are no longer common, as they too have largely been superseded by automated systems and newer technology.

Stocking the Order

Once a shipment has been delivered and verified and the inventory has been updated, it is time to stock the order (see Figure 11-4). Medications must be stored according to the specifications of each manufacturer. Stored medications may be refrigerated, frozen, or kept at room temperature.

Most pharmacies organize stocked medications by route of administration, such as injectables, topicals, and orals. Medications are then further organized by name, either alphabetically by brand name, in which case generic equivalents are stocked next to alphabetically organized brand-name drugs, or by generic name, in which case all drugs are alphabetically arranged by the generic drug name, whether the medication is a branded or generic product.

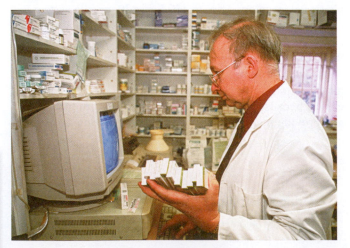

FIGURE 11-3 The adjustment of inventory for a delivered shipment can be handled manually or electronically.
Source: Josh Sher/Science Source

■ Procedure 11-2

Receiving an Order

1. Accept delivery of the order.
2. Verify the order.
3. Adjust the inventory.
4. Stock the order.
5. File the paperwork pertaining to the order.

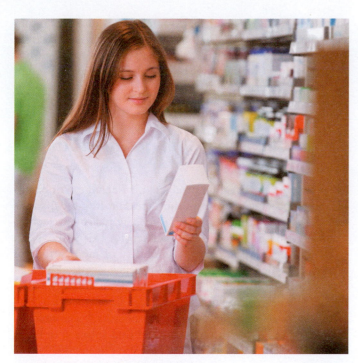

FIGURE 11-4 Stocking an order.
Source: Tyler Olson/Shutterstock

Recordkeeping

The pharmacy must keep records of each order placed and received, both for internal purposes and for regulatory accountability; regulatory agencies, such as the State Board of Pharmacy and the DEA, often carefully scrutinize pharmacy records and inventory. Although most pharmacies use an automated system to manage and track inventory, paper reports must still be generated and maintained. The specific format and frequency of reports vary by facility; the task of generating reports is typically handled by a designated pharmacy buyer or the pharmacy manager.

In addition to inventory reports, the pharmacy should maintain copies of the packaging slips for each order, as a manual backup to electronic files (see Figure 11-5).

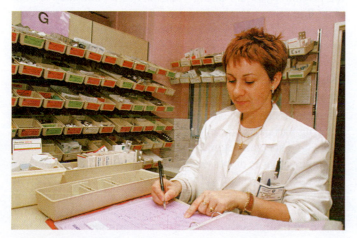

FIGURE 11-5 The pharmacy buyer maintains records for inventory management.
Source: PHANIE/Science Source

Ordering Atypical Products

Many times pharmacies need to place orders for atypical products or products that are less commonly needed by their customers. The pharmacy's ultimate goal is to order what the customer needs no matter the call for the product. Customers can also make suggestions or order special products from a pharmacy. However, it is sometimes necessary for the customer to go to another pharmacy or choose another product similar to the one he or she needs. Most pharmacies will do their best to meet the customer's needs. Because ordering atypical products may cost more for both the pharmacy customer and the pharmacy, take care when ordering special products. The customer may need to pay more to get the product he or she wants, or the pharmacy may have to absorb the cost of the product—something most businesses do not wish to do.

Biologics

Biologics, or immunotherapy, are biological therapies used to treat cancer by using either natural or synthetic substances. Such substances work by stimulating the body's immune system to help treat different cancers. Biologics are often used in conjunction with chemotherapy and radiation therapy. This type of treatment may be used to treat various conditions other than cancer. Hospital pharmacies generally carry biologics and also work in preparing and compounding these drug treatments.

Interferon

Another form of cancer drug is called interferons, or hormone-like proteins produced by the body's white blood cells that assist the immune system in fighting harmful infections. Once considered the cancer "wonder drug," interferon drugs have many side effects that increase at higher doses. Possible side effects are severe fatigue, chills, fever, muscle aches, headaches, joint aches, and possible mood changes. Pharmacy technicians often come in contact with interferon medications in the hospital setting.

HIV Medications

AIDS or acquired immunodeficiency syndrome continues to be a worldwide epidemic. Strides have been made, however, in the treatment of AIDS, and hopefully someday a cure will be found. Recently, HIV home test kits have gone under review with the Food and Drug Administration (FDA) and new medications continue to be approved for AIDS. Because AIDS is such a serious illness, technicians may find they will come in contact with those who have the illness and medications used to treat the condition will most often be found in hospital pharmacies.

Investigational Drugs

Investigational drugs are not available in the traditional sense of obtaining drugs from a retail or hospital pharmacy. Investigational drugs or experimental drugs are medications that have not been approved by the FDA and/or have not been approved for new use. These are also drugs that are still in the stages of testing for effectiveness and safety. These special drugs can be obtained in two ways.

- Through a clinical trial—by participating in a clinical trial, patients can gain access to experimental drugs. Safety and effectiveness have not been tested with these special drugs, and patients are taking a chance with these medications.
- Through an outlet outside of clinical trials—this method is called expanded access or compassionate use. Drugs will need to meet certain criteria to be used as a compassionate use drug. Clinical evidence must show that the drug will benefit a cancer patient and the drug will need to be given safely outside of clinical trials. Drugs will also need to be in adequate supply for ongoing clinical trials to be considered a compassionate use drug.

Nonformulary Drugs

As discussed in Chapter 9, drugs not included in the drug formulary can and will be dispensed by a pharmacy, but the cost of the drug will be higher to beneficiaries (unless the health care provider can deem the prescription a medical necessity). Proving the drug is a medical necessity for an individual usually means justifying the reason the patient needs the medication and how the medication will help or cure his or her condition or disease. The pharmacist, technician, or doctor may need to make calls to insurance providers and fill out forms to get the drug classified as an override and approved for the patient so it is covered by his or her insurance or at least most of the cost is covered by a co-pay. In addition, if the medical necessity is not approved, then the patient may have to pay out of pocket for the drug if it is not covered by insurance or if he or she wants brand-name drugs instead of the generic equivalent.

Back-Ordered Products

Back-ordered medications are drugs that are currently unavailable from the supplier. Back orders may cause a customer who needs the drug in a hurry to seek it from a different pharmacy, or the pharmacy to order it from a different manufacturer. Prescription orders can sometimes take as little as two days to a week depending on the needed medication. A common reason for back-ordered products can be drug

---

recall the process in which a drug manufacturer or the FDA requires that specific drugs or devices be returned to the manufacturer because of a specific concern about the recalled product.

expired drugs drugs that have not been dispensed as of the manufacturer's printed expiration date.

shortages. If the product is back-ordered, it is possible to substitute certain prescriptions for the one that is needed right away. Some items or drugs can be substituted for appropriate drugs, and some cannot be switched out for a different equivalent prescription, as this depends on the medication or supplies needed.

Communicating Changes in Product Availability

The availability of certain products may change. For example, formulary changes, drug shortages, or drug recalls may make a certain product unavailable. The pharmacy technician must possess strong customer service skills to explain such changes related to the availability of medications or medical supplies to customers and pharmacy staff. Although customers may be unhappy about the unavailability of their medication or a certain product, you can usually work to find a solution. Part of being a successful pharmacy employee is being able to deal with problems and find solution to those issues.

Communicating Changes to Patients

Because the pharmacy world changes so quickly, pharmacy technicians need to communicate drug changes to patients in the proper manner. When communicating drug changes such as strength variances, recalls, special orders, specialty drugs, and hard-to-order items, a pharmacy technician should remember the following:

1. State the specific change in the drug order.
2. State why there is a change in the drug order.
3. Communicate what decisions need to be made to solve the problem.
4. Discuss alternatives to the problem or drug alternatives.
5. Give a time frame as to when the problem can be solved or the drug can be ordered.

By communicating clearly and offering solutions to the problem, you are doing your best as a pharmacy technician. Sometimes the best communicators are the employees who can look at the whole picture when it comes to solving problems.

Communicating Changes to Health Care Providers

When communicating changes to health care providers concerning drug variances, strength, recalls, special orders, specialty drugs, and specialty items, follow the basic rules of effective communication as discussed in Chapter 3. Basic modes of communication are written, verbal, and nonverbal communication. Written communication can take the form of an e-mail, letter, or memo. Verbal communication is in-person communication, phone communication, or webcam communication (such as

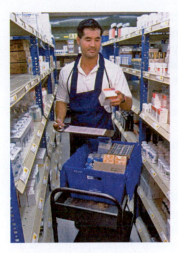

FIGURE 11-6 Handling returns is part of inventory management.
Source: Mark Richards/PhotoEdit, Inc.

Skype). The best communication comes from remembering the following: Being open, listening, repeating, respecting, and sharing are the best ways to be successful at your job and in relaying information to health care providers. Pharmacy technician's errors can be costly, even deadly. All pharmacy communication should be clear, concise, and free of error.

Returns

The last basic component of inventory management is handling returns (see Figure 11-6). In pharmacy, returns are typically made for one of the following reasons: expired drugs, manufacturer recalls, overstocked/undesired products, incorrect product sent by the wholesaler, or incorrectly ordered item.

Product Returns

Occasionally, a pharmacy needs to return products that have neither expired nor been recalled. It may be that the pharmacy has become overstocked with a particular product, or that an item was ordered accidentally, or even that the pharmacy is trying to reduce the amount of money invested in inventory sitting on its shelves. In any of these cases, to be returnable to the original supplier, the product must be in its original condition, unopened and unmarked. Each supplier has its own specific procedure for handling returns, so the pharmacy technician must be familiar with each vendor's process.

Recalls

Prescription and over-the-counter medications can be recalled directly by the manufacturer or by the FDA, as authorized by the Food, Drug, and Cosmetic Act. In most cases, manufacturers work closely with the FDA and, therefore, issue product recalls voluntarily.

Recalls are classified as Class I, Class II, or Class III. Class I recalls are the most dangerous and are designated for products that are defective and could cause serious adverse health conditions or death. Class II recalls are for products that could cause temporary or moderate adverse health conditions. Class III recalls are for products that would not cause harm, but have been mislabeled or are otherwise not in compliance with FDA regulations.

Recalled products are returned to their manufacturers directly from the pharmacy. Manufacturers prepare and distribute precise details and instructions on how pharmacies are to respond to a recall. Recalled products are identified by their NDC and lot numbers.

Expired Drugs

Except for medical devices, every product in a pharmacy comes with an expiration date, which indicates when the product is no longer considered safe for use. Expiration dates must be monitored manually, which is typically done by checking the expiration date on all inventory regularly, such as once a month.

Inventory should be rotated so that drugs with shorter expiration dates are used before those with longer shelf lives. Drugs that are set to expire within six months are typically marked or labeled with an expiration sticker to draw the attention of pharmacy staff. **Expired drugs** must never be dispensed, so it is critical to monitor the stock and remove expired medications from the shelf.

Once a drug expires (reaches its expiration date), it must be returned to the manufacturer or destroyed, with proper documentation of the destruction. Most pharmacies opt to return expired drugs, because manufacturers provide a rebate or credit in most cases.

Problem with Excessive Inventory

Excessive inventory can cause many problems for all types of pharmacies. The major problems with excessive inventory are discussed next.

- High costs—too much inventory can lead to profit loss, more drugs to keep up with, and the need to pay pharmacy employees for keeping track of the inventory. Excess product can also expire, get damaged, stolen, or lost.

PROFILE IN PRACTICE

Helen is a pharmacy technician who works in a long-term care facility. When reviewing her inventory order, Helen notices that a pint of liquid medication is damaged and leaked during shipment.

▶ *How should Helen handle this matter?*

 Return Companies

Numerous companies, such as Guaranteed Returns, are available that can handle the entire return process on expired drugs for a pharmacy. Such a company will send employees to physically process the return and complete all the required paperwork. The company keeps a percentage of the refund as its fee for this service.

- Sales—the pharmacy will make less money if it has waste or excess inventory. Additional space is needed to store more products and more time and money is needed by employees to keep track of the overstock. Drugs may be recalled at any time, and this can create stock that is outdated or no longer needed. Narcotic drugs can go bad after a certain period of time, and this will create an overstock as well.
- Finances—the drug seller may not be selling its product correctly, marketing or advertising effectively, or ordering the product inaccurately. Time, effort, and resources are needed to properly stock products or medications, and these three ideals are compromised when excess stock is carried in the pharmacy.

Importance of Cash Flow

Cash flow is payment for medications including receipts for cash, credit, disbursements, gift card sales, and payments for co-pays. A purchase journal will record the purchases of merchandise for sale. Positive cash flow means the pharmacy is making money and profiting from its sales and doing well. Negative cash flow means the pharmacy is not making money from its sales and is not doing well financially.

Medication Disposal

Medications that are expired, deteriorated, contaminated, or dropped should be disposed of properly. Drug disposing should never be done carelessly. For example, never flush drugs down the toilet because this can harm the environment and also get into drinking water systems. Pharmacies can get credit for returning broken, damaged, or tainted products. These medications should be marked for credit and returned to the drug manufacturer. Many states have drug take-back programs, which allow individuals to bring their medications back to the pharmacy or to their local police department for proper disposal. Each pharmacy will have its own set of rules, regulations, and proper disposal protocol. Pharmacy technicians may be responsible for the returning of products to drug manufacturers and also for proper *final* disposal of drugs that are no longer needed or considered to be *bad*. These medications should be labeled either "Expired Drugs—Do Not Use" or "Returned for Store Credit—Do Not Use." Pharmacy technicians must follow the lead of their pharmacist and pharmacy manager concerning the specific disposal of medications.

Disposal of Controlled Substances

Controlled substances that are no longer needed or are considered tainted, damaged, broken, chipped, melted, or expired should be disposed of properly. Controlled substances should be marked for store credit and returned to the manufacturer

or marked as damaged products. Proper disposal depends on each individual pharmacy. Controlled substances should be kept under proper lock and key so they are not accessed easily. Controlled substances are often coveted drugs and wanted by improper individuals who wish to steal or abuse medications. They must be monitored and kept track of carefully. The pharmacist or pharmacy manager must file a report concerning controlled substances every 10 days, and a list of these prescriptions should be kept at all times.

Dropped Drugs

Prescriptions that are dropped cannot be given to patients under any circumstances. These drugs are to be considered tainted drugs. Dropped pills should be swept up right away and packaged for store credit or proper disposal depending on the specific rules of the pharmacy and the wishes of the pharmacist or pharmacy manager.

Theft and Diversion

Theft and diversion are a reality in any hospital or retail pharmacy. How a pharmacy handles theft and diversion differs from pharmacy to pharmacy. Training classes should be given to properly train technicians on how to handle robbery and theft. Remembering to stay calm during a robbery is key, and theft or robbery should be reported to proper authorities and the DEA (if narcotics are stolen) immediately following the incident. Unfortunately, pharmacy employees who are not upstanding will take or steal medications. Those who commit such crimes will face termination from their job, and criminal consequences will also be a reality for those who take prescriptions from the workplace. Deterrence (diversion) can be handled in many ways. Installing security systems, alarms, locked pull-down gates, and securing narcotics in a safe place can also deter criminals or drug addicts. Having security guards in store can also help keep criminals and addicts from stealing money and drugs from the pharmacy.

Counterfeit Medications, Theft, and Chemical Dependency

Counterfeit drugs are simply fake medications. Pharmacists and pharmacy technicians should be aware of counterfeit medications and follow FDA announcements concerning fake medications. Counterfeit drugs should immediately be reported to supervisors, appropriate authorities, and the FDA. Pharmacy employees should also look out for altered prescriptions. Those addicted to prescription drugs will sometimes result in theft or robbery. The coveted drugs are often controlled substances. Controlled substances should always be kept under lock and key, as those who are addicts will do anything to get the medications they crave.

Summary

Evaluating costs and sources is a large part of pharmacists' and pharmacy technician's job duties. Cost analysis and cost control are used to realize cost objectives. Evaluating medication costs depends on whether the medication is a brand-name drug or in generic form. Drug strength, manufacturer, supplier, volume sold, and availability of the drug also matter in inventory management. Being familiar with ordering practices is part of the pharmacy technician's job, and he or she can be a great help in making sure that the right prescription and medical products are ordered correctly. Automated ordering systems make a technician's job easier and enable the technician to work more efficiently in the long run.

Sometimes the technician must deal with insurance providers and may also need the pharmacist to override medications when they are not automatically covered by certain insurance providers. Special approvals are often needed to get brand-name drugs when a generic is not in order for the patient.

Damaged drugs should never be used. They should be discarded and destroyed in a proper manner. Narcotic medications must be kept track of carefully under lock and key. Dropped pills must be discarded along with damaged medications.

Theft is a reality along with deterring the act. Pharmacies can take certain measures to keep criminals out as well as protecting their products in a careful and safe manner. Counterfeit drugs are also a form of theft. The pharmacist and pharmacy technician can keep abreast of fake medications by following FDA alerts and news reports concerning mock medications. Inventory management is just a small part of a pharmacy technician's duties.

Chapter Review Questions

1. Which of the following is *not* considered an atypical drug for inventory management?
   a. biologics
   b. interferons
   c. investigational drugs
   d. nonformulary drugs

2. Which class recalls are for products that would not cause harm, but have been mislabeled or are otherwise not in compliance with FDA regulations?
   a. I
   b. II
   c. III
   d. IV

3. Which method of purchasing requires a dollar-volume commitment and may have restrictions on additional, outside agreements?
   a. primary vendor
   b. purchasing direct
   c. wholesale
   d. secondary vendor

4. Order confirmations are normally provided through any of the following, *except* _____.
   a. e-mail
   b. telephone
   c. reports
   d. written letter

5. The most common method for delivery of orders is _____.
   a. a courier
   b. FedEx
   c. UPS
   d. USPS

6. All of the following are considered problems with excessive inventory, *except* _____.
   a. finances
   b. high costs
   c. product shortages
   d. sales

7. A _____ is a listing of preapproved drugs for specific purposes.
   a. formulary
   b. GPO
   c. purchasing system
   d. wholesaler

8. If narcotics are stolen from the pharmacy, the _____ should be notified immediately.
   a. CDC
   b. FDA
   c. DEA
   d. SBOP

9. The discovery of counterfeit drugs should be notified to the _____ immediately.
   a. CDC
   b. FDA
   c. DEA
   d. SBOP

10. Which of the following is a condition for which an outside company, such as Guaranteed Returns, will handle product returns?
    a. expired drugs
    b. drug recalls
    c. overstocked drugs
    d. nonformulary drugs

Critical Thinking Questions

1. What are the advantages and disadvantages of each method of purchasing for a pharmacy?

2. Why must expired drugs be destroyed or returned to the manufacturer?

3. If you observe the pharmacy manager is diverting drugs from the pharmacy, what are your responsibilities and obligations, if any? How would you handle the situation?

Web Challenge

1. Visit Pharmacy Purchasing Outlook's website (www.pharmacypurchasing.com) and research information on the role of pharmacy buyers. Write a brief report on your findings.

2. Go to the FDA website (www.fda.gov) and research information on current counterfeit drug warnings. Prepare a brief written report of your findings, including tips on how to distinguish the counterfeits.

References and Resources

"Access to Investigational Drugs." *National Cancer Institute*. Web. 1 June 2012.

"Communicating with Other Healthcare Professionals." *Pharmacy Technician's Letter*. Web. 12 June 2012.

"Counterfeit Medication." *FDA*. Web. 31 May 2012.

"Formulary & Non-Formulary Medications." *TRICARE*. Web. 1 June 2012.

"HDMA White Paper on Product Availability: Communication Guidelines for Managing Product Shortages in the Healthcare Supply Chain." *Healthcare Distribution Management Association*. Web. 1 June 2012.

Gore, Mary Jane. "Automation Aids Prescription Processing—But Professional Judgment Remains Indispensable." *JMCP*. Web. 1 June 2012.

Kokemuller, Neil. "Problems with Retail and Over-Inventory." *The Houston Chronicle & Demand Media*. Web. 31 May 2012.

The Department of Defense Pharmacoeconomic Center. Web. 1 June 2012.

"What is Cancer?" *American Cancer Society*. Web. 1 June 2012.

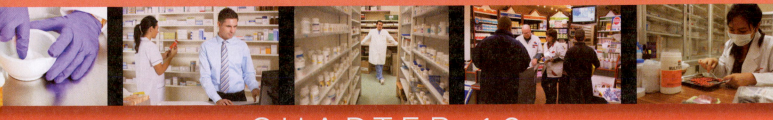

CHAPTER 12

Insurance and Third-Party Billing

LEARNING OBJECTIVES

After completing this chapter, you should be able to:

- Define and describe drug utilization reviews (evaluations).
- List and describe the various types of insurance.
- Describe and differentiate Medicare and Medicaid.
- Recognize and define terms commonly used in insurance billing.
- Describe and perform the steps required in collecting data for insurance purposes.
- Describe and perform the steps necessary to transmit a prescription for insurance.
- List and explain common insurance billing errors and their solutions.
- Define fraud as it pertains to insurance billing.

KEY TERMS

adjudication, p. 200

carrier/insurer/provider, p. 200

claim, p. 200

co-pay, p. 200

days supply, p. 200

deductible, p. 200

dispense as written (DAW), p. 200

Medicaid, p. 198

Medicare, p. 198

processor, p. 200

INTRODUCTION

Insurance and third-party billing is another critical responsibility managed by pharmacy technicians. The pharmacy must be properly reimbursed by insurance carriers in a timely fashion if the pharmacy is to operate. Insurance billing requires specific knowledge and training, but with practice and experience, the pharmacy technician will be able to manage this important task.

Insurance Billing

We hear almost every day about the high cost of health care. Prescription costs are a contributing factor in that equation. To help defray the costs of prescriptions, many Americans have purchased or have employer-subsidized prescription insurance. One of the responsibilities of an ambulatory pharmacy technician is to process insurance claims for patients. Remembering a few basic points, along with some computer experience, will set technicians on their way to competence.

Formularies

The Food and Drug Administration (FDA) maintains a national formulary of prescription medications. This formulary is similar to those established by pharmacies and insurance companies, except the FDA's formulary includes all approved prescription and generic drugs. The formulary is important in utilizing the pharmacy benefit manager (PBM). According to MedicineNet.com, the PBM is under contract through managed care organizations, companies that are self-insured, and government programs that are used to manage various pharmacy networks, management, drug utilization review, outcome management, and also disease management. Some additional important terms go along with understanding the pharmacy formulary. An open formulary generally covers drugs not listed in the formulary. Closed formularies are formularies where drugs are not listed in the formulary and are not covered without a doctor stating and authorizing the need for a certain drug to treat a patient's illness or condition. These special drugs may require special written authorization, verbal approval, and/or a pharmacists' and doctors' override. Restricted formularies restrict and limit the types of drugs to generics or specific drugs within a certain class.

Another term to remember in the realm of formularies is a tier. A tier is a very particular list of prescription drugs. Formularies are part of the PBM and divide into what is called a tier. Each tier is associated with a certain amount a patient will pay or co-pay. Three-tiered formularies will generally consist of generic drugs, preferred brand mediations, and nonpreferred drugs. Compounding drugs fall into the nonpreferred drug list. Biologics and specialty drugs come under a different category and are gaining demand concerning PMBs and the inclusion of these drugs into a generic drug category. These drugs may also be considered into a biogenerics category.

Drug Utilization Reviews/Evaluations

Drug utilization reviews work by improving quality health care, patient safety, and ensuring the formulary is used in a mandatory manner. One step in the drug utilization review is

Medicare the health insurance program for individuals aged 65 years or older, younger people with disabilities, and people with end-stage renal disease.

Medicaid the health insurance program for individuals and families with low income or individuals with disabilities.

gaining prior (or pre) authorization or getting approval for the medication before the drug is prescribed and dispensed. Prescriptions that need prior approval are often narcotics, drugs that are highly addictive, specialty drugs, and costly drugs. Another step in the drug utilization review process is the checking of the drug against the formulary, patient's eligibility, correct dosage, medication interactions, disease interactions, and other issues pertaining to the prescription. Pharmacy technicians and pharmacists will also receive any edits or changes to the prescription at this time. In addition, the doctor who prescribed the drug is contacted if there are any special questions or if there is an issue regarding the approval of the prescription before it is filled by the pharmacist. There may be issues with insurance, Medicaid, or Medicare, and those issues need to be cleared up before the patient actually gets the drug in his or her hand. Pharmacists may also practice therapeutic interchange. This practice is the substitution of one drug for another, but the drug is in the same class. Formulary compliance can increase if therapeutic interchange is practiced. Doctors, however, need special permission to change out drugs in the same class (due to the fact that drugs contain many different chemical compounds).

Types of Insurance

There are a number of health insurance options and many different insurers. This section discusses each type very briefly.

Health Maintenance Organizations

A health maintenance organization (HMO) is a type of health insurance coverage in the United States that is fulfilled through hospitals, doctors, pharmacies, and other providers with which the HMO has a contract.

Patients must select a primary care physician (PCP), who has contracted with the HMO, to be their first or primary point of medical care. To ensure benefit coverage, the PCP must make referrals to specialists in advance; the HMO usually has a list of approved specialists. HMO policies are generally the least expensive insurance plan option, because of their restrictions and conditions.

> **❝ Workplace Wisdom HMOs**
>
> Common HMO providers include Aetna, Cigna, Humana, Kaiser, and TRICARE (CHAMPUS). **❞**

Preferred Provider Organizations

A preferred provider organization (PPO) differs from an HMO in that patients have greater choice in selecting their physicians and other care providers. Patients can choose to be seen by in-network providers, which have a direct contract with the PPO, or out-of-network providers, although it is more expensive to visit out-of-network providers. In addition, patients generally can elect to go to a specialist without a referral or prior authorization. A PPO may maintain lists of in-network specialists as well as PCPs.

> ❝ **Workplace Wisdom** PPOs
>
> Common PPO providers include BlueCross/BlueShield (BCBS), Pacificare, and United Healthcare (UHC). ❞

Drug Discount/Coupon Cards

Drug discounts and coupon cards usually offer patients a small amount off of the cost of prescriptions. Such discounts may take the form of chain retail discount cards with store discounts that include discounts on pharmacy drugs and items. Pharmacies can also offer drug manufacturer vouchers and coupons. Other organizations and companies offer patient-assistance programs to help defer the cost of medications as well. Such discounts may be a lifesaver for many patients, especially if they take more than one drug. Drug costs are high for brand-name drugs, and generic equivalents, if any, can be prescribed for the drug. Patient-assistance programs can take the form of enrolling in a savings program at no cost to the patient, or the medication may be provided by filling out assistance paperwork that is sent directly from the drug company. Senior prescription discount cards are also another way pharmacy customers can save on their prescriptions. Various pharmacies offer the cards to older people to save a certain percentage off of their medications.

Medicare

Medicare is the health insurance program for individuals aged 65 years or older, younger people with disabilities, and persons with end-stage renal disease. It is funded by the federal government, in part through payroll taxes. Medicare is made up of several parts: Part A, which provides hospital insurance; Part B, which provides medical insurance; Part C, also known as Medicare Advantage, which allows patients to receive all of their health care services through a provider organization; and Part D, which provides prescription drug insurance.

Medicaid

Medicaid is the health insurance program for individuals and families with low income or individuals with disabilities; it is managed by the state and funded jointly by the state and federal government. Among the patients on Medicaid are eligible low-income parents, children, seniors, and persons with disabilities. Medicaid eligibility requirements are determined and vary by each state.

Patients who meet eligibility requirements may have both Medicaid and Medicare coverage.

TRICARE

TRICARE is a medical insurance plan for U.S. uniformed servicemen's and service women's families. The plan is a Department of Defense health insurance plan. Benefits are offered to service people of all branches of the armed services and those employed by public health service and National Oceanic and Atmospheric Administration (NOAA).

There are five different types of TRICARE.

TRICARE Standard

TRICARE Standard is a fee-based medical insurance program. It covers those individuals who cannot obtain services offered by a military treatment facility (MTF). With TRICARE Standard, patient's medical expenses are shared by both the service person's family and TRICARE. An important term to remember along with TRICARE is cost share. Cost-share payments are limited to a catastrophic cap. This cap is a limit on medical expenses the individual pays annually. After the coverage year is up, then TRICARE pays 100%.

TRICARE Prime

TRICARE Prime can be thought of as an HMO. TRICARE Prime enrollees are given a primary care manager, and this manager handles management of the patient's full care. Under TRICARE Prime, patients and beneficiaries must pay yearly enrollment fees, but no deductible and no payment is required at military facilities for medical treatments. Active servicemen and servicewomen do not pay to go to civilian network providers. Co-payments are made by beneficiaries, and the amount of the co-pay depends on the scope of services a patient receives.

TRICARE Reserve Select

This premium-based plan is available for particular National Guard service people and (Reserve Activated) employees. The plan applies to military personnel who started working in the military on or after September 11, 2001.

TRICARE for Life

TRICARE for Life is a program and promise to military personnel in regards to their military health care and a guarantee that coverage would always be there for them in times of need, specifically for a lifetime. TRICARE for Life was established in October 2001 and provides coverage for those over 65 years. With TRICARE for Life, the following protocol is followed in payment for services:

1. Medicare pays first.
2. Secondary insurance picks up after Medicare.
3. TRICARE picks up where these services leave off and covers the unpaid balance.

TRICARE Drug Programs

TRICARE provides many options and services to beneficiaries of all eligible U.S. uniformed service members. TRICARE for Life (TFL) beneficiaries are entitled to Medicare Part A/B and are based on age, disability, and end-stage renal disease. TRICARE beneficiaries can fill their prescriptions at any of the MTF pharmacies, through mail order, at TRICARE retail network pharmacies, or through non-network pharmacies. Military treatment facilities are the cheapest way to fill medications for service people and their families. TRICARE mail order pharmacy (TMOP) is easy and cost effective. Mail ordering medications take about 10–14 days. The most expensive option for beneficiaries is to go to a non-network pharmacy.

Civilian Health and Medical Program of the Veterans Administration

Civilian Health and Medical Program of the Veterans Administration (CHAMPVA) is now the Department of Veterans Affairs. CHAMPVA covers those families of disabled veterans (who are totally and permanently disabled) due to injuries sustained in acts of war or service-related injuries. Those servicemen and servicewomen who died in the service will have coverage for surviving spouses and their children. In 1996, The Veterans Healthcare Eligibility Reform Act was passed, and it requires those with a 100% disability to be included in CHAMPVA to be able to get their health care costs covered.

Worker's Compensation

Worker's compensation is a form of insurance for employees who are injured while at work. Patients are not responsible for any payments, as all costs are covered by the employer. Worker's compensation, however, requires that providers complete extensive and tedious paperwork to receive payment.

Understanding the Insurance Billing Process

Most ambulatory pharmacies bill their patients' insurance carriers for them. The responsibility for collecting, maintaining, and transmitting insurance claims thus rests on the shoulders of the pharmacy technician (see Figure 12-1). The entire process is usually done by computer. Through the Internet, the pharmacy electronically submits a claim to the insurance provider's computer, or a third-party claims processor; after that (one hopes), there is an exchange of funds. This exchange takes mere moments in most cases, so the patients can be on their way.

Insurance Terms

Just as in pharmacy, the insurance world has its own set of terms used in conducting its business. The following are some of the more common terms:

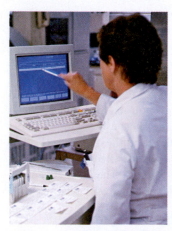

FIGURE 12-1 The insurance billing process is usually done by computer.
Source: Keith Brofsky/Getty Images, Inc.

- **Adjudication**—the process of transmitting a prescription electronically to the proper insurance company or third-party biller for approval and billing.
- **Carrier/insurer/ provider**—the insurance company.
- **Processor**—a company hired by the insurer to process claims.

- **Claim**—a request for reimbursement, for products or services rendered, from a health care provider to an insurance provider.
- **Co-pay**—a portion of the cost of a service or product that a patient pays out of pocket each time it is provided. For example, Mrs. Brown pays $5.00 for each prescription regardless of the actual cost of the medication.
- **Deductible**—a set amount a client pays up front before insurance coverage applies. This may be paid all at once or in increments. For example, Mrs. Brown has a $100 deductible. Her insurer may pay only 80% of each claim until she has paid $100; thereafter, her carrier pays 100%.
- **Dispense as written (DAW)**—a notation by the prescriber instructing the pharmacy to use the exact drug written (usually brand). Insurance providers may request the prescriber to state, in writing, the medical reasoning for this choice.
- **Days supply**—the number of days a dispensed quantity of medication will last.

Collecting Insurance Data

Just as the pharmacy keeps a confidential patient profile of all the clients it serves, so too do insurance providers, whether public or private. When an insurance provider hires a third party to process claims, the insurer provides the necessary client information to the adjustors (see Figure 12-2). Whether it be the government (Medicaid and Medicare) or a private insurer (Blue Cross, Aetna, etc.), all providers keep records of their customers. These records contain much of the same information as the pharmacy patient profile.

Before a claim can be paid, the information in the claim has to match—exactly—the insurance company's information on file, starting with the correct name; the insurer may also provide an account number and possibly a personal code. Marriages, divorces, and births all can affect the continuation of insurance coverage. It is the technician's responsibility to collect all the current relevant information required for insurance billing for the pharmacy, but it is the patient's responsibility to keep the insurance provider's information updated.

Here is an example of this process: When Mary Smith got married, she changed her surname to Brown. The new Mrs. Brown dutifully changed her credit cards, address, and driver's license. When she came to the pharmacy, the astute technician also updated her profile in the computer. However, when her insurance claim was submitted, it was refused! Why? Because Mrs. Brown neglected to update her records with her insurance provider; thus, the information submitted by the pharmacy, though correct, did not match the information in the insurance provider's records. *Claim denied.* For insurance billing to work, the two profiles (pharmacy and insurance) must match exactly.

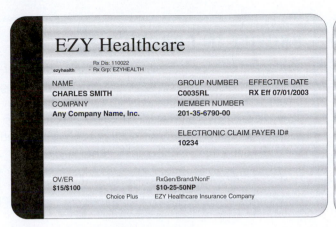

FIGURE 12-2 Insurance information.

Transmitting Prescriptions

Assuming that the patient profiles match, the billing technician's job is just starting. The insurance provider will need to know the name of the medication being dispensed. Providers may have formularies just as pharmacies do; in other words, the insurance provider will pay only for approved medications. Along with the strength and dose, there is the question of brand or generic.

Providers usually pay much more of the cost of a generic medication and shift more of the cost of a brand-name drug back to the patient. The exception to this rule is when a provider includes a DAW code for medical reasons. For example, Mrs. Brown requested a brand-name drug be used in filling her prescription. Her normal co-pay is $5.00, but this time it costs her $72.00. This is because Mrs. Brown's insurance provider will not pay for brand-name drugs unless her doctor states that it is medically necessary by placing "DAW" on her prescription.

If a technician writes the DAW code on a prescription, even in error, he could be charged with insurance fraud. If Mrs. Brown did not request the brand-name drug, but the prescriber did, and the technician forgot to put DAW in the claim, Mrs. Brown may end up paying way too much.

❝ Workplace Wisdom Common DAW Codes

DAW Code	Meaning
0	Physician authorized generic substitution and (a) patient accepts the generic substitution or (b) a generic equivalent is not available.
1	Physician requires that the prescription be filled exactly as written—no substitution permitted.
2	Physician authorized generic substitution and (a) a generic equivalent is available, but (b) the patient refuses generic substitution.

Troubleshooting Insurance

There are times when an insurance issue cannot be handled by computers. A good example is the case of an older woman whose doctor orders birth control pills as a hormone replacement. The insurance computer automatically refuses to pay for the prescription, because birth control expenses are not covered. In this case, the technician may have to call the provider and explain that the medication is not being used for birth control, but for hormone replacement, which is a covered therapy.

As noted earlier, insurance computers simply match information coming in with the information in their databases. The case of twins can be an insurance billing challenge, because the computers simply match the parents' policy number with the eligible member number (e.g., Dad—01, Mom—02, and Children—03) and birth dates. Unfortunately, twins have the same birth dates. If they are both to receive a prescription, the provider may have to be contacted by phone before the proper payment can be made (see Figure 12-3).

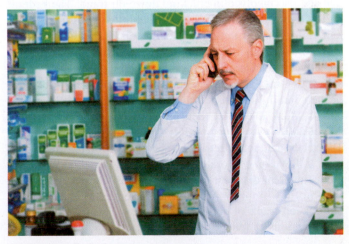

FIGURE 12-3 There are times when an insurance issue cannot be handled by computers.
Source: Minerva Studio/Shutterstock

Common Errors/Messages

The following are some of the error messages most commonly encountered in insurance billing rejections:

- Incorrect name—may be due to use of a nickname, marriage, or divorce.
- Incorrect days supply—will affect refill times and insurance reimbursements.
- Incorrect provider—because of changes in employment or employer-provided benefits.
- Incorrect birth date—may be entered incorrectly for a number of reasons.

These errors will trigger the following refusal messages:

- "Patient not covered"—the patient was not recognized, possibly because of incorrect name, wrong birth date, incorrect provider, or new coverage.
- "Too early to refill" —the wrong days supply may have been entered.

A technician should never take these types of messages at face value or as the last word on the subject; rather, he or she should continue investigating. This is part of good patient service. There are times, however, when the insurance carrier will still refuse, even though you have done all you can to get a payment on behalf of your patient.

Insurance billing is a customer service that pharmacy technicians provide for their patients each day. Insurance billing is done electronically. When machines talk to machines, they communicate only as well as the people operating them. Human intervention can save the day and humanize what can be a very cold process.

Fraud

HIPAA formed the Healthcare Fraud and Abuse Control Program to catch and prosecute any fraud or abuse in health care and insurance claims. The Office of the Inspector General enforces all related laws. The FBI and Department of Justice are also involved in cracking down on fraud. The Federal False Claims Act and USC 3729 prohibit submitting fraudulent claims and making false statements in conjunction with claims. The anti-kickback statute makes it illegal to give incentives for referents for services paid by government health care programs. The Stark statute makes it illegal for doctors or their family members to have financial relationships with clinics where they refer their patients. The "Sarbanes–Oxley Act of 2002" was signed on July 30, 2002, by President Bush. The act created many reforms to ensure corporate responsibility, cut down on corporate and accounting fraud, and compliment financial disclosures. The Sarbanes–Oxley Act created the Public Company Accounting Oversight Board, which helps keep track of auditing activities. Twenty states have their versions of federal false claims act. Claim fraud occurs

PROFILE IN PRACTICE

Dave is a pharmacy technician working in a retail pharmacy. He is processing a prescription for 90 Zoloft 100 mg tablets to be taken one at bedtime. The insurance company has rejected the prescription, citing "Incorrect Days Supply," but the patient insists that her paperwork stated she could get a three-month supply of her medications.

▸ *How should Dave assist his patient?*

when pharmacies or others falsely report charges to payers. Abuse means an action that misuses the money that government allocated.

Pharmacists can be charged for employees' actions and should always be updated on fraudulent activities and practices and watch out for fraudulent issues as they can take many forms. Pharmacy practices carry out compliance plans for protection against compliance problems and liability.

Billing

The pricing of medication can change often, and these changes are updated in a computer database. The cost of medication seems to be going up every day, and it is the job of the pharmacy technician to keep the medication database updated as this will affect ordering and restocking in the pharmacy. Reports can be run for the pharmacy manager so that he or she can see the rise and fall of different prices. These rises and falls can affect drug ordering, product ordering, and also the decision as to which drug manufacturer the pharmacy will utilize. Pricing systems are generally pharmacy-specific programs that allow pricing to be updated and cost changes that reflect the ups and downs of drug manufacturer's cost variances. There are a variety of companies that make pricing systems for pharmacy billing. Some of the features of these programs are:

- Increased billing speed and accuracy
- File management via paperless systems
- Better customer service for the patient
- User-friendly programs
- Training manuals or the option to receive training from a program specialist
- Less medication errors

Without computerized pharmacy billing systems, there would not be a way to track pricing and billing issues. Virtually every pharmacy runs on computerized billing systems, and the need for error-free work is essential to the proper functioning of any pharmacy.

Information Systems

A pharmacy system should provide support for the following activities performed in the pharmacy:

- Inpatient order entry, management, and dispensing
- Outpatient order entry
- Management and dispensing
- Inventory and purchasing management
- Reports of utilization, workload, and financial reports
- Clinical monitoring
- Manufacturing and compounding
- Intervention management
- Medication administration
- Connectivity to other systems
- Pricing, charging, and billing

Order entry in the pharmacy identifies a pharmaceutical drug the doctor ordered. Aspects of order entry are the item strength, package size, method of administration, and ingredients the pharmacy prepares. Efficient ongoing automated resupply of the medication is a must.

A pharmacy information system facilitates the definition of the order and the resupply of ordering. During order entry, the information should provide assistance in reviewing the order for drug interactions and allergies. The patient profile is the primary order review screen used in most pharmacies. The status of an order is one of the most important pieces of information in the pharmacy. In addition to status changes, there are several other types of edits that can be performed on pharmacy drug orders. Computer dispensing worklists are among the most important outputs of a pharmacy system. The use of automation in the inpatient setting performs routine dispensing.

The pharmacy system must allow for quick online claims while the prescription is filled. The system must recognize and display administration instructions clearly. Pharmacy systems handle inventory ordering, and reporting capabilities are also important in systems handling. Most pharmacy systems track active costs and patient care information. The system also monitors for clinical issues such as:

- Drug interaction allergies
- Food interactions
- Lab test interactions
- Dosing
- Disease state side effects

Medication and administration forms can be printed through different pharmacy systems, and a continual interchange within systems is needed. Security is also another important aspect of pharmacy systems.

Price Updates

Wholesalers and software management vendors will notify pharmacies of price changes and availability on a regular basis. Many computerized info management systems offer automatic pricing and updates as inventory quantity and pricing change. The price of certain medications will depend on whether the drug is a brand-name or generic medication. This price can vary greatly. For example, an independent pharmacy may charge $70.00 for a brand-name antidepressant medication, while a chain store charges $90.00. If a patient is paying out of pocket for his or her prescription, the patient will likely choose the pharmacy offering the cheaper price. So, with this said, it is to the advantage of pharmacies to keep their prices low. Price updates can be done either automatically in computerized systems or using data entry software and organization—with the final results being transferred into spreadsheet programs for review. Billing programs will vary greatly depending on whether the technician works in a hospital or retail setting.

Report Generation

Report generation of pharmacy facts, figures, and billing can be produced in a variety of programs that store, compile, and print data based on information entry. Pharmacy technicians may complete data entry in a variety of computer programs, and this data can then be imported into a spreadsheet and then reviewed or printed. Pharmacists and pharmacy technicians can use these reports to make decisions concerning product ordering, medical supply ordering, and financial gains and losses for the pharmacy.

Summary

Insurance billing requires a comprehensive knowledge of billing terms, codes, and policies, such as DAW codes, authorized days supply, and formularies. Many insurance claim rejections can be prevented by ensuring that all information is correctly entered into the pharmacy's computer system before a claim is submitted.

When properly trained, pharmacy technicians are able to assist the pharmacist by handling these responsibilities and allowing the pharmacist to focus on more clinical aspects of providing pharmaceutical care. These responsibilities vary by facility, but with time and experience, pharmacy technicians can effectively manage these aspects of pharmacy practice.

Chapter Review Questions

1. Medicare is the federally funded insurance program for people, including those _____.
   a. aged 60 or older
   b. with disabilities
   c. with cardiac disease
   d. in active duty in the military

2. What is the correct DAW code for a prescription on which the physician does not permit generic substitution?
   a. 0
   b. 1
   c. 2
   d. 3

3. All of the following contain regulations pertaining to fraud, *except* _____.
   a. Federal False Claims Act
   b. HIPAA
   c. Sarbanes–Oxley Act
   d. USC 2739

4. The medical insurance plan for U.S. military personnel and their families is _____.
   a. Aetna
   b. Humana
   c. TRICARE
   d. United Health Care

5. _____ is the health insurance program for individuals and families with low incomes or individuals with disabilities.
   a. CHAMPV
   b. Medicaid
   c. Medicare
   d. TRICARE

6. An error code of "Patient Not Covered" means _____.
   a. the insurance coverage has been terminated
   b. the name is entered incorrectly
   c. the date of birth is incorrect
   d. any of the above

7. Aetna is an example of a(n) _____.
   a. HMO
   b. PPO
   c. drug discount card
   d. worker's compensation plan

8. Which of the following actions would *not* affect continuation of insurance coverage?
   a. a birth
   b. a divorce
   c. a marriage
   d. work promotion

9. The co-pay is the portion of the cost of a prescription that is paid by the _____.
   a. insurance carrier
   b. patient
   c. pharmacy
   d. wholesaler

10. BlueCross/BlueShield is an example of a(n) _____.
    a. HMO
    b. PPO
    c. drug discount card
    d. workers compensation plan

Critical Thinking Questions

1. What incentive do drug manufacturers have to establish patient-assistance programs?

2. If an individual has a worker's compensation claim, yet requests to use his or her personal insurance plan, what are the potential consequences?

3. Why would January typically be the month with the most insurance rejections? What strategies could a pharmacy implement to reduce rejections?

Web Challenge

1. Using the Internet, research various prescription insurance plans and write a brief report on an HMO plan, a PPO plan, and a drug discount card program that you find.

2. To learn more about both Medicare prescription drug coverage and formularies, review the CMS Medicare Formulary at http://www.cms.gov Search under the Medicare tab from the home page, and then review the options under Prescription Drug Coverage.

References and Resources

"A Primer on Pharmacy Information Systems." *Journal of Healthcare Information Management*. Web. 6 June 2012.

American Society of Health-System Pharmacists. "ASHP Guidelines on Medication-Use Evaluation." *American Journal of Health-System Pharmacy*. 53 (1996): 1953–1955. Print.

"Definition of Pharmacy Benefit Manager." MedicineNet .com. Web. 20 September 2012.

Johnston, Mike. *The Pharmacy Technician: Foundations and Practices*. 1st ed. Upper Saddle River, NJ: Pearson, 2009. Print.

"Retail Pharmacies." *Prodigy Systems*. Web. 13 June 2012.

"The Laws That Govern The Securities Act." *Securities and Exchange Commission*. Web. 30 August 2012.

"What are Drug Utilization Reviews (DUR)?" *The Academy of Managed Care Pharmacy's Concepts in Managed Care Pharmacy*. Web. 6 June 2012.

"What do pharmacy system costs?" *Pharmacy Management Software*. Web. 6 June 2012.

"What is CHAMPVA?" *U.S. Department of Veterans Affairs*. Web. 6 June 2012.

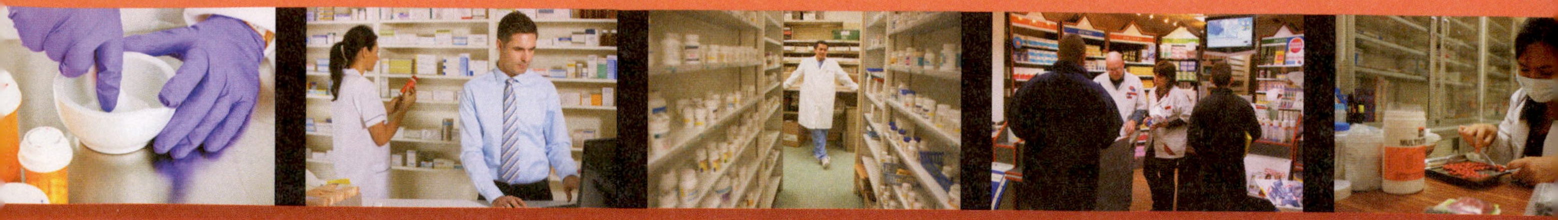

CHAPTER 13

Over-the-Counter (OTC) Products

LEARNING OBJECTIVES

After completing this chapter, you should be able to:

- Define and describe the FDA categories and regulations pertaining to OTC products.
- Outline the process for prescription drugs to become approved for OTC classification.
- List and describe common OTC analgesics and antipyretics.
- List and describe common OTC respiratory agents.
- List and describe common gastrointestinal system agents.
- List and describe common OTC integumentary system agents.
- List and describe common OTC central nervous system agents.
- List and describe common OTC ophthalmic, otic, and oral agents.
- List and describe common OTC contraceptive products.
- List and describe common smoking cessation products.
- List and describe common behind-the-counter (BTC) products.
- List and describe common herbal and alternative treatments.
- List and describe common vitamins and supplements.
- List and describe common OTC medical devices and diagnostic agents.
- List and describe common OTC fertility and pregnancy tests.
- Describe the use of nebulizers.
- List and describe common OTC test screening kits.
- List and describe common OTC medical supplies.
- Define and describe the pharmacy technician's role with OTC products, devices, and supplies.

KEY TERMS

alopecia, p. 216
analgesic, p. 208
antacid, p. 214
antidiarrheal, p. 214
antiemetic, p. 214
antiflatulent, p. 214
antihemorrhoidal, p. 214
antihistamine, p. 210
antipyretic, p. 208
antitussive, p. 210
decongestant, p. 210
dermatitis, p. 218
expectorant, p. 210
laxative, p. 214
over-the-counter (OTC), p. 207

INTRODUCTION

Over-the–counter (OTC) products are items that the Food and Drug Administration (FDA) has ruled safe for common consumer use and therefore do not need a written prescription. The FDA labels OTC products as self-medicating, meaning the average consumer can read and understand the product information and directions and administer the product in a way that does not cause harm to the consumer. Still, OTCs come with some warnings and precautions. Pharmacy technicians who understand how OTC products affect prescription medications, or know how to educate patients on the use of medical devices, help to alleviate patient concerns and build avenues of trust. Although providing patients with the best possible route of care is important, the pharmacy technician must also remember what information is within their lawful scope of practice. It cannot be said enough; it is unlawful for pharmacy technicians to provide medical advice or medication information, whether it is prescription or OTC. If a patient requests information concerning OTC medications, the technician should refer the patient to the pharmacist. Above all, concern for the patient's safety must be the pharmacy technician's main priority. A technician who not only understands this but also mimics it in their career will not only have a long career in pharmacy, but gain the respect of other health care professionals.

Transition from Prescription to OTC

It takes several years and millions, sometimes billions, of dollars for a new drug to become available to the consumer. The drug manufacturer must first seek approval from the FDA, and in order to do that it must prove the drug has potential benefit to the general public as well as a limited risk of safety. The drug company then files a new drug application (NDA) with the FDA. Once the application is approved and is past this hurdle, it is on to a three-phase clinical stage, most of which involves rigorous studies and data collection. Volunteers who fit the drug's profile are tested for benefits and side effects of the drug, and even after this information is collected, the FDA may require the drug manufacturer to make changes to the drug or place restrictive conditions on its release to market—a very long and expensive road.

Once everything is in place and the FDA has given its approval, the drug manufacturer may proceed in marketing the drug in the United States. The drug manufacturer holds a 20-year patent on the drug, but the clock starts ticking from the time the drug was developed, not from the time the drug is marketed. So how does a drug make it from these steps to OTC status?

In 1951 the Durham–Humphrey Amendment to the Food, Drug, and Cosmetic Act of 1938 created two distinct classes of drugs: prescription and nonprescription. Before this amendment there was no real distinction between prescription and nonprescription drugs. In accordance with the stipulations set forth by Durham–Humphrey, any drug that has the potential to be highly habit forming or could impose harm on the patient would need to be prescribed under the supervision of a physician and would be labeled as a prescription drug by the FDA. The amendment also required these drugs to carry a warning from the manufacturer, which stated, "Caution: Federal law prohibits dispensing without a prescription." Any drugs that did not fall within the confines of these restrictions could be labeled as nonprescription or OTC.

There are more than 700 nonprescription products in the U.S. market today, and the number continues to climb. For a drug to make it to nonprescription status, the drug manufacturer must file an NDA with the FDA. This process normally begins after a prescription drug has been in the U.S. market for several years, allowing the drug manufacturers to compile data relating to the drug's efficacy and safety. If there is substantiated reason to believe the drug would be not only safe, but beneficial on the nonprescription market, the drug manufacturer will begin the process of taking the drug from a prescription to nonprescription status with the FDA. This process is known as "Rx to OTC switch."

Still it is not just as simple as the drug manufacturer turning over its data to the FDA and filing an application. It takes a minimum of 10 months and quite often longer, for the FDA to approve a drug switch to OTC status. There are a few key questions the FDA must be able to answer, before it will approve the OTC status:

- Is the product safe for consumer use based upon market research and data collected by the drug manufacturer?
- What is the potential for abuse?
- Are the drug's benefits greater than its risks?
- How easily would the average consumer be able to administer the drug in relation to self-diagnosis and the drug's intended use?

Only after all of these questions are answered and sound, and reliable data is collected, can a drug make the switch from prescription to nonprescription status. The FDA is a governing body whose job is to protect the citizens of the United States from harm. If regulations are not followed or are done so in a haphazard manner, then processes will be questioned and the safety of the consumer is compromised. While the steps involved in bringing a drug to nonprescription status may seem arduous, they are of extreme necessity and importance; convenience should never be substituted for safety.

One final note: If at any time the FDA finds a nonprescription drug to be unsafe or without benefit to the average consumer, it may remove the drug's nonprescription status. A recent example of this came into play in 2011 when the FDA required all combination cold medications marketed for infants and toddlers to be removed from store shelves, a risk that the FDA felt outweighed the benefit.

Over-the-Counter (OTC) A drug or device that has been approved by the FDA to be purchased without a prescription.

Common OTC Products

There are an estimated 700 FDA-approved nonprescription drugs available in the U.S. market. The sales from OTC products reached a staggering 17 billion in 2010, and the prediction for future sales will not decrease any time soon. The average consumer walking into a local drug store is overwhelmed by row after row of OTC drugs and the difficult task of deciding which product to purchase.

Some of the most common reasons consumers purchase OTC products include pain relief; fever reduction; sleep aid; relief from the symptoms associated with allergies—runny nose, sneezing, and watery eyes; elimination of conditions associated with constipation or diarrhea; and reduction of cold symptoms, particularly cough and mucosal buildup. Whatever the reason for the consumer's purchase of an OTC product, the consumer must keep in mind that although the FDA has gone to great lengths to reduce risk to the consumer, there are still precautions and warnings, which need to be followed.

It is clear OTC-marketed drugs have had a tremendous effect when it comes to the ability of self-medication for the general public. Although regulations have been set in place to protect consumers, it is always a good idea to read drug facts labels and, if necessary, present any questions or concerns to a licensed pharmacist. As more prescription drugs make the switch to OTC status, pharmacy technicians should familiarize themselves with these changes, keeping up to date with industry standards and changes. Knowledge is an invaluable tool, but knowing the limits of that knowledge is even more important. A pharmacy technician should always refer medical-based questions concerning OTCs to the pharmacist, encouraging drug safety and protecting the consumer.

Analgesics and Antipyretics

There are over 80 classifications of OTC medications; to understand each and everyone would, to say the least, be mind boggling. Yet, understanding the classification an OTC drug might fall into may help explain its purpose. Analgesics and antipyretics are two classifications of OTC drugs that most people have purchased sometime within their life. These two classifications have specific function, which oftentimes usefully coincide with one another.

Analgesics and **antipyretics** are some of the most routinely purchased OTC products on the U.S. consumer market. Today, there are over 100 FDA-approved OTC analgesic and antipyretic drugs on pharmacy shelves (see Figure 13-1). While the FDA has deemed these drugs to be safe and effective for consumers, they do not come without warning. Acetaminophen, one of three categories of analgesics, has recently come under fire from the FDA and consumer advocate groups; primary concerns deal with insufficient administration directions on product labels and overdosing by consumers who do not understand or

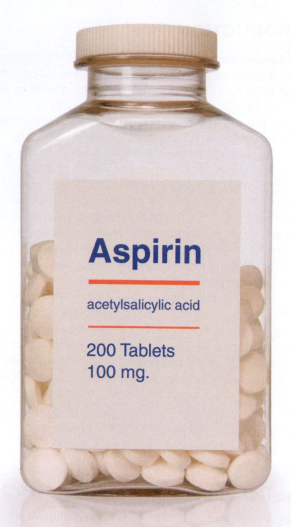

FIGURE 13-1 Aspirin is an OTC analgesic
Source: James Steidl/Shutterstock

Aspirin and OTC Analgesics

Aspirin, which is often used to relieve pain or reduce inflammation, is not appropriate to give to children under the age of 19 years. Research has found children under the age of 19 years who have a fever associated with the chicken pox or flu and are given aspirin are at greater risk for contracting Reyes syndrome, a disease that primarily attacks the liver and brain and ultimately leads to death. While aspirin may not be appropriate in most cases to give to children, it is quite useful for adults. Aspirin also has antiplatelet properties and is often prescribed as a low dose daily maintenance drug for those who are at risk for heart attack or stroke.

Analgesics and antipyretics are available on OTC shelves in various forms, from oral tablets and solutions to gums, suppositories, and topical creams. Products are also associated with various types of release mechanisms: immediate release, chewable tablets, extended release tablets and capsules, enteric-coated tablets, and quick-dissolving tablets. Pharmacy technicians should take the time to familiarize themselves with these products as well as the warning that comes with the product's key ingredient.

Analgesic A drug that is used to help reduce pain.

Antipyretic A drug that is used to help reduce or eliminate fever.

do not follow recommended daily allowances. Extended use of acetaminophen at greater than 4 gm a day can cause liver damage and even death. This becomes even further complicated by combination products that already have acetaminophen listed as a main ingredient.

Analgesics

Analgesics are drugs that help to reduce pain. In fact, the term *analgesic* is derived directly from the Greek: *an = without and algesis = sense of pain*. Pain, which is completely subjective, is built upon several underlying factors. Physical, mental, emotional, biochemical, physiological, and even cultural factors influence the feeling and intensity of pain. No matter what the reason, each of us has felt pain. Headaches, backaches, and pain felt from an injury or postoperative surgery are some of the more common reasons we feel pain; analgesics are the first line of defense against pain.

Analgesics are drugs that help to reduce or eliminate mild to moderate pain. They are further classified into three recognized categories: acetaminophen, salicylate, and nonsteroidal anti-inflammatory (NSAIDs). Each category has properties specific to the drugs within it and often overlaps with other drug classifications.

Analgesics are available in as many varieties and forms as the pain they treat. Safety and precautions should always be observed when using any OTC drug, but nowhere is it more important than when administering an analgesic to an infant or a child. Drug manufacturers have taken steps to make the process of self-diagnosis and administration safer by changing labels and dosing instructions. Pharmacy technicians who stay informed of industry standards and changes are better equipped to make the necessary changes in their own department or pharmacy, taking the element of risk out of the equation for the pharmacy and the patient.

Acetaminophen

Acetaminophen is the most common analgesic. It is relatively inexpensive and is available in a variety of forms for ease of consumer use. Tylenol, manufactured by the McNeil Company, is perhaps the most recognizable brand acetaminophen produced in the U.S. market, but is also manufactured under many generic names, such as Genapap, Feverall, Actamin Maximum Strength, Altenol, Aminofen, Anacin Aspirin Free, Apra, which are all FDA-approved U.S. trade names.

Acetaminophen is available as a 325-mg and 500-mg tablet/caplet; a 650-mg extended release tablet/caplet; 160-mg/5-ml children's oral elixir; 80-mg/0.8-ml infant solution; 120-mg, 325-mg, and 650-mg suppositories; and an 80-mg children's and 160-mg junior disintegrating tablet. It is also important to recognize acetaminophen is often one of the primary ingredients in multisymptom products marketed for cold and flu.

While acetaminophen is effective in reducing pain, it has warnings attached to its use. FDA standards state more than 4 gm of acetaminophen a day has the potential for increased liver damage. Patients who routinely drink more than three alcoholic beverages a day and use acetaminophen also increase their potential for liver damage. The FDA has begun a campaign to

> ### info Acetaminophen
>
> While acetaminophen is safe to use for mild to moderate pain for infants and children, parents or caregivers should take special caution by reading all drug fact labels and dosing instructions. In May 2011 manufacturers of infant's and children's acetaminophen products proposed one standard concentration for their oral solution and elixir products. Across the broad FDA-approved standard concentration is 160 mg/5 ml oral elixir for children and 80 mg/0.8 ml for infants. Further packaging changes include weight-based dosing for children 2–12 years of age and the addition of the words "fever reducer" for infant solutions. Further proposed safety measures require calibrated oral syringes for infant's packaging and oral dosing cups for children's packaging. All necessary changes need to prevent and protect infants and children from accidental overdose from acetaminophen.

improve consumer compliance when self-administering acetaminophen. Poor product labeling, unclear dosing instructions, and uneducated consumers are all pieces of the problem that leads to consumer acetaminophen toxicity.

McNeil, the manufacturer of Tylenol, has voluntarily taken steps to help reduce the incidence of acetaminophen toxicity by not only making product labeling friendlier to consumers, but warning them of the potential for liver toxicity when more than 4 gm a day is ingested. The FDA recommended daily dosing of acetaminophen for an adult is 325–650 mg every 4–6 hours or 100 mg every 3–4 hours and not to exceed 4 gm total. Anyone who may have renal or liver disease should talk with their physician before using acetaminophen, as their dosing may need to be adjusted.

Salicylate

Aspirin is also classified as an analgesic and falls under the category of a salicylate. It also has anti-inflammatory and anti-platelet properties, meaning it falls within those classifications. Long used to combat pain, aspirin is sometimes used in conjunction with acetaminophen. A good example of this would be Excedrin Migraine and Excedrin Extra Strength; it should be noted these products also contain caffeine as part of their active ingredients.

Aspirin, which can be used for mild to moderate pain, also carries warnings for the consumer, which include restricted use in children under 16 years of age, increased incidence for peptic ulcer, tinnitus (ringing in the ears) or hearing impairment with extended use, should not be used in patients with bleeding or platelet disorders, and increased risk for renal damage in patients who already have renal impairment.

Aspirin is marketed in the United States under the following trade names: Ecotrin, Bayer, Ascription, Aspergum, Aspirtab, Easprin, Ecpirin, and Entercote. Aspirin, like acetaminophen, is available in various forms and dosages. Aspirin is available in the U.S. consumer market as an 81-mg (chewable and oral), 162-mg, and 325-mg tablet; 500-mg extra strength tablet; 81-mg, 325-mg, 500-mg, and 650-mg enteric-coated tablet; a 227-mg gum; as well as a 120-mg, 300-mg, and 600-mg suppository.

FDA-approved dosing recommendations are as follows: Oral adult usage as an analgesic or antipyretic should be 325–650 mg every 4–6 hours a day and only up to 4 gm total daily. Recommendations for adult rectal usage include 300–600 mg every 4–6 hours and no more than 4 gm total daily. Patients using aspirin for its anti-inflammatory or anti-platelet properties will need to consult their physician. Aspirin dosing for children under the age of 16 years, due to the increased risk for Reyes Syndrome, is not recommended, but can be done under the supervision of a physician.

While acetaminophen has few possible drug-to-drug interactions, aspirin can carry quite a few. One well-established drug-to-drug interaction associated with aspirin is its contraindication to the anticoagulant (prevents clotting of the blood) drug, Coumadin (warfarin). Since Coumadin and aspirin are both known agents that prevent and delay clotting of the blood, the combination of these two drugs given together increases a patient's chance for excessive bleeding, ulceration, gastrointestinal irritation, and perforation. If a patient is known to be taking Coumadin or any other anticoagulant drug, the patient should consult their physician before taking any form of aspirin.

Nonsteroidal Anti-Inflammatory Drugs

The final category of analgesics belongs to nonsteroidal anti-inflammatory drugs (NSAIDs). This category of OTC analgesics includes ibuprofen, naproxen, and magnesium salicylate; some would also say aspirin falls within this category, because of its anti-inflammatory properties. NSAIDs, like aspirin and acetaminophen, have properties that make them classifications of other drug categories. As well as being an analgesic, NSAIDs are antipyretics. NSAIDs carry some similar warnings as aspirin, primarily potential for gastrointestinal occurrences and dosing adjustment for those who may have renal impairment. NSAIDs also carry a FDA black box warning regarding the increased risk for stroke, myocardial infarction, and cardiovascular thrombotic events in those patients who are already at risk for cardiovascular disease.

OTC NSAIDs as an analgesic are used to treat mild to moderate pain and also pain associated with migraine, osteoarthritis, and rheumatoid arthritis. Ibuprofen, the most commonly used NSAID, is available under the following U.S. trade names: Advil, Motrin, A-G Profen, Addaprin, Bufen, Genpril, Haltran, and I-Prin. While ibuprofen is available in strengths greater than 200 mg, 200 mg is the only strength that is available for OTC sale.

OTC-strength ibuprofen is available as a tablet, a capsule, liquid capsules, chewable tablets, suspension, and liquid drops. Adult dosing recommendations are 200–400 mg every 4–6 hours and no more than 1,200 mg a day. It is not recommended that ibuprofen be taken for extended periods of time due to its incidence for gastrointestinal bleeding and ulcers. Ibuprofen that needs to be taken for extended for periods of time should be done so under the watchful eye of a physician. Furthermore, those patients who may already be compromised by renal disease should consult their physicians for dosing instructions as adjustments in dosing may have to be made.

Ibuprofen is safe to use in children and infants, but is not recommended for use in infants under the age of six months unless authorized by a physician. Ibuprofen is available as a 100-mg/5-ml oral suspension, 50-mg/1.25-ml liquid drops, and 100-mg chewable tablets. Parents and caregivers should use caution when administering ibuprofen to infants and children, taking special care to read all drug fact labels, dosing instructions, and warnings. OTC administration of ibuprofen for pediatric treatment is not recommended for more than 10 days. Parents and caregivers who have questions concerning continuing ibuprofen for more than 10 days should contact their physician or pharmacist.

Naproxen sodium can also be labeled as analgesic and is the newest of the NSAIDs approved for the OTC market. Naproxen sodium 220 mg is the only strength available in the United States for sale as an OTC. Clinical uses for naproxen include headache, gout, bursitis, osteoarthritis, rheumatoid arthritis, as well as tendonitis and fever. When looking for naproxen on the pharmacy shelves, you might find it under one of these FDA-approved trade names: Alaxen, Aleve, Aleve Arthritis, Anaprox, Midol Extended Relief, and Naproxen Sodium. Naproxen is available as 220-mg tablet, caplet, gelcap, and liquid cap. The recommended adult dosing of naproxen is 220 mg every 8–12 hours, with no more than 660 mg a day. However, in patients over the age of 65 years, naproxen is recommended only as 220 mg every 12 hours and no more than 440 mg a day. This degree in dosage is due to the increased risk of ulceration and gastrointestinal bleeding after the age of 65 years. Naproxen is not recommended for use in children under the age of 12 years, and after the age of 12 years dosing should follow the same recommendations as adults.

Magnesium salicylate is an analgesic NSAID whose primary use includes relief for pain associated with rheumatoid arthritis and osteoarthritis. Magnesium salicylate is available under the following U.S. trade names: Doan's Extra Strength, Doan's Regular, Keygesic-10, MST 600, Momentum, and Novasal. The available strength of magnesium salicylate varies depending upon the trade product, but can be found in as a 325-mg, 580-mg, 600-mg, and 650-mg tablet.

Magnesium salicylate carries a warning for those with renal impairment as well as those who consume more than two alcoholic beverages a day. Magnesium salicylate, because it is a cousin to aspirin, should not be given to children younger than 19 years of age due to the advanced risk for Reyes Syndrome.

Antihistamine A drug that blocks histamine and leukotriene receptors and relieves common allergy symptoms.

Antitussive A drug that suppresses unproductive coughs.

Decongestant A drug that aides in reducing sinus and mucosal buildup.

Expectorant A drug that loosens and thins mucus and phlegm build up in the chest.

As with other NSAIDs, magnesium salicylate has the potential for gastrointestinal bleeding and ulcerations with extended use. Anyone using magnesium salicylate for longer periods of time should consult with his or her physician on a regular basis.

Adult dosing when being used for pain relief from rheumatoid arthritis and osteoarthritis is 600 mg every 3–4 hours as needed, with a maximum of eight tablets a day. Magnesium salicylate dosing has not been proven safe for use in children less than 19 years of age.

Antipyretics

Antipyretics are drugs that help to reduce or eliminate fever. Most analgesics are considered to also be antipyretics and therefore often serve a dual purpose in patient care. Antipyretics, which are also sometimes referred to as antifebrile or antithermic, are generally considered safe to use and are the most common drug used to rid an infant or child of fever. Antipyretic, like analgesics, gets its meaning from the Greek: *anti = against and pyretos = fever or fire.*

Antipyretics are drugs that relieve or reduce fever, and as you may already know many analgesics are also antipyretics. In keeping with the knowledge that some analgesics can also be antipyretics, it would stand to reason the same warnings and precautions that are taken with analgesics should be taken with antipyretics.

Unlike pain, fever is not subjective and oftentimes have a more defined root cause. Fevers are usually caused by a viral or bacterial pathogen and are not uncommonly the first symptom of illness. Fever from viral pathogens, for the most part, is relatively benign and can often be extinguished with an OTC antipyretic such as acetaminophen or ibuprofen. Fever from bacterial pathogens can be more serious, requiring the use of not only an OTC antipyretic but an antibiotic as well.

The body's temperature is controlled by the part of the brain known as the hypothalamus. The hypothalamus acts as an internal thermostat for the body, producing functions like sweating and shivering to regulate the body's temperature to a baseline 98.7 degrees. Fever is the body's response to excessive production of prostaglandin. As the buildup of prostaglandin increases, the hypothalamus's ability to control the body's temperature decreases, and the end result, of course, is fever. Antipyretics work off of these mechanics, blocking the buildup of prostaglandin and restoring the body's temperature to normal.

Acetaminophen and ibuprofen are the two most often used antipyretics, but aspirin and naproxen can also be used as fever relievers, although use of either of these drugs is not recommended in children. While acetaminophen and ibuprofen are both capable of reducing fever and can be categorized as antipyretics, they do maintain some individual differences.

Acetaminophen use in children younger than six months of age is acceptable, but dosage should be weight based at 10–15 mg/kg/dose on a schedule of every 4–6 hours as needed. Daily doses of acetaminophen for children who have fever should not exceed five doses in a 24-hour period. If the fever spikes above 104 degrees or lasts for more than a few days, particularly for children, older adults, or someone whose health is comprised, then it may be necessary to see a physician. Adults who may have a fever should follow the same recommended dosing used for pain, always remembering it is critical to not exceed more than 4,000 gm daily, due to the increased risk for liver damage if taken above the recommended dose.

Ibuprofen, unlike acetaminophen, is not recommended for use in children less than two years of age. Ibuprofen used to reduce fever in children six months of age and older should be administered by the following recommendations: Fever that is less than 102.5 degrees should have a dosage based on 5 mg/kg/dose, fever that is greater than 102.5 should have a dosage based on 10 mg/kg/dose. Scheduling should be done on every 6–8 hours as needed, and the maximum daily allowed dose should not exceed more than 40 mg/kg/day. Adults who use ibuprofen due to fever should follow the same dosing instructions when taken for pain, using caution in cases of renal impairment and gastrointestinal issues. The maximum daily allowance for adults using ibuprofen unless supervised by a physician is 1.2 gm.

Aspirin and naproxen may also be used as an antipyretic for adults, but must never be used as an antipyretic for children younger than 19 years old. The use of aspirin in children younger than 19 years of age has been linked to Reyes Syndrome, and naproxen has not been proven safe for use in children younger than 12 years old. Still, adults must use caution when using aspirin or naproxen in cases of fever due to drug properties, which may lead to gastrointestinal bleeding, peptic ulcers, or contraindications to prescription medications such as Coumadin (warfarin).

Acetaminophen and ibuprofen are the two most commonly used antipyretics for children as well as adults. Aspirin and naproxen do have antipyretic properties, but are more commonly used as analgesics. Magnesium salicylate has no antipyretic properties, but remains an effective analgesic for rheumatoid arthritis and osteoarthritis.

Respiratory System Agents

Symptoms like a stuffy nose, cough, or sore throat can be contributed to a number of ailments, such as cold, flu, and seasonal allergies. Respiratory system agents are the class of OTC drugs used to combat the symptoms associated with these conditions (Figure 13-2). Most of these remedies have long been available on the pharmacy shelf and considered safe and effective by the FDA; yet caution should be used when administering any OTC medication. Paying attention to drug fact labels, dosing instructions, as well as warnings and precautions helps to eliminate complications later.

The class of OTC drugs known as respiratory agents can be broken down further into four separate categories: **antihistamines**, **antitussives**, **decongestants**, and **expectorants**. Each one of these categories plays an individual role, and some can play a dual role, but they all help to cure the symptoms that are associated with the respiratory system.

Antihistamines help control allergy symptoms, antitussives calm coughs, decongestants relieve stuffy nose and chest congestion, and expectorants help expel the mucus associated with chest congestion and/or a stuffy nose, making breathing easier. Many of these OTC drug categories work together to defeat the same or multiple symptoms.

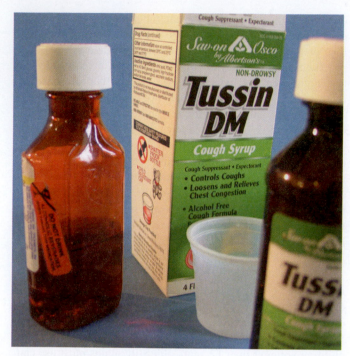

FIGURE 13-2 OTC respiratory agents
Source: Custom Medical Stock Photo

Many respiratory system agents are safe for use in children and older adults, but still others carry warnings for those who use blood pressure medications or have heart disease. Even with the warnings and precautions, the fact remains that these drugs are generally safe and effective for OTC consumer use. Respiratory system agents that have made the leap from prescription to OTC not only create availability for the masses, but also provide a less expensive route of health care for many others. While it may seem difficult at best, to stay up to date with the changes that happen within this OTC classification, pharmacy technicians should strive to familiarize themselves with this information. Staying informed is one of the best ways a pharmacy technician can use to recognize a patient who may need an OTC medication consultation with the pharmacist and in turn potentially save the patient from harm.

Pharmacy technicians should know the difference between antitussives and expectorants as well as the differences between antihistamines and decongestants; being able to separate the drug that aids in curing or calming respiratory system ailments gives the pharmacy technician a larger knowledge base and a greater understanding of OTC respiratory system agents.

Antihistamines

Sneezing is the body's reaction to foreign substances, which can aggravate the lining of the nose, mouth, and throat. It is essentially a reflex action. When irritants like pollen or animal dander enter through the nose, histamines or leukotrienes create a chemical that allows the blood vessels in the nose to open and the brain in turn tells the nose these chemicals do not belong here and expels them by sneezing. Antihistamines help to block histamine and leukotriene receptors, alleviating symptoms like sneezing, runny nose, and watery eyes.

The pharmacy aisle contains numerous OTC antihistamines. When choosing an antihistamine, consider the following questions. What are the side effects? Does it cause drowsiness? Is it safe for people with glaucoma or high blood pressure? Is it safe for children? Are there any drug interactions? Not all antihistamines work the same for everyone, so many people need to try a few before finding the one that works for them.

Most antihistamines are manufactured as a tablet, capsule, or liquid. They may be sold as a single product or a combination product, such as an analgesic/antihistamine, like Tylenol PM (acetaminophen and diphenhydramine). Antihistamines may also be a key ingredient in multisymptom products, so it is always good to check the label before purchasing or using one of these types of OTC products.

While the majority of consumers purchase antihistamines for symptoms related to seasonal allergies or cold and flu, antihistamines can also be used to abate allergic reactions, hives, or itchy irritated eyes and skin. Some of the most commonly purchased OTC antihistamines are:

- Cetirizine, sold under the trade name Zyrtec
- Chlorpheniramine, sold under the trade names Aller-Chlor, Chlorphen, and Chlor-Trimeton Allergy
- Clemastine, sold under the trade names Tavist, Tavist-1, and Dayhist Allergy
- DimenhyDRINATE, sold under the trade names Dramamine, Driminate, and Trip Tone
- Diphenhydramine, sold under the trade names Benadryl, Nytol Quick Caps, Nytol Quick Gels, Geridryl, Genahist, Diphenyl, and Diphenhist
- Fexofenadine, sold under the trade names Allegra and Allegra ODT
- Loratadine, sold under the trade names Alavert, Claritin, Claritin Reditabs, Clear-Atadine, Triaminic Allerchews, Children's Clear-Atadine, Children's Dimetapp ND Allergy, and Children's Claritin

Most of the OTC antihistamines listed here are available as a tablet, capsule, disintegrating tab, chewable tab, and/or an oral elixir/solution. Diphenhydramine is also available as a topical 2% gel or cream or as a 0.5% lotion. Those who are already compromised due to renal or liver function should consult with their physician before using any antihistamines, because of the potential need for dosing adjustment. Alcohol and nutritional and herbal supplements carry a warning of increased drug effects and should be taken with caution when using an antihistamine. Consumers should always thoroughly read drug fact labels as well as dosing, administration, side effect, and warning information.

OTC antihistamines are commonly used OTC products that are deemed safe and effective by the FDA; however, should a question arise concerning an antihistamine it should be brought to the pharmacist's attention. If after speaking to the pharmacist the patient still has questions or concerns, the pharmacist may refer the patient back to their physician or prescriber.

When using an antihistamine in a pediatric patient, parents and caregivers should consult their child's physician before beginning any OTC antihistamine therapy. Diphenhydramine, cetirizine, fexofenadine, loratadine, and chlorpheniramine have been proven to be the safest and most effective for children 6 to 12 years of age. Cetirizine and fexofenadine are the only OTC antihistamines recommended for children two to six years of age. Children younger than two years of age should not be administered an OTC antihistamine without first consulting their physician or prescriber.

Antihistamines can help ease the symptoms associated with seasonal allergies, colds, and flu as well as abate allergic reactions and itchy skin and eyes. The OTC market for antihistamine drugs continues to grow and may become increasingly confusing, but the pharmacy technician who stays abreast of continued changes can help aid the pharmacist in the best treatment for the patient.

Antitussives

Antitussives are OTC drugs that suppress unproductive coughs. Quite often they are used in combination with another category of respiratory system agent such as an expectorant or decongestant. While antitussives have long been considered safe for consumer OTC use, safe administration in children under the age of six years has been called into question by consumer groups and the FDA. In 2008, the Consumer Health Care Products Association and manufacturers were ready to voluntarily change drug labeling to state "not for use in children 4 years of age and younger." The FDA did not reject this change, but also did not make the change a mandate. The FDA later went on to advise manufacturers of OTC antitussive products to not include dosing instructions for children six years old and younger.

Dextromethrophan is the only marketed OTC antitussive in the U.S. market. Dextromethrophan is available as a liquid, suspension, extended release suspension, a liquid gel cap, an oral spray, a disintegrating strip, or a throat lozenge. Dextromethrophan is marketed under the following U.S. trade names:

- Delsym 12-hour Cough Relief
- Theraflu long-acting Cough
- Vicks 44 Cough

Finally, while dextromethrophan is currently considered safe for consumer use by the FDA, speculation regarding its regulatory status has been some cause of concern. In September 2010 the FDA formed a committee to question whether dextromethrophan should be delegated back to prescription-only status; no final decision has been made.

Decongestants

Decongestants or a decongestant combination that might use a decongestant and analgesic is usually used for relief from the symptoms associated with a stuffy nose. They work by narrowing swollen nasal passages, allowing sinus drainage and mucosal buildup to be freely expelled from the nose.

OTC decongestants are available as oral (tablets, caplets, and liquids) and nasal sprays. OTC decongestants available in oral form are limited to pseudoephedrine and phenylephrine. Both pseudoephedrine and phenylephrine have formulations acceptable to use in adults as well as children but neither pseudoephedrine nor phenylephrine is recommended for use in children under the age of four.

As with pseudoephedrine, phenylephrine comes with interactions, which needed to be mentioned. MAOIs and tricyclic antidepressants increase the level and effects of phenylephrine, so it is always best to check with your prescriber before beginning any medication that may have phenylephrine listed. Also, it is best to avoid the herbal medications ephedra and yohimbe when using products with phenylephrine due to the potential for central nervous system (CNS) stimulation.

OTC decongestants are also offered as nasal sprays and solutions, often offering the patient more immediate relief from congestion. Ephedrine, naphazoline, oxymetazoline, phenylephrine, and xylometazoline are available as primary, OTC, decongestant ingredients for nasal sprays and solutions. OTC nasal decongestants are safe to use, but extended periods of use are not recommended; three to five days is the best course of action so as not to cause rebound. The FDA also does not recommend the use of OTC nasal decongestant in children younger than 12 years of age, until administered under the recommendation of a physician.

There are several important factors involved in choosing a decongestant; whether it is oral or nasal careful consideration must be paid not only to the patient's need, but to age, prescribed medications, and duration of therapy. Any request for information concerning decongestants should be presented to the pharmacist or the patient's physician, first and foremost is the patient's safety.

Expectorants

Chest congestion is often a symptom associated with a cold, and where there is chest congestion, there is a cough; but a cough is not always just a cough. A cough that needs to be suppressed would call for an antitussive, like dextromethrophan. A cough that is caused by a buildup of phlegm or mucus and needs to be expelled from the lung would benefit from an expectorant.

Expectorants help to loosen and thin the mucus and phlegm, which may build up in the lung, because of nasal or other mucosal drainage. A cough due to chest congestion is oftentimes referred to as a *nonproductive cough*; this simply means, when you cough you are unable to rid your lungs of the mucus and phlegm, and in turn the mucus and phlegm continue

info

DM and MAOIs

One more important note concerning dextromethrophan and monoamine oxidase inhibitors (MAOIs): MAOIs, a class of drugs used to treat depression, may lose their effectiveness when used in conjunction with dextromethrophan, causing high blood pressure, arrhythmias (irregular heart beat), hyperpyrexia (elevated body temperature), or myoclonus (muscle spasms). For these reasons, it is strongly recommended any MAOIs be discontinued for 14 days before administering dextromethrophan.

to build up in your lungs. Chest congestion that continues without any relief can eventually turn to pneumonia, and a situation like this may be fatal for an infant or child, a person whose health is already compromised, or an older person.

Guaifenesin is the OTC expectorant most people recognize on the pharmacy shelf and the only FDA-approved expectorant available. Guaifenesin is indicated for chest congestion and cough due to colds or flu; it is not indicated for chronic coughs, which may come from chronic obstructive pulmonary disease (COPD), asthma, smoker's cough, or emphysema.

Guaifenesin is commercially available as an oral liquid, syrup, as well as an immediate and extended release tablet. Gauifenesin is also often an ingredient in combination or multisymptom medications, which are meant to combat colds and flu, so it is always best to read drug facts labels before taking gauifenesin in addition to a combination or multisymptom OTC medication.

As previously mentioned, guaifenesin can be packaged as a combination drug. Guaifenesin DM is guaifenesin with the antitussive dextromethrophan, helping to not only clear chest congestion, but calm the cough as well. Guaifenesin with codeine or guaifenesin AC is a combination expectorant, antitussive narcotic. Guaifenesin AC is a class 5 narcotic and is a prescription medication in most states, but there are a few states where guaifenesin AC in low dose is allowed as an OTC sale; so it is worth mentioning.

Robitussin is the most recognized trade name on the U.S. market, but Humibid, Tussin EX, Mucinex, Vicks Chest Congestion Relief, Vicks DayQuil Mucus Control, and Benylin E are also available trade-name drugs. Guaifenesin is an effective cough expectorant, which aids to disperse phlegm and mucus from the lungs. Ridding the lungs of phlegm and mucus helps to prevent a more serious illness, such as pneumonia, later in the patient's care.

Gastrointestinal System Agents

OTC gastrointestinal system agents aid in conditions related to hampered gastrointestinal processes: heartburn, nausea/vomiting, and diarrhea (Figure 13-3). While the OTC preparations used to treat these conditions are plentiful, choosing the right one can be confusing. What may work for heartburn will not work for nausea or vomiting, and what works for diarrhea may not be effective for conditions with intestinal gas. Questions

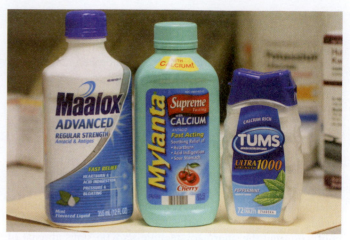

FIGURE 13-3 OTC gastrointestinal agents
Source: Martin/Custom Medical Stock Photo

may also arise concerning which products are safe for use in children and older people as well as contraindications to prescription medications.

Reading drug facts label provides the most information about a product including indication, active ingredients, administration directions, and warning, but, if after reading the drug facts label, questions still remain, then it is always best to speak with a pharmacist. A pharmacy technician who believes a patient may need additional help understanding which gastrointestinal system product is right for them should suggest consultation with the pharmacist.

OTC gastrointestinal system drugs can be further separated into one of six different categories: **antacids**, **antidiarrheals**, **antiemetics**, **antiflatulents**, **antihemorrhoidals**, and **laxatives**. Most of these categories have drugs available for use in children as well as in older people, but precaution should always be taken by reading the product's drug facts label.

Antacids

Antacids are the category of OTC gastrointestinal system drugs that deals with reducing stomach acid and calming the effects of a sour stomach. Antacids can actually be further separated by their mechanism of action: antacids (neutralize stomach acid), H2 receptor antagonist (blocks stomach acid and helps to prevent gastroesophageal reflux disease), and proton pump inhibitors (PPI) (reduce stomach acid and aid in the healing of peptic ulcers).

Antacids, first of this subcategory, neutralize stomach acid and are often used for heartburn, a burning and often painful feeling associated with an excessive buildup of stomach acid. Heartburn can be caused by any number of reasons: spicy foods, carbonated or caffeinated drinks, poor dietary habits, or obesity. Antacids offer immediate relief, but do not cure the conditions associated with heartburn.

Calcium carbonate is the primary ingredient used in antacids like Tums and Rolaids. Calcium carbonate–based antacids should not be given to children younger than two years of age, and the maximum daily dose for children two to five years should not exceed 483 mg. Children ages 6–11 years may have a

---

Antacid A drug that reduces stomach acid.

Antidiarrheal A drug that is used to help eliminate diarrhea.

Antiemetic A drug used to subside or reduce nausea and vomiting.

Antiflatulent A drug used to rid the intestinal tract and stomach of excess gas or air.

Antihemorrhoidal A drug used to help reduce or eliminate hemorrhoids.

Laxative A drug used to reduce or eliminate constipation.

daily intake of 996 mg per day, and children older than 11 years and adults may have a maximum daily allowance of 7,000 mg.

Antacids may have magnesium hydroxide, aluminum hydroxide, or magnesium carbonate, or a combination of these ingredients, as their primary base of action. Sodium bicarbonate and citric acid are also ingredients found in antacids. Compounds that have any of these as their key ingredients are generally not recommended for use in children less than 12 years of age, and consultation with the child's physician should be done before administration.

H2 receptor antagonist and PPI are the next two categories of antacids that are available in OTC formulations. They work to reduce the buildup of stomach acid, which causes heartburn and sour stomach, as well as treat ulcers and prevent them from returning. H2 receptor antagonist such as Zantac 75 can be taken in advance of heartburn occurring, minimizing its effects. PPIs work to lessen the chance of peptic ulcers by blocking the stomach's production of acid. PPIs, Prilosec OTC or Prevacid 24 hours, are not intended for extended usage and should never be taken longer than 14 days; in addition, therapy should not be reported more frequently than every four months. Any therapy needed longer than the intended recommendations should be under the supervision of a physician. H2 receptor antagonist should not be given to children younger than 12 years of age, and PPIs should not be given to children younger than 18 years of age; if treatment is needed for a patient younger than the recommended ages, it must be done under the supervision of a physician.

Questions or concerns about antacids, H2 receptor inhibitors, or PPIs should be brought to the attention of the pharmacist for further consultation and evaluation. Pharmacy technicians who can understand the category classifications of antacids are better equipped to research information the pharmacist may need for patient consultation and will ultimately have a hand in the safety and care of the patient.

Antidiarrheals

Diarrhea is defined as having three or more loose or free-flowing stools a day. It is most notably a symptom of gastroenteritis (inflammation that involves the stomach and the small intestines), but can be caused by poor nutrition, irritable bowel syndrome, viral infections, and dysentery, or medication side effects. Diarrhea can cause dehydration and malabsorption of much-needed nutrients. In some cases, if left untreated, it may be fatal.

Several OTC antidiarrheals are available on the U.S. market today. Before using any antidiarrheal, always read the product's drug facts label. Antidiarrheals are not recommended for use in children under the age of five years, and extreme caution must be taken when administering them to older people, due to the increased risk for dehydration.

Antidiarrheals can be broken down into three subcategories: loperamide, bismuth subsalicylate, and digestive enzymes. It should be noted that since diarrhea is often accompanied by intestinal gas, one or more of these ingredients may be produced as a combination antidiarrheals/antiflatulents. Also, antidiarrheals should not be taken for more than a period of three days, and patients who use OTC antidiarrheals usually see improvement within two days. If diarrhea does not improve or continues beyond the third day, patients should see their physician.

Antidiarrheals are effective in controlling diarrhea symptoms associated with illness or infection, but part of recovery includes hydration. Caution should be taken when administering them to older people, because of the heightened risk for dehydration, and the FDA does not recommend administration of antidiarrheals in children under the age of five years. If diarrhea persists beyond three days or does not become better in less than two days, then the patient should consult a physician.

Antiemetics

Nausea and vomiting are unpleasant responses to gastrointestinal discomfort and irritability. OTC antiemetics are drugs that are used to subside or reduce the incidence of nausea and vomiting. They are available in a variety of forms: liquid, tablets, chew tablets, and acupressure bands. Nausea and vomiting typically occur due to a viral illness, but can also be caused by dizziness associated with seasickness, food poisoning, emotional stress, symptoms of gallbladder disease, or extreme pain. OTC antiemetics have proven to be useful in these instances, but should not be used in nausea and vomiting associated with pregnancy.

OTC antiemetics have been proven to be safe and effective, but only when used under specified guidelines. Antiemetics are not recommended for use in children under the age of six years. If nausea and vomiting last longer than 24–48 hours or has worsened after 24 hours, even while using OTC antiemetics, the patient should see their physician.

Finally, hydration during nausea and vomiting is essential for preventing dehydration, which is often associated with excessive nausea and vomiting. Chronic nausea and vomiting may be a precursor to a larger medical issue and should never be treated continually with OTC antiemetics. Should a question arise concerning the proper administration of or indication for antiemetics, it is best to consult your pharmacist or physician.

Antiflatulents

OTC antiflatulents are drugs that rid the intestinal tract and stomach of excessive gas and air. Some antiflatulents give the gastrointestinal system relief once gas has already formed; these include simethacone and activated charcoal. Others help to stop the formation of gas when taken prior to eating: alpha-galactosidase replacements and lactase replacement.

Simethacone and activated charcoal are the two most readily available OTC drugs for intestinal gas. Alpha-galactosidase replacements and lactase replacement are still fairly young by pharmacy standards and work to eliminate intestinal gas in a manner different from simethacone or activated charcoal.

Simethacone is the only OTC antiflatulent approved for use in infants and children. Activated charcoal is not approved for intestinal gas relief, but it does have some intestinal gas release properties, which drug manufacturers continue to develop. Alpha-galactosidase replacements have had some marketed success as an antiflatulent, but come with a caution when used in patients who have diabetes. Alpha-galactosidase replacements like Beano can produce 2 to 6 gm of carbohydrates per 100 gm of food, which is counterproductive for a diabetic. Alpha-galactosidase replacements are a naturally produced enzyme which reduces gas in the digestive tract. Lactase replacement products are OTC drugs used for gas associated with the inability to digest lactose; dairy products are a common enemy for someone who cannot tolerate lactose.

Probiotic products such as Align Digestive Care, Culturelle Probiotic Digestive Health Capsule and Florastor are also considered to be effective OTC antiflatulent treatments. Probiotics are also found in food products like yogurt, and while they certainly are not considered to be an oral drug product, some pharmacies may stock them in their store, especially if there is customer-accessible refrigerated section.

Intestinal gas, while not a topic anyone likes to discuss, is a very real problem and if left untreated can cause life interruptions and embarrassment for those who become its victim. Dietary changes, exercise, and using OTC antiflatulents are some of the easiest ways to handle this problem. As with any issue where self-medication is used, if relief or improvement is not accomplished with the OTC drug, then it is time to see a physician.

Antihemorrhoidals

OTC antihemorrhoidals are preparations that can be purchased over the counter to treat the complications associated with hemorrhoids. Hemorrhoids are the result of stress and strain placed upon the veins and tissues surrounding the anus and lower portion of the rectum; constipation is usually the underlying reason hemorrhoids form.

When strain and stress are placed upon the veins and tissues surrounding the anus and lower rectum, blood flow accumulates to this area during defecation, causing burning, swelling, itching, and discomfort. Most hemorrhoids can be eased by OTC preparations, offering relief and reducing burning, itching, and swelling.

There are, however, hemorrhoids that should not be handled by self-medicating products; nonhemorrhoidal anorectal disorders have a greater risk factor and may include conditions such as polyps, fissures, inflammatory bowel disease, or abscesses. If any of these conditions are present, a physician should be consulted for further treatment and evaluation.

Antihemorrhoidals are available in a variety of forms and product packaging for ease of consumer application. Foams, creams, ointments, suppositories, and wipes are all forms produced for the consumer's self-medicating use of antihemorrhoidal preparations. Preparations may contain local topical anesthetics like benzocaine or a vasoconstrictor (reduces swelling) such as witch hazel. Still others will have hydrocortisone as a main ingredient or a combination of ingredients, which may include pramoxine, zinc oxide, glycerin, or mineral oil. While antihemorrhoidal products are safe to use for most consumers, they should not be used for children 12 years or younger. Any issues relating to the rectal area in a child should be relayed to a physician for evaluation and treatment.

There are several FDA-approved antihemorrhoidal products for the consumer's self-medicating use; choosing the best one to fit the consumer's needs depends upon the symptoms and their severity. Bleeding associated with hemorrhoids should not be handled by self-medication and should always be left to the professional judgment of a physician. Remember to read drug facts labels as well as warnings and administration directions. If questions still remain concerning the product, a pharmacist is the best choice for answers.

Laxatives

Laxatives are OTC drugs used to treat constipation. Constipation is the result of the buildup of stool due to hard or infrequent bowel movements. Constipation can be caused by a number of reasons: poor dietary habits, lack of exercise, or side effects from prescription medications. Most cases of constipation can be treated with OTC laxatives.

OTC laxatives are self-medicating drugs, which allow the stool to either soften or lubricate in order for defecation and relief to occur. Chronic constipation can be a cause for concern and should not be treated with repeated use of laxatives. Diverticulitis, bowel obstructions, or intestinal tumors may be more serious underlying factors for constipation, and a physician should be consulted for further treatment.

Laxatives not only soften stool so it can pass, but also help reduce other symptoms associated with constipation like abdominal pain, flatulence, and rectal pressure and pain. Laxatives are available to the consumer as tablets, capsules, powders, suppositories, and enemas. Laxatives should not be given to children younger than six years of age, and if a laxative is necessary for a child younger than six years, consult a physician. Laxatives should not be taken two hours prior to or after any other medication is taken and should not be taken above recommended dosing. Patients who take medications for heart disease, blood pressure, or potassium levels as well as some antibiotic treatment should consult a pharmacist or their physician before beginning any laxative treatment.

Most laxatives work within a 3- to 72-hour window and should not be taken for chronic constipation lasting more than 7 days. If there is no improvement after using a laxative for the recommended period of time, then a physician should be consulted. Oral OTC laxatives should be taken with a full glass of water, and powdered laxatives can oftentimes be mixed in juices as well, but be certain to read administration instructions first.

Laxatives are categorized by their mechanism of action: bulk forming, emollient (softening), lubricant, saline, hyperosmotic, stimulant, or combination. If confusion exists concerning which OTC laxative best fits the patient's needs, the pharmacy technician should suggest a consultation with the pharmacist.

One final note concerning laxatives: Laxative abuse is a serious issue and should be handled as such. It is part of an eating disorder issue, when a person becomes dependent on laxatives because the person feels they will help him or her "keep the weight off." Unfortunately, this is not the case and can lead to some very serious consequences: dehydrations, kidney

---

Alopecia Hair loss.

damage (from severe dehydration), perforated bowels, possible colon cancer, and, if not treated, death.

Laxatives are approved only for temporary bouts of constipation and should never be used for chronic situations and certainly never for weight loss.

Integumentary System Agents

The integumentary system is the largest system in the human body and encompasses skin, hair, fingernails, and toenails (see Chapter 25). OTC integumentary system agents are drugs used to treat conditions related to the integumentary system such as sunburn, dandruff, head lice, warts, and skin rashes. Integumentary system drug categories are:

- Acne—dermatological use
- Alopecia—thinning or receding hair lines
- Anti-infectives—minor cuts and scraps
- Corns, calluses, and warts—dermatological use
- Dandruff—hair products
- Dermatitis—dermatological use (itchy, flaky skin, and rash)
- Head lice—hair product for microscopic infestation
- Sunscreen and sunburn—preventive and relief measures

The volume of OTC products available to the consumer under these categories is too numerous to contain within just a few pages, but as with any OTC drug, if help is required in decision making, a pharmacist should be consulted (Figure 13-4). Many OTC integumentary system agents are formulated specifically for children, and few have any notable side effects.

Acne

Acne is a dermatological condition that typically affects teenagers. Chapter 25 provides additional information about acne and prescription medications that are used in its treatment.

In many cases, acne may be treated with OTC products, which vary by ingredient and are often used as a combination of ingredients. Choosing the correct acne product may simply come down to what works best for the patient in an effective

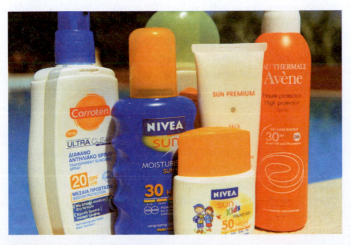

FIGURE 13-4 Integumentary system agents
Source: © Lynne Sutherland/Alamy

and cost-containing manner. Some of the key ingredients in OTC acne products include benzyl peroxide, salicylic acid, sulfur, alpha-hydroxyl acid, or a combination of several of these ingredients in one product. Acne that becomes chronic or whose effects are not lessened by OTC acne products may need a prescription medication and should be handled by a dermatologist or family physician.

Alopecia

Alopecia is the loss of hair. Most of us would relate alopecia to male pattern baldness, but the truth is alopecia can happen in both men and women. Alopecia can be divided into two different groups: androgenetic alopecia, which is inherited; and areata alopecia, which is essentially the body attacking itself, resulting in the loss of hair follicles. While areata alopecia is called by the same name in both men and women, androgenetic alopecia is called female diffuse hair loss in women.

OTC alopecia drugs have proved useful for those who have both types of alopecia, but largely are marketed toward androgenetic alopecia. There are no preventive measures to stop androgenetic alopecia from occurring, but it is thought that the decrease in stress levels may help lessen the effects of areata alopecia. While OTC alopecia products, or any product for alopecia, will not completely restore hair to its original volume, they do help to enhance hair growth and have had encouraging results. Currently the only OTC ingredient is minoxidil, and it is available in a generic as well as brand name.

Minoxidil should be applied twice a day and over a period of four months. While minoxidil is safe for topical OTC use, it should not be used in children or women who are pregnant or may become pregnant. As with any medication, you should read all administration instructions before beginning to use. If questions or concerns are unanswered after reading the drug facts label, a pharmacist or a physician should be consulted.

Anti-Infectives

OTC anti-infectives are topical ointments, creams, and powders, which help to prevent infections due to minor cuts and scrapes. Anti-infectives have three central ingredients that combine to make one product: bacitracin, neomycin, and polymyxin B sulfate. Anti-infectives may also have a local anesthetic agent, used to numb the affected area, as part of the product's ingredients.

Anti-infectives have long been the standard for first-aid kits and medicine cabinets; safe and effective in combating the possibility of infection, anti-infectives carry very little risks or precautions. Anti-infectives are useful in healing minor cuts and scrapes as well as uncomplicated burns, including burns associated with sunburn. Injuries being treated with anti-infectives should be cleaned thoroughly before applying the anti-infective; in addition a daily assessment should be done so as to evaluate the healing process of the injury. If healing does not seem to be occurring after using an anti-infective for at least seven days, then the wound may require a visit to a physician.

Anti-infectives should be kept out of the reach of small children and properly discarded after the expiration date.

Applications of anti-infectives are suggested at an interval of two to four times a day, discontinuing use once the wound has sufficiently healed. Any wounds that do not heal properly or look as if they have gotten worse should be attended to by a physician. Questions concerning the right anti-infective to use can be answered by the pharmacist.

Corns, Calluses, and Warts

Corns, calluses, and warts are conditions that typically affect the skin on the hands and feet. Corns and calluses are abnormal growths of skin formed from repeated friction on certain areas of the skin like between fingers and toes. They occur more frequently in women than in men and are common among people whose shoes do not fit properly—too big or too small. It is unusual for corns and calluses to be painful, but they can become sore and irritating, particularly if they grow too large.

Warts are caused by the human papillomavirus (HPV). They normally form on the hands and feet; being noncancerous warts is more an issue of irritation than pain. Wart growth is due to a protein, keratin, which builds too quickly on the epidermis of the skin.

OTC products for corns, calluses, and warts commonly include salicylic acid as a key ingredient and can, oftentimes, be easily treated, although some treatments may need to be repeated several times to achieve the desired result. OTC products for corns, calluses, and warts should be kept out of the reach of young children and properly discarded once the product reaches expiration.

OTC products to remove corns, calluses, and warts are safe to use and can be effective, but should always be used as directed. Read all drug facts label information before beginning any corn, callus, or wart removal therapy. Children who are in need of wart removal therapy should be administered drugs formulated for children. If after the directed treatment is completed, the preferred result is not achieved, it may be necessary to see a physician.

Dandruff

Dandruff, or seborrhea, is a form of eczema or dry, itchy, flaking skin, which is primarily seen on the head and around hair follicles. Formed in areas which tend to be oily, dandruff is more embarrassing and bothersome, than harmful.

Several OTC integumentary system agents on the market treat dandruff quite safely and can be used daily, and are effective as well. OTC dandruff formulations usually contain a few common elements in a variety of combinations; coal tar, salicylic acid, selenium sulfide, and ketoconazole are a few of the most familiar used. Dandruff ingredients can be broken down into three different categories: antimalassezia products, cytostatic products, or keratolytics, and a possible fourth category, combination products.

Antimalassezia formulations of dandruff products have a base of action, which attacks the growth of yeast cells, which is believed to be one of the causes behind the symptoms associated with dandruff; pyrithione zinc is the primary ingredient used in these products.

Selenium sulfide formulation's mechanism is very much like that of antimalassezia, but with one precaution—it needs to be washed thoroughly from hair in order to avoid discoloring; blonde, gray, or dyed hair sees the most issues.

Ketoconazole is a synthetic or manmade, antifungal agent and works to combat fungal infections, which may fester and cause eczema or dermatitis to turn into conditions related to dandruff. Patients who use ketoconazole-based dandruff shampoo should do so no more than twice a week, allowing two days between shampooing and a four-week period of therapy.

Coal tar dandruff shampoos are used to treat dermatitis and psoriasis associated with dandruff's itching and flaking skin. Over the years coal tar has been an effective combatant for dandruff, but can cause hair discoloring and contact dermatitis if left on the skin for any period of time; hair must be thoroughly rinsed in order to prevent these reactions from happening.

The treatments that are presently available for self-medicating dandruff have had various results; which one is the best to use depends on the severity of the dandruff as well as on possible side effects and reactions. Dandruff that does not get better with OTC treatment therapies should be brought to the attention of a dermatologist.

Dermatitis

Dermatitis is yet one more issue that can commonly affect the integumentary system. Better known as dry skin, dermatitis can leave the outer layer of skin feeling dry, flaky, and itchy. Seasons and climates can affect the incidence of dermatitis as can bath water that is too warm and poor bathing habits. Dermatitis can affect anyone, but older people are more susceptible because the aging process tends to dry out skin faster, making it harder to keep moisturized.

OTC products used for dermatitis commonly have petrolatum, mineral, urea, and camphor as ingredients. The best product for dermatitis is usually based on trial and error, which leads to personal preference.

Children younger than two years of age should be taken to a physician for conditions of dermatitis. Changing habits to lessen irritations include using products with an absence of perfume, drying thoroughly after a bath or shower, remaining properly hydrated, not using excessive amounts of moisturizers, and using mild soaps for bathing. If chronic dermatitis is not improved with OTC products, it may mean a larger issue needs to be treated; it would be best to consult a physician.

Head Lice

Head lice are spread by close contact or by sharing hair brushes, combs, and even hats. The height of "lice season" is between August and November when children are typically returning to school and starting bad habits all over again. Lice are tiny creatures, which are very difficult to detect with the naked eye. Lice spread themselves by laying eggs or nits close to the scalp. Nits usually reach adulthood by the ninth day and if not fed immediately upon hatching will die in

---

Dermatitis A condition that results in dry, flaky or itchy skin.

24 hours. A head lice infestation that goes untreated can repeat its cycle every three weeks.

When the hair is inspected for head lice, the area around the crown will show the most evidence of an infestation. A lice comb is oftentimes needed to rake away nits and their casings as well as any feces they may have left behind. The primary OTC ingredient for treatment of head lice is pyrethrins 0.33%/piperonyl butoxide 4%.

Although the thought of a head lice infestation might be distressful, it is treatable. It is important to read all drug facts label information and directions. Also, always follow product directions exactly as they are explained in order to properly kill the current infestation and prevent another one from happening.

The best way to keep a head lice infestation from happening is by not sharing combs, hair brushes, or hats and if an infestation is found begin treatment immediately. Most head lice–ridding products have the same active ingredient, so personal preference and cost may be the only factors needed in choosing the correct product.

Sunscreen and Sunburn

Sunscreen is an FDA-regulated OTC product to protect your skin from sunburn. Sunburn occurs when the skin is exposed to too many harmful rays, causing a burn. Numerous OTC sunscreens and sunburn aids are available.

Sunscreen is rated by the FDA on its efficiency and safety. In June 2011 the FDA allowed any sunscreen product with an SPF (standardized sun protection factor) above 15 to be labeled as having the ability to aid against the prevention of skin cancer. Products which have an SPF of 2–14 may not make this claim, but may state they are effective against ultraviolet broad spectrum (UVB) rays. Currently there is a purposed rule in limbo at the FDA, which would allow no sunscreen product to be labeled greater than 50 SPF.

Choosing the right sunscreen depends mainly upon personnel circumstances. If the sunscreen is for a child an SPF of 30+ is recommended, and infants younger than six months should use a sunscreen specifically formulated for them; also consultation with a physician before using sunscreen for an infant is recommended.

Sunburns can be mild or very severe, and the more severe they are the more painful they become. The affects of sunburn are not immediate, but are usually felt in full force a few hours later. Relief from sunburn will usually require a topical product with properties to reduce pain and swelling. One of the most important things you can do for sunburn healing is to stay out of the sun.

Treat sunburn immediately and stay out of the sun, so skin has a chance to heal. Topical OTC products can help reduce pain and swelling, making it much more tolerable. While most topical OTC sunburn products have an anesthetic element, Aloe Vera gel can help cool a burn and an NSAID like ibuprofen can be useful in reducing swelling and easing pain. All in all the best sunburn remedy to use is proper protection from the beginning.

Central Nervous System Agents

OTC central nervous system agents have a direct effect on the central nervous system. Drugs that fall under the classification of antihistamines like Benadryl (diphenhydramine) or decongestants like pseudoephedrine can have an effect on the central nervous system.

Side effects from central nervous system agents can include confusion, loss of balance, dizziness, or anxiety. OTC sleep remedies like Tylenol PM (acetaminophen/diphenhydramine) are central nervous system agents that relieve insomnia due to pain. An OTC medication that causes central nervous system interruption or side effects should be carefully monitored by the patient, being certain to discontinue medications that make symptoms worse.

Patients should read all drug fact labels and follow dosing and administration directions as the label prescribes. Any further concerns about potential side effects should be directed to the attention of the pharmacist or the physician. Pharmacy technicians should never attempt to answer questions concerning medications or give medical advice; doing so puts the patient's safety at risk.

Ophthalmic Agents

Ophthalmic agents are drugs specially formulated to treat disorders and conditions of the eye. Ophthalmic agents are available as eye drops, which go directly in the eye, and eye ointments, which are normally used along the eyelid. OTC ophthalmic agents are used to treat seasonal allergies; dry eye, a condition where the eyes produce few tears and often feel as if they are dry; and conjunctivitis, a contagious viral infection, which is more readily known as "pink eye" because of the redness and swelling associated with the condition; allergic conjunctivitis is associated with seasonal allergies.

OTC ophthalmic agents can be broken down into three main categories: antihistamines, decongestants, and artificial tears. When choosing the right eye drop, an evaluation of the

info   Choosing Sunscreens

Protecting yourself from the harmful rays of the sun is essential in preventing skin cancer: wearing clothing that protects your skin, not being exposed to the sun for longer periods of time, and use of a sunscreen with an SPF of 15 or higher. Remember to reapply sunscreen after being in the water or out in the sun for periods longer than 40 minutes. Water and the body's natural sweating process will eventually wash away sunscreen. Protect arms, legs, and face, being careful not to spray into eyes or mouth. Wearing a hat and sunglass protection are also good ideas. When choosing a sunscreen, choose one that best fits your needs: Will you be in the water, will it be used on a child, or will you be participating in sports? Remember to reapply sunscreen several times a day, especially if you are in and out of the water. Sunscreens with an SPF of 15+ are best for providing protection against rays of the sun and help decrease the chances for skin cancer later.

symptom should be made. If you have eyes that are dry, red, and itchy, you may need to choose an artificial tear ophthalmic solution. If you have allergic conjunctivitis, you may need an ophthalmic antihistamine; viral conjunctivitis will probably require the use of a ophthalmic decongestant.

Most self-medicating ophthalmic treatments revolve around the eyelid. If there is an issue with the eyeball itself, it should never be self-medicated. Issues involving the eyeball need to be seen by an ophthalmologist or optometrist to rule out any serious issue that may need treatment. It is also recommended that OTC eye preparations not be used on a regular basis. If there is an ophthalmic issue that needs chronic attention, then it needs to be taken to the attention of an ophthalmologist or optometrist.

OTC ophthalmic products are safe, but only when they are used as directed. Reading important drug fact labels and directions can answer questions and save potential treatment problems later on. It is important to keep all ophthalmic medications in a place where they are not accessible to children. If questions remain concerning OTC ophthalmics, consult the pharmacist.

Ophthalmic Antihistamines

Watery eyes, itching, burning, and redness are all symptoms associated with allergic rhinitis or seasonal allergies. Taking oral antihistamines for seasonal allergies is common, but allergy symptoms that are severe may need a little more help with relief. Ophthalmic antihistamines are drugs that provide relief from seasonal allergy symptoms when they concern the eye.

Most OTC ophthalmic products have pheniramine maleate or antazoline phosphate (antihistamine) in combination with the decongestant naphazoline. The only single ophthalmic ingredient available on the OTC market contains ketotifen.

Most ophthalmic antihistamines are indicated for the temporary relief from symptoms associated with seasonal allergies (allergic conjunctivitis) and should be taken only when needed to reduce the chance of drug rebound. Ophthalmic antihistamines like ketotifen have been FDA approved for use in children three years of age and older. It is also recommended that pregnant women not use any type of medicated eye drop or ointment.

Symptoms of allergic conjunctivitis may include red watery eyes with drainage and itching. Treatment for allergic conjunctivitis may include the use of an artificial tear ophthalmic solution as well to ward off the symptom of dry irritation.

Ophthalmic antihistamines offer relief from seasonal allergy symptoms as well as viral conjunctivitis, but should not be used on a chronic basis. Questions concerning which ophthalmic antihistamine should be used need to be answered by a pharmacist. While ophthalmic antihistamines are approved for use in children older than three years, it is still best practice to consult a physician before use. Always be sure to store ophthalmic antihistamine (and all other) drops in a place not easily accessible to children.

Ophthalmic Decongestants

Ophthalmic decongestants are the second category of OTC ophthalmics available on the U.S. market today. Ophthalmic decongestants are most commonly used to treat viral conjunctivitis

(pink eye). Symptoms of viral conjunctivitis (which is contagious for up to one week) include draining, pink, watery discharge; dry, itching eye; and eye discomfort. Viral conjunctivitis may take up to three weeks to cure and is usually incited due to a recent cold or other viral infection. Viral conjunctivitis may benefit from a combination of an ophthalmic antihistamine and an artificial tear ophthalmic solution.

The four primary ingredients available as OTC ophthalmic decongestants are naphazoline (often seen in combination with ophthalmic antihistamine), oxymetazoline, phenylephrine, and tetrahydrozoline. While all of these product ingredients are approved safe and effective by the FDA, it is recommended they not be used by pregnant women, and their use in children may be questionable. If use is needed in a pregnant woman or a child, it is best to consult a physician first.

OTC ophthalmic decongestants are available as combination drops as well, either in combination with an antihistamine or an astringent (cleans the eye).

OTC ophthalmic decongestants should not be used for extended periods of time due to the increased risk for rebound. If a problem persists after using an ophthalmic decongestant for three days, it is best to seek the advice of an optometrist or ophthalmologist. If aid is needed when choosing a self-medicating ophthalmic decongestant, the pharmacist is the only pharmacy professional with the knowledge needed to choose the correct ophthalmic decongestant.

Artificial Tears

Artificial tears are used to treat a variety of eye ailments and are oftentimes used in conjunction with an ophthalmic antihistamine or an ophthalmic decongestant. Artificial tears lubricate and cleanse the eye. Possible reasons for using an ophthalmic artificial tear include viral conjunctivitis, allergic conjunctivitis, dry eyes, or irritations of the eye such as redness.

Dry eye, a condition that causes red eye irritation, a feeling like something foreign is in the eye, and dryness of the eye, is the most common condition that require the use of artificial tears. Use of artificial tears for dry eye is often seen in older people, who may already have an ocular condition; or in those who wear contact lens daily, due to the drying effect the contact lens may have on the eye; as well as irritants which may invade the eye.

There are numerous OTC artificial tear products on the market today, most of which have a lubricant such as hydroxypropyl methylcellulose or carboxymethylcellulose (CMC) as a main ingredient. Artificial tears work best when used once or twice a day; in the morning and at bedtime are best. Artificial tears can be used more frequently, three to four times daily, for more severe cases of dry eye, but a physician should be consulted first. Artificial tears are safe enough to use in pregnant women and children, but a physician should be consulted first.

OTC artificial tears are quite effective in conditions such as viral and allergic conjunctivitis or dry eye, but if the problem persists or does not improve with self-medication, then it should be taken to the attention of a physician. The wide array of OTC artificial tear products can be confusing; help from a pharmacist when choosing an artificial tear ophthalmic may be the best available choice.

Otic Agents

Otic agents are OTC products that involve the ear. One important rule of them involves the use of eye drops in the ear. It is acceptable to use an eye drop in the ear, but never an ear drop in the eye. Ear wax removal, swimmer's ear, and mild ear pain are some of the most common conditions that require the use of OTC otic agents. Chronic conditions such as otitis media, an infection of the ear, which is quite painful and usually needs an antibiotic to resolve, should be handled by a physician.

The three different categories of OTC otic products available on the U.S. market today are the following:

- Cerumen-softening product—helps to remove excessive ear wax; carbamide peroxide is usually found in these types of products.
- Ear-drying products—helps to dry out the ear, which may have water or fluid trapped inside the ear canal; isopropyl alcohol and anhydrous glycerin are common ingredients.
- Botanical and homeopathic products—have some proven qualities for easing mild ear pain; typically will have olive oil or vitamin E oil as a main ingredient.

Choosing the correct OTC otic agents depends greatly on the condition needed to be treated. Ear drainage and pain may result from an excessive buildup of ear wax; removal of the ear wax brings almost immediate relief. Long days of swimming in summer often create bouts of swimmer's ear; drying the ear with an OTC otic agent eliminates pain and the internal ear pressure feeling often associated with this issue. Ear pain, no matter the age, is an unpleasant experience; botanicals and homeopathic products may provide relief from pain or at the very least stabilize the pain until an appointment can be made with a physician.

❝ Workplace Wisdom

Never place anything foreign into the ear. Products like Q-tips are meant for cleaning the outside of the ear and should never be placed directly into the ear. Placing a Q-tip or other cotton swab can force earwax further into the canal and cause permanent hearing damage or loss. Ear pain that is associated with a fever should be treated by a physician as this can sometimes be a sign of an ear infection. Swimmer's ear can be prevented by wearing ear plugs or a swimmer's cap.

Always follow drug facts label directions when using an OTC otic agent. Further questions concerning OTC otic agents should be answered only by the pharmacist. If a problem persists after the use of an OTC otic agent, do not hesitate to seek the advice of a physician; speaking with the right professional may help to eliminate the chance for permanent hearing loss or damage. ❞

Oral Agents

Oral OTC agents are ones that are used for conditions of the mouth or oral cavity. Oral OTC agents can range from products to relieve tooth pain and cold sores to even mouthwashes and toothpaste. The number of oral OTC agents available is too numerous to count. OTC oral agents can be in the form of a liquid, solution, paste, or even dissolvable strip.

OTC oral agents have very few safety concerns and can often be used in children and pregnant women. There are several OTC products formulated specifically for children. Some OTC products like mouthwash or rinse aids may have alcohol as a main ingredient, so it is always best to read the product label before administering them to a child. Mouthwash and oral fluoride aids should never be swallowed, but rather swished around the mouth for one to two minutes and then spit out. It is not recommended that children younger than six years use these products.

Dental creams, paste, and effervescent tablets meant for cleaning dentures are also part of OTC oral products. While those with dentures may purchase the majority of these products, they can also be used to clean orthodontic equipment such as mouth retainers.

Oral rehydration products may also fall under the category of OTC oral agents. Oral rehydration products are an essential part of rehydrating the body after a bout with a viral illness such as the flu. Products like Pedialyte and Cerelyte are available in a drinkable oral solution as well as an "ice pop" form and are useful in rehydrating children who have mild dehydration due to vomiting or diarrhea associated with a viral illness.

Choosing the best OTC oral treatment involves knowing what needs to be treated, the age of the person receiving the treatment, and perhaps some personal product preference.

Cold Sores

Cold sores (herpes simplex labialis) are a condition that can successfully be treated with OTC oral agents. Cold sores are caused by a virus known as herpes simplex. Herpes simplex labialis is contagious and is spread by direct contact. Herpes simplex can lay dormant once it is transmitted and then show itself with a cold, virus, dental work, or even menstruation.

It is estimated that 84% of the population, over the age of 40, has had some kind of contact with herpes simplex labialis, but only 30–40% of the population will actually develop a reaction. Herpes simplex labialis can be painful and is oftentimes recurrent. Found embarrassing by most, herpes simplex labialis starts by forming small red pustules on the mouth (usually around the lip area) then eventually crusting over toward the end of the illness.

Ways to prevent herpes simplex labialis from spreading include thorough hand washing (during cold and flu season), keeping a distance from others if you are infected, washing the area with a mild soap and hot water to reduce the infection and using an OTC oral agent to expedite the healing process. Currently the only FDA-approved OTC oral agent for herpes simplex labialis is docosanol 10%, which is marketed under the brand name Abreva.

Abreva, which helps to ease the pain of cold sores as well as reduces itching and swelling, should be used at the onset of herpes simplex labialis, applying up to five times a day until the lesion is gone. It is important not to use Abreva for a period longer than 10 days. If a second breakout occurs an application of triple antibiotic, along with Abreva, applied three to four times a day is recommended. Use of Abreva in children should be directed to a physician.

Cold sores can be painful and bothersome, but can be healed successfully by OTC oral products like Abreva. It is important to follow all recommended directions concerning the application of Abreva. Questions concerning Abreva should be answered by a pharmacist. Persistent cold sore issues may need to be treated by a physician and should not be treated by self-medicating means for more than a period of 10 days.

Oral Pain

For most of us oral pain causes significant interruption in our lives. Eating, sleeping, and even talking can be difficult when you have oral pain. The most common forms of oral pain involve issues related to tooth pain, teething in infants, irritations from dental equipment such as braces or retainers, pain from ill-fitting dentures, and sores in or on the mouth—canker or cold sores.

The OTC products available to treat these conditions are abundant and should be chosen considering a number of factors: age, source of pain, and severity of pain. OTC oral pain product can be found as topical solutions, cleaning agents, rinses, and protectants. While some OTC oral pain products are formulated specifically for infants and children, checking with a pharmacist or physician may first eliminate concern of safety. Dental pain that lasts any length of time should be handled by a dentist, so as to prevent possible infection or tooth extraction.

OTC oral pain agents when needed for use in infants and children should be suggested by a physician. Oral pain associated with tooth pain needs to be treated by a dentist to prevent further tooth damage. Abreva is the only FDA-approved OTC drug available to treat cold sores, but should be used as directed in order to receive the most benefit. Remember to keep all OTC oral pain agents out to the reach of children. If after reading an oral pain agent's drug facts label, questions still exist, a pharmacist is the best equipped to handle any additional questions.

Contraceptives

Contraceptives are OTC products that help to prevent pregnancy, and some contraceptive methods can be used as ways to prevent the spread of sexually transmitted diseases (STDs). Most people are familiar with prescription birth control, but there are several safe, effective, and reliable FDA-approved OTC contraceptives available today. Of course the best way to prevent pregnancy is abstinence, but there are other methods of birth control that have proven to be effective; most of them have been around much longer than prescription contraceptives and can prove to be sometimes safer.

OTC contraceptives can be in the form of foams, jellies, creams, and, of course, condoms. Condoms have proven their worth when it comes to OTC contraceptives; not only is using condoms a proven method for birth control, but it can also help prevent the spread of STDs. Condoms, which are now available as a female anatomy contraceptive, are available in many forms and are most effective when used with a spermicidal jelly or foam. Male condoms fit over the penis and collect sperm after ejaculation and before it has a chance to cross over into the female's vagina. Female condoms work very much the same

way, fitting inside the female's vagina like a hallow tube and allowing the ejaculated sperm to collect inside. Personal lubricants are not a form of contraceptive, but they do aid in the application of condoms and work to reduce friction and stress during sexual intercourse.

Spermicidal foams, creams, and jellies may also be effective forms of contraceptive agents. These types of contraceptives are used as immobilizers, blocking sperm before it reaches the female's cervix. Users of spermicides are at greater risk for pregnancy than users of condoms, but spermicides are still an effective method.

Female contraceptive sponges are another form of FDA-approved contraceptive agents. Contraceptive sponges are barrier agents, which are placed into the female's vagina prior to sexual intercourse. This method is usually accompanied by a spermicidal foam or jelly. Again, this method is not as effective as using condoms, increasing the risk for pregnancy.

Instructional use for these products is readily available on the packaging. Both male and female condoms have a greater success rate when used with a spermicide. Condoms are available in many materials, but latex is the primary material used. Those who have allergies related to latex may want to choose condoms manufactured from a different material sources such as natural membrane (lamb skin), nonlatex natural rubber, or polyurethane.

Smoking Cessation

OTC smoking cessation products are drugs that help someone to stop smoking. Smoking cessation products are available as gum, transdermal patches, sprays, and lozenges. Each year more than 35 million people attempt to quit smoking, but only about 5% make it past the first year.

The benefits of quitting smoking far outweigh any pleasure derived from smoking:

- Decreased risk of heart disease
- Improvement for lung and heart circulation by almost 30%
- Reduced chance of premature death due to smoking
- Less chance of developing lung cancer or other cancers
- Reduced risk of COPD or other lung diseases as well as improvement in COPD
- Less chance of having a baby with a low birth weight or abnormality

Nicotine lozenges are some of the most common smoking cessation tools available over the counter. Lozenges are available in a 2-mg and 4-mg strength. Therapy guidelines suggest a person who normally begins smoking within 30 minutes of waking to begin therapy with 4-mg lozenge and if it is more than 30 minutes begin with a 2-mg lozenge. Therapy is a 6-week scheduled program beginning with 1 lozenge a day every 1–2 hours, with no more than 5 lozenges in a 6-hour period or 20 in a 24-hour period. Lozenges should be slowly sucked on and never chewed.

Nicotine gum is a smoking cessation agent others find convenient. Nicotine gum, like the lozenges, is available as a 2-mg and 4-mg gum piece. Therapy guidelines suggest starting with a 2-mg piece if you smoke fewer than 25 cigarettes a day and 4 mg if you smoke more than 25 cigarettes a day. Begin with 1 piece every 1–2 hours for the first 6 weeks, then step down to 1 piece every 2–4 hours on weeks 7–9, and 1 piece every 4–8 hours on weeks 10–12. Never use more than 24 pieces a day. Nicotine gum should not be chewed 15 minutes prior to or after eating food or water. It is also suggested nicotine gum be used by chewing and then letting the gum sit between your gum line and mouth.

Finally, nicotine transdermal patches are the newest form of smoking cessation OTC product and work on step-down therapy. Nicotine transdermal patches are available in a 21-mg, 14-mg, and 7-mg strength. Therapy guidelines suggest if you smoke more than 10 cigarettes in a day start with the 21-mg patch for six weeks, then 14-mg patch for two weeks, and finally 7-mg patch for two more weeks. If you smoke fewer than 10 cigarettes start with the 14-mg patch for six weeks and step down to the 7-mg patch for two weeks. Patches should be placed on the arm in the morning (trying not to use the same place twice) and taken off at bedtime. When taking off the patch make sure to fold the patch onto itself and wash hands thoroughly after discarding. One caution to make note of is abnormal or vivid dreams have been reported as a potential side effect of the patch; if this occurs you may need to look at using a different method.

OTC smoking cessation products are not for patients younger than 18 years of age and are not recommended for use in patients who may have an underlying heart defect or who may have another medical condition that compromises their health. OTC smoking cessation products are also not recommended for pregnant or breast-feeding women. Before any smoking cessation therapy is begun, it is always best to first consult a physician or a pharmacist.

Behind-the-Counter Products

Behind-the-counter (BTC) products are nonprescription products that carry an element of risk, but are still technically classified as an OTC product. The FDA and consumer groups have long been debating whether or not this third category of drug status should be added to FDA standards. Countries like Great Britain and Australia have long had laws requiring a BTC status for certain medications. Initial debate over BTC products began in the 1980s with the OTC release status of ibuprofen. Some consumer groups felt releasing ibuprofen to an OTC status was too risky and suggested a third category status for BTC products.

Products that could be labeled as BTC include cough medications with codeine, any product containing pseudoephedrine, insulin syringes, and emergency contraception. Pseudoephedrine was relegated to BTC status in 2006 in an effort to control the illegal compounding of "street meth." As part of the Bush administration's Patriot Act of 2006, consumers must show government ID before purchasing pseudoephedrine products, and pharmacies must keep a record of purchases for at least two years.

Insulin syringe distribution is a program in some large cities aimed at stopping the spread of HIV and hepatitis C. Under this program pharmacists may give out 10 insulin syringes as long as certain conditions are met; pharmacy must provide written or oral instructions on safe usage and disposal of syringe, and it may not dispense syringes to anyone less than 18 years of age.

Emergency contraceptives may be another product found behind the pharmacy counter. Emergency contraceptives are meant to be given within 72 hours in order to prevent pregnancy. Situations that may call for an emergency contraceptive might include rape and/or sexual assault, females who have forgotten to take their prescribed contraceptive and had intercourse, or if a condom breaks. Pharmacists must follow some strict rules before dispensing emergency contraceptives; no one under the age of 17 years may purchase emergency contraceptives, and in addition IDs (driver's license) must be presented and a record needs to be kept in the pharmacy.

As the debate about BTC products continues between the FDA and consumer advocacy groups, it is clear to see there may very well be a need for a third drug status category. Any product currently behind pharmacy counters needs careful consideration before dispensing and more than likely consultation with the pharmacist in order to purchase.

Herbal and Alternative Treatments

Herbals are any product made from a botanical or plant; they are not regulated by the FDA and are not technically considered tablets or pills because they are plant-based. According to the 1994 Dietary Supplement Health and Education Act, herbals are considered to be dietary supplements. Dietary supplements are meant to supplement dietary nutrition and not to cure ailments.

Herbals can be found on pharmacy shelves as teas, powders, skin gels, liquids, and capsules (Figure 13-5). The use of herbals as treatments has been documented for thousands of years, and recently more and more people are finding these treatments useful. Because the FDA does not regulate herbals (remember they are not considered drugs), they do not have the same monitoring standards as prescription and nonprescription drugs. In 2000 the FDA updated laws regarding labeling placed on herbals; according to the new law no herbal could claim it was a known treatment for a specific ailment or disease. For example, ginkgo biloba is thought to be useful in retaining memory, but it cannot claim it is a cure for Alzheimer's disease on its label.

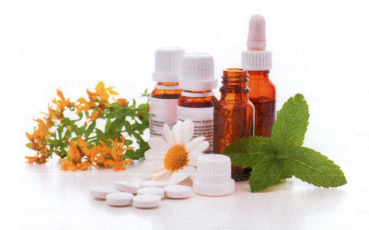

FIGURE 13-5 OTC herbal treatments
Source: Alexander Raths/Shutterstock

❝ Workplace Wisdom

Special care should be taken when using herbals and prescription medication as many have interactions with prescription drugs, which can be harmful or even cause death. Keep all herbals out of the reach of children and pets. Patients should know that if while using a herbal treatment they begin to experience side effects, they should stop taking the treatment. Most important, patients should check with the pharmacist or a physician before beginning any herbal or alternative treatment. Finally, many people find herbal and alternative treatment methods to be a safer and more natural form of treatment, but education about a product may make a big difference to its success. Consulting the pharmacist is always the best route of action for patients who should be certain to let the pharmacist know of all the medications they are currently taking. ❞

❝ Workplace Wisdom

Although vitamins and supplements can be beneficial in some instances, they can be harmful in others. For instance, vitamins E and K have a negative effect on the prescription blood thinner Coumadin and should never be used while taking Coumadin. Antacid tablets have a negative effect on iron or ferrous sulfate, decreasing the absorption and stability of iron. Vitamin C is easily destroyed by heat and light, rendering it useless if exposed to either. ❞

PROFILE IN PRACTICE

Scott is a pharmacy technician working at a grocery store pharmacy. After processing multiple prescriptions for Mrs. Nguyen, Scott notices that she has seven large bottles of various herbal remedies in her shopping cart. Scott remembers reviewing Mrs. Nguyen's patient profile and there were no OTC or herbal treatments listed.

▶ What action is appropriate for Scott to take, if any, regarding Mrs. Nguyen's potential use of herbal products along with her prescription medications?

▶ Why is it important to ensure OTC products are listed in a patient's profile?

Vitamins and Supplements

Vitamins and supplements are an 18 billion dollar industry. Many pharmacies have several shelves dedicated to just these products. Most people meet their daily nutritional allowance simply by the food they take in every day; yet thousands of people start their day with a daily vitamin or perhaps give their children a chewable multivitamin. In fact, almost 50% of all Americans take some form of vitamin or nutritional supplement. So the question might be, Are vitamins and supplements really beneficial? The jury may still be out on this answer. Most dieticians and physicians may say a daily vitamin supplement is not necessary, but yet others, will disagree.

There are circumstances where a daily vitamin supplement is beneficial. Poor dietary habits or food sources that inadequately provide proper nutrition is the number one reason a daily vitamin supplement may be needed. Oftentimes this problem will arise in lower social classes where resources are not available to purchase food, which provides the proper daily nutrition. Older people may also benefit from a daily vitamin supplement. It is well known that as we age our body loses its storage of calcium; many daily vitamin supplements contain added doses of calcium for just this reason. People whose health is already compromised may benefit from a daily vitamin in order to supplement nutritional needs.

Vitamin formulations are available for infants as well as children and adults. Vitamin supplements are available as tablet, capsules, liquids, and even lozenges (Figure 13-6). It is important to speak with a physician or pharmacist before taking any vitamin supplement therapy. Keep vitamin supplements out of the reach of children and pets; too many vitamin supplements resemble candy in the eyes of a child.

Finally, vitamin supplements are not under the same strict regulations as prescription and nonprescription drugs. In the eyes of the FDA, vitamins and supplements are dietary substances, not drugs. Vitamins and supplements may not make claims that they can cure a specific disease or suggest that they may have the ability to do so. Labels should be read carefully before purchasing, and questions should be directed to the pharmacist.

Medical Devices and Diagnostics

Medical devices and diagnostics are items that aid in care or monitor care for the health of the patient. Many of the medical devices and diagnostics available today are not reimbursable through insurance or flexible spending accounts, but are items that many people use throughout their day.

Walkers, canes, crutches, and arm slings would all be considered medical devices. Blood pressure cuffs and glucometers

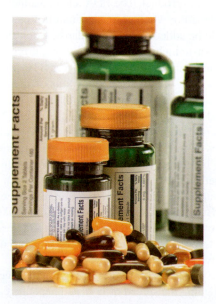

FIGURE 13-6 Vitamins
Source: Monticello/Shutterstock

would be considered diagnostics, because they are monitoring, in this case, blood pressure and blood sugar. Hearing aids and hearing aid batteries are medical devices, because they help to aid a person in hearing. Eyeglasses would be a medical device as well, an aid for sight. It is hard to imagine, but even bandages are considered medical devices.

Urological supplies like catheters and urine bags as well as products for stoma care are another type of medical device found in a pharmacy. TED hose and support hose stocking are special-order items found in a pharmacy.

Pharmacy technicians are usually the first point of contact for medical devices and diagnostics, and many pharmacies have technicians who specialize in assisting patients with their medical device needs. Many medical devices and diagnostics require detailed attention to insurance forms and billing; pharmacy technicians are best suited to fulfill this need, freeing the pharmacy for consultation duties.

Pharmacy technicians should familiarize themselves with their pharmacy's medical devices and diagnostics in order to provide the best care and service available for the patient. If there is a need concerning a medical device or diagnostic that a pharmacy technician cannot fulfill, a helping hand from the pharmacist may be what is needed to complete the care of the patient.

Cholesterol

Home cholesterol monitoring tests are a diagnostic test that can be purchased over the counter to monitor cholesterol. Home cholesterol monitoring tests have been on the OTC pharmacy market since 1993; yet there is a great deal of debate as to whether these tests help or hinder the monitoring of cholesterol. One thing that is certain is that a home diagnostic cholesterol test should never substitute for a full laboratory test.

The majority of home cholesterol monitoring tests measure only the total cholesterol, although there are a few on the market that now measure high-density lipoproteins (HDLs) and low-density-lipoproteins (LDLs) (Figure 13-7). Cholesterol monitoring tests can cost anywhere from $14 for the simplest tests to $125 for the more sophisticated test. In order to use most home cholesterol monitoring test, you simply prick your finger with the provided lancet, place a drop of blood on the chemical slip, and wait for the results. It usually takes about 10 minutes for the chemical paper change, and then it gets matched with the color scale on the bottle, which tells the level of cholesterol in the blood.

One thing to take into consideration when using home cholesterol monitoring tests is the inability of the test to use factors like age, weight, and family history. In thorough cholesterol screenings these factors and oftentimes many more need to be taken into consideration. There is also a fear that patients will not comply because they feel their cholesterol has already been tested within the bound of where it should. Conversely, some patients may use home cholesterol testing as a litmus test for further cholesterol screening.

Use of home cholesterol test monitoring comes down to personal preference and physician recommendations. Any questions concerning cholesterol or test monitor need to be directed to the pharmacist.

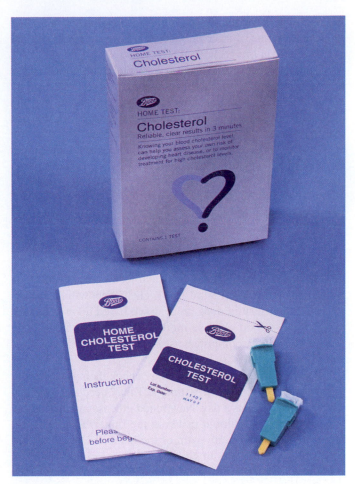

FIGURE 13-7 Cholesterol monitoring test
Source: Mark Thomas/Science Source

Diabetes

There are three different types of diabetes: type 1, type 2, and gestational. Type 1 diabetes is sometimes referred to as juvenile diabetes and always needs insulin for treatment. Type 1 diabetes is normally diagnosed in children and young adults. In type 1 diabetes the body has no ability to produce insulin. Only 5% of people diagnosed with diabetes have type 1. Through proper diet and insulin controls, people with type 1 diabetes can live a normal, healthy life.

Type 2 diabetes is the diabetes that is diagnosed in most people. People who have a greater risk for being diagnosed with type 2 diabetes include those who are overweight or obese, over the age of 65, have a family history, or come from a specific culture group: African Americans, Latinos, Native Hawaiians, Asian Americans, and Pacific Islanders. Type 2 can be controlled by diet, exercise, as well as insulin and medication therapy.

The final type of diabetes is gestational diabetes. Gestational diabetes happens when a women is pregnant. Gestational diabetes usually happens around the 24th week of gestation. Having gestational diabetes does not mean you will have diabetes after you give birth or that you had it prior to conceiving. Gestational diabetes, which can be controlled by diet and exercise, does not put the mother or the baby at risk, but if the sugar level cannot be controlled, insulin therapy may be necessary.

Women, who have gestational diabetes, especially if it is seen in more than one of their pregnancies, have a greater risk for diabetes later in life.

Type 2 diabetes is becoming a serious issue in the United States, but through diet and exercise as well as education its numbers can be decreased. Pharmacists are equipped with the knowledge necessary to help patients avoid drug formulations that may have an adverse effect on their diabetes. If a question or consultation is needed concerning diabetes and medication, the pharmacist should be consulted.

Blood Glucose Monitor

Blood glucose monitors are used to take readings of blood sugar for those who have diabetes. Blood glucose monitors measure the amount or concentration of glucose in the blood. The patient will prick their finger with a lancet, then place a drop of blood on the glucose strip, and feed it into the machine for an instant reading (Figure 13-8). The patient will then know to adjust their insulin dose up or down based upon this reading. Today's blood glucose monitors are as technologically advanced as most computers; some require downloading of software and updates.

People with type 2 diabetes may check their glucose only one time a day while those with type 1 may need to repeat this process several times a day. New blood glucose monitors allow the patient to test without pricking the finger. Some glucose monitors fit neatly in the palm of the hand and never need to be calibrated. Advances in glucose monitors continue to grow, becoming friendly or less painful for the patient.

Choosing a blood glucose monitor to fit the needs of the patient can be a daunting task, but pharmacy technicians who educated themselves about blood glucose monitors are

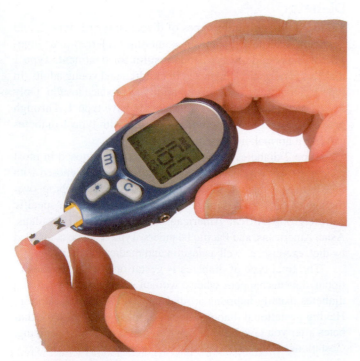

FIGURE 13-8 Blood glucose monitor
Source: arka38/Shutterstock

better equipped to help the patient make the choice that is right for them.

Insulin Supplies

Along with a blood glucose monitor, a diabetic patient may need to have glucose-monitoring strips, batteries to run the glucose monitor, insulin syringes if the patient needs to use insulin, and sharps container to discard insulin needles after use. If travel is part of the patient's daily routine, a container or case to carry supplies and insulin may also be necessary.

Glucose test strips are usually machine specific and vary in price. Some machines do not need to be machine specific, allowing the patient to purchase a less expensive glucose-monitoring strip, if necessary. Insta-Glucose is a product that aids in increasing low blood sugar levels and may be part of diabetes insulin supplies.

Once again pharmacy technicians who arm themselves with this knowledge are better equipped when it comes to helping patients obtain the insulin supplies that best fit their needs. Many pharmacies have a specialty area where patients have questions concerning supplies and billing concerns answered by a pharmacy technician who has been trained for just this purpose. Of course, any questions concerning medication or insulin dosing need to be referred to the pharmacist.

Urinary Ketones

Urinary ketone tests are performed to check for rising sugar levels in the urine. Ketone testing is important in type 1 diabetes patients and in women who have gestational diabetes. Diabetic ketoacidosis is an emergency situation, which left untreated can cause serious illness and even death. Ketones are made from broken-down fat storage, as more ketones are made when blood sugar rises and are detected in the urine.

Urinary ketone tests are the most common way to check for ketone levels. In order to use a ketone test, the patient must collect a clean urine sample and then dip the strip into the urine and wait the specified amount of time. Once the allotted time has passed, the patient can check the strip against the color level on the bottle, which will show how high the ketone levels are in the urine.

Ketone testing strips can be compromised by drugs such as Capoten or if the testing strips are old or exposed to air. Ketone strips can also produce a negative result if the patient drinks a very acidic drink—any citric drink. Ketone strips can be purchased over the counter at any pharmacy and should be found in the same area as other diabetic supplies.

Pharmacy technicians who understand the reasons behind testing, such as ketone testing, help the patient retain better control over their diabetes, which may help to reduce future complications.

Fertility and Pregnancy Tests

Fertility and pregnancy test kits will be found in the same OTC section of the pharmacy. Fertility test helps a woman predict when she is ovulating in order to be able to conceive. Pregnancy test tells a woman whether she has conceived. Both tests work in similar ways and with similar test indicators.

Fertility and pregnancy tests are relatively easy to use and surprisingly accurate. The test checks for rises in female hormones normally seen during ovulation; the woman urinates across the test and waits the required time for the test to complete. Once the test is complete, it will indicate either positive (ovulation/pregnancy) or negative (no ovulation/pregnancy). While these tests are accurate, a follow-up blood test with a physician is the only positive way to test for pregnancy.

Fertility and pregnancy tests can be up to 99% accurate. One pregnancy test states if conception has occurred after one day of a missed menses cycle. Still, as with many things, there are false positives, and it is recommended to take the test twice; most kits include two testing strips for just this reason. Pharmacy technicians may be able to help patients decide on which brand is best for their situations based upon customer preference, cost, and ease of product use.

Nebulizers

Nebulizers are machines that vaporize medication into the air in order to open up airways. Nebulizers are common pieces of equipment for those who have asthma, especially a child who has chronic asthmas. Safe and effective, nebulizers speed prescription asthma medication such as albuterol in a mist of air so it can be brought into the lung faster and more easily. This method of treatment is usually needed for emergent situations and allows the patient to have more relief from their asthma symptoms.

Most pharmacies do not typically stock nebulizers and will often need to order them for the patient. The patient may also need a prescription from their physician in order for some insurance companies to cover the cost associated with purchasing a nebulizer. A mast, tubing, and peak flow meter (to measure lung capacity) may also be needed to be ordered; a prescription may be necessary for these items as well.

Choosing a nebulizer may be based on physician preference, but should most certainly fit the patient's needs (Figure 13-9). Portable nebulizers may require battery packs, and nebulizers for small children will need to have size-appropriate mask in order to give the most benefit.

Pharmacy technicians should remember to ask appropriate questions when ordering a nebulizer for a patient: size of the patient, need, portability, possible physician preference request, and insurance needs. Remembering these things will make the transaction much smoother for the patient as well as the technician.

Test Screening Kits

Test kits are just as their name suggests—kits that test for something. In an OTC pharmacy today you can find test kits for just about everything, from predictions of ovulation to paternity testing. The first thing that should be known about these test kits is that, even though most of them are accurate, cost-effective, and easy to use, these tests are only a marker for a problem that may or may not need medical attention. Positive test results or even suspicion of a condition should be directed to a physician.

Home test kits offer reassurance and verification while providing privacy and cost-effectiveness for the patient. OTC

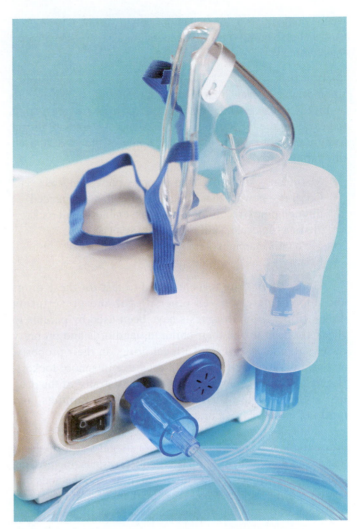

FIGURE 13-9 Nebulizer
Source: Galina Mikhalishina/Shutterstock

pharmacies often have a variety of these tests, including ones that can test for:

- Cholesterol
- Illicit drug use
- STIs
- Pregnancy
- Paternity
- Ovulation

Choosing the test that best meets the patient's needs may be confusing, so a pharmacy technician who is able to sift through the patient's questions can often offer the best suggestion, always remembering to take the patient's issue into consideration above all other things. Patients rely on pharmacy technicians and pharmacists to not only aid them in decision making, but also protect their privacy. Many of these tests involve sensitive matters and should always be handled as such.

HIPAA provides for a patient's privacy concerning all matters relating to the patient's health care. Pharmacy staff should carry forward these regulations just as any other health care system or professional. Pharmacy technicians are often the first person contact; professionalism not only gives the patient your trust, but also builds a positive reputation as a representative of the pharmacy.

Illicit Drugs

Illicit drugs are drugs that are illegal to use and considered to be highly abusive and addictive. Illicit drugs are considered to be C-I on the DEA controlled substance list and are illegal to purchase, use, or manufacture. Some of the most abused illicit drugs are:

- Marijuana—smoked, baked in foods, brewed in teas
- Cocaine—powder that is inhaled through nose, inhaled through pipe (freebasing), crack (resembles small rocks)
- Heroin—injected, sniffed, snorted, smoked
- Methamphetamines—smoked, snorted, injected
- Ecstasy—tablet, capsule, powder

Home illicit drug tests are used to test for these drugs and approximately seven other illegal and prescription drugs. Home illicit drug tests have been used by parents to check for drug use in their children, landlords and property owners to check for use of illegal drugs on their property, and schools to check for illegal drug use in school lockers. Home drug tests often provide the administrator of the drug test with quick results, approximately five minutes, and most are up to 99% accurate.

Home illicit drug tests can check for several specific illegal drugs at one time, and some check for illegal and legal drugs that are commonly abused such as antidepressants, methadone, and benzodiazepines. Home illicit drug tests use methods that test hair, urine, saliva, and as a wipe that can validate traces of illegal drugs on objects like backpacks, door knobs, locker doors, or door handles.

Home illicit drug tests cost from approximately $9.00 for simpler test to $150.00 for tests that are more complicated. Home illicit drug tests can be purchased at the local pharmacy and are approved by the FDA.

Home illicit drug tests may be a good choice for parents who feel they need to confirm their children's illegal drug use or for a landlord who may need to confirm a tenant's illegal drug use. Relatively inexpensive, accurate, and quick to use, these tests are a good marker for determining if there is a larger issue that needs to be dealt with. Pharmacy technicians may be able to assist the customer by knowledgably providing information, which may help the customer make the decision that best suits their needs.

Sexually Transmitted Infections

STIs are sexual transmitted infections, which can be bacterial or viral in nature. STIs are primarily spread from unprotected sexual intercourse. Bacterial infections often go undetected because the infected person does not realize they are infected with the bacteria. Symptoms from a bacterial STI might include:

- Discharge from vagina, penis, or anus
- Bleeding after sexual intercourse
- Pelvic or lower abdominal pain
- Pain with intercourse

Common bacterial infections are chlamydia, syphilis, gonorrhea, and trichomoniasis. Bacterial STIs can be treated with antibiotics and are curable.

Patients who are infected with a viral STI often do show signs of the disease; some of the most common symptoms are:

- Viral genital warts
- Genital herpes
- Ulcers or sores around the anus or groin area
- Lower abdominal pain

Common viral STIs include herpes, hepatitis B, HIV (human immunodeficiency virus), and HPV. Viral STIs are not curable and will always remain in the patient's system, sometimes going dormant for periods of time.

Home STI tests can be used in the privacy of a person's home. These tests use a person's urine to check for infection and cost approximately $60.00. Home STI tests offer people privacy in matters that can be embarrassing, while diagnosing a very risky health concern.

Home STI tests can offer confirmation of a disease, which may need further treatment or help those who are infected from spreading the STI. Pharmacy technicians are able to help patients who need the use of these tests in a manner of professionalism, which is knowledge based and also one that takes into consideration the patient's initial reason for their visit to the pharmacy, building a reputation as a health professional whose first concern is the patient.

Medical Supplies

Medical supplies are anything that aids a person in the care of their medical needs or condition. For some people, like those who are diabetic, it may be insulin needles, a glucometer, and testing strips. A person who has had a hip replacement may need to temporarily rely on the use of a cane or walker. A child with severe asthma may not be able to find relief without a nebulizer. Medical supplies are many different things to many different people.

Medical supplies are such a thriving business; some pharmacies have specialty areas dedicated to singularly helping people with these needs; many times pharmacy technicians are entrusted to supervise these departments. A pharmacy technician who has firsthand knowledge concerning medical supplies must also have knowledge concerning medical billing and insurance.

Insurance companies all have their own set of rules when it comes to what they will and will not pay for when matters turn to medical supplies. Medicare, for example, will not pay for a medical supply item that does not meet its definition of durable medical supplies.

- Supply needs to be useful in the patient's home.
- Supply must be able to withstand repeated use.
- Supply must be needed for the patient's care.
- Medical supplies must be provided by a Medicare-approved supplier.
- Item must serve a medical purpose.

Of course, each patient's insurance will vary, so it is always best practice to contact the patient's insurance company, before ordering or selling any large medical supplies to a patient.

It is also important to remember, even though a product may be defined as being an OTC product by the FDA, the patient's insurance company may still require a written prescription from the patient's physician in order to process the payment for the medical supplies.

Pharmacy technicians often have a great deal of knowledge when it comes to matters of medical supplies, and it certainly is well within pharmacy technicians' scope of practice to assist patients in these matters, taking into consideration the operational rules of their pharmacy.

Pharmacy technicians are trusted professionals who have a valuable service to offer to patients. Helping a patient complete a transaction for medical supplies, whether it is ordering the supply or dealing with insurance and billing issues, only reiterates the need for their specialized skill set.

The Pharmacy Technician's Role with OTC Products, Devices, and Supplies

Pharmacy technicians are an invaluable member of the pharmacy team. As roles for pharmacists continue to change, pharmacy technicians will be entrusted with more responsibilities. The number of categories of OTC drugs can be monstrous, but pharmacy technicians who take the time to familiarize themselves with these products are more adaptable to situations and able to assist patients with their needs. Still, pharmacy technicians must always remember their legal limitations; technicians are not allowed by law to offer medical advice or give advice concerning medications; consultation is a job for the pharmacist only.

Pharmacists and patients both rely on the technician to have the knowledge necessary to deal with billing and ordering issues concerning OTC products, devices, and supplies. As we have seen from this chapter, the number of OTC products and categories seems to be endless. New products make it to the pharmacy market each year, bringing with them new advancements, which need to be learned. Prescription medications make the switch to OTC almost as fast as new products come to the market.

Billing and insurance payment laws change on a regular basis. Medicare and other insurances regularly evaluate what they will and will not pay for when it comes to the OTC products and devices, which line store shelves. Pharmacy technicians are relied upon from not only the pharmacist, but the patient as well, to understand the process behind billing and insurance. Needless to say, the possibilities for pharmacy technicians might just be considered endless.

Pharmacy technicians who arm themselves with the most up-to-date information and seek to learn more about new products and devices prove time and again how invaluable a member of the pharmacy team they really are. Patients grow to trust technicians, and pharmacists see them as the professionals they really are and can be.

As health care goes into another decade and another stage, so will rules and regulations concerning pharmacy. Technicians will take a larger role, requiring more education and tighter regulations from State Boards of Pharmacies. It is the technician who sees these advancements coming and learns to benefit from them, who ultimately gains the most.

Summary

OTC pharmacy is a much more involved specialty of pharmacy than most people realize. The limit of most people's understanding is what they see when they walk through the door of their local pharmacy. Pharmacy technicians who learn the in and out of OTC products, devices, and medical equipment, including billing and ordering of these products, help to wipe away a little of the confusion when it comes to decision making. On the other hand, a superior pharmacy technician also knows the limits of the law and never crosses that line. Patient safety and the pharmacy technician's professional position within the pharmacy are far too important to step across the lines of written regulation.

Pharmacy is changing by leaps and bounds; OTC products and devices are a monumental part of this change, and pharmacy technicians will be the ones who help carry over change to the next decade. For a comprehensive table of OTC products, see Appendix A.

Chapter Review Questions

1. There are more than _____ nonprescription (OTC) products approved by the FDA today, classified into one of _____ recognized therapeutic classes.
   a. 500; 45
   b. 1,100; 26
   c. 900; 64
   d. 700; 80

2. The generic name for Claritin, an OTC antihistamine, is _____.
   a. cetirizine
   b. fexophenadine
   c. loratadine
   d. pseudoephedrine

3. Which of the following is an OTC antitussive?
   a. Delsym
   b. Zyrtec
   c. Mucinex
   d. Sudafed

4. Minoxidil is indicated for the treatment of _____.
   a. alopecia
   b. dandruff
   c. cough
   d. dry eyes

5. Analgesics are classified into the following categories, *except* _____.
   a. acetaminophen
   b. antipyretics
   c. NSAIDs
   d. salicylate

6. The only OTC FDA-approved drug for cold sores is _____.
   a. Abreva
   b. Anbesol
   c. Orabase
   d. Zilactin B

7. Which of the following is not a BTC product?
   a. emergency contraception
   b. insulin syringes
   c. pseudoephedrine
   d. selenium sulfide

8. Which of the following is *not* considered a BTC product?
   a. Cheratussin AC
   b. Nizoral AD
   c. Plan B One
   d. Sudafed

9. Aspirin is classified as a(n) _____-based analgesic.
   a. acetaminophen
   b. salicylate
   c. NSAID
   d. none of the above

10. Individuals who smoke more than 10 cigarettes a day and want to quit smoking using OTC nicotine patches are recommended to start with the _____ patch for the first six weeks.
    a. 28 mg
    b. 21 mg
    c. 14 mg
    d. 7 mg

Critical Thinking Questions

1. Why are pharmacy technicians prohibited from making recommendations to patients for OTC products?

2. What are the benefits and disadvantages of OTC screening tests for illicit drug use and STIs?

3. Why is it important for pharmacy technicians to be knowledgeable on OTC products, devices, and supplies?

Web Challenge

1. Using the Internet, select one herbal supplement and research recommended daily intake and purported health benefits. Write a review of your findings in two or three paragraphs.

2. Using the Internet, research three different brands of glucometers, including their key features. Write a two or three paragraph review of your findings, including which category of patients would be most suitable for each product (i.e., older people, children, and business people who travel frequently).

References

American Diabetes Association. 2012. Web. 15 June 2012.

Behrenbeck, T. "Are Home Cholesterol Test Kits Accurate?" *Mayo Clinic.* October 2010. Web. 15 June 2012.

Centers for Disease Control. 2012. Web. 15 June 2012.

"Components of the Gastrointestinal System." *Virtual Medical Centre.* 2012. Web. 12 June 2012.

"Constipation Symptoms." *Mayo Clinic.* January 2011. Web. 13 June 2012.

Consumer Healthcare Products Association. "FAQs About Rx to OTC Switch." *CHPA.* 2012. Web. 8 June 2012.

"Decongestants: OTC Relief of Congestion." *FamilyDoctor. org.* February 2012. Web. 11 June 2012.

Dilulio, R. "The Right Fit: Choosing the Best Nebulizer for Your Patient." *RT Magazine.* January 2008. Web. 15 June 2012.

Dlugosz, C. *The Practitioner's Quick Reference to Non-Prescription Drugs.* Washington, DC: APhA. 2009. Print.

Drug Information Handbook. 21st ed. Hudson, OH: Lexicomp. 2012. Print.Food and Drug Administration. "FDA Intends to Remove Unapproved Drugs from Market."*FDA.* December 2011. Web. 8 June 2012.

Food and Drug Administration. "OTC Drug Facts Labeling." *FDA.* May 2009. Web. June 2012.

Food and Drug Administration. "Over-the-Counter (OTC) Monograph Process." *FDA.* 2012. Web. 7 June 2012.

Food and Drug Administration. "This Week in FDA History— Oct. 26, 1951." *FDA.* May 2009. Web. 8 June 2012.

Georgeson, P. "Why Do We Sneeze?" *Scientific American.* April 2000. Web. 11 June 2012.

Heper, M. "Solving the Drug Patent Problem." *Forbes.* May 2002. Web. 8 June 2012.

"Illicit Home Drug Tests." *CVS Pharmacy.* n.p. Web. 16 June 2012.

Institutes for the Study of Healthcare Organizations and Transactions. "Switching: Should Prescription Drugs be Available Over-the-Counter (OTC)?" *ISHT.* 2000. Web. 8 June 2012.

Jacobs, L. "Prescription to Over-the-Counter Drug Reclassification." *American Family Physician.* May 1998. Web. 8 June 2012.

Johnston, Mike. *The Pharmacy Technician: Foundations and Practices.* 1st ed. Upper Saddle River, NJ: Pearson, 2009. Print.

Krinsky, D., Berardi, R., Ferreri, S., Hume, A., Newton, G., Rollins, C., and Tietze, K. *Handbook of Nonprescription Drugs: An Interactive Approach to Self-Care.* 17th ed. Washington, DC: APhA. 2012. Print.

"Laxative Abuse: Some Basic Facts." *National Eating Disorders Association.* 2005. Web. 14 June 2012.

"Medicare Coverage of Durable Medical Equipment." *Medicare Interactive.* 2011. Web. 16 June 2012.

Morgan H. *STIs Home Test: A Method for Diagnosing STI's.* August 2011. Web. 16 June 2012.

Mosby's Dictionary of Medicine, Nursing, and Health Professionals. 8th ed. St. Louis, MO: Mosby Elsevier. 2009. Print.

News Medical. "Removal of OTC Drugs for Toddlers from Market Reduces Therapeutic Errors." *News Medical.* August 2011. Web. 8 June 2012.

PR Web. "US Allergy Drugs Market to Exceed $14.7 Billion by 2015, According to New Report by Global Industry Analysts, Inc."*PR Web.* February 2010. Web. 8 June 2012.

Pray, W. and Pray, G. "Behind the Pharmacy Counter: A Third Class of Drugs." *US Pharmacist.* September 2011. Web. 15 June 2012.

"Regulation of Pseudoephedrine." *FDA.* April 2010. Web. 11 June 2012.

Sanchez, A. *Sexually Transmitted Infections: Bacterial STI's.* 2009. Web. 16 June 2012.

"Sexual Transmitted Disease." *Centers for Disease Control.* June 2012. Web. 16 June 2012.

Terrie, Y. "OTC Products for Smoking Cessation." *Pharmacy Times.* August 2010. Web. 15 June 2012.

Tietze, K. *Handbook of Nonprescription Drugs: An Interactive Approach to Self-Care.* 17th ed. Washington, DC: APhA. 2012. Print.

"Types of Nebulizers." *Steady Health Community Home.* April 2011. Web. 15 June 2012.

University of Arizona. "Over-the-Counter-Drugs (Ch. 14)" *UofA.* n.p. Web. 7 June 2012.

"What Are Herbal Supplements?" *John Hopkins Medicine.* 2012. Web. 15 June 2012.

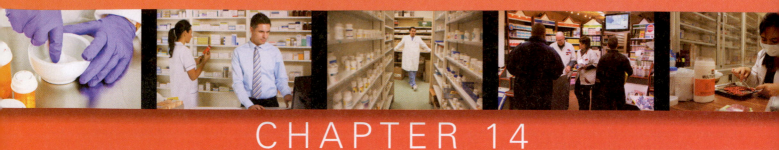

Introduction to Compounding

INTRODUCTION

Webster's New World Dictionary defines the word *compound* as a verb meaning "1. to mix or combine, 2. to make by combining parts, and 3. to intensify by adding new elements." In pharmacy practice, the term *compounding* refers to the sterile and nonsterile preparation of many types of made-to-order suspensions, capsules, suppositories, topically applied medications, intravenous admixtures, and parenteral nutrition solutions. In essence, pharmaceutical **compounding** is the practice of extemporaneously preparing medications to meet the unique

---

compounding the practice of extemporaneously preparing medications to meet the unique need of an individual patient according to the specific order of a prescriber.
excipients any substance added to a prescription to confer a suitable consistency or form to the duig.

info

To Learn More

This chapter is just an overview of the specialty practice of compounding in community pharmacy. Specific techniques have not been included, as they are too advanced and detailed for the scope of this book. For an in-depth look at extemporaneous compounding and step-by-step procedures, please review *The Pharmacy Technician Series: Compounding* by Mike Johnston (Pearson/Prentice Hall, 2005).

need of an individual patient according to the specific order of a prescriber. This differs from the traditional practice of pharmacy in that it involves a special relationship between patient, prescriber, and pharmacist.

Compounding medications for patients' specific needs is an integral part of the 5,000-year history of pharmacy. As recently as 1938, when the Food, Drug, and Cosmetic Act was introduced, 50% of prescriptions were compounded. During that time, pharmacists did most of the drug preparation and distribution. Today, as pharmacists become part of a multidisciplinary, multiskilled team to provide quality patient care, they rely more and more on pharmacy technicians. Technicians have now assumed many of the duties that were once performed by the pharmacist. One such duty is drug preparation: specifically, compounding and preparation of intravenous drugs.

Overview of Compounding

Pharmacy is the only profession that allows the extemporaneous compounding of chemicals for therapeutic care. Over the past 20 years, the need for compounded prescriptions has increased. Several reasons for this increase include the discontinuation of certain drugs by the original manufacturers, the removal of some drugs from the market by the Food and Drug Administration (FDA), and the unavailability of drugs in a strength or dosage form appropriate for a specific patient. Patients with sensitivities or allergies to preservatives or certain other **excipients** (substances) must often have their medications compounded, so that the offending agent or agents are omitted. A combination therapy that a prescriber desires, but that is not currently commercially available, can also be successfully compounded.

Pharmacy technicians, who have been adequately educated and trained, can play a vital role in the practice of extemporaneous compounding, including research, actual compounding of medications, and marketing (see Figure 14-1).

The physical properties of the prescribed drug and the dosage form desired by either the prescriber or the patient determine the level of difficulty in preparing the compounded prescription. In some cases, compounding will be a simple two-step process, whereas in others, it will require extensive knowledge and the performance of many steps.

Regardless of the procedure, pharmacists must consider certain criteria for all compounded prescriptions. They must

perform research on the active ingredient to determine cost-effectiveness, availability, solubility, stability, and possible dosage forms. Every pharmacy that compounds prescriptions should have access to quality reference resources. Some of these valuable resources include the following books and journals:

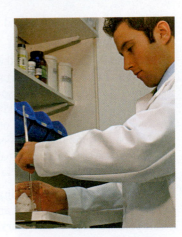

FIGURE 14-1 A pharmacy technician compounding a prescription.

- *Remington's Pharmaceutical Sciences*
- *The Merck Manual*
- *The Merck Veterinary Manual*
- *Trissel's Stability of Compounded Formulations*
- *Drug Facts and Comparisons*
- *United States Pharmacopeia*
- *Veterinary Drug Handbook*
- *International Journal of Compounding Pharmacists*

Regulations and Accreditation

USP 795

The United States Pharmacopeia (USP) regulates compounding pharmacy by setting standards for compounded medicines under the guidance of volunteer pharmacy compounding experts, and offers resources and support for the work of compounding practitioners. USP's official standards for pharmacy compounding of sterile and nonsterile preparations are available through general chapters 797 and 795, respectively, and monographs published in the USP–NF. USP is also a founding member of the Pharmacy Compounding Accreditation Board (PCAB), which is committed to uniform accreditation standards for the compounding profession.

USP developed chapter 795 to provide guidance on applying good compounding practices in the preparation of nonsterile compounded formulations for dispensing and/or administration to humans or animals. USP 795 was recently revised, and the chapter now includes new material, such as categories of compounding (simple, moderate, and complex); new definitions for terms (e.g., beyond-use date, hazardous drug, and stability); and criteria for compounding each drug preparation (e.g., suitable compounding environment and use of appropriate equipment).

PCAB Accreditation

The PCAB was founded when eight of the nation's leading pharmacy organizations joined together to create a voluntary quality accreditation designation for the compounding industry.

Organizations that founded PCAB and make up the board of directors include:

- American College of Apothecaries (ACA)
- National Community Pharmacists Association (NCPA)
- American Pharmacists Association (APhA)
- National Alliance of State Pharmacy Associations (NASPA)
- International Academy of Compounding Pharmacists (IACP)
- National Home Infusion Association (NHIA)
- National Association of Boards of Pharmacy (NABP)
- United States Pharmacopeia (USP)

The goals of PCAB accreditation are to (1) improve quality of compounding operations and preparations, (2) provide a competitive edge in the marketplace and ability to secure new business, (3) offer validation for compounding pharmacies to meet national standards, and (4) strengthen community confidence. PCAB's standards focus on a set of best quality practices and demonstrate quality, distinction, confidence, credibility, and security for prescribers and patients alike.

Compounding a Prescription

In addition to researching the active ingredients and excipients needed in a compounded prescription, the preparer must also know how to do pharmaceutical calculations. The potential for error is great in this area of compounding. Something as simple as a misplaced decimal point can have devastating results for the patient. Only a properly trained individual should perform the critical calculations involved in formulating a compounded prescription, and all calculations and measurements should be checked by the pharmacist.

The first step in compounding a prescription is to obtain a formula or recipe, prepared by a pharmacist, that includes all the necessary ingredients and explicit instructions for the preparer. The formula may be one that has already been published, or it may be created by the pharmacist in the compounding facility. If a formula is handwritten, it must be written legibly, with instructions communicated clearly to the preparer.

From the formula or recipe, the pharmacy technician then creates a worksheet that contains a list of active ingredients and excipients and the exact amounts needed of each to prepare the particular prescription. This worksheet should first be double-checked for error and then referred to as a checkpoint throughout preparation of the prescription. As the preparer weighs each ingredient, she can check it off the worksheet. (This is especially necessary when a formula calls for multiple active ingredients and excipients.) The pharmacist should confirm the weights of all active ingredients. In some states, however, technicians may be allowed to check the work of other technicians during this step, with the authorization of the pharmacist.

Pharmaceutical compounding requires an extensive amount of equipment. When performing any task, you must be

---

geometric dilution technique of starting with the ingredient of the smallest amount and doubling the portion by adding the other ingredients, in order of quantity, until fully mixed.

Procedure 14-1

General Compounding Process

1. Obtain the recipe or formula.
2. Write up a compounding worksheet based on the formula.
3. Collect all ingredients and equipment necessary to prepare the compound.
4. Weigh each ingredient and have the measurements verified by the pharmacist.
5. Following the directions of the formula, prepare the compounded medication.
6. Package and label the compounded medication in an appropriate container.
7. Have the pharmacist do a final check on the compound.
8. Clean the workstation and equipment used.

---

info Industry Insights

It is estimated that 1% of all prescriptions dispensed in the United States are compounded prescriptions; thus, this is a niche market. Most community pharmacies do basic compounding on occasion, but the majority of compounded prescriptions are dispensed by independent, niche pharmacies dedicated to compounding. Pharmacy technicians who are educated on and trained in the principles and skills of compounding have greater career opportunities available and typically earn higher salaries.

---

able to choose the appropriate tool needed to prepare a quality product. It is important for you as the compounding technician to be familiar with the tools available and their functions.

Equipment and Supplies

Table 14-1 shows a partial list of compounding equipment and the basic functions of each tool.

Compounding Facilities

An area suitable for compounding must be established before you begin preparing a compounded prescription (see Figure 14-2). The area should be separate from all other work areas and away from heavy traffic flow. The workspace should be large enough to accommodate all the necessary supplies. It should be clean and free of any clutter. Any object not directly involved in compound preparation should be removed. All tools and surface areas should be cleaned just prior to use and again when the compounding is complete. This can be accomplished by wiping everything down with 70% isopropyl alcohol or another suitable cleaning solution. This will safeguard the compounded prescription from possible cross-contamination, as well as preventing microbial growth within the final product.

When mixing the active ingredient(s) with the excipient(s), practice the principle of **geometric dilution**. This means that

TABLE 14-1 Examples of Compounding Equipment

Equipment Name	Use
Balance	Measuring ingredients; can be either digital/electronic or manual
Beakers	Measuring ingredients and mixing or heating ingredients
Capsule-filling equipment	Preparing capsules
Chopper/grinder	Breaking up solids or ingredients of large particle size
Electronic mortar and pestle	Mixing creams and ointments and reducing particle size
Filter paper	Removing particulate matter from a liquid
Funnels	Transferring liquids and powders
Graduates	Measuring liquids
Heat gun	Melting bases and smoothing the tops of troches and suppositories
Homogenizer	Reducing particle size and evenly suspending liquids
Hot plates	Melting bases
Liquid blender	Mixing liquids
Magnetic stir plate	Continuous stirring
Magnetic stirrers	Continuous stirring
Molds	Making troches and suppositories
Mortars and pestles	Mixing powders and reducing particle size
Glass	Liquids
Wedgwood	Powders
Porcelain	Powders
Ointment tile	Making creams and ointments
Powder blender	Mixing powders
Refrigerator	Storing ingredients and prescriptions that require cold temperatures
Safety glasses	Protecting the preparer's eyes from debris
Sieves in various mesh sizes	Reducing particle size
Spatulas	Mixing creams and ointments and retrieving chemicals from bottles
Spray bottles	Dispensing cleaning solutions or distilled water
Stirring rods	Stirring liquids by hand
Strainers	Removing particulate from a liquid
Thermometers	Controlling and checking temperature
Tongs	Picking up items that should not be handled
Tube crimper	Sealing ointment tubes
Tubes	Dispensing creams and ointments
Wash bottles	Washing
Weigh boats/papers	Weighing ingredients on a balance
Weights for calibration	Calibrating balances

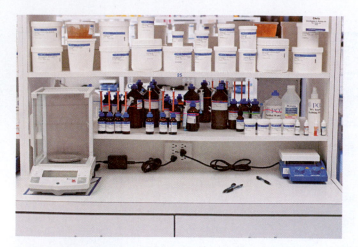

FIGURE 14-2 A typical compounding area.

you start with the ingredient of which the smallest amount is needed and double the portion by adding the rest of the ingredients in ascending order of quantity. Each addition should result in a *doubled* amount until all the ingredients are mixed in. This process ensures even distribution of the active ingredient throughout the final product.

The most appropriate dosage form will depend not only on the drug that is being compounded, but also on the patient. The patient is probably the most important factor in the decision as to which dosage form to use for a compounded prescription. Some common dosage forms that can be effectively compounded are capsules, liquids, transdermal gels, creams, ointments, suppositories, and chewables. For each form, you must follow precise instructions if you are to prepare a quality, efficacious product. Although pharmacists can recommend an appropriate dosage form, the prescriber's approval is required.

Quality Assurance

Although compounded products are prepared on an individual basis to meet the special needs of a patient or patient population, the pharmacy must have a good **quality assurance (QA)** program and maintain proper records to ensure that patients are receiving safe, stable, and properly compounded medications. In regard to compounding, QA is a program of activities used to ensure that the procedures used in the preparation of compounded products lead to products that meet certain specifications and standards.

In October 2012, a serious meningitis outbreak claimed the life of 233 individuals in 15 states according to the Centers for Disease Control and Prevention. The outbreak was due to contaminated steroid shots distributed by New England Compounding Pharmacy (NECC), located in Framingham, Massachusetts. Such horrible incidents illustrate the need for QA in compounding medications.

quality assurance (QA) a program of activities used to ensure that the procedures used in the preparation of compounded products meet specific standards.

Typical components of a good QA program include standard operating procedures (SOPs), formulation records, compounding worksheets, ingredient record forms, material safety data sheets (MSDS), documented training, and quality control (QC) tests for each compound.

Standard Operating Procedures

An SOP is a set of step-by-step written instructions on how to do a certain task. All important tasks performed in a compounding pharmacy should be covered by SOPs and documentation. SOPs should be developed for facility maintenance; equipment calibration and maintenance; personnel training and validation; and the preparation, packaging, and storage of compounded items. SOPs should also include sign-off or log sheets to document that the SOPs have been followed.

SOPs are necessary because there may be more than one way to do a particular task. For example, each technician or pharmacist may clean the room in a different manner. One person may prefer to clean all the shelving and countertops with 70% isopropyl alcohol, while another person would clean the area weekly with a different type of disinfectant. An SOP for this task would clearly define, step by step, how to consistently perform this routine task and possibly prevent bacterial resistance by using the same **disinfectant** all the time.

All tasks completed need to be documented on a sign-off or log sheet. If a problem arises with the task, the logs or records may provide information that can be used to correct the problem.

SOPs can assure that:

- The equipment is properly maintained and calibrated (Figure 14-3).
- Supplies and chemicals are received, inventoried, compliant with compounding standards, stored properly, and disposed of correctly.
- All procedures and tasks are performed consistently and documented.

Since SOPs require logs and sign-off sheets to maintain proper records, a notebook or file should be kept for each SOP to organize and maintain these records for easy retrieval. Depending on the pharmacy or organization, SOPs generally follow a uniform format:

1. SOP number—a unique number assigned to distinguish between SOPs.
2. Date effective—the date that the SOP is implemented.
3. Author—the name of the person who wrote the SOP.
4. Authorization signature—signature of the pharmacy administrator who approves the SOP.
5. Purpose of procedure—one or two brief sentences explaining why the task or procedure is being done.
6. Equipment/materials—list of equipment or materials needed to perform the SOP.
7. Procedure—a detailed step-by-step explanation that can be easily followed by different individuals to obtain the same results.

SOP # A-505-01-069Y	**STANDARD OPERATING PROCEDURES**	Page: 1 of 3.

CALIBRATION REQUIREMENTS for LABORATORY EQUIPMENT

1. PURPOSE

The purpose of this Standard Operational Procedure is to provide a standard calibration procedure and standard calibration sheets for the calibration of all types of laboratory equipment.

2. Responsibility

❶- Symbol indicates routine calibration performed by the departmental staff.

❷- Symbol indicates twice annual calibration performed by metrology department

❸- Symbol indicates annual or biannual calibration performed by an external contracted third party metrology firm.

3. Equipment

As defined on the calibration sheet and equipment specific SOPs

4. Frequency

Internal laboratory calibration ; Prior to **routine** use of equipment (e.g. daily balance calibration, system suitability test, pH meter etc.) ❶

Metrology department ❷ calibration; Monthly (Analytical balances only)

Metrology department ❷ calibration; Twice per year

Metrology department ❷; and after equipment maintenance or relocation

Metrology department ❷; and after repair of critical part replacement

External calibration ❸; Annually or biannually calibration by contracted Third Party according to equipment specific SOP

5. Procedure

5.1 Operate the equipment in accordance with the relevant Operating instructions.

5.2 Perform the equipment calibration according to the equipment specific SOP

5.3 Fill out form "Calibration Record" Sheet, see Attachment 2.

5.4 Evaluate if "SUITABILITY Sticker" has been compromised, [Attachment 1].

5.5 In cases where the SUITABILITY of equipment has been compromised (e.g dissolution equipment) due to the re-calibration the technician will deface and cross-out the "SUITABILITY Sticker" and attach a note stating "Performance Verification Invalidated Due To Re-Calibration"

5.6 Attach "Calibration Sticker", to equipment [Attachment 1].

5.7 The performance verification of the equipment (only where necessary) shall be repeated prior to routine laboratory use.

ED.NO: 02 Replaces Ed 01.	Effective Date :	APPROVED:			
Ed. Status: Operational	June 2013	Laboratory	Maintenance	Metrology	QA

FIGURE 14-3 Sample SOP—balance calibration.

8. Documentation forms—sheets that record the results of the SOP. The information documented should include the date that the SOP is performed, the operator's signature, and the results. A comment line is optional, but can be used to explain and document unusual results.

PCAB accreditation requires SOPs regarding the cleaning, maintenance, calibration and verification of each piece of equipment.

Dosage Forms and Basic Guidelines

There are many types of dosage forms. They include capsules, tablets, powders, lozenges, troches, sticks, suppositories, solutions, suspensions, emulsions, ointments, pastes, creams, gels, and ophthalmic, otic, and nasal preparations. This section briefly discusses each type.

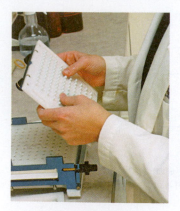

FIGURE 14-4 A capsule-filling machine.

Capsules

Capsules, as an oral dosage form, have been used for more than a century (see Figure 14-4). The capsule has an important role in drug delivery in that it is extremely versatile and offers a broad range of dosage options for patients. The apsule offers flexibility in dosing to the prescriber, as well as to the patient with specific needs.

Capsules can be prepared either by hand or by using a capsule machine. The method used will depend on the quantity needed and the physical characteristics of the powders included in the formula. Using a capsule machine saves time and produces a number of capsules at a time, depending on the size of the machine and the desired quantity. Capsules are available in many sizes, as shown in Figure 14-5.

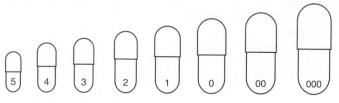

FIGURE 14-5 Capsule size chart.

Tablets

Tablets are a solid dosage form that can be administered orally, **sublingually**, vaginally, or as an implant under the skin. Several different forms of tablets can be compounded.

Compressed tablets, made by pharmaceutical manufacturers, are the most commonly prescribed dosage form; they are

---

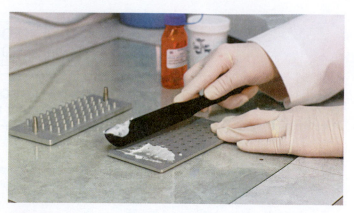

FIGURE 14-6 A technician prepares tablets using a mold.

convenient, portable, stable, and easy to administer. The single disadvantage of commercially made tablets is that they are available only in fixed dosage strengths and combinations.

The compounding pharmacy has always had the ability to compound molded tablets, and now, with the advent of pellet presses and single-punch tablet presses, compressed tablets can be prepared according to the requirements of specific patients (see Figure 14-6).

Powders

Powders are a solid dosage form made from a thoroughly blended mixture of one or more active ingredients and excipients (see Figure 14-7). As a pharmaceutical dosage form, powders may be used either internally (such as BC Powder) or externally, like talcum powder.

Although the use of powders has declined, there is still an occasional need for a prescription powder. Patients who are either unable to swallow or have extreme difficulty in swallowing tablets or capsules (such as some pediatric and geriatric patients) can benefit from having their medication in powder form.

Lozenges and Troches

Lozenges and **troches** are both oral dosage forms that are placed in the oral cavity, either onto the tongue or into the cheek

---

capsule a solid dosage form in which the active ingredient and any excipients are enclosed in a soluble gelatin shell that will dissolve in the stomach.

tablet a solid dosage form that may be administered orally, sublingually, vaginally, or under the skin.

sublingually under the tongue; preparations may be administered by placing them under the tongue and allowing them to dissolve.

powder a solid dosage form made from blended active ingredients and excipients.

lozenge a solid dosage form administered orally to be dissolved in the mouth.

troche an interchangeable term for lozenge, but sometimes prepared in soft form.

suppository a solid dosage form used to administer medication by way of the rectum, vagina, or urethral tract.

aqueous water soluble.

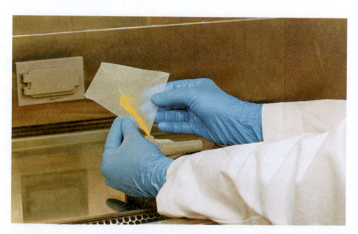

FIGURE 14-7 Powders are a solid dosage form made from a thoroughly blended mixture of one or more active ingredients and excipients.

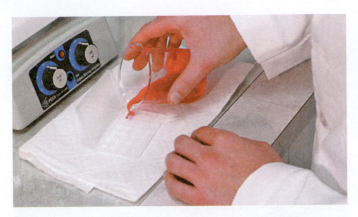

FIGURE 14-8 A technician makes troches using a mold.

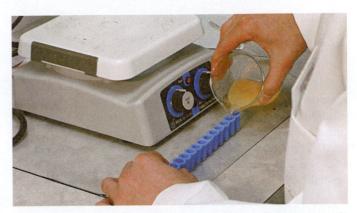

FIGURE 14-10 A technician prepares suppositories.

pouch, and allowed to dissolve; they are usually meant to disintegrate over time (see Figure 14-8). Recently, soft, chewable troches have been developed that are intended to be chewed and swallowed, to deliver medication to the gastrointestinal tract.

Some of the advantages of using troches and lozenges are that they are easy to handle and administer to a variety of patients. Because their base is made of sugar, troches generally have a pleasant taste, which makes them popular with pediatric, geriatric, and hospice patients.

Sticks

Medicated sticks are a unique dosage form used for topical application of local anesthetics, sunscreens, antivirals, antibiotics, and, of course, cosmetics. Sticks offer patients, physicians, and pharmacists a dosage form that is convenient, relatively stable, and fairly easy to prepare. Although relatively simple, the process of properly preparing medicated sticks can be a bit time consuming (see Figure 14-9).

Suppositories

A **suppository** is a solid dosage form that is inserted into the rectum or vagina. The suppository melts and softens or dissolves at body temperature, thus allowing absorption of the medication into the surrounding tissues. Suppositories can have either a systemic effect or a local effect, depending on the

desired effect expected by the prescriber or on the drug being used. Suppositories can be made in several different shapes and sizes, depending on the patient and the disease state being treated.

When determining which base is the most appropriate to use in compounding a suppository, the pharmacy staff will have to consider the physical characteristics of the drug ordered as well as the patient (see Figure 14-10). Some of the common bases used for preparing suppositories include fattibase, polybase, and cocoa butter. A drug may be dissolved in the base, or it may have to be suspended, depending on the physical characteristics of the drug ordered. Whether the drug is dissolved or suspended, the active ingredients and excipients should be added in geometric proportion to ensure that the active ingredient is equally dispersed throughout the suppository product.

Solutions

In an **aqueous** solution, a water-soluble chemical is dissolved in the water phase of the compound. This may consist of just enough distilled or preserved water to dissolve the drug, or water may be as much as 50% of the final volume. After the drug is completely dissolved in the water, the preparer may complete the compound by adding flavoring agents and bringing it to the final volume with a sweetening agent such as Ora-Sweet, Simple Syrup, or Karo Syrup (see Figures 14-11

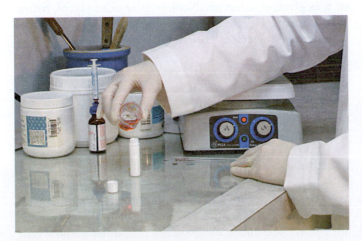

FIGURE 14-9 A technician prepares a stick.

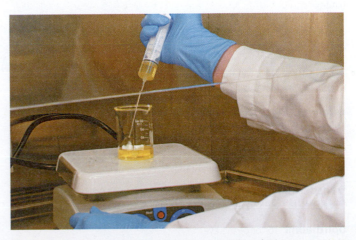

FIGURE 14-11 A technician prepares a sterile solution.

and 14-12). Although the drug is in solution, it may be necessary for the patient to shake the liquid before use to evenly distribute the flavor.

Suspensions

A **suspension** is a liquid preparation that contains insoluble solid particles uniformly dispersed throughout the vehicle. A suspension must be shaken prior to administration to ensure that the proper dose is dispensed. If a drug is to be suspended, a suspending agent such as Ora-Plus or Karo Syrup will be needed (see Figure 14-13).

Emulsions

An **emulsion** is another type of liquid or semisolid preparation that can be taken orally or applied topically. Emulsions are prepared whenever two immiscible liquids must be dispensed in the same preparation. An emulsifying agent is used to hold the two liquids together. One part is oil and the other part is aqueous. Emulsions are either water-in-oil or oil-in-water, depending on the external phase of the final product. Generally, emulsions that are to be used internally are of the oil-in-water type, whereas emulsions for topical use may be of either type.

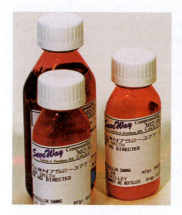

FIGURE 14-12 Examples of packaged liquids.

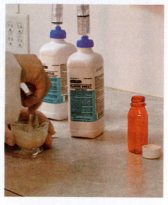

FIGURE 14-13 Working with a suspension.

---

suspension liquid containing ingredients that are not soluble in the vehicle.

emulsion a suspension that consists of two immiscible liquids and an emulsifying agent to hold them together.

ointment a semisolid topical preparation that is applied to the skin or mucous membranes.

comminuting the process of reducing the particle size of a substance by grinding; also known as trituration.

trituration the process of reducing the particle size of a substance by grinding; also known as comminuting.

transdermal gel a gel that penetrates the skin and allows the active ingredient to be easily absorbed into the body; also known as a PLO gel.

ophthalmic for or of the eye.

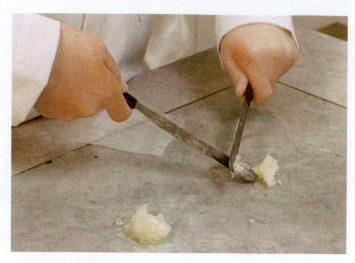

FIGURE 14-14 Preparing an ointment.

As with a suspension, the patient should be instructed to shake an emulsion well before use to temporarily suspend the aqueous phase into the oil phase and equally distribute the active ingredient(s).

Ointments

An **ointment** is a semisolid preparation that is usually applied to the skin or to mucosal tissue. An ointment does not penetrate into the skin; rather, it stays on top of the skin. Ointments should be soft and easily spreadable. They should also be smooth in texture, not gritty. Common ointment bases used in compounding include white petrolatum, hydrophilic petrolatum, Aquaphor, hydrous lanolin, and PEG ointments.

To ensure a smooth ointment, the particle size of the powder being incorporated into the base should be reduced to an impalpable form by **comminuting** or **triturating**, which is the process of reducing particle size to a fine powder. This can be achieved by using a Wedgwood or porcelain mortar and pestle or by forcing the powder(s) through a size 100 mesh sieve (see Figure 14-14). Once the particle size is reduced, the powder can then be mixed into the base, using geometric dilution. At times, it will be necessary to "wet" the powder with a solvent, such as glycerin, ethoxydiglycol, or propylene glycol, before incorporating it into the base. Other times, the drug is dissolved in oil, such as mineral oil, before it is mixed with the base.

Pastes

Pastes are stiff, or very viscous, ointments that do not melt or soften at body temperature. They are intended to be used as protective coverings over the areas where they are applied, such as diaper rash preparations.

Creams

A *cream* is a soft, opaque solid that is usually applied externally (see Figure 14-15). Creams dissipate into the skin, healing the affected area from the inner layers of the dermis. Medications are usually suspended or dissolved in a water-soluble base

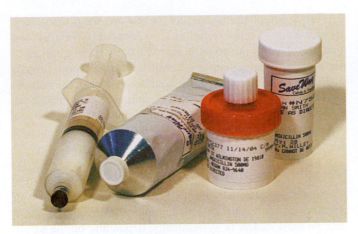

FIGURE 14-15 Examples of packaged topical creams.

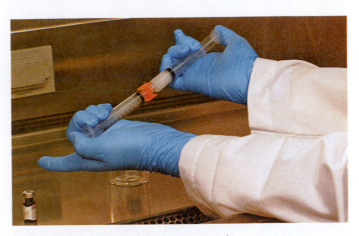

FIGURE 14-17 A technician loading a gel.

when a cream is compounded (see Figure 14-16). A cream must be smooth, and the active ingredients should be dissolved completely so that they will be totally absorbed into the skin. Cream bases available for compounding include vanishing cream base and HRT base, as well as some commercially prepared creams such as Cetaphil, Eucerin, and Lubriderm.

When adding active ingredients to creams, it is critical to practice the principles of geometric dilution to ensure even dispersion. A wetting agent may be necessary; and, again, the volume required to wet the powder should be calculated into the formula when determining the amount of base needed to bring the product to the final desired quantity.

Gels

Gels are semisolid systems consisting of suspensions made up of small inorganic particles or large organic molecules interpenetrated by a liquid.

The **transdermal gel** is a unique, semisolid dosage form that is becoming increasingly popular. Transdermal gels have special absorption enhancers that "push" the medication through the layers of the skin so that the medication can be absorbed into the bloodstream. The transdermal gel is an especially desirable alternative for pediatric patients, animals that are difficult to "pill" or otherwise medicate, older people, and patients who are physically or mentally disabled.

The most common form of compounded transdermal gel therapy is a two-phase vehicle made from pluronic lecithin organogel (PLO). It consists of both an oil phase and an aqueous phase, making it a suitable choice for many chemicals. The oil phase, which is lecithin isopropyl palmitate, is generally used in a concentration of 22%; the balance is made of poloxamer. Oil-soluble drugs

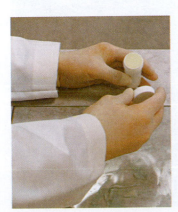

FIGURE 14-16 An example of a cream.

should be dissolved in the oil phase, whereas water-soluble drugs should be dissolved in the aqueous phase. The determined amount of drug is dissolved in the appropriate phase, and then the two components are mixed together using a shearing action (see Figure 14-17). This shear force is necessary for proper micelle formation in the gel. The poloxamer gel is a liquid, which is stored in the refrigerator. When brought to room temperature, it will form a gel. It is important for the final product to be stored at room temperature. Auxiliary labels to this effect (as well as other instructions for the patient, not included on the prescription label) should be placed on the package prior to dispensing.

Ophthalmic Preparations

Ophthalmic preparations, or preparations for the eye, may be in the form of a solution, a suspension, or an ointment; all forms must be sterile (see Figure 14-18). Solutions, which must be clear and particulate-free, are the ophthalmic dosage form most commonly prepared in compounding pharmacies.

In addition to the active drug, ophthalmic preparations require several different ingredients to make them nonirritating to and compatible with the tissues of the eye. The eye

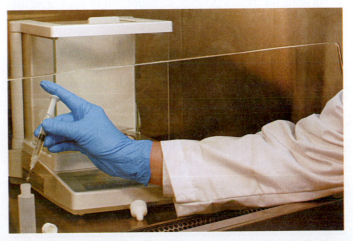

FIGURE 14-18 A technician prepares an ophthalmic preparation.

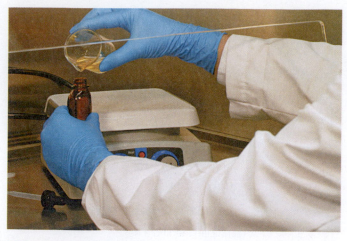

FIGURE 14-19 A technician prepares a liquid otic preparation.

generally tolerates a pH range of 4 to 11. Buffers are used in ophthalmic preparations to maintain the pH of the product within the desired range during storage and administration to the eye.

Preservatives are necessary when the ophthalmic preparation is intended for multiple uses. They prevent contamination of the preparation from microbial growth.

Otic Preparations

Preparations for the ear, or **otic** preparations, are made in liquid, powder, or ointment form (see Figure 14-19). Solutions and suspensions are instilled into the ear, whereas ointments are applied to the external ear. Powders are used infrequently, but are usually administered to the ear canal by a physician. Otic preparations are generally used to treat local infections and the pain associated with them. Other otic products are used to dissolve or remove blockages that can lead to infection.

The vehicles most often used when compounding otic liquids are propylene glycol, glycerin, polyethylene glycol, vegetable oil (especially olive oil), and, occasionally, mineral oil. It is necessary to use a viscous liquid such as one of these, because the compound should adhere to the ear canal. Water and alcohol may be used as a vehicle, but typically are used as solvents for the drugs being compounded or used in an irrigating solution. The physical characteristics of the ingredients used in otic preparations that must be considered include solubility, viscosity, and tonicity. Almost always, a preservative is used in an otic preparation. Although otic preparations need not be sterile, it is important for the pharmacy technician to follow QC procedures to prevent cross-contamination or microbial growth in the compound. Many chemicals used in otic preparations are soluble in the vehicles used in compounding them. Because of the general viscosity of these products, a suspending agent is usually not necessary if the drug is insoluble.

When compounding a liquid for otic use, the drug and any preservatives or other excipients are accurately weighed and then dissolved or mixed with approximately three-quarters of the vehicle. When the drug is completely dissolved or evenly suspended, the preparation is then brought to final volume with more of the vehicle. When an ointment is being prepared, the drug and any other ingredients are accurately weighed and then mixed into the base using the principles of geometric dilution.

Nasal Preparations

Preparations for nasal administration may take the form of solutions, suspensions, gels, or ointments. These preparations may be used locally or systemically, depending on the nature of the drug and the vehicle it is in.

In addition to the active ingredient, several excipients will most likely be used. These include the vehicle, buffers, preservatives, and tonicity-adjusting agents. Because nasal preparations are generally dispensed in multiuse containers, it is necessary to include a preservative. The pH must be adjusted so that maximum stability is obtained. Two common vehicles used for nasal solutions are sodium chloride 0.9% and sterile water for injection.

Ingredients for nasal preparations should be sterile, and aseptic technique should be used to make them. Sterility may be obtained by filtration or autoclaving (see Figure 14-20). If a drug is water soluble, it will be dissolved in a portion of the vehicle and the liquid will be brought to final volume with the vehicle. A suspension will require that the active ingredient and any excipients be mixed by using geometric dilution with a suspending agent and then brought to final volume with the appropriate vehicle. Nasal gels or ointments are made by mixing the active ingredient and any excipients with the base, using the principles of geometric dilution.

QA procedures should be observed when making nasal preparations. Before the compound is dispensed, the pharmacist should determine clarity, pH, and correct volume or weight.

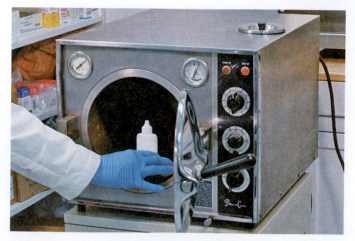

FIGURE 14-20 A technician places a nasal preparation in an autoclave for sterilization.

otic for or of the ear.

Veterinary Compounding

Veterinary compounding is one of the fastest growing areas of pharmaceutical compounding. Medication doses are usually calculated on the basis of milligrams per kilogram of body weight. Because of the vast differences in the sizes and physiology of animals, this makes appropriate dosing nearly impossible when using manufactured products.

The same principles used in compounding of human medications apply to veterinary compounding. Stability, solubility, drug availability, dosage form choices, cost-effectiveness of drug sources, and quality of final product are all factors to be considered before attempting to compound for animals.

In addition to capsules, flavored liquids, transdermal gels, and suppositories, the chewable treat is another dosage form available for veterinary pharmaceutical compounding. A chewable form, made from a base of ground food product and gelatin mixed with the active ingredient, is an excellent choice for animals. Some flavor choices for these chewable forms include liver, tuna, salmon, shrimp, chicken, and beef. Again, solubility is taken into consideration when preparing the treat form. If a drug is water soluble, it can be incorporated into the gelatin phase of the compound. If insoluble, it will be mixed in geometric proportion with the solid, or food, phase of the compound and then mixed with the gelatin. The mixture is then forced into precalibrated molds by way of a syringe or other means. The final product is a soft, chewable form that can be offered to the animal as a treat, or mixed in with a small amount of the animal's favorite food, for consumption.

Medication Flavoring

Successfully flavoring a medication is a critical step in the process of properly preparing a prescription, especially when the taste of a particular drug is such that it will not be tolerated by the patient when administered orally.

Psychological Impact

Although no therapeutic benefit is evident, using the proper coloring and flavoring for medicinal substances is of considerable psychological importance. For example, a patient or the caregiver may think a liquid medication that is as clear as water and has no smell lacks the active ingredient(s). Conversely, a liquid that has been flavored, for example, with bubblegum and slightly tinged with a pink color will be thought to be more effective. A medication that is disagreeable, in appearance, texture, or taste, can be made more attractive and palatable by the careful choice of the most appropriate flavoring, sweetening, diluting, suspending, or coloring agent. Selection of the proper agent is important in preparing the best formulation and in ensuring patient compliance in medication administration. This selection is typically made by the pharmacist, or by the compounding technician subject to the pharmacist's review.

Sensory Roles in Flavoring

Taste, smell, sight, touch, and even sound are complex experiences that may influence the flavor sensation. In general, individuals are usually more sensitive to the aroma of a preparation than to the actual taste. Older adult patients may require added amounts of flavor to achieve the desired result. Females tend to be more sensitive to smell than males. Certain diseases will alter a patient's ability to taste and smell. For example, a patient suffering from a cold or influenza may have a dulled sense of smell and/or taste. When the nostrils are held closed, raw onions will taste sweet; likewise, bad-smelling medications will be much easier to ingest.

Psychological factors such as sight and sound play an important role in flavor experience, as certain reflexes become conditioned through association. In the classic experiments by Pavlov, the ringing of a bell caused the gastric juices of a habituated dog to begin to flow, even though no food was placed in front of the animal. Part of the enjoyment of eating crunchy foods, such as raw celery or carrots, is the sound they make as they are being chewed. Furthermore, the color of a preparation and the flavor should coincide. For example, cherry-flavored substances should be red and grape-flavored substances should be purple.

Flavoring Considerations

Consider each prescription that requires flavoring on an individual basis. It is important to be aware of any allergies or sensitivities a patient may have to particular ingredients, such as chocolate, peanuts, or possibly a particular preservative or dye. It is also helpful to know the patient's likes and dislikes, as well as any idiosyncrasies he or she may have. One should not rely on what is traditionally used or a flavor choice that is popular among a general group. For example, although most pediatric patients like flavors such as grape, bubblegum, and cherry, some patients may not tolerate the tannins or a specific dye contained in the flavoring agent, or they simply may not care for these flavors.

Pediatric Flavoring

Children have more taste buds than adults and, therefore, are more sensitive to taste. Infants and children tend to prefer sweet tastes, and do not respond well to bitter flavors. Appropriate flavor choices for children include raspberry, bubblegum, marshmallow, butterscotch, citrus, berry, and vanilla. The palate of a newborn or an infant typically has not been exposed to a wide variety of tastes; therefore, this young patient will not require as strong a flavor as an older patient. A patient who is required to take a medication for a long period of time may require a milder flavor to avoid flavor fatigue.

Adult Flavoring

Adults are usually more tolerant of bitter flavors, so with extremely bitter drugs a flavoring agent such as coffee, chocolate, cherry, anise, grapefruit, or mint will be acceptable. These bitter flavors are generally an acquired taste. Their own "bite" is helpful in cutting the bitterness of the drug.

Impact on Stability, Solubility, and pH

Other factors to be considered when choosing an appropriate flavoring agent include stability, solubility, pH, and the physical properties of the flavors available. Some flavors can negatively affect the compounded prescription, such as raising or lowering the pH of the final product, and possibly cause instability. Aqueous solutions should be flavored with water-miscible flavors, whereas oil preparations will require the use of an oil-based flavor. These factors may limit a patient's choice of available flavors. Some flavoring agents or the preservatives in the flavor may affect the active ingredient in the compound and cause degradation of the drug.

Compounded medications that are stable only at a certain pH should be flavored with an agent that will not affect the pH or one that will enhance the pH of the final product. Although pH values may be equal to or within close range from manufacturer to manufacturer, the exact pH should be obtained from the company that is the source of the flavoring agent. Most chemical companies that offer products for medicinal flavoring will be able to provide a list of their flavors and the relative pH values. This is a reference that every pharmacy that offers flavoring as a service should have.

Four Taste Types

There are four basic taste experiences: sour, sweet, bitter, and salty (see Figure 14-21), plus a recently discovered fifth sense, called *umami*, which tastes glutamates and cannot be duplicated by the combination of any of the other four tastes. Each of these four taste types is experienced in a specific area of the tongue that contains taste buds with specialized functions. Taste receptors for all tastes are located in a narrow area surrounding the entire tongue. Sweet, salty, and sour taste receptors are in a region just inside the outer edge of the tongue. Salty and sour receptors are located in a small region toward the back of the tongue. Sour-only receptors are located approximately in the center of the tongue. There is an area toward the center and front of the tongue where no sensation of taste is experienced. Sweet and sour taste receptors are located just in front of this region, with bitter, sweet, and sour tastes being experienced near the tip of the tongue just inside the area containing the receptors for all tastes. The brain, however, is not able to distinguish different taste components; rather, it perceives taste as a composite sensation.

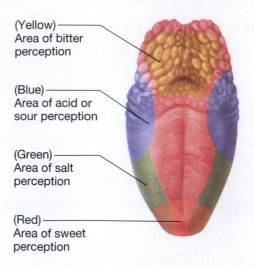

(Yellow)
Area of bitter perception

(Blue)
Area of acid or sour perception

(Green)
Area of salt perception

(Red)
Area of sweet perception

FIGURE 14-21 The four basic taste experiences are sour, sweet, bitter, and salty.

Flavoring Techniques

Flavoring of medications can be seen as both a challenge and an opportunity. The challenge lies in the fact that there are no general or definite rules for what is right. There are no absolutes when it comes to flavoring, especially when working with an extemporaneously compounded prescription. Every formula that requires flavoring should be analyzed individually. The challenge of flavoring is further complicated by the individual preferences of each patient. The opportunity in flavoring lies in the ability to produce a quality product that the patient is willing to take or, at the very least, that the patient will tolerate.

Five basic flavoring techniques are used in preparing an acceptable product that minimizes a negative experience with regard to taste:

1. Blending uses a flavor that will blend with the drug taste. Citrus flavors blend with sour tastes; bitter tastes can be blended with salty, sweet, and sour tastes; salt reduces bitterness and sourness and increases sweetness. Chemicals such as vanillin, monosodium glutamate (MSG), and benzaldehyde are used for blending.
2. Overshadowing or overpowering involves the use of a flavor with a stronger intensity than the original product. Examples of intense flavoring vehicles are wintergreen, methyl salicylate, glycyrrhiza (licorice), and oleoresins.
3. Physical methods include the formulation of insoluble ingredients into a suspension; and emulsification of oils, where the offensive-tasting ingredient is placed in the oil phase and the flavoring or sweetening agent is placed in the aqueous phase. Effervescent additives are used in the preparation of salty-tasting drugs. The use of a high-viscosity fluid such as a syrup will limit contact of the offensive element with the tongue.
4. Chemical methods include absorption of the drug with an ingredient that eliminates the taste of the offensive drug.

5. Physiological methods involve using an additive such as menthol, peppermint, spearmint, or a spice such as cinnamon or clove to anesthetize the taste buds within the tongue. These flavor products reduce the sensitivity of the taste buds to bitterness.

In addition, flavor enhancers, such as MSG, may be added to ensure the intensity of flavor. It is important to note, however, that many patients are hypersensitive or allergic to MSG. The most used flavor enhancer is vanilla. It can be added along with almost any flavoring agent to stimulate and intensify the desired flavor without altering the flavor or adding its own taste.

Coloring

Proper coloring of the prescription is equally important when making a compounded medication. The color should be appealing and appropriate for the dosage form. It is not always necessary to color a product, but if a coloring agent is used, it should match the flavor of the product. Some patients may have sensitivities or allergies to certain dyes. This should be determined before compounding begins. There are sources of dye-free flavoring agents, and these should be considered for the patient who cannot tolerate a certain dye. In any case, the amount of color added to the formulation should be minimal, so that the final product is moderately light in color.

Summary

Extemporaneous compounding is a special service provided by a number of community-based pharmacies. Additional training, skills, and practice are required for a pharmacy technician to assist in compounding, but compounding also provides a number of advanced professional opportunities for those who pursue these skills.

Chapter Review Questions

1. What are some of the factors that must be considered before compounding a prescription medication?
   a. cost-effectiveness, availability, solubility, and stability
   b. suspending agent, profit margin, and ease of preparation
   c. proper tools, adequate support personnel, and time
   d. insurance reimbursement, available flavoring agents, active ingredient, and source

2. A set of step-by-step written instructions on how to do a certain task is referred to as the _____.
   a. MSDS
   b. SOP
   c. QA
   d. QC

3. Pharmacy is the only profession that allows the extemporaneous compounding of chemicals for _____.
   a. resale
   b. veterinarians
   c. therapeutic care
   d. use in physicians' offices

4. Of the following reference materials, which would not be necessary in a compounding facility?
   a. *Remington's Pharmaceutical Sciences*
   b. *The Merck Manual*
   c. *Drug Facts and Comparisons*
   d. *Pharmacy Times Magazine*

5. Which part of the compounding procedure has the greatest potential for error?
   a. pharmaceutical calculations
   b. retrieving the proper chemical
   c. selecting the proper vehicle
   d. choosing the best flavor

6. All of the following are flavoring techniques *except* _____.
   a. absorbing
   b. blending
   c. physiological methods
   d. overshadowing

7. The compilation of ingredients and instructions is known as the _____.
   a. worksheet
   b. menu
   c. formula
   d. list

8. To avoid cross-contamination, the compounding area should be cleaned _____.
   a. before the procedure
   b. after the procedure
   c. daily
   d. both before and after the procedure

9. A semisolid preparation that is usually applied to the skin or mucosal tissue is known as a(n)_____.
   a. emulsion
   b. ointment
   c. cream
   d. suspension

10. Which of the following types of mortar and pestle would be the ideal choice when working with liquids?
   a. porcelain
   b. glass
   c. Wedgwood
   d. any of the above

Critical Thinking Questions

1. What are three reasons extemporaneous compounding is important to pharmaceutical care?

2. Why is compounding considered a specialty?

3. Why does medication flavoring have an impact on patient compliance?

Web Challenge

1. Go to the following websites and print out information on obtaining advanced training, or certification, as a compounding pharmacy technician:
   http://fagron.us
   http://www.pccarx.org
   http://www.pharmacytechnician.org
   http://www.letcomedical.com

2. Go to http://www.compoundingtoday.com and print out an archived e-newsletter to discuss in class.

References and Resources

Allen, Lloyd V. Jr. "A History of Pharmaceutical Compounding." *Secundum Artem*. 11 (3). Web. 15 June 2012.

Allen, Lloyd V. Jr. "Pharmaceutical Compounding Calculations." *Secundum Artem*. 5 (2). Web. 15 June 2012.

Allen, Lloyd V. Jr. "Pharmacy Compounding Equipment." *Secundum Artem*. 4 (3). Web. 15 June 2012.

Allen, Lloyd V. Jr. *The Art, Science, and Technology of Pharmaceutical Compounding*. Washington, DC: APhA, 1998. Print.

Associated Press. "Meningitis Outbreak: Lawmakers Seeking Justice Dept. Probe of Pharmacy." Associated Press. Web. 17 October 2012.

Colbert, B., Ankney, J., and Lee, K. *Anatomy, Physiology, and Disease: An Interactive Journey for Health Professionals*. Upper Saddle River, NJ: Pearson Education, 2009.

Johnston, Mike. *The Pharmacy Technician: Foundations and Practices*. 1st ed. Upper Saddle River, NJ: Prentice Hall Health, 2009. Print.

Johnston, Mike. *The Pharmacy Technician Series: Compounding*. Upper Saddle River, NJ: Prentice Hall Health, 2006. Print.

Pharmacy Compounding Accreditation Board. 2012. Web. 18 June 2012.

Stobbe, Mike. "Meningitis Outbreak: Unsanitary Conditions, Worker Sloppiness Could Be to Blame." Detroit Free Press. Web. 17 October 2012.

United States Pharmacopeia. 2012. Web. 18 June 2012.

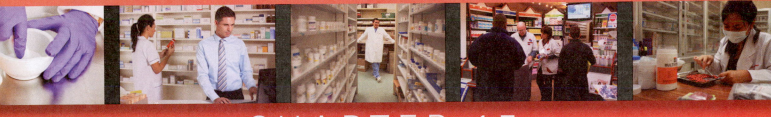

CHAPTER 15

Introduction to Sterile Products

LEARNING OBJECTIVES

After completing this chapter, you should be able to:

- Outline and describe the key regulations and guidelines pertaining to sterile product preparations.

- Identify and list the equipment and supplies used in preparing sterile products.

- Demonstrate proper cleaning of laminar flow hoods.

- List the routes of administration associated with sterile products.

- List and describe key characteristics of sterile products.

- Discuss special concerns regarding total parenteral nutrition (TPN).

- Discuss special concerns regarding chemotherapy and cytotoxic drugs.

- Demonstrate proper garbing procedures.

- Demonstrate proper hand-washing techniques.

- Demonstrate how to withdraw from a vial.

- Demonstrate how to reconstitute a powder vial.

- Demonstrate how to remove fluid from an ampule.

KEY TERMS

antineoplastics, p. 256

aseptic technique, p. 248

bench or countertop model, p. 250

bevel, p. 250

biological safety cabinet, p. 250

buffer capacity, p. 256

chemotherapy, p. 256

class 100 environment, p. 248

console model, p. 250

cytotoxic, p. 258

HEPA, p. 250

infusion, p. 254

intradermal, p. 254

intramuscular, p. 254

intrathecal, p. 254

intravenous, p. 254

isotonicity, p. 254

IV admixture, p. 250

laminar flow hood, p. 250

lumen, p. 250

parenteral nutrition, p. 256

pH, p. 254

piggyback bags, p. 252

precipitate, p. 254

sterile, p. 248

subcutaneous, p. 254

tonicity, p. 254

INTRODUCTION

As pharmacy practice moves to a more patient-centered concept of pharmaceutical care, pharmacists rely on pharmacy technicians to take on new and expanded roles. Technicians have assumed many of the drug distribution responsibilities, traditionally performed by pharmacists, to free pharmacists to provide direct patient care; however, technicians need proper training to be qualified to perform these responsibilities. This chapter introduces pharmacy technicians to sterile products and aseptic technique.

As you learned in Chapter 14, nonsterile compounding requires knowledge of numerous dosage formulations, such as capsules, solutions, suspensions, suppositories, and topicals. Sterile compounding requires, in addition, a command of aseptic technique. The more complex the compounding, the more precautions and steps must be added to guidelines to ensure proper aseptic technique.

Aseptic Technique

Aseptic technique is a way to perform a procedure under controlled conditions in a manner that minimizes the chance of contamination of the preparation (see Figure 15-1). Contamination can be caused by the following factors:

- Environment—conditions, such as the air, where the compounding is being performed must be controlled.
- Equipment—all objects that come in contact with the drug(s) must be sterile.
- Personnel—touch contamination is the most frequent cause of contamination.

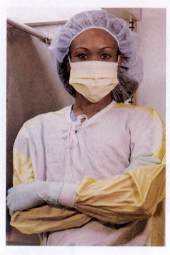

FIGURE 15-1 A technician dressed in sterile clothing.

We address each of these causes of contamination in detail, because each plays a key role in proper aseptic compounding.

The preparation of **sterile** drug compounds requires the utmost diligence to ensure final product integrity and sterility. Sterile products must be prepared with aseptic technique in a **class 100 environment**. This is a type of airflow unit capable of producing an environment containing no more than 100 airborne particles of a size 0.5 micron or larger, per cubic foot of air. Such an environment exists inside a certified horizontal or vertical laminar flow hood, a class 100 clean room, and a barrier isolator. A *barrier isolator* is a closed system made up of four solid walls, an air-handling system, and a transfer and interaction compartment.

Regulations and Guidelines

Various agencies issue guidelines to help establish standard practices and ensure universal testing procedures. Many regulatory agencies and professional associations have published guidelines for aseptic procedures and quality control programs for pharmacy. These evolving standards cover both good manufacturing practices (GMPs) and quality assurance programs.

Food and Drug Administration

The FDA publishes GMPs, a regularly updated set of standards that offers guidelines for the compounding of sterile products. Another FDA document states guidelines on the manufacture of sterile products by aseptic processing. Included in these documents are quality system regulations, which will make standards consistent with quality system requirements.

The Joint Commission

The Joint Commission publishes many general standards regarding pharmaceuticals and the facilities that manufacture, store, and deliver them. Similar to the FDA, the Joint Commission constantly revises its standards to improve compliance and keep up with the ever-evolving field of drugs and their manufacturing processes.

Through stringent inspections performed at timed intervals, the Joint Commission offers a highly respected and often necessary accreditation for health care organizations. Its focus is on the current state of health care and the potential for safer, higher quality care. In addition to its published set of guidelines, the Joint Commission offers support to help organizations understand, participate, and comply with the accreditation process.

---

info

To Learn More

This chapter is just an overview of this specialty practice in institutional pharmacy. Specific techniques are not included, as they are too advanced and detailed for the scope of this book. For an in-depth look at sterile products and step-by-step procedures for aseptic technique, review *Sterile Products and Aseptic Technique for Pharmacy Technicians*, 2nd edition, by Mike Johnston (Prentice-Hall Health, 2010).

---

aseptic technique the process of performing a procedure under controlled conditions in a manner that minimizes the chance of contamination of the preparation.

sterile free from bacteria and other microorganisms.

class 100 environment the classification of an airflow unit capable of producing an environment containing no more than 100 airborne particles of a size 0.5 micron or larger, per cubic foot of air.

Centers for Disease Control and Prevention

The Centers for Disease Control and Prevention (CDC) publishes guidelines to assist in the prevention of spreading disease or infection. Since the primary goal of aseptic compounding mirrors these guidelines, it is easy to see why the CDC documents would be important to understand and put into practice. CDC guidelines also provide invaluable information for hospital environment controls, especially where infection prevention is concerned.

USP 797

The United States Pharmacopeia (USP) has published the first enforceable national standards for sterile compounding, USP 797. This major publication has gained the attention of numerous pharmacy regulatory entities, such as state boards of pharmacy (SBOPs), the Joint Commission, the FDA, and many others. Agencies such as these are using USP 797 as a universal guide, while amending and revising their own current publications.

USP 797 defines the responsibilities of many areas subjected to quality control and offers a virtually unquestionable view as to what is necessary for the quality control process. It is important as a pharmacy technician compounding sterile products that you understand their impact on your pharmacy career.

USP 797 classifies compounded sterile products (CSPs) as low risk level, medium risk level, or high risk level. Risk levels define where a particular prepared product might be grouped based on the type of CSP, compounding processes, and environments. Each risk level has variant recommendations and guidelines as well, which aid in reducing contamination of all sorts.

ASHP Guidelines

Some of the most widely and longest recognized publications regarding quality assurance with sterile products, as well as all other pharmaceuticals and related information, are the guidelines established by the American Society of Health-System Pharmacists (ASHP). ASHP has taken an active role in producing documents addressing quality assurance. The ASHP guidelines on quality assurance for pharmacy-prepared sterile products outline the numerous considerations that are subjected to quality testing and assurance. It is a comprehensive document that addresses all areas impacted by quality assurance.

ASHP guidelines cover policies and procedures, personnel training, storage, handling, facilities, equipment, garb, aseptic technique, product preparation, process validation, documentation, expiration dating, labeling, and end-product evaluations. ASHP guidelines are divided into three risk levels as follows.

Risk Level 1

Risk level 1 includes products that are stored at room temperature and completely administered within 28 hours of preparation; unpreserved, sterile, and prepared for administration to more than one patient and contain suitable preservatives; or prepared by a closed-system aseptic transfer of

> ### info Specialty Certification
> Many health-system pharmacy settings require IV certification and/or prior experience for employment consideration, and it is also a requirement to practice aseptic technique in numerous states. So, in an effort to meet various SBOP regulations, as well as to provide potential employers with assurance of competency and technique mastery, the National Pharmacy Technician Association (NPTA) offers specialty certification programs in sterile products/IV admixture and chemotherapy. To learn more about NPTA's specialized certification programs, go to **www.pharmacytechnician.org/sterile** or **www.pharmacytechnician.org/chemo** for details on the specific programs.

sterile, nonpyrogenic, finished pharmaceuticals obtained from licensed manufacturers into sterile final containers obtained from licensed manufacturers.

Examples that fall in this category include the following: single-patient admixtures, sterile ophthalmics, syringes without preservatives used within 28 hours, batch-prefilled syringes with preservatives, and TPN solutions made by gravity transfer of carbohydrates and amino acids into an empty container with the addition of sterile additives with a needle and syringe.

Risk Level 2

Risk level 2 includes products that are administered beyond 28 hours after preparation and storage at room temperature; batch-prepared without preservatives and intended for use by more than one patient; or compounded by complex or numerous manipulations of sterile ingredients obtained from licensed manufacturers by using a closed-system aseptic transfer. Examples that fall in this category include the following: injections for use in a portable pump or reservoir over multiple days, batch-reconstituted antibiotics without preservatives, batch-prefilled syringes without preservatives, and TPN solutions mixed with an automatic compounding device.

Risk Level 3

Risk level 3 includes products that are compounded from non-sterile ingredients or components, containers, or equipment before terminal sterilization; or prepared by combining multiple ingredients, sterile or nonsterile, by using an open-system transfer before terminal sterilization.

Examples that fall in this category include the following: alum bladder irrigation, morphine injection made from powder or tablets, TPN solutions made from dry amino acids or sterilized by final filtration, and autoclaved IV solutions.

Basic Equipment and Supplies

Basic equipment and supplies used in sterile compounding include laminar flow hoods, vertical flow hoods, biological safety cabinets, needles, syringes, and IV bags. This section introduces each one briefly.

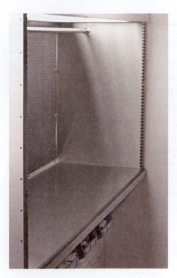

FIGURE 15-2 A laminar flow hood.

Laminar Flow Hoods

Laminar flow hoods are designed to reduce the risk of airborne contamination during the preparation of **IV admixtures** by providing an ultraclean environment (see Figure 15-2). The most important part of a laminar flow hood is a high-efficiency, bacteria-retentive filter, commonly called a **HEPA** (high-efficiency particulate air) filter. Room air is taken into the unit and passed through a prefilter to remove relatively large contaminants such as dust and lint. The air is then compressed and channeled up behind and through the HEPA filter, which removes virtually all bacteria. The purified air then flows out over the entire work surface in parallel streams at a uniform velocity.

A laminar flow hood has three basic functions. The first is to provide clean air in the working area. This is done by passing room air through the bacteria-retentive filter to provide a continuous flow of clean air in the work area. Second, the constant flow of air out of the laminar flow hood prevents room air from entering the work area. Last, the air flowing out suspends and removes contaminants introduced into the work area by material (such as IV bags, syringes, or drug packaging) or personnel. Thus, a laminar flow hood provides an environment virtually free of airborne contaminants, in which sterile procedures can be safely performed. Laminar flow hoods may be used in the pharmacy to perform the following procedures:

- Preparation of IV admixtures
- Preparation of ophthalmic solutions

---

laminar flow hood a device containing a HEPA filter; used for preparing sterile products.

IV admixture a mixture of a solution and drug(s) prepared aseptically to be administered via a vein.

HEPA a high-efficiency particulate air filter; used in flow hoods.

console model a horizontal laminar flow hood that sits on the floor.

bench (countertop) model a horizontal laminar flow hood that sits on top of a counter; the space underneath it can be used for storage.

biological safety cabinet a vertical laminar flow hood used to provide protection for the worker, the work environment, and the drug.

bevel the sharp, pointed, diagonally cut end of a needle.

lumen the hollow space inside a needle.

■ Procedure 15-1

Cleaning a Horizontal Laminar Flow Hood

The technician should always clean the horizontal laminar airflow workbench from top to bottom, from the back to the front opening.

1. Wash the entire hood walls and surface with sterile water to remove salt, starch, sugar, and/or proteins.
2. Soak stubborn spots for 10–15 minutes, and then wipe clean.
3. To disinfect, wipe all the surfaces of the hood with sterile 70% isopropyl alcohol (IPA) using lint-free fabric.
4. Starting at the IV pole, wipe all surfaces of the pole from left to right with sterile 70% IPA.
5. After you clean the pole, clean the sides of the hood. Starting at the back of the hood, wipe sides in a vertical fashion (top to bottom) using overlapping strokes. Repeat on the opposite side.
6. To clean the work surface, or work bench, start at the back corner and clean the surface using horizontal (right to left) overlapping strokes from the back of the work surface to the outer edge.
7. Document the hood cleaning as required by the facility.

- Reconstitution of powdered drugs
- Filling of unit-dose syringes
- Preparation of miscellaneous sterile products

Laminar flow hoods come in various sizes and models. One model, called a **console model**, sits on the floor. The other common model is called a **bench or countertop model**, because it sits on top of a counter; the space underneath it can be used for storage. Laminar airflow hoods are usually kept running continuously. If the hood has been turned off, it is recommended that it be run for at least 30 minutes before the work surface area is used again, so that the room air will be replaced with clean, filtered air. Laminar flow hoods should be inspected and certified every six months to ensure that the HEPA filter is intact, unclogged, and has no holes in it. The prefilters in the hoods should be changed monthly.

Vertical Flow Hoods

Both console and bench models are available with vertical rather than horizontal airflow. With vertical flow, room air enters at the top of the unit, is channeled through the bacteria-retentive filter (which forms the ceiling of the unit), and down vertically across the work surface area. Neither of these models of laminar flow hoods should be used when preparing chemotherapy drugs. Although they protect the drug product from microbial contamination, they do not protect personnel or the environment from the hazards of these drug agents. These laminar flow hoods blow air across the work surface toward the operator and into the work environment. Drug particles or aerosols of these hazardous agents can easily contaminate both workers and the work environment.

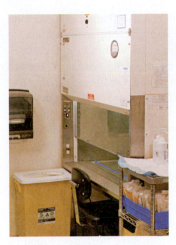

FIGURE 15-3 An example of a biological safety cabinet.

Biological Safety Cabinets

Rather than a horizontal laminar flow hood, a **biological safety cabinet (BSC)** is recommended to provide protection for the worker, the work environment, and the drug (see Figure 15-3). In a BSC, air enters the unit at the top, where it passes through a prefilter to remove large contaminants. Air then passes through a HEPA filter and is directed down toward the work surface, just as with a vertical laminar flow hood. The filter forms the ceiling of the work area in the BSC and removes bacteria to provide ultraclean air. Unlike the mechanism in a vertical laminar flow hood, however, as air approaches the work surface, it is pulled through vents at the front, back, and sides of the unit. A major portion of the contaminated air is recirculated back into the cabinet, and only a minor portion is passed through a HEPA filter before being exhausted into the room. BSCs may also contain a partition on the front of the hood to help protect the user from exposure to hazardous substances.

BSCs are of two basic types. A class 2, type A, which was just described, represents the minimum recommended environment for preparing chemotherapy agents. Class 2, type B BSCs have greater intake flow velocities and are vented outside the building rather than back into the room. This type of safety cabinet is preferred, but the need to vent the filtered air to the outside can carry with it a substantial construction/installation cost.

It is important that BSCs run continuously. If turned off for any reason, such as for maintenance or filter changes, the cabinet must be thoroughly cleaned with a detergent, and the exhaust area must be covered with impermeable plastic and sealed to prevent any contaminants from escaping from the unit.

Workplace Wisdom USP 797

Although introduced in 2004, revisions continue to be made to USP 797. The most current information on these regulations can be found at www.usp.org.

Needles

A *needle* consists of two parts: the shaft and the hub. The *shaft* is the long, slender stem of the needle that is beveled (diagonal cut) at one end to form a point. The cut end of the needle is the **bevel**. The hollow bore of the needle shaft is known as the **lumen**. At the other end of the needle is the *hub*, to which a syringe can be attached (see Figure 15-4).

Needle size is designated by length and gauge. The length of a needle is measured in inches from the juncture of the hub and the shaft to the tip of the point. Needle lengths range from

■ Procedure 15-2

Cleaning a Vertical Laminar Flow Hood or BSC

1. Wash the entire hood walls and surface with sterile water to remove salt, starch, sugar, and/or proteins.
2. Soak stubborn spots for 10–15 minutes, and then wipe clean.
3. To disinfect, wipe all the surfaces of the hood with sterile 70% IPA using lint-free fabric.
4. Starting at the IV pole, wipe all surfaces of the pole from left to right with sterile 70% IPA.
5. After you clean the IV pole, clean the back surface of the hood from top to bottom with overlapping horizontal strokes.
6. Starting at the back of the hood, wipe sides from top to bottom with overlapping horizontal strokes. Repeat on the opposite side.
7. To clean the work surface, or work bench, start in the back corner and clean the surface using horizontal (right to left) overlapping strokes from the back of the work surface to the outer edge.
8. Document the hood cleaning as required by the facility.

info Facility Guidelines

For facilities, USP 797 states that the surfaces of all ceilings, walls, floors, shelving, cabinets, and work surfaces in the buffer room and/or anteroom should be smooth, free from cracks and crevices, and nonshedding, so that they are easy to clean and sanitize. Junctures of ceilings and walls, walls and walls, and floors and walls must be covered or caulked to make them easier to clean. The areas may not have any dust-collecting ledges, pipes, or similar surfaces. Work surfaces must be durable, smooth, and made of stainless steel or molded plastic. Carts should be made of stainless steel wire or sheet construction, with good-quality, cleanable caster wheels, and should be restricted to use in the controlled area only.

3/8 inch to 3½ inches or longer. The gauge of a needle, used to designate the size of the lumen, ranges from 27, the finest, to 13, the largest. The finer the needle, the higher the gauge number. In some disposable needles, the gauge is designated by the color of the hub (to facilitate recognition). One factor in choosing a needle size is the thickness (viscosity) of the solution to be injected. A fine needle with a relatively small lumen may be acceptable for most solutions, but a needle with a larger lumen and a smaller gauge number may be needed for more viscous solutions. Another factor in selecting the proper needle is the nature of the rubber closure to be penetrated. A fine needle with a smaller lumen may be preferred for rubber closures that core easily; *coring* means that part of the rubber closure gets carried into the drug solution when the needle penetrates the rubber

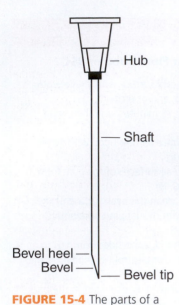

FIGURE 15-4 The parts of a needle.

closure. Needles are sterilized, individually wrapped, and disposable. Never reuse a used needle.

Filter needles are similar to other needles, except that they have a filter in the hub to catch any particles from an ampule or vial. They are used to vent small-volume vials. Dispensing pins, which can be attached to the syringe directly for multiple draws, rather than attaching multiple needles, are just one example of the various styles of equipment available from the many different distributors. Each works in the same fashion, by providing a venting system that traps any particles larger than the pores of the dispensing pin. A variety of different pore sizes are available. A 0.22-micron pore size is considered to be a sterilizing filter capable of removing all microorganisms. Other sizes commonly used in the pharmacy and suitable for clarifying solutions have porosities of 0.45 micron, 1 micron, 5 microns, or 10 microns. The choice of which needle to use depends on your ability to manipulate the pin and the cost of the device.

Syringes

The two basic parts of a syringe are the barrel and the plunger (see Figure 15-5). The *barrel* is a tube that is open at one end and tapers into a hollow tip at the other end. The open end is extended radially outward to form a rim, or flange, to prevent the barrel from slipping through the fingers during manipulation.

The *plunger* is a piston-type rod with a slightly cone-shaped tip that passes inside the barrel of the syringe. The other end of the plunger is shaped into a flat knob for easy manipulation. The plunger must be able to move freely throughout the barrel, yet its surface must be so close to the barrel that the fluid cannot pass in between, even when under considerable pressure.

The tip of the syringe provides the point of attachment for a needle. The tip may be tapered to allow the needle hub to be slipped over it and held on by friction. With a system that uses this method, the needle is reasonably secure, but it may slip off if not properly attached or if considerable pressure is used to inject the solution. Locking devices have been developed to secure the needle more firmly onto the tip of the syringe; one such device has the trade name Luer-Lok. These devices incorporate a collar with a circular internal groove into which the needle hub is inserted. A half-turn locks the needle in place. This capability is especially valuable when pressure is required.

Graduation lines on the barrel of the syringe indicate the volume of solution inside. It is easier to make accurate readings, if the color of the tip of the plunger is different from that of the syringe itself. Syringes are disposable and have a capacity range of 0.5–60 mL. Graduation lines may be in milliliters or other measures, depending on the capacity and intended uses of the syringe; for example, the larger the capacity of the syringe, the larger the interval between graduation lines. Special-purpose syringes, such as insulin syringes, have graduation lines in both milliliters and insulin units to reflect their intended use.

To select an appropriate syringe, use the rule that the capacity of the syringe should be the next size larger than the volume to be measured. For example, use a 3-mL syringe to measure a 2.3-mL dose; select a 5-mL syringe to measure a 3.8-mL dose. This way, the graduation marks on the syringe will be in the smallest possible increments for the dose measured. Syringes should not be filled to capacity, because the plunger can easily be dislodged. It is recommended that syringes containing chemotherapy drugs not be filled to more than three-quarters of capacity.

Sterile, disposable syringes are discarded after one use and have the same advantages as disposable needles. Although syringes today are made of plastic, because it costs less, glass syringes are still available for drugs that are incompatible with plastic. Both syringes and needles must be disposed of in a sharps container. Do not recap needles after they have been used.

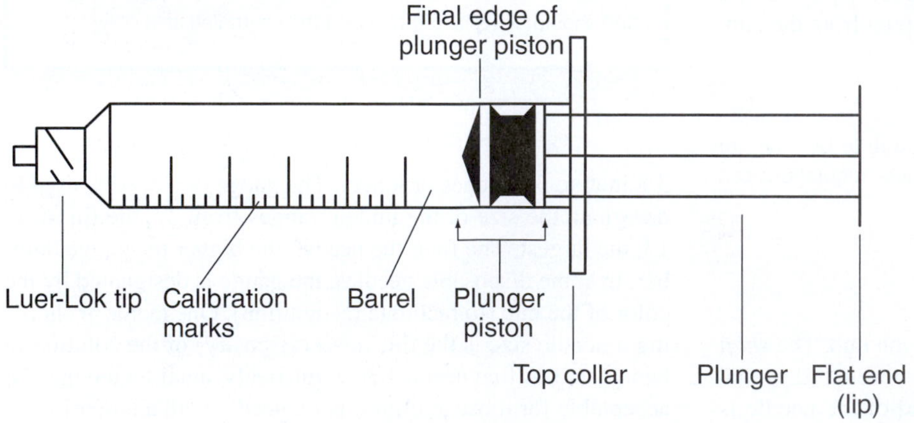

Prefilled Syringes

Some pharmaceutical manufacturers supply common doses of frequently used or emergency-use drugs in prefilled syringes. Prefilled syringes eliminate the need to measure doses, thus saving valuable time in compounding admixtures. Prefilled syringes are commonly

Final edge of plunger piston

Luer-Lok tip | Calibration marks | Barrel | Plunger piston | Top collar | Plunger | Flat end (lip)

FIGURE 15-5 The parts of a syringe.

piggyback bags minibags that hold 50 mL or 100 mL of solution and are used to administer drugs intermittently.

placed in emergency carts, or are used in emergency rooms when it is critical to get medication to patients as quickly as possible.

Most prefilled syringes are supplied in a syringe that does not have a plunger. This is to prevent the drug from accidentally squirting out if pressure is applied to the plunger during storage or transferring. A device called a *tubex holder* is screwed onto the back of the syringe (where the plunger would have been), and a locking ring is then tightened around the end of the syringe.

IV Bags

Plastic bags are used for dilution of a solution, and are the most common containers used in administering IV medications to patients. Plastic bags are available in many different sizes, with 50 mL, 100 mL, 250 mL, 500 mL, and 1,000 mL being the most common. Special bags for compounding parenteral nutrition are available in 2,000-mL and 3,000-mL sizes. Most IV bags are made of polyvinyl chloride (PVC). More expensive than PVC bags are non-PVC bags, which are used for specific drugs (such as Taxol) that can adhere to the plastic of PVC IV bags. Figure 15-6 shows the parts of an IV administration setup.

At the top of the bag is a flat plastic extension with a hole to allow the bag to be hung on an administration pole. At the other end of the bag are two ports of about the same length. The administration set port has a blue plastic cover that maintains the sterility of the port. The cover is easily removed by pulling on it. Once it is pulled off, the sterile port of the administration set is exposed. Solution will not drip from the plastic bag at this point, because a plastic diaphragm of about ½ inch inside the port seals in the liquid. When the spike of the administration set is inserted into this port, it punctures the inner diaphragm, allowing the solution to flow from the flexible plastic bag into the administration set. When the solution has filled the administration set (this process is called *priming* the set), make sure to clamp the administration set so that the solution does not leak out. Once the inner diaphragm is punctured, it is not resealable.

The other port is the medication port. It is covered by a protective rubber tip. Medication is added to the solution through the medication port by means of a needle and syringe. The rubber tip is self-sealing, thus preventing solution from leaking when the needle punctures the tip.

Approximately ½ inch inside this port is a plastic diaphragm that must be punctured for solution to enter the bag. The inner diaphragm is not self-sealing when punctured by a needle, so the rubber tip must stay attached to the bag.

Graduation marks at 25–100 mL intervals, which indicate the volume of solution infused, are located on both sides of the front of some plastic bags, depending on the capacity of the bags.

When you label a plastic bag, it does not matter which side of the bag you place the label on; however, many institutions place the label on the printed side of the bag, beneath the solution name, and offset slightly to one side so that the graduation marks near the side can still be read. This procedure has the advantage of providing a convenient cross-check between the actual solution and the name appearing on the admixture label.

Some IV solutions, such as 5% dextrose injection and 0.9% sodium chloride injection, are available in minibags, or **piggyback bags**. These bags typically hold 50 mL or 100 mL of solution and are used to administer drugs (such as antibiotics) intermittently rather than continuously.

The plastic bag system is completely closed to air. It does not depend on air to displace the solution as it leaves the bag. The bag collapses as the solution is administered, so a vacuum is not created inside.

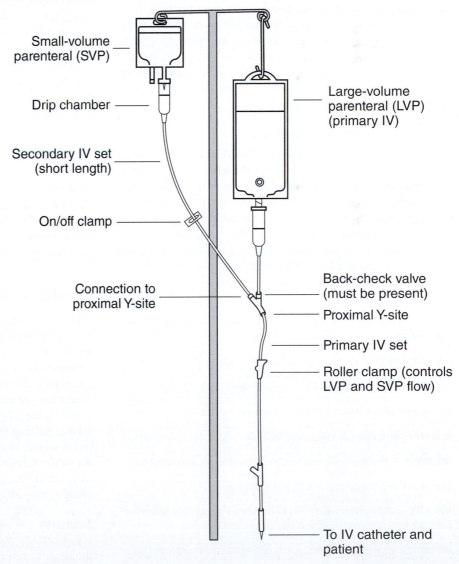

FIGURE 15-6 The parts of an IV.

Routes of Administration

When drugs must be injected, any one of several routes can be used to administer them. Often, certain drugs can be administered only through specific routes, and this will be listed in the package insert. The most common injectable routes of administration are **intravenous** (in the vein), **intramuscular** (in the muscle), and **subcutaneous** (in the skin). Other, less frequently used routes include **intradermal** (in the dermis of the skin) and **intrathecal** (in the spine).

IV administration of drugs has advantages over other routes, because it provides the fastest route to the bloodstream. There are no barriers, like skin or muscle, to absorb the drug first, so the IV route allows the most rapid onset of action. If someone cannot take medication by mouth because he is unconscious or vomiting, then IV administration is the best route. Because the inner lining of a vein is relatively insensitive to pain, drugs that can be irritating if given by another route can be given intravenously at a slow rate without causing pain. Drugs that can be diluted to reduce irritation can be given only intravenously, because the tissues around the other routes cannot accommodate the large volume. Figure 15-7 shows some commonly used IV sites.

Intravenous Administration

There are two types of IV administration. The first, an IV push, is an intravenous injection in which the prepared medication is drawn up into a syringe and administered over a short time. The amount of medication is usually a small volume pushed through an IV line that is already in place on the patient. Before a medication is pushed into the vein, the syringe is pulled slightly back to draw blood out (*aspirated*) to make sure that the tip of the needle is in the vein.

Intravenous sites

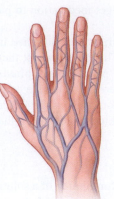 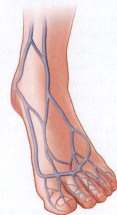

Several sites on the body are used to intravenously administer drugs: the veins of the antecubital area (in front of the elbow), back of the hand, and some of the larger veins of the foot. On some occasions, a vein must be exposed by a surgical cut.

FIGURE 15-7 Intravenous administration sites.

The second type of administration is an IV **infusion**. Infusions are given to overcome dehydration, to build up depleted blood volumes, and to aid in the administration of medications. An infusion allows a larger volume of solution to be given at a constant rate (which depends on the drug being administered). Infusions can be administered continuously or intermittently. Continuous infusions are used to administer larger volumes of solutions over several hours at a slow, constant rate. Intermittent infusions are used to administer a relatively small volume over a short time at specific intervals.

Risks

There are some risks involved in IV administration. A primary problem is that if there is an error in the dose, it is difficult to stop the drug, because it is very quickly dispersed throughout the body and will start working within a few minutes. Another risk is the possibility of infection anytime the skin is punctured. These risks are why the pharmacy technician must have the knowledge and skills to prepare sterile products correctly.

Sterile Products

Sterile products, such as IV solutions and TPN, are medications compounded using aseptic technique. Sterility is the focus for making these products, because of the way they are administered. When a patient takes a capsule or tablet, the body has built-in defense mechanisms to filter the product before it enters the patient's bloodstream. IV solutions and TPNs, in contrast, are administered directly, bypassing many of these natural defense mechanisms. Use of aseptic technique ensures that products being administered directly into a patient's veins are sterile and do not introduce any particles or *pyrogens*, such as bacteria, fungi, or viruses, which can produce a fever or cause sepsis, a blood infection.

Sterility

Sterility is freedom from bacteria and other microorganisms. Solutions to be injected must be sterile. A product is either sterile or nonsterile; products cannot be partially sterile. Sterility

---

intravenous parenteral injection in the vein.

intramuscular parenteral injection in the muscle.

subcutaneous parenteral injection in the skin.

intradermal parenteral injection in the dermis of the skin.

intrathecal parenteral injection in the spine.

infusion a relatively large volume of solution given at a constant rate.

pH describing the degree of acidity of a solution.

tonicity a state of normal tension of the tissues by virtue of which the parts are kept in shape, alert, and able to function properly.

isotonic containing the same tonicity concentration as red blood cells.

precipitate a solid that forms within a solution.

info Sterile Products

The word *aseptic* comes from the Latin prefix *a*, meaning "without," and the Latin word *sepsis*, meaning "infection." When we use the term *aseptic*, we are talking about making or compounding a product without infection, also referred to as *sterile*.

Certain characteristics are desired in an IV solution. Some of the characteristics can be seen by visual inspection, whereas others cannot. The solution must be clear—which should not be confused with colorless—to indicate that the drug added has dissolved completely. IV fat emulsions (which are mostly used in conjunction with TPN solutions) are an exception to this rule, because they look like milk. A solution must also be free of any visible particulate matter (such as rubber cores from vials).

cannot be determined visually, but proper aseptic technique can maintain the sterility of solutions, drugs, and supplies during preparation.

pH

The term **pH** is used to describe the degree of acidity of a solution. pH values range from 0 to 14, with values below 7 representing greater acidity of the solution; values above 7 represent less acidity or greater alkalinity. A solution having a pH of 7 is neither acidic nor alkaline; it is considered neutral. Plasma in the human body has a pH of about 7.4, and solutions should be around that same pH. pH is another characteristic that cannot be seen, but it can be tested after a drug is prepared.

Tonicity

A final characteristic that cannot be determined visually is **tonicity**, which refers to a state of normal tension of the tissues by virtue of which the body tissues and parts are kept in shape, alert, and able to function properly. An **isotonic** solution has the same concentration as red blood cells. Isotonic IV solutions minimize patient discomfort and damage to red blood cells. The stinging caused by either a hypertonic solution (which may cause shrinkage of red blood cells) or a hypotonic solution (which may cause swelling of red blood cells) is not experienced with an isotonic solution. IV solutions should be as close to isotonic as possible. A good reference point to remember is that 0.9% sodium chloride injection and 5% dextrose injection are both approximately isotonic.

Storage

When storing sterile products, try to avoid places that are exposed to extreme hot or cold temperatures. Exposing products to cold could cause some drugs in a solution to **precipitate**. Solutions that contain drugs should also not be exposed to high temperatures, because the heat may accelerate decomposition of the drug. IV solutions should be kept at room temperature or in a cool place.

Common Products

Many different types of solutions are commercially available; however, three types are most frequently used: sodium chloride injection, dextrose injection, and Ringer's injection. These three most resemble the plasma in the blood. Sodium chloride 0.9% and dextrose 5% are isotonic, as mentioned earlier, but both provide a source of fluid and electrolyte replacement. Ringer's injection can be modified with the addition of sodium lactate to produce lactated Ringer's injection. Ringer's solutions are primarily used for fluid replacement and as a source of electrolytes.

Compatibility

Not all drugs are compatible with each other. The incompatibility may be between two drugs or between a drug and an IV solution. The possibility of an unexpected or undesirable combination is relatively low compared with the number of IV admixtures prepared, but incompatibility is always possible. An incompatibility can lead to a patient not receiving the full therapeutic dose of a medication or, even worse, to an adverse reaction. Some incompatibilities, such as a color change or hazy appearance, can be detected. Precipitate can form in the solution, or an evolution of a gas may even be smelled.

Be aware that sometimes when drugs are combined, an expected and harmless visible change may occur. Reading the package insert or checking with the pharmacist can confirm the reason for a change in appearance. Other incompatibilities cannot be detected visually. If two drugs are mixed that are incompatible with each other, one drug can cause the degradation of the other drug. Many factors can affect the compatibility and stability of drugs in IV admixtures. The following subsections describe each of the factors that may cause incompatibility.

Workplace Wisdom The Handbook on Injectable Drugs

The Handbook on Injectable Drugs, by Lawrence A. Trissel, is an excellent reference book commonly used by pharmacy personnel when they are preparing sterile products. The text provides extensive compatibility information on the medications used in sterile products.

pH

pH is one of the most common causes of incompatibility. Combining two drugs that require two different pH values for the final solution can cause one or both drugs to either degrade or precipitate.

Light

Some drugs will start to break down and lose their therapeutic effect if exposed to light. Medications that are sensitive to light are supplied by the manufacturer in dark-colored (generally amber or brown), vials or ampules, and are dispensed in amber, light-sensitive bags.

Dilution

The concentration of a drug in solution may be a factor in its compatibility with other drugs. A problem can be avoided by ensuring that the drug in question is properly diluted before it is combined with the other drug.

Chemical Composition

The chemical composition of one drug can cause a change in the therapeutic effect of the other drug. When the two drugs combine, the new chemical combination may initiate adverse events.

Time

Most drugs start to degrade within a short time after being added to an IV solution.

Solutions

Some drugs require a specific solution or diluent to be used for reconstitution and further dilution. Choosing the wrong solution can cause the drug to break down more quickly, or can cause precipitate to form. Some drugs are packaged with a specific diluent for reconstitution; an example of this is Herceptin (trastuzumab).

Temperature

Heat increases the rate of most chemical reactions. Because the degradation of a drug in solution can be considered a chemical reaction, care must be taken to keep admixtures at a stable temperature. Some drugs remain more stable refrigerated than at room temperature. Some drugs, however, should never be refrigerated, because a precipitate can form. Not many experts recommend freezing drugs after reconstitution, and sometimes freezing actually reduces the stability of the drug.

Buffer Capacity

Buffer capacity is the ability of a solution to resist a change in pH when either an acidic or an alkaline substance is added to the solution. Many drugs contain buffers to increase their stability. IV solutions, in general, do not have high buffer capacities. Therefore, when a drug with a high buffer capacity is added, the resulting solution will have a pH closest to the drug added.

Order of Mixing

The order in which drugs are added to a solution may be a factor in compatibility. Drugs that are concentrated and combined may react to form precipitate, whereas those same drugs in diluted

---

buffer capacity the ability of a solution to resist a change in pH when either an acidic or an alkaline substance is added to the solution.

parenteral nutrition complex admixtures used to provide nutritional support to patients who are unable to take in adequate nutrients through the gastrointestinal tract.

chemotherapy drug therapy used to treat cancer and other diseases.

antineoplastics agents, such as medications, that prevent the growth of malignant cells.

---

solutions may be combined acceptably. This is very important when mixing parenteral nutrition solutions (discussed in detail later in this chapter). Electrolytes are commonly prescribed with phosphates, but this causes a problem with parenteral solutions if they are not mixed correctly. To avoid the problem, it is important to mix the solution well after each addition is made and to add the electrolytes last, after the phosphate has been well diluted.

> ❝ **Workplace Wisdom** **Calcium Gluconate**
>
> The additive calcium gluconate tends to precipitate easily when mixed with other electrolytes, so many facilities recommend adding this component last. ❞

Plastic

As mentioned earlier, some drugs are incompatible with the plastic container that will hold the solution. Certain chemicals in PVC plastic can leach out of the bag, or the drug may adhere to the bag. It is recommended that one use a non-PVC container for these particular drugs.

Filters

Filters, also mentioned earlier, represent a possible problem in effective administration of a drug to a patient. Filters can cause a reduction in concentration of the drug to be administered.

Minimizing Incompatibilities

To minimize incompatibilities, follow these general guidelines:

1. Use solutions promptly after preparation to ensure administration of the most stable product; drugs tend to degrade in a relatively short time. If a newly made admixture is not to be used immediately, it should be placed in the refrigerator.
2. Minimize the number of drugs added to a solution. As the number of drugs added increases, the chance of an incompatibility rises. It becomes increasingly difficult to find information on compatibilities when more than two drugs are added to a solution.
3. Check incompatibility resources to verify which drugs have a very high or very low pH. Most drugs are acidic, so combining them with a drug having a very high pH is more likely to result in an incompatibility.

The most often used resources for information on incompatibilities are the manufacturers' drug package inserts. The package inserts have a wealth of information about the drug. Each package insert is developed by the manufacturer and approved by the FDA when the drug is marketed. The package insert generally is not as good a reference for incompatibilities; however, many other excellent resources are available, such as incompatibility charts, articles in professional magazines, reference books, and the Internet. These can give you more accurate and up-to-date information.

Incompatibility charts list drugs that can and cannot be mixed in particular solutions. Some charts list drugs horizontally across the top and vertically down one side. You find one drug in the top list and the other drug in the side list; then you follow along the lines for the two constituents of the admixture from the top and the side until the lines intersect. A notation in the space where the lines intersect denotes whether the mixture is compatible. (One problem with this kind of chart is that it does not list the reason the two drugs are incompatible.)

The *American Journal of Health-System Pharmacy* frequently has detailed research articles on IV incompatibilities. Some very useful reference books are the *Handbook on Injectable Drugs* and the *Drug Facts and Comparisons*. Many pharmacy departments also maintain a file that categorizes drugs, to make looking up drug information quicker and easier. Some pharmacy computer systems screen IV admixture incompatibilities as well as drug interactions, alerting the pharmacist or pharmacy technician to these issues when the order is entered, before it is prepared.

Total Parenteral Nutrition

Parenteral nutrition solutions are complex admixtures used to provide nutritional support to patients who are unable to take in adequate nutrients through the gastrointestinal tract. These admixtures are composed of such things as fat, protein, dextrose, electrolytes, vitamins, and water. Parenteral solutions can be formulated and calculated to match an individual's nutritional requirements. Parenteral nutrition solutions are also referred to as *TPN solutions* or *TPNs*. Due to the complexity of and time needed to prepare a TPN solution, many pharmacies that compound a large number of parenteral nutrition solutions use high-speed compounders, automixers, or micromixers. These machines prepare complex solutions safely, accurately, and quickly. Automixers can hold from two to ten different components of the appropriate solution to be mixed. Figure 15-8 shows an intravenous (IV) solution.

These compounders consist of two principal parts: the pump module and the control module. The pump module is placed in the laminar flow hood along with the components, which hang from hangers in the hood. A disposable transfer set is hooked up to the machine, and then each tubing, or lead, is inserted into the source of each component. Each lead is color-coded to its specific spot on the compounder. All the leads come together at a junction and are connected to the final solution, which hangs from a hanger hooked up to an electronic scale that measures fluid by weight. This method is more accurate than measuring fluid volume, because it is not adversely affected by air entering the system.

The control module is the computer that controls how much of each component goes into the final solution. The control module is kept outside the laminar flow hood and is controlled by using the keypad to enter data for each component. Some pharmacies have installed a bar-code system in their automixers to detect when a lead is not correctly attached to the right station. The bar code is scanned against the lead tubing and then scanned at the corresponding station; if they match, the correct attachment is assured. If the bar codes do not match when scanned, an alarm sounds and an error display appears on the control module.

Parenteral nutrition solutions must be administered with caution. There are two ways to administer parenteral nutrition solutions intravenously. The first is through a central vein; the second is through a peripheral vein. They are most commonly infused into a large central vein that leads directly to the heart. The subclavian vein, under the collarbone, is used most often. The route of administration may affect the concentration of certain ingredients in the TPN solution.

Chemotherapy

The use of **chemotherapy** or **antineoplastics** to treat cancer began in the late 1940s. It was not until the late 1970s that health professionals became aware of potential hazards associated with the handling of antineoplastic drugs (see Figure 15-9). Concern has been mounting steadily over the risks incurred by pharmacy staff members who prepare and dispose of cytotoxic agents. Most of these agents were designed to damage the DNA of rapidly dividing cancer cells. However, because they lack specificity, any rapidly dividing cells in the body, whether normal or cancerous, become damaged. Repeated exposure to DNA-active drugs over a long period of time could potentially lead to irreparable DNA damage and might cause mutations, whether cancerous or not, to occur in unborn babies.

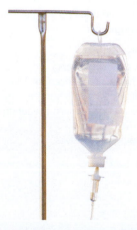

FIGURE 15-8 An example of an intravenous (IV) solution.
Source: © arztsamui/Fotolia

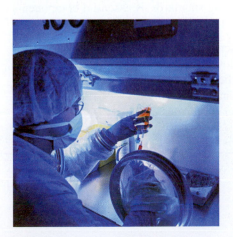

FIGURE 15-9 Preparing an antineoplastic drug.
Source: Colin Cuthbert/Science Source

Health problems caused by acute exposure to **cytotoxic** agents include sensitivity, coughing, dizziness, headaches, caustic vesicant-like marks, and eye reactions. These can be caused by direct skin contact, inhalation, ingestion, or accidental injection of agents. The long-term consequences of low-dose exposure to antineoplastic agents are also a serious concern. To date, there is no conclusive proof that the potential problems associated with preparing these drugs will occur in professionals who have minimal exposure from handling these products. Furthermore, there is neither a known threshold of danger nor a reliable method of monitoring health care workers' exposure.

❝ Workplace Wisdom   Cytotoxic Agents

Personnel working with or around cytotoxic agents should always wear appropriate personal protective equipment (PPE), such as gloves, gowns, masks, and face shields. ❞

Several agencies, including the Occupational Safety and Health Administration, the National Institutes of Health, and the ASHP, have issued guidelines regarding the safe handling of drugs. Common sense dictates that, regardless of the type or size of the facility, practical measures are necessary for employee protection. Any organization handling cancer chemotherapy or other hazardous drugs must accept the following standards as essential components of occupational safety:

- Written policies and procedures
- Employee education
- Certification
- Continuing education
- Proper aseptic technique

---

cytotoxic poisonous or destructive to cells.

- Access to medical attention for employees exposed to hazardous drugs
- Appropriate documentation of exposure incidents

Employees must be informed of the possible risks and controversies at the time of hire and should be given the option of reassignment at vulnerable periods in their lives. For women, these times may include documented pregnancy and during breast-feeding. Some pregnant women choose to continue handling chemotherapeutic agents, because they are confident that their workplace provides adequate protection. Some men may request a transfer away from drug preparation when planning for a family, because of the possible impact of cytotoxic agents on a male's sperm count.

An employee's competence and understanding of good work practices should be tested not only before hire, but also periodically throughout employment, through observation and written evaluation. Up-to-date policies and procedures for compounding sterile products should be written and available to all personnel involved in IV preparation. When policies and procedures are changed and additions or deletions are made, these updates should be communicated to all employees involved in drug preparation. The policies and procedures should address education and training requirements, competency evaluations, storage and handling of products and supplies, storage and delivery of final products, maintenance of facilities and equipment used in drug preparation, appropriate protective garments to be worn, validation of proper preparation technique, labeling of final products, documentation, quality control, and conduct for personnel working in the controlled area.

Basic Procedures

The following are basic procedures necessary for proper aseptic technique.

▌ Procedure 15-3

Dressing/Garbing Up

Pharmacy technicians should don PPE and perform actions in the anteroom in the following order:

1. Put on shoe covers.
2. Put on face mask and hair covers.
3. Aseptically wash hands (see Procedure 15.4).
4. Put on nonshedding gown with snug-fitting cuffs.
5. Put on eye shields (optional unless preparing hazardous drugs).
6. Put on sterile, powder-free gloves.

■ Procedure 15-4

Proper Hand Washing

The following procedure should be completed for preparing sterile products with aseptic technique:

1. Remove all jewelry, watches, and objects up to the elbow (acrylic nails and nail polish are also prohibited).
2. Adjust water to the appropriate temperature.
3. Using an approved disinfecting agent/cleanser, clear all four surfaces of each finger, all surfaces of hands, wrists, and arms up to the elbows in a circular motion. No part of your fingers, hands, wrists, or arms should touch the sink, faucet, or any other object; otherwise, it will be considered contaminated.
4. Rinse off all soap and residue, starting with the fingers and working down to the arms, by holding hands and arms upright and allowing the water to run off and drip to the elbow.
5. Dry fingers, hands, wrists, and arms with lint-free paper towels without touching anything.
6. Turn off the water faucet using a lint-free paper towel and avoid touching any surface.

■ Procedure 15-6

Reconstituting a Powder Vial

You must reconstitute a powdered vial in the primary engineering control (PEC) using proper aseptic technique.

1. Follow the proper procedures for dressing, hand washing, and cleaning the hood. Gather all necessary materials for the manipulation.
2. Swab all rubber tops with alcohol and allow the alcohol to dry.
3. Make sure that the needle is firmly attached to the syringe.
4. Draw up the correct amount of diluent needed for the reconstitution, using the procedure described in Procedure 15.5.
5. Pull back on the plunger to clear the neck of the syringe.
6. Remove the needle and replace it with a vented needle.
7. Carefully add diluent to the powdered vial.
8. Gently swirl or shake to dissolve. The powder must dissolve completely.
9. Change the vented needle back to a regular needle and carefully remove the desired amount from the vial.
10. Remove any air bubbles.
11. Withdraw the needle and carefully recap.

■ Procedure 15-5

Withdrawing from a Vial

This type of manipulation is the easiest and most common. It can be used in almost all manipulations in one form or another.

1. Follow the proper procedures for dressing, hand washing, and cleaning the hood.
2. Gather all necessary materials for the manipulation.
3. Swab all rubber tops with alcohol and allow the alcohol to dry.
4. Make sure that the needle is firmly attached to the syringe.
5. Pull the plunger back on the syringe to slightly less than the amount needed to be drawn up.
6. Remove the needle cap. Find the center of the stopper and position the needle with the bevel end up.
7. Holding the needle at approximately a 45-degree angle, insert the needle through the stopper.
8. Gently push the air from the syringe into the vial.
9. Invert the vial and release the plunger. The air in the vial will push the plunger out of the syringe on its own. If needed, pull back on the plunger until the desired amount is withdrawn.
10. Withdraw the needle and carefully recap.

■ Procedure 15-7

Removing Fluid from an Ampule

This procedure must be performed in the clear air space using proper aseptic technique.

1. Follow the proper procedures for dressing, hand washing, and cleaning the hood.
2. Gather all necessary materials for the manipulation.
3. Remove any fluid from the neck of the ampule, by tapping or thumping the top of the ampule.
4. Swab the neck of the ampule with alcohol.
5. Hold the ampule at a 20-degree angle toward the side of the hood.
6. Using your thumbs, apply pressure, on the indicated mark if provided, on the neck of the ampule, pressing away from yourself and towards the side of the hood.
7. Using a filter needle, withdraw the necessary volume.
8. Remove any air bubbles from the syringe.
9. Change the needle to a regular needle prior to injecting into a vial or bag.
10. Remove any air bubbles from the syringe.
11. Insert the needle into the additive port of the IV bag, or the appropriate vial, and slowly inject.

Summary

Sterile products must be prepared using proper aseptic technique to ensure that all products remain free of bacteria, fungi, pyrogens, infections, and other microorganisms. To ensure sterility, these products are prepared in laminar flow hoods (including horizontal flow hoods and biological safety cabinets) that contain HEPA filters.

Sterile products are most commonly administered parenterally through various administration sites, such as veins (IV) and muscle tissue (IM). Other sterile products, however, are administered via other routes; these include total parenteral nutrition, ophthalmic preparations, and otic preparations. Sterile product preparation can be a complex, high-risk process in the health care setting. Pharmacy technicians play an integral role in the procurement, storage, preparation, and distribution of these products. Training, education, and competency measurement are critical to ensure a safe chemotherapy process for patients and employees. Increasing pharmacy technicians' awareness of safety standards for preparing sterile products will ensure a safe work environment and reduce potential medication errors.

Chapter Review Questions

1. The following are the basic functions of the air flow in a laminar flow hood, *except* _____.
   a. preventing room air from entering the hood
   b. providing clean air in the hood
   c. suspending and removing contaminants introduced into the hood
   d. providing personnel with protection from hazardous agents

2. Laminar flow hoods may be used to perform the following procedures, *except* _____.
   a. reconstitution of powdered drugs
   b. preparation of ophthalmic solutions
   c. preparation of hazardous drugs
   d. filling of unit-dose syringes

3. What does HEPA stand for?
   a. huge effective particulate aerolizer
   b. high-efficiency particulate air
   c. highly effective particulate air
   d. high-efficiency particular airborne

4. What micron pore size is considered to be a sterilizing filter?
   a. 0.45
   b. 0.22
   c. 5
   d. 1

5. Which route of administration is given in the spine?
   a. intramuscular
   b. intradermal
   c. intrathecal
   d. intravenous

6. The desired characteristics of an intravenous solution include all of the following *except* _____.
   a. clarity (except fat emulsions)
   b. freedom from particulates
   c. hypotonicity
   d. sterility

7. When an intravenous solution is considered neutral, what is its pH?
   a. 0
   b. 7
   c. 14
   d. 7.4

8. The following are factors that can affect compatibility or stability of drugs, *except* _____.
   a. strength of the drug
   b. dilution of the drug in a solution
   c. chemical composition of the drugs
   d. pH of the drugs

9. The following are the essential components of occupational safety for any organization, *except* _____.
   a. proper aseptic technique
   b. continuing education
   c. DNA samples from all employees
   d. certification

10. Which of the following is *not* a form of personal protective equipment?
    a. scrubs
    b. gloves
    c. gown
    d. face shield

Critical Thinking Questions

1. Why are certain compounded medications required to be sterile?

2. Can aseptic technique guarantee 100% sterility? Why or why not?

3. What risks are posed to pharmacy technicians who prepare chemotherapy drugs?

Web Challenge

1. Go to the United States Pharmacopeia (USP) website at www.usp.org and search for information on USP 797. Select one of the risk categories and prepare a one-page summary of the information that you find.

2. Visit the American Society of Health-System Pharmacists (ASHP) website and search for their *Guidelines for Handling Hazardous Drugs*. Prepare a one-page summary of the information that you find: http://www.ashp.org

References and Resources

ASHP. "ASHP Guidelines on Quality Assurance for Pharmacy-Prepared Sterile Products." *American Journal of Health-System Pharmacists*. 57 (2000): 1150–1169. Print.

Attolio, R.M. "Caring Enough to Understand: The Road to Oncology Medication Error Prevention." *Hospital Pharmacy*. 31 (1996): 17–26. Print.

Bergemann, Don A. "Handling Antineoplastic Agents." *American Journal of Intravenous Therapy and Clinical Nutrition*. January 1983: 13–17. Print.

Blecher, C.S., Glynn-Tucker, E.M., McDiarmid, M., and Newton, S.A., eds. *Safe Handling of Hazardous Drugs*. Pittsburgh: ONS Publishing, 2003. Print.

Buchanan, E. *Sterile Compounding Facilities. Principles of Sterile Product Preparation*. Bethesda, MD: ASHP. 1995. Print.

Buchanan, E. Clyde and Philip J. Schneider. Compounding Sterile Preparations. 3rd ed. Bethesda, MD: ASHP. 2009. Print.

Dorr, R.T. *Practical Safety Precautions for Handling Cytotoxic Agents in Hospital Pharmacies*. Tucson, AZ: The University of Arizona Health Sciences Center, 1990. Print.

Hunt, Max L. Jr., ed. *Training Manual for Intravenous Admixture Personnel*. Chicago, IL: Precept Press, 1995. Print.

Johnston, Mike. *The Pharmacy Technician: Foundations and Practices*. 1st ed. Upper Saddle River, NJ: Prentice Hall Health, 2009. Print.

Johnston, Mike. *The Pharmacy Technician Series: Sterile Products*. Upper Saddle River, NJ: Prentice Hall Health, 2006. Print.

Johnston, Mike. Sterile Products and Aseptic Technique for the Pharmacy Technician. 2nd ed. Upper Saddle River, NJ: Pearson. 2011. Print

King, L.D. "Considering Compounding." *America's Pharmacist*. September 2002: 16–20. Print.

Talley, C. Richard. *Sterile Compounding in Hospital Pharmacies*. Bethesda, MD: American Journal of Health-System Pharmacists, 2003. Print.

Thompson, C.A. "USP Publishes Enforceable Chapter on Sterile Compounding." *American Journal of Health-System Pharmacists*. 60 (2003): 814–817. Print.

Trissel, Lawerence A. Handbook on Injectable Drugs. 17th ed. Bethesda, MD: AHP. 2013. Print.

SECTION III

Pharmacy
Calculations

16. Basic Math Skills

17. Measurement Systems

18. Dosage Calculations

19. Concentrations and Dilutions

20. Alligations

21. Parenteral Calculations

22. Business Math

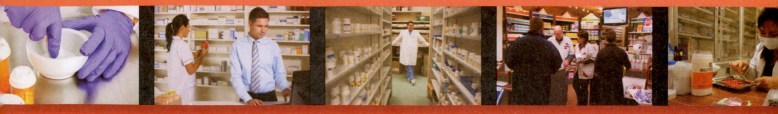

CHAPTER 16

Basic Math Skills

LEARNING OBJECTIVES

After completing this chapter, you should be able to:

- Determine the value of a decimal.

- Add, subtract, multiply, and divide decimals.

- Recognize and interpret Roman numerals.

- Change Roman numerals to Arabic numerals.

- Change Arabic numerals to Roman numerals.

- Describe the different types of common fractions.

- Add, subtract, multiply, and divide fractions.

- Define a ratio.

- Define a proportion.

- Solve math problems by using ratios and proportions.

KEY TERMS

common fraction, p. 268

complex fraction, p. 268

cross-multiplication, p. 272

decimal fraction, p. 264

denominator, p. 268

fraction line, p. 268

improper fraction, p. 268

numerator, p. 268

proper fraction, p. 268

proportion, p. 272

ratio, p. 270

Roman numeral, p. 266

simple fraction, p. 268

INTRODUCTION

Knowledge of basic arithmetic is essential for today's pharmacy technician. You must have basic skills in mathematics to understand and perform drug preparations. Nearly every aspect of drug dispensing requires a consideration of numbers. All advanced pharmacy calculations, which are explained throughout this text, rely on a solid understanding of basic math principles. This chapter will serve as a review of these general principles and as an assessment of your basic math skills.

Basic Math Pretest

The following diagnostic pretest will help guide your review and determine your strengths and weaknesses in basic math skills. The test should take approximately one hour. Decimals should be rounded to the thousandths. You will need scratch paper.

Circle the decimal with the highest value in each group.

1. 2.1, 1.87, 0.31

2. 1.37, 1.33, 1.89

3. 0.4, 0.44, 0.41

Circle the decimal with the lowest value in each group.

4. 40.4, 40.0, 40.003

5. 0.10, 0.11, 0.012

6. 7.01, 7.71, 7.76

Add the following decimals.

7. 2.25 + 5.89 = _____

8. 15.89 + 61.128 = _____

9. 4.004 + 4.24 + 0.007 = _____

Subtract the following decimals.

10. 6.25 − 0.80 = _____

11. 6.665 − 0.007 = _____

12. 18.64 − 2.11 = _____

Multiply the following decimals.

13. 1.4 × 2.16 = _____

14. 5.47 × 1.15 = _____

15. 4.4 × 3.875 = _____

Divide the following decimals.

16. 0.87 ÷ 0.2 = _____

17. 4.4 ÷ 0.3 = _____

18. 4.0 ÷ 3.5 = _____

19. A pharmacy had 20.9 gm of hydrocortisone powder in stock. Preparation of a prescription required 2.5 gm. How much hydrocortisone powder remained in stock after the prescription was made? _____

20. Missy Jones earned $725.78 last week. Her payroll deductions totaled $169.47. How much remained after payroll deductions? _____

21. Ray Wilhelm earned $371.64 for working 38 hours. How much did he earn per hour? _____

Identify the value of each of the following Roman numerals.

22. X _____

23. M _____

24. C _____

Give the equivalent Arabic numbers for each of the following Roman numerals.

25. XXIII _____

26. VIII _____

27. XLVII _____

Add the following fractions. Reduce to the lowest possible terms.

28. $\frac{2}{3} + \frac{1}{8} =$ _____

29. $\frac{4}{9} + \frac{1}{5} =$ _____

30. $\frac{2}{7} + \frac{1}{3} =$ _____

Subtract the following fractions. Reduce to the lowest possible terms.

31. $\frac{1}{8} - \frac{1}{12} =$ _____

32. $\frac{4}{4} - \frac{1}{8} =$ _____

33. $\frac{6}{7} - \frac{1}{8} =$ _____

Multiply the following fractions. Reduce to the lowest possible terms.

34. $\frac{1}{10} \times \frac{2}{3} =$ _____

35. $\frac{250}{1} \times \frac{6}{9} =$ _____

36. $\frac{5}{20} \times \frac{6}{40} =$ _____

Divide the following fractions. Reduce to the lowest possible terms.

37. $\frac{1}{15} \div \frac{1}{10} =$ _____

38. $\frac{2}{5} \div \frac{4}{6} =$ _____

39. $\frac{1}{7} \div \frac{2}{3} =$ _____

40. A jigsaw puzzle contains 5,240 pieces. Joan estimates that the puzzle is $\frac{1}{4}$ completed. How many pieces have been put in place in the puzzle? _____

41. There were 10,240 attendees at a conference. If $\frac{3}{4}$ of the audience were women, how many women attended the conference? _____

42. A computer sells for $3,000. The company charges $\frac{1}{5}$ of the purchase price as a maintenance fee. How much is the maintenance fee for this computer? _____

Solve the following problems for x.

43. $\frac{3}{x} = \frac{5}{20}$ _____

44. $\dfrac{15}{1} = \dfrac{30}{x}$ _____

45. $\dfrac{6}{12} = \dfrac{x}{144}$ _____

Convert as indicated.

46. 0.09 to a percent _____

47. $\dfrac{4}{5}$ to a percent _____

48. 37% to a fraction _____

49. $\dfrac{1}{3}$ to a ratio _____

50. $\dfrac{1}{500}$ to a ratio _____

TABLE 16-1 Decimals as Fractions

Decimal Number	Read	Fraction
3.2	Three and two-tenths	$3\dfrac{2}{10}$
0.9	Nine-tenths	$\dfrac{9}{10}$
0.04	Four-hundredths	$\dfrac{4}{100}$
2.15	Two and fifteen-hundredths	$2\dfrac{15}{100}$
0.357	Three hundred fifty-seven-thousandths	$\dfrac{357}{1000}$

Decimals

A clear understanding of decimals is critical to drug dispensing. A decimal point can mean the difference between a correct dose and a serious overdose or underdose. To determine the value of a decimal, you must first recognize that every digit in a decimal has a place value.

Decimals as Fractions

Decimals are fractions with a denominator that is a multiple of 10, such as 10, 100, and 1,000. The value of the denominator is determined by the number of digits to the right of the decimal point. **Decimal fractions** are written as a whole number with a zero and a decimal point in front of the value (Table 16-1). For example, $\dfrac{8}{10}$ represents the decimal 0.8, $\dfrac{8}{100}$ represents the decimal 0.08, and $\dfrac{8}{1,000}$ is equivalent to 0.008. It is often helpful to read decimals as their fraction equivalent.

Zeros placed either before or after a decimal number do not change the value of the number. For example, 0.8 could be written as 0.80, 00.8, or 0.80000; however, in health care professions such as pharmacy, you should always place a zero before the decimal point to avoid misreading a number. For example, .8 should be written as 0.8 to prevent it being read as the whole number 8. It is easy to miss a lone decimal point!

Key Points for Working with Decimals

Remember these points when working with decimals:

- Moving the decimal point one place to the right multiplies the number by 10 (Figure 16-1). For example, 80.65 becomes 806.5 when you move the decimal point one place to the right, and 80.65 × 10 = 806.5.
- Moving the decimal point one place to the left divides the number by 10. For example, 80.65 becomes 8.065 when you move the decimal point one place to the left, and 80.65 ÷ 10 = 8.065.
- When calculating dosages, you need to consider only three places to the right of the decimal (thousandths), because drug dosages are not measured beyond this point.

Practice Problems 16-1

Use the following problems to practice working with decimals.

Circle the number with the highest value in each group.

1. 2.45, 2.09, 2.54
2. 4.37, 6.05, 3.34
3. 1.4, 1.63, 11.19
4. 5.4, 3.86, 10.04
5. 6.23, 7.5, 12.19

Circle the number with the lowest value in each group.

6. 0.08, 0.15, 0.21
7. 7.53, 7.54, 7.05
8. 0.1, 0.32, 0.17
9. 1.125, 0.125, 1.1
10. 5.75, 2.95, 0.06

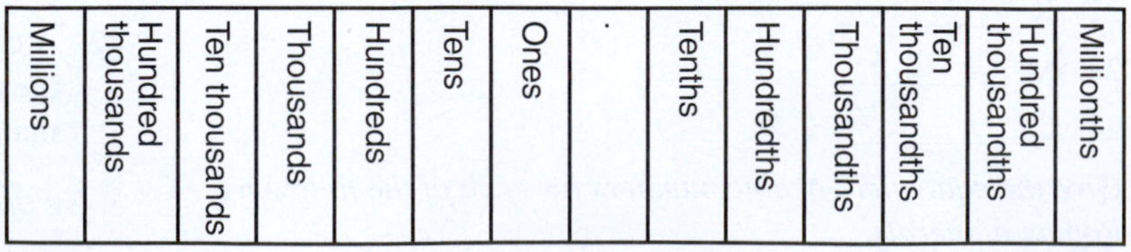

decimal fractions fractions written as a whole number with a zero and a decimal point in front of the value.

Millions	Hundred thousands	Ten thousands	Thousands	Hundreds	Tens	Ones	.	Tenths	Hundredths	Thousandths	Ten thousandths	Hundred thousandths	Millionths

FIGURE 16-1 Place value.

Rounding

As previously mentioned, in pharmacy practice, decimals are considered at most to the thousandth, or third decimal, place, which means that some numbers must be rounded to the nearest tenth, hundredth, or thousandth for practical application. When rounding decimals, you should assume that you are rounding to the thousandth, unless instructed otherwise. Consider the following three steps:

1. Determine the appropriate decimal place to round to.
2. Look at the number directly to the right of the decimal place being rounded to.
3. If the number is 0, 1, 2, 3, or 4, the answer should be rounded down by simply removing the additional decimal places. If the number is 5, 6, 7, 8, or 9, the answer should be rounded up by removing the additional decimal places and increasing the number in the decimal place being rounded to by 1.

EXAMPLE 16.1

Round 24.2609 to the nearest:

Thousandth 24.261

> There is a 0 in the thousandth place and a 9 to its right—round up.

Hundredth 24.26

> There is a 6 in the hundredth place and a 0 to its right—round down.

Tenth 24.3

> There is a 2 in the tenth place and a 6 to its right—round up.

Whole number 24

> There is a 4 in the ones' place and a 2 to its right—round down.

 Practice Problems 16-2

Use the following problems to practice rounding numbers.

Round 13.42891 to the nearest:

1. Thousandth
2. Tenth
3. Hundredth

Round 0.96235 to the nearest:

4. Whole number
5. Thousandth

Adding and Subtracting Decimals

Although adding and subtracting decimals is a simple and basic skill, you must still pay attention to avoid making careless errors that can lead to significant adverse effects when dispensing medications. Consider the following three steps when adding or subtracting decimals:

1. Write the numbers vertically and line up the decimal points.
2. Add zero placeholders, if necessary.
3. Add/subtract from right to left.

EXAMPLE 16.2

0.89 + 0.76 = _____

```
  0.89
+0.76    Add the 9 and 6 first, then the 8, the 7,
  1.65    and the 1 that was carried over.
```

So, 0.89 + 0.76 = 1.65

EXAMPLE 16.3

Add 1.25 and 0.8 and 1.32.

```
  1.25    Add a zero after the 8 as a placeholder to keep
  0.80    all of the numbers in line. Add the 5, 0, and 2;
+1.32    then the 2, 8, and 3; then the 1, 1, and the 1 that
  3.37    was carried.
```

So, 1.25 + 0.8 + 1.32 = 3.37.

EXAMPLE 16.4

4.45 − 2.25 = _____

```
  4.45
−2.25    Subtract the 5 from the 5, the 2 from the 4,
  2.20    and the 2 from the 4.
```

So, 4.45 − 2.25 = 2.20 or 2.2.

EXAMPLE 16.5

Subtract 0.43 from 0.67.

```
   0.67    In word problems, the "from" figure should
              always be on top.
−  0.43    Subtract the 3 from the 7, then subtract the 4
   0.24    from the 6.
```

So, 0.43 subtracted from 0.67 is 0.24.

Practice Problems 16-3

Use the following problems to practice adding and subtracting decimals.

Add the following decimals.

1. 3.34 + 9.98 = _____

2. 0.65 + 2.57 = _____

3. 3.065 + 30.30 = _____

4. 75.456 + 789.2 = _____

5. 5.002 + 7.28 + 0.012 = _____

Subtract the following decimals.

6. 4.44 − 3.34 = _____

7. 8.1 − 0.056 = _____

8. 1.99 − 0.5 − 0.5 = _____

9. 2.7 − 1.0024 = _____

10. 19.57 − 6.04 = _____

Multiplying Decimals

Multiplying decimals is a very simple process. The multiplication process is exactly the same as it is for whole numbers, with just one additional step at the end.

1. Multiply the numbers, ignoring the decimal points.
2. Add the total number of decimal places from the original numbers and then place a decimal point that number of places by moving from the right to the left of the answer. If there are not enough numbers for correct placement of the decimal point, add as many zeros as necessary.

EXAMPLE 16.6

1.8 × 2 = _____

$$
\begin{array}{r}
1.8 \\
\times\, 2 \\
\hline
36
\end{array}
$$ Multiply the top number by 2.

Now, add the total number of decimal point places in the original two numbers, which in this example is one.

Starting from the right, move one place to the left and add the decimal.

3.6

So, 1.8 × 2 = 3.6

Roman numerals letters and symbols used to represent numbers.

EXAMPLE 16.7

0.56 × 0.12 = _____.

$$
\begin{array}{r}
0.56 \\
\times\, 0.12 \\
\hline
112 \\
+\, 560 \\
\hline
672
\end{array}
$$

112   Multiply the top number by 2.
+ 560   Add a zero placeholder, then multiply the top number by 1.

Now, add the total number of decimal point places in the original two numbers—four.

Starting from the right, move four places to the left and add the decimal. A leading zero must be added, because the answer is only three digits.

0.0672

So, 0.56 × 0.12 = 0.0672.

 Practice Problems 16-4

Use the following problems to practice multiplying decimals.

Multiply the following decimals.

1. 5.56 × 6.78 = _____

2. 1.75 × 3.4 = _____

3. 5.88 × 1.25 = _____

4. 500 × 0.015 = _____

5. 1.3 × 4.7 = _____

Dividing Decimals

The division of decimal numbers requires several more steps than multiplication. This procedure must be done properly, and in order, to eliminate errors. The five steps you should follow to divide decimals are the following:

1. Place the dividend, or number to be divided, inside the division bracket.
2. Place the divisor, or number you are dividing by, outside the division bracket.
3. Change the divisor to a whole number by moving the decimal point all the way to the right.
4. Move the decimal point in the dividend the same number of places to the right as you did with the divisor.
5. Place a decimal point directly above the decimal in the dividend and divide as normal.

EXAMPLE 16.8

$10.08 \div 2.4 =$ _____

$2.4\overline{)10.08}$ Place the dividend in the division bracket and the divisor outside of it.

$24\overline{)100.8}$ Make the divisor a whole number by moving its decimal point to the right; then, adjust the decimal point in the dividend by the same number of places.

$$
\begin{array}{r}
4.2 \\
24\overline{)100.8} \\
\underline{96.} \\
48 \\
\underline{48} \\
0
\end{array}
$$

Place a decimal point above the decimal point in the dividend and divide as normal.

So, $10.08 \div 2.4 = 4.2$.

Practice Problems 16-5

Use the following problems to practice division of decimals.

Divide the following decimals.

1. $0.82 \div 0.2 =$ _____

2. $73 \div 13.40 =$ _____

3. $0.02 \div 0.006 =$ _____

4. $14.8 \div 2 =$ _____

5. $176 \div 2.2 =$ _____

Roman Numerals

Roman numerals are used in health care to designate drug quantities. In the Roman system, letters or symbols are used to represent numbers. The symbols and their position are critical to your understanding and accurate deciphering of them. Study the Roman numerals and their Arabic equivalents shown in Table 16-2.

Rules for Roman Numerals

When working with Roman numerals, you must observe specific rules to ensure accuracy.

Rule 1.   Roman numerals are never repeated more than three times in a row.

EXAMPLE 16.9

Five is not represented as IIII. It is represented as V.

TABLE 16-2 Roman Numerals

Roman Numeral	Arabic Equivalent
I	1
V	5
X	10
L	50
C	100
D	500
M	1,000

Rule 2.   When a Roman numeral is repeated, or when a smaller numeral follows a larger numeral, their values are added together.

EXAMPLE 16.10

$III = 1 + 1 + 1 = 3$
$XXXI = 10 + 10 + 10 + 1 = 31$
$MDC = 1,000 + 500 + 100 = 1,600$
$VII = 5 + 1 + 1 = 7$

Rule 3.   When a smaller numeral comes before a larger numeral, the one of lesser value is subtracted from the larger value.

EXAMPLE 16.11

$IV = 5 - 1 = 4$
$XL = 50 - 10 = 40$
$CM = 1,000 - 100 = 900$
$VL = 50 - 5 = 45$

Rule 4.   When a numeral of smaller value comes between two numerals of larger value, the subtraction rule is always applied first, and then the addition rule.

EXAMPLE 16.12

$XIV = 10 + (5 - 1) = 14$
$XLIX = (50 - 10) + (10 - 1) = 49$
$CVL = 100 + (50 - 5) = 145$

❝ Workplace Wisdom Roman Numerals

- Ones (I) may only be subtracted from fives (V) and tens (X).
- Tens (X) may only be subtracted from fifties (L) and hundreds (C).
- Hundreds (C) may only be subtracted from five hundreds (D) and thousands (M).

❞

Practice Problems 16-6

Use the following problems to practice converting Roman to Arabic numerals.

Convert the following Arabic numbers to Roman numerals.

1. 81 = _____

2. 367 = _____

3. 23 = _____

4. 2,650 = _____

5. 368 = _____

Convert the following Roman numerals to Arabic numerals.

6. XI = _____

7. CCXIX = _____

8. DCCCXCVIII = _____

9. MCMXCIV = _____

10. DC = _____

Perform the indicated operations. Record the answers in Arabic numerals.

11. CX + DC = _____

12. MMXL − DCCIX = _____

---

proper fraction a fraction in which the value of the numerator is smaller than the value of the denominator.

common fraction a fraction written with a numerator that is separated by a fraction line and positioned above a denominator.

denominator the bottom value of a fraction; placed beneath the fraction line.

numerator the top value of a fraction; placed above the fraction line.

fraction line a symbol representing the division of two values; placed between the numerator and the denominator of a fraction.

improper fraction a fraction in which the value of the numerator is larger than the value of the denominator.

simple fraction a proper fraction, with both the numerator and the denominator reduced to their lowest terms.

complex fraction a fraction in which both the numerator and the denominator are themselves common fractions.

13. XIII × IV = _____

14. LXVIII ÷ II = _____

15. IX − V = _____

Fractions

A **proper fraction** is a quantity that is less than a whole number. There are two types of fractions: **common fractions**, such as $\frac{1}{2}$ and $\frac{3}{8}$; and decimal fractions, such as 0.5 and 0.78. We covered decimal fractions earlier in this chapter, so this section focuses on common fractions.

A common fraction consists of three parts: the **denominator**, which is the number below the fraction line; the **numerator**, which is the number above the fraction line; and the **fraction line**, which separates the numerator and denominator. Technically, the fraction line represents a division symbol, because $\frac{1}{2}$ translates to $1 \div 2$.

$$\text{Numerator} \rightarrow \frac{1}{2} \leftarrow \text{Denominator}$$

The denominator indicates the total number of parts into which the whole is divided. The numerator indicates the number of parts used or being considered.

There are four basic types, or categories, of common fractions: proper fractions, improper fractions, simple fractions, and complex fractions.

Proper Fractions

A *proper fraction* is a fraction in which the value of the numerator is smaller than the value of the denominator.

EXAMPLE 16.13 PROPER FRACTIONS

$$\frac{1}{2} \qquad \frac{4}{8} \qquad \frac{9}{10}$$

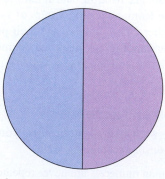

$\frac{1}{2}$ is a proper fraction

Improper Fractions

An **improper fraction** is a fraction in which the value of the numerator is larger than the value of the denominator.

EXAMPLE 16.14 IMPROPER FRACTIONS

$$\frac{3}{2} \qquad \frac{7}{3} \qquad \frac{12}{11}$$

Simple Fractions

When a proper fraction is reduced to its lowest terms, it is considered a **simple fraction**.

EXAMPLE 16.15 SIMPLE FRACTIONS

$\frac{4}{8}$ is a proper fraction, but it can be reduced by dividing both the numerator and the denominator by 4, producing $\frac{1}{2}$, which is a simple fraction. That is, it cannot be reduced any further.

Complex Fractions

A **complex fraction** is a fraction in which both the numerator and the denominator are themselves fractions.

EXAMPLE 16.16 COMPLEX FRACTIONS

$$\frac{\frac{1}{6}}{\frac{1}{4}}$$

Rules for Calculating with Fractions

Certain rules must be observed when working with, and calculating, fractions. Understanding of these rules is a necessary foundation; you will use them when you later learn to solve ratios and proportions and do most pharmacy calculations.

Rule: Reducing Fractions to Lowest Terms

To reduce a fraction to its lowest terms, thereby making it a simple fraction, you simply divide both the numerator and the denominator by the largest whole number that will go evenly into them both.

EXAMPLE 16.17 REDUCING FRACTIONS

Reduce $\frac{4}{16}$ to its lowest terms.

The largest whole number that will divide evenly into both 4 (the numerator) and 16 (the denominator) is 4.

$4 \div 4 = 1$

$16 \div 4 = 4$

So, $\frac{4}{16}$ reduces to $\frac{1}{4}$.

Rule: Converting Improper Fractions

Improper fractions can be converted to an equivalent whole number or mixed number by dividing the numerator by the denominator. Any remainder should be expressed as a proper fraction and reduced to lowest terms.

EXAMPLE 16.18 CONVERTING IMPROPER FRACTIONS

$\frac{21}{7}$ is an improper fraction.

If you divide the numerator (21) by the denominator (7), you get 3, a whole number.

$$\frac{21}{7} = 21 \div 7 = 3$$

$\frac{4}{3}$ is also an improper fraction.

The denominator (3) will go into the numerator (4) only one time, with a remainder of 1, which becomes $\frac{1}{3}$ when you place the remainder over the original denominator.

$$\frac{4}{3} = 4 \div 3 = 1\frac{1}{3}$$

Workplace Wisdom Converting Mixed Fractions

To convert a mixed fraction to an improper fraction, simply multiply the whole number by the denominator and add that number to the numerator. For example, $1\frac{2}{3}$ would be converted to $\frac{5}{3}$, by multiplying 1×2, which equals 3, and then adding that to the numerator, which is 2. Upon adding 3 to the numerator (3 + 2), the new numerator becomes 5, the denominator stays the same, and the whole number can be removed.

Rule: Adding and Subtracting Fractions

To add or subtract fractions, all the fractions must have the same denominator. If necessary, each fraction can be converted to a fraction with the least common denominator; then, you can add or subtract the numerators.

EXAMPLE 16.19 ADDING FRACTIONS

$$\frac{1}{4} + \frac{1}{4} = \rule{2cm}{0.4pt}$$

Because both fractions have the same denominator, simply add the numerators (1 + 1) and place this over the common denominator.

$$\frac{1}{4} + \frac{1}{4} = \frac{2}{4}$$

$\frac{2}{4}$ can then be reduced to $\frac{1}{2}$.

$$\frac{1}{2} + \frac{1}{3} = \rule{2cm}{0.4pt}$$

These two fractions have different denominators, so the least common denominator must first be determined, which in this case is 6.

Now, both fractions must be converted to contain a denominator of 6.

$$\frac{1}{2} \times \frac{3}{3} = \frac{3}{6}$$

$$\frac{1}{3} \times \frac{2}{2} = \frac{2}{6}$$

$$\frac{3}{6} + \frac{2}{6} = \frac{5}{6}$$

EXAMPLE 16.20 SUBTRACTING FRACTIONS

$$\frac{9}{10} - \frac{7}{10} \underline{\hspace{2cm}}$$

These two fractions have the same denominator, so you can subtract the numerators $(9 - 7)$ to get 2.

$$\frac{9}{10} - \frac{7}{10} = \frac{2}{10}$$

$\frac{2}{10}$ can be further reduced to $\frac{1}{5}$.

$$\frac{4}{5} - \frac{1}{10} = \underline{\hspace{2cm}}$$

Because these two fractions do not have the same denominator, the least common denominator must be established, which in this case is 10.

$$\frac{4}{5} \times \frac{2}{2} = \frac{8}{10}$$

$$\frac{8}{10} - \frac{1}{10} = \frac{7}{10}$$

Rule: Multiplying Fractions

When multiplying fractions, multiply the numerators by the numerators and then the denominators by the denominators. Reduce to lowest terms.

EXAMPLE 16.21 MULTIPLYING FRACTIONS

$$\frac{4}{9} \times \frac{6}{8} = \underline{\hspace{2cm}}$$

$4 \times 6 = 24$

$9 \times 8 = 72$

So, $\frac{4}{9} \times \frac{6}{8} = \frac{24}{72}$, which can be reduced to $\frac{1}{3}$.

---

ratio the expression of a relationship of two numbers, separated by a colon (:).

proportion two, or more, equivalent ratios or fractions that both represent the same value.

Rule: Dividing Fractions

To divide fractions, invert (flip upside down) the divisor, and then multiply the two fractions. Reduce to lowest terms.

EXAMPLE 16.22 DIVIDING FRACTIONS

$$\frac{2}{8} \div \frac{3}{7} = \underline{\hspace{2cm}}$$

$$\frac{2}{8} \times \frac{7}{3} = \underline{\hspace{2cm}}$$

$2 \times 7 = 14$

$8 \times 3 = 24$

So, $\frac{2}{8} \div \frac{3}{7} = \frac{14}{24}$, which can be reduced to $\frac{7}{12}$.

❝ Workplace Wisdom Reciprocals

The inverted fraction used when dividing fractions is referred to as the *reciprocal*. ❞

Practice Problems 16-7

Calculating Fractions

Add the following fractions.

1. $\frac{1}{6} + \frac{3}{4} + \frac{2}{12} = \underline{\hspace{2cm}}$

2. $\frac{2}{3} + \frac{1}{2} + \frac{1}{4} = \underline{\hspace{2cm}}$

3. $1\frac{3}{8} + 1\frac{4}{5} = \underline{\hspace{2cm}}$

Subtract the following fractions.

4. $\frac{5}{16} - \frac{1}{8} = \underline{\hspace{2cm}}$

5. $6\frac{5}{12} - 3\frac{2}{12} = \underline{\hspace{2cm}}$

6. $\frac{1}{2} - \frac{1}{5} = \underline{\hspace{2cm}}$

Multiply the following fractions.

7. $\frac{3}{8} \times \frac{5}{12} = \underline{\hspace{2cm}}$

8. $\frac{2}{3} \times \frac{5}{8} = \underline{\hspace{2cm}}$

9. $1\frac{1}{5} \times \frac{2}{3} = \underline{\hspace{2cm}}$

Divide the following fractions.

10. $\dfrac{7}{8} \div \dfrac{5}{6} =$ _____

11. $\dfrac{1}{4} \div \dfrac{1}{2} =$ _____

12. $7 \div \dfrac{2}{3} =$ _____

Ratios and Proportions

Ratios and proportions are basic math skills that can be effective in solving the majority of pharmacy calculations. The rest of the chapters in this book rely heavily on a solid comprehension of working with ratios and proportions, so it is very important that you understand the following information.

Ratios

A **ratio** expresses the relationship of two numbers and is separated by a colon (:), just as a fraction expresses the relationship of two numbers and is separated by a fraction line. For example, if an ointment contained 1 gm of active ingredient for every 10 gm of ointment base, a relationship, or ratio, is established regarding the amount of active ingredient compared to the amount of inactive ingredient (1:10).

EXAMPLE 16.23 RATIOS AS FRACTIONS

1:2 is a ratio and is read as "1 to 2."

This ratio can be rewritten as a fraction, $\frac{1}{2}$, read as "1 over 2."

The ratio 3:8 can be rewritten as the fraction $\frac{3}{8}$.

 Practice Problems 16-8
Ratios as Fractions

Convert the following ratios to fractions and reduce to lowest terms.

1. 4:6 = _____

2. 6:8 = _____

3. 1:25 = _____

Fractions can just as easily be converted to ratios. Rewrite the numerator as the first number followed by a colon (:) and then the denominator as the second number in the ratio.

EXAMPLE 16.24 FRACTIONS AS RATIOS

The fraction $\frac{5}{8}$, stated as 5 over 8, can be restated as 5:8, or 5 to 8.

 Practice Problems 16-9
Fractions as Ratios

Convert the following fractions to ratios.

1. $\dfrac{4}{5} =$ _____

2. $\dfrac{9}{10} =$ _____

3. $\dfrac{1}{400} =$ _____

To convert a ratio to a percentage, rewrite the ratio as a fraction, divide the numerator by the denominator, then multiply by 100, and add the percentage sign (%) to the answer.

EXAMPLE 16.25 RATIOS AS PERCENTAGES

1:4 = _____%

$1:4 = \dfrac{1}{4}$

$1 \div 4 = 0.25$

$0.25 \times 100 = 25$

1:4 = 25%

Practice Problems 16-10
Ratios as Percentages

Convert the following ratios to percentages.

1. 6:8 = _____

2. 1:25 = _____

3. 1:250 = _____

4. 1:10 = _____

5. 4:16 = _____

Proportions

Proportions are two, or more, equivalent ratios or fractions that both represent the same value. The majority of pharmacy calculations are performed by establishing a proportion and then solving for the unknown. This can be illustrated by referring back to our previous example of the ointment that contains 1 gm of active ingredient per 10 gm of ointment base. If you know that you need 10 gm of active ingredient, you can use a proportion to determine the amount of inactive ointment base required.

Proportions are written as two ratios or fractions separated by a double colon symbol (::). The double colon symbol translates to "equals" or "is equal to," so the equal sign (=) is sometimes used in place of the double colon symbol.

info

Percentages

A percentage is another format used to represent a ratio, as a fraction of 100. Percentages are noted by using the percent sign (%). For example, 5% is equivalent to:

- 5/100
- 0.05
- 1:20

To convert a percentage to a fraction, simply remove the percent sign and place the number over 100. To convert it to a decimal, divide the percent number by 100. To convert a percentage to a ratio, change the ratio to a fraction (over 100) and then reduce it to lowest terms.

When working with pharmacy calculations, it is imperative that you are comfortable converting back and forth between decimals, fractions, percentages, and ratios.

EXAMPLE 16.26 SAMPLES OF PROPORTIONS

1:4::2:8

2:3 = 6:9

$\dfrac{3}{5} :: \dfrac{6}{10}$

$\dfrac{4}{7} = \dfrac{8}{14}$

Solving for X

Cross-multiplication is a critical principle to understand in solving pharmacy calculations. Once you have set up two ratios or fractions in relationship to each other as a proportion, you can cross-multiply to solve for the unknown (X).

There are two approaches to using cross-multiplication to solve for X. You should practice using both methods and then use the approach you are most comfortable with.

In the first approach, you set the proportion up as fractions, making sure to keep units of measurement the same across from one another. Cross-multiply along the diagonal with two numbers, and divide that value by the remaining number to solve for X.

EXAMPLE 16.27 SOLVING FOR X

2:10::X:30

First, set up the proportion as fractions.

cross-multiplication   a principle used in solving pharmacy calculations; you set up two ratios or fractions in relationship to each other as a proportion and solve for the unknown variable.

$\dfrac{2}{10} = \dfrac{X}{30}$

Multiply along the diagonal with two numbers (2 and 30).

$2 \times 30 = 60$

Divide that value by the remaining number to solve for X.

$60 \div 10 = 6$

$X = 6$

So, 2:10::6:30

In the second approach, you again set the proportion up as fractions, making sure to keep units of measurement the same across from one another. This time, however, you cross-multiply along both diagonals to establish an equation, which you can solve for X.

EXAMPLE 16.28 SOLVING FOR X

3:5::12:X

First, set up the proportion as fractions.

$\dfrac{3}{5} = \dfrac{12}{X}$

Then, cross-multiply both diagonals to establish an equation.

$3 \times X = 3X$

$5 \times 12 = 60$

$3X = 60$

Now, you can use basic algebra to solve for X. In this example, that is done by dividing both sides of the equation by 3.

$\dfrac{3X}{3} = \dfrac{60}{3}$

$X = 20$

So, 3:5::12:20

Practice Problems 16-11
Solving for X

Using cross-multiplication, solve for X.

1. 3:9::X:27

2. 233:1::X:15

3. 4:9 = X:81

4. X:10::25:50

5. 12.5:X = 75:600

RQWQCQ

Consider the following tips for working with word problems.

RQWQCQ is a useful strategy when solving math word problems. Each of the letters in RQWQCQ stands for a step in the strategy.

Read—First, read the entire problem to fully understand it. You may find it helpful to read the problem out loud, visualize the problem in your mind, or even draw a picture of the problem.

Question—Determine the question to be answered in the problem. Often the question is directly stated. When it is not stated, you will have to identify the question to be answered.

Write—List all the facts provided in the problem. Then, cross out any facts presented in the problem that are not needed to answer the question. Often, you will not need all the facts presented in the problem to answer the question; the extraneous details can simply cause confusion.

Question—Ask yourself, "What computations must I do to answer the problem?"

Compute—Set up the problem on paper and do the computations. Check your computations for accuracy and make any needed corrections.

Question—Look at your answer and then ask yourself, "Is this answer possible?" You may find that your answer is not possible, because it does not fit the facts presented in the problem. If this happens, go back through the steps of RQWQCQ until you arrive at an answer that is possible.

PROFILE IN PRACTICE

Paul is currently a pharmacy technician student. His grades are good, but he is frustrated with pharmacy calculations. He wonders why he must learn this material, since he assumes the computers handle all of the calculations anyways.

▸ *Why is it important for students, like Paul, to have a strong knowledge of math to practice as pharmacy technicians?*

Summary

Although none of the material covered in this chapter should have been new to you, sometimes, you need a solid, basic math review. As you prepare to learn and understand the calculations performed in the pharmacy, remember that all the calculations you will learn are based on the basic skills covered in this chapter. If you find that you are still having difficulty with the problems presented in this chapter, you should continue to go over this material before proceeding to the other chapters in Section III.

Chapter Review Questions

Carry answers to three decimal places and round to two places. Express fractions in lowest terms.

Circle the decimal with the highest value in each group.

1. 4.1, 4.01, 4.001

2. 3.0, 1.5, 2.8

3. 0.2, 0.5, 0.8

4. 0.2, 0.13, 0.26

5. 3.7, 3.6, 2.35

Circle the decimal with the lowest value in each group.

6. 1.233, 1.844, 1.999

7. 2.5, 1.8, 10.8

8. 0.05, 0.5, 0.115

9. 14.03, 16.03, 12.01

10. 1.25, 3.5, 1.26

Complete the operations indicated.

11. $1.233 + 12.01 =$ _____

12. $40.25 - 16.37 =$ _____

13. $0.65 \times 10.467 =$ _____

14. $18.6 \times 3.42 =$ _____

15. $1.25 \div 0.5 =$ _____

Convert to Roman numerals.

16. 7 _____

17. 25 _____

18. 89 _____

19. 67 _____

20. 472 _____

Convert to Arabic numbers.

21. XL _____

22. MMLV _____

23. LXXXVI _____

24. MCMXCV _____

25. LXXVIII _____

Complete the operations indicated.

26. $\dfrac{2}{4} + \dfrac{1}{3} =$ _____

27. $3\dfrac{1}{5} + 2\dfrac{2}{10} =$ _____

28. $\dfrac{4}{5} - \dfrac{1}{10} =$ _____

29. $\dfrac{6}{8} - \dfrac{1}{4} =$ _____

30. $\dfrac{5}{6} + \dfrac{3}{30} + \dfrac{3}{5} =$ _____

31. $\dfrac{2}{3} \times \dfrac{5}{8} =$ _____

32. $4\dfrac{2}{3} \times 3 =$ _____

33. $\dfrac{1}{15} \times \dfrac{6}{30} =$ _____

34. $4 \div \dfrac{3}{4} =$ _____

35. $\dfrac{25}{100} \times \dfrac{6}{10} =$ _____

36. $\dfrac{7}{8} \div \dfrac{5}{6} =$ _____

37. $8 \div \dfrac{1}{3} =$ _____

38. $\dfrac{3}{4} \div 20 =$ _____

39. $6\dfrac{1}{2} + 3\dfrac{2}{4} =$ _____

40. $4\dfrac{3}{8} \div 2\dfrac{2}{4} =$ _____

Solve the following word problems.

41. A patient is to take a medication that contains 0.25 mg per tablet. The patient is to take one tablet every two hours until pain is relieved. If it takes five tablets to obtain the desired effect, the patient took how many milligrams of drug? _____

42. Human blood has a pH of 7.4. A urine test shows a pH of 4.6 for the patient's urine. What is the difference in pH between the blood and the urine? _____

43. A patient takes 250 mg of drug twice a day for seven days. What is the total dose? _____

44. A patient is taking 0.5 oz. of cough syrup per dose. If the bottle contains 20.5 oz., how many doses are in the bottle? _____

45. The cornerstone of the hospital shows the date when the hospital was built as MCMLXV. When was the hospital built? _____

46. A child is to receive X grains of a medication that is available in V-grain tablets. How many tablets should the child receive? _____

47. A laboratory technician uses $\frac{1}{4}$ oz, $\frac{2}{3}$ oz, and $\frac{3}{8}$ oz of solution to prepare an IV admixture. How much total solution does she use? _____

48. A pediatric nurse measures a one-year-old child and finds that the child is $40\frac{1}{4}$-inch tall. At birth the child was $20\frac{3}{4}$-inch tall. How much did the child grow in one year? _____

49. A pharmacy technician uses a 480-mL bottle of cough syrup to fill unit-dose vials. If each vial holds $\frac{1}{15}$ of the volume of the stock bottle of cough syrup, how many milliliters of cough syrup are in each vial? _____

50. How many $\frac{1}{3}$ gm doses can be dispensed from a stock bottle containing 12 gm? _____

References and Resources

Hegstad, Lorrie N. and Wilma Hayek. *Essential Drug Dosage Calculations*. 4th ed. Upper Saddle River, NJ: Pearson, 2001. Print.

Johnston, Mike. *Pharmacy Calculations: The Pharmacy Technician Series*. Upper Saddle River, NJ: Pearson, 2005. Print.

Lesmeister, Michelle Benjamin. *Math Basics for the Healthcare Professional*. 4th ed. Upper Saddle River, NJ: Pearson, 2013. Print.

Mikolah, Alan A. *Drug Dosage Calculations for the Emergency Care Provider*. 2nd ed. Upper Saddle River, NJ: Prentice Hall, 2003. Print.

Olsen, June, Anthony Giangrasso, and Dolores Shrimpton. *Medical Dosage Calculations*. 10th ed. Upper Saddle River, NJ: Pearson, 2011. Print.

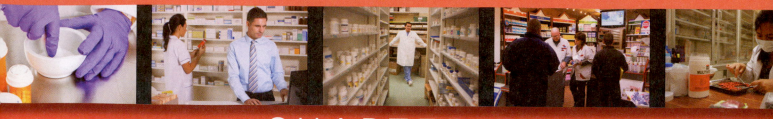

CHAPTER 17

Measurement Systems

LEARNING OBJECTIVES

After completing this chapter, you should be able to:

- List the three fundamental systems of measurement.
- List the three primary units of the metric system.
- Define the various prefixes used in the metric system.
- Recognize abbreviations used in measurements.
- Explain the use of international units and milliequivalents.
- Convert measurements between the household system and the metric system.
- Convert measurements between the apothecary system and the metric system.
- Perform temperature conversions.

KEY TERMS

apothecary system, p. 280
avoirdupois system, p. 280
Celsius, p. 284
Fahrenheit, p. 284
grain, p. 280
gram, p. 277
household system, p. 280
international units (IU), p. 279
liter, p. 277
meter, p. 277
metric system, p. 277
milliequivalent (mEq), p. 279

INTRODUCTION

Three fundamental systems of measurement are used to calculate dosages: the metric, apothecary, and household systems. Pharmacy technicians must understand each system and how to convert from one system to another. Most prescriptions are written using the metric system.

---

metric system the international and scientific standard system of measurement; based on the meter, the gram, and the liter.

meter metric system's primary unit of length.

liter metric system's primary unit of volume.

gram metric system's primary unit of weight.

The Metric System

The need for an international measurement system was recognized more than 300 years ago. In 1670, Gabriel Mouton proposed a measurement system based on the length of one minute of arc of a great circle of the earth. In 1671, Jean Picard suggested the length of a pendulum beating seconds as the unit of length. Other proposals were also made, but it was more than 100 years before any decisions were made.

In 1790, the National Assembly of France asked the French Academy of Sciences to deduce an invariable standard for all the measures and all the weights. The commission developed the **metric system**, a system that was both simple and scientific. The unit of length was set as a portion of the earth's circumference. Measures for volume and mass were derived from the unit of length, so that all units of measurement in the system would be related.

The metric system uses decimals to indicate tenths, hundredths, and thousandths; larger and smaller versions of each unit were created by multiplying or dividing the basic units by 10. This feature provides great convenience to users of the system. Similar calculations in the metric system can be performed simply by shifting the decimal point; therefore, the metric system is a *base 10* or *decimal* system.

The metric system is the most widely used system of measurement in the world today. It is more accurate than the household and apothecary systems and is preferred for health care applications, because it is more precise and more common.

The metric system is based on these three primary units:

- **meter**—measures length
- **liter**—measures volume
- **gram**—measures weight

Prefixes are added, when necessary, to indicate larger or smaller units. The four prefixes most commonly used in pharmaceutical calculations are the following:

- kilo- = 1,000, or one thousand of the base unit
- centi- = 0.01, or one-hundredth of the base unit
- milli- = 0.001, or one-thousandth of the base unit
- micro- = 0.000001, or one-millionth of the base unit

Tables 17-1 and 17-2 show the metric measurements and abbreviations you will encounter most frequently in everyday pharmacy practice.

TABLE 17-1 Metric Units of Measurement

Length	Weight	Volume
meter (m)	gram (g or gm)	liter (l or L)
centimeter (cm)	milligram (mg)	milliliter (ml or mL)
millimeter (mm)	microgram (mcg)	
	kilogram (kg or Kg)	

Remember: Although less frequently used, a cubic centimeter (cc) is sometimes used to denote a milliliter.

TABLE 17-2 Metric System Prefixes with Standard Measures

	Unit	Abbreviation	Equivalents
Weight	gram	g or gm	1 gm = 1,000 mg
	milligram	mg	1 mg = 1,000 mcg = 0.001 gm
	microgram	mcg	1 mcg = 0.001 mg = 0.000001 gm
	kilogram	kg	1 kg = 1,000 gm
Volume	liter	L or l	1 L = 1,000 mL
	milliliter	mL or ml	1 mL = 1 cc = 0.001 L
	cubic centimeter	cc or mL	1 cc = 1 mL = 0.001 L
Length	meter	m	1 m = 100 cm = 1,000 mm
	centimeter	cm	1 cm = 0.01 m = 10 mm
	millimeter	mm	1 mm = 0.001 m = 0.1 cm

Guidelines for Metric Notation

Use the following guidelines when working with metric notations.

1. Always place the number before the abbreviation. For example, write:
   4 mg, not mg 4
2. Place a zero to the left of the decimal when the decimal is less than 1. For example, write:
   Synthroid 0.2 mg, not Synthroid .2 mg
   This is a critical rule, as it will help prevent confusion and possible dosage error; in this case, 2 mg might be given if the decimal is not noticed.
3. Never place a zero to the right of the decimal place when you have a whole number. For example, write:
   A patient weighs 20 kg, not 20.0 kg
4. Always use decimals to reflect fractions when using the metric system. For example, write:
   6.5 mL, not 6 1/2 mL
5. Avoid unnecessary (trailing) zeros. For example, write:
   3.2 gm, not 3.20000 gm
6. When converting from small units to larger units, make sure your number decreases proportionally. For example, write:
   2,000 mg = 2 gm

7. When converting from large units to smaller units, make sure your number increases proportionately. For example, write:
   20 kg = 20,000 g

8. When multiplying metric values by multiples of 10, move the decimal point one place to the right for each zero in the multiplier.

9. When dividing metric values by multiples of 10, move the decimal point one place to the left for each zero in the divisor.

10. When in doubt, do not guess about the correct meaning. Always check when clarification is needed. A one-decimal-place error in dosing can be fatal to a patient!

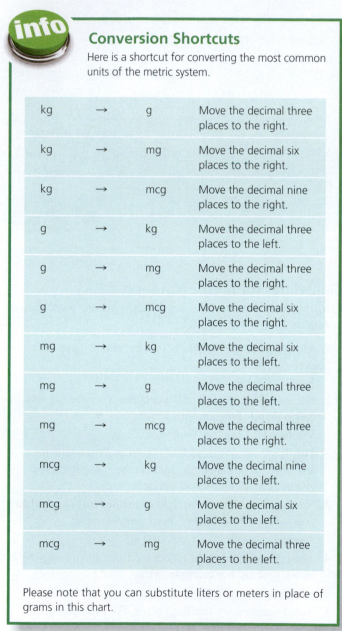

info Conversion Shortcuts

Here is a shortcut for converting the most common units of the metric system.

kg	→	g	Move the decimal three places to the right.
kg	→	mg	Move the decimal six places to the right.
kg	→	mcg	Move the decimal nine places to the right.
g	→	kg	Move the decimal three places to the left.
g	→	mg	Move the decimal three places to the right.
g	→	mcg	Move the decimal six places to the right.
mg	→	kg	Move the decimal six places to the left.
mg	→	g	Move the decimal three places to the left.
mg	→	mcg	Move the decimal three places to the right.
mcg	→	kg	Move the decimal nine places to the left.
mcg	→	g	Move the decimal six places to the left.
mcg	→	mg	Move the decimal three places to the left.

Please note that you can substitute liters or meters in place of grams in this chart.

---

international units measurement of a drug in terms of its action, not its physical weight.

milliequivalent (mEq) unit of measurement based on the number of grams of a drug in 1 mL of a normal solution.

Practice Problems 17-1

Write the following metric measures using correct abbreviations denoting units of measure.

1. seven micrograms _____
2. two-tenths of a milligram _____
3. nine grams _____
4. five-hundredths of a kilogram _____
5. ten milliliters _____
6. three and one-tenth liters _____
7. two-tenths of a microgram _____
8. five hundred milligrams _____
9. six-hundredths of a gram _____
10. one hundred milliliters _____
11. thirty-one liters _____
12. seven-tenths of a microgram _____
13. eight-hundredths of a milligram _____
14. three kilograms _____
15. four and one-tenth milliliters _____
16. three hundred fifty liters _____
17. seven and four-tenths grams _____
18. one thousand micrograms _____
19. fifteen hundred milligrams _____
20. one and one-fifth kilograms _____

Convert the following metric units.

21. 30 mcg = _____ mg
22. 100 mg = _____ gm
23. 0.6 gm = _____ kg
24. 2.5 kg = _____ gm
25. 0.22 gm = _____ mg
26. 1,500 mg = _____ mcg
27. 1,000 mcg = _____ mg
28. 15.6 L = _____ mL
29. 1,500 mL = _____ L
30. 0.2008 kg = _____ mcg
31. 2,650 mL = _____ L
32. 988 mg = _____ gm
33. 0.0125 gm = _____ mg

34. 7,550 mL = _____ L

35. 0.789 L = _____ mL

36. 100 mcg = _____ gm

37. 6,000,000 gm = _____ kg

38. 1.18 L = _____ mL

39. 2,000 gm = _____ mcg

40. 1 L = _____ mL

PROFILE IN PRACTICE

Danielle works at a high-volume pharmacy and sometimes feels overwhelmed. When translating a prescription for data entry, she mistook 10 mcg for 10 mg.

▶ *What effect will Danielle's mistake, if not caught, have on the patient?*

Practice Problems 17-2

When solving the following problems, convert all measurements to the same units.

1. A newborn weighs 2,800 gm. What is her weight in kilograms? _____

2. A patient receives a prescription for 2.5 gm of an antibiotic. The strength of tablets on the shelf is 250 mg. How many tablets should the patient take? _____

3. A patient is to receive 1.5 gm of cephalexin per day divided into three equal doses.

   a. If the capsules are available in 100-mg, 250-mg, and 500-mg strengths, which dosage should be used? _____

   b. If the dosage is increased to 2 gm per day divided into four equal doses, what dosage should be used? _____

4. A pharmacy technician must combine four partially filled bottles of powder into one. How many grams of powder does she have if the bottles contain 240 gm, 0.45 kg, 2,300 mg, and 22,000 mcg? _____

5. How many grams of aminophylline would be required to prepare 100 capsules of 7.5 mg each? _____

6. How many 180-mL bottles can be filled with 6.5 L of cough syrup? _____

7. A technician is preparing a compound. The prescription requires 350 mg of dextrose, 500 mg of sodium, and 150 mcg of potassium per 1,000 mL. What is the total weight in grams of the dry ingredients? _____

8. If the total dose is 0.85 gm and the drug has to be given in four equal doses, what is the amount of each dose in milligrams? _____

9. A wholesaler is selling 250 gm of a compounding powder for $6.79. How many grams can you get for $40? _____

10. You have acetaminophen tablets in 500-mg strength. If the prescription calls for 250 mg twice daily for five days, how many tablets would you give? _____

International Units

A number of drugs, such as insulin, heparin, and penicillin, are measured in **international units (IU)**. Therefore, pharmacy technicians must be able to recognize unit dosages and their official abbreviations. An IU measures a drug in terms of its action, not its physical weight.

When writing IUs, do not use commas in the unit value unless it has at least five numbers (e.g., 25,000 units). Remember to write out the word *unit*(s) and do not use the abbreviation IU, as it could be easily misread as a Roman numeral or as an abbreviation for *intravenous*.

Practice Problems 17-3

Express the following unit dosages using the correct numeric notation and abbreviation(s).

1. one hundred fifteen units _____

2. ten thousand units _____

3. one million units _____

4. fifty-three units _____

5. two hundred thousand units _____

6. three hundred seventy-five units _____

7. one hundred units _____

8. one thousand units _____

9. eighty-five units _____

10. seven hundred units _____

Milliequivalent

A **milliequivalent (mEq)** is the number of grams of a drug in 1 mL of a normal solution. Potassium chloride is a common example of a drug expressed in milliequivalents. Dosages are written with the number followed by the abbreviation (e.g., 20 mEq).

Practice Problems 17-4

Express the following milliequivalent dosages using the correct numeric notation and abbreviation(s).

1. seventy-five milliequivalents _____
2. thirty milliequivalents _____
3. forty milliequivalents _____
4. twenty-five milliequivalents _____
5. fifteen milliequivalents _____
6. twenty milliequivalents _____
7. eighty-five milliequivalents _____
8. one hundred fifty milliequivalents _____
9. ten milliequivalents _____
10. fifty-five milliequivalents _____

The Apothecary System

The **apothecary system** is an old English system of measurement. Even though it will probably be replaced exclusively by the metric system at some point, it is still used for certain medications. The **grain** is the primary unit of weight in this system. The abbreviation for grain is *gr*. The basic units for volume or liquid measurement are the minim, the fluid dram, and the fluid ounce, as shown in Tables 17-3 and 17-4.

TABLE 17-3 Apothecary Weights

20 grains (gr) = 1 scruple
3 scruples = 1 dram = 60 grains
8 drams = 1 ounce (oz.) = 480 grains
12 ounces = 1 pound = 5,760 grains

TABLE 17-4 Apothecary Fluid Measures

60 minims = 1 fluid dram
8 fluid drams = 1 fluid ounce = 480 minims
16 fluid ounces = 1 pint
2 pints = 1 quart = 32 fluid ounces
4 quarts = 1 gallon = 128 fluid ounces

apothecary system an old English system of measurement of weight, based on the grain.

grain the primary unit of weight in the apothecary system.

avoirdupois system the current American system of measurement of weight, based on a pound being equivalent to 16 ounces.

household system the system of measurement commonly used in American households, usually related to food and beverages.

The Avoirdupois System

The **avoirdupois system** (see Table 17-5) is another system used only for measuring weight; it is also being replaced by the metric system. The name is derived from the old French term *avoir de pois*, meaning "goods of weight" and referring to goods sold by weight rather than by the piece. This system, which is based on a pound being equivalent to 16 ounces, is the weight system most commonly used in the United States, and it is still used extensively in Canada and the United Kingdom as well.

TABLE 17-5 Avoirdupois Weights

1 ounce (oz.) = 437.5 grains (gr) = 28.4 g
16oz.=1 pound (lb.) = 7,000 gr

The Household System

Household units are used primarily to assist the patient with measuring while at home. Pharmacy technicians should be familiar with **household system** measurements, so that they can explain medication directions easily in understandable terms, such as simply telling the patient to take 1 teaspoon (tsp.) instead of 5 mL (see Tables 17-6 and 17-7).

TABLE 17-6 Household Measure Equivalents

3 teaspoons (tsp.) = 1 tablespoon (Tbsp.)
2 tablespoons = 1 fluid ounce (fl. oz.)
8 fluid ounces = 1 cup
2 cups = 1 pint (pt.)
2 pints = 1 quart (qt.)
4 quarts = 1 gallon (gal.)

TABLE 17-7 Household Measures and Metric Equivalents

1 tsp.=5 mL
1 Tbsp.=15 mL
1 fl. oz.=30 mL
1 cup = 240 mL
2.2 lb.=1 kg
1 mL = 20 drops (gtt)

Practice Problems 17-5

Express the following measurements using the correct abbreviation.

1. 75 milliequivalents _____
2. 10 teaspoons _____
3. 20 ounces _____
4. 10 tablespoons _____
5. one hundred units _____
6. seven drops _____
7. two pints _____
8. three quarts _____
9. six gallons _____
10. five hundred units _____
11. twelve grains _____
12. one-half ounce _____
13. sixteen pints _____
14. two and one-half grains _____
15. thirty ounces _____

Converting Measurements

Although the metric system is used almost exclusively in pharmacy, the other systems of measurement, including the apothecary system, the avoirdupois system, and the household system, are used in certain cases. As a pharmacy technician, you will need to convert units of measure from one system of measurement to another.

Because pharmacies stock only a fraction of the drugs and dosage forms available, it is sometimes necessary to convert an order to match the stock on hand. Several conversion factors will help you convert apothecary and household values to the metric system (see Tables 17-8 and 17-9). However, these conversion factors are not absolute; the relationships are considered approximate equivalents. Therefore, you should choose the most direct route through a calculation. Remember, your job is to be sure the prescribed drug is delivered to the patient accurately calculated.

Converting the Household System

Converting between the metric and household systems is just a matter of memorizing the conversion factors and using them. Because the metric system is the most widely used (and preferred for accuracy), you should perform conversions to and from the metric system (see Table 17-8). Be aware that there are minor differences between the various systems. One example to note is the pound. In the apothecary system, 1 lb.=12 oz., whereas in the household system, 1 lb. = 16 oz.

Converting lbs. and ozs.

Converting lbs. and ozs. If the system is not stated, assume that 16 oz.=1 lb.

TABLE 17-8 Household to Metric Conversions

Household Measure		Metric Equivalent
1 teaspoon	=	5 mL
1 tablespoon	=	15 mL
1 fluid ounce	=	30 mL
1 pint	=	480 mL
1 gallon	=	3,840 mL
1 cup	=	240 mL
1 ounce	=	28.4 gm
1 pound	=	454 gm
1 pound	=	16 oz.

TABLE 17-9 Apothecary to Metric Conversion

Apothecary Measure		Metric Equivalent
15 minims	=	1 mL
1 fluid dram	=	4 mL
1 fluid ounce	=	30 mL
1 ounce	=	8 drams
1 dram	=	60 grains
6 fluid ounces	=	180 mL
8 fluid ounces	=	240 mL
16 fluid ounces	=	500 mL
32 fluid ounces	=	1,000 mL
1 grain	=	65 mg
1 ounce	=	140 grains
15 grains	=	1 gm
1 pound	=	12 oz.
2.2 pounds	=	1 kg

You can perform conversions between the household and metric systems by setting up proportions as fractions and then multiplying the fractions to get the correct answer.

Formula—Conversion of Systems

This formula can be used to convert measurements between the various systems discussed.

$$\text{Units that you have} \times \frac{\text{Number of units that you want}}{\text{Units that you have}}$$

EXAMPLE 17.1

Convert 5 tsp. to milliliters.

$$5 \text{ tsp.} \times \frac{5 \text{ mL}}{1 \text{ tsp.}} = 25 \text{ mL}$$

EXAMPLE 17.2

Convert 3 Tbsp. to milliliters.

$$3 \text{ Tbsp.} \times \frac{15 \text{ mL}}{1 \text{ Tbsp.}} = 45 \text{ mL}$$

EXAMPLE 17.3

Convert 4 oz. to milliliters.

$$4 \text{ oz.} \times \frac{30 \text{ mL}}{1 \text{ oz.}} = 120 \text{ mL}$$

EXAMPLE 17.4

Convert 6.5 cups to milliliters.

$$6.5 \text{ cups} \times \frac{240 \text{ mL}}{1 \text{ cup}} = 1,560 \text{ mL}$$

EXAMPLE 17.5

Convert 60 mL to teaspoons.

$$60 \text{ mL} \times \frac{1 \text{ tsp.}}{5 \text{ mL}} = 12 \text{ tsp.}$$

Celsius (centigrade) international unit of measurement for temperature.

Fahrenheit American unit of measurement for temperature.

Practice Problems 17-6

Convert the following measurements.

1. 4 Tbsp. = _____ mL
2. 4 pints = _____ mL
3. 1 Tbsp. = _____ mL
4. 3 fl. oz. = _____ mL
5. 3 gal. = _____ mL
6. 8 mL = _____ tsp.
7. 6 pt. = _____ mL
8. 5 lb. = _____ gm
9. 2,365 mL = _____ pt.
10. 90 Tbsp. = _____ mL
11. 4.5 gal. = _____ pt.
12. 45 mL = _____ fl. oz.
13. 60 kg = _____ lb.
14. 15 mL = _____ tsp.
15. 6 oz. = _____ mL
16. 3 qt. = _____ pt.
17. 5 cups = _____ oz.
18. 1.5 gal. = _____ qt.
19. 12 oz. = _____ cups
20. 4 cups = _____ mL.

21. You need to give 2 mg of a drug. The drug on hand has a concentration of 8 mg per ounce. How many teaspoons will you give? _____

22. The prescription calls for a dosage of 2 tsp. Your stock bottle contains 16 oz. How many teaspoons are in this bottle? _____

23. You are to reconstitute a particular drug. Each vial will get 6 oz. of sterile water. You have 1.5 gal. of sterile water. How many vials can you prepare? _____

24. You need to prepare three prescriptions containing the following volumes: 1 gal., 2 qt., and 10 oz. How many tablespoons were dispensed in the three prescriptions? _____

25. How many teaspoons are in a pint? _____

Converting the Apothecary System

The apothecary system is an ancient system of measurement based on grains of wheat, and it produces more approximate than exact values. Some prescribers still order medications using the apothecary system. The most commonly used apothecary measures are grains for solids and drams for liquids.

EXAMPLE 17.6

Convert 180 gr to ounces.

Using the conversion value, set up a proportion to solve for the number of ounces:

1 oz.=480 gr

$$\frac{1 \text{ oz.}}{480 \text{ gr}} \quad \frac{X \text{ oz.}}{180 \text{ gr}}$$

Then, cross-multiply and solve for X. (See Chapter 16 for a review of cross-multiplication.)

$$480X = 180$$

$$X = \frac{180}{480} = 0.375$$

So, 180 gr = 0.375 oz.

Practice Problems 17-7

Convert the following measurements.

1. 5 gr = _____ mg

2. 30 mL = _____ drams

3. 15 gr = _____ mg

4. 4 oz. = _____ gm

5. 300 mg = _____ gr

6. $\frac{1}{2}$ oz. = _____ mL

7. 7 drams = _____ oz.

8. 9 kg = _____ lb.

9. $\frac{1}{6}$ gr = _____ mg

10. 40 mL = _____ drams

11. 360 mL = _____ oz.

12. 50 gr = _____ mg

13. 3.5 kg = _____ lb.

14. 60 drams = _____ oz.

15. 150 lb. = _____ oz.

16. 680 gm = _____ lb.

17. 99 lb. = _____ kg

18. 0.5 gr = _____ mg

19. 300 mg = _____ gr

20. 10 dram = _____ mL

21. A child weighs 42 lb. and is to receive 2 mg/kg/day. How much of the drug should the child receive per day? _____

22. A medication order calls for a potassium supplement to be administered in at least 150 mL of juice. How many ounces of juice should the patient pour? _____

23. A baby weighs 9.6 lb. What is the baby's weight in kilograms? _____

24. A doctor orders $\frac{1}{5}$ gr of codeine. How many milligrams is this dose equivalent to? _____

25. A cancer patient is given $\frac{1}{4}$ gr of morphine sulfate every two hours. How many milligrams of morphine does he receive in eight hours? _____

26. A pharmacy technician is to fill a prescription for 10 gr of aminophylline. Tablets are available in 500–mg strength. How many tablets should the technician give? _____

27. A bottle of medication contains 45 drams. How many milliliters does it contain? _____

28. A prescription calls for the patient to take 3 drams. How many ounces is that? _____

29. Twenty-three grains equals how many grams? _____

30. How many milliliters of cough medicine are in 12 drams? _____

Temperature Conversions

Another important conversion in health care involves conversion between **Celsius** and **Fahrenheit** temperatures. The temperature measurement most commonly used in the United States is the Fahrenheit (°F) scale. In most other countries, the metric measurement of Celsius (°C) or **centigrade** is used. In the Fahrenheit system, the freezing point is 32° and the boiling point is 212°. In the Celsius system, the freezing point is 0° and the boiling point is 100°.

Simple formulas are used to convert between the two temperature scales. There is a 180° difference between the boiling and the freezing points on the Fahrenheit thermometer, and a 100° difference on the Celsius thermometer. Therefore, each Celsius degree is 180/100 or 1.8 the size of a Fahrenheit degree.

Workplace Wisdom Calculating Temperature Conversions

You may find it easier to perform temperature conversions using the following formula. It can be used with basic algebra to solve for either °C or °F.

$9C = 5F - 160$

To convert from Fahrenheit temperature to Celsius, use the following formula:

$$°C = \frac{°F - 32}{1.8}$$

EXAMPLE 17.7

Convert 80 °F to °C.

$$°C = \frac{80 - 32}{1.8}$$

$$°C = \frac{48}{1.8}$$

$$°C = 26.7°$$

To convert Celsius temperature to Fahrenheit, multiply by 1.8 and add 32.

$$°F = 1.8 \times °C + 32$$

EXAMPLE 17.8

Convert 60 °C to °F.

$$°F = 1.8 \times 60 + 32$$

$$°F = 108 + 32$$

$$°F = 140°$$

Practice Problems 17-8

Convert the following temperatures. Round your answers to tenths.

1. 70°F = _____ °C
2. 99°F = _____ °C
3. 100°F = _____ °C
4. 80°F = _____ °C
5. 45°F = _____ °C
6. 4°C = _____ °F
7. 32°C = _____ °F
8. 15°C = _____ °F
9. 38.4°C = _____ °F
10. 26°C = _____ °F
11. The normal temperature of hot water is 115°F. What is the temperature in Celsius? _____ °C
12. The normal body temperature range is 96.8°F to 100°F. What is the range in Celsius? _____ °C to _____ °C
13. The normal oral temperature is 37°C. What is the temperature in Fahrenheit? _____ °F
14. If a child has a fever of 101°F, what is his temperature in Celsius? _____ °C
15. If a drug is to be kept at 56°F, what is the storage temperature in Celsius? _____ °C

Workplace Wisdom Converting Temperatures Using the 9C = 5F − 160 Formula

Another option for converting temperatures is the formula $9C = 5F - 160$. This algebraic formula works for converting between both units. Simply replace the "C" or "F," where C = Celsius and F = Fahrenheit, with the known temperature, and solve algebraically.

Summary

Regardless of your practice setting, a solid knowledge of the systems of measurement and their units and abbreviations is the foundation for all pharmacy calculations. You must have a comprehensive understanding of this material before attempting pharmacy calculations.

Every practice setting is individual and unique; the conversions that you need to calculate on a regular basis at your practice setting will become second nature to you. Until such time, use the charts and formulas from this chapter. Although miscalculation of a conversion may seem to be a minor issue, it could have drastic and irrevocable effects on a patient's health.

Chapter Review Questions

1. 545 gm = _____.
   a. 1.2 lb.
   b. 12 lb.
   c. 0.54 lb.
   d. 0.12 lb.

2. 2 cups = _____.
   a. 120 mL
   b. 240 mL
   c. 480 mL
   d. 160 mL

3. 240 oz. = _____.
   a. 15 pt.
   b. 5 pt.
   c. 1.5 pt.
   d. 0.5 pt.

4. 2.5 cups = _____.
   a. 2.0 oz.
   b. 20 oz.
   c. 3.0 oz.
   d. 30 oz.

5. 2°F = _____.
   a. 32.4°C
   b. 28.6°C
   c. −12.4°C
   d. −16.7°C

6. How many 8 oz. bottles can be filled from 5 gal. of medicine? _____
   a. 80
   b. 20
   c. 30
   d. 110

7. A child weighs 34.1 kg. What is his weight in pounds?
   a. 16
   b. 34
   c. 52
   d. 75

8. A medication has 300 mg in 50 mL. How many milligrams are in 3 oz.?
   a. 900
   b. 1,500
   c. 540
   d. 450

9. If there are 30 mg in a teaspoon, how many grams are in a fluid ounce?
   a. 6.0
   b. 1.5
   c. 0.18
   d. 0.15

10. If a prescription reads "Take 2 tablespoons 3 times a day for 10 days," how many total tablespoons will the patient take?
    a. 30
    b. 300
    c. 80
    d. 60

Critical Thinking Questions

1. Why is proper decimal notation so critical in pharmacy calculations?

2. Why does pharmacy continue to use both the metric system and the household system of measurement extensively?

3. When would a pharmacy technician need to perform temperature conversions?

References and Resources

Hegstad, Lorrie N. and Wilma Hayek. *Essential Drug Dosage Calculations*. 4th ed. Upper Saddle River, NJ: Pearson, 2001. Print.

Johnston, Mike. *Pharmacy Calculations: The Pharmacy Technician Series.* Upper Saddle River, NJ: Pearson, 2005. Print.

Lesmeister, Michelle Benjamin. *Math Basics for the Healthcare Professional*. 4th ed. Upper Saddle River, NJ: Pearson, 2013. Print.

Mikolah, Alan A. *Drug Dosage Calculations for the Emergency Care Provider*. 2nd ed. Upper Saddle River, NJ: Prentice Hall, 2003. Print.

Olsen, June, Anthony Giangrasso, and Dolores Shrimpton. *Medical Dosage Calculations*. 10th ed. Upper Saddle River, NJ: Pearson, 2011. Print.

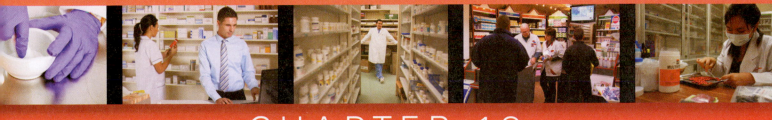

CHAPTER 18

Dosage Calculations

LEARNING OBJECTIVES

After completing this chapter, you should be able to:

- Calculate the correct number of doses in a prescription.
- Determine the quantity to dispense for a prescription.
- Calculate the amount of active ingredient in a prescription.
- Determine the correct days supply for a prescription.
- Perform multiple dosage calculations for a single prescription.
- Calculate accurate dosages for pediatric patients.
- Convert a patient's weight from pounds to kilograms.
- Perform dosage calculations based upon mg/kg/day.

INTRODUCTION

Proper dosing of medications is important to ensure patient safety. **Dosage calculations** include calculation of the number of doses, dispensing quantities, and ingredient quantities. These calculations are performed in the pharmacy on a daily basis. Therefore, the pharmacy technician must have a full working knowledge of how to perform these calculations.

To perform dosage calculations, you will utilize the information and principles introduced in previous chapters of this book. You can perform these calculations by setting up ratios and proportions, keeping like-units consistent, and cross-multiplying to solve for the unknown.

---

dosage calculations pharmacy calculations pertaining to the number of doses, dispensing quantities, and/or ingredient quantities.

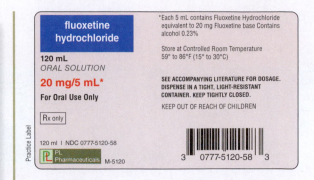

SIG Code Refresher

These are some of the most common abbreviated directions, or SIG codes, that you will need to be familiar with when processing prescriptions and calculating dosages.

qd—every day
qod—every other day
bid—twice a day
tid—three times a day
qid—four times a day
q4h—every four hours, or six times a day
q6h—every six hours, or four times a day
q8h—every eight hours, or three times a day
q12h—every 12 hours, or twice a day
q4–6h—every four to six hours, or four to six times a day
prn—as needed

Middots

For the purpose of this text, middots (·) are sometimes used to indicate multiplication and to avoid confusion with the unknown "X".

Calculating the Number of Doses

Determining the correct number of **doses** to be dispensed, or available in stock, is an important dosage calculation. In this section, you will learn how to calculate the number of doses.

EXAMPLE 18.1

How many 1 tsp. doses are in a 4 oz. bottle of fluoxetine HCl liquid solution 20 mg/5 mL? (See Figure 18-1.)

To calculate the number of doses, you should first determine which information presented is actually applicable to the question. Too often, we make mistakes in dosage calculations because we overcomplicate them.

Let us look at the information that has been provided:

✓ 1 tsp. po—*the dose*
✗ qd—*the frequency*
  4 oz. —*the quantity dispensed*
✗ Fluoxetine HCl solution 20 mg/5 mL—*the drug name and strength*
✗ 120 mL—*the quantity of the stock bottle*

The question is simply asking how many doses make up the total amount being dispensed. The strength of the drug, frequency of dosage, and quantity of the stock bottle have no relevance in performing this calculation.

So now we know that we are working with 1 tsp. doses and a total quantity of 4 oz. To perform this calculation using a ratio/proportion, we need to have similar units of measure—in this case, mL.

dose the amount of medication prescribed to be taken at one time.

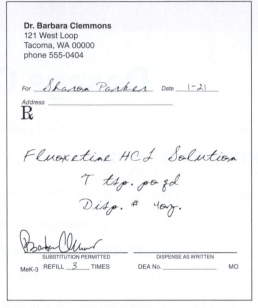

FIGURE 18-1 Drug label for fluoxetine hydrochloride oral solution.

You could also solve the problem by using a ratio/proportion.

$$\frac{1 \text{ oz.}}{30 \text{ mL}} = \frac{4 \text{ oz.}}{X \text{ mL}}$$

Cross-multiply and solve the equation for X.

$$30 \cdot 4 = 120 \text{ and } 1 \cdot X = (1)X$$
$$(1)X = 120$$

Now that we have both quantities converted to units in mL, we can set up our ratio/proportion and solve.

$$\frac{1 \text{ dose}}{5 \text{ mL}} = \frac{X \text{ doses}}{120 \text{ mL}}$$

Cross-multiply.

Now set up your equation and solve for X.

$$5X = 120$$

To solve for X, divide both sides by 5.

$$\frac{5X}{5} = \frac{120}{5}$$
$$120 \div 5 = 24$$
$$X = 24$$

So, there are 24 doses (of 5 mL each) in a 4-oz. (120-mL) bottle.

EXAMPLE 18.2

How many doses are provided in the prescription shown in Figure 18-2?

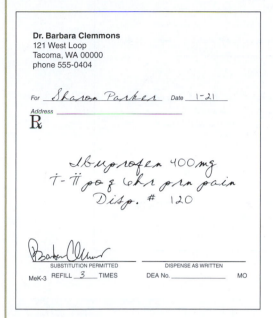

```
Dr. Barbara Clemmons
121 West Loop
Tacoma, WA 00000
phone 555-0404

For  Sharon Parker      Date  1-21
Address _____
Rx

          Ibuprofen 400mg
     i-ii po q 6hr prn pain
          Disp. # 120



[signature]
        SUBSTITUTION PERMITTED        DISPENSE AS WRITTEN
MeK-3  REFILL _3_ TIMES    DEA No. _____    MO
```

FIGURE 18-2

Let us look at the information that has been provided:

✓ 1–2 po—*the dose*

✗ q6h prn pain—*the frequency*

✓ 120—*the quantity dispensed*

✗ Ibuprofen 400 mg—*the drug name and strength*

❝ Workplace Wisdom Conservative Calculations

Always use the higher dosage amount when performing dosage calculations on prescriptions that have a range for the dose, as in Example 18.2. This will provide the most conservative solution and ensure the most accurate potential for days supply. ❞

Using the information provided, set up the ratio/proportion and solve.

$$\frac{1 \text{ dose}}{2 \text{ tabs}} = \frac{X \text{ doses}}{120 \text{ tabs}}$$

Cross-multiply.

Now set up your equation and solve for X.

$$2X = 120$$

To solve for X, divide both sides by 2.

$$\frac{2X}{2} = \frac{120}{2}$$

$$120 \div 2 = 60$$

So, a minimum of 60 doses have been prescribed.

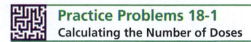

Practice Problems 18-1
Calculating the Number of Doses

1. How many dosages are provided in the prescription shown in Figure 18-3?

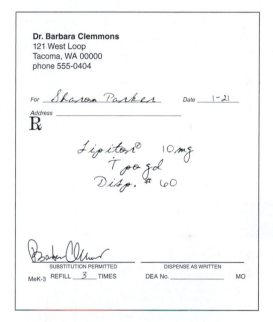

```
Dr. Barbara Clemmons
121 West Loop
Tacoma, WA 00000
phone 555-0404

For  Sharon Parker      Date  1-21
Address _____
Rx

         Lipitor® 10mg
            i po qd
          Disp. # 60



[signature]
        SUBSTITUTION PERMITTED        DISPENSE AS WRITTEN
MeK-3  REFILL _3_ TIMES    DEA No. _____    MO
```

FIGURE 18-3

2. How many dosages are in this 50-mL bottle of erythromycin drops, if the dosage is for two dropperfuls? (See Figure 18-4.)

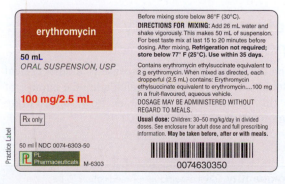

```
erythromycin

50 mL
ORAL SUSPENSION, USP

100 mg/2.5 mL

Rx only

50 ml  NDC 0074-6303-50
PL Pharmaceuticals   M-6303

Before mixing store below 86°F (30°C).
DIRECTIONS FOR MIXING: Add 26 mL water and
shake vigorously. This makes 50 mL of suspension.
For best taste mix at last 15 to 20 minutes before
dosing. After mixing, Refrigeration not required;
store below 77° F (25°C). Use within 35 days.

Contains erythromycin ethylsuccinate equivalent to
2 g erythromycin. When mixed as directed, each
dropperful (2.5 mL) contains: Erythromycin
ethylsuccinate equivalent to erythromycin....100 mg
in a fruit-flavoured, aqueous vehicle.
DOSAGE MAY BE ADMINISTERED WITHOUT
REGARD TO MEALS.

Usual dose: Children: 30–50 mg/kg/day in divided
doses. See enclosure for adult dose and full prescribing
information. May be taken before, after or with meals.

0074630350
```

Practice Label

FIGURE 18-4

3. How many doses are provided in the prescription shown in Figure 18-5?

Dr. Barbara Clemmons
121 West Loop
Tacoma, WA 00000
phone 555-0404

For Sharon Parker Date 1-21
Address
℞
Vicodin® 5/500
i po q8hr
Disp. # 50

SUBSTITUTION PERMITTED DISPENSE AS WRITTEN
MeK-3 REFILL ______ TIMES DEA No. ______ MO

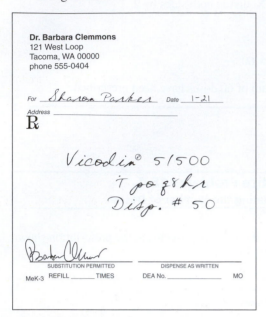

FIGURE 18-5

4. How many 1 tsp. doses are in each bottle of azithromycin 200 mg/5 mL, as shown in Figure 18-6, when mixed?

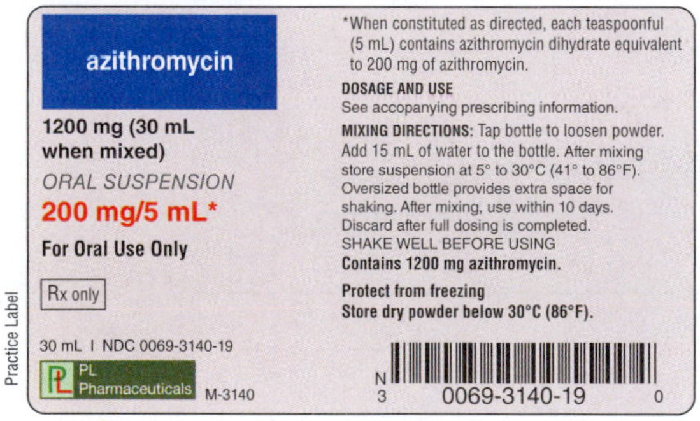

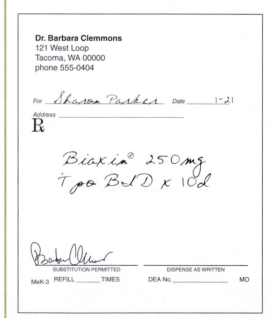

FIGURE 18-6

Calculating the Quantity to Dispense

Determining the proper quantity to dispense is another critical dosage calculation, and is similar to calculating the number of doses. In this section, you will learn how to calculate **dispensing quantities**.

dispensing quantity the total amount of medication to be dispensed.

5. How many doses are provided in the prescription shown in Figure 18-7?

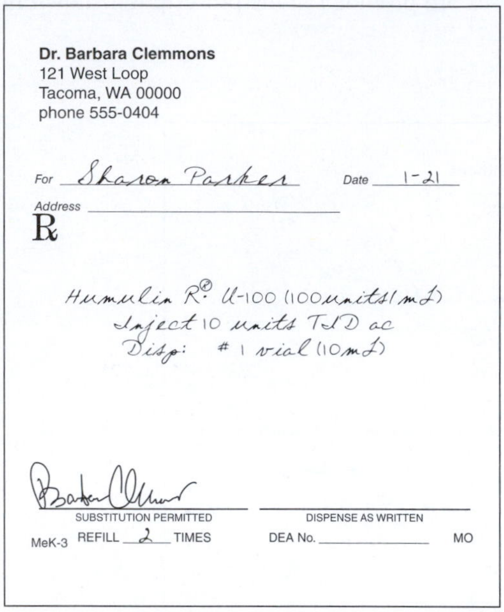

Dr. Barbara Clemmons
121 West Loop
Tacoma, WA 00000
phone 555-0404

For Sharon Parker Date 1-21
Address
℞
Humulin R® U-100 (100 units/mL)
Inject 10 units TID ac
Disp: # 1 vial (10 mL)

SUBSTITUTION PERMITTED DISPENSE AS WRITTEN
MeK-3 REFILL 2 TIMES DEA No. ______ MO

FIGURE 18-7

EXAMPLE 18.3

How many Biaxin 250 mg tablets should be dispensed, according to the prescription shown in Figure 18-8?

Dr. Barbara Clemmons
121 West Loop
Tacoma, WA 00000
phone 555-0404

For Sharon Parker Date 1-21
Address
℞
Biaxin® 250mg
i po BID x 10d

SUBSTITUTION PERMITTED DISPENSE AS WRITTEN
MeK-3 REFILL ______ TIMES DEA No. ______ MO

FIGURE 18-8

To solve this dosage calculation, it is important first to determine which information is necessary; it is also critical to know the common SIG codes to perform dosage calculations. Let us look at the information that has been provided:

✓ 1 po—*the dose*

✓ BID—*the frequency*

✓   × 10d—*the duration*

✗   Biaxin 250 mg—*the drug name and strength*

✗   100 tablets—*the quantity of the stock bottle*

To calculate the appropriate quantity to dispense, use the following formula:

Dose × frequency × duration = quantity to dispense

Using the information provided in the prescription, you can set up the calculation as follows:

1·2·10 = X

1 · 2 · 10 = 20

20 = X

So, 20 tablets of Biaxin 250 mg should be dispensed.

EXAMPLE 18.4 CALCULATING THE QUANTITY TO DISPENSE

How much promethazine with codeine syrup should be dispensed, according to the prescription shown in Figure 18-9?

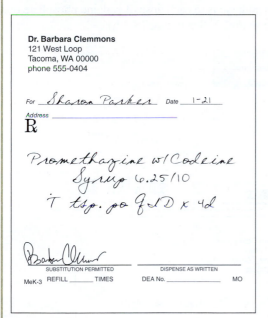

FIGURE 18-9

Let us look at the information that has been provided:

✓   1 tsp. po—*the dose*

✓   qid—*the frequency*

✓   × 4d—*the duration*

✗   Promethazine with codeine syrup 6.25/10—*the drug name and strength*

To calculate the appropriate quantity to dispense, use the following formula:

Dose × frequency × duration = quantity to dispense

Using the information provided in the prescription, you can set up the calculation as follows:

1 tsp. · 4 · 4 = X

1 · 4 · 4 = 16

16 = X

So, 16 tsp., or 80 mL, of promethazine with codeine should be dispensed.

Practice Problems 18-2
Calculating the Quantity to Dispense

1. What quantity should be dispensed for the prescription shown in Figure 18-10?

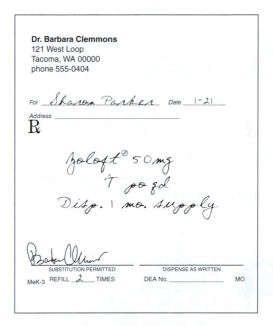

FIGURE 18-10

2. What quantity should be dispensed, using the stock medication shown in Figure 18-11, to provide 20 mg of diazepam prior to the procedure and 10 mg following the procedure?

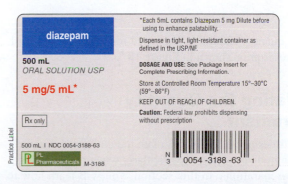

FIGURE 18-11

3. What quantity should be dispensed for a three-month supply of the prescription shown in Figure 18-12?

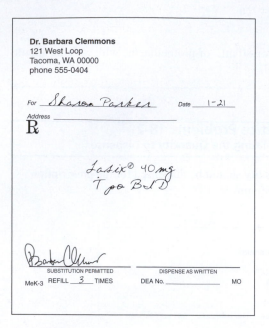

Dr. Barbara Clemmons
121 West Loop
Tacoma, WA 00000
phone 555-0404

For _Sharon Parker_   Date _1-21_

Address _____

R

Lasix® 40 mg
T po BID

SUBSTITUTION PERMITTED   DISPENSE AS WRITTEN

MeK-3   REFILL _3_ TIMES   DEA No. _____   MO

FIGURE 18-12

4. What quantity should be dispensed when 50 mg of amitryptyline has been prescribed daily for three weeks, if the medication shown in Figure 18-13 is all that is available?

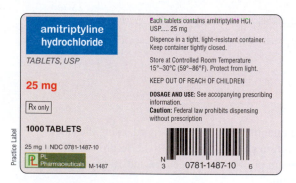

amitriptyline hydrochloride

TABLETS, USP

25 mg

Rx only

1000 TABLETS

25 mg | NDC 0781-1487-10

PL Pharmaceuticals M-1487

N 3   0781-1487-10   6

Each tablets contains amitriptyline HCl, USP..... 25 mg

Dispence in a tight. light-resistant container. Keep container tightly closed.

Store at Controlled Room Temperature 15°–30°C (59°–86°F). Protect from light.

KEEP OUT OF REACH OF CHILDREN

DOSAGE AND USE: See accompanying prescribing information.
Caution: Federal law prohibits dispensing without prescription

FIGURE 18-13

5. What quantity should be dispensed for a 30-day supply of the prescription shown in Figure 18-14?

Calculating the Quantity of Ingredient

It is sometimes necessary to calculate the amount, or quantity, of active ingredient required, particularly when preparing compounded preparations. In this section, you will learn how to accurately determine the quantity of active ingredient.

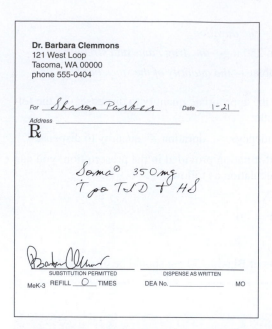

Dr. Barbara Clemmons
121 West Loop
Tacoma, WA 00000
phone 555-0404

For _Sharon Parker_   Date _1-21_

Address _____

R

Soma® 350 mg
T po TID + HS

SUBSTITUTION PERMITTED   DISPENSE AS WRITTEN

MeK-3   REFILL _O_ TIMES   DEA No. _____   MO

FIGURE 18-14

EXAMPLE 18.5

How much codeine is in each dose of codeine phosphate oral solution 15 mg/mL? (See Figure 18-15.)

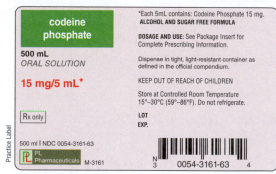

codeine phosphate

500 mL
ORAL SOLUTION

15 mg/5 mL*

Rx only

500 ml | NDC 0054-3161-63

PL Pharmaceuticals M-3161

*Each 5mL contains: Codeine Phosphate 15 mg.
ALCOHOL AND SUGAR FREE FORMULA

DOSAGE AND USE: See Package Insert for Complete Prescribing Information.

Dispense in tight, light-resistant container as defined in the official compendium.

KEEP OUT OF REACH OF CHILDREN

Store at Controlled Room Temperature 15°–30°C (59°–86°F). Do not refrigerate.

LOT
EXP.

N 3   0054-3161-63   4

Dr. Barbara Clemmons
121 West Loop
Tacoma, WA 00000
phone 555-0404

For _Sharon Parker_   Date _1-21_

Address _____

R

Codeine Oral Soln. 15 mg/mL
T tt sp. po prn pain
Disp. # 4 oz.

SUBSTITUTION PERMITTED   DISPENSE AS WRITTEN

MeK-3   REFILL _____ TIMES   DEA No. _____   MO

FIGURE 18-15

Let us first look at all the information provided to determine which facts we will use in solving the problem:

✓   1 Tbsp. po—*the dose*

✗   prn—*the frequency*

✗   4 oz.—*the quantity to dispense*

✓   Codeine phosphate oral solution 15 mg/mL—*the drug name and strength*

✗   500 mL—*the quantity of the stock bottle*

To solve this problem, we need to set up a ratio/proportion using the dose and strength—but remember that units of measure must be the same. The dose (1 Tbsp.) is equivalent to 15 mL. (You should know this by memory.)

Now, we can set up the ratio/proportion.

$$\frac{15 \text{ mg}}{1 \text{ mL}} = \frac{X \text{ mg}}{15 \text{ mL}}$$

Cross-multiply and then set up the equation to solve for X.

15 · 15 = 225 and 1 · X = 5X

1X = 225

X = 225

So, there is 225 mg of codeine in each 1 Tbsp. dose.

Let us first look at all the information provided to determine which facts we will use in solving the problem:

✓   400 mg—*the dose*

✗   500 mL—*the quantity to dispense*

✓   Dopamine HCl injection 80 mg/mL—*the drug name and strength*

To solve this problem, we must determine how many milliliters of the stock dopamine must be added to the normal saline IV solution bag. We must set up a ratio/proportion.

$$\frac{80 \text{ mg}}{1 \text{ mL}} = \frac{400 \text{ mg}}{X \text{ mL}}$$

Cross-multiply and then set up the equation to solve for X.

1 · 400 = 400 and 80 · X = 80X

400 = 80X

Now divide both sides by 80 to solve for X.

$$\frac{400}{80} = \frac{\cancel{80}X}{\cancel{80}}$$

X = 5

So, we must add 5 mL of the stock dopamine HCl injection to the IV solution.

EXAMPLE 18.6 CALCULATING THE QUANTITY OF INGREDIENT

How many milliliters of stock dopamine must be added to the IV solution? (See Figure 18-16.)

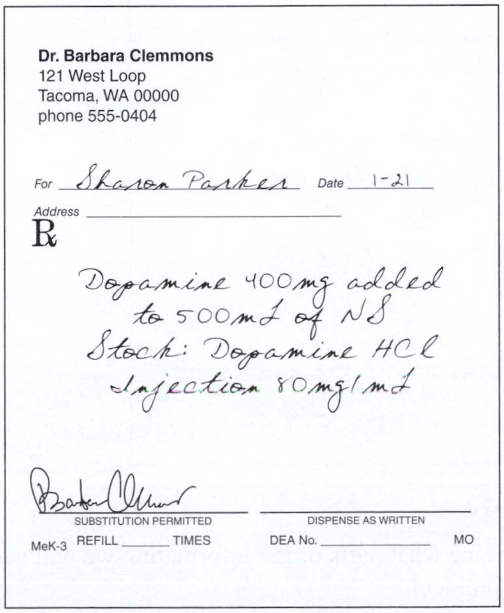

Dr. Barbara Clemmons
121 West Loop
Tacoma, WA 00000
phone 555-0404

For *Sharon Parker*   Date 1-21

Address _____

℞

Dopamine 400mg added to 500mL of NS
Stock: Dopamine HCl Injection 80mg/mL

SUBSTITUTION PERMITTED   DISPENSE AS WRITTEN

MeK-3   REFILL _____ TIMES   DEA No. _____   MO

FIGURE 18-16

Practice Problems 18-3
Calculating the Quantity of Ingredient

1. Z-Pak contains six tablets of azithromycin 250 mg, which are taken over the course of five days. How many total milligrams of active ingredient are contained in a Z-Pak?

2. How many micrograms of Fentanyl would be contained in 1.5 mL? (See Figure 18-17.)

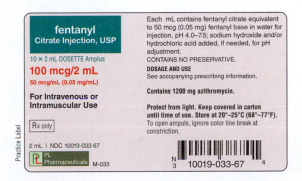

FIGURE 18-17

3. How many milligrams of acetaminophen are contained in two Lortab 2.5 tablets (2.5 mg hydrocodone/500 mg acetaminophen)?

4. How many milligrams of dexamethasone are contained in 1 tsp., based on the label shown in Figure 18-18?

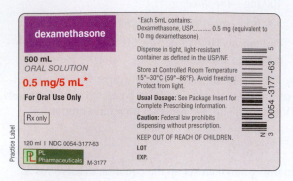

FIGURE 18-18

5. How many milligrams of hydrocortisone are found in 1 Tbsp. of Cortef 10 mg/5 mL?

Calculating the Correct Days Supply

Accurate calculation of the number of days a prescription should last, or **days supply**, is important, especially when billing through a third-party insurance provider. If an incorrect days supply is entered, the original prescription could be denied, the co-pay may be miscalculated, or refill coverage could be affected. In this section, you will learn how to calculate the correct days supply.

EXAMPLE 18.7

How many days should the prescription shown in Figure 18-19 last?

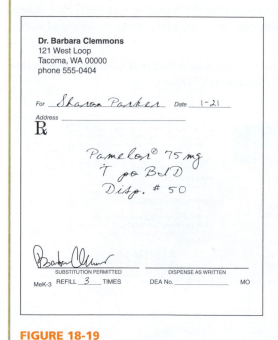

FIGURE 18-19

days supply the expected duration for a prescription being dispensed; how long the amount of medication dispensed will last if taken as directed.

Let us determine what parts of the information we will need to solve the problem.

✓   1 po—*the dose*
✓   bid—*the frequency*
✓   50—*the quantity to dispense*
✗   Pamelor 75 mg—*the drug name and strength*
✗   100 capsules—*the quantity of the stock bottle*

To calculate the appropriate days supply, use the following formula:

$$\text{Days supply} = \frac{\text{quantity dispensed}}{\text{dose} \times \text{frequency}}$$

Using the information provided, set up the formula as follows.

$$X = \frac{50 \text{ (quantity dispensed)}}{1 \times 2 \text{ (dose} \times \text{frequency)}}$$

This becomes:

$$X = \frac{50}{2} \text{ or } X = 25$$

So, this prescription should last for 25 days.

EXAMPLE 18.8

How many days should the prescription shown in Figure 18-20 last?

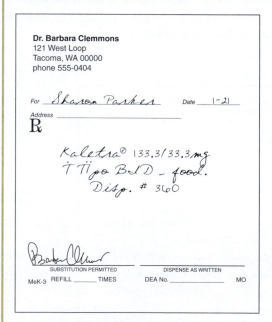

FIGURE 18-20

Let us determine what parts of the information we will need to solve the problem.

✓   1–2 po—*the dose*
✓   BID—*the frequency*

✓   360—*the quantity to dispense*

✗   Kaletra 133.3/33.3 mg—*the drug name and strength*

To calculate the appropriate days supply, use the following formula:

$$\text{Days supply} = \frac{\text{quantity dispensed}}{\text{dose} \times \text{frequency}}$$

Using the information provided, set up the formula as follows:

$$X = \frac{360 \text{ (quantity dispensed)}}{2 \times 2 \text{ (dose} \times \text{frequency)}}$$

This becomes:

$$X = \frac{360}{4} \text{ or } X = 90$$

So, this prescription should last for 3 months, or 90 days.

Practice Problems 18-4
Calculating the Correct Days Supply

1. How many days will the prescription shown in Figure 18-21 last?

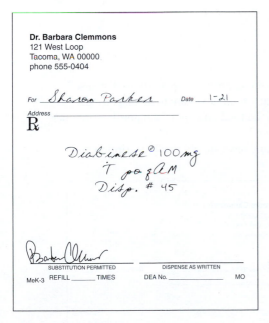

FIGURE 18-21

2. How many days will a 150-mL bottle of cefaclor 125 mg/5 mL last, if the patient is to take 2 tsp. three times daily? (See Figure 18-22.)

3. How many days will the prescription shown in Figure 18-23 last?

4. How many days should five tablets of Cialis 5 mg last, if the prescription directs the patient to use a maximum of one tablet every three days?

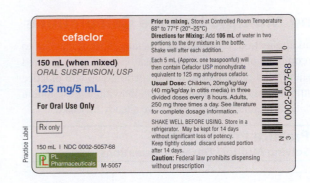

FIGURE 18-22

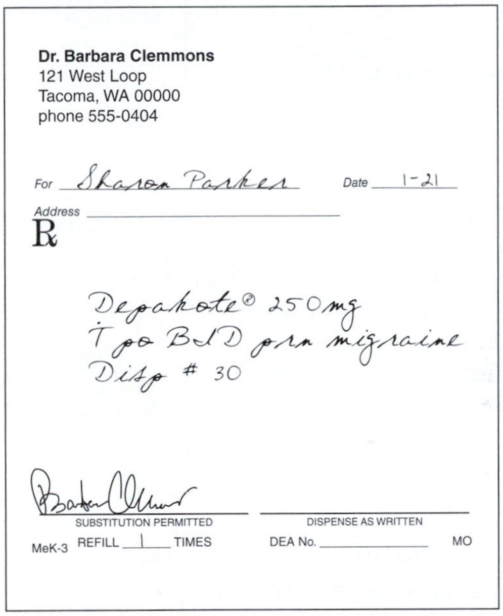

FIGURE 18-23

5. How many days will the prescription shown in Figure 18-24 last?

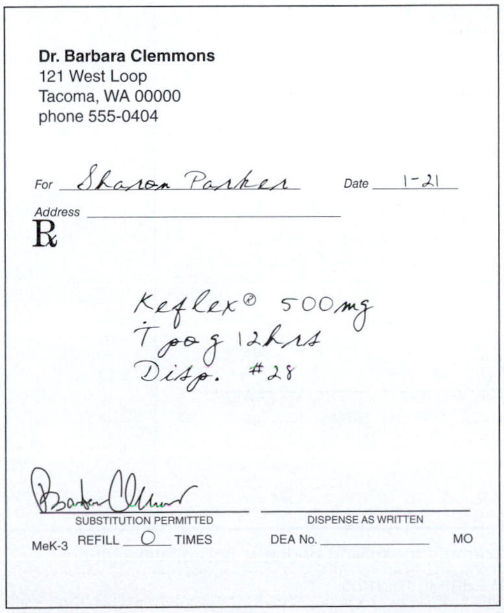

FIGURE 18-24

Solving Multiple Dosage Calculations

In practical application, pharmacy technicians most often need to perform a combination of the dosage calculations previously covered to prepare and fill a prescription. In this section, you will practice solving multiple dosage calculations for an individual prescription. The calculations required are those we have already reviewed.

Practice Problems 18-5
Solving Multiple Dosage Calculations

1.

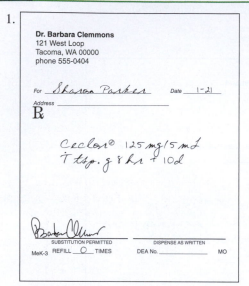

Dr. Barbara Clemmons
121 West Loop
Tacoma, WA 00000
phone 555-0404

For _Sharon Parker_   Date _1-21_

Address _____

℞

Ceclor® 125 mg/5 mL
Ť tsp. q 8 hr ⨯ 10 d

SUBSTITUTION PERMITTED   DISPENSE AS WRITTEN

MeK-3   REFILL _0_ TIMES   DEA No. _____ MO

FIGURE 18-25

a. What is the appropriate quantity to dispense?
b. How many total doses are to be dispensed?
c. What is the total amount of amoxicillin, in mg, to be dispensed?
d. How many days should this prescription last?

2.

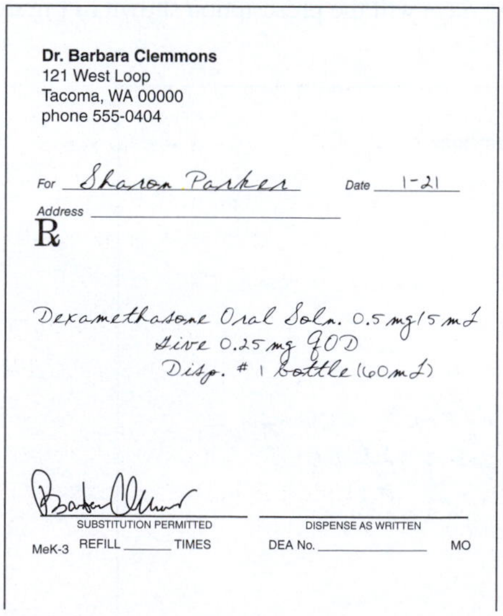

Dr. Barbara Clemmons
121 West Loop
Tacoma, WA 00000
phone 555-0404

For _Sharon Parker_   Date _1-21_

Address _____

℞

Dexamethasone Oral Soln. 0.5 mg/5 mL
Give 0.25 mg QOD
Disp. # 1 bottle (60 mL)

SUBSTITUTION PERMITTED   DISPENSE AS WRITTEN

MeK-3   REFILL _____ TIMES   DEA No. _____ MO

FIGURE 18-26

Fried's Rule is a formula for solving pediatric dosage calculations based on the patient's age in months.

Young's Rule a formula for solving pediatric dosage calculations based on the patient's age in years.

a. What is the appropriate quantity to dispense?
b. How many total doses are to be dispensed?
c. What is the total amount of dexamethasone, in mg, to be dispensed?
d. How many days should this prescription last?

3.

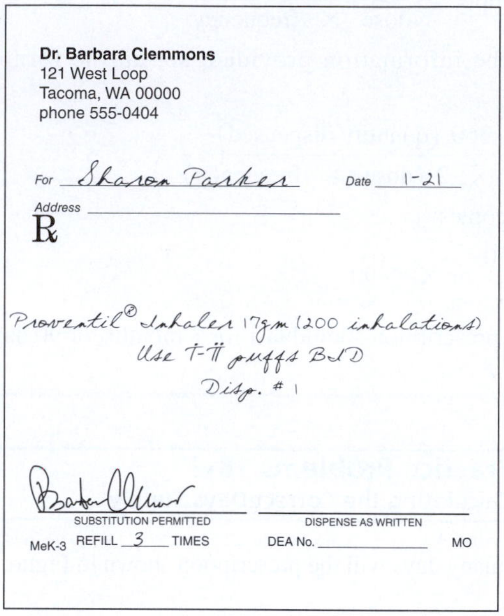

Dr. Barbara Clemmons
121 West Loop
Tacoma, WA 00000
phone 555-0404

For _Sharon Parker_   Date _1-21_

Address _____

℞

Proventil® Inhaler 17gm (200 inhalations)
Use Ť-Ŧ puffs BID
Disp. # 1

SUBSTITUTION PERMITTED   DISPENSE AS WRITTEN

MeK-3   REFILL _3_ TIMES   DEA No. _____ MO

FIGURE 18-27

a. What is the appropriate quantity to dispense?
b. How many total doses are to be dispensed?
c. What is the total amount of albuterol, in mg, per inhalation?
d. How many days should this prescription last?

4.

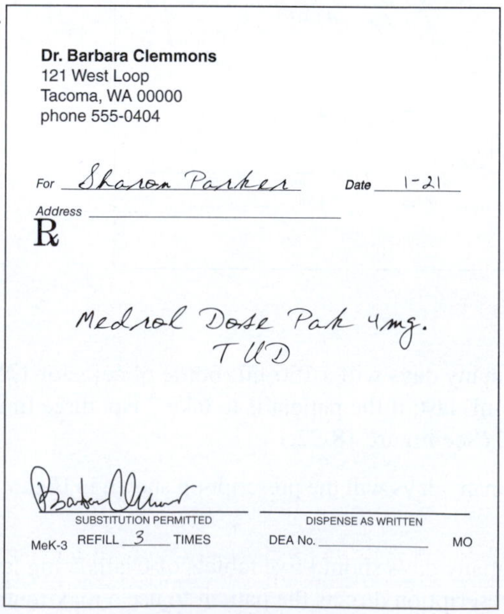

Dr. Barbara Clemmons
121 West Loop
Tacoma, WA 00000
phone 555-0404

For _Sharon Parker_   Date _1-21_

Address _____

℞

Medrol Dose Pak 4mg.
T UD

SUBSTITUTION PERMITTED   DISPENSE AS WRITTEN

MeK-3   REFILL _3_ TIMES   DEA No. _____ MO

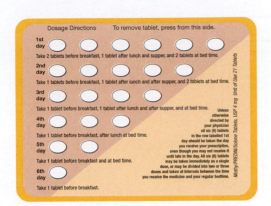

FIGURE 18-28

a. What is the appropriate quantity to dispense?
b. How many total doses are to be dispensed?
c. What is the total amount of methylprednisolone, in mg, to be dispensed in the pack?
d. How many days should this prescription last?

5.

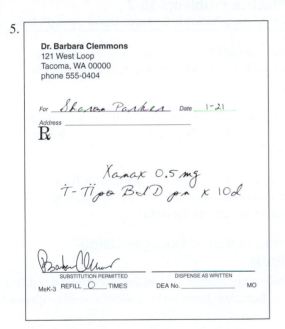

Dr. Barbara Clemmons
121 West Loop
Tacoma, WA 00000
phone 555-0404

For *Sharon Parker* Date *1-21*

Address

℞

Xanax 0.5 mg
T-Tipo BID prn × 10d

SUBSTITUTION PERMITTED   DISPENSE AS WRITTEN

MeK-3   REFILL _O_ TIMES   DEA No. _____ MO

FIGURE 18-29

a. What is the appropriate quantity to dispense?
b. What is the maximum number of doses available if 60 tablets are dispensed?
c. What is the maximum amount of alprazolam, in mg, to be taken daily?
d. How many days could this prescription last if 60 tablets are dispensed?

Calculating Pediatric Dosages

Pediatric patients (a group that includes both infants and children) require special dosing that is adjusted for their age and body weight (Figure 18-30). A number of formulas have been used throughout the years to determine the best dosage for pediatric patients; the most common are reviewed in this section. Chapter 32 reviews additional special considerations concerning pediatric patients.

Calculating Pediatric Dosages Using Fried's Rule

Fried's Rule is a formula used in calculating pediatric dosages based on the child's age, stated in months.

EXAMPLE 18.9

An infant, 15 months old and weighing 20 lb., needs streptomycin sulfate, which is usually administered to adults as 1 gm (1,000 mg) in a daily IM injection. What is the appropriate dosage for the infant?

To calculate the pediatric dosage based on a child's age, in months, simply use the formula for Fried's Rule. Using the information provided, set up the calculation as follows:

$$\text{Pediatric dose} = \frac{15\,(\text{age in months})}{150} \times 1{,}000\text{ mg (adult dose)}$$

$$\text{Pediatric dose} = \frac{15}{150} \times 1{,}000$$

$$\text{Pediatric dose} = 0.1 \times 1{,}000$$

$$\text{Pediatric dose} = 100\text{ mg}$$

So, according to Fried's Rule, the pediatric dosage appropriate for a 15-month-old would be 100 mg.

Practice Problems 18-6
Calculating Pediatric Dosages Using Fried's Rule

1. A 20-month-old child needs acetaminophen; the normal adult dose is 650 mg. What is the appropriate dosage for the child?

2. An 18-month-old needs amikacin sulfate; the normal adult dose is 250 mg. What is the appropriate dosage for the child?

3. A 28-month-old child needs erythromycin; the normal adult dose is 250 mg qid. What is the appropriate dosage for the child?

Calculating Pediatric Dosages Using Young's Rule

Young's Rule is another formula used in calculating pediatric dosages; it too is based on age. The difference between Young's Rule and Fried's Rule is that Young's Rule uses a formula based on the age expressed in years rather than months.

FORMULA	Pediatric Dosing

Fried's Rule

$$\text{Child's dosage} = \frac{\text{Age in months}}{150} \times \text{Adult dosage}$$

Young's Rule

$$\text{Child's dosage} = \frac{\text{Age of child in years}}{\text{Age of child in years} + 12} \times \text{Adult dosage}$$

Clark's Rule

$$\text{Child's dosage} = \frac{\text{Child's weight in pounds}}{150} \times \text{Adult dosage}$$

FIGURE 18-30 Pediatric dosing.

EXAMPLE 18.10

Let us reexamine Example 18.9 in light of Young's Rule, which uses the child's age in years. The age of a 15-month-old could be expressed as 1.25 years, since the child has lived for

12 months (1 year) + 3 months ($\frac{1}{4}$ or 0.25 of a year).

Using an age of 1.25 years and the information provided in Example 18.9, set up the calculation, using Young's Rule, as follows:

$$\text{Pediatric dose} = \frac{1.25 \ (\text{age in years})}{13.25 \ (\text{age of child} + 12)} \times$$
$$1{,}000 \text{ mg (adult dose)}$$

$$\text{Pediatric dose} = \frac{1.25}{13.25} \times 1{,}000$$

$$\text{Pediatric dose} = 0.094 \times 1{,}000$$

$$\text{Pediatric dose} = 94 \text{ mg}$$

So, according to Young's Rule, the pediatric dosage appropriate for a 15-month-old would be 94 mg.

Clark's Rule a formula for solving pediatric dosage calculations based on the patient's weight in pounds.

mg/kg/day a formula for solving dosage calculations based on the patient's weight in kilograms.

Practice Problems 18-7
Calculating Pediatric Dosages Using Young's Rule

1. A three-year-old child is prescribed amoxicillin; the normal adult dose is 500 mg. What is the appropriate dosage for the child?

2. A six-year-old needs propylthiouracil; the normal adult daily dose is 150 mg. What is the appropriate dosage for the child?

3. A child who is nine years old is prescribed Tavist syrup; the normal adult dose is 1.34 mg bid. What is the appropriate dosage for the child?

Calculating Pediatric Dosages Using Clark's Rule

Clark's Rule is yet another method for calculating a pediatric dosage. This formula is based on the patient's weight expressed in pounds.

EXAMPLE 18.11

Let's reexamine Example 18.9 in light of Clark's Rule, which uses the child's weight in pounds.

Using a weight of 20 lb. and the information provided in Example 18.9, set up the calculation using Young's Rule, as follows:

$$\text{Pediatric dose} = \frac{20 \ (\text{weight in pounds})}{150} \times$$
$$1{,}000 \text{ mg (adult dose)}$$

Pediatric dose $= \dfrac{20}{150} \times 1{,}000$

Pediatric dose $= 0.133 \times 1{,}000$

Pediatric dose $= 133$ mg

So, according to Clark's Rule, the pediatric dosage appropriate for a 15-month-old who weighs 20 lb. would be 133 mg.

Practice Problems 18-8
Calculating Pediatric Dosages Using Clark's Rule

1. A child weighing 80 lb. is prescribed hydrochlorothiazide; the normal adult dose is 50 mg. What is the appropriate dosage for the child?

2. A child weighing 76 lb. is prescribed quinine sulfate; the normal adult dose is 325 mg tid. What is the appropriate dosage for the child?

3. A child weighing 98 lb. is prescribed Kaletra, a protease-inhibitor combination therapy; the normal adult dose is 400 mg lopinavir/100 mg ritonavir. What is the appropriate dosage for the child?

Converting Weight from Pounds to Kilograms

Although it is not technically a dosage calculation, the conversion of a patient's weight from pounds to kilograms is a calculation needed when performing dosage calculations based on mg/kg, which is discussed in the next section.

EXAMPLE 18.12

If an infant weighs 20 lb., what is her weight in kilograms?

Using the weight conversion formula, you divide the patient's weight, which in this case is 20 lb., by 2.2 to convert the weight from pounds to kilograms.

$20 \div 2.2 = 9.09$

So, the infant weighs 9.09 kg.

Practice Problems 18-9
Converting Weight

Convert the following:

1. 12,012 lb. = _____ kg

2. 18 kg = _____ lb.

3. 74 lb. = _____ kg

4. 41 kg = _____ lb.

5. 38 kg = _____ lb.

6. 60 lb. = _____ kg

7. 24 kg = _____ lb.

8. 100 lb. = _____ kg

Calculating Dosages Using mg/kg/day

The most precise, and preferred, method of calculating dosages is based on the number of milligrams suggested per kilogram per day, or **mg/kg/day**. This method is also the most accurate and preferred method when calculating pediatric dosages.

EXAMPLE 18.13

Using the infant example from Examples 18.9 to 18.11, determine the pediatric dosage if it is recommended to administer 20 mg/kg/day (maximum of 1 gm) of streptomycin sulfate to this infant.

We have already calculated this infant's weight as 9.09 kg; so now we will multiply the recommended number of milligrams by her weight in kilograms to calculate the appropriate daily pediatric dosage.

20 mg $\times$ 9.09 kg $\times$ 1 day = pediatric daily dosage

20 $\times$ 9.09 $\times$ 1 = pediatric daily dosage

181.8 = pediatric daily dosage

So, according to the mg/kg/day formula, the patient should be given 181.8 mg of streptomycin sulfate as a daily IM injection.

Practice Problems 18-10
Calculating Dosages Using mg/kg/day

1. A dose of 4 mg/kg/day of Plaquenil can be recommended for certain children suffering from lupus. What would be the appropriate dosage for a patient who weighs 40 kg?

2. For children, the daily dose of Omnicef is 18 mg/kg, up to a maximum dose of 600 mg/day. What is the appropriate daily dosage for a patient who weighs 87 lb.?

3. The recommended dosage of fluconazole for oropharyngeal candidiasis is 6 mg/kg on day 1, followed by 3 mg/kg/day thereafter. What are the appropriate dosages for a child weighing 32 kg?

4. A child who weighs 76 lb. is prescribed the antibiotic cefaclor. It is recommended that children receive 20 mg/kg/day in divided doses every eight hours. How many milligrams should this child take per dose?

5. Acute lymphatic leukemia in children can respond well to methotrexate given 2.5 mg/kg every 18 days intravenously. What would be the appropriate dosage of methotrexate to administer biweekly to a child weighing 110 lb.?

PROFILE IN PRACTICE

Sheree is a pharmacy technician who works at a chain drugstore pharmacy. Recently she has filled a prescription for a patient that contained 60 tablets, with directions to take one to two tablets twice daily. Sheree entered the prescription as a 30-day supply. After two weeks, the patient requested a refill, and it was denied by the insurance company.

▶ *What mistake did Sheree make?*
▶ *What steps can she take to resolve the problem?*

Summary

Dosage calculations are varied and more than likely will be the pharmacy calculations you perform most often. Dosage calculations include determining the number of doses, dispensing quantities, and amount of active ingredients required, for both adult and pediatric patients.

Chapter Review Questions

1. How many 1 Tbsp. doses are in 1 pt. of lactulose solution, USP 10 gm/15 mL?
   a. 32
   b. 64
   c. 128
   d. 192

2. How many milligrams of estradiol are delivered over 48 hours by one 0.075 mg/day patch?
   a. 0.225
   b. 0.150
   c. 333
   d. 0.075

3. You are asked to compound maldroxyl 60 mL, diphenhydramine elixir 60 mL, and viscous lidocaine 2%, qs to 200 mL. How much viscous lidocaine 2% will you need to prepare the order?
   a. 60 mL
   b. 4 mL
   c. 80 mL
   d. 200 mL

4. The recommended pediatric dose of ampicillin is 25 mg/kg/day q8h. Your patient is a four-week-old infant who weighs 7.5 lb. Which is the best dose for this patient?
   a. 15 mg
   b. 25 mg
   c. 28 mg
   d. 45 mg

5. How many days will 4 oz. of clemastine fumarate syrup 0.5 mg/5 mL last if the dose is 1 tsp. tid?
   a. 24
   b. 8
   c. 30
   d. 12

6. How many grams of drug are in 480 mL of docusate sodium syrup 60 mg/15 mL?
   a. 28.8
   b. 1.92
   c. 1,920
   d. 2.88

7. How many milligrams are in a 2-mL dose of prochlorperazine injection 5 mg/mL given IM for severe nausea and vomiting?
   a. 10
   b. 5
   c. 2.5
   d. 15

8. How many milliliters of chloral hydrate syrup 500 mg/5 mL are required for a dose of 200 mg?
   a. 2.5
   b. 5
   c. 2
   d. 1

9. The recommended pediatric dose for promethazine is 0.25 mg/kg qid. What is the best dose for a 12-year-old boy who weighs 95 lb.?
   a. 2.5 mg
   b. 10 mg
   c. 12.5 mg
   d. 15 mg

10. How many total grams of active ingredient are in three syringes of testosterone 2% topical gel containing 3 gm of gel each?
    a. 0.18
    b. 0.6
    c. 666
    d. 1.81

Critical Thinking Questions

1. How do dosage calculations affect the insurance billing process?

2. Why is the mg/kg/day method preferred over the other pediatric dosage formulations?

3. List the various types of dosage calculations, along with an explanation of how to solve each type.

References and Resources

Hegstad, Lorrie N. and Wilma Hayek. *Essential Drug Dosage Calculations*. 4th ed. Upper Saddle River, NJ: Pearson, 2001. Print.

Johnston, Mike. *Pharmacy Calculations: The Pharmacy Technician Series*. Upper Saddle River, NJ: Pearson, 2005. Print.

Lesmeister, Michelle Benjamin. *Math Basics for the Healthcare Professional*. 4th ed. Upper Saddle River, NJ: Pearson, 2013. Print.

Mikolah, Alan A. *Drug Dosage Calculations for the Emergency Care Provider*. 2nd ed. Upper Saddle River, NJ: Prentice Hall, 2003. Print.

Olsen, June, Anthony Giangrasso, and Dolores Shrimpton. *Medical Dosage Calculations*. 10th ed. Upper Saddle River, NJ: Pearson, 2011. Print.

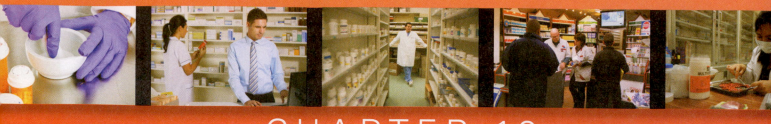

CHAPTER 19

Concentrations and Dilutions

LEARNING OBJECTIVES

After completing this chapter, you should be able to:

- Calculate weight/weight concentrations.
- Calculate weight/volume concentrations.
- Calculate volume/volume concentrations.
- Calculate dilutions of stock solutions.

KEY TERMS

concentration, p. 302

diluent, p. 310

percent strength, p. 302

% volume/volume (%v/v), p. 302

% weight/volume (%w/v), p. 302

% weight/weight (%w/w), p. 302

INTRODUCTION

Concentrations of many pharmaceutical preparations are expressed as a **percent strength**. This is an important concept. Percent strength represents how many grams of active ingredient are in 100 mL. In the case of solids such as ointments, percent strength represents the number of grams of active ingredient present in

---

concentration a term for the strength of active pharmaceutical ingredient in a medication.

percent strength representation of the number of grams of active ingredient contained in 100 mL.

% weight/weight (%w/w) percent strength concentration of a solid active ingredient contained within a solid base.

% weight/volume (%w/v) percent strength concentration of a solid active ingredient contained within a liquid base.

% volume/volume (%v/v) percent strength concentration of a liquid active ingredient contained within a liquid base.

100 gm. Percent strength can be reduced to a fraction or a decimal, which may be useful in solving these calculations. It is best to convert any ratio strengths to percents.

Workplace Wisdom Equivalents

Grams and milliliters are used interchangeably in concentration problems, as they are considered equivalent measures. With which you are dealing depends on whether you are working with solids in grams, or liquids in milliliters.

Concentrations

Concentration problems are classified into three categories:

- **Weight/weight** concentrations are those in which a solid active ingredient (e.g., a powder) is mixed with a solid base (e.g., an ointment).
- **Weight/volume** concentrations are those in which a solid active ingredient (e.g., a powder) is mixed with a liquid base (e.g., a syrup).
- **Volume/volume** concentrations are those in which a liquid active ingredient is mixed with a liquid base (e.g., an emulsion).

Weight/Weight Concentrations

Calculation of weight/weight concentrations can be easily and accurately performed by following these steps:

1. Set up a proportion with the amount of active ingredient listed over the total quantity, as grams over grams.
2. Convert the proportion to a decimal (by dividing the numerator by the denominator).
3. Multiply the converted number by 100 to express the final concentration as a percentage.

EXAMPLE 19.1

If 1 gm of active ingredient powder is mixed with 99 gm of white petrolatum, what is the final concentration (w/w)?

Let's look at the information that has been provided and is critical to solving the calculation:

1 gm	Amount of active ingredient
99 gm white petrolatum	Amount of base
100 gm*	Total quantity (1 gm of active ingredient + 99 gm of base)

*It is important to be careful in determining the amount for the total quantity. If you do not add both the active ingredient and base quantities for the total quantity—even if they are not both listed—the calculation will be set up incorrectly from the very start!

The first step is to set up a proportion with the amount of active ingredient listed over the total quantity.

$$\frac{1 \text{ gm (active)}}{100 \text{ gm (total)}}$$

Next, convert the proportion to a decimal by dividing the numerator by the denominator.

$$1 \text{ gm} \div 100 \text{ gm} = 0.01$$

Now, multiply the converted number by 100 to express the final concentration as a percentage.

$$0.01 \times 100 = 1\%$$

So, the final weight/weight concentration is 1%.

EXAMPLE 19.2

A 120-gm compounded cream contains 12 gm of active ingredient powder. What is the concentration (w/w)?

Let us look at the information that has been provided and is critical to solving the calculation:

12 gm	Amount of active ingredient
Not provided	Amount of base
120 gm*	Total quantity

*In this example, we are not given the amount of base, only the amount of active ingredient and the total quantity.

First, set up a proportion with the amount of active ingredient listed over the total quantity.

$$\frac{12 \text{ gm (active)}}{120 \text{ gm (total)}}$$

Now, convert the proportion to a decimal by dividing the numerator by the denominator.

$$12 \text{ gm} \div 120 \text{ gm} = 0.1$$

Finally, multiply the converted number by 100 to express the final concentration as a percentage.

$$0.1 \times 100 = 10\%$$

Therefore, the final weight/weight concentration of the compounded cream is 10%.

EXAMPLE 19.3

A 30-gm compounded ointment contains 105 mg of neomycin sulfate in 30 gm. What is the final concentration (w/w)?

Let us look at the information that has been provided and is critical to solving the calculation:

0.105 gm	Amount of active ingredient
Not provided	Amount of base
30 gm	Total quantity

Set up a proportion with the amount of active ingredient listed over the total quantity.

$$\frac{0.105 \text{ gm (active)}}{30 \text{ gm (total)}}$$

Then, convert the proportion to a decimal by dividing the numerator by the denominator.

$$0.105 \text{ gm} \div 30 \text{ gm} = 0.0035$$

Now, multiply the converted number by 100 to express the final concentration as a percentage.

$$0.0035 \times 100 = 0.35\%$$

Therefore, the final weight/weight concentration is 0.35%.

❝ Workplace Wisdom Calculating Concentrations

For accurate concentration calculations, the proportion must be set up as grams over grams. Example 19.3 provides the amount of active ingredient in milligrams, which must first be converted to grams. ❞

EXAMPLE 19.4

If you add 3 gm of salicylic acid to 97 gm of an ointment base, what is the final concentration (w/w) of the product?

Let's look at the information that has been provided and is critical to solving the calculation:

3 gm	Amount of active ingredient
97 gm	Amount of base
100 gm	Total quantity (3 gm + 97 gm)

Set up a proportion with the amount of active ingredient listed over the total quantity.

$$\frac{3 \text{ gm (active)}}{100 \text{ gm (total)}}$$

Now, convert the proportion to a decimal by dividing the numerator by the denominator.

$$3 \text{ gm} \div 100 \text{ gm} = 0.03$$

Multiply the converted number by 100 to express the final concentration as a percentage.

$$0.03 \times 100 = 3\%$$

Therefore, the final weight/weight concentration of the ointment is 3%.

EXAMPLE 19.5

How much oxiconazole nitrate powder is required to prepare the following order?

Dr. Barbara Clemmons
121 West Loop
Tacoma, WA 00000
phone 555-0404

For _Sharon Parker_   Date _1-21_
Address _____

℞

1% Oxiconazole
Nitrate Ointment
Disp. 45g

_____   _____
SUBSTITUTION PERMITTED   DISPENSE AS WRITTEN

MeK-3 REFILL _____ TIMES   DEA No. _____ MO

Let's look at the information that has been provided and find out what is missing:

Not provided	Amount of active ingredient
Not provided	Amount of base
45 gm	Total quantity
1%	Final

In this problem, we have been given the final concentration and asked to determine the amount of active ingredient needed. Notice that, in essence, the previous examples could have been solved by using the following formula:

$$\frac{\text{gm active ingredient}}{\text{gm total quantity}} \times 100 = \text{final percent strength}$$

Up to this point, we have been able to calculate the final percent strength (% strength) by filling in the other amounts and solving. We will take the same approach to solving this problem; the only difference is that we will solve for the number of grams of active ingredient.

Using the information we know and the preceding formula, let us fill in everything we can.

$$\frac{X \text{ gm (active)}}{45 \text{ gm (total)}} \times 100 = 1\%$$

To solve for X, the unknown quantity of active ingredient, we can divide both sides of the equation by 100. This will cancel it out on the left side and create a fraction on the right side.

$$\frac{X \text{ gm (active)}}{45 \text{ gm (total)}} \times \frac{100}{100} = \frac{1}{100}$$

Now, we have a ratio and proportion, which can be cross-multiplied and solved for X.

$$\frac{X \text{ gm (active)}}{45 \text{ gm (total)}} = \frac{1}{100}$$

Cross-multiply.

$$X \times 100 = 100X$$

$$1 \times 45 = 45$$

So, $100X = 45$

Now we can divide both sides by 100 to solve for X (the quantity of active ingredient needed).

$$\frac{100X}{100} = \frac{45}{100}$$

$$X = 0.45$$

So, 0.45 gm or 450 mg of oxiconazole nitrate powder is needed for this order.

EXAMPLE 19.6

How much fluorouracil powder is in 25 gm of 5% Efudex cream?

Let's look at the information that has been provided:

Not provided   Amount of active
Not provided   Amount of base
25 gm   Total quantity
5%   Final

Again, we have been given the final concentration and asked to determine the amount of active ingredient needed.

Using the information known and the formula, fill in everything you can.

$$\frac{X \text{ gm (active)}}{25 \text{ gm (total)}} \times 100 = 5\%$$

Divide both sides of the equation by 100 to set up a ratio and proportion that can be solved.

$$\frac{X \text{ gm (active)}}{25 \text{ gm (total)}} \times \frac{100}{100} = \frac{5}{100}$$

Now we have a ratio and proportion, which can be cross-multiplied and solved for X.

$$\frac{X \text{ gm (active)}}{25 \text{ gm (total)}} = \frac{5}{100}$$

Cross-multiply.

$$X \times 100 = 100X$$

$$5 \times 25 = 125$$

So, $100X = 125$

Now, divide both sides by 100 to solve for X (the quantity of active ingredient needed).

$$\frac{100X}{100} = \frac{125}{100}$$

$$X = 1.25$$

So, 1.25 gm of fluorouracil powder is contained in 25 gm of 5% Efudex cream.

Practice Problems 19-1
Weight/Weight Concentrations

1. Zovirax contains 200 mg of acyclovir in 4 gm. What is the concentration of this product?

2. Tinactin contains 0.15 gm of tolnaftate powder in 15 gm. What is the percent strength of this cream?

3. Bactroban ointment contains 0.6 gm of mupirocin per 30-gm tube. What is the percent strength of this product?

4. Zonalon cream contains 1.5 gm of doxepin HCl with 28.5 gm of a cream base. What is the concentration of Zonalon?

5. To prepare a topical cream, you add 150 mg of metronidazole to 14.85 gm of a cream base. What is the final percent strength of this cream?

6. If 6 gm of azelaic acid is added to 24 gm of a cream base to produce Azelex cream, what is the concentration of this product?

7. Hytone contains 500 mg of hydrocortisone powder with 19.5 gm of an emollient base. What is the percent strength of Hytone?

8. How much boric acid is contained in 50 gm of a 20% boric acid ointment?

9. How much sulfur is contained in 160 gm of a 5% Plexion SCT cream?

10. Vaniqa cream contains 13.9% eflornithine HCl. How many grams of active ingredient are contained in 30 gm of Vaniqa?

Weight/Volume Concentrations

Calculation of weight/volume concentrations can be easily and accurately performed by following these steps:

1. Set up a proportion with the amount of active ingredient listed over the total quantity, as grams over milliliters.
2. Convert the proportion to a decimal (by dividing the numerator by the denominator).
3. Multiply the converted number by 100 to express the final concentration as a percentage.

If 100 gm of active ingredient powder is mixed with 500 mL of normal saline, what is the final concentration (w/v)?

Let's look at the information that has been provided and is critical to solving the calculation:

100 gm	Amount of active ingredient
500 mL normal saline	Amount of base
500 mL	Total quantity

" Workplace Wisdom Weight/Volume Concentrations

When mixing powders with liquids, the liquid (base) quantity is considered the total quantity, because the powder will either dissolve or suspend within the base liquid. **"**

The first step is to set up a proportion with the amount of active ingredient listed over the total quantity.

$$\frac{100 \text{ gm (active)}}{500 \text{ mL (total)}}$$

Next, convert the proportion to a decimal by dividing the numerator by the denominator.

$$100 \text{ gm} \div 500 \text{ mL} = 0.2$$

Now, multiply the converted number by 100 to express the final concentration as a percentage.

$$0.2 \times 100 = 20\%$$

So, the final weight/volume concentration is 20%.

Example 19.9 provides the formula for normal saline: 0.9% NaCl.

If 25 gm of active ingredient powder is mixed with 250 mL of distilled water, what is the final percent strength (w/v)?

Let's look at the information that has been provided and is critical to solving the calculation:

25 gm	Amount of active ingredient
250 mL	Total quantity

First, set up a proportion with the amount of active ingredient listed over the total quantity.

$$\frac{25 \text{ gm (active)}}{250 \text{ mL (total)}}$$

Next, convert the proportion to a decimal by dividing the numerator by the denominator.

$$25 \text{ gm} \div 250 \text{ mL} = 0.1$$

Now, multiply the converted number by 100 to express the final concentration as a percentage.

$$0.1 \times 100 = 10\%$$

So, the final weight/volume percent strength is 10%.

If 9 gm of sodium chloride is diluted in 1 L of sterile water for injection (SWFI), what is the final percent strength (w/v)?

Let's look at the information that has been provided and is critical to solving the calculation:

9 gm	Amount of active ingredient
1,000 mL*	Total quantity

*Remember that the total quantity must be expressed as milliliters, so the 1 L given in the original problem statement is converted to 1,000 mL.

Set up a proportion with the amount of active ingredient listed over the total quantity.

$$\frac{9 \text{ gm (active)}}{1,000 \text{ mL (total)}}$$

Next, convert the proportion to a decimal by dividing the numerator by the denominator.

$$9 \text{ gm} \div 1000 \text{ mL} = 0.009$$

Now, multiply the converted number by 100 to express the final concentration as a percentage.

$0.009 \times 100 = 0.9\%$

So, the final weight/volume percent strength is 0.9%.

EXAMPLE 19.10

Xylocaine liquid contains 1.5 gm of lidocaine HCl in 30 mL. What is the final concentration (w/v)?

Let's look at the information that has been provided and is critical to solving the calculation:

1.5 gm   Amount of active ingredient

30 mL   Total quantity

Set up a proportion with the amount of active ingredient listed over the total quantity.

$$\frac{1.5 \text{ gm (active)}}{30 \text{ mL (total)}}$$

Now, convert the proportion to a decimal by dividing the numerator by the denominator.

$1.5 \text{ gm} \div 30 \text{ mL} = 0.05$

Finally, multiply the converted number by 100 to express the final concentration as a percentage.

$0.05 \times 100 = 5\%$

So, the final weight/volume concentration is 5%.

EXAMPLE 19.11

Melanex solution contains 0.9 gm of hydroquinone in every 1-oz. bottle. What is the final percent strength (w/v)?

Let's look at the information that has been provided and is critical to solving the calculation:

0.9 gm   Amount of active ingredient

30 mL*   Total quantity

*Remember that the total quantity must be expressed as milliliters, so the 1 oz. is converted to 30 mL.

Set up a proportion with the amount of active ingredient listed over the total quantity.

$$\frac{0.9 \text{ gm (active)}}{30 \text{ mL (total)}}$$

Next, convert the proportion to a decimal by dividing the numerator by the denominator.

$0.9 \text{ gm} \div 30 \text{ mL} = 0.03$

Now, multiply the converted number by 100 to express the final concentration as a percentage.

$0.03 \times 100 = 3\%$

So, the final weight/volume percent strength is 3%.

EXAMPLE 19.12

Rogaine Extra Strength is a 5% solution of minoxidil in alcohol. How much active ingredient is in a 60-mL bottle?

Let's look at the information that has been provided and find out what is missing:

Not provided   Amount of active ingredient

60 mL   Total quantity

5%   Final strength

In this problem, we have been given the final concentration and asked to determine the amount of active ingredient needed. Notice that, in essence, the previous examples could be solved by using the following formula:

$$\frac{\text{gm active}}{\text{mL total quantity}} \times 100 = \text{final percent strength}$$

Using the information we know and the preceding formula, let us fill in everything we can.

$$\frac{\text{X gm (active)}}{60 \text{ mL (total)}} \times 100 = 5\%$$

To solve for X, the unknown quantity of active ingredient, we can divide both sides of the equation by 100. This will cancel it out on the left side and create a fraction on the right side.

$$\frac{\text{X gm (active)}}{60 \text{ mL (total)}} \times \frac{\cancel{100}}{\cancel{100}} = \frac{5}{100}$$

Now we have a ratio and proportion, which can be cross-multiplied and solved for X.

$$\frac{\text{X gm (active)}}{60 \text{ mL (total)}} = \frac{5}{100}$$

Cross-multiply.

$\text{X} \times 100 = 100\text{X}$

$60 \times 5 = 300$

So, $100\text{X} = 300$

Now we can divide both sides by 100 to solve for X (the quantity of active ingredient needed).

$$\frac{\cancel{100}\text{X}}{\cancel{100}} = \frac{300}{100}$$

$\text{X} = 3$

So, a 60-mL bottle of 5% Rogaine Extra Strength contains 3 gm of minoxidil powder.

Practice Problems 19-2
Weight/Volume Concentrations

1. Betagan Liquifilm contains 25 mg of levobunolol HCl in 10 mL of solution. What is the percent strength?

2. If 250 gm of dextrose is added to 1 L of SWFI, what is the final concentration?

3. Cleocin T contains 10 mg of clindamycin phosphate per mL of solution. What is the percent strength of this product?

4. Pred Forte contains 0.15 gm of prednisolone in 15 mL of ophthalmic suspension. What is the concentration of this product?

5. How much sodium chloride powder is needed to prepare 1 L of a 0.45% NaCl solution?

6. How much phenylephrine HCl would be needed to prepare 20 mL of a 2.5% ophthalmic solution?

7. Sebizon lotion contains 8.5 gm of sulfacetamide sodium in 85 mL of solution. What is the final concentration of this product?

8. How much silver nitrate is needed to prepare 2 oz. of a 30% silver nitrate solution?

9. How much albuterol sulfate is needed to compound 120 unit-dose vials (3 mL) of 0.042% albuterol for nebulization?

10. Drysol contains 7.5 gm of aluminum chloride hexahydrate in 37.5 mL of an alcohol base. What is the final percent strength of Drysol?

Volume/Volume Concentrations

Calculation of volume/volume concentrations can be easily and accurately performed by following these steps:

1. Set up a proportion with the amount of active ingredient listed over the total quantity, as milliliters over milliliters.
2. Convert the proportion to a decimal (by dividing the numerator by the denominator).
3. Multiply the converted number by 100 to express the final concentration as a percentage.

EXAMPLE 19.13

If 10 mL of active ingredient is mixed with distilled water to make a total of 200 mL, what is the final concentration (v/v)?

Let's look at the information that has been provided and is critical to solving the calculation:

10 mL	Amount of active ingredient
200 mL	Total quantity

The first step is to set up a proportion with the amount of active ingredient listed over the total quantity.

$$\frac{10 \text{ mL (active)}}{200 \text{ mL (total)}}$$

Next, convert the proportion to a decimal by dividing the numerator by the denominator.

$$10 \text{ mL} \div 200 \text{ mL} = 0.05$$

Now, multiply the converted number by 100 to express the final concentration as a percentage.

$$0.05 \times 100 = 5\%$$

So, the final volume/volume concentration is 5%.

EXAMPLE 19.14

If 180 mL of active ingredient is added to 820 mL of an alcohol-based solution, what is the final strength (v/v)?

Let's look at the information that has been provided and is critical to solving the calculation:

180 mL	Amount of active ingredient
820 mL	Amount of base
1,000 mL	Total quantity

" Workplace Wisdom Volume/Volume Concentrations

It is important to be careful when determining the amount for the total quantity. If you do not add both the active and base quantities for the total quantity, even if they are not both listed, the calculation will be set up incorrectly from the very start!

The first step is to set up a proportion with the amount of active ingredient listed over the total quantity.

$$\frac{180 \text{ mL (active)}}{1,000 \text{ mL (total)}}$$

Next, convert the proportion to a decimal by dividing the numerator by the denominator.

$$180 \text{ mL} \div 1,000 \text{ mL} = 0.18$$

Now, multiply the converted number by 100 to express the final concentration as a percentage.

$$0.18 \times 100 = 18\%$$

So, the final volume/volume strength is 18%.

EXAMPLE 19.15

If 36 mL of bezoin tincture is combined with 84 mL of an 80% alcohol solution, what is the final strength (v/v)?

Let's look at the information that has been provided and is critical to solving the calculation:

36 mL	Amount of active ingredient
84 mL	Amount of base
120 mL	Total quantity

Be careful: 80% is not a factor in solving this problem. It is simply describing the base product.

The first step is to set up a proportion with the amount of active ingredient listed over the total quantity.

$$\frac{36 \text{ mL (active)}}{120 \text{ mL (total)}}$$

Next, convert the proportion to a decimal by dividing the numerator by the denominator.

$$36 \text{ mL} \div 120 \text{ mL} = 0.3$$

Now, multiply the converted number by 100 to express the final concentration as a percentage.

$$0.3 \times 100 = 30\%$$

So, the final volume/volume strength is 30%.

EXAMPLE 19.16

How many milliliters of active ingredient must be added to distilled water to produce 60 mL of a 25% solution (v/v)?

Let's look at the information that has been provided and find out what is missing:

Not provided	Amount of active ingredient
60 mL	Total quantity
25%	Final strength

In this problem, we have been given the final concentration and asked to determine the amount of active ingredient needed. Notice that, in essence, the previous examples could have been solved by using the following formula:

$$\frac{\text{mL active}}{\text{mL total quantity}} \times 100 = \text{final percent strength}$$

Using the information we know and the preceding formula, let us fill in everything we can.

$$\frac{X \text{ mL (active)}}{60 \text{ mL (total)}} \times 100 = 25\%$$

To solve for X, the unknown quantity of active ingredient, we can divide both sides of the equation by 100. This will

cancel it out on the left side and create a fraction on the right side.

$$\frac{X \text{ mL (active)}}{60 \text{ mL (total)}} \times \frac{\cancel{100}}{\cancel{100}} = \frac{25}{100}$$

Now we have a ratio and proportion, which can be cross-multiplied and solved for X.

$$\frac{X \text{ mL (active)}}{60 \text{ mL (total)}} = \frac{25}{100}$$

Cross-multiply.

$$X \times 100 = 100X$$

$$60 \times 25 = 1,500$$

So, $100X = 1,500$

Now we can divide both sides by 100 to solve for X (the quantity of active ingredient needed).

$$\frac{\cancel{100}X}{\cancel{100}} = \frac{1,500}{100}$$

$$X = 15$$

So, 15 mL of active ingredient is necessary to produce 60 mL of a 25% solution.

Practice Problems 19-3
Volume/Volume Concentrations

1. If 20 mL of alcohol is combined with 80 mL of distilled water, what is the percent of v/v concentration?

2. If 200 mL of active ingredient is combined with 300 mL of normal saline, what is the final percent strength?

3. If 2 Tbsp. of extract is mixed with 120 mL of oral suspension base, what is the final concentration of the suspension?

4. If 5 mL of medicated tincture is combined with simple syrup to make a total of 2 oz, what is the final percent strength of the product?

5. If 48 mL of lidocaine is mixed with 552 mL of a suspension base, what is the final percent v/v concentration?

6. How many milliliters of active ingredient are required to be added to normal saline to produce a total of 250 mL of a 15% solution?

7. How much gentian violet should be added to alcohol to produce a total of 1 L of a 5% solution?

8. How much active ingredient must be added to distilled water to produce a total of 20 mL of a 70% solution?

9. If 20 mL of butyl stearate is mixed with 380 mL of alcohol, what is the final percent strength?

10. If 20 mL of artificial flavor concentrate is mixed with 105 mL of SWFI, what is the final concentration of this product?

Dilutions

Stock solutions are strong (very concentrated) solutions that you can later dilute to the strength ordered or desired. The larger volume that you mix with the stock solution is called the **diluent**. You can use the following formula to calculate dilutions, where Q represents the quantity, expressed in milliliters or grams, and C represents the concentration listed as a percent strength:

$$Q1 \times C1 = Q2 \times C2$$

The equation may also be written this way, as a ratio and proportion:

$$\frac{Q1}{Q2} :: \frac{C2}{C1}$$

❝ Workplace Wisdom Dilutions

Some pharmacy technicians and instructors use the formula C1V1 = C2V2, or C1 × V1 = C2 × V2, where C = concentration and V = volume. Either terminology works fine, so use what is easiest for you to remember. ❞

Notice that the quantities are shown on one side and the concentrations on the other. Note also that the initial values, represented by the number 1, are diagonal to each other and that the final values, represented by the number 2, are on the opposite diagonal.

Calculating dilution problems requires you to place the provided elements in the formula appropriately before solving.

Q1 = initial quantity or volume
Q2 = final, or desired, quantity or volume
C1 = initial concentration expressed as a percentage (stock solution)
C2 = final, or desired, concentration expressed as a percentage (final solution)

When solving dilutions, three of these four elements will be provided; you must place them appropriately in the formula and then solve for the unknown.

EXAMPLE 19.17

How much stock solution of hydrogen peroxide 12% solution will you need to make 480 mL of hydrogen peroxide 3% solution?

Q1 = X

C1 = 12%

Q2 = 480 mL

C2 = 3

Use the formula by plugging in the known elements:

X × 12 = 480 × 3

12X = 1,440

To solve for X, divide both sides by 12.

$$\frac{\cancel{12}X}{\cancel{12}} = \frac{1,440}{12}$$

X = 120 mL

So, you would need 120 mL of the 12% solution to dilute to 480 mL of a 3% solution.

EXAMPLE 19.18

You had 60 gm of a 20% coal tar solution, which you diluted to produce 100 gm. What is the strength of the final product?

Q1 = 60 g

C1 = 20%

Q2 = 100 g

C2 = X

Use the formula by plugging in the known elements:

60 × 20 = 100 × X

1,200 = 100X

To solve for X, divide both sides by 100.

$$\frac{1,200}{100} = \frac{\cancel{100}X}{\cancel{100}}$$

12 = X

So, the final product is a 12% coal tar solution.

EXAMPLE 19.19

If you diluted 90 mL of an 8% benzocaine lotion to 6%, how much could you produce?

Q1 = 90 mL

C1 = 8%

Q2 = X

C2 = 6%

Use the formula by plugging in the known elements:

90 × 8 = X × 6

720 = 6X

To solve for X, divide both sides by 6.

$$\frac{720}{6} = \frac{\cancel{6}X}{\cancel{6}}$$

120 = X

So, you would be able to produce 120 mL of the diluted 6% lotion.

---

diluent a substance used to dilute another substance.

Practice Problems 19-4
Dilutions

1. How much of a 12% solution will you need to produce 150 mL of a 6% solution?

2. How much of a 50% silver nitrate solution do you need to produce 1 oz. of a 10% silver nitrate solution?

3. How much of a 6% solution can you make by diluting 500 mL of a 20% solution?

4. How much prostaglandin 500 mcg/mL solution is needed to prepare 10 cc of prostaglandin 20 mcg/mL solution?

5. How much doxepin 10 mg/mL concentrate should you dilute to prepare 240 mL of doxepin 25 mg/5 mL?

6. Rx: povidone iodine 2% soaking solution 1 L. How much povidone iodine 12% solution should you dilute to prepare the order?

7. You have a stock solution of lidocaine HCl 4% solution. How much of the stock solution is needed to prepare 1 oz. of lidocaine HCl 2% nasal spray?

8. Rx: hydrochloric acid 1% solution 4 oz. You have a stock solution of hydrochloric acid 50%. How much of the stock solution is required to prepare the order?

9. You have a stock solution of hydroxycobalamin 10 mg/mL. How much of the stock solution is needed to prepare 30 mL of a hydroxycobalamin 5,000 mcg/mL solution?

10. Rx: vancomycin 50 mg/100 mL Disp: 100 mL. In stock, you have vials that contain vancomycin 50 mg/10 mL. How many milliliters of stock solution will you need to prepare this order?

PROFILE IN PRACTICE

Bonnie works as a pharmacy technician at St. Joseph's Hospital inpatient pharmacy. The pharmacist asks Bonnie to dilute a stock solution to 25% of the original strength. Bonnie determines that the easiest way to do this is to take one-fourth of the volume of the original stock solution and q.s. to the original volume with SWFI.

▶ *Will Bonnie obtain the desired dilution using this method?*

Summary

The calculation of concentrations and dilutions, which can appear overwhelming and intimidating, is in essence no more than a series of simple ratios and proportions. You will use concentrations and dilutions in a variety of pharmacy practice settings, so it is important that you master this skill.

Chapter Review Questions

1. 35% w/w contains how many grams of active ingredient per 100 gm?
   a. 35
   b. 3.5
   c. 100
   d. 0.35

2. How many milligrams of active ingredient will you need to prepare 120 mL of a product that contains 4 mg/mL of active ingredient?
   a. 120
   b. 4
   c. 480
   d. 400

3. What is the percent strength of clemastine fumarate syrup 0.5 mg/5 mL?
   a. 0.05
   b. 0.01
   c. 0.025
   d. 0.5

4. Which of the following has the lowest concentration?
   a. 4 mg/mL
   b. 4%
   c. 2 mg/mL
   d. 2%

5. What is the final volume when you dilute 10 mL of a lidocaine 6% nasal spray to a lidocaine 2% nasal spray?
   a. 10 mL
   b. 12 mL
   c. 15 mL
   d. 30 mL

6. How many milliliters of gentian violet 2% solution will you need to make 240 mL of a 0.5% solution?
   a. 5
   b. 20
   c. 60
   d. 120

7. What is the final strength when you dilute 25 mL of a 12% solution with 100 mL water (final volume 125 mL)?
   a. 5.0%
   b. 2.0%
   c. 2.4%
   d. 3.0%

8. What is the resulting ratio strength when you dilute 12 mL of liquid coal tar to make 240 mL of coal tar solution?
   a. 1:5
   b. 1:10
   c. 1:12
   d. 1:20

9. How many grams of thymol should you dilute to make 30 mL of a 4% thymol in alcohol topical nail solution?
   a. 0.12
   b. 1.2
   c. 4.0
   d. 7.5

10. What is the final volume when you dilute 50 mL of a sorbitol 50% solution to a 20% solution?
   a. 125 mL
   b. 150 mL
   c. 250 mL
   d. 200 mL

Critical Thinking Questions

1. Can a solution ever be diluted to a strength higher than the starting solution? Why or why not?

2. Why is it important to determine whether the active ingredient is contained within, or being added to, the base when calculating w/w and v/v concentrations?

3. How much normal saline (NS) would be needed to produce 1 L of a 0.45% sodium chloride solution?

References and Resources

Lesmeister, Michelle Benjamin. *Math Basics for the Healthcare Professional*. 4th ed. Upper Saddle River, NJ: Pearson, 2013. Print.

Lorrie N. and Wilma Hayek. *Essential Drug Dosage Calculations*. 4th ed. Upper Saddle River, NJ: Pearson, 2001. Print.

Johnston, Mike. *Pharmacy Calculations: The Pharmacy Technician Series*. Upper Saddle River, NJ: Pearson, 2005. Print.

Mikolah, Alan A. *Drug Dosage Calculations for the Emergency Care Provider*. 2nd ed. Upper Saddle River, NJ: Prentice Hall, 2003. Print.

Olsen, June, Anthony Giangrasso, and Dolores Shrimpton. *Medical Dosage Calculations*. 10th ed. Upper Saddle River, NJ: Pearson, 2011. Print.

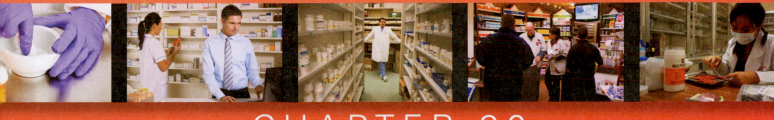

CHAPTER 20

Alligations

INTRODUCTION

Alligations are used when mixing two products with different percent strengths of the same active ingredient. The strength of the final product will fall between the strengths of each original product.

Solving Alligations

You can use the alligation method to determine how many parts of the same product, with different strengths, you will need to create the final strength requested. Further, you can calculate exactly how many milliliters or grams you need of each constituent (beginning) product.

The Alligation Grid

The alligation grid shown in Figure 20-1, which is also referred to as a tic-tac-toe board, is simply a tool that makes it easier to solve pharmacy alligation problems. In the following examples, you will learn what each segment of the grid represents.

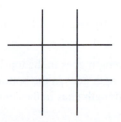

FIGURE 20-1 The alligation grid.

---

alligation a principle relating to the solution of questions concerning the compounding or mixing of different ingredients.

Key Points to Solving Alligations

It is critical that you understand the following points when working alligation problems.

- Solvents and diluents, such as water, vanishing cream base, and white petrolatum, are considered to have a percent strength of zero.
- Liquids, including solutions, syrups, elixirs, and even lotions, are expressed in milliliters.
- Solids, including powders, creams, and ointments, are expressed in grams.
- The alligation formula requires that you express the strength as a percentage when setting up the problem. You must convert any ratio strength in the initial question to a percent strength.
- When writing percents or using decimals, always use a leading zero (e.g., 0.25%). This helps prevent errors in interpretation. It would be a terrible error—possibly even fatal—to dispense something in 25% strength that was really supposed to be 0.25% strength.
- 1 fl. oz. = 29.57 mL This is commonly rounded to 30 mL.
- 1 avoirdupois oz. = 28.35 gm. This measurement, used for solids, is also commonly rounded to 30 gm.

EXAMPLE 20.1

Rx: Prepare 120 gm of a 2% hydrocortisone ointment using a 1% ointment and a 2.5% ointment.

Let us look at the information that has been provided:

2.5%	Higher strength
1%	Lower strength
2%	Desired strength
120 gm	Desired quantity

First, draw the alligation grid.

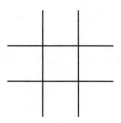

Now, fill in the alligation grid with the information provided in the problem.

- The higher strength goes in the top-left box.
- The lower strength goes in the bottom-left box.
- The desired strength goes in the center box.

Higher 2.5

Desired 2

Lower 1

Next, we calculate the numbers that should go into the top-right and bottom-right boxes.

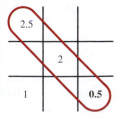

Higher 2.5

Desired 2

Lower 1

This is done by working diagonally and taking the difference between the two numbers that are already in place.

Let us look at the first diagonal, which contains 2.5 and 2. The difference between these two numbers goes in the bottom-right box.

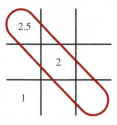

The difference between 2.5 and 2 is 0.5, so 0.5 goes in the bottom-right box.

$$2.5 - 2 = 0.5$$

Now, we can work on the other diagonal, which contains 1 and 2. The difference between these two numbers goes in the top-right box.

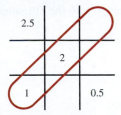

The difference between 1 and 2 is 1, so 1 goes in the top-right box.

$$1 - 2 = -1$$

Only positive numbers can go into the alligation grid, so –1 is changed to 1.

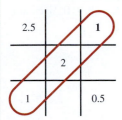

The numbers on the right-hand side of the alligation grid represent the number of parts per ingredient, when read straight across. This means that there should be 1 part of the 2.5% (higher-strength) ointment and 0.5 parts of the 1% (lower-strength) ointment to make the 2% ointment.

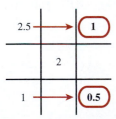

Now, by adding the numbers in the right column, we can determine the total number of parts necessary. In other words,

1 part (2.5%) + 0.5 parts (1%) = 1.5 parts total

Now that we have determined the number of parts needed for each ingredient and the total number of parts to be used, we can set these up as proportions.

$$\frac{\text{Parts needed}}{\text{Total parts}}$$

2.5% ointment

$$\frac{1 \text{ part}}{1.5 \text{ parts}} \text{ or } \frac{1}{1.5}$$

1% ointment

$$\frac{0.5 \text{ parts}}{1.5 \text{ parts}} \text{ or } \frac{0.5}{1.5}$$

Finally, we can take the proportion of parts needed of each ointment and multiply it by the desired quantity to determine the quantity of each ingredient needed.

2.5% ointment

$$\frac{120 \text{ gm}}{1.5} \times 1 = 80 \text{ gm}$$

1% ointment

$$\frac{120 \text{ gm}}{1.5} \times 0.5 = 40 \text{ gm}$$

So, we would combine 80 gm of the 2.5% ointment and 40 gm of the 1% ointment to produce 120 gm of a 2% ointment.

❝ Workplace Wisdom Positive Numbers Only

Remember that only positive numbers can be used within the alligation grid. If you are working with a negative number, remove the minus sign. ❞

EXAMPLE 20.2

Rx: Prepare 90 gm of triamcinolone 0.05% cream. In stock, you have 454 gm each of triamcinolone 0.025% cream and triamcinolone 0.1% cream.

Let us look at the information that has been provided:

0.1%	Higher strength
0.025	Lower strength
0.05%	Desired strength
90 gm	Desired quantity

First, draw the alligation grid.

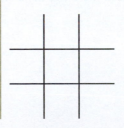

Now, fill in the alligation grid with the information provided in the problem.

- The higher strength goes in the top-left box.
- The lower strength goes in the bottom-left box.
- The desired strength goes in the center box.

Higher 0.1

Desired 0.05

Lower 0.025

Next, we calculate the numbers that should go into the top-right and bottom-right boxes.

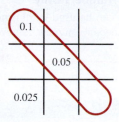

Higher 0.1

Desired 0.05

Lower 0.025

This is done by working diagonally and taking the difference between the two numbers that are already in place.

Let us look at the first diagonal, which contains 0.1 and 0.05. The difference between these two numbers goes in the bottom-right box.

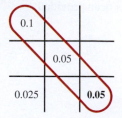

The difference between 0.1 and 0.05 is 0.05, so 0.05 goes in the bottom-right box.

$$0.1 - 0.05 = 0.05$$

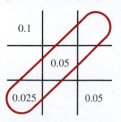

Now, we can work on the other diagonal, which contains 0.025 and 0.05. The difference between these two numbers goes in the top-right box.

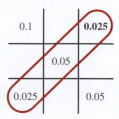

The difference between 0.025 and 0.05 is 0.025, so 0.025 goes in the top-right box.

$$0.025 - 0.05 = -0.025$$

Remember, only positive numbers can go into the alligation grid, so −0.025 is changed to 0.025.

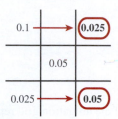

The numbers on the right-hand side of the alligation grid represent the number of parts per ingredient, when read straight across. This means that there should be 0.025 parts of the 0.1% cream and 0.05 parts of the 0.025% cream to make the 0.05% cream.

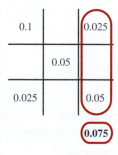

Now, by adding the numbers in the right-hand column, we can determine the total number of parts necessary. In other words,

$$0.025 \text{ parts } (0.1\%) + 0.05 \text{ parts } (0.025\%) = 0.075 \text{ parts total}$$

Now that we have determined the number of parts needed for each ingredient and the total number of parts to be used, we can set these up as proportions.

$$\frac{\text{Parts needed}}{\text{Total parts}}$$

0.1% cream

$$\frac{0.025 \text{ parts}}{0.075 \text{ parts}} \text{ or } \frac{0.025}{0.075}$$

0.025% cream

Finally, we can take the proportion of parts needed of each cream and multiply it by the desired quantity to determine the quantity of each ingredient needed.

0.1% cream

$$\frac{90 \text{ gm}}{0.075} \times 0.025 = 30 \text{ gm}$$

0.025% cream

$$\frac{90 \text{ gm}}{0.075} \times 0.05 = 60 \text{ gm}$$

So, we would combine 30 gm of the 0.1% cream and 60 gm of the 0.025% cream to produce 90 gm of a 0.5% cream.

EXAMPLE 20.3

Rx: How much of a 2.5% cream and a 0.5% cream would be required to compound 100 gm of a 1% cream?

Let us look at the information that has been provided:

2.5%	Higher strength
0.5%	Lower strength
1%	Desired strength
100 gm	Desired quantity

First, draw the alligation grid.

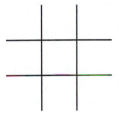

Now, fill in the alligation grid with the information provided in the problem.

- The higher strength goes in the top-left box.
- The lower strength goes in the bottom-left box.
- The desired strength goes in the center box.

Higher 2.5

Desired 1

Lower 0.5

Next, we calculate the numbers that should go into the top-right and bottom-right boxes.

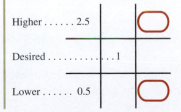

Higher 2.5

Desired 1

Lower 0.5

This is done by working diagonally and taking the difference between the two numbers that are already in place.

Let us look at the first diagonal, which contains 2.5 and 1. The difference between these two numbers goes in the bottom-right box.

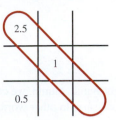

The difference between 2.5 and 1 is 1.5, so 1.5 goes in the bottom-right box.

$$2.5 - 1 = 1.5$$

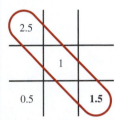

Now we can work on the other diagonal, which contains 0.5 and 1. The difference between these two numbers goes in the top-right box.

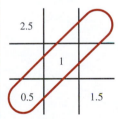

The difference between 0.5 and 1 is 0.5, so 0.5 goes in the top-right box.

$$0.5 - 1 = -0.5$$

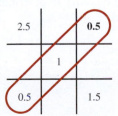

Remember, only positive numbers can go into the alligation grid, so −0.5 is changed to 0.5.

The numbers on the right-hand side of the alligation grid represent the number of parts per ingredient, when read straight across. This means that there should be 0.5 parts of the 2.5% cream and 1.5 parts of the 0.5% cream to make the 1% cream.

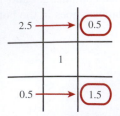

Now, by adding the numbers in the right-hand column, we can determine the total number of parts necessary. In other words,

0.5 parts (2.5%) + 1.5 parts (0.5%) = 2 parts total

Now that we have determined the number of parts needed for each ingredient and the total number of parts to be used, we can set these up as proportions.

$$\frac{\text{Parts needed}}{\text{Total parts}}$$

2.5% cream

$$\frac{0.5 \text{ parts}}{2 \text{ parts}} \text{ or } \frac{0.5}{2}$$

0.5% cream

$$\frac{0.5 \text{ parts}}{2 \text{ parts}} \text{ or } \frac{0.5}{2}$$

Finally, we can take the proportion of parts needed of each cream and multiply it by the desired quantity to determine the quantity of each ingredient needed.

2.5% cream

$$\frac{100 \text{ gm}}{2} \times 0.5 = 25 \text{ gm}$$

0.5% cream

$$\frac{100 \text{ gm}}{2.0} \times 1.5 = 75 \text{ gm}$$

So, we would combine 25 gm of the 2.5% cream and 75 gm of the 0.5% cream to produce 100 gm of a 1% cream.

EXAMPLE 20.4

Rx: Prepare 500 mL of a 7.5% dextrose solution using SWFI and D10W.

Let us look at the information that has been provided:

10%	Higher strength
0%	Lower strength
7.5%	Desired strength
500 mL	Desired quantity

D10W stands for dextrose 10% in water, thus making it a 10% strength.

Remember that bases, such as SWFI, have 0% strength, because they contain no active ingredient.

Now, fill in the alligation grid with the information provided in the problem.

- The higher strength goes in the top-left box.
- The lower strength goes in the bottom-left box.
- The desired strength goes in the center box.

Higher 10

Desired 7.5

Lower 0

Next, we will calculate the numbers that should go into the top-right and bottom-right boxes. This is done by working diagonally and taking the difference between the two numbers that are already in place.

Let us look at the first diagonal, which contains 10 and 7.5. The difference between these two numbers goes in the bottom-right box.

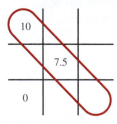

The difference between 10 and 7.5 is 2.5, so 2.5 goes in the bottom-right box.

10 − 7.5 = 2.5

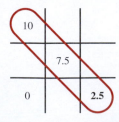

Now we can work on the other diagonal, which contains 0 and 7.5. The difference between these two numbers goes in the top-right box.

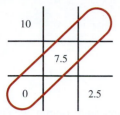

The difference between 0 and 7.5 is 7.5, so 7.5 goes in the top-right box.

$$0 - 7.5 = -7.5$$

Remember, any negative number must be changed to a positive number to be used in the grid.

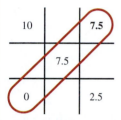

The numbers on the right-hand side of the alligation grid represent the number of parts per ingredient, when read straight across. This means that there should be 7.5 parts of the D10W and 2.5 parts of the SWFI in a 7.5% dextrose solution.

(grid)

Now, by adding the numbers in the right-hand column, we can determine the total number of parts necessary. In other words,

7.5 parts (10%) + 2.5 parts (0%) = 10 parts total

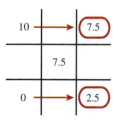

Now that we have determined the number of parts needed for each ingredient and the total number of parts to be used, we can set these up as proportions.

Parts needed
──────────
Total parts

D10W

• $\dfrac{7.5 \text{ parts}}{10 \text{ parts}}$ or $\dfrac{7.5}{10}$

SWFI

• $\dfrac{2.5 \text{ parts}}{10 \text{ parts}}$ or $\dfrac{2.5}{10}$

Finally, we can take the proportion of parts needed of each cream and multiply it by the desired quantity to determine the quantity of each ingredient needed.

D10W

$$\frac{500 \text{ mL}}{10} \times 7.5 = 375 \text{ mL}$$

SWFI

$$\frac{500 \text{ mL}}{10} \times 2.5 = 125 \text{ mL}$$

So, we would combine 375 mL of the D10W and 125 mL of the SWFI to prepare 500 mL of a 7.5% dextrose solution.

EXAMPLE 20.5

Rx: Prepare 1 L of a 20% alcohol solution using a 90% alcohol and a 10% alcohol.

Let us look at the information that has been provided:

90%	Higher strength
10%	Lower strength
20%	Desired strength
1 L (1,000 mL)	Desired quantity

Now, fill in the alligation grid with the information provided in the problem.

• The higher strength goes in the top-left box.
• The lower strength goes in the bottom-left box.
• The desired strength goes in the center box.

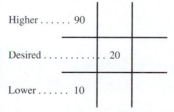

Next, we calculate the numbers that should go into the top-right and bottom-right boxes. This is done by working diagonally and taking the difference between the two numbers that are already in place.

Let us look at the first diagonal, which contains 90 and 20. The difference between these two numbers goes in the bottom-right box.

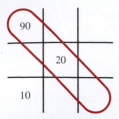

The difference between 90 and 20 is 70, so 70 goes in the bottom-right box.

$$90 - 20 = 70$$

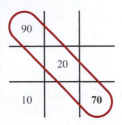

Now we can work on the other diagonal, which contains 10 and 20. The difference between these two numbers goes in the top-right box.

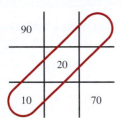

The difference between 10 and 20 is 10, so 10 goes in the top-right box.

$$10 - 20 = -10$$

Remember, any negative number must be changed to a positive number to be used in the grid.

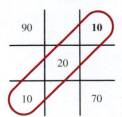

The numbers on the right-hand side of the alligation grid represent the number of parts per ingredient, when read straight across. This means that there should be 10 parts of the 90%

alcohol and 70 parts of the 10% alcohol to prepare a 20% alcohol solution.

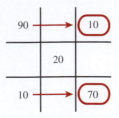

Now, by adding the numbers in the right-hand column, we can determine the total number of parts necessary. In other words,

10 parts (90%) + 70 parts (10%) = 80 parts total

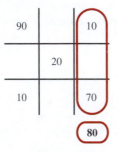

Now that we have determined the number of parts needed for each ingredient and the total number of parts to be used, we can set these up as proportions.

$$\frac{\text{Parts needed}}{\text{Total parts}}$$

90% alcohol

$$\frac{10 \text{ parts}}{80 \text{ parts}} \text{ or } \frac{10}{80}$$

10% alcohol

$$\frac{70 \text{ parts}}{80 \text{ parts}} \text{ or } \frac{70}{80}$$

Finally, we can take the proportion of parts needed of each cream and multiply it by the desired quantity to determine the quantity of each ingredient needed.

90% alcohol

$$\frac{1,000 \text{ mL}}{80} \times 10 = 125 \text{ mL}$$

10% alcohol

$$\frac{1,000 \text{ mL}}{80} \times 70 = 875 \text{ mL}$$

So, we would combine 125 mL of the 90% alcohol and 875 mL of the 10% alcohol to prepare 1 L of a 20% alcohol.

Practice Problems 20-1
Solve the following alligation problems using an alligation grid.

1. Rx: silver nitrate 0.25% solution 1% 1 L. You have 1 gal. of silver nitrate 1% stock solution, which you can dilute with distilled water. How many milliliters of each will you need to make the final product?

2. Rx: 1 L of a 1:200 soaking solution. You have a 1:45 stock solution and water. How many milliliters each will you need to prepare the order?

3. Rx: coal tar 5% ointment 120 gm. You have coal tar 10% ointment and coal tar 2% ointment. How many grams of each will you use to prepare the final product?

4. You are instructed to prepare 454 gm of a 15% ointment. In stock you have 5% and 30%. How much of each will you need to prepare the order?

5. Rx: Prepare 480 mL of a 1:30 solution using a 1:10 solution and a 1:50 solution. What quantities will be used of each stock solution to make the 1:30 solution?

6. You need to prepare 80 gm of a 9% cream using a 20% stock cream and a cream base. How much is needed of each?

7. You are asked to prepare 1 L of a 1:200 soaking solution, using a 1:50 stock soaking solution and distilled water. How much of each will you need to use?

8. How much SWFI would you need to add to 1,500 mL of a stock normal saline (0.9% NaCl) to produce a 0.45% sodium chloride solution?

9. Rx: alcohol 30%. How many milliliters of 90% alcohol should you add to 25 mL of 10% alcohol to make 30% alcohol?

10. Rx: hydrocortisone 2% ointment. How many grams of petrolatum should you add to 30 gm of hydrocortisone 2.5% ointment to reduce its strength to 2.0%? (The percent strength of petrolatum is zero.)

11. Rx: normal saline. How many milliliters of water must you add to 500 mL of a 10% stock solution of sodium chloride to make a batch of normal saline (sodium chloride 0.9% solution)?

12. Rx: ichthammol, 10% ointment. How many grams of ichthammol 20% ointment should you add to 40 gm of ichthammol 4% ointment to make ichthammol 10% ointment?

13. Rx: benzalkonium chloride 1:1,000 solution. How many milliliters of water should you add to 50 mL of benzalkonium chloride 0.25% solution to prepare the order?

14. Rx: zinc oxide 10% ointment 45 gm. How many grams of zinc oxide 20% ointment and zinc oxide 5% ointment should you mix to prepare the order?

15. Rx: aluminum acetate 1:400 solution 1 gal. How many milliliters of Burrow's solution (aluminum acetate 5%) should you use to prepare the order?

16. Rx: histamine phosphate 1:10,000 solution 10 mL. How many milliliters of a histamine phosphate 1:10 solution do you need to prepare the order?

17. Rx: benzocaine 2.5% ointment 2 oz. How many grams of benzocaine 2% ointment should you mix with 22.5 gm of benzocaine 10% ointment to prepare the order?

18. When using a 0.5% cream and a 2% cream to produce a 1.25% cream, how many parts of each initial ingredient are needed?

19. In what proportion would you add SWFI to D10W to produce D6W?

20. Rx: Prepare a 750 mL solution of a 2:50 solution, and a 3:50 solution. What quantities will be used of each stock solution to make the 2:50 solution?

PROFILE IN PRACTICE

Kim is a pharmacy technician who works at a specialty compounding pharmacy. A dermatologist has prescribed a topical ointment in precisely 0.45%, to accommodate the patient's sensitivities. After researching the substance, Kim discovers that the lowest strength available for the medication is 2%.

▶ *What can Kim compound the stock medication with to produce 60 gm of the 0.45% ointment, and with what quantities?*

Summary

In certain situations, a pharmacy must use the alligation method to combine two varying strengths of a drug, or combine a drug with a base or diluent, to achieve the prescribed strength. Although these calculations can be confusing at first, once you master the alligation grid, you should be able to perform these calculations easily.

Chapter Review Questions

1. How much of a 20% cream should you add to 26 gm of 1% cream to make a 4% cream?
   a. 6.00 gm
   b. 5.20 gm
   c. 4.88 gm
   d. 3.00 gm

2. How much of 25% stock solution and distilled water will you need to make 1 L of a 1:400 solution?
   a. 10 mL of the 25% solution and 990 mL of water
   b. 100 mL of the 25% solution and 900 mL of water
   c. 990 mL of the 25% solution and 10 mL of water
   d. 900 mL of the 25% solution and 10 mL of water

3. How much of a 10% cream and a 0.5% cream will you need to prepare 120 gm of a 2.5% cream?
   a. 20 gm of the 10% cream and 100 gm of the 0.5% cream
   b. 100 gm of the 10% cream and 20 gm of the 0.5% cream
   c. 25 gm of the 10% cream and 95 gm of the 0.5% cream
   d. 95 gm of the 10% cream and 25 gm of the 0.5% cream

4. How much of povidone iodine 20% solution and water will you need to make 120 mL of a povidone iodine 3% rinse?
   a. 18 mL of the 20% solution and 102 mL of water
   b. 102 mL of the 20% solution and 18 mL of water
   c. 24 mL of the 20% solution and 96 mL of water
   d. 96 mL of the 20% solution and 24 mL of water

5. How much of lidocaine 0.5% topical gel should you mix with lidocaine 10% topical gel to make 15 gm of a lidocaine 2% topical gel?
   a. 2.4 gm
   b. 5.0 gm
   c. 9.5 gm
   d. 12.6 gm

6. How much of 1:25 solution and 1:500 solution should you mix to make 1 L of a 1:250 soaking solution?
   a. 947 mL of the 1:25 solution and 53 mL of the 1:500 solution
   b. 53 mL of the 1:25 solution and 947 mL of the 1:500 solution
   c. 250 mL of the 1:25 solution and 750 of the 1:500 solution
   d. 750 mL of the 1:25 solution and 250 mL of the 1:500 solution

7. Which of the following is the ratio strength for 12.5%?
   a. 1:2
   b. 1:4
   c. 1:6
   d. 1:8

8. How much of NaCl 10% stock solution should you add to 100 mL of NaCl 0.45% solution to make normal saline?
   a. 1 mL
   b. 2 mL
   c. 5 mL
   d. 10 mL

9. How many grams of 0.1% cream should you mix with 24 gm of 12% cream to make a 6% cream?
   a. 10.4
   b. 12.2
   c. 24.4
   d. 33

10. How many parts of each of a 1% product and a 3% product do you need to make a 2.5% product?
    a. 2.5 parts of the 1% product and 1 part of the 3% product
    b. 1 part of the 1% product and 2.5 parts of the 3% product
    c. 1.5 parts of the 1% product and 0.5 part of the 3% product
    d. 0.5 part of the 1% product and 1.5 parts of the 3% product

Critical Thinking Questions

1. Why are bases, such as vanishing cream, considered to have 0% strength?

2. How can alligation problems be double-checked after solving, to ensure accuracy?

3. In what scenario might a pharmacy technician be required to perform an alligation problem, outside of an independent, compounding pharmacy?

References and Resources

Hegstad, Lorrie N. and Wilma Hayek. *Essential Drug Dosage Calculations*. 4th ed. Upper Saddle River, NJ: Pearson, 2001. Print.

Johnston, Mike. *Pharmacy Calculations: The Pharmacy Technician Series*. Upper Saddle River, NJ: Pearson, 2005. Print.

Lesmeister, Michelle Benjamin, Michelle. *Math Basics for the Healthcare Professional*. 4th ed. Upper Saddle River, NJ: Pearson, 2013. Print.

Mikolah, Alan A. *Drug Dosage Calculations for the Emergency Care Provider*. 2nd ed. Upper Saddle River, NJ: Prentice Hall, 2003. Print.

Olsen, June, Anthony Giangrasso, and Dolores Shrimpton. *Medical Dosage Calculations*. 10th ed. Upper Saddle River, NJ: Pearson, 2011. Print.

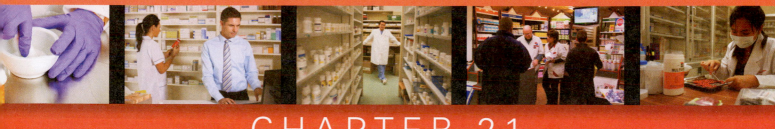

CHAPTER 21

Parenteral Calculations

LEARNING OBJECTIVES

After completing this chapter, you should be able to:

- Illustrate the principle of basic dimensional analysis.
- Calculate flow duration for parenteral products.
- Calculate the volume per hour for parenteral orders.
- Calculate the drug per hour for parenteral products.
- Calculate drip rates in both drops/minute and milliliters/hour.
- Calculate TPN milliequivalents.

KEY TERMS

drop factor, p. 332

drops per minute (gtts/ minute), p. 331

drug per hour (mg/hour), p. 330

flow rate duration, p. 326

flow rates, p. 325

hypertonic solutions, p. 334

hypotonic solutions, p. 334

isotonic solutions, p. 334

IV infusion, p. 325

microdrip, p. 332

total parenteral nutrition (TPN), p. 323

volume per hour (mL/hour), p. 328

INTRODUCTION

The preparation and administration of parenteral products, such as IV infusions, **total parenteral nutrition (TPN)**, and chemotherapy drugs, require specific calculations. It is common for individuals to become overwhelmed and confused when approaching complex pharmacy calculations. The truth is, however, that although many pharmacy calculations may appear to be complex, they are in actuality very simple. This chapter explains parenteral calculations using the principle of basic dimensional analysis.

Basic Dimensional Analysis

Calculations regarding sterile product and flow rates are typically viewed as among the most difficult in pharmacy practice, but each problem can be solved by using either basic dimensional analysis or ratios/proportions. We covered ratios/proportions

---

total parenteral nutrition (TPN) a solution made to supply many of the body's basic nutritional needs via parenteral administration.

extensively in earlier chapters of this book, so now we investigate the basics of dimensional analysis.

Before moving forward, however, let us review several fundamental math principles.

1. Any number multiplied by 1 retains the same value.
   Example: $4 \times 1 = 4$
   Example: $\frac{1}{2} \times 1 = \frac{1}{2}$

2. Any whole number can be expressed as a fraction by placing a 1 as the denominator.
   Example: $3 = \frac{3}{1}$
   Example: $18 = \frac{18}{1}$

3. Any number divided by itself equals 1.
   Example: $4 \div 4 = 1$
   Example: $\frac{2}{2} = 1$

The first set of examples (Examples 21.1–21.5) and practice problem (Practice Problem 21.1) in this chapter will not appear to have anything at all to do with sterile product calculations, but be patient: These early examples are laying a foundation so that you can better comprehend and perform more advanced flow rate calculations.

EXAMPLE 21.1 BASIC DIMENSIONAL ANALYSIS

How many hours are there in six days?

In this problem, we are working with days and hours. What information, or facts, do we know about days and hours?

- There are 24 hours in 1 day.

This could be written as:

- 24 hours = 1 day

- $\dfrac{1 \text{ day}}{24 \text{ hours}}$

- $\dfrac{24 \text{ hours}}{1 \text{ day}}$

Using the principle of dimensional analysis, we can solve the problem.

$$6 \text{ days} = \frac{6 \text{ days}}{1} \times \frac{24 \text{ hours}}{1 \text{ day}} = ?$$

After setting the problem up, we cancel out like-units and/or numbers.

$$6 \text{ days} = \frac{6 \text{ days}}{1} \times \frac{24 \text{ hours}}{1 \text{ day}} = ?$$

which can now be written as:

$$6 \text{ days} = 6 \times 24 = ?$$

Therefore, six days is equivalent to 144 hours.

$$6 \text{ days} = 6 \times 24 = 144$$

EXAMPLE 21.2 BASIC DIMENSIONAL ANALYSIS

How many minutes are in five hours?

In this problem, we are working with minutes and hours. What information, or facts, do we know about minutes and hours?

- There are 60 minutes in 1 hour.

This could be written as:

- 1 hour = 60 minutes

- $\dfrac{1 \text{ hour}}{60 \text{ minutes}}$

- $\dfrac{60 \text{ minutes}}{1 \text{ hour}}$

Using the principle of dimensional analysis, we can solve the problem.

$$5 \text{ hours} = \frac{5 \text{ hours}}{1} \times \frac{60 \text{ minutes}}{1 \text{ hour}} = ?$$

After setting the problem up, we cancel out like-units and/or numbers.

$$5 \text{ hours} = \frac{5 \text{ hours}}{1} \times \frac{60 \text{ minutes}}{1 \text{ hour}} = ?$$

which can now be written as:

$$5 \text{ hours} = 5 \times 60 = ?$$

Therefore, 5 hours is equivalent to 300 minutes.

$$5 \text{ hours} = 5 \times 60 = 300$$

EXAMPLE 21.3 BASIC DIMENSIONAL ANALYSIS

How many seconds are in 45 minutes?

We know that there are 60 seconds in every 1 minute. This could be written as:

- 1 minute = 60 seconds

---

flow rate a term used to describe a number of common pharmacy calculations used in the preparation of IV infusions.

IV infusion a compounded solution that provides fluids, specific medications, nutrients, electrolytes, and minerals to a patient.

- $\dfrac{1\ \text{minute}}{60\ \text{seconds}}$

- $\dfrac{60\ \text{seconds}}{1\ \text{minute}}$

Using the principle of dimensional analysis, we can solve the problem.

$$45\ \text{minutes} = \frac{45\ \text{minutes}}{1} \times \frac{60\ \text{seconds}}{1\ \text{minute}} = ?$$

After setting the problem up, we cancel out like units and/or numbers.

$$45\ \text{minutes} = \frac{45\ \cancel{\text{minutes}}}{1} \times \frac{60\ \text{seconds}}{1\ \cancel{\text{minute}}} = ?$$

which can now be written as:

$$45\ \text{minutes} = 45 \times 60 = ?$$

Therefore, 45 minutes is equivalent to 2,700 seconds.

$$45\ \text{minutes} = 45 \times 60 = 2{,}700$$

EXAMPLE 21.5 BASIC DIMENSIONAL ANALYSIS

How many seconds are in four days?

We know that there are 60 seconds in every 1 minute, 60 minutes in every 1 hour, and 24 hours in every 1 day. Using the principle of dimensional analysis, we can solve the problem—but once again, we need to add an additional component not present in previous examples.

$$4\ \text{days} = \frac{4\ \text{days}}{1} \times \frac{24\ \text{hours}}{1\ \text{day}} \times \frac{60\ \text{minutes}}{1\ \text{hour}} \times \frac{60\ \text{seconds}}{1\ \text{minute}} = ?$$

After setting the problem up, we cancel out like-units and/or numbers.

$$4\ \text{days} = \frac{4\ \cancel{\text{days}}}{1} \times \frac{24\ \cancel{\text{hours}}}{1\ \cancel{\text{day}}} \times \frac{60\ \cancel{\text{minutes}}}{1\ \cancel{\text{hour}}} \times \frac{60\ \text{seconds}}{1\ \cancel{\text{minute}}} = ?$$

which can now be written as:

$$4\ \text{days} = 4 \times 24 \times 60 \times 60 = ?$$

$$4\ \text{days} = 4 \times 24 \times 60 \times 60 = 345{,}600$$

Now, we know that there are 345,600 seconds in 4 days.

EXAMPLE 21.4 BASIC DIMENSIONAL ANALYSIS

How many seconds are in three hours?

We know that there are 60 seconds in every 1 minute and that there are 60 minutes in every 1 hour. Using the principle of dimensional analysis, we can solve the problem—but to solve this problem, we now have to add a third component.

$$3\ \text{hours} = \frac{3\ \text{hours}}{1} \times \frac{60\ \text{minutes}}{1\ \text{hour}} \times \frac{60\ \text{seconds}}{1\ \text{minute}} = ?$$

After setting the problem up, we cancel out like-units and/or numbers.

$$3\ \text{hours} = \frac{3\ \cancel{\text{hours}}}{1} \times \frac{60\ \cancel{\text{minutes}}}{1\ \cancel{\text{hour}}} \times \frac{60\ \text{seconds}}{1\ \cancel{\text{minute}}} = ?$$

which can now be written as:

$$3\ \text{hours} = 3 \times 60 \times 60 = ?$$

$$3\ \text{hours} = 3 \times 60 \times 60 = 10{,}800$$

Therefore, there are 10,800 seconds in 3 hours.

Practice Problems 21-1
Basic Dimensional Analysis

1. How many hours are in six days?
2. How many minutes are in 14 hours?
3. How many minutes are in a day?
4. Forty minutes is equivalent to how many seconds?
5. How many seconds are in 50 minutes?
6. How many hours are in 1.5 days?
7. There are _____ minutes in 2.1 hours.
8. How many seconds are in 10 hours?
9. One hour is equal to _____ seconds.
10. How many seconds make up a full day?

Flow Rates

Flow rates is a term used to describe a number of common pharmacy calculations used in the preparation of **IV infusions** (compounded solutions that provide fluids, specific medications, nutrients, electrolytes, and minerals to a patient). Precise calculations are required for IV infusions to ensure that the fluid and medication(s) are being delivered at the right speed, at the right strength, and for the right amount of time.

Flow Rate Duration

Flow rate duration refers to the length of time over which an IV will be administered, or how long an IV bag will last before it must be changed.

EXAMPLE 21.6 FLOW RATE DURATION

A 1-L IV bag is being administered at a rate of 200 mL/hour. How long will this IV bag last?

Do not get overwhelmed or confused now that the problems are talking about IV bags instead of days, hours, and seconds. Just as before, we can use dimensional analysis to solve this problem. In essence, the problem being asked is, 1 L is equal to how many hours?

Again, we should start by looking at the information, or facts, that we know. We know that there are 1,000 mL in every 1 L, which could be written as:

- 1 L = 1,000 mL

- $\dfrac{1\ L}{1,000\ mL}$

- $\dfrac{1,000\ mL}{1\ L}$

We also know, according to the problem, that 200 mL is being administered per hour, which can be written as:

- 1 hour = 200 mL

- $\dfrac{1\ hour}{200\ mL}$

- $\dfrac{200\ mL}{1\ hour}$

Using the principle of dimensional analysis, we can solve the problem.

$$1\ L = \frac{1\ L}{1} \times \frac{1,000\ mL}{1\ L} \times \frac{1\ hour}{200\ mL} = ?$$

After setting the problem up, we cancel out like-units and/or numbers.

$$1\ L = \frac{1\ \cancel{L}}{1} \times \frac{1,000\ \cancel{mL}}{1\ \cancel{L}} \times \frac{1\ hour}{200\ \cancel{mL}} = ?$$

which can now be written as:

$$1\ L = \frac{1 \times 1,000 \times 1\ hour}{200} = ?$$

$$1\ L = \frac{1,000}{200} = 5\ hours$$

Therefore, the 1-L bag will last five hours.

EXAMPLE 21.7 FLOW RATE DURATION

A 2-L IV bag is to be administered at 250 mL/hour. How long will the IV bag last?

Let us start by looking at the information, or facts, that we know. We know that there are 1,000 mL in every 1 L, which could be written as:

- 1 L = 1,000 mL

- $\dfrac{1\ L}{1,000\ mL}$

- $\dfrac{1,000\ mL}{1\ L}$

We also know, according to the problem, that 250 mL is being administered per hour, which can be written as:

- 1 hour = 250 mL

- $\dfrac{1\ hour}{250\ mL}$

- $\dfrac{250\ mL}{1\ hour}$

Using the principle of dimensional analysis, we can solve the problem.

$$2\ L = \frac{2\ L}{1} \times \frac{1,000\ mL}{1\ L} \times \frac{1\ hour}{250\ mL} = ?$$

After setting the problem up, we cancel out like-units and/or numbers.

$$2\ L = \frac{2\ \cancel{L}}{1} \times \frac{1,000\ \cancel{mL}}{1\ \cancel{L}} \times \frac{1\ hour}{250\ \cancel{mL}} = ?$$

which can now be written as:

$$2\ L = \frac{2 \times 1,000 \times 1\ hour}{250} = ?$$

$$2\ L = \frac{2,000}{250} = 8\ hours$$

Therefore, the 2-L bag will last 8 hours.

---

flow rate duration length of time over which an IV will be administered, or how long an IV bag will last before it must be changed.

EXAMPLE 21.8 FLOW RATE DURATION

A patient is set to get a 500-mL infusion of cimetidine in lactated Ringer's (LR) 5% at 10:00 a.m. The bag is to be administered at a rate of 125 mL/hour. At what time will the infusion be complete?

This example provides us with additional information, such as the drug name, solution strength, and administration start time. As always, let us start by looking at the information that we know and that we will need to calculate the problem. We know that:

- The bag contains a total of 500 mL.
- The bag is being administered at a rate of 125 mL/hour.
- The infusion is scheduled to start at 10:00 a.m.

Using the principle of dimensional analysis, we can determine how long the infusion will last.

$$500 \text{ mL} = \frac{500 \text{ mL}}{1} \times \frac{1 \text{ hour}}{125 \text{ mL}} = ?$$

After setting the problem up, we cancel out like-units and/or numbers.

$$500 \text{ mL} = \frac{500 \text{ m\cancel{L}}}{1} \times \frac{1 \text{ hour}}{125 \text{ m\cancel{L}}} = ?$$

which can now be written as:

$$500 \text{ mL} = \frac{500 \times 1 \text{ hour}}{125} = ?$$

$$500 \text{ mL} = \frac{500 \times 1 \text{ hour}}{125} = 4$$

Therefore, the 500-mL bag will last 4 hours.

The question being asked, however, is at what time will the infusion be completed?

To answer this, simply take the start time (10:00 a.m.) and add the length of duration (4 hours).

10:00 a.m. + 4 hours = 14:00 hours, or 2:00 p.m.

EXAMPLE 21.9 FLOW RATE DURATION

Three 1-L IV bags are to be infused at a rate of 150 mL/hour. How long will these three bags last?

Let us start by looking at the information, or facts, that we know. We know that:

- There are three IV bags to be administered.
- One IV bag contains 1 L.

- There are 1,000 mL in every 1 L.
- The bags are being administered at a rate of 150 mL/hour.

Using the principle of dimensional analysis, we can solve the problem.

$$3 \text{ bags} = \frac{3 \text{ bags}}{1} \times \frac{1 \text{ L}}{1 \text{ bag}} \times \frac{1{,}000 \text{ mL}}{1 \text{ L}} \times \frac{1 \text{ hour}}{150 \text{ mL}} = ?$$

After setting the problem up, we cancel out like-units and/or numbers.

$$3 \text{ bags} = \frac{3 \text{ ba\cancel{gs}}}{1} \times \frac{1 \text{ \cancel{L}}}{1 \text{ ba\cancel{g}}} \times \frac{1{,}000 \text{ m\cancel{L}}}{1 \text{ \cancel{L}}} \times \frac{1 \text{ hour}}{150 \text{ m\cancel{L}}} = ?$$

which can now be written as:

$$3 \text{ bags} = \frac{3 \times 1 \times 1{,}000 \times 1 \text{ hour}}{150} = ?$$

$$3 \text{ bags} = \frac{3 \times 1 \times 1{,}000 \times 1 \text{ hour}}{150} = 20$$

Therefore, the three bags will last 20 hours.

EXAMPLE 21.10 FLOW RATE DURATION

Two 2-L IV bags containing heparin sodium and normal saline (NS) are set for administration at a rate of 250 mL/hour at 7:00 a.m. When will both bags be completely administered?

Let us start by looking at the information, or facts, that we know. We know that:

- One IV bag contains 2 L.
- There is 1,000 mL in every 1 L.
- The bags are being administered at a rate of 250 mL/hour.

Using the principle of dimensional analysis, we can solve the problem.

$$2 \text{ bags} = \frac{2 \text{ bags}}{1} \times \frac{2 \text{ L}}{1 \text{ bag}} \times \frac{1{,}000 \text{ mL}}{1 \text{ L}} \times \frac{1 \text{ hour}}{250 \text{ mL}} = ?$$

After setting the problem up, we cancel out like-units and/or numbers.

$$2 \text{ bags} = \frac{2 \text{ ba\cancel{gs}}}{1} \times \frac{2 \text{ \cancel{L}}}{1 \text{ ba\cancel{g}}} \times \frac{1{,}000 \text{ m\cancel{L}}}{1 \text{ \cancel{L}}} \times \frac{1 \text{ hour}}{250 \text{ m\cancel{L}}} = ?$$

which can now be written as:

$$2 \text{ bags} = \frac{2 \times 2 \times 1{,}000 \times 1 \text{ hour}}{250} = ?$$

$$2 \text{ bags} = \frac{2 \times 2 \times 1,000 \times 1 \text{ hour}}{250} = 16$$

Therefore, the two bags will last 16 hours.

The question being asked, however, is at what time will the infusion be completed?

To answer this, simply take the start time (7:00 a.m.) and add the length of duration (16 hours).

7:00 a.m. + 16 hours = 23:00 hours, or 11:00 p.m.

Practice Problems 21-2
Flow Rate Duration

1. A 500-mL bag is to be administered at a rate of 100 mL/hour. How long will the IV bag last?

2. A 1-L IV bag is running at a rate of 250 mL/hour. How long will the infusion last?

3. 500 mL of NS is being infused at a rate of 200 mL/hour. What will be the duration of the infusion?

4. 500 mg cefazolin in 100 mL D5W is being administered at a rate of 200 mL/hour. How long will the IV last?

5. A 500-mL bag with Diamox is being infused at a rate of 250 mL/hour. How long will it take to infuse the entire bag?

6. A 1-L bag is being infused at a rate of 200 mL/hour. If the infusion began at 8:15 a.m., when will it be finished?

7. A 1-L bag is being infused at a rate of 250 mL/hour. How long will the bag last?

8. 750 mL of NS is set to be administered at a rate of 150 mL/hour, starting at 11:00 a.m. At what time will the infusion be finished?

9. Two 1-L IV bags with ascorbic acid are being administered at a rate of 200 mL/hour. How long will it take to infuse both bags?

10. A 250-mL bag with ranitidine is being administered at the maximum rate of 10.7 mL/hour. How long will the bag last?

Volume per Hour

Volume per hour, or **mL/hour**, refers to the amount of fluid, or solution, that will be administered to the patient intravenously per hour.

---

volume per hour (mL/hour) the amount of fluid, or solution, that will be administered to the patient intravenously per hour.

EXAMPLE 21.11 VOLUME PER HOUR

A patient is to receive 750-mL infusion over 3 hours. What is the rate of infusion in mL/hour?

Unlike the previous IV flow rate problems, solving volume per hour is easily done by setting up a ratio and proportion and then solving for the unknown, as illustrated here.

$$\frac{\text{Total mL}}{\text{Total hours}} = \frac{X}{1 \text{ hour}}$$

Using the information provided in the problem, set up a ratio and proportion.

$$\frac{750 \text{ mL}}{3 \text{ hours}} = \frac{X}{1 \text{ hour}}$$

Now, we must cross-multiply.

$$3 \times X = 750 \times 1$$

$$3X = 750$$

Using basic algebra principles, isolate the unknown (X) to solve. In this example, we must divide both sides of the equation by 3 to isolate X.

$$\frac{3X}{3} = \frac{750}{3}$$

$$X = 250$$

This infusion will be administered at 250 mL/hour.

EXAMPLE 21.12 VOLUME PER HOUR

A 250-mL IV, containing 1 mg of Isuprel, is to be given over 100 minutes. What is the rate of infusion in mL/hour?

Using the information provided in the problem, set up a ratio and proportion. Since the administration time is given in minutes, we can substitute 60 minutes for 1 hour beneath the unknown (X).

$$\frac{250 \text{ mL}}{100 \text{ minutes}} = \frac{X}{60 \text{ minutes}}$$

Next, cross-multiply.

$$100 \times X = 250 \times 60$$

$$100X = 15,000$$

Now, solve for X.

$$\frac{100 X}{100} = \frac{15,000}{100}$$

So, X = 150

This infusion will be administered at a rate of 150 mL/hour (60 minutes).

EXAMPLE 21.13 VOLUME PER HOUR

500 mL of D5W containing 1 gm of lidocaine hydrochloride is to be given over 250 minutes. What is the infusion rate in mL/hour?

First, set up the ratio and proportion.

$$\frac{500 \text{ mL}}{250 \text{ minutes}} = \frac{X}{60 \text{ minutes}}$$

Next, cross-multiply.

$250 \times X = 500 \times 60$

$250X = 30,000$

Now, solve for X.

$$\frac{250 \, X}{250} = \frac{30,000}{250}$$

$X = 120$

This infusion will be administered at 120 mL/hour (60 minutes).

EXAMPLE 21.14 VOLUME PER HOUR

A 250-mL IV is to be administered over 50 minutes. What is the infusion rate in mL/hour?

First, set up the ratio and proportion.

$$\frac{250 \text{ mL}}{50 \text{ minutes}} = \frac{X}{60 \text{ minutes}}$$

Next, cross-multiply.

$50 \times X = 250 \times 60$

$50X = 15,000$

Now, solve for X.

$$\frac{50 \, X}{50} = \frac{15,000}{50}$$

$X = 300$

This infusion will be administered at a rate of 300 mL/hour (60 minutes).

Notice that the actual IV is being administered in less than an hour, so the rate per hour should logically contain more volume than the actual IV.

EXAMPLE 21.15 VOLUME PER HOUR

1,000 mL NS containing 50 mg nitroprusside sodium is to be administered over 50 minutes. What is the infusion rate in mL/hour?

First, set up the ratio and proportion.

$$\frac{1,000 \text{ mL}}{50 \text{ minutes}} = \frac{X}{60 \text{ minutes}}$$

Next, cross-multiply.

$50 \times X = 1,000 \times 60$

$50X = 60,000$

Now, solve for X.

$$\frac{50 \, X}{50} = \frac{60,000}{50}$$

$X = 1,200$

This infusion will be administered at a rate of 1,200 mL/hour, or 1.2 L/hour (60 minutes).

Practice Problems 21-3
Volume per Hour

1. 1 L is being infused over 4 hours. What is the rate of infusion in mL/hour?

2. 400 mL is being administered over 4 hours. What is the administration rate per hour?

3. 2 L is to be given via IV over 8 hours. What is the rate of infusion per hour?

4. 480 mL of D5W containing dobutamine is being given over 8 hours. What is the administration rate per hour?

5. 1 gm of Gemzar in 25 mL of NS is to be administered over 30 minutes. What is the rate of infusion in mL/hour?

6. 150 mL is being infused over 30 minutes. What is the rate of infusion in mL/hour?

7. 250 mL is being given over 100 minutes. What is the administration rate per hour?

8. 500 mL of NS is being administered over 6 hours. What is the rate in mL/hour?

9. 50 mL of SWFI containing folic acid is to be infused over 30 minutes. What is the infusion rate per hour?

10. 100 mL of Iveegam is infused over 100 minutes. What is the rate of infusion per hour?

Drug per Hour

Drug per hour, or **mg/hour**, refers to the dosage, or amount of medication in milligrams, that will be administered per hour of infusion.

EXAMPLE 21.16 DRUG PER HOUR

100 mg of medication is to be administered in 500 mL of LR over 2 hours. How much drug will be administered per hour?

Like solving volume per hour, calculating the amount of medication administered per hour is easily done by setting up a ratio and proportion and then solving for the unknown, as illustrated here.

$$\frac{\text{Total mg}}{\text{Total hours}} = \frac{X}{1 \text{ hour}}$$

Using the information provided in the problem, set up a ratio and proportion.

$$\frac{100 \text{ mg}}{2 \text{ hours}} = \frac{X}{1 \text{ hour}}$$

Now, we must cross-multiply.

$$2 \times X = 100 \times 1$$

$$2X = 100$$

Using basic algebra principles, isolate the unknown (X) to solve. In this example, we must divide both sides of the equation by 2 to isolate X.

$$\frac{2 X}{2} = \frac{100}{2}$$

$$X = 50$$

This infusion will provide 50 mg/hour.

EXAMPLE 21.17 DRUG PER HOUR

600 mg of fluorouracil is to be administered by continuous infusion over 24 hours. How much drug will be administered per hour?

---

drug per hour (mg/hour) the dosage, or amount of medication in milligrams, that will be administered per hour of infusion.

drops per minute (gtts/minute) the volume of medication to be administered each minute.

drop factor an abbreviated form referring to a specific drip rate.

microdrip the most commonly used drip rate, 60 gtts/mL.

Using the information provided in the problem, set up a ratio and proportion.

$$\frac{600 \text{ mg}}{24 \text{ hours}} = \frac{X}{1 \text{ hour}}$$

Now, cross-multiply.

$$24 \times X = 600 \times 1$$

$$24X = 600$$

Using basic algebra principles, isolate the unknown (X) to solve. In this example, we must divide both sides of the equation by 24 to isolate X.

$$\frac{24 X}{24} = \frac{600}{24}$$

$$X = 25$$

This infusion will provide 25 mg/hour.

EXAMPLE 21.18 DRUG PER HOUR

200 mg of Vibramycin IV is diluted in 400 mL of LR to be administered over 4 hours. How much drug will be administered per hour?

First, set up a ratio and proportion.

$$\frac{200 \text{ mg}}{4 \text{ hours}} = \frac{X}{1 \text{ hour}}$$

Next, cross-multiply.

$$4 \times X = 200 \times 1$$

$$4X = 200$$

Now, solve for X.

$$\frac{4 X}{4} = \frac{200}{4}$$

$$X = 50$$

This infusion will provide 50 mg/hour.

EXAMPLE 21.19 DRUG PER HOUR

125 mg of Cardizem is being infused in 125 mL over 12.5 hours. How much drug will be administered per hour?

First, set up a ratio and proportion.

$$\frac{125 \text{ mg}}{12.5 \text{ hours}} = \frac{X}{1 \text{ hour}}$$

Next, cross-multiply.

$$12.5 \times X = 125 \times 1$$

$$12.5X = 125$$

Now, solve for X.

$$\frac{12.5X}{12.5} = \frac{125}{12.5}$$

$$X = 10$$

This infusion will provide 10 mg/hour.

EXAMPLE 21.20 DRUG PER HOUR

5 million units of Penicillin G Aqueous are being delivered in 1 L of D5W over 12 hours. How much drug will be administered per hour?

First, set up a ratio and proportion.

$$\frac{5,000,000 \text{ units}}{12 \text{ hours}} = \frac{X}{1 \text{ hour}}$$

Next, cross-multiply.

$$12 \times X = 5,000,000 \times 1$$

$$12X = 5,000,000$$

Now, solve for X.

$$\frac{12 X}{12} = \frac{5,000,000}{12}$$

$$X = 416,666.67$$

Therefore, this infusion will provide 416,667 units per hour.

Practice Problems 21-4
Drug per Hour

1. 200 mg of medication in 1 L is administered over 4 hours. How much drug will be administered per hour?

2. 750 mg of medication in 2 L is to be infused over 4 hours. How much drug will be administered per hour?

3. 500 mg of medication in 500 mL is to be given over 4 hours. How much drug will be administered per hour?

4. 250 mL of Plasmanate, which contains 25 gm of plasma protein, is to be administered over 250 minutes. How much drug will be administered per hour?

5. 500 mg of nafcillin sodium in 150 mL is to be infused over 30 minutes. How much drug will be administered per hour?

6. A 100-mL bag contains 150 mg of medication to be given over 30 minutes. How much drug will be administered per hour?

7. 25 mcg of medication in 250 mL is to be infused over 2 hours. How much drug will be administered per hour?

8. 250,000 units of medication in 1 L are administered over 8 hours. How much drug will be administered per hour?

9. 100 mg teniposide in 500 mL is given over 45 minutes. How much drug will be administered per hour?

10. 75 mg of Demadex in D5W is to be administered over 24 hours. How much drug will be administered per hour?

Drop Factors

When preparing sterile products, pharmacy personnel are often responsible for calculating the rate of IV administration, expressed as **drops per minute (gtts/minute)**. Literally, this drip rate will determine how the IV pump is calibrated and the volume of medication to be administered each minute.

Various IV administration sets release specific drops per milliliter. Microdrip sets are calibrated to deliver 60 gtts/mL, whereas macrodrip sets might be calibrated to deliver 10 gtts/mL, 15 gtts/mL, or 20 gtts/mL (see Figure 21-1). The larger the number of drops per milliliter, the smaller the drops will be—because, of course, 1 mL is 1 mL.

In pharmacy, you will work with four common IV drip rates: 10 gtts/mL, 15 gtts/mL, 20 gtts/mL, and 60 gtts/mL. Drip rates can be expressed by their **drop factor**, which is just a simpler way of stating a drip rate (see Table 21-1).

❝ Workplace Wisdom Always Assume 60 gtts/mL

The most commonly used drip rate is the **microdrip**, 60 gtts/mL. Therefore, if a problem does not indicate a specific drip rate or drop factor, you should always assume 60 gtts/mL. ❞

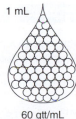

1 mL — 10 gtt/mL   1 mL — 15 gtt/mL   1 mL — 20 gtt/mL   1 mL — 60 gtt/mL

Standard or Macrodrop Calibration   Microdrop Calibration

FIGURE 21-1 Illustration of drip sets.

TABLE 21-1 Drip Rates Expressed by Drop Factor

Drop Factor	Drip Rate (gtts/mL)
60	60
20	20
15	15
10	10

EXAMPLE 21.21 DRIP RATES

A 1-L bag of D5W is to be administered at a drop factor of 60 over 6 hours. What is the flow rate in gtts/minute?

Let us start by looking at the information, or facts, that we know. We know that:

- One IV bag contains 1 L.
- There are 1,000 mL in every 1 L.
- The drop factor is 60, so there are 60 gtts/mL.
- The duration of administration is 6 hours.
- There are 60 minutes in 1 hour.

Using the principle of dimensional analysis, we can solve the problem.

$$1 \text{ bag} = \frac{1,000 \text{ mL}}{6 \text{ hours}} \times \frac{60 \text{ gtts}}{1 \text{ mL}} \times \frac{1 \text{ hour}}{60 \text{ minutes}} = ?$$

After setting the problem up, we cancel out like-units and/or numbers.

$$1 \text{ bag} = \frac{1,000 \text{ mL}}{6 \text{ hours}} \times \frac{60 \text{ gtts}}{1 \text{ mL}} \times \frac{1 \text{ hour}}{60 \text{ minutes}} = ?$$

which can now be written as:

$$1 \text{ bag} = \frac{1,000 \times 1 \text{ gtts}}{6 \text{ minutes}} = ?$$

$$1 \text{ bag} = \frac{1,000 \times 1 \text{ gtts}}{6 \text{ minutes}} = 166.66$$

So, the infusion rate is 167 gtts/minute.

EXAMPLE 21.22 DRIP RATES

500 mL is to be administered to a patient over 5 hours, using a drop factor of 15. What is the flow rate in gtts/minute?

Let us start by looking at the information, or facts, that we know. We know that:

- One IV bag contains 500 mL.
- The drop factor is 15, so there are 15 gtts/mL.
- The duration of administration is 5 hours.
- There are 60 minutes in 1 hour.

Using the principle of dimensional analysis, we can solve the problem.

$$1 \text{ bag} = \frac{500 \text{ mL}}{5 \text{ hours}} \times \frac{15 \text{ gtts}}{1 \text{ mL}} \times \frac{1 \text{ hour}}{60 \text{ minutes}} = ?$$

After setting the problem up, we cancel out like-units and/or numbers.

$$1 \text{ bag} = \frac{500 \text{ mL}}{5 \text{ hours}} \times \frac{15 \text{ gtts}}{1 \text{ mL}} \times \frac{1 \text{ hour}}{60 \text{ minutes}} = ?$$

which can now be written as:

$$1 \text{ bag} = \frac{500 \times 15 \text{ gtts}}{300 \text{ minutes}} = ?$$

$$1 \text{ bag} = \frac{7,500 \text{ gtts}}{300 \text{ minutes}} = 25$$

So, the infusion rate is 25 gtts/minute.

EXAMPLE 21.23 DRIP RATES

Rx: Vancomycin 250 mg/250 mL Disp. 500 mg over 3 hours q8h. What is the flow rate in gtts/minute?

Let us start by looking at the information, or facts, that we know. We know that:

- One IV bag contains 500 mL.
- The drop factor is not stated, so we must assume 60 gtts/mL.
- The duration of administration is 3 hours.
- There are 60 minutes in 1 hour.

Notice that the additional information provided is not necessary in solving this problem.

Using the principle of dimensional analysis, we can solve the problem.

$$1 \text{ bag} = \frac{500 \text{ mL}}{3 \text{ hours}} \times \frac{60 \text{ gtts}}{1 \text{ mL}} \times \frac{1 \text{ hour}}{60 \text{ minutes}} = ?$$

After setting the problem up, we cancel out like-units and/or numbers.

$$1 \text{ bag} = \frac{500 \text{ mL}}{3 \text{ hours}} \times \frac{60 \text{ gtts}}{1 \text{ mL}} \times \frac{1 \text{ hour}}{60 \text{ minutes}} = ?$$

which can now be written as:

$$1 \text{ bag} = \frac{500 \times 1 \text{ gtts}}{3 \text{ minutes}} = ?$$

$$1 \text{ bag} = \frac{500 \text{ gtts}}{3 \text{ minutes}} = 166.66$$

So, the infusion rate is 167 gtts/minute.

EXAMPLE 21.24 DRIP RATES

A 100-mL bag containing 1 gm of Zanosar is to be infused, with a drop factor of 15, over 1 hour. What is the flow rate in gtts/minute?

We know that:

- One IV bag contains 100 mL.
- The drop factor is 15, so there are 15 gtts/Ml.
- The duration of administration is 1 hour.
- There are 60 minutes in 1 hour.

Using the principle of dimensional analysis, we can solve the problem.

$$1 \text{ bag} = \frac{100 \text{ mL}}{1 \text{ hour}} \times \frac{15 \text{ gtts}}{1 \text{ mL}} \times \frac{1 \text{ hour}}{60 \text{ minutes}} = ?$$

After setting the problem up, we cancel out like-units and/or numbers.

$$1 \text{ bag} = \frac{100 \text{ mL}}{1 \text{ hour}} \times \frac{15 \text{ gtts}}{1 \text{ mL}} \times \frac{1 \text{ hour}}{60 \text{ minutes}} = ?$$

which can now be written as:

$$1 \text{ bag} = \frac{100 \times 15 \text{ gtts}}{60 \text{ minutes}} = ?$$

$$1 \text{ bag} = \frac{1,500 \text{ gtts}}{60 \text{ minutes}} = 25$$

So, the infusion rate is 25 gtts/minute.

EXAMPLE 21.25 DRIP RATES

Rx: 2 gm Mandol in 1 L of D10W over 4 hours tid. What is the flow rate in gtts/minute?

Let us start by looking at the information, or facts, that we know. We know that:

- One IV bag contains 1,000 mL (1 L).
- The drop factor is not stated, so we must assume 60 gtts/mL.
- The duration of administration is 4 hours.
- There are 60 minutes in 1 hour.

Notice that the additional information provided is not necessary in solving this problem.

Using the principle of dimensional analysis, we can solve the problem.

$$1 \text{ bag} = \frac{1,000 \text{ mL}}{4 \text{ hours}} \times \frac{60 \text{ gtts}}{1 \text{ mL}} \times \frac{1 \text{ hour}}{60 \text{ minutes}} = ?$$

After setting the problem up, we cancel out like-units and/or numbers.

$$1 \text{ bag} = \frac{1,000 \text{ mL}}{4 \text{ hours}} \times \frac{60 \text{ gtts}}{1 \text{ mL}} \times \frac{1 \text{ hour}}{60 \text{ minutes}} = ?$$

which can now be written as:

$$1 \text{ bag} = \frac{1,000 \times 1 \text{ gtts}}{4 \text{ minutes}} = ?$$

$$1 \text{ bag} = \frac{1,000 \times 1 \text{ gtts}}{4 \text{ minutes}} = 250$$

So, the infusion rate is 250 gtts/minute.

Practice Problems 21-5
Drip Rates

1. Rx: Claforan (cefotaxime) 500 mg/50 mL IV over 60 minutes. What is the flow rate in gtts/minute?

2. Rx: ampicillin 0.5 gm/100 mL 50 mg/kg/day q8h over 90 minutes. The patient weighs 30 kg. What is the flow rate in mL/hour?

3. Rx: penicillin G potassium 20,000,000 units/L over 24 hours. What is the flow rate in mL/hour?

4. Rx: dexamethasone sodium phosphate 0.25 mg/kg/dose q8h over 30 minutes. The patient weighs 14 lb. You have a stock vial containing 4 mg/mL in a 10-mL vial; the IV bag holds 50 mL, and the IV administration set delivers 30 gtts/mL. What is the flow rate in gtts/minute?

5. Rx: Ringer's Solution 500 mL over 6 hours. What is the flow rate in mL/hour?

6. Rx: D5W 1.44 L over 24 hours. What is the flow rate in gtts/minute?

7. Rx: electrolyte solution 500 mL over 250 minutes. What is the flow rate in mL/hour?

8. Rx: antibiotic 250 mL over 2 hours. The IV administration set delivers 15 gtts/mL. What is the flow rate in gtts/minute?

9. Rx: Rocephin 2 gm/100 mL over 1 hour. The IV administration set delivers 30 gtts/mL. What is the flow rate in mL/hour?

10. Rx: insulin 100 units/250 mL over 2.5 hours. The IV administration set delivers 30 gtts/mL. What is the flow rate in gtts/minute?

TPN Milliequivalents

Total parenteral nutrition (TPN) is a solution made to supply many of the body's basic nutritional needs. It also contains necessary fluids, vitamins, and lipids. In essence, it is everything needed to sustain a human body nutritionally.

Electrolyte Solutions

Electrolytes in solution conduct electricity. When electrolytes are dissolved in water, they split into charged particles known as *ions*, which carry an electric charge. Electrolytes are important in maintaining acid–base balance in body fluids, controlling body water volume, and regulating metabolism.

Electrolytes are commonly added to TPN solutions according to the needs of the patient as indicated by the physician on the order. *Parenteral* indicates that the solution is delivered into the bloodstream via IV infusion.

Milliequivalents are used to express the concentration of electrolytes in solution. Solutions can be isotonic, hypertonic, or hypotonic, depending on their concentration as it relates to the osmotic pressure of human red blood cells. Solutions, therefore, are classified as one of the three following types, depending upon the tonicity:

Isotonic solutions—solutions that have an osmotic pressure equal to that of cell contents. NS (sodium chloride 0.9% solution) is considered isotonic with human red blood cells.

Hypertonic solutions—solutions that have greater osmotic pressure than cell contents. Hypertonic solutions cause cells to dehydrate and shrink.

Hypotonic solutions—solutions that have a lower osmotic pressure than cell contents. Hypotonic solutions cause cells to take on water and expand.

After receiving a TPN order, the pharmacy technician must determine how many milliliters will be extracted from the stock vial and injected into the TPN bag. Each item is extracted from the stock vial and injected into the TPN bag separately; that is, only one item is added at a time. TPNs are prepared in the clean room using aseptic technique.

❝ Workplace Wisdom TPN Automixers

Most health-system pharmacies now use automated machines called *automixers* to prepare TPN orders. The user needs to enter only the Rx order. These machines are connected to common stock solutions and automatically perform the necessary calculations and fluid draws. However, pharmacy technicians are still required to be proficient in performing these calculations. ❞

EXAMPLE 21.26 TPN MILLIEQUIVALENTS

Electrolyte	Stock Vial (mEq/mL)	Rx Order (mEq)	Volume Required
NaCl	4	60	X

---

isotonic solutions solutions that have an osmotic pressure equal to that of cell contents.

hypertonic solutions solutions that have greater osmotic pressure than cell contents. Hypertonic solutions cause cells to dehydrate and shrink.

hypotonic solutions solutions that have a lower osmotic pressure than cell contents. Hypotonic solutions cause cells to take on water and expand.

To calculate the volume required for electrolyte milliequivalents, you could set up a proportion and solve for X; you could set up a basic algebraic equation; or, most easily, you can divide the ordered amount of milliequivalents by the stock vial concentration, as long as the concentration is stated as X mEq/mL.

$$60 \div 4 = 15$$

So, you need to add 15 mL of the stock NaCl to the TPN.

EXAMPLE 21.27 TPN MILLIEQUIVALENTS

Electrolyte	Stock Vial (mEq/mL)	Rx Order (mEq)	Volume Required
K acetate	2	20	X

Again, because the stock concentration is listed as "per 1 mL," it is not necessary to set up a proportion or equation. Simply divide the quantity ordered by the stock concentration.

$$20 \div 2 = 10$$

10 mL of K acetate 2 mEq/mL must be added to the TPN.

Practice Problems 21-6
Milliequivalents

Electrolyte	Stock Vial (mEq/mL)	Rx Order (mEq)	Volume Required
Na phosphate	4	30	X
MgSO4	4	36	X
Na acetate	2	10	X
KCl	2	40	X
Ca gluconate	0.465	20	X

PROFILE IN PRACTICE

Robin is a pharmacy technician who works at an infusion clinic pharmacy. When preparing a TPN, Robin makes a mistake and withdraws the *strengths* of the electrolytes listed, rather than the calculated volumes needed.

▸ *The error is caught by the pharmacist, but what would have been the consequences had this error gone unchecked?*

Summary

Often described as the most difficult and challenging calculations used in pharmacy, parenteral calculations, drip rates, and TPN milliequivalents are all solved with basic, fundamental mathematics. If you properly use proportions, cross-multiplication, and dimensional analysis, you will be able to perform virtually all parenteral calculations that are done by pharmacy technicians.

Chapter Review Questions

1. You have a stock vial of cefotaxime 1 gm/50 mL. The dose is 1 gm over 30 minutes. How many mg/minute will the patient receive?
   a. 13
   b. 27
   c. 33
   d. 67

2. You have a stock vial of cefotaxime 500 mg/10 mL. The dose is 2 gm over 30 minutes. What is the flow rate in mL/hour?
   a. 40
   b. 60
   c. 80
   d. 100

3. You have a stock vial of cefotaxime 1 gm/50 mL. The dose is 2 gm over 30 minutes. What is the flow rate in gtts/minute, if the administration set is calibrated to 20 gtts/mL?
   a. 27
   b. 67
   c. 80
   d. 87

4. What is the flow rate, in gtts/minute, for a 1 L TPN over 12 hours, if the IV administration set is calibrated to deliver 30 gtts/mL?
   a. 42
   b. 30
   c. 12
   d. 60

5. What is the flow rate in gtts/minute for 100 mL of an antibiotic administered over 30 minutes?
   a. 200
   b. 100
   c. 60
   d. 83

6. You have an order for cefuroxime 1.5 gm/50 mL with a maximum dose of 1.5 gm q8h. The patient weighs 200 lb. What is the flow rate in gtts/minute, if his dose is administered over 90 minutes?
   a. 90
   b. 50
   c. 40
   d. 33

7. You have a stock vial of product 30 mg/mL. How many milliliters will you need to prepare an IV infusion containing a dose of 150 mg/50 mL?
   a. 5
   b. 10
   c. 20
   d. 30

8. You have a stock vial of sodium bicarbonate 0.5 mEq/mL. How many milliliters do you need to provide 60 mEq?
   a. 40
   b. 80
   c. 120
   d. 160

9. You have a stock vial of magnesium sulfate 4 mEq/mL. How many milliliters do you need to provide 24 mEq?
   a. 4
   b. 6
   c. 8
   d. 12

10. You have a stock vial of calcium gluconate injection 4.65 mEq/10 mL. How many milliliters do you need to provide 70 mEq?
    a. 70
    b. 120
    c. 150
    d. 32

Critical Thinking Questions

1. In what ways are calculations using milliequivalents similar to ratio and proportion calculations?

2. Why does pharmacy assume a drop factor of 60 unless notified otherwise?

3. What impact can miscalculated flow rates have on the nursing staff, and ultimately the patient?

References and Resources

Hegstad, Lorrie N. and Wilma Hayek. *Essential Drug Dosage Calculations*. 4th ed. Upper Saddle River, NJ: Pearson, 2001. Print.

Johnston, Mike. *Pharmacy Calculations: The Pharmacy Technician Series*. Upper Saddle River, NJ: Pearson, 2005. Print.

Lesmeister, Michelle Benjamin. *Math Basics for the Healthcare Professional*. 4th ed. Upper Saddle River, NJ: Pearson, 2013. Print.

Mikolah, Alan A. *Drug Dosage Calculations for the Emergency Care Provider*. 2nd ed. Upper Saddle River, NJ: Prentice Hall, 2003. Print.

Olsen, June, Anthony Giangrasso, and Dolores Shrimpton. *Medical Dosage Calculations*. 10th ed. Upper Saddle River, NJ: Pearson, 2011. Print.

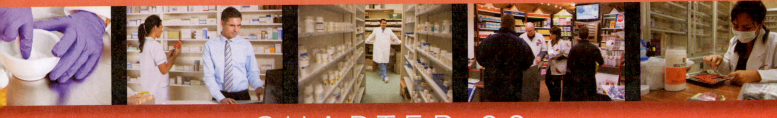

CHAPTER 22

Business Math

LEARNING OBJECTIVES

After completing this chapter, you should be able to:

- Define and understand how to calculate cost, selling price, and markup.

- Explain co-payments and average wholesale price (AWP).

- Define and understand how to determine markup and markup percent.

- Define and understand how to calculate gross profit and net profit.

KEY TERMS

cost, p. 338
gross profit, p. 340
markup, p. 338
net profit, p. 340
profit, p. 340

INTRODUCTION

The goal of any business is to make a profit; pharmacy is no different. It is necessary to maintain enough profit in the business model to be able to take care of obligations such as rent and inventory expense and have a positive net income at the end of the fiscal year. Profits help pay salaries of employees, so it is important to keep a certain profit margin above supply costs so that the business can afford to keep and pay its employees.

Pharmacy is a Business

In order to maintain a profitable business, many pharmacies have had to diversify their products and services. In addition to dispensing prescriptions, many pharmacies now offer immunizations, specialty compounds, nutritional counseling, and disease state management services, and some offer other items, such as health and beauty aids, gifts, and even food. There is an art to managing a pharmacy in a way that cares for patients and the prices they pay for medicines while providing a business model that results in a positive net income. Controlling inventory, accounts receivable, cash flow, and variable expenses is a vital component of a successful business.

Cost, Selling Price, and Markup

Every product sold in a pharmacy has three essential numbers—cost, markup, and selling price. Accuracy is critical when working with these figures, as they directly impact the profitability of the pharmacy. A minor mistake could cost the pharmacy a significant financial loss.

Cost

Every product in a pharmacy, whether it is a bottle of prescription antibiotics or an over-the-counter (OTC) product, is purchased from a wholesaler or manufacturer for a specific cost. This cost, or cost of goods sold, can be $0.20 or $2,000, depending on the product, but it is always less than the amount that the pharmacy charges the customer. Cost is sometimes referred to as *invoice cost* or *acquisition cost*, and it is of particular importance when taking quarterly or annual inventory.

❝ Workplace Wisdom

In order to note the cost of products, many pharmacies have created a coding system in which each letter in the code represents a number. This invoice cost is then printed on the wholesaler sticker by using the code or numerals. An example of a code might be:

P H A R M O C I S T
1 2 3 4 5 6 7 8 9 0

The code shown here is not misspelled—10 different letters are necessary for the code to work properly. For example, if the cost of a product was $8.45, the sticker would be marked *IRM*. This method allows for the actual cost to be placed on products, for staff use, without the customer knowing about it.

Selling Price

While cost refers to the amount of money the pharmacy paid for a product, the selling price is the total amount of money the pharmacy receives from the sale of the product. For OTC products, the selling, or retail, price is noted on a price sticker placed on the product or, more commonly, is programmed into the product's bar code. When you ring up the sale, the selling price is the amount that you key or scan into the cash register. Wholesalers provide price stickers to be attached to each OTC product. Some stores use bar code scanning and show the price on a shelf tag. Selling price, however, does not always refer only to the amount of money the customer pays. For prescription products, the total selling price includes the amount to be paid by the third-party insurer and the patient's co-payment.

---

cost the amount of money the pharmacy pays to acquire a product

markup the amount of money that the pharmacy adds to the cost to establish the selling price

Patient Co-Payments

Many prescriptions are filled under third-party prescription plans for which the patient must make a co-payment. Co-payments vary; they may be a standard amount or a percentage of the total prescription price. Many third-party plans operate under a tiered co-payment system. For example, generic products might be $15.00, preferred brand-name products $30.00, and nonpreferred brand-name products $50.00; some products may be excluded from coverage.

Third-Party Insurance Coverage

Reimbursement formulas set by the plan are used to calculate the total price for each prescription. Pharmacy computer systems communicate with the insurer through a computer data switch. Total price and the customer co-payment are transmitted back to the pharmacy system at the time of processing.

info · Calculating Third-Party Insurance Coverage

The amount an insurance company will contribute to the selling price of a product can be calculated so long as you are provided with the reimbursement pricing formula and the AWP.

Let us consider a plan that reimburses AWP−14%+$2.50, and the AWP for a product is $58.00.

First, you need to calculate the AWP percentage discount. In this case, it is 14%. If you convert the percentage to a decimal (0.14 in this example) and multiply it by the AWP, you will get the AWP percentage discount. Therefore, $58.00 (AWP) × 0.14 (discount percentage stated as a decimal) equals $8.12. This means that the insurance company will reimburse $49.88 ($58.00 × 0.14). Then, you have to add any necessary flat processing fees included in the pricing formula, which in this case is $2.50. So, for this example, the pharmacy will be reimbursed 52.38 (49.88 + 2.50) from the insurance company, in addition to the patient's co-payment.

It is always important to make sure that the AWP is calculated for the proper quantity before calculating third-party insurance coverage. For example, if the AWP is $58.00 for a bottle of 100 capsules, but the prescription is only for 30, the AWP for the prescription would actually be $17.40, prior to the pricing formula's AWP discount. To calculate this, simply divide the AWP by the AWP's stated quantity ($58.00/100), and then multiply it by the amount being dispensed (30).

Once the price is calculated according to the plan formula, the patient is responsible for the designated co-payment, and the insurance company is responsible for the balance. The balance due to the pharmacy is batched with other claims from the same processor, and payment is transmitted to the pharmacy by check or electronic funds transfer along with a reconciliation statement. Many states have implemented prompt-payment legislation to help pharmacies collect payment in a timely manner. Some plans provide reconciliation statements through the Internet.

■ Formulas—Selling Price, Markup, and Cost

When you need to calculate the selling price, markup, or cost, any variation of the following formula can be used, so long as you know at least two of the three amounts.

Selling price = cost + markup

or

Markup = selling price − cost

or

Cost = selling price − markup

Note that all three versions are, in essence, the exact same formula. Choose one version to learn, and you will be able to calculate selling price, markup, or cost.

Most pharmacy systems perform a price update function weekly to update all drug files to the most current average wholesale price (AWP) data. This is critical, because nearly all third-party plans use a pricing formula based on AWP—for example, AWP − 14% + 2.50.

❝ Workplace Wisdom Calculating the Total Price with Insurance

Never forget to include both the third-party insurance adjusted reimbursement amount and the patient's co-payment to calculate the accurate selling price for prescription products. ❞

Markup

The difference between the selling price and the cost, stated in dollars and cents, is the **markup**. The markup should always be a positive number; otherwise, you are selling a product for less than what the pharmacy has paid for it, thus losing money on the transaction.

EXAMPLE 22.1

At what price should a bottle of vitamins be sold for, if the acquisition cost is $6.15 and there is a $3.00 markup?

First, determine that this question is asking you to calculate the selling price.

Selling price = cost + markup

X = $6.15 + $3.00

X = $9.15

Therefore, the vitamins should be sold for $9.15

EXAMPLE 22.2

If a thermometer sells for $9.95 and the pharmacy paid $4.25 for it, what is the amount of markup?

Markup = selling price − cost

X = $9.95 − $4.25

X = $5.70

Therefore, the amount of markup on the thermometer is $5.70.

EXAMPLE 22.3

If a package of syringes sells for $5.98 and a $2.10 markup is included, what is the invoice cost of the syringes?

Cost = selling price − markup

X = $5.98 − $2.10

X = $3.88

The insulin syringes cost the pharmacy $3.88.

Markup Percent

In most situations, markup is calculated and discussed as a percentage, rather than a specific amount. Calculating the markup percent is very simple, all you have to do is to divide the markup amount by the cost and then multiply by 100 to get the markup percent.

PROFILES IN PRACTICE

Romaine is asked to put a variety of products that have not sold in six months on clearance. She is instructed to clear items at 5% less than the cost. Romaine knows that the products being cleared have a standard markup of 100%, but she does not have the invoices that list the original costs.

1 *Can Romaine accurately determine the clearance prices with the information available to her?*
2 *If one of the items she is putting on clearance normally sells for $10.00, what would be the clearance price?*

■ Formula—Markup Percent

Use the following formula to calculate markup percent:

$$\frac{Markup}{Cost} \times 100 = \text{markup percent}$$

or

$$\frac{(Selling\ price - cost)}{Cost} \times 100 = \text{markup percent}$$

Note that the second formula includes the markup amount formula as the numerator. These are the exact same formula, just two different ways of looking at it, depending upon the information you are provided with.

EXAMPLE 22.4

If an item that costs $70.00 is marked up to $100.00, what is the markup percent?

The selling price minus the cost is placed as the numerator and then divided by the cost. The result is then multiplied by 100 to determine the markup percent.

In this example, the cost ($70) is subtracted from the selling price ($100), which equals $30, and $30 is divided by the cost ($70), equaling 0.4286.

0.4286 is multiplied by 100 to get 42.86%, the markup percent.

$$\frac{(100 - 70)}{70} \times 100 = 42.86\%$$

This can be verified as: $70.00 × 1.4286 = $100.0

Profit—Gross and Net

Profit refers to the difference between the selling price and the costs associated with a product. There are two types of profit calculated by businesses—gross profit and net profit.

■ Formula—Gross Profit

This is calculated the same way as markup:

Gross profit = selling price − cost

---

profit the difference between the selling price and the costs associated with a product

gross profit the difference between the selling price and the cost, or costs of goods sold, for a product

net profit the difference between the selling price and all costs for a product (the cost of goods sold + overhead costs)

■ Formula—Gross Profit Percent

$$\frac{Gross\ profit}{Selling\ price} \times 100 = \text{gross profit percent}$$

Gross Profit

When considering price and markup on prescription products, the industry uses the term **gross profit** to mean how much above cost the pharmacy is paid for a given product.

EXAMPLE 22.5

If a prescription costs the pharmacy $14.85 and sells for $38.20, what is the amount of gross profit?

Gross profit = selling price − cost

X = $38.20 − $14.85

X = $23.35

The pharmacy makes a gross profit of $23.35 on this prescription.

So, to the extent that pharmacy technicians are involved in business calculations, gross profit and markup are one in the same; however, gross profit percent is calculated differently than the markup percent. Whereas markup percent is calculated by dividing against the product's cost, gross profit percent is calculated by dividing against the product's selling price.

EXAMPLE 22.6

Determine the gross profit percent based on the information provided in Example 22.5 .

In Example 22.5, a prescription cost the pharmacy $14.85 and it was sold for $38.20, providing a gross profit of $23.35.

To calculate the gross profit percent, simply divide the gross profit amount ($23.35) by the selling price ($38.20) and multiply by 100.

$23.35/$38.20 = 0.611

0.611 × 100 = 61.1%

The gross profit percent on this prescription is 61.1%.

Overhead

Gross profit for the particular prescription or product, however, does not consider a number of other factors related to the cost of doing business. These costs, known as overhead, are added

■ Formula—Net Profit

Net profit = selling price − (cost + overhead)

■ Formula—Net Profit Percent

$$\frac{\text{Net profit}}{\text{Selling price}} \times 100 = \text{net profit percent}$$

costs needed to maintain and operate the business. Overhead expenses include items such as rent, electricity, phone lines, insurance, pharmacy supplies, and payroll, just to name a few. Cost of goods sold, that is the acquisition cost of a drug or product, is not a part of overhead.

Net Profit

Net profit refers to the money left over after you have paid invoice cost (cost of goods sold) and overhead. As the bottom line number, net profit is generally what most people are referring to when they discuss profit. Net profit is the last line found on a standard accounting income statement. A negative number reflects a net loss.

EXAMPLE 22.7

A bottle of OTC cough syrup sells for $7.49. The pharmacy paid $3.40 for the product and has $2.10 in associated overhead. What is the net profit?

Net profit = selling price − (cost + overhead)

X = $7.49 − ($3.40 + $2.10)

X = $7.49 − ($5.50)

X = $1.90

Therefore, the pharmacy makes $1.90 net profit on each bottle of that OTC cough syrup.

EXAMPLE 22.8

Determine the net profit percent on the information provided in Example 22.7.

In Example 22.7, a bottle of OTC cough syrup cost the pharmacy $3.40 in costs of goods sold and $2.10 in overhead; it was sold for $7.49, providing a net profit of $1.90.

To calculate the net profit percent, simply divide the net profit amount ($1.90) by the selling price ($7.49) and multiply by 100.

$1.90/$7.49 = 0.25367

0.25367 × 100 = 25.37%

The net profit percent on this cough syrup is 25.37%.

❝ Workplace Wisdom Improving the Bottom Line

Let us compare two different income statements. Notice how much the net profit is improved when holding down expenses.

	Store #1		Store #2	
Income	$1,500,00	100%	$1,500,000	100%
− Cost of goods sold	$1,050,00	70%	$1,050,000	70%
− Overhead and expenses	$300,000	20%	$270,000	8%
= Net profit	$150,000	10%	$180,000	12%

Improving net profit by 2%, through either better purchasing or reducing expenses, resulted in an additional $30,000 per year. ❞

Income Statement

A simplified accounting income statement looks like this:

Income	100%	All the money that comes in
− Cost of goods sold	70%	Cost for inventory purchases
− Overhead and expenses	20%	Cost for overhead and salaries
= Net profit	10%	What is left over

Businesses increase their net profit by negotiating the lowest possible cost of goods and reducing overhead expenses. This explains why pharmacies hire more pharmacy technicians than pharmacists, consider the difference in salary, and routinely review and reduce total staff hours, to reduce the payroll overhead expense. If purchases and expenses are minimized, the only other way to increase net profit is through increased prices. This is difficult in today's market due to the large volume of third-party plans that have a contract formula for calculating selling price.

Many pharmacies have 80% or more of their volume tied to third-party plans. The cost of goods sold percentage shown, 70%, is a sample target. In today's market, very few stores actually achieve a 30% margin. However, average overhead and expenses for most businesses run around 18–20% of sales. This creates a strain on net profit. Therefore, pharmacies should be diligent in controlling inventory.

Accounting Formulas

The following common accounting formulas are included here as a reference:

Formula	Selling Price
Selling price = cost + markup	

Formula	Markup
Markup = selling price − cost	

Formula	Cost
Cost = selling price − markup	

Formula	Markup Percent
$\text{Markup percent} = \dfrac{(\text{selling price} - \text{cost})}{\text{cost}} \times 100$	
or	
$\text{Markup percent} = \dfrac{\text{markup}}{\text{cost}} \times 100$	

Formula	Gross Profit
Gross profit = selling price − cost	

Formula	Gross Profit percent
$\dfrac{\text{Gross profit}}{\text{Selling price}} \times 100 = \text{gross profit percent}$	

Formula	Net Profit
Net gross profit = selling price − (cost + overhead)	

Formula	Net Profit percent
$\dfrac{\text{Net profit}}{\text{Selling price}} \times 100 = \text{net profit percent}$	

 Practice Problems 22-1

Perform the following pricing calculations:

1. If special-order items are marked up at 25% above AWP, what is the selling price for an item that has an AWP of $13.29?

2. If invoice cost of an item is $7.00 and the selling price is $13.89, how much is the markup? What is the markup percent?

3. Advanced herbal and vitamin formulations are marked up at 50% over invoice cost. If the invoice cost is $12.30, what is the selling price? How much is the markup?

4. Hemorrhoid suppositories are priced at $3.29, and their invoice cost is $1.80. What is the amount of the markup? What is the markup percent?

5. Weekly medication planners are marked up at 96% above invoice cost. A new display has arrived with an invoice, and no suggested retail pricing stickers have been provided. What is the selling price for each item?

    a. 7-day pill pack, invoice cost $3.50

    b. 7-day pill pack with alarm, invoice cost $4.84

    c. 1-day pill box, invoice cost $0.64

    d. 28-day pill organizer tray, invoice cost $7.64

6. Glucometer test strips are sold for $98.00 per box of 100 strips. The net profit on the strips is $22.00. Store overhead per box of strips is $4.30. What is the invoice cost for the box of strips?

7. High-protein nutrition drink packets have an invoice cost of $32.00 per box. The selling price is $52.95. Overhead is $3.90. What is the net profit for the item?

8. Digital blood pressure monitors are priced at your pharmacy for $42.89, and the cost is $34.59. Overhead is 4% of cost. What is the net profit?

    Use the following sample plan formulas to solve the following problems:

    Brand-name product formula: AWP − 14% − $2.50

    Generic product formula: AWP − 35% + 1.75

9. Product ABC has an invoice cost of $18.00/C. This means $18.00/100 capsules. The AWP is $36.30/C. The prescription calls for 42 capsules. ABC is a generic antibiotic.

    a. What is the selling price according to the plan formula?

    b. What is the gross profit?

    c. What is the gross profit percent?

10. Brand-name product XYZ nasal spray has an invoice cost of *PRSTT*, using the cost code provided at the beginning of the chapter. The AWP for the product is $175.65.

    a. What is the selling price?

    b. What is the gross profit?

    c. What is the gross profit percent?

    For each of the following price stickers, use the sample third-party formulas to calculate the selling price for 30 units, the gross profit, and the gross profit percent.

11. Accupril sticker

    Cost: $97.05/90

    AWP: $122.31/90

12. Xenical sticker

    Cost: $108.01/100

    AWP: $132.86/100

13. Diltiazem sticker

    Cost: $63.00

    AWP: $130.10

14. Tri-sprintec sticker

    Generic birth control

    7/7/7 pack

    Packaged 6 × 28

    Cost: $140.02

    AWP: $218.68

15. If invoice cost of an item is $26.14 and the selling price is $46.92, how much is the markup? What is the markup percent? What is the gross profit? What is the gross profit percent?

Summary

As with all businesses, pharmacies must give special attention to accounting and operational calculations. Inventory mismanagement, improper pricing, and inadequate reimbursement can quickly cause a pharmacy to lose money.

Chapter Review Questions

1. What is the selling price for a product that costs $8.50 and has a 29% markup?
   a. $8.79
   b. $10.97
   c. $17.00
   d. $24.65

2. What is the markup percent for a product that costs $20.00 and sells for $39.95?
   a. 19.95
   b. 20
   c. 50
   d. 99.75

3. Which of the following is an example of overhead?
   a. payroll
   b. markup
   c. inventory
   d. cost of goods sold

4. Using the formula AWP − 14% + $2.50, what is the gross profit percent for 30 tablets of a product that has an AWP of $87.00/C and an invoice cost of $62.34/C?
   a. 18.7
   b. 33.4
   c. 24.9
   d. 6.2

5. Using the formula AWP − 35% + $2.50, what is the gross profit for 30 tablets of a generic product that has an acquisition cost of $42.60/C and an AWP of $164.35/C?
   a. $2.50
   b. $12.78
   c. $21.77
   d. $34.55

6. Determine the overhead for a product with a selling price of $89.00, cost of $62.00, and net profit of $8.50.
   a. $8.50
   b. $18.50
   c. $28.50
   d. $38.50

7. Determine the selling price for a product with a cost of $6.42, overhead of $1.89, and net profit of $2.00.
   a. $10.31
   b. $6.42
   c. $1.89
   d. $2.00

8. Determine the cost for a product with a selling price of $29.38, overhead of $4.50, and net profit of $8.00.
   a. $12.50
   b. $21.38
   c. $24.88
   d. $16.88

9. Determine the gross profit for a product with a selling price of $68.49, cost of $42.00, and overhead of $7.50.
   a. $18.99
   b. $34.50
   c. $49.50
   d. $26.49

10. What is the markup percent for a product that costs $10.00 and sells for $13.99?
    a. 3.99
    b. 39.9
    c. 10
    d. 13.9

Critical Thinking Questions

1. Give an example of a tiered co-payment system.

2. Describe markup and how it can be calculated.

3. List three items that are present in overhead.

References and Resources

Hegstad, Lorrie N. and Wilma Hayek. *Essential Drug Dosage Calculations*. 4th ed. Upper Saddle River, NJ: Pearson, 2001. Print.

Johnston, Mike. *Pharmacy Calculations: The Pharmacy Technician Series*. Upper Saddle River, NJ: Pearson, 2005. Print.

Lesmeister, Michelle Benjamin. *Math Basics for the Healthcare Professional*. 4th ed. Upper Saddle River, NJ: Pearson, 2013. Print.

Mikolah, Alan A. *Drug Dosage Calculations for the Emergency Care Provider*. 2nd ed. Upper Saddle River, NJ: Prentice Hall, 2003. Print.

Olsen, June, Anthony Giangrasso, and Dolores Shrimpton. *Medical Dosage Calculations*. 10th ed. Upper Saddle River, NJ: Pearson, 2011. Print.

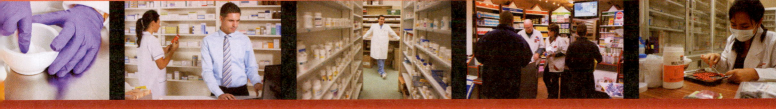

CHAPTER 23

The Body and Drugs

LEARNING OBJECTIVES

After completing this chapter, you should be able to:

- Explain the differences between pharmacodynamics and pharmacokinetics.
- Understand the ways in which cell receptors react to drugs.
- Describe the mechanism of action of drugs and identify and understand its key factor.
- Explain how drugs are absorbed, distributed, metabolized, and cleared by the body.
- Explain the difference between fat-soluble and water-soluble drugs and give examples of each.
- Identify and explain the effect of bioavailability and its relationship to drug effectiveness.
- Understand addiction and addictive behavior.
- Describe the role of a pharmacy technician in identifying drug-abusing patients.
- List and identify some drugs that interact with alcohol.

KEY TERMS

absorption, p. 350
addiction, p. 355
agonist, p. 347
antagonist, p. 347
bioavailability, p. 352
clearance, p. 354
dependency, p. 354
distribution, p. 357
drug–drug interaction, p. 349
excretion, p. 350
half-life, p. 349
metabolism, p. 352
metabolites, p. 350
pharmacodynamics, p. 346
pharmacokinetics, p. 350
receptor, p. 346
site of action, p. 346
target cell, p. 348
tolerance, p. 355

INTRODUCTION

Pharmacists expect competent pharmacy technicians to know more than how to count, pour, and prepare medications. Although the pharmacist is responsible for providing pharmaceutical care to patients using his or her specialized knowledge, technicians too must understand the basics of pharmacology. *Pharmacology* can be defined as the study of drugs, including their composition, uses, application, and effects.

This chapter introduces some basic concepts of pharmacology, including pharmacodynamics and pharmacokinetics. You will learn how the body absorbs, distributes, transforms, and eliminates medications. You will also review the effects of drug and chemical abuse.

Pharmacodynamics

Most drugs affect the cells in the body by interacting with specific drug **receptors**. One way to understand this process is to use a lock-and-key analogy. Consider each cell in the body as having locks (the receptors), each of which requires a specific key that can lock or unlock it to produce an effect. Specific drugs "unlock" certain receptors in the body. In other words, drugs are developed to interact with certain unique receptors to produce a certain effect on the body. Ideally, this effect can be measured. The study of how drugs produce their effects on the desired cells and how a drug is processed by the body is called **pharmacodynamics**.

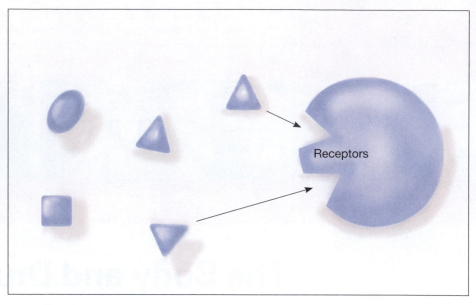

FIGURE 23-1 Receptor site.

Receptor Complex

A receptor (again, think of it as a lock requiring a key) on a cell interacts with a specific drug because the drug "fits" the specific structure of the receptor. The drug is often designed to have a structure that is the same as or similar to that of the cells intended to be affected. Once the "key" is "turned," the chemical structure of the drug is permitted into the cell, where it can exert its effect on the particular function of the cell (see Figure 23-1).

As an example, let us look at a class of drugs that can reduce allergy symptoms. *Histamine* is a chemical released by certain cells; it is responsible for the common symptoms of allergic reactions, like burning, itchy eyes, and a runny nose. Drugs called *antihistamines* interact or bind with histamine receptors on cells, effectively turning them off and thus reducing the action of histamine. The result is a reduction of the allergic symptoms.

Drugs have specific shapes and structures that match up with the shapes of the receptors on specific cells. In many instances, because of its characteristics, a drug can interact with more than one cell receptor. A classic example is diphenhydramine, which reacts with both histamine receptors and receptors in the nervous system. The interaction with the nervous system causes the main side effect of diphenhydramine, drowsiness.

Site of Action

When first developing a pharmaceutical agent, the scientists researching it usually do not merely stumble upon a receptor (although that can happen). More commonly, they create a new drug based on the knowledge that there is a specific **site of action** for each class of drug.

It is true that the specific site of action of some drugs is unknown. However, the FDA requires drug-manufacturing companies to prove two things: The drug works (is effective), and it is safe. If the manufacturer can prove efficacy and safety, it need not always describe or specify the site of action.

Chemistry is a science and sometimes an art as well. Aspirin is a classic example of understanding where a specific drug exerts its effects. There are specific sites located in an area of the brain called the *hypothalamus*, which is, among other things, the body's temperature regulator (see Figure 23-2). By matching some of the sites (receptors) on the cells of the hypothalamus, aspirin helps reduce the body's temperature.

Mechanism of Action

The term *mechanism of action* refers to how a drug works and produces its desirable (and sometimes undesirable) effects. For example, when a patient undergoes anesthesia for surgery, the

---

receptor a molecular structure located on the surface of the cell that binds with a particular chemical or chemicals. When a chemical binds with a receptor, the receptor is stimulated to either produce or inhibit a specific action.

pharmacodynamics the study of the biochemical and physiologic effects of drugs and their mechanisms of action.

site of action the location where a drug will exert its effect.

agonist a type of drug that activates the receptor to produce a predicted action.

antagonist a type of drug that prevents receptor activation.

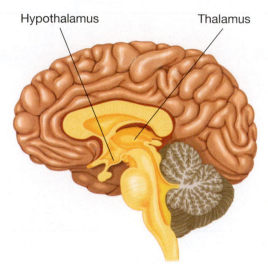

FIGURE 23-2 The hypothalamus.

drugs used for pain reduction interrupt the pathway between the central nervous system and the peripheral nervous system so that the person is no longer capable of sensing pain. Without this mechanism of action, patients who undergo massive surgical procedures would go into shock.

Receptor Site

The *receptor site* is the location where the drug (chemical) binds to the cell. Once the drug develops a bond with a body cell (at the receptor site), specific molecular changes can occur. For example, when opioids (narcotics) are used, they bind to cells and cause the changes to occur within the cell itself; the cellular changes reduce the amount of perceived pain. The pain still exists—in surgery, for example, cells are necessarily damaged in some areas—but the brain does not perceive the pain, because specific qualities of the cells that normally send pain signals are turned off. (Recall the analogy of the key that turns a lock, which in turn produces a specific response.)

The known receptors are so numerous that it would be difficult to describe every one of them. New receptors are always being discovered; hence, the market for new, more powerful, and more specific drugs is enormous.

Agonists and Antagonists

An **agonist** is a specific type of drug that produces a certain, predicted action when it binds to the correct receptor (i.e., to the receptor for which it was designed). In this situation, the drug is doing exactly what it has been designed to do, although there may or may not be side effects as well (both

predicted and unpredicted). Agonists bind with cells and produce cellular responses resulting in a therapeutic effect. Many hormones and neurotransmitters (e.g. acetylcholine, histamine, and norepinephrine) and many drugs (e.g. morphine, phenylephrine, and isoproterenol) act as agonists. For example, the agonist isoproterenol is used to treat asthma because it mimics the effects of catecholamines (hormones and neurotransmitters such as adrenaline, noradrenaline, and dopamine) in relaxing bronchial muscles in the lung. It does this by interacting with one specific class of adrenergic receptor.

In contrast, an **antagonist** is a drug that does not produce any noticeable effect when it binds to a specific receptor on the cell. Its function is to block the action of that receptor, often by physically blocking other chemicals from attaching to the receptor. However, because a drug is a chemical, an antagonist may or may not have predictable side effects.

Antagonists interact selectively with receptors. They reduce or prevent the action of another substance (agonist) at the receptor site. For example, propranolol, a drug used to control blood pressure and pulse rate in cardiac patients, is an antagonist of a class of adrenergic receptors that control blood pressure and heartbeat rate.

Agonists have two main properties. The first is *affinity*— the ability of the agonist to actually bind to the cell receptor structure. (Again, if you imagine this as a lock and a key, it will make more sense.) The other property is the *efficacy* of the agonist, or the ability of the drug to affect the cell and cellular structure and change the way the cell behaves. In essence, if the drug is an agonist, and it does what it is designed for and intended to do, it is considered *efficacious*.

There are useful aspects of both kinds of drugs (see Figure 23-3). Just because an antagonist does not produce a noticeable effect, one cannot conclude that the drug is not useful. Remember that the function of an antagonist is to prevent action of another substance, rather than to produce its own effect. Antagonists have important uses; otherwise, such drugs would not exist.

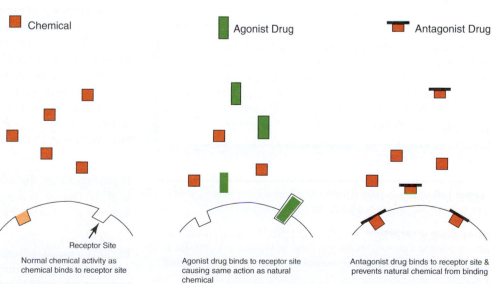

FIGURE 23-3 Example of agonistic and antagonistic drug action.

Even though antagonists bind to certain receptors without producing any noticeable action, they could be advantageous to the life of the cell as well as the life of the organism. Think about a person who has used the wrong drug, or a patient who is brought into the emergency room because he has overdosed on one of the morphine-derivative drugs. Emergency-room staff can administer a classic antagonist, called *naloxone*, which binds to the exact sites where the illicit drug attaches; the result is a prompt reversal of what would otherwise be a life-threatening situation.

There are thousands of other reasons for using antagonists as pharmacological agents, and just as many ways in which they are used. As a pharmacy technician, will you be able to identify the agonists and the antagonists? Well, maybe if you are a chemistry buff, but knowing all of them is not a specific requirement for the technician job. Knowing that they exist, how they work, and how to identify them is far more important.

Remember the **target cell**. This term actually refers to a large number of cells, all of which are similar to each other. Target cells include the nerve cells and cells that are involved with the heart or the vascular system, especially with respect to circulation and blood pressure. These and many others make up what chemists and pharmacologists think of as target cells—the cells and receptors that become involved when a specific medication is used.

The Dose–Response Curve

A relatively simple principle of pharmacology and pharmacodynamics is that the patient's response is directly related to the amount of the drug administered. If the dose–response relationship was plotted on a chart, you would see a curve that graphically depicts this relationship, as shown in Figure 23-4. As simple as this basic principle might seem, it is probably one of

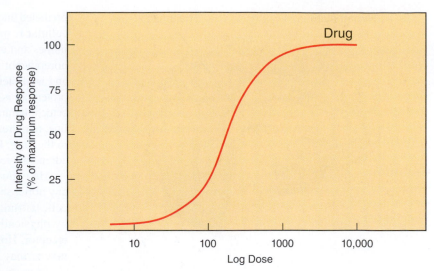

FIGURE 23-4 The dose–response curve.

the most important aspects of pharmacology you will encounter as a technician. With respect to this curve, a *dose* is defined as the specific amount of the drug required to achieve a desired effect, which is referred to as the *response to the drug*.

If you think about how a graph might represent the way a drug reacts with a cell (and with all cells that are similar to the target cell), you can easily grasp the idea that, in time, a maximal response will be attained (see Figure 23-4). After that point, adding more of the same drug will be of no benefit. That does *not* mean, however, that adding more drug will not cause harm; in fact, in most such cases, harm *does* occur, especially when people abuse drugs.

The point on the graph that represents the maximal response is called the *ceiling*. Beyond that point, drugs often become toxic, especially to the liver and the kidneys. Knowing that there are drugs that do not have a ceiling is important in pharmacodynamics; this is where your knowledge about what you do in the facility where you are employed counts the most. The pharmacy technician is slowly and quite effectively moving from being just a cashier to being an expert about certain classes of drugs.

Although you probably will not learn the mechanisms of action of drugs at the chemical level, your knowledge of how the drugs work generally, and why specific chemicals can be dangerous, can be an asset to the pharmacist for whom you work. It is really that simple—but it is not necessarily easy. Because the science of medicine is always producing new results, your job requirements will always be changing, and there will always be new things to learn.

Potency

In pharmacology, the word *potency* means exactly what it does in general usage. It is a measurement of the strength of a drug that is required to produce a specific effect on the body.

ED50

ED50 is a measurement of the specific amount of a drug that will achieve 50% of the maximal response. This is an important concept, because it is used to measure the full potency of some drugs without having to achieve such a level.

---

info

Agonists and Antagonists

Agonists and antagonists have been useful in studies of binding sites on receptors. Such investigations are useful in drug design, when researchers' goal is to activate or inactivate certain classes of receptors. The terms *agonist* and *antagonist* simply define the exact action of a substance.

---

target cell a general term referring to a large number of cells, all of which are similar, on which a particular drug is intended to act.

drug–drug interaction an interaction between two or more drugs administered to a patient, resulting in either an increase or a decrease in the therapeutic effects of one or more of the drugs, or an adverse effect.

half-life the time required for serum concentration levels of an absorbed and distributed drug to decrease by one-half.

Half-Life

Half-life, written $T_{\frac{1}{2}}$ is the time required for plasma serum concentration levels of an absorbed and distributed drug to decrease by one-half. Once the drug is at a serum concentration of less than 3%, it is considered to have been removed from the body. Half-life is applicable to those drugs that follow through with the first bypass of elimination, which means that they go through the liver as well as the gastrointestinal (GI) tract. The half-life of a drug determines how many times a day a drug is dosed. Patients on drugs with longer half-lives, such as digoxin or coumadin, take fewer doses per day. In contrast, drugs with shorter half-lives, such as ibuprofen and acetaminophen, must be taken more frequently to maintain therapeutic serum levels.

Time–Response Curve

The time–response curve provides a means to determine the length of time for which a specific drug will continue to have the same degree of effect. The effect may be on a class of cells, an organ, or the entire body, depending on the relationship between the body, the drug, and what is being treated. Ideally, when no other drugs (or foods) have an adverse effect on a drug, the time–response curve will be a bell curve, showing a specific onset of action (which can be measured), the entire duration of action, and the termination of action (see Figure 23-5).

Pharmacodynamic Mechanisms

Much is known about the interactions between the many different drugs that can be taken into the human body. These pharmacologic drug interactions are an important aspect of pharmacology. If discovered by the pharmacy technician, any potential interactions should be brought to the attention of the pharmacist on duty.

Many of the problems related to **drug–drug interactions** occur when an antagonistic drug is added to one that is not, or an antagonistic drug is added to a number of other antagonistic drugs. This duplication of action can start a process by which a drug is either able to compete for specific sites on cells or to prevent other chemicals from binding on other cells.

As you will learn in the next section, specific sites on a cell, when turned on, will cause the cell to act in one way; in contrast, a chemical can be used to turn off or block a cellular mechanism. The chemicals in the drug connect to the cell and become the key that locks or unlocks a series of systems, which

PROFILE IN PRACTICE

Juanita is a pharmacy technician who works in a neighborhood retail pharmacy. Mrs. Jones comes in to pick up her prescriptions. When ringing up the order, Juanita notices that Mrs. Jones has a prescription for warfarin and is also purchasing aspirin. Juanita knows that a serious drug interaction occurs between warfarin and aspirin.

▸ *What should Juanita do?*

then work together to make the cell react in a specific way. An excellent example of a drug–drug interaction is when a specific kind of medication, such as a tricyclic antidepressant, is used along with a specific kind of blood pressure medication, such as clonidine. When mixed, these two drugs tend to counteract each other, and the effect can be a severe drop in blood pressure.

Think about an older patient who is being treated for neuropathic pain (the tricyclics are sometimes used to help control pain in certain conditions) and is also using a patch called Catapress (which is available in a number of dose strengths). If the older patient were to stand up quickly, she could have a sudden problem with her blood pressure because this combination of medications can cause *postural hypotension*. If a patient's profile changes, and you notice that a health care provider (such as a pain management physician) has added a tricyclic antidepressant without realizing that the patient is also on clonidine, your job is to alert the pharmacist, to ensure that the physician is notified of the potential problem.

❝ Workplace Wisdom Medication Experts

Physicians are not necessarily medication experts. The medication expert is the pharmacist. Pharmacists have knowledge of all of the medications that a patient is taking, via the patient's profile. Therefore, it is important that, as a competent pharmacy technician, you alert the pharmacist whenever you suspect a problem (drug interactions, therapeutic duplication, etc.). With your help, the pharmacist can ensure that the patient receives the best, safest, and most effective drug regimen available. ❞

Keep in mind the following specific, and important, issues about drug–drug interactions:

- **Time**—the time needed for a drug to take effect is important. Some drugs take effect immediately, whereas other drugs take a much longer time to act. This depends, of course, on the kind of drug, how it is absorbed, and the dosage form or packaging (which also affects absorption). Some drugs, because of the way they are constituted, take a long time to become fully effective—sometimes

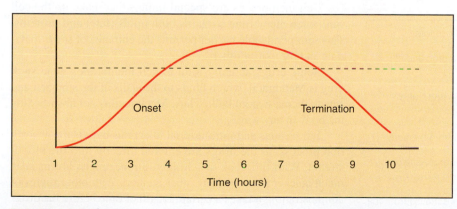

FIGURE 23-5 The time–response curve.

weeks or even longer. Just because a patient has recently begun taking a new drug does not mean that the effect will be immediate. Some drugs must first be processed through the liver. Some drugs even build up **metabolites** that will not have an immediate effect on the body. Therefore, the patient could be on the way home, on the way to a supermarket, or on vacation when the individual effects of the two drugs finally merge. The result can be very dangerous, particularly if the patient is driving at the time.

- **Drug testing**—In many instances, drug-testing procedures are performed on healthy people. There may be significant differences in the effects of drugs in real patients, however. Suppose that a patient is taking an antibiotic; one of the drugs used to control acid secretion in the stomach (the H2 blockers); and warfarin, the chief drug used to keep blood from coagulating (clotting). This patient then undergoes a heart valve transplant. The danger of using an antibiotic, such as erythromycin, along with warfarin might not have shown up in drug studies; however, in the clinical world—that is, in real life—there have been many instances in which the combination of these two drugs has caused severe problems, such as an increase in prothrombin time, which measures how well the drug warfarin is working.

Pharmacokinetics

Pharmacology is a very broad topic, and there are many books that explain the ways in which drugs are absorbed, used, and excreted by the body. Many readers, however, are scared off when they encounter words such as **pharmacokinetics**. A broad definition of the term is "the study of the time course of a drug and its metabolites in the body following drug administration by any route."

In simple terms, *pharmacokinetics* is the study of how the body handles drugs (whether they are administered orally, by way of IV, or any other means), how drugs are changed from their original form into something that the body can use (typically by way of the liver or other organs), and how drugs are eliminated from the body. This section focuses on medications once they are inside the body, rather than their presentation (dosage form) or the particulars of administration.

Plasma Concentration

Suppose that a patient takes a pill or a nurse injects a patient with a medication. These are two different methods of intake, and the drugs administered follow two different pathways, but both drugs end up being absorbed into the body. After absorption is complete, the bloodstream becomes the vehicle that actually delivers the drug to the parts of the body requiring treatment. One factor that determines the amount of the drug needed to do any good (have any effect in the body) is the affinity of the drug to be bound to proteins that are available in the bloodstream.

The level and concentration of a specific drug in the patient's body can be measured through certain tests done in a laboratory setting. The tests actually involve a combination of the measurement of the drug that is bound to the cells of the body and the amount of the drug that is not bound to the cells in the body (in this case, blood cells). This is a simplified version of what happens, but the entire concept of plasma concentration (Cp) is well beyond the scope of this text, and it has very little to do with the real clinical picture. Knowing that there is a way to measure the amount of a specific drug in a person's body also has little to do with pharmacy practice. So, this section presents only a bare-bones overview of drug absorption, distribution, **metabolism**, and **excretion**, in discussing how drugs do the jobs for which they are designed.

Drug Absorption

Drug **absorption** refers to how a drug enters the body. In order for a drug, such as a pill taken by mouth, to enter the body, it must first be swallowed. Then a process begins by which the drug eventually enters the body's fluids, mainly the bloodstream. For example, a drug contained in a pill passes into the bloodstream by getting through specific membranes, such as the membranes inside the stomach and the intestines. Absorption depends largely on the type of drug, how it is designed, and the condition it is intended to treat; these are all reasons why a prescriber uses a particular drug or type of drug. Liquids are more readily absorbed than tablets or capsules, because they are already broken down to some extent.

Cell membranes are special linings that make up the cell wall; each membrane contains both lipids (fats) and proteins. This semipermeable barrier permits the entrance of some materials and the exit of others.

Some drugs actually bind to cell membranes. One such drug is Metamucil, which binds to the walls of the stomach and acts to increase stool bulk. Thus, Metamucil is not absorbed by the body in any way.

Intravenous and intra-arterial injections bypass the absorption process, as the drugs are entered directly into the bloodstream. With this type of administration, results are usually much quicker than with any other method. With other routes of administration, it takes a certain length of time before the drugs start to act on the body.

---

metabolite any substance produced by the metabolic process.

pharmacokinetics the study of the time course of a drug and its metabolites in the body following drug administration.

metabolism the process of transforming drugs in the body; also known as *biotransformation*.

excretion the process by which drugs are eliminated from the body.

absorption the process by which a drug is moved from the site of administration into the bloodstream.

distribution the process by which an absorbed drug is moved from the bloodstream to body tissues or receptors.

Absorption of a drug does not always occur by way of the stomach and bloodstream. Inhaled medications, for example, enter through the mouth and go to the lungs. The mucous membranes of the alveoli absorb the medication and send it into the capillaries and then to the bloodstream. Medications administered rectally or vaginally have a very slow release rate, as the medications dissolve and are absorbed gradually through the rectal or vaginal mucous membranes (such drugs are actually considered to be applied topically).

Topical medications (with the exception of transdermal patches) are not necessarily absorbed through the skin into the bloodstream; some display only a topical effect. An example is hydrocortisone cream used for inflammatory skin conditions. The transdermal patch, in contrast, enhances penetration through the skin by reducing the particle size of the medication.

Drug Distribution

Drug **distribution** refers to the movement of an absorbed drug from the bloodstream into body tissues. Once a drug is absorbed, it is then distributed throughout the body by way of the circulatory system. Some of the drug molecules bind to plasma proteins. Others that do not bind to plasma proteins float through the bloodstream and may interact with various receptors, producing a therapeutic effect. Plasma proteins, such as albumin, do not provide any therapeutic effect in and of themselves.

Membrane Transport Mechanisms

All cells in the human body have specialized transport mechanisms (recall the earlier discussion of cell membranes) by which all materials, including pharmaceuticals, are moved into and out of the cells; normally, drugs must pass into cells in order to perform their functions. The types of transport include filtration, passive transport, and active transport. The type of transport merely describes the ways in which a drug gets from the outside of a cell into the cell properly.

It is important, at least for academic purposes, to understand how these mechanisms work. Following are more specific definitions of each of the mechanisms.

Passive Diffusion

Passive diffusion is another term for *passive transport* across a cell membrane. The force that permits a substance to be transported into the cell from outside depends largely on the concentration differences between the two environments (extracellular and intracellular). If an equilibrium state does not exist between the two environments, the specific differences between two *gradients* will enable certain substances to pass through the membranes; that is, the drug molecules move from an area of high concentration into an area of low concentration (see Figure 23-6).

Facilitated Diffusion

In *facilitated diffusion*, a carrier protein permits specific molecules, such as glucose (sugar), to pass through certain parts of the cells. This is far different from the preceding process, in that it does not require the expenditure of energy. This is an important consideration with some drugs because of the rate at

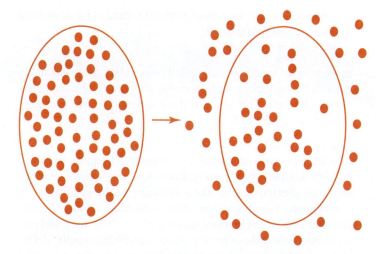

FIGURE 23-6 In passive diffusion, molecules cross to the outside of the cell membrane into an area with a lower concentration of molecules.

which the drug or other substance is permitted to pass through a membrane; there must be enough of a carrier or facilitator protein to allow the process to occur.

Active Transport

Active transport is a special kind of transportation system between the two environments (intracellular and extracellular). This process costs the cells energy; it uses the fact that certain substances are permitted to accumulate outside the cells (see Figure 23-7). After a time, the accumulation of these substances generates a special sort of concentration gradient that,

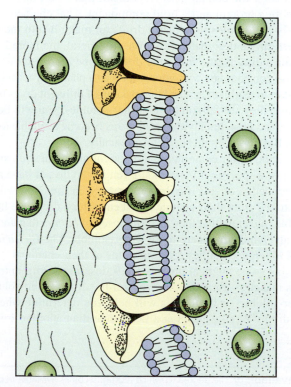

FIGURE 23-7 Active transport.

in time, will enable the transportation of these substances from outside the cell into the cell.

Pinocytosis

In the form of transportation called *pinocytosis*, the cell actually engulfs the substance and, in doing so, permits the substance to enter the cell. This process also requires a degree of energy expenditure by the cell.

Bioavailability

The transport mechanisms just discussed enable drugs to become available to the body. Each drug has its own qualities and characteristics that take advantage of the specific body mechanisms for absorption; drug researchers and designers consider these aspects when shaping what a drug does, and prescribers consider these factors when prescribing specific drugs. However, there are other specific factors that also determine how well or how fast a drug becomes available to the body, such as *gastric emptying*—the ability of the stomach to permit the passage of materials from the stomach to the small intestine. (Most drugs and foods are absorbed at a much faster rate in the small intestine than in the stomach. One exception to this rule is alcohol.) So, there is a great deal more involved in the transport of a drug into the body than just swallowing a pill and expecting it to work. For various reasons, the **bioavailability** of drugs is time restricted—some drugs require immediate access to the body's cells to become effective, whereas other drugs can survive the longer time it takes for them to become available to the body.

The Quality of Drugs—Solubility

Getting back to the cell membrane and its structure, and how drugs enter the cells themselves, recall that a cell membrane has both a protein and a lipid component. That characteristic largely determines how fast a drug can make it into the cell to perform its designated function. In general, the more lipid-soluble a drug is, the faster the drug will be absorbed into the cell. As you continue with your studies as a pharmacy technician and start to really understand the makeup of different drugs (e.g., whether they are fat-soluble or water-soluble), you will better understand how quickly different drugs become available to the body. But how does this help you clinically?

Suppose, for example, that a patient has a question about how fast a specific drug works. Even if you do not have a lot of knowledge of specific drug chemistry, in time you will be able to tell from their chemical makeup which drugs are lipid-soluble (meaning that they are composed of *buffers* that are lipids) and which drugs are more water-soluble. The *Physician's Desk Reference* defines drugs in terms of their chemical structure, but some medical professionals describe a drug in terms of its makeup—for example, whether the drug is lipid-soluble, water-soluble, or both. This will help you determine whether one drug will take effect at a faster rate than another drug or

a different kind of drug. This applies to most over-the-counter (OTC) drugs as well; the labels will tell you about the basic chemical makeup, and you need not be a chemistry major to understand and use some of these concepts.

By and large (with the exception of highly soluble general anesthetics used during surgery), drugs are water-soluble and only partially soluble—and there are reasons for that. First, the human body is made up mostly of water; hence, water-soluble drugs are more liable to be absorbed well and have good bio-availability. Second, except for medications used in emergencies, drugs do not have to work immediately; hence, the partial solubility of most drugs is not problematic. Because of the different cellular transport mechanisms, there are specific reasons for drugs to be both water- and lipid-soluble. Because we know a good deal about the cell membrane, drugs are manufactured to handle both the process of absorption into the body and the process of transport and use at the cellular level.

For a drug to be absorbed via the GI tract, it must be both water- and lipid-soluble. If a drug contains too much water, it cannot pass through the very fatty (lipid) layers of the GI tract. In contrast, absorption of drugs that have too much lipid in their makeup will be delayed. (This is why some medications, such as Dilantin, do not work as effectively in some people as in others.)

Drugs and Their Ionization

Generally speaking, chemicals that are *ionized* (positively or negatively charged) do not readily cross the cell membrane barrier. In contrast, the unionized forms of chemicals—chemicals that do not carry a positive or negative electrical charge—are more readily absorbed into the cell.

Electrically charged molecules cannot readily cross the barrier of a cell wall because most cell walls are composed of proteins and lipids (as well as other components) that are also electrically charged. Therefore, like two magnets placed with the same poles adjacent to one another, these molecules repel each other.

A basic understanding of cell characteristics and the transport of chemicals across cell membrane barriers will make you better able to comprehend the makeup of drugs (without having to go through a lot of physiology and chemistry courses). Thus, you will function more effectively and be more valuable as a pharmacy technician.

Drug Distribution and Metabolism

You now know some of the basics about how drugs enter the human body. But what happens to medications once they are absorbed? With few exceptions, most medications must undergo a number of changes in the body to become effective. It is not quite as simple as most people think—their ability to take that pill this morning and have it work is the result of many, many years of research and development. The people who work behind the scenes in the pharmaceutical companies are responsible for ensuring that the medications work and are safe.

---

bioavailability the degree to which a drug becomes available to body tissue(s) after administration.

The Path

For a medication to become absorbed into the body, it must first undergo what is called the *first-pass process*, which is completed in the liver. This process applies only to medications taken orally, not to those that are administered through other routes; these latter medications are manufactured in such a way that the body can more readily use them (see Figure 23-8).

After a patient takes a pill, it goes through the many different processes that ultimately lead to its entering the bloodstream. From that point, the medication is delivered to the various organs in the body. There are several factors involved in the transportation of the drug by the blood to the body tissues, and these are discussed next.

Plasma-Binding Protein

Several large proteins are responsible for delivering many substances from the intestines, through the blood, and then to the body tissues. These proteins are albumins and the several different types of globulins. They have many different functions and capabilities, including the ability to transport chemicals through the blood. Some drugs are transported after undergoing a process called *protein binding*, in which they are attracted to and physically or chemically attached to these proteins; other drugs float freely through the blood.

The chemicals that are not bound to plasma proteins work their specific pharmacologic effects on the target organs (such as a sore, inflamed throat treated by an antibiotic). Some drugs are highly bound to the proteins, but a good majority of them are unbound. It is the free-floating part of the drug that makes the difference. After a drug uses all available protein-binding sites, the amount of chemical available for use can be determined by measuring the portion of the drug that remains unbound. Two issues determine the degree to which a drug becomes bound to a protein site (e.g., to cells in the bloodstream): (1) the binding affinity of the drug and (2) the number of available sites on the cells. As long as the volume of the drug is adequate, the amount of unbound drug will remain sufficient to get the job done.

Many equations and laws govern the pharmacokinetics of drugs, and a pharmacological chemist can tell you exactly how all of this works. Although you do not need an extensive knowledge of these laws and equations, it is helpful to understand, for example, why some drugs should be taken with food, some drugs should not be taken with milk, and some drugs should be taken only on an empty stomach. The point is to get a dosage where as much of that drug as is necessary to do the job remains unbound to plasma proteins.

Absorption

The absorption of a drug governs the bioavailability of that drug—the amount of drug that is available for use. Several factors influence absorption. As mentioned previously, a drug must be both lipid-(fat) and water-soluble to enter the body through the GI tract. There is more to it than just what gets through the gut, however; how the drug is manufactured also plays a part. This is why some patients demand the "real thing," the non-generic form of a drug—because, they claim, it works better. And, to some extent, they are right.

Some drugs on which the original manufacturer has lost patent protection are still manufactured by the original maker,

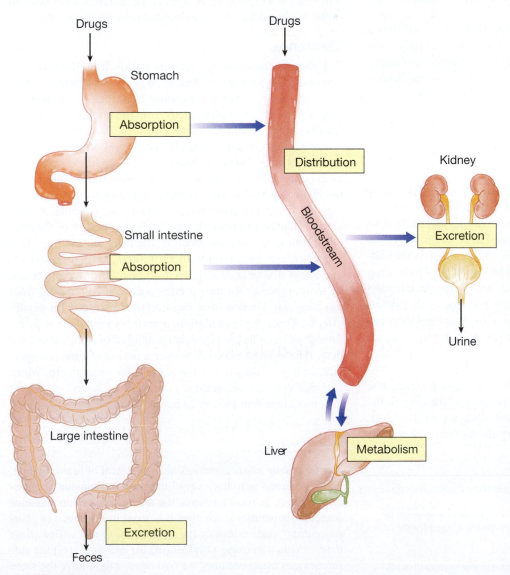

FIGURE 23-8 The path.

but other versions may be produced by other drug companies owned by the original brand-name manufacturer or by entirely separate companies. These other versions may contain the same amount and strength of the active ingredient (drug), but not be the same in terms of bioavailability. It's not always the active chemical that determines absorption; the buffer into which the drug has been instilled can make a huge difference. Different buffers can completely change the degree to which the drugs are made available to the body.

These considerations pertain mostly to orally administered drugs. When a drug enters the body via the IV or IM routes, whether it is a brand-name or generic drug, it is usually almost completely available within minutes.

Salt Forms

A drug may be available in more than one salt form, such as hydroxyzine HCl and hydroxyzine pamoate. When a drug is available in more than one salt form, each form is considered a separate chemical entity, with its own clinical profile and uses. Although the active ingredient may be the same, the drugs are not considered pharmaceutical equivalents. Instead, they are pharmaceutical alternatives.

Consider the drug theophylline, which, by itself, has a bioavailability factor of 1.0 (meaning that it is completely available). However, this drug is often dispensed not as theophylline, but as aminophylline, which is only 80% theophylline—it contains only 80% of the fraction of the drug salt, or *ester*, that is the "parent" compound. The ratio of the two factors, bioavailability (F) and the salt (S), will determine how well the drug is absorbed.

Rate of Administration

The rate at which a drug is administered is not measured by the time it takes to swallow a pill, but by a formula that uses the two fractions identified previously with respect to the dosing interval. Certain drugs are designed to be taken every four hours, for example, for many reasons, one of which is the half-life of the drug; another reason is the rate at which the drug can be absorbed over a given period. This helps the chemists (during the research and development process) as they determine the average rate of administration, to ensure that there is a certain amount of the drug in the system at all times.

Volume of Distribution

Theoretically, if you consider the body as a single entity, you can assume that there is a specific amount of the drug in the body at any given time. This is not always true, however, because of many factors, including the different chemicals

Two Compartments for Drugs in the Body

Most of the time a pharmacist considers a drug as being taken into one compartment or entity: the entire body. However, within the body the drug is actually in two compartments: (1) part of the drug is in the blood and in organs that have a relatively high rate of blood flow, such as the heart; (2) part of the drug is in the other, minute tissues of the body. (At a certain point, there will be an equilibrium; clinically speaking, though, this concept is not relevant to you or the pharmacist unless you are working in an environment where there is compounding of drugs.)

in the bloodstream, the bioavailability of the drug, the initial plasma concentration, and the amount of drug that is freely available at any given time. The actual volume of distribution, therefore, is determined by a number of factors, including the *loading dose*, which is often higher than the dose the patient will take on a regular basis. This is the difference between an initial loading dose and the subsequent *maintenance dose*.

Clearance

The **clearance** of a drug—its elimination from the body—is determined by a number of factors. When a manufacturer develops a new drug, one of the questions it must answer is how the drug will be cleared (eliminated) from the body, and how fast. Ideally, a drug would be eliminated at the same rate at which it is absorbed, yielding a "steady-state" level of the drug in the body at all times. However, because of the varied absorption and availability of the drug in the various bodily tissues (remember the two-compartment model), this is not always the case.

The rates of distribution, absorption, and elimination must all be balanced to ensure that the body has enough of the drug at all times, and not too much of the drug at any time. This is particularly important with antibiotics, antihypertensives, and drugs that treat cancer, because many of these drugs can be toxic. Ignoring the time it takes a drug to be removed from the body can allow a toxic buildup of the drug, with deadly effects. Through a calculation, a *maintenance dose* is determined, which tells the physician a number of things about the drug. The amount to be given over a period of time is important, as is your duty to tell the patient, for example, to "Make sure that you take one of these pills every six hours" or, "Don't take more than four pills in 24 hours."

Addiction

The term *drug abuse* is subject to a great deal of interpretation, and is so broad as to have very little meaning outside of a specific context. In most contexts, the term carries many negative societal connotations, whether it is used in reference to pharmaceutical medications or the agents commonly called *street drugs*. Although using OxyContin, for example, is quite different from using cocaine, the two drugs might have the same potential for abuse, depending on the user and the prescriber.

---

clearance the time it takes a drug to be eliminated from the body.

addiction a pattern of compulsive substance abuse characterized by a continued psychological and physiological craving or need for the substance and its effects.

tolerance when a person requires (psychologically or physiologically) larger doses of a drug to achieve the same effect.

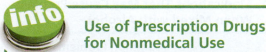

Use of Prescription Drugs for Nonmedical Use

According to the National Institute for Drug Abuse, approximately 48 million people (aged 12 years and over) have used prescription drugs for nonmedical reasons. This is almost 20% of the U.S. population.

There are specific reasons for the variety of definitions, as the term *drug abuse* is actually an overly broad term applied to a large array of problems, including addiction, dependency, and even the occasional use of certain drugs. Although these problems might all present in the same way, in terms of how the patient or user acts, it is important to understand the differences between dependency and addiction, as they involve two clearly different mechanisms and have different consequences.

Characteristics of Addiction

Addiction is a disease and should not be thought of in the same way as chemical dependency. *Addiction* is defined as both a psychological and physiological dependency. For a drug or a chemical to be addictive, specific withdrawal symptoms must arise following an abrupt change in the practice of use. Specific signs of addiction, typically seen in persons addicted to a specific substance, include:

- **An absorbing focus**—all addictions consume some time, thought, and energy.
- **Increasing tolerance**—to achieve the same effect as when the person first started using the agent, he or she must ingest more of the chemical over time; later, there is a loss of control over the use of the agent.
- **A growing denial**—typically, users become so sensitive to the thought of using the agent that they tend to deny any interest in the agent, in order to sustain their previous pattern of life.
- **Damaging consequences**—there is no such thing as a harmless addiction, whether it is an addiction to a substance or to any other thing. All addicts eventually bring some form of destruction on themselves and their families. Typically, they lose three things: employment, interest in self, and previous reputation. Addictions are enslaving and destructive dependencies on an agent such as a drug or a pharmaceutical chemical.
- **Painful withdrawal**—almost always, there is a painful physical and psychological withdrawal for some time after the agent is abruptly stopped, for whatever reason. (This is sometimes also true with chemical dependency.) The addict usually has angry, uncontrollable outbursts; periods of anxiety; panic attacks; tremors; severe depression; and a sense of loss of anything good in life.

Causes of Addiction

Specific addictive street drugs, such as cocaine, heroin, and morphine, cause the release of *dopamine*, a neurotransmitting chemical in the brain. Dopamine is only one of the many different neurotransmitters in the brain that control such attributes as thought, actions, and emotions. When these neurotransmitters are functioning normally, the person is also considered normal. Dopamine has been linked to some of the more common problems seen in those who are addicted. For example, a proven link exists between dopamine and other catecholamines found in the brain and the adrenal system; imbalances can lead to hypertension and other diseases.

Each higher dose of the abused drug causes higher dopamine levels, which is why people who are addicted to drugs are also depressed. In the addict's brain, the higher doses of dopamine activate a negative feedback system that, in time, causes the nervous system to be less sensitive to the neurotransmitter. The first high, therefore, is never duplicated by subsequent doses. Drug abusers increase the dose of a drug in an attempt to achieve the same effect as they achieved previously; this repeated effort causes the disease. Finally, the addict requires such high doses that his or her body can no longer adapt. The results are sometimes fatal.

The Criteria for Addiction

Specific criteria exist to help identify if a person is addicted to a specific chemical or drug. Depending on the level of addiction, nine different items are present in varying degrees:

1. The patient takes the drug (or drugs) in larger amounts than are needed to achieve the expected results. Patients taking narcotics for pain relief reach this threshold when they take more than they need to achieve pain relief and instead are seeking other effects of the medications. The patient develops a high tolerance for the drug.
2. There have been many unsuccessful attempts to quit taking the medication, accompanied by a persistent period of craving and a desire to obtain the medication, sometimes at any cost to the patient or others involved, such as family members or friends.
3. Excessive time is used in obtaining the medication; a patient, for example, uses many different health care providers and pharmacies to obtain a specific medication.
4. There are periods when the patient feels intoxicated (or appears to be intoxicated or acting strangely or unusually compared with previous encounters).
5. The patient thinks about giving up other things in life for the purpose of drug seeking and use.
6. The patient continues to use the drug or medication, even after he and his family have been told of the potential damage to his life or vital organs—or danger to others in his life.
7. The marked **tolerance** for the medication leaves a trail of information that can sometimes be determined by checking databases or talking with other providers or pharmacists.
8. The patient manifests characteristic withdrawal symptoms with any attempt to stop taking the specific drug, particularly during times when pharmacies are closed (such as holidays or weekends), or any other periods when the drug is not available.
9. The patient consistently uses the drug to prevent withdrawal symptoms.

Alcohol

Alcohol (EtOH), although legal in certain circumstances, is a depressant. One of the largest problems associated with the use of alcohol is its concomitant use with prescribed medications. Typically, a pharmaceutical label will include instructions indicating if a medication should not be used with alcohol. Because alcohol is a highly addictive substance, it is prudent and appropriate to discuss this drug and list some of the more commonly abused drugs associated with the consumption of alcohol.

Workplace Wisdom Drug–Alcohol Interactions

A complete list of drugs that can have interactions with alcohol is too long to include here. Comprehensive lists of drugs and their interactions with alcohol can be found in pharmacy references such as *Drug Facts and Comparisons*.

Alcohol, Other Drugs, and Their Effects on the Body

Alcohol and some of the more common drugs that are addictive or cause harm to the body have an immediate and altering effect on specific perceptions and emotions. After repeated use of these substances, some form of dependence often develops—symptoms are produced that are consistent with tolerance and withdrawal.

It is essential that you, as a pharmacy technician, realize that many commonly prescribed drugs can cause devastating effects when mixed with alcohol. Certainly, an auxiliary label containing such information should be placed on the vial for that particular medication, but it might also be in your best interest to personally call a patient's attention to the warning.

According to the American Society of Addiction Medicine, alcoholism is a "primary, *chronic* disease with genetic, psychosocial, and environmental factors influencing its development and manifestations." Alcoholism is a disease, pure and simple. It refers to consuming ethanol in a potentially hazardous or harmful manner. You are not responsible for the patient's problem with this disease, but you are responsible for the types of medications that are dispensed from your institution—and the list of medications that can cause problems when alcoholics take them is long. Table 23-1 lists many medications that are potentially problematic when mixed with other medications. This list should be posted somewhere in your pharmacy to ensure that patients can review what they are currently buying and what they have at home.

Immediate Effects of Alcohol

Like some of the drugs that are dispensed from any typical pharmacy, alcohol has a number of effects. Alcohol has specific mood-altering and mind-altering effects. Alcohol and some other drugs alter the levels of dopamine in the brain. As

TABLE 23-1 Medications That May Cause Problems When Mixed with Alcohol

Drug	Common Problems Associated with the Use of Alcohol
Alprazolam, diazepam	Drowsiness, dizziness, an increased risk of overdose
Aspirin, Advil, Tylenol	Stomach upset, bleeding ulcers, liver damage, increased heart rate
Clonazepam, phenytoin	Drowsiness, increased risk of seizures
Cimetidine, nizatidine	Rapid heart rate, sudden changes in blood pressure
Diphenhydramine, temazepam	Drowsiness, dizziness, an increased risk of overdose
Glyburide, metformin	Rapid heart rate, sudden changes in blood pressure, convulsions, possibly coma
Griseofulvin, Flagyl	Rapid heart rate, sudden changes in blood pressure, liver damage
Herbal preparations	Increased drowsiness
Hydrocodone, oxycodone	Drowsiness, dizziness, risk of overdose
Isosorbide, nitroglycerine (NTG)	Rapid heartbeat, sudden changes in blood pressure
Warfarin	Occasional drinking may lead to internal bleeding; heavier drinking may have the opposite effect, resulting in clots

discussed earlier in this chapter, this neurotransmitter affects the degree to which synapses interact with each other. Alcohol raises the level of dopamine in the brain; according to some recent research, even the anticipation of alcohol ingestion can have an effect on dopamine levels. Drugs such as amphetamines increase the action of dopamine by blocking the molecule that normally transports it away from the specific centers of the brain where most of its activity is centered. Another neurotransmitter, serotonin, is thought to have an even more immediate effect from the use of alcohol and some other drugs, particularly those currently prescribed for the treatment of depression (the serotonin-secretion reuptake inhibitors, or SSRIs).

Long-Term Effects of Alcohol

Cells in the brain, like cells in other parts of the body, are subject to change, given the right conditions. Over time, drugs and alcohol can actually change the chemical composition of the brain, altering the way the cells react to each other and resulting in *neuroadaptation*; in other words, over time the brain learns other ways to function because of the damage drugs and alcohol have done to it. For example, excessive consumption of alcohol can cause a sudden change in the amount of neurotransmitters, which can decrease the number of dopamine receptors in the brain. In time, this can have a long-term effect on the ways in which the abuser makes decisions and exercises judgment.

Neurotoxic Effect

Over the long term, chronic abuse of drugs or alcohol (or both) can affect the brain to the point that a person develops dementia (loss of memory). Long-term use of such drugs as methamphetamine and cocaine can produce such effects as altered ability to see and impaired hearing. One of the most common problems associated with long-term use of alcohol is a disease called Weicke-Korsakoff's syndrome, which is a type of dementia that is often accompanied by specific nutritional problems. This disease is often associated with an inability to learn new things, recall details such as people's names and addresses, or even remember a subject that was just mentioned.

Alcoholism

According to the American Society of Addiction Medicine, alcoholism is a "primary, *chronic* disease" characterized by the following four symptoms:

1. Craving or urge to drink—described by some as a need.
2. Loss of control—the alcoholic person is unable to stop once the person has begun drinking.
3. Physical dependence—the alcoholic person experiences symptoms of withdrawal, such as nausea, shakiness, sweating, and anxiety, after the person stops drinking.
4. Tolerance—the alcoholic person must drink greater amounts of alcohol to get the same "buzz" or "high."

Several withdrawal syndromes are observed during the first 48 hours of cessation of drinking, or alcohol withdrawal:

- Seizures
- Blood pressure changes
- Delirium tremens (hallucinations, tremors, and shaking caused by alcohol withdrawal; may be fatal)
- Dehydration
- Malnutrition
- Ataxia
- Nystagmus
- Cognitive changes

Treatment of Alcoholism

A 12-step group support program, such as Alcoholics Anonymous, in conjunction with individual therapy and counseling, is essential in the treatment of alcohol addiction. Thiamine and folate are routinely used to reverse common nutritional deficiencies, and a few benzodiazepines that are used to combat anxiety may also be used for alcohol withdrawal. Benzodiazepines are sometimes used during the first few days after a person stops drinking to help him or her safely withdraw from alcohol. Extreme agitation during withdrawal may require the use of other drugs, such as barbiturates, antipsychotics, anticonvulsants, and antihypertensives. The smallest dosage necessary to manage symptoms should be given. The liver may suffer severe benzodiazepine toxicity if the patient is given a long-acting benzodiazepine for alcohol withdrawal. The antipsychotic Haldol (haloperidol) IV and the benzodiazepine Ativan (lorazepam) can be given together to help control delirium tremens (the DTs). However, haloperidol must be used with caution because of the risk of torsade de pointes (an uncommon type of ventricular tachycardia in which the QT interval increases markedly, causing sudden death).

Some drugs, such as ReVia (naltrexone), can help people remain sober. The combination of counseling and naltrexone can reduce the craving for alcohol and help prevent a return to alcohol abuse and a relapse into heavy drinking, but only *after* the patient stops drinking. Naltrexone works by blocking the same receptors and areas that narcotics and alcohol block in the brain: the mu receptors, limbic system, and reticular formation. This action lessens the feeling of needing to drink alcohol, so the patient can stop drinking more easily. Side effects of naltrexone include nausea, headache, constipation, dizziness, nervousness, insomnia, drowsiness, and anxiety. Recommended dose is 50 mg daily.

Antabuse (disulfiram) discourages drinking by making patients feel nauseated and flushed and develop sudden stomach cramps, headache, and vomiting when or if they drink alcohol. This type of management of alcoholism is called *aversion therapy*.

A new drug used in the management of alcoholism to support abstinence from alcohol is Campral (acamprosate calcium). Studies have shown that this drug reduces alcohol intake in alcohol-dependent animals. This drug does not have disulfiram-like side effects.

Table 23-2 lists some drugs commonly used to treat withdrawal symptoms.

Smoking Withdrawal and Cessation

Statistics show that almost 23.4% of all adult males and 18.5% of all adult females in the United States continue to smoke, despite all the recognition and acknowledgment that smoking is detrimental to health. Although many people find that support groups or therapy help them quit smoking, others quit cold turkey. Still others use some of the pharmaceutical agents on the market to help them curb the urge to smoke. The pharmaceutical agents available include:

Nicotine inhalers—a nicotine oral inhalation system called Nicotrol Inhaler is available by prescription, but requires the use of four inhalers a day, totaling 2,000 puffs per day, to achieve adequate nicotine levels. This poses compliance problems. Side effects include mouth and throat irritation due to the oral delivery.

Nicotine nasal spray—Nicotrol NS, available by prescription, requires four sprays per hour, or a maximum

TABLE 23-2 Alcohol Withdrawal Treatment

Benzodiazepines	Indications	Usual Adult Dose
Ativan (lorazepam)	Alcohol withdrawal and DTs; short-acting	2–4 mg IV q one hour prn until calm
Librium (chlordiazepoxide)	Alcohol withdrawal, DTs; long-acting	25–100 mg every one to two hours as needed
Serax (oxazepam)	Alcohol withdrawal; short-acting	15–30 mg, three or four times daily
Valium (diazepam)	Alcohol and cocaine withdrawal; long-acting	10–20 mg every one to three hours for first three doses
Antipsychotics		
Haldol (haloperidol)	Extreme agitation during withdrawal	2–4 mg IV q one hour prn, until calm
Miscellaneous Antialcoholic Agents (Detoxification Helpers)		
Antabuse (disulfiram)	Management of enforced sobriety	Initial dose: 500 mg po qd for one to two weeks
		Maintenance dose: 125–500 mg po qd (not to exceed 500 mg/day)
Campral (acamprosate calcium)	Maintenance of abstinence from alcohol	Dose: two 333 mg tablets (666 mg) po tid
ReVia (naltrexone)	Treatment for alcohol dependency	Dose: 50 mg po qd

of 80 sprays per day. Common side effects are nasal and throat irritation and rhinorrhea.

Nicotine gum—Nicorette (nicotine polacrilex) is available OTC in 2-mg and 4-mg strengths. The most effective dose is the use of 10 to 15 pieces of 4-mg gum per day initially; after two weeks, most patients benefit

dependency the state of being dependent.

from use of the 2-mg strength. Nicotine gum should be chewed once or twice every few minutes and then placed between the cheek and the gum (buccal placement) until the next "chew." GI upset, caused by chewing the gum too quickly and swallowing nicotine with saliva, is a common side effect.

Nicotine patch—once prescription-only, Habitrol, Nicoderm CQ, and Nicotrol are now available OTC. The Fagerstrom test score determines which strength of patch the patient should begin using. A score of 5 to 6 indicates that the patient should use the 21-mg nicotine patch, a score of 3 to 4 means that the 14-mg nicotine patch is appropriate for initial therapy, and a score of 0 to 2 indicates initial use of the 7-mg nicotine patch. Side effects are mild skin irritation just under the patch and possible sleep disruption. The patient may be able to alleviate these problems by rotating the patch site and removing the patch at bedtime. People who use the patch should know that concomitant smoking and nicotine patch use may cause sudden cardiac death.

❝ Workplace Wisdom Smoking—No Longer a Habit

In 2000, the American Psychiatric Association updated its stance on smoking: It is considered a mental disorder, not a habit. **❞**

Medications Used in Smoking Cessation

The immediate-release form of the antidepressant bupropion inhibits the uptake of the monoamine neurotransmitters norepinephrine and serotonin and weakly blocks the reuptake of dopamine. The sustained-release form weakly inhibits the neuronal uptake of norepinephrine, serotonin, and dopamine. It is believed that this monoamine inhibition causes the reduction in the urge to smoke. The most common side effects of bupropion include dry mouth and sleep interruptions. If depression is also present, the patient will benefit from the antidepressant effects of this drug. Note that bupropion is sold as antidepressant Wellbutrin XL for anxiety/GAD, Wellbutrin for depression, and Zyban for smoking cessation. The combined use of antidepressant, bupropion, and nicotine replacement agents appears to be the most effective treatment for nicotine dependence (nicotine withdrawal/smoking cessation). Zyban (bupropion) should be dosed as follows: 150 mg per day for 3 days, and then 150 mg twice daily for 8 to 12 weeks.

Varenicline (Chantix) is a new smoking-cessation medication that does not contain nicotine but helps patients by reducing their urge to smoke. It targets the same receptors that nicotine does and blocks nicotine from attaching to these receptors. Chantix is available in 0.5-mg and 1-mg tablets and is dosed as follows:

Days 1 through 3—0.5 mg po once daily

Days 4 through 7—0.5 mg po twice daily

Day 8 through the end of treatment—1 mg po twice daily

Side effects include nausea and vomiting, sleep disturbances, constipation, and gas/flatulence.

Antianxiety agents are also used to reduce the symptoms of anxiety associated with nicotine withdrawal and smoking cessation. Benzodiazepines enhance the effects of a brain chemical called gamma aminobutyric acid (GABA). This chemical slows down nerve cell activity and decreases nerve excitement, thus causing relaxation and quieting the anxiety symptoms that accompany smoking withdrawal. Maintenance drug therapy may include Xanax (alprazolam) and other benzodiazepines. Alprazolam may be dosed 0.25 to 0.5 mg po bid to tid, with a maximum daily dose of 4 mg.

Drug Dependency

A great deal of confusion exists, even among clinicians, about the differences between dependency and addiction. As discussed earlier in this chapter, drug addiction involves compulsive behavior coupled with psychological and physiological dependence on a drug. Drug **dependency** is different. Drug dependency is characterized by physiological dependence and tolerance to the drug. Drug dependency does not necessarily always lead to addiction.

Controlled Medications

According to the United States Controlled Substances Act of 1970, each medication that has a potential for abuse is identified by a number ranging from I through V, determined by the medication's ability to influence behavior and its potential for abuse. The following considerations apply when, for example, a new medication for pain control is released into the market: the degree to which the medication has a potential for abuse; whether the substance has been determined to have a current and acceptable medical use; and whether the use of the medication, under medical supervision, is safe. Let us look at some medications generally classified for pain relief and their properties that can lead to abuse.

An *opiate* is a drug that has its origin in the opium poppy, from which such substances as cocaine and morphine are manufactured. *Opioid* is a scientific term used to describe a large number of medications and substances, including the opiates, medications made synthetically (such as methadone), and medications having properties that

interfere with specific receptors in the brain that "turn off" pain in the body.

The list of opioids also includes a number of other drugs that either compete with specific receptors or antagonize other receptors in the brain. The ultimate effect for the normal user is an eradication of the problem. The abuser is actually looking for some of the side effects of these drugs, most of which, over time, can cause damage to the brain, the kidneys, and the liver, to mention a few of the important organs that keep the body alive. The federal government controls these substances for the safety and well-being of society.

Workplace Wisdom Fraudulent Prescriptions

It is the pharmacist's duty to counsel patients on the correct ways to take their medications, the effects of the medications, and drug interactions. However, as a technician, you play a vital role in helping the pharmacist prevent drug misuse and abuse. You can help prevent prescription fraud by identifying prescriptions that appear to be fake, be altered, or look false. Some pharmacies have even implemented hotlines to alert other pharmacies in the area when a prescription fraud is detected.

Without doubt, inconsistent use of the terms *addiction*, *dependency*, and *tolerance* leads to many misunderstandings among those who regulate the system for dispensing narcotics and other medications that have a potential for chemical dependence or addiction. Most of these misconceptions concern patients who are taking medications designed for pain relief and labeled as narcotics. Because of the many misunderstandings, a good number of patients suffer with untreated pain. It is true that a small percentage of patients have been identified as using such medications for reasons other than pain relief, but many pain patients suffer needlessly because of the mistaken idea that everyone who takes narcotics is an addict or will inevitably become addicted.

The Role of the Pharmacy Technician

Certainly, it is not within your jurisdiction to take prescription counseling into your own hands. However, it *is* your responsibility to bring possible abuse and other questionable situations to the attention of your pharmacist so that he or she can take the appropriate actions. Your pharmacist might know other information about the patient; after all, a pharmacist's license depends on what is dispensed, when it is dispensed, and for what reasons. Your position, however, does have its advantages, in that you may know something about the patient that the pharmacist does not know. A discussion between you and the pharmacist is, therefore, justified whenever you have questions or concerns of this nature.

Summary

As you have discovered, being a knowledgeable pharmacy technician involves more than counting out pills to fill a patient's prescription. No employer should expect you to have the same background in pharmacology as your pharmacist, but they will expect you to have an understanding of basic pharmacological concepts.

If drugs are to produce their desired effects, they must be available to the cell receptors. Many variables influence how efficiently drugs are carried through the bloodstream to the target organ they are intended to affect. Of course, the route of administration plays an important part; other factors include the affinity of the drug, the transport mechanism of the target cell, and the solubility of the drug. Factors such as absorption, distribution, and ionization of the drug all contribute to how the body handles the drug once it is administered.

It is important to remember that liver function can have a significant impact on the efficacy of a drug. In addition, bioavailability, rate of administration, half-life, and clearance of the drug, as well as other factors, play a large role in ensuring that a sufficient amount of drug is available to produce the desired therapeutic effect. This is the main goal of pharmacotherapeutics.

Although the lines are sometimes blurred, there is a difference between drug addiction and drug dependency. Drug addiction is a disease, and it involves compulsive behavior as well as psychological and physiological dependence. Drug dependency, in contrast, usually involves only physiological dependence.

All of this knowledge is of no value unless you can utilize it. Knowing the trade and generic name for a drug is important; knowing the intended action of the drug and how the drug interacts with other drugs is far more important.

Chapter Review Questions

1. To ensure the body has enough of a drug at all times, all of the following must be balanced, *except* _____.
   a. rate of absorption
   b. rate of action
   c. rate of distribution
   d. rate of elimination

2. How a drug works, or produces a desired or undesired effect, is referred to as _____.
   a. the first-pass effect
   b. mechanism of action
   c. potency
   d. dose–response curve

3. The amount of the drug that is actually available for use by the body is known as _____.
   a. bioavailability
   b. affinity
   c. processing
   d. solubility

4. All of the following drugs are indicated for alcohol withdrawal treatment, *except* _____.
   a. Ativan
   b. Antabuse
   c. Chantix
   d. Haldol

5. An initial dose that may be a higher dose than the patient will take on a regular basis is called a(n) _____.
   a. intermittent dose
   b. STAT dose
   c. loading dose
   d. subtherapeutic dose

6. The measurement of the specific amount of a drug that will achieve half of the maximal response is _____.
   a. ED50
   b. drug clearance
   c. volume of distribution
   d. half-life

7. The amount of time it takes for a drug serum level to decrease by 50% is _____.
   a. ED50
   b. drug clearance
   c. volume of distribution
   d. half-life

8. Addiction is characterized by _____.
   a. compulsive behavior
   b. physiological dependence
   c. psychological dependence
   d. all of the above

9. The function of a(n) _____ is to block the action of the receptor and prevent activation.
   a. agonist
   b. antagonist
   c. receptor site
   d. target cell

10. In general, which of the following chemical forms more readily crosses the cell membrane barrier?
    a. ionized
    b. positively charged
    c. unionized
    d. deionized

Critical Thinking Questions

1. Explain why it is important for you, as a pharmacy technician, to understand not only how to prepare customer prescriptions, but also the effects that the prescription drugs have on your customer's body.

2. Explain why drugs that have shorter half-lives must be dosed at more frequent intervals than drugs with longer half-lives.

3. Using what you have learned in this chapter, and drawing from your own personal experiences, how much responsibility do you believe drug-addicted persons have for causing their own drug addiction?

Web Challenge

1. Go to http://www.youtube.com and and search for a video about drug absorption. Write a brief summary about what you learned.

2. Go to http://www.mayoclinic.com to research more about drug addiction. Choose three different drugs and discuss the signs and symptoms of addiction to each.

References and Resources

Adams, M.P., D.L. Josephson, and L.N. Holland, Jr. *Pharmacology for Nurses—A Pathophysiologic Approach*. 4th ed. Upper Saddle River, NJ: Pearson Education, 2013. Print.

"Addiction Criteria." http://www.druglibrary.org/schaffer/library/addcrit.htm. Web. 21 June 2007.

Advocacy and Policy. Definitions Related to the Use of Opioids for the Treatment of Pain. A Consensus Document from the American Academy of Pain Medicine, the American Pain Society, and the American Society of Addiction Medicine. http://www.ampainsoc.org. Web. 21 June 2007.

"Alcohol, Drugs and the Brain." http://www.open.org/tahana/ADA/twfadbr.htm. Web. 22 June 2007.

"Alcoholism Statistics." http://www.alcoholism-statistics.com. Web. 21 June 2007.

"Alcoholism Statistics." http://www.stopaddiction.com. Web. 21 June 2007.

Andreoli, T., C. Carpenter, C. Bennett, and F. Plum. *Essentials of Medicine* (4th ed.). Philadelphia: W.B. Saunders, 1997. Print.

"Anxiety-Management." http://health.usnews.com/usnews/health/brain/anxiety/anx.manage.htm. Web. 22 June 2007.

Baker, R., R. Rakel, and E. Bope, eds. "Psychiatric Disorders: Alcoholism." In *Conn's Current Therapy 2002*. Philadelphia: W.B. Saunders, 2002. Print.

Carmichael, B.P. *Drug Abuse: Addiction vs. Dependency.* "Glossary of Terms." http://www.medsch.wisc.edu/painpolicy/glossary.htm. Web. 20 June 2007.

Harmful Interactions: Mixing Alcohol with Medicines. (Publication Number 03-5329). Bethesda, MD: National Institute on Alcohol Abuse and Alcoholism, February 2003.

Holland, N., and M.P. Adams. *Core Concepts in Pharmacology (3rd ed.).* Upper Saddle River, NJ: Pearson Education, 2010. Print.

Koda-Kimble, M.A. *Applied Therapeutics: The Clinical Use of Drugs* (5th ed.). Vancouver, WA: Applied Therapeutics, 1992. Print.

Porter, R.S. *The Merck Manual* (9th ed.). Rahway, NJ: Merck Research Laboratories, 2011. Print.

"Prescription Drugs: Abuse and Addiction." http://www.nida.nih.gov. Web. 22 June 2007.

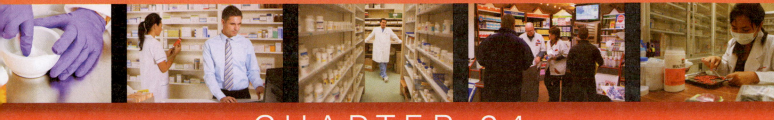

CHAPTER 24

The Skin

LEARNING OBJECTIVES

After completing this chapter, you should be able to:

- List, identify, and diagram the basic anatomical structure of the skin.

- Explain the function or physiology of the skin.

- List and define common diseases affecting the skin and understand the causes, symptoms, and pharmaceutical treatments associated with each disease.

KEY TERMS

acne, p. 365

adipose, p.364

bactericidal, p. 365

bacteriostatic, p. 365

carcinoma, p. 368

cellulitis, p. 367

eczema, p. 364

infection, p. 365

mitigate, p. 370

parasite, p. 368

pathogen, p. 365

pigmentation, p. 369

psoriasis, p. 364

rash, p. 364

rosacea, p. 369

sebum, p. 365

INTRODUCTION

The skin is the largest organ of the body and has several functions. It also is subject to a wide variety (more than 1,000) of medical conditions and diseases. Skin conditions and diseases range from minor irritations to severe infections. Although creams and ointments are widely used to treat skin conditions, treatment options include oral and injectable medications as well. This chapter discusses several common skin conditions and diseases and the treatments available for these disorders.

Anatomy

Considered the largest organ of the body, the skin performs several functions:

- It acts as a mechanical barrier to infection.
- It enables and enhances the sense of touch.
- It assists in the regulation of body temperature.
- It allows excretion of waste products and salt from the body.
- Through exposure to sunlight, it enables synthesis of vitamin D for the absorption of calcium.

The skin has three main layers: the epidermis, the dermis, and the subcutaneous (SC) layers. The skin provides protection from heat, ultraviolet (UV) radiation, and infection. Exposure of the skin to sunlight helps the body to produce vitamin D, which is needed to make cholesterol and to absorb the calcium and phosphorus that build strong bones. As the largest sensory organ, the skin also plays a large role in the ability to feel heat, cold, pain, and pleasure (see Figure 24-1).

The *epidermis* is the outermost layer of the skin and contains *melanocytes*, where pigment is stored. It is the thinnest skin layer and is also known as the *scarfskin* or *cuticle layer*.

The *dermis* contains fibroblasts that are responsible for secreting the proteins collagen and elastin. These proteins provide the support for and elasticity of the skin. These proteins are surrounded by a jelly-like substance called the *ground substance*, which also plays a substantial role in maintaining the

hydration of the skin. The dermal layer contains immune cells involved in the defense against foreign invaders that may pass through the epidermis; it also houses hair follicles; blood vessels; sweat and oil glands; and the sensory receptors for touch, pain, heat, and cold. It has an important role in maintaining body temperature at the norm of about 98.6 °F.

The dermis is attached to an underlying SC layer, also called the *hypodermis*, where the outermost part of the muscle is located. The SC layer stores **adipose** (fat) tissue and contains the connective tissue.

Diseases and Conditions of the Skin

As noted earlier, the skin is prone to more than 1,000 common problems, which may be organized into one of the ten categories discussed briefly in this section.

Rash

A **rash** is an area of red, inflamed skin, or a group of red spots, caused by irritation, allergy, infection, or defects in the skin structure, such as blocked pores or malfunctioning oil glands. Examples of rashes are contact dermatitis and hives.

Eczema

Eczema is a skin inflammation that manifests with red pimple-like bumps and is characterized by itching, blistering, or oozing areas that progress to scaly, brownish, or thickened skin. Some of the drugs that have recently been developed for eczema are also used to treat chronic plaque psoriasis. They include two FDA-approved immunomodulator creams and ointments: Elidel (pimecrolimus) cream, used for mild-to-moderate atopic eczema; and Protopic (tacrolimus), used for severe atopic eczema. *Immunomodulators* are agents that affect the body's immune system in some way. These creams and ointments are not steroids but are used to treat the itch and inflammation associated with atopic eczema and psoriasis.

Psoriasis

Psoriasis is a noncontagious, chronic immune disorder in which specific immune cells become overactive and release excessive amounts of proteins called *cytokines*. One of these cytokines is called tumor necrosis factor (TNF), which normally helps regulate the body's immune response to infection and inflammation. However, in patients with psoriasis, TNF causes inflammation instead of preventing it. This leads to the formation of painful, often disfiguring, psoriasis plaques. The turnover of skin cells is rapid, and the affected skin becomes thick, red, and scaly.

Until recently, treatment for psoriasis managed only the patient's pain and skin inflammation. Some of the greatest discoveries—"breakthrough drugs"—in the treatment of skin disorders and diseases have been drugs for chronic plaque psoriasis and psoriatic arthritis. Some of these drugs have also been approved for use with rheumatoid arthritis. Some of the most recent drug discoveries that have changed the way psoriasis is treated and managed are reviewed next.

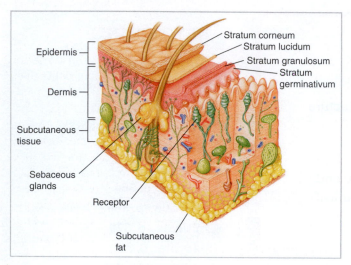

Epidermis
Dermis
Subcutaneous tissue
Sebaceous glands
Receptor
Subcutaneous fat

Stratum corneum
Stratum lucidum
Stratum granulosum
Stratum germinativum

FIGURE 24-1 Structure of the skin.

---

adipose fat.

rash a skin condition characterized by redness and inflammation.

eczema an inflammatory skin condition characterized by itching, redness, blistering, and oozing.

psoriasis a noncontagious, chronic skin disease characterized by rapid turnover of skin cells, resulting in thick, red, and scaly skin.

infection an invasion of pathogens into the body; an infection occurs when a pathogenic microbe is able to multiply in the tissues (*colonize*).

pathogen a disease-causing microorganism.

bactericidal kills microorganisms.

bacteriostatic inhibits the growth and/or reproduction of microorganisms.

acne a bacterial infection accompanied by an overproduction of sebum.

sebum an oily substance produced by the sebaceous glands in the skin.

Treatments for Psoriasis

Enbrel (etanercept), a SC injectable drug for psoriasis, is an anti-TNF therapy agent that works by binding to the over-produced TNF. This attachment causes the TNF to become biologically inactive, resulting in a significant reduction in inflammation. This SC injection can be self-administered.

Remicade (infliximab) is administered by intravenous infusion under the supervision of a specialist and in combination with methotrexate (MTX), a potent antineoplastic agent used in the treatment of rheumatoid arthritis. MTX is given with infliximab to help prevent the formation of anti-infliximab antibodies.

Amevive (alefacept), which is given IM or as an infusion by a doctor, has the severe adverse reaction of lowering the T-cell count, which lessens the immune system's ability to fight cancer, infections, and other diseases. Amevive works by binding to a specific lymphocyte antigen, CD2, and then inhibiting LFA-3/CD2 interaction, thus reducing lymphocyte (T-cell) counts and thereby treating the cause of psoriasis.

Raptiva (efalizumab), indicated for plaque psoriasis, is an antibody that prevents activated T-cells from entering the skin. This drug is administered by SC injection once a week. Common side effects include headache, chills, fever, nausea, muscle aches, and thrombocytopenia. Efalizumab is technically described as an "immunosuppressive recombinant humanized IgG1 kappa isotype monoclonal antibody." This drug binds to a receptor that is expressed on all leukocytes. This attachment inhibits or blocks the adhesion of leukocytes to other cell types. The final result is that Raptiva decreases the activation of T-lymphocytes and, therefore, the inflammation of psoriatic skin.

Oral Elidel (pimecrolimus), made by Novartis, selectively inhibits inflammatory cytokine release. Limited evidence suggests the potential efficacy of 20 or 30 mg Oral Elidel, taken orally twice daily, in the treatment of chronic plaque psoriasis (also see Table 24-1).

> **❝ Workplace Wisdom** Psoriasis
>
> Psoriasis reportedly affects up to 2% of the U.S. population. ❞

Skin Infections

Skin **infections** may be categorized by the causative agent into three types: viral, bacterial, and fungal. The following sections provide a brief overview of each type.

Viral Infections

A viral skin infection occurs when a virus penetrates the stratum corneum and infects the inner layers of the skin. Examples include herpes simplex, warts, and shingles (herpes zoster). Temporary viral infections, such as chicken pox and measles, also affect the skin. Antibiotics (ABX) and antibacterial agents cannot cure viral infections; antiviral medications and time are the only two treatments.

A new drug for treating sexually transmitted external genital and anal warts, an immunomodulator known as Aldara (imiquimod) 5% cream, is now available. Although the warts are caused by the human papilloma virus (HPV) and are not curable, the drug can decrease their size and therefore the severity of pain. HPV is the most common sexually transmitted disease (STD).

Bacterial Infections

Bacterial skin infections are caused by many different bacteria, but the most common bacterial **pathogens** are *Staphylococcus*, *Streptococcus*, and *Pseudomonas*. If left untreated, these infections may spread throughout the body, becoming more serious and possibly causing systemic infections. Examples include Lyme disease, impetigo, folliculitis, and cellulitis.

ABX can be topically or orally administered, depending upon the microorganism and the specific ABX. Antibacterial agents are either **bactericidal** or **bacteriostatic**. Their main mechanism of action is to stop cell wall protein synthesis within the bacterium, which prevents the growth of the cell wall. The inside of the cell continues to grow and eventually bursts through the cell wall, leaking out the cytoplasm and nucleus. Thus, the microorganism explodes, collapses in on itself, and dies.

Fungal Infections

Fungal skin infections, also known as *mycoses*, occur when normally harmless fungi gain entry into the skin, rather than staying on the outer layer of the skin (epidermis). These infections are usually external, affecting the skin, hair, and nails. Yeasts are a subtype of fungus, characterized by clusters of round or oval cells. Fungal infections occur in damp, dark, and warm places on the body. Examples include athlete's foot, jock itch, and ringworm. Fungal infections such as athlete's foot typically create itchy red areas that may crack or blister. These infections are common and generally mild; however, people with suppressed immune systems, or who have been taking ABX for a long time, are more susceptible to fungi spreading deep within the body, which causes more serious systemic disease. Patients with diabetes are also at highest risk.

Acne

Acne is an infection caused by a bacterium and an overproduction of **sebum** that clogs the hair follicles. The extra sebum accompanies an increase in the number and activity of hair follicles during puberty. Acne can be categorized as either noninflammatory or inflammatory.

Noninflammatory acne consists of the following:

- **Whiteheads**—occur when the trapped sebum and bacteria remain under the skin; may manifest as small white spots.
- **Blackheads**—occur when the trapped sebum and bacteria partially break through the surface of the skin and turn black (this is due to pigmentation, not dirt).

Inflammatory acne consists of the following:

- **Papules**—formed when the wall of a follicle breaks; white blood cells rush to the site and inflammation occurs.
- **Pustules**—occur following the formation of a papule as the white blood cells move to the surface of the skin.

TABLE 24-1 Prescription and OTC Treatments for Psoriasis

Generic Name	Brand Name	Dosage Forms and Availability	Route of Administration	Common Adult Dosage
acitretin	Soriatane	10 mg, 17.5 mg, 22.5 mg, 25 mg capsules	Oral	25–50 mg daily
adalimumab	Humira	20 mg, 40 mg pre-filled syringe (PFS)	SC	Initial dose of 80 mg, followed by 40 mg every other week
alefacept	Amevive	15 mg SDV	IM	15 mg IM weekly for 12 weeks
anthralin	Dritho-Scalp	0.5% cream	Topical	Apply daily
betamethasone	Diprolene (AF)	0.5% cream, 0.5% lotion, 0.5% ointment	Topical	Apply once or twice daily
calcipotriene	Dovonex	0.005% cream, 0.005% ointment, 0.005% topical solution	Topical	Apply once or twice daily
clobetasol propionate	Temovate	0.5% cream, 0.5% ointment, 0.5% gel	Topical	Apply twice daily
coal tar	DHS tar, Doak tar, Theraplex T	Foam, ointment, lotion, shampoo	Topical	As directed
cyclosporine	Sandimmune, Neoral	25 mg, 100 mg capsules; 100 mg/mL solution	Oral	Initially 2.5 mg/kg, given in two divided doses; maximum 4 mg/kg/day in divided doses
desoximetasone	Topicort	0.05% ointment	Topical	Apply twice daily
etanercept	Enbrel	25 mg, 50 mg PFS; 25 mg MDV	Injection	50 mg twice weekly
fluocinolone	Synalar	0.025% cream	Topical	Apply two to four times daily
fluocinonide	Lidex	0.5% cream	Topical	Apply two to four times daily
fluticasone propionate	Cutivate	0.05% cream, 0.05% lotion, 0.05% ointment	Topical	Apply twice daily
hydrocortisone	Aveeno anti-itch cream, Cortaid	1% cream, 1% ointment	Topical	Apply two to four times daily
hydrocortisone valerate	Westcort	0.2% cream, 0.2% ointment	Topical	Apply twice or thrice daily
infliximab	Remicade	100 mg SDV	IV	5 mg/kg at zero, two, and six weeks, followed by 5 mg/kg every six weeks
methotrexate	Rheumatrex	2.5 mg tablets— dose paks	Oral	7.5 mg once weekly, divided into three doses
tazarotene	Tazorac	0.5%, 0.1% gel; 0.5%, 0.1% cream	Topical	Apply daily
ustekinumab	Stelara	45 mg, 90 mg PFS; 45 mg, 90 mg SDV	SC	45–90 mg initially and four weeks later, followed by 45–90 mg every 12 weeks

- **Nodules**—occur when the follicle wall breaks and causes deep tissue inflammation. A nodule can be painful and may cause tissue damage with scarring.
- **Cysts**—consist of a liquid- or semi-liquid-filled lesion accompanied by severe inflammation, pain, and scarring.

The exact cause of acne has not been determined, but it is *not* brought on by eating chocolate or greasy foods, as some people believe. However, several factors may increase a person's risk of developing acne:

- **Heredity**—if the parents had acne, the chances of their children developing acne are higher.

- **Hormones**—changes during puberty and pregnancy can cause glands to plug up more frequently.
- **Medications**—some drugs, such as oral or injectable steroids, can cause or worsen acne.
- **Makeup**—greasy, oily, and pore-clogging makeup can lead to acne.

See Tables 24-2 and 24-3.

Cellulitis

Cellulitis is an acute, deep infection of the connective tissue accompanied by inflammation. The causative agent is

TABLE 24-2 Prescription Treatments for Acne

Generic Name	Brand Name	Dosage Forms and Availability	Route of Administration	Common Adult Dosage
clindamycin topical	Cleocin T	10 mg/mL gel, 10 mg/mL lotion	Topical	Apply twice daily
doxyclycline	Monodox, Oracea	50 mg, 75 mg, 100 mg capsule	Oral	100–200 mg daily
erythromycin topical	Erygel, Staticin	1.5% solution; 2% gel	Topical	Apply once or twice daily
isotretinoin	Accutane	10 mg, 20 mg, 40 mg capsule	Oral	0.5 to 1 mg/kg/day for 15 to 20 weeks
minocycline	Minocin	50 mg, 100 mg capsule	Oral	100–200 mg daily
tetracycline	Sumycin	250 mg, 500 mg tablets	Oral	125–250 mg four times daily for one to two weeks, then decrease to 125–500 mg daily
tretinoin	Retin-A, Renova	Cream	Topical	Apply once daily

TABLE 24-3 OTC Treatments for Acne

Generic Name	Brand Name	Dosage Forms and Availability	Route of Administration	Common Adult Dosage
benzoyl peroxide	Clearasil, Desquam, Oxy, Neutrogena	3.5–10%, cream, gel, topical solution	Topical	Apply once or twice daily
salicylic acid	Noxema, Stridex	Varies	Topical	Apply once or twice daily
sulfur and resorcinol	Clearasil	Varies	Topical	Apply once or twice daily

info

Statistics on Acne

Acne, the most common skin disease, occurs in approximately 85% of all people between the ages of 12 and 24 years.

cellulitis an inflammation of the connective tissue of the skin.

Staphylococcus, Streptococcus, or another bacterium. Enzymes produced by the bacteria destroy skin cells. The skin tissues of the infected area show all the cardinal signs of inflammation—redness, irritation, and pain. People most prone to cellulitis include those with a break in the skin from an insect bite or injury; those with a history of peripheral vascular disease diabetes, or ischemic ulcers; those who have recently had cardiovascular, pulmonary, or dental procedures or surgeries; and those who use immunosuppressive or corticosteroid medications. Prescription treatment for cellulitis includes oral ABX, such as cefazolin (Ancef) or dicloxicillin (Dynapen), or intravenous ABX, such as cefazolin, oxacillin, or nafcillin.

Hives

Hives are a very uncomfortable skin condition that can appear on a small part of the body or all over the body. They appear as elevated red bumps on the skin's surface. Hives itch, burn, and usually sting. The more an individual scratches the hives, the more they can be spread. Hives can also lead to contact dermatitis and other skin conditions. To relieve itching, patients can use creams, such as hydrocortisone or pramoxine/zinc acetate (Caladryl, Calamine) and also take antihistamines, such as diphenhydramine, depending on how serious the case starts out or develops. Hives can accompany breathing difficulty or a patient's throat closing up. Such cases should be treated as an emergency, and individuals should seek treatment right away if serious symptoms occur or persist.

Parasitic Infestations

Parasitic infestations are caused by insects or worms that burrow into the skin to live and/or lay their eggs. Some infestations caused by **parasites** are scabies and lice. Parasites may enter and infect an injured or open wound or may be transferred from one infested person or object to another person. *Scabies* is characterized by small red bumps and intense itching; it is caused by mites that burrow into the skin from bedding and mattresses.

> ❝ **Workplace Wisdom** Parasitic Infestations
>
> Any patient who has a prescription to treat a parasitic infestation should be told to wash in very hot water (or dry-clean) all recently worn clothing, underwear, sheets, pillowcases, and towels. ❞

---

parasite an organism that lives on or inside another organism.

carcinoma a malignant tumor.

pigmentation color.

rosacea a facial skin disorder accompanied by chronic redness and inflammation and/or acne.

Tumors and Cancerous Growths

Tumors and cancerous growths occur when skin cells multiply or reproduce faster than normal. Those without cell mutation are considered *benign* or noncancerous, even though they may grow rapidly. In contrast, tumors or skin growths characterized by rapid reproduction and mutation of cells are considered *malignant* or cancerous.

There are three main types of skin cancer: basal cell carcinoma, squamous cell cancer, and malignant melanoma.

Basal Cell Carcinoma

Basal cell **carcinoma** is the most common and most curable skin cancer. It occurs in the epidermis, usually on the face and scalp (see Figure 24-2).

The main cause of basal cell carcinoma is early, frequent, and extended sun exposure; this accounts for 25% of all new cancers.

Squamous Cell Cancer

Squamous cell is the second most common skin cancer, accounting for about 20% of all skin cancers. It can grow and spread rapidly, often appearing on the back of the hands, on the ears, or on the edges of the lips. It usually develops in the outer layer of the epidermis. When this cancer spreads or *metastasizes*, it can invade distant organs and tissues and become fatal.

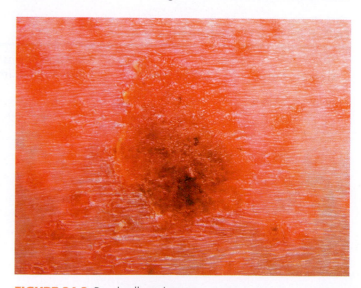

FIGURE 24-2 Basal cell carcinoma.
Source: Vizual Studio/Shutterstock

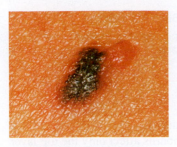

FIGURE 24-3 Malignant melanoma.
Source: Dr. P. Marazzi/Science Source

Malignant Melanoma

Malignant melanoma is the deadliest form of skin cancer; often, the signal is a mole that changes shape or color and may begin to bleed (see Figure 24-3). However, it can be cured if caught when the tumor is still thin and localized in the outermost layer of the skin. At first, a melanoma is localized and usually spreads across the skin before it moves into the deeper skin layers.

Precancerous Conditions

An *actinic keratosis* (AK), also called a *solar keratosis*, is a scaly or crusty bump that originates on the skin surface. It may be light or dark and tan, pink, or red, and is usually rough. Although it may develop slowly, about 5% of AKs become squamous cell carcinomas; therefore, AK is considered a *precursor* to cancer or a precancerous growth. It may also spread to other organs and tissues on its own (see Table 24-4).

Pigmentation Disorders

The color of the skin is determined by the amount of melanin produced by the body and, to some extent, genetics. Melanocytes produce melanin. Melanocyte malfunction or absence, exposure to cold or chemicals, infections, or severe skin burns can contribute to a loss of skin **pigmentation** or hypopigmentation. An example of hypopigmentation is vitiligo. Additional or excess skin pigmentation is known as *hyperpigmentation*.

Causes of hyperpigmentations include hormonal changes (especially in women using systemic birth control), aging, and metabolic disorders. Examples are freckles and age spots or "liver spots."

Miscellaneous Skin Conditions and Diseases

The skin conditions and diseases discussed next do not fall into any of the preceding nine categories.

Hyperkeratosis

Hyperkeratosis is a condition that results from having too much keratin, which is a protein of the skin, hair, and nails. It causes the skin to harden and thicken. Examples of hyperkeratosis include calluses, corns, and warts. *Warts* are small bumps on the skin surface that are caused by an HPV.

Wrinkles

Wrinkles are caused by the combination of a breakdown of the collagen and elastin within the dermis and a reduction in the size of the fat cells in the skin; these two factors result in sagging skin. Reduced production of sebum causes the moisture barrier of the skin to become thinner; consequently, more moisture is released, which results in dryer skin. When sagging, loose skin becomes dry and wrinkles are more pronounced.

Rosacea

Rosacea is a chronic disorder of unknown cause in which the skin of the face becomes red and develops pimples and lesions; these symptoms may be accompanied by enlargement of the nose. In oily, acne-prone areas, deep-seated papules and pustules cause small blood vessels to enlarge (*telangiectasia*),

TABLE 24-4 Prescription Treatments for Skin Cancer

Generic Name	Brand Name	Dosage forms and Availability	Route of Administration	Common Adult Dosage
fluorouracil	Efudex, Fluoroplex, Carac	2% topical solution, 5% topical solution, 5% cream	Topical	Apply once a day to the skin where lesions appear, using enough to cover the entire area with a thin film
imiquimod	Aldara	5% cream	Topical	Apply as directed by physician once daily or thrice per week at bedtime; allow medication to stay on skin for 6–10 hours and then wash the area thoroughly with soap and water; repeat until warts are gone (up to 16 weeks)

resulting in a flushed appearance that may last for long periods of time. There is no cure for rosacea, but with proper treatment, the symptoms can be **mitigated** (controlled). Prescription treatment includes topical ABX, such as sodium sulfacetamide, and oral ABX, such as tetracycline or metronidazole.

Spider Veins

Spider veins are broken blood vessels, such as capillaries, which then enlarge. As they enlarge, they become visible through the surface of the skin, varying in color from blue, purple, and orchid to bright red. The cause may be obesity, tight stockings, exposure to sun, or natural or drug-induced hormonal changes in women.

Burns

Burns can be categorized by cause, as:

- *Thermal*—resulting from contact with fire or heat.
- *Chemical*—resulting from contact with acids, bases, or vesicants.
- *Electrical*—resulting from contact with an electrical current.
- *Friction*—resulting from harsh rubbing of the skin.
- *Sunburn*— resulting from overexposure to sunlight.

Burns are also classified by the severity, depth, or degree of injury to the skin:

- *First-degree* burns—limited damage to the epidermis; characterized by redness and pain. Considered superficial burns.
- *Second-degree* burns—damage to both the epidermis and the dermis; characterized by redness, blisters, mild-to-moderate edema, and pain. Considered moderate burns.
- *Third-degree* burns—destruction of all the epidermis, dermis, and SC tissue; characterized by a leathery or dry white, brown, or black appearance. Blistering does not occur. These are considered critical burns, and skin grafting is usually recommended.
- *Fourth-degree* burns—destruction of the skin and underlying tissues (muscles, tendons, ligaments, and bones). Considered critical burns; skin grafts are required.

The "Rule of Nines" is used when estimating the amount of body surface area that has been burned. For an adult, the percentage of the body burned can be calculated as follows:

If one arm (9%), the groin (1%), and one leg (18%) were affected, the patient would be burned over 28% of the body.

The major cause of death among burn patients is not the burn itself, but the complication of infections caused by prolonged treatment and skin grafts. Burned areas are highly susceptible to infection due to the open lesions. Silver sulfadiazine (Silvadene) is a topical burn cream that works by acting on the cell membrane wall to inhibit microbial activity and some yeast. In addition, when applied at the recommended $\frac{1}{16}$-inch thickness, it allows oxygen to pass through to promote healing. The cream is applied once every 12 hours, along with a dressing change. Mafenide acetate (Sulfamylon) is another topical anti-infective used to treat burns.

> ## ❝ Workplace Wisdom Burn Statistics
>
> Approximately 2.4 million people report burn injuries each year. Burns result in between 8,000 and 12,000 deaths annually in the United States. ❞

Sunburn

When someone gets sunburn, they have visible damage from sun exposure and UV rays. Sunburns affect only the top layer of the skin, but are very painful to the touch. Patients experience not only pain, but also itching, peeling, and redness. Sunburns in which the skin blisters and swells are a much more serious type of sunburn. The sunburn takes longer to heel, as nerve endings and deeper skin layers have been affected. Sunburns can also include heatstroke, an allergic reaction, vision problems, and discoloration and damage to the skin's surface or deeper layers. Long-term peeling and cracking of the skin can also be due to bad sunburn.

Decubitus Ulcers

A *decubitus ulcer*, also known as a *pressure* or *bed sore*, is an ulceration of the skin due to pressure. These ulcers can also be caused by prolonged friction or exposure to cold. Pressure sores can range from mild (redness and/or blistering, often disappearing soon after pressure is relieved) to severe (deep tissue wounds extending to the bone or through the bone into internal organs). Sixty-seven percent of all pressure sores occur on the hip and buttock regions. The following factors increase the risk of decubitus ulcers:

- Fragile skin
- Being bedridden or in a wheelchair
- Chronic conditions, such as diabetes or cardiovascular disease, in which circulation is impaired
- Malnourishment
- Older age
- Urinary or bowel incontinence
- Inability to move body parts without assistance

Decubitus ulcers are classified into stages by the depth or degree of injury to the tissues:

- Stage I—characterized by reddening of unbroken skin; this is an early warning that a problem exists. It is usually treated by alleviating pressure, avoiding exposure to the cause, and protecting and padding the area.
- Stage II—characterized by an abrasion, blister, or superficial ulceration of the skin resulting from damage to the epidermis. Treatments include applying skin lotions to hydrate the tissues around the sore, as well as additional padding and relief of pressure.
- Stage III—characterized by a crater-like lesion that extends through the SC tissue. Medical care is needed to treat the sore and prevent infection.
- Stage IV—characterized by a lesion that extends through the skin into the muscle, bone, tendon, or ligaments. It can cause life-threatening infections and will not heal without proper treatment (see Table 24-5).

TABLE 24-5 Prescription and OTC Treatments for Ulcers

Generic Name	Brand Name	Dosage forms and Availability	Route of Administration	Common Adult Dosage
bacitracin zinc	Bacitracin Zinc	Ointment	Topical	Apply as directed
metronidazole acquired	MetroGel	0.75% topical gel	Topical	Apply daily
mupirocin	Bactroban, Centany	2% cream, 2% ointment	Topical	Apply thrice daily
polymyxin b sulfate, neomycin, bacitracin	Neosporin	2% cream, 2% ointment	Topical	Apply as directed
retapamulin	Altabax	1% ointment	Topical	Apply as directed

Warts

Warts can be both unsightly and painful. They are hard, bumpy, rough pieces of skin that have accelerated growth. Warts carry an HPV that is highly contagious and can be spread from person to person. Warts can grow virtually anywhere on the human body such as the genitals, hands, fingers, toes, palms, and feet. A wart is treatable and curable. It may appear brown or pink, or in the color of the affected person's flesh. The treatment for warts depends on the type of wart the patient has developed. Treatment options can range from no treatment where the wart goes away by itself to treatment by a doctor. Topical medications and injections can also help clear up warts. Over-the-counter (OTC) treatments are also another option for banishing the unsightly very hard bumps of skin (see Table 24-6).

Athlete's Foot

Athlete's foot is a common fungal infection of the extremities, specifically the foot. This type of fungal infection can be treated by most OTC remedies. Athlete's foot is not a serious condition but causes painful itching, burning, and possible skin peeling. The fungi often live in moist areas that are warm such as hot tubs, pools, gym's showers, and tubs. Athlete's foot can also be caused by wearing stockings, not changing socks often when sweating a lot or after exercising, or not changing your shoes out often. Athlete's foot is more of an annoyance than a serious condition (see Table 24-7).

Herpes

There are many different types of herpes viruses. Herpes can generally be defined as many viral diseases that include blister-like sores or vesicles present on mucous membranes. Herpes can take a variety of forms and should be treated as soon as an outbreak happens. Treatment for the herpes virus depends on the type of herpes a patient has contracted.

Herpes simplex 1 is oral herpes. It causes sores around the mouth and can be spread through kissing and sharing toothbrushes or eating utensils. Herpes typ. 2 is contracted through sexual contact with another person who has the disease. Those individuals with herpes can go through dormant periods or outbreaks that can be brought on by various factors such as

TABLE 24-6 Prescription and OTC Treatments for Warts

Generic Name	Brand Name	Dosage Forms and Availability	Route of Administration	Common Adult Dosage
fluorouracil	Efudex, Fluoroplex, Carac	2% topical solution, 5% topical solution, 5% cream	Topical	Apply once a day to the skin where lesions appear, using enough to cover the entire area with a thin film
salicylic acid	Wart Off, Compound D, Dr. Schools Freeze Away Wart Remover, Compound W Freeze	17% gel, liquid, pads, strips	Topical	Follow skin preparation instructions on product label; this product is applied once or twice daily as needed (until wart is removed) for up to 12 weeks

TABLE 24-7 Prescription and OTC Treatments for Athlete's Foot

Generic Name	Brand Name	Dosage Forms	Route of Administration	Common Adult Dosage
clotrimazole	Desenex AF, Lotrimin AF	Cream, lotion, topical solution	Topical	Apply twice daily
ketoconazole	Nizoral	2% cream	Topical	Apply twice daily
miconazole	Desenex, Croex Powder	Powder, spray	Topical	Apply twice daily
tolnaftate	Lamisil AF, Tinactin	Cream, powder, ointment, spray, topical solution	Topical	Apply twice daily

emotional stress, menstruation, physical stress, immunosuppression due to AIDS, or medications. Chemotherapy drugs and steroids can also bring on an outbreak. The condition cannot be cured, but pain and outbreaks can be controlled with medication (see Table 24-8).

Impetigo

Impetigo is common mostly in children, but adults can also be infected. The condition is caused by a streptococcal bacterium. Impetigo is extremely contagious and can be passed on to others through skin contact, sheets, towels, clothing, toys, and other items. Scratching and picking at the sores can cause the infection to spread on the affected patient or to others. Impetigo appears as small red sores and then develops into blisters that break open. The sores ooze, are crusty, and are coated with a yellow crust. They can increase in number, diameter, and intensity. Medical treatment includes ABX, topical ointments, and isolation due to the contagious nature of the condition (see Table 24-9).

Lice

Lice are common and are caused by a parasite named *Pediculus humanus capitis*. There are head lice and also genital lice. The bugs can be fully treated and are curable. Symptoms of lice are sores on the scalp, itching, and a feeling like something is moving within the hair. Lice can live on areas of the body such as the legs, armpits, mustache, eyebrows, beards, and anywhere they can latch on to hairy areas of the body. Lice can be cured with OTC treatments and also prescription medication.

TABLE 24-8 Prescription and OTC Treatments for Herpes

Generic Name	Brand Name	Dosage Forms and Availability	Route of Administration	Common Adult Dosage
acyclovir	Zovirax	200 mg capsule; 400 mg, 800 mg tablets; 200 mg/5 mL suspension	Oral	200–800 mg five times daily for 10 days
docosanol	Abreva	Cream	Topical	Apply as directed
famciclovir	Famvir	125 mg, 250 mg, 500 mg tablets	Oral	Two 1-gm doses
penciclovir	Denavir	1% cream	Topical	Apply every two hours
valacyclovir	Valtrex	500 mg, 1 gm caplets	Oral	Two 2-gm doses

TABLE 24-9 Prescription Treatments for Impetigo

Generic Name	Brand Name	Dosage Forms and Availability	Route of Administration	Common Adult Dosage
mupirocin	Bactroban	2% cream, 2% ointment	Topical	Apply thrice daily
retapamulin	Altabax	1% ointment	Topical	Apply twice daily for five days

TABLE 24-10 Prescription Treatments for Lice

Generic Name	Brand Name	Dosage forms and Availability	Route of Administration	Common Adult Dosage
benzyl alcohol	Ulesfia	5% lotion	Topical	Apply to dry hair, leave on for 10 minutes, and then rinse; repeat after seven days if still present.
lindane	Kwell	1% shampoo	Topical	Apply directly to dry hair without adding water. Work thoroughly into the hair and allow to remain in place for four minutes, and then add small quantities of water to hair until a good lather forms. Immediately rinse all lather away.
malathion	Ovide	0.5% lotion	Topical	Apply to dry hair and allow to dry naturally. Shampoo after 8–12 hours; repeat after seven to nine days if still present.
permethrin	Acticin, Elimite, Nix	5% cream	Topical	Use enough solution to saturate hair and scalp; leave on for 10 minutes and then rinse with water; remove eggs (nits) with comb provided; apply second treatment in 7–10 days if needed
pyrethrins and piperonyl butoxide	A-200, Pronto, Rid, Tegrin-LT	0.33%/4% shampoo, 0.33%/4% spray	Topical	Apply as directed

Bedding, clothes, towels, washcloths, toys, stuffed animals, clothes, hats, and all other items that have come in contact with a person who is affected by lice should be washed in very hot water and detergent, disinfected, and/or dry-cleaned (see Table 24-10).

PROFILE IN PRACTICE

Travis is a pharmacy technician at Mercy General Hospital. A patient arrives in the emergency room with third-degree burns on his head, torso, left arm, groin, and both legs.

▸ *What percentage of the patient's body has been burned?*

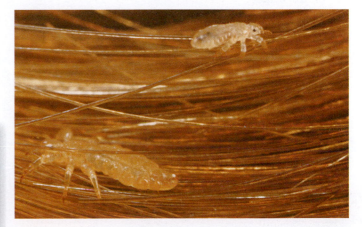

FIGURE 24-4 Parasitic infestation—head lice.
Source: Darlyne A. Murawski/National Geographic Stock

Summary

The skin, considered the largest body organ, consists of three main layers: the epidermis, the dermis, and the SC layer. The skin performs several important functions, such as serving as a barrier to foreign organisms and debris, managing and regulating the body temperature, excreting salts and excess water, and acting as a shock absorber to protect the underlying organs.

Diseases of the skin can range from simple rashes to deadly cancers (malignant melanoma). The most common skin disease, acne, affects approximately 17 million Americans. Fortunately, a large array of pharmaceuticals are available to treat skin conditions and diseases.

Chapter Review Questions

1. Which layer of the skin contains blood vessels and hair follicles?
   a. dermis
   b. epidermis
   c. subcutaneous layer
   d. both b and c

2. According to the "Rule of Nines," what would be the percentage of body burned on an individual who had burns on both arms and one leg?
   a. 9
   b. 18
   c. 27
   d. 36

3. Cellulitis is characterized by inflammation of the
   _____.
   a. dermis
   b. epidermis
   c. subcutaneous layer
   d. deep connective tissue

4. Which of the following is considered the deadliest form of skin cancer?
   a. basal cell carcinoma
   b. malignant melanoma
   c. squamous cell cancer
   d. benign skin tumors

5. The cause of the skin condition _____ is unknown.
   a. cellulitis
   b. hyperkeratosis
   c. rosacea
   d. spider veins

6. Elidel cream is used to treat which of the following skin conditions?
   a. acne
   b. rosacea
   c. eczema
   d. urticaria

7. Herpes simplex, herpes zoster, and warts are classified as what type of skin infection?
   a. bacterial
   b. fungal
   c. parasitic
   d. viral

8. Which of the following ingredients is *not* found in Neosporin?
   a. bacitracin
   b. mupirocin
   c. neomycin
   d. polymyxin B sulfate

9. More than _____ of all skin cancer cases in the United States are caused by continuous or early-life sun exposure?
   a. 15%
   b. 30%
   c. 60%
   d. 90%

10. Which of the following drugs is used to treat lice infestations in children?
    a. griseofulvin
    b. lindane
    c. miconazole
    d. pyrethrins

Critical Thinking Questions

1. What type of precautions should a caregiver take when administering treatment to a patient with severe burns, or when applying medication to burns?

2. Discuss what can be done to prevent the spread of parasite infestations?

3. Why do you believe acne affects so many people? What do you think can be done (outside of medication) to help reduce the number and severity of acne outbreaks?

Web Challenge

1. Visit the American Cancer Society's website at http://www.cancer.org to learn more about skin cancer. Write a summary of ways to prevent basal and squamous cell cancers.

2. To learn more about adult and pediatric dermatological conditions, go to http://www.healthsystem.virginia.edu. At the home page, click on the "Patients & Visitors" tab and then choose *patient information*. Then, from the drop-down menu (under adult or children health topics), choose dermatology. Write a short summary of three conditions you find discussed at this website; include treatment options.

3. Visit http://www.acne.org to learn more about the causes of acne.

References and Resources

"About Aldara® (imiquimod)—Package Insert for Both External Genital Warts and Actinic Keratoses." http://www.3m.com/us/healthcare/pharma/aldara/AKPI.pdf. 7 July 2007. Web.

"About Amevive® (Alefacept) Doctor's Guide: Amevive (Alefacept), Treatment for Psoriasis, Approved in Israel, Receives 'Positive Opinion' from Swiss Regulatory Authority, May 3, 2004." http://www.pslgroup.com/dg/243fd2.htm; http://www.rxlist.com/cgi/generic3/amevive.htm; http://www.centerwatch.com/patient/drugs/dru820.html. 7 July 2007. Web.

"About Commonly Sexually Transmitted Diseases: HPV." http://www.princeton.edu/puhs/SECH/hpv.html. 7 July 2007. Web.

"About Elidel® 1% (Pimecrolimus) Cream for Eczema by National Eczema Society." http://www.eczema.org/PIMECROLIMUSCREAM.pdf. 7 July 2007. Web.

"About Enbrel® (Etanercept) FDA Approval of Enbrel (Etanercept) for Psoriasis on April 30, 2004." http://www.amgen.com/news/viewPR.jsp?id=521767; http://www.enbrel.com/news/pdf/Enbrel_Psoriasis_Approval.pdf; http://my.webmd.com/content/article/86/99063.htm. 3 July 2007. Web.

"About Raptiva® (Efalizumab)." http://www.thedrugdatabase.com/directory/R/Raptiva; http://www.raptiva.com/about/faqs.jsp#Q7. 1 July 2007. Web.

"About Raptiva: Genetech Patient and Professional Information Website." http://www.drugs.com/raptiva.html. 29 June 2007. Web.

"About Remicade® (Infliximab)." http://www.dermnetnz.org/dna.psoriasis/infliximab.html. 29 June 2007. Web.

"About Skin Anatomy and Physiology." http://www.essential-dayspa.com/Skin_Anathomy_and_Physiology.htm. 29 June 2007. Web.

"About Skin Cancer: The Skin Cancer Foundation." http://www.skincancer.org. 20 June 2007. Web.

"About Tacrolimus for Eczema and Psoriasis: AAD: Tacrolimus Ointment Safe and Effective in All Ages for Mild to Moderate Eczema, by Bruce Sylvester." http://www.docguide.com/news/content.nsf/news/85256977005 73E1885256E37006578F2?OpenDocument&id=48dde4a 73e09a969852568880078c249&c=Dermatitis&count=10. 29 June 2007. Web.

"Acne." http://www.medicinenet.com. 17 September 2007. Web.

Adams, M.P., D.L. Josephson, and L.N. Holland Jr. *Pharmacology for Nurses: A Pathophysiologic Approach.* (4th ed.). Upper Saddle River, NJ: Pearson, 2013.

American Association of Family Physicians. "Common Bacterial Skin Infections." http://www.aafp.org/afp/20020701/119.html. 29 June 2007. Web.

"Decubitus Ulcer Information and Wound Stages." LDHP Medication Review Services Corporation, December 1999. http://www.expertlaw.com. 17 September 2007. Web.

"Degree of Burns." http://www.burnsurvivorsttw.org. 3 August 2013. Web.

"Food, Drug and Cosmetic Act." http://www.fda.gov/opacom/laws/fdcact/fdcact1.htm. 7 July 2007. Web.

"Healthepic Anatomy of Skin." http://www.healthepic.com/hers/static/hers_beauty_skindeep_anatomy.htm. 29 June 2007. Web.

Holland, N. and M.P. Adams. *Core Concepts in Pharmacology.* (3rd ed.). Upper Saddle River, NJ: Pearson, 2010.

"How to Treat Burns of All Degrees." http://www.med-help.net. 15 September 2007. Web.

Kamel, M.N. "Anatomy of the Skin." http://www.telemedicine.org/anatomy.htm#functions. 27 June 2007. Web.

Moyer, P. "About ORAL Elidel® AAD: Oral Pimecrolimus Effective in Treating Psoriasis." http://www.pslgroup.com/dg/22ebd2.htm. 29 June 2007. Web.

"Pressure Ulcer." http://www.nlm.nih.gov. 2 August 2013. Web.

Revis, D.R. "Decubitus Ulcers." October 25, 2005. http://www.emedicine.com. 17 September 2007. Web.

"Web MD Reports." *Herpes Simplex: Herpes Type 1 and 2.* Web MD. 6 August 2012. Web.

"What Is Acne?" http://www.skincarephysicians.com. 17 September 2007. Web.

"What Is Acne? Fast Facts: An Easy-to-Read Series of Publications for the Public." http://www.niams.nih.gov. 2 August 2013. Web.

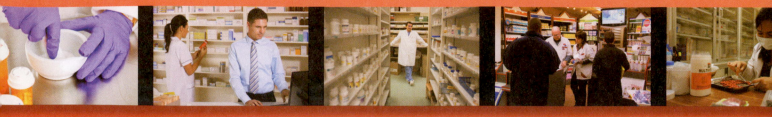

CHAPTER 25

The Eyes and Ears

LEARNING OBJECTIVES

After completing this chapter, you should be able to:

- List, identify, and diagram the basic anatomical structure and parts of the eye and ear.

- Describe the function or physiology of the ears and eyes.

- List and define common diseases affecting the eyes, and understand the causes, symptoms, and pharmaceutical treatments associated with each disease.

- List and define common diseases affecting the ears, and understand the causes, symptoms, and pharmaceutical treatments associated with each disease.

KEY TERMS

asymptomatic, p. 382

blepharitis, p. 378

cataract, p. 385

conjunctivitis, p. 378

cycloplegic, p. 387

glaucoma, p. 383

hordeolum, p. 378

humor, p. 377

intraocular, p. 383

iridotomy, p. 385

macular degeneration, p. 387

mucopurulent, p. 379

mydriatic, p. 387

ophthalmic, p. 378

otitis media, p. 393

retinopathy, p. 385

stye, p. 378

tinnitus, p. 392

INTRODUCTION

Chapter 24 discussed the largest sensory organ, the skin. This chapter explores the sense of sight; the sense of hearing; and the respective sensory organs, the eye and the ear. Vision is the most basic and primary of our senses, and we tend to value it more than any other sense. Loss of sight usually means that a person will rely more acutely on the sense of hearing. Many parts of the eye contribute to the perception of a good image, but it is the retina, a piece of brain tissue, that is most vital for vision; it takes direct stimulation from the world outside the body, in the form of light, and begins the process of translating that stimulation into images.

The ear is responsible for hearing. Sound waves travel from the outer ear down the external auditory canal, striking the eardrum and making it vibrate. These vibrations cause three tiny bones in the middle ear to amplify the sound to the cochlea of the inner ear. From here, nerves ultimately transmit the sound to the brain where it is interpreted. Disorders of the ear include infection of the eustachian tube, or serous otitis media, complications of earwax buildup, and types of hearing loss.

humor a body fluid.

Anatomy and Physiology of the Eye

The main structures of the eye include the cornea, sclera, conjunctiva, iris, pupil, lens, retina, optic nerve, macula, vitreous humor, choroid, and the extraocular muscles (see Figure 25-1).

- The *cornea* is the clear or transparent outer "window" of the eye, made up primarily of connective tissue. It focuses light as the light enters the eye.
- The opaque, white portion around the circumference of the cornea is the *sclera*.
- The thin, transparent layer that extends from the edge of the cornea and covers the sclera and lines the inside of the eyelids is the *conjunctiva*.
- The colored disc visible through the cornea is the *iris*. The opening in the iris is the *pupil*.
- The *lens* (or *crystalline lens*) is located directly behind the iris. The lens focuses light onto the retina.
- Often referred to as the "film" of the camera, the *retina* lines the back of the eye. The retina is composed of sensory tissue that converts light rays into impulses that move along the optic nerve.
- The *optic nerve* is the visual pathway by which electrical impulses move from the retina to the brain and back.
- The *macula* is a small yellowish area in the retina that provides the most central and acute vision.

- The *vitreous* **humor**, composed mostly of water, occupies about 80% of the interior of the eye between the lens and the retina.
- The *choroid* is the layer between the sclera and the retina. The choroid is composed of layers of nourishing blood vessels.

Three pairs of extraocular muscles regulate the motion of each eye: the medial/lateral rectus muscles, the superior/inferior rectus muscles, and the superior/inferior oblique muscles. Cranial nerve III stimulates four of the six extraocular muscles: medial rectus, superior rectus, inferior rectus, and inferior oblique. The eye orbit is surrounded in layers of soft, fatty tissue, which protect and cushion the eye and enable it to turn easily.

How the Eye Works

Understanding of specific eye diseases begins with knowledge of how the eye works. As you know, the function of the eyes is to allow the person to see. Vision occurs as light waves reflected from an object, such as a building, enter the eye through the cornea and then through the pupil. The light waves *converge*, or come together, first at the cornea, and then are further focused by the crystalline lens to a nodal point called "N" that is located on the immediate backside surface of the lens. This is the point where the image becomes *inverted*

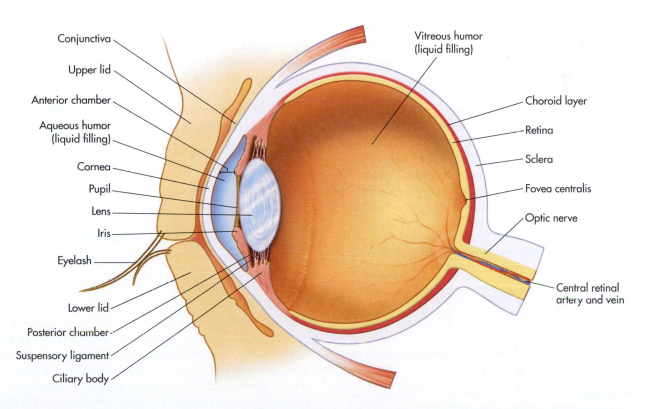

Conjunctiva
Upper lid
Anterior chamber
Aqueous humor (liquid filling)
Cornea
Pupil
Lens
Iris
Eyelash
Lower lid
Posterior chamber
Suspensory ligament
Ciliary body

Vitreous humor (liquid filling)
Choroid layer
Retina
Sclera
Fovea centralis
Optic nerve
Central retinal artery and vein

FIGURE 25-1 Anatomy of the eye.

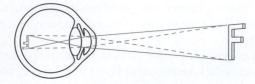

FIGURE 25-2 The eye as a camera.

(turned upside down). In a young pair of eyes, the lens of the eye can modify its shape to change focus from far distance to near distance.

The light progresses through the vitreous humor and then back to a clear focus on the retina and macula (see Figure 25-2).

If the eye is comparable to a camera, the retina would be considered the film inside the camera, registering the tiny photons of light that interact with it. Inside the retina, millions of tiny receptor cells, called *photoreceptors*, absorb the light energy and trigger nerve impulses.

The two types of photoreceptors are called rods and cones. *Rods* are the elongated, rod-shaped receptor cells that function best in low light. They are used for peripheral and night vision as well as in the perception of shape, size, and brightness. *Cones* are conical receptor cells that function best in bright light; they enhance the perception of fine detail and color.

Nerve impulses from the cones and rods are sent as electrical signals along the optic nerve to the occipital lobe at the posterior of the brain. This part of the brain interprets the electrical signals as visual images. Therefore, it is actually the brain that "sees"; the eyes only aid in the visual process (primarily as light collectors).

Diseases of the Eyes

The eyes are prone to many diseases and disorders, including infection, vision problems, and allergic reactions. With most common **ophthalmic** products, side effects are minimal, but may include localized ocular toxicity and hypersensitivity, including eyelid itching and swelling, and conjunctival redness. Ophthalmic products must be sterile, pH-balanced, clear, and particle-free; they are typically used for dry eyes, infection, inflammation, and allergies. This chapter discusses infections and vision disorders. The treatment of allergic reactions involving the eyes, with antiallergenic agents, antihistamines, artificial tears, and anti-inflammatory products, is addressed in a later chapter.

---

ophthalmic pertaining to the eye.

stye an infection of one (or more) of the sebaceous glands of the eye.

hordeolum an infection of one (or more) of the sebaceous glands of the eye.

blepharitis an inflammation of the eyelid margins accompanied by redness.

conjunctivitis an acute or chronic inflammation of the conjunctiva.

mucopurulent containing or composed of mucus and pus.

Eye Infections and Pharmaceutical Treatment

This section describes some common infections of the eye and the pharmaceutical treatment of those infections.

Stye

A **stye** or **hordeolum** is a localized infection of the sebaceous gland in a hair follicle at the base of an eyelash. Although visual acuity is unchanged, a stye is accompanied by redness, swelling, and eyelid pain. If the infection is deep within the lid, it is called a *meibomianitis* or *internal hordeolum*, and is sometimes accompanied by conjunctivitis and purulent drainage. Anti-infective eye drops are instilled into the lower conjunctival sac, and warm tap water or cold compresses can be applied for 10 minutes per hour, or 20 minutes four times a day, to control inflammation.

Staphylococcus aureus and *Staphylococcus epidermidis* are the most likely causative agents, so treatment is with antibiotics. Topical antibiotics are usually ineffective. Styes typically disappear on their own, and therefore oral antibiotic therapy is usually not warranted. In rare cases, though, oral antibiotic therapy could include a 10-day course of one of the following:

- Dicloxacillin 250 mg po q6h
- Erythromycin 250 mg po qid
- Tetracycline 250 mg po qid
- Amoxicillin 500 mg po tid

Blepharitis

Blepharitis is an inflammation of the eyelid margins, accompanied by redness, thickening, and possibly the formation of scales and crusts or shallow marginal ulcers. Ulcerative blepharitis is considered acute, whereas seborrheic blepharitis and meibomian gland dysfunction (meibomitis) are chronic types of blepharitis. The latter is often associated with acne rosacea. To treat ulcerative blepharitis, use one of the following antibiotic ointments for seven to ten days:

- Bacitracin/polymyxin B
- Gentamicin 0.3% qid

To treat seborrheic blepharitis, improve hygiene, use diluted baby shampoo to clean the eyelids, and remove greasy buildup.

To treat meibomian gland dysfunction, use oral antibiotic: doxycycline 100 mg po bid, over three to four months tapered down over the course of therapy.

Conjunctivitis

Conjunctivitis is the acute or chronic inflammation of the conjunctiva caused by a virus, bacteria, allergy, or irritant wind, smoke, or snow. Conjunctivitis has four major causes: allergies, bacteria, viruses, and chlamydia. Conjunctivitis can accompany the common cold and *exanthems* (viral rashes), such as rubella, measles, chicken pox (varicella), and mumps.

Allergic Conjunctivitis

Allergic conjunctivitis, or *redeye,* is caused by hay fever, dust, mite dander, or animal dander. Allergic conjunctivitis usually affects both eyes; symptoms include itching, swelling, and tearing (see Figure 25-3). Allergic conjunctivitis is usually seasonal and is not contagious.

Bacterial Conjunctivitis

Bacterial conjunctivitis often starts in one eye but soon spreads to the other. It usually includes a thick, sticky **mucopurulent** discharge that causes the eyelids and eyelashes to be matted or pasted shut upon awakening. There may be mild sensitivity to light (*photophobia*) with some discomfort, but usually no pain. Visual function is normal in most cases. The eye creates its own bacteriostatic lysozymes and immunoglobulins in the tear film, contributing to its strong immune defense. The eye will fight to return to homeostasis, and the infecting bacteria will eventually be destroyed.

However, an extra-heavy load of external organisms can overpower the immune system, causing a conjunctival infection and setting the eye up for potential corneal infection. Therefore, antibiotics should be given to avoid such a possibility.

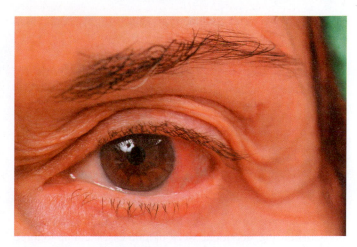

FIGURE 25-3 Bacterial conjunctivitis.
Source: Levent Konuk/Shutterstock

A broad-spectrum ophthalmic antibiotic, treating both gram-positive and gram-negative organisms, and an anti-inflammatory agent will treat both the infection and the inflammation (see Table 25-1). A wet, sticky, matted-shut eyelid is usually

TABLE 25-1 Prescription Treatments for Conjunctivitis

Generic Name	Brand Name	Dosage Forms and Availability	Route of Administration	Common Adult Dosage
erythromycin	Ilotycin	3.5-gm tube, 1-gm plastic container	Ophthalmic	$^1/_2$ inch two to eight times daily; in neonates, the ointment is applied once within one hour of birth
gentamicin	Genoptic (solution) Garamycin (ophthalmic ointment)	1 mL in 5-mL bottle	Ophthalmic	Solution: one to two gtts q2-3h; ointment: apply $^1/_2$ inch q3–4h, bid-tid
idoxuridine	Dendrid (Viroptic, Vira-A, VIGIV)	7.5-mL bottle	Ophthalmic	Initially, 1 gtt q1h during day and q2h at night; may decrease over time
natamycin	Natacyn (suspension)	15-mL fill packaged in 15-mL bottle	Ophthalmic	1 gtt four to six times daily or a minimum of 14 days
sulfacetamide sodium	Bleph-10	5 mL in 10-mL bottle	Ophthalmic	1-2 gtts q1-4h initially; for ointment, apply a thin ribbon qid and hs
tobramycin	(solution and ointment)	2.5-mL, 5-mL, 10-mL drop-container dispenser	Ophthalmic	Solution: 1-2 gtts q 4 h; ointment: apply bid-tid
trifluridine	Viroptic	7.5-mL bottle	Ophthalmic	1 gtt q 2 h while awake for a maximum of 9 gtts; may decrease to 1 gtt q 4 h while awake (for seven days) for a maximum of 7 gtts/day
vidarabine	Vira-A (ointment)	3.5-gm tube	Ophthalmic	Apply thin ribbon to lower eyelid five times daily at three-hour intervals

indicative of bacterial conjunctivitis that is highly contagious (see Table 25-1).

Viral Conjunctivitis

Viral conjunctivitis or *pinkeye* has a short duration and is usually self-limiting, about one week in mild cases and up to three weeks in severe cases. It usually follows an upper respiratory infection or results from contact with someone who is infected. No treatment or cure is currently available. Symptoms, however, can often be relieved with lubricants and cold compresses. If it is suspected that a bacterial infection is also present, treat with ophthalmic antibiotics, such as sulfacetamide sodium 10% drops or trimethoprim/polymyxin B for seven to ten days. A matted-down, shut eyelid with a crust is indicative of viral conjunctivitis, which is contagious.

Conjunctivitis Caused by Chlamydia

Conjunctivitis may be caused by the sexually transmitted disease chlamydia. Often referred to as *neonatal inclusion conjunctivitis* or *swimming pool conjunctivitis*, newborns can acquire the infection from their mothers as they pass through the birth canal. Neonates are treated with erythromycin 12.5 mg/kg po or IV qid for 14 days, because pneumonia and other complications may result from untreated conjunctivitis.

Infected mothers and their sexual partners are also treated to cure the conjunctivitis and concomitant genital infection with one of the following:

- Azithromycin 1 gm po once
- Doxycycline 100 mg po bid for one week
- Erythromycin 500 mg po qid for one week

Table 25-2 lists various topical ophthalmics used for ocular infections.

TABLE 25-2 Various Topical Ophthalmics Used for Ocular Infections

Trade Name	Generic Name	Indication	SIG
Antibacterials (ABs)			
Aminoglycosides			
Tobrex	tobramycin, 0.3% solution or ointment	Bacterial conjunctivitis, corneal infections	1 to 2 gtts q4h
			Severe infections: 2 gtts q1h until improvement, then the above regimen. Apply ribbon ung q3–4h
Genoptic	gentamicin	Bacterial conjunctivitis, corneal infections	1 to 2 gtts q4h
Garamycin Ophthalmic	gentamicin, 0.3% ophthalmic solution	Bacterial conjunctivitis, corneal ulcers, blepharitis	Severe infections: 2 gtts q1h
Erythromycins			
Ilotycin	erythromycin, 0.5% ophthalmic ointment	Neonatal inclusion or chlamydial, *Neisseria gonorrhea*, or swimming pool conjunctivitis	Apply approximately 1-cm ribbon ung not to exceed (NTE) six times daily
Sulfur-Based			
Bleph-10	sulfacetamide sodium, 10% ophthalmic solution	Bacterial infections that may or may not accompany viral infection (secondary infections)	1 to 2 gtts q2–3h, tapered down for 7 to 10 days
Combination Antibiotics			
Maxitrol	polymixin B sulfate, neomycin, and bacitracin zinc (ointment)	Blepharitis, nongonococcal bacterial and adult gonococcal conjunctivitis	Apply 1-cm ribbon ung, q2h qid

TABLE 25-2 Various Topical Ophthalmics Used for Ocular Infections (*Continued*)

Trade Name	Generic Name	Indication	SIG
			In addition, single dose of ceftriaxone 1 gm IM or ciprofloxacin 500 mg bid po for five days
Polytrim	polymixin B sulfate, trimethoprim sulfate, and gentamicin 0.3%	Bacterial infections, blepharitis, nongonococcal bacterial and adult gonococcal conjunctivitis	Apply 1-cm ribbon ung, q2h qid
Fluoroquinalones (ABs)			
Ciloxan	ciprofloxacin	Bacterial infections caused by stubborn resistant *Pseudomonas*	1 to 2 gtts qid q1h for the first few days
Ocuflox	ofloxacin, 0.3% solution	Same as above	1 to 2 gtts q2–4h for two days, then 1 to 2 gtts q4h for seven days
Chibroxin	norfloxacin, 0.3%	Same as above	1 to 2 gtts q4h for seven days
Combination Drugs			
Tobradex	tobramycin and dexamethasone; antibacterial and steroid combinations for infection and inflammation	Bacterial conjunctivitis, corneal ulcers	Apply approximately ribbon ung, NTE qid
			1 to 2 gtts q4–6h
Antivirals			
Viroptic	trifluridine, 1% solution (a pyrimidine [thymidine] analog activated by cellular thymidine kinase)	Epithelial keratitis caused by herpes simplex virus and keratoconjunctivitis (works by inhibition of DNA polymerase; DOC in the United States for topical ophthalmic antiviral therapy as it is least vulnerable to resistant strains)	To cornea: 1 gtt q2h NTE 9 gtts/day, then 1 gtt q4h and tapered thereafter
Vira-A	vidarabine, 3% ointment	Acute keratoconjunctivitis, epithelial keratitis caused by herpes simplex virus 1 and 2 (interferes with early steps of viral DNA synthesis; rapidly metabolizes to Ara-Hx)	Ribbon q3h, NTE five doses per day
Herplex (halogenated pyrimidine derivatives)	idoxuridine, 0.1% solution and ointment	Acute keratoconjunctivitis, epithelial keratitis caused by herpes simplex virus 1 and 2 (slows growth of viruses by blocking reproduction; produces incorrect DNA copies, thus preventing the virus from replicating and infecting or destroying tissue)	Ointment: ribbon q4h. Solution: 1 gtt q1h in morning, q2h in evening

TABLE 25-2 Various Topical Ophthalmics Used for Ocular Infections (*Continued*)

Trade Name	Generic Name	Indication	SIG
Antihistamines			
Emadine	emedastine difumarate, 0.05% ophthalmic solution	Allergic conjunctivitis (antihistamine prevents H-1 from binding on the eye cell, thus preventing itching, watering, and redness)	1 gtt in the affected eye, NTE qid
Livostin 0.05%	levocabastine, 0.05% suspension	Allergic conjunctivitis (antihistamine for seasonal allergic conjunctivitis. MOA—same as above)	1 gtt qid
Patanol	olopatadine, 0.1%	Allergic conjunctivitis (antihistamine. MOA—same as above)	1 gtt bid or q6–8h
Mast Cell Stabilizers			
Alomide	lodoxamide, 0.1% solution	Allergic conjunctivitis (mast cell inhibitors prevent allergic reactions) and for vernal keratoconjunctivitis, vernal conjunctivitis	1–2 gtts qid, NTE three months
Crolom	cromolyn sodium, 4%	Allergic conjunctivitis	1–2 gtts qid
Alamast	pemirolast potassium, 0.01%	Allergic conjunctivitis	1–2 gtts qid
Anti-Inflammatory Agents			
Acular	ketorolac	Any conjunctivitis (for NSAID anti-inflammatories MOA, see Chapter 23 regarding inflammation process and site of action of ASA, NSAIDs, and COX-2 inhibitors)	1 gtt qid
Eflone, Forte Liquifilm, FML Liquifilm, FML S.O.P. 0.1% ointment	fluorometholone, 0.1% suspension or ointment	Any conjunctivitis (MOA of topical corticosteroids for inflammation in stubborn cases of conjunctivitis, keratitis, iritis—inducing phospholipase A2 inhibitory proteins responsible for controlling the biosynthesis of prostaglandins and leukotrienes, thereby reducing or inhibiting the release of arachidonic acid and interfering with the inflammation cycle)	1–2 gtts bid, tid, and qid
Pred Forte	prednisolone acetate, 0.12% to 1.0%	Any conjunctivitis (MOA of topical corticosteroids for inflammation in stubborn cases—same as above)	1 gtt q1–6h (Caution: Use may cause glaucoma)

TABLE 25-2 Various Topical Ophthalmics Used for Ocular Infections (*Continued*)

Trade Name	Generic Name	Indication	SIG
Decongestants/Vasoconstrictors			
Naphcon, Allerest, Clear Eyes	naphazoline HCl, 0.1% solution	Allergic conjunctivitis (decongestant vasoconstrictor returns blood to its origin, reducing redness)	1 gtt bid to qid, NTE five days
OcuClear, Visine LR	oxymetazolone, 0.025% solution	Same as above	1–2 gtts qid
Visine, Murine Plus	tetrahydrozoline, 0.05% solution	Same as above	1–2 gtts bid to tid
Combination Drugs			
Naphcon-A	naphazoline HCl/pheniramine maleate, 0.1% solution (decongestant with an antihistamine)	Allergic conjunctivitis (MOA—vasoconstriction, while antihistamine prevents H1 binding on eye cells)	1 gtt bid to qid NTE five days
Zaditor	ketotifen fumarate, 0.025% (antihistamine—mast cell stabilizer with anti-inflammatory properties)	Allergic conjunctivitis (MOA—antihistamine binds to H-1 receptors of the eyes, preventing allergic response; mast cell stabilizer prevents H-1 release, decreasing chemotaxis and activation of eosinophils; inhibits proinflammatory mediators)	1 gtt q8–12h (patients over three years of age)

Eye Disorders That Affect Vision

Eye infections are usually self-limiting; only severe infections require treatment with antibiotics. Infections rarely contribute to vision problems. This section addresses eye diseases that affect the function of the eye and contribute to irreversible vision problems; we also discuss treatments available for these diseases and conditions.

Glaucoma

Glaucoma is one of the leading causes of permanent blindness, affecting more than 2 million Americans. Glaucoma is a slow, progressive disease that increases the **intraocular** pressure and decreases the outflow of the aqueous humor. Visual impairment is irreversible and permanent. Blindness from glaucoma is inevitable, as there is no cure for glaucoma. However, its progress can be slowed with proper care.

---

glaucoma a group of eye diseases characterized by an increase in intraocular pressure.

intraocular within the eye.

asymptomatic showing no evidence of disease or disordered condition.

Groups at high risk include the following:

- African-Americans
- Asians
- Patients who have family members with glaucoma
- Patients who have had eye injury
- Steroid users
- Persons over the age of 60

Other risk factors include the following:

- Nearsightedness
- Diabetes
- Hypertension (HTN)

Glaucoma is usually **asymptomatic**. In most cases, detection and prevention of the disease is through glaucoma screening during routine eye examinations (see Figure 25-4).

There are two main types of glaucoma: open angle and closed angle. Patients with glaucoma should consult with their physician before taking any OTC medication. Antihistamines, decongestants, and vasoconstrictors may worsen their condition, as these drugs can increase intraocular pressure (IOP).

Open-Angle Glaucoma

Open-angle glaucoma, or *wide-angle glaucoma*, constitutes about 90% of all cases of glaucoma.

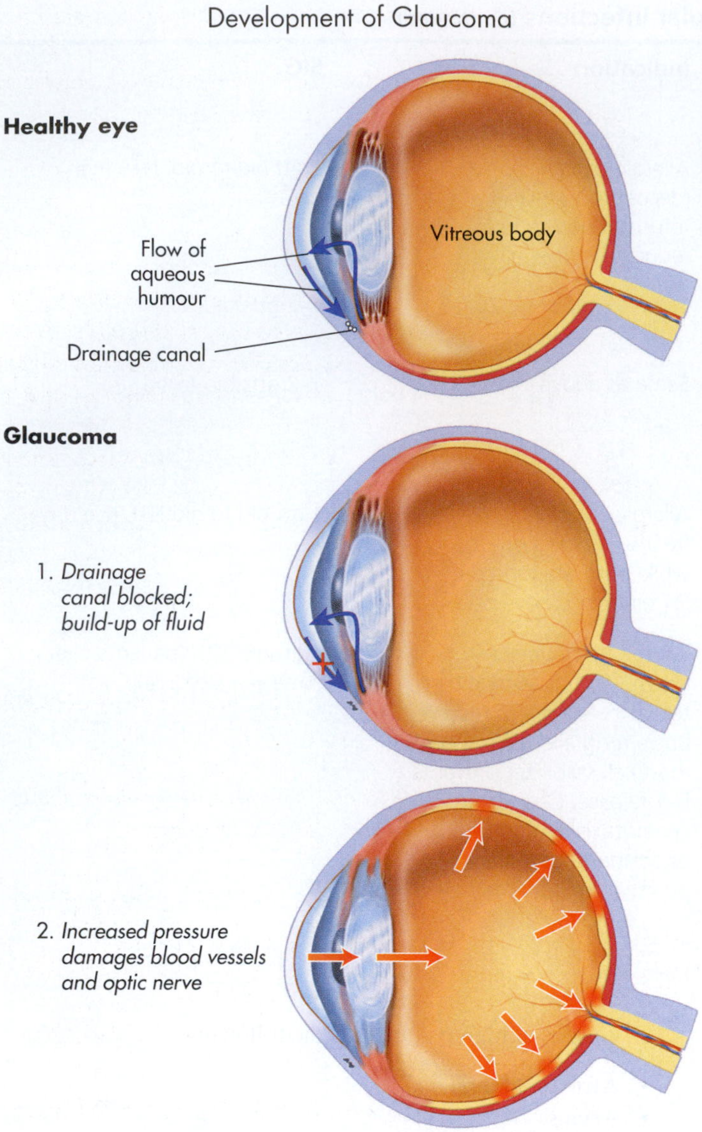

Development of Glaucoma

Healthy eye

Flow of aqueous humour

Drainage canal

Vitreous body

Glaucoma

1. *Drainage canal blocked; build-up of fluid*

2. *Increased pressure damages blood vessels and optic nerve*

FIGURE 25-4 The development of glaucoma.

It is defined as an increase in IOP due to abnormality in the trabecular meshwork that controls flow of aqueous humor between the anterior chamber and the canal of Schlemm. In this disorder, the canal is impaired and does not allow the fluid to return to the blood system. Because the fluid does not drain fast enough, IOP builds up and creates pressure against the optic nerve. If not treated, the condition can lead to a gradual loss of vision. Three basic treatments are available: medication, laser surgery, and filtration surgery. The goal of treatment is to lower the pressure in the eye.

iridotomy an incision made in the iris of the eye to enlarge the pupil.

cataract a condition in which the lens becomes opaque and interferes with the transmission of light to the retina

retinopathy a noninflammatory disease in which the retina has become damaged

Closed-Angle Glaucoma

In *closed-angle* or *narrow-angle glaucoma*, the anterior chamber of the eye (the space between the cornea and iris) fills with aqueous humor and the iris becomes misshapen. The edge of the iris blocks drainage of the humor, causing an increase in pressure. Closed-angle is the least common and most devastating form of glaucoma.

Although patients with open-angle glaucoma do not experience symptoms, those with closed-angle glaucoma may. Symptoms can come on rapidly, and should be considered an emergency, as blindness can occur within three to five days if left untreated. Symptoms include the following:

- Sudden intermittent changes in IOP due to extensive and prolonged pupil dilation
- Ocular pain or inflammation
- Blurred vision
- Headache
- Pressure over the eye
- A cloudy cornea
- Extreme sensitivity to light, or seeing halos around lights
- Nausea and/or vomiting
- Moderate pupil dilation that is not reactive to light

The cause is usually an inherited anatomic deformity of the anterior chamber, which predisposes it to be or to become narrow so that aqueous humor cannot freely flow or drain. In addition to heredity, any one of the following may precipitate closure of the anterior chamber:

- Defect in the eye chamber
- Anything that causes the pupil to dilate (dim lighting, dilation, drops for eye examinations)
- Certain oral or injected medications
- Blow to the eye
- Diabetes-related growth of abnormal blood vessels over the angle
- Most at risk are those who are Asians, farsighted, or over the age of 60. People in these groups should have their pressure checked every year or two.

Secondary Glaucoma

Secondary glaucoma occurs as the result of an eye injury, inflammation, tumor, advanced cases of cataracts, or diabetes, or it can be induced by use of drugs such as steroids. This form of glaucoma may be mild or severe, and may be either open-angle or closed-angle glaucoma. Treatment is the same as that for primary glaucoma.

Many cortisone-like drugs are widely used to treat a variety of conditions, such as asthma, poison ivy, arthritis, and other inflammatory conditions. Such drugs as ingredients in eyedrops

info

Glaucoma Statistics

Glaucoma has caused more than 5 million people to lose their vision worldwide (50,000 in the United States alone). It is most prevalent in those over 60 years of age.

or eye ointments may cause secondary glaucoma; people with existing primary glaucoma must be sure not to use them. Corticosteroids that are injectable, oral, or topically applied to the skin are not a danger to most patients. However, after glaucoma patients undergo a guarded filtration procedure, in which a new drain is made, postsurgical use of such corticosteroids will be required for approximately one month to reduce inflammation and prevent scarring that could close the new drain.

Oral medications taken for high blood pressure can cause problems for people with glaucoma. Therefore, it is advisable for glaucoma patients to try to control their blood pressure by nonmedicinal means, such as weight reduction and exercise. When lifestyle changes are not effective, antihypertensive medications will be indicated, but the glaucoma must be carefully monitored because it can worsen.

Fluid is constantly flowing into and out of the eye. If that flow is blocked, the pressure inside the eye rises. Oral cold remedies may contain drugs that enlarge or dilate the pupil by causing the iris to constrict. These prescription drugs are atropine or atropine-like products. (The same compound can be found in Lomotil for diarrhea.) The dilated pupil places pressure on the drain, preventing the release of aqueous humor, because outflow channels are blocked by the iris when the pupil is enlarged. Psychotropic agents and *tranquilizers* also dilate the pupil. Therefore, people with narrow anterior chamber angles are at risk for developing elevated IOP when their pupils are dilated (as in the dark, or from the use of eyedrops or oral medications that dilate the pupil). The FDA requires labels on these agents to warn consumers that the medications may cause glaucoma and should not be used by persons with existing glaucoma. Those who have had **iridotomy** are not at risk of new closure by such drugs.

Drugs for glaucoma either decrease the formation of aqueous humor, increase the outflow of aqueous humor, or both (see Table 25-3). The newest type of antiglaucoma agent, a prostanoid selective FP receptor agonist, works by increasing the outflow of aqueous humor by two routes: the canal of Schlemm and trabecular meshwork, and the uveoscleral route (see Table 25-3).

Cataracts

A **cataract** is a condition in which the lens becomes opaque and interferes with the transmission of light to the retina; the vision becomes less sharp, less colorful, and less intense. It is a myth that a *film* grows on the eyes; rather, a cataract develops within the eye. The lens becomes opaque when old cells of the lens die and become trapped within the capsule that contains the lens. The cells then accumulate over time, causing the lens to cloud and images to look blurred or doubled. Cataracts are usually a natural result of aging; however, eye injuries, diseases (diabetes and alcoholism), and certain medications can cause cataracts. They can be treated only with surgery in which the clouded lens is replaced with a clear, plastic lens. The four causes of cataracts are the following:

1. Congenital—hereditary, or measles infection during the first trimester.
2. Trauma—injury to the lens.

3. Age—85% of people over 80 years of age have some clouding of the lens.
4. Metabolic and toxic agents—induced by diabetes, smoking, or taking certain drugs (digoxin, alcohol).

Table 25-4 lists the prescription treatments for cataracts.

Vascular Retinopathies

Vascular **retinopathy** is a noninflammatory disease in which the retina has become damaged. It is important to understand that there are many causes, including diabetes and HTN. There is no pharmaceutical treatment for the many different types of retinopathies; however, some retinopathies may respond to laser treatment.

A technician should pay attention and listen to a patient who mentions visual disturbances while taking specific medications. Report all discussions to the pharmacist, who has better knowledge and understanding of the side effects and interactions of the drugs and may contact the patient's physician about further observation and testing.

Types of Retinopathies

1. *Simple* or *nonproliferative* retinopathies are characterized by defective bulging of vessel walls, which causes bleeding into the eye. The bulging is caused by small clumps of dead retinal cells, called *cotton wool exudates*, and by closed vessels. This form of retinopathy is considered mild.
2. *Proliferative* retinopathies are severe forms characterized by newly grown blood vessels and scar tissue formed within the eye, by closed-off blood vessels that are badly damaged, and by the retina breaking away or detaching from the surrounding mesh of blood vessels that nourish it.

In general, many retinopathies occur due to the following sequence of events. Blood flow to the retina is disrupted, by either blockage or breakdown of the various vessels. Bleeding or hemorrhage occurs, and fluid, cells, and proteins known as *exudates* leak into the area. A lack of oxygen to surrounding tissues (*hypoxia*) or decreased blood flow results; ischemia may lead to necrosis of the retina or other ocular tissue. This stimulates production of certain chemicals by the body, which in turn causes new blood vessels to grow. This new growth is called *neovascularization*. However, these new vessels generally leak blood, causing further problems. The retina may swell, and adversely affect vision, or the retina may detach completely. The following are common causes of retinopathies:

- Certain medications—medications such as chloroquine, thioridazine, and large doses of tamoxifen, can cause the arteries and veins to become blocked, resulting in a retinal artery or vein occlusion.
- Microaneurysms or bleeding into the vitreous humor.
- Direct sunlight exposure—for example, looking directly at the sun during an eclipse can cause *solar retinopathy*.

TABLE 25-3 Prescription Treatments for Glaucoma

Generic Name	Brand Name	Dosage Forms and Availability	Route of Administration	Common Adult Dosage
betaxolol	Betoptic	2.5-mL, 5-mL, 10-mL, 15-mL bottle	Ophthalmic	1 gtt bid
bimatoprost	Lumigan	2.5-mL fill in a 5-mL container, 5-mL fill in a 10-mL container, 7.5-mL fill in a 10-mL container	Ophthalmic	1 gtt qd in evening
brimonidine	Alphagan P	5-mL fill in 10-mL bottle, 10-mL fill in 15-mL bottle	Ophthalmic	1 gtt tid
brinzolamide	Azopt	5-mL, 10-mL, 15-mL plastic DROP-TAINER dispensers	Ophthalmic	1 gtt of 1% tid
carbachol	Miostat	2.0-mL glass vial with a 1.5-mL fill	Ophthalmic	No more than ½ mL instilled before or after securing sutures
carteolol	Octupress, carteolol hyrochloride	5-mL, 10-mL, 15-mL bottle	Ophthalmic	1 gtt bid
dipivefrin	Propine	5-mL, 10-mL, 15-mL bottle	Ophthalmic	1 gtt q12h
dorzolamide	Trusopt	10 mL in 18-mL bottle	Ophthalmic	1 gtt tid
latanoprost	Xalatan	2.5-mL bottle	Ophthalmic	1 gtt qd in evening
levobunolol	OptiPranolol, Betagan	2.5-mL, 5-mL, 10-mL, 15-mL bottle	Ophthalmic	1-2 gtts qd
methazolamide	Neptazane	25-mg, 50-mg tablets	Oral	50 mg to 100 mg bid-tid
metipranolol	Optipranolol	5-mL, 10-mL bottle	Ophthalmic	1 gtt bid
pilocarpine	Isopto Carpine	15-mL bottle	Ophthalmic	1 gtt of 1%, 2%, or 4% up to qid
timolol maleate	Timoptic,	5 mL in 7.5-mL bottle; 10 mL in 18-mL bottle	Ophthalmic	1 gtt of 0.25% bid. If clinical response is not adequate, the dosage may be changed to 1 gtt of 0.5% bid
travoprost	Travatan	2.5-mL fill, 5-mL fill	Ophthalmic	1 gtt qd in evening

TABLE 25-4 Prescription Treatments for Cataracts

Generic Name	Brand Name	Dosage Forms and Availability	Route of Administration	Common Adult Dosage
acetylcholine	Miochol-E	Vial of 20-mg acetylcholine chloride powder for intraocular solution, ampoule of 2-mL diluents	Ophthalmic	5-mg to 20-mg injection before or after suture is in place
diclofenac 1% solution	Voltaren	2.5-mL, 5-mL bottles	Ophthalmic	1–2 gtts within one hour before surgery; after surgery, 1 gtt qid for two weeks

- Neovascularizations or the formation of new blood vessels—these tend to be fragile, leak protein, and bleed.
- Diabetes—diabetic retinopathies are confined to the retina and involve thickening of capillary walls and microaneurysm formation, followed by rupture and bleeding into the retina. In proliferative diabetic retinopathies, the retina bleeds into the vitreous humor.
- Central vein occlusion—this is often secondary to HTN, diabetes mellitus, or sickle cell anemia; it causes a rapid deterioration of visual acuity.
- Atherosclerosis—*atherosclerotic retinopathy* is the hardening or thickening of the retinal arteries.
- Retinal artery occlusion—the complete blockage of an artery to the retina; it results in sudden, unilateral blindness (one-eye or one-sided anopsia).
- Hypertension—*hypertensive retinopathy* is damage to the retinal arteries caused by high blood pressure.
- Syphilis—*syphilitic retinopathy* occurs when the retina becomes infected by the spirochete that causes syphilis.

Macular Degeneration

Macular degeneration is the deterioration of the macula, the small central portion of the eye. The condition generally occurs in older individuals. Treatments can include antiangiogenic drugs, laser therapy, photodynamic therapy, vitamins, and low-vision aids.

Cycloplegic Drugs, Mydriatic Drugs, and Lubricants

Certain drugs help ophthalmologists examine their patients' eyes. Drugs that relax the ciliary muscle are called **cycloplegic** drugs. Drugs that dilate the pupils are known as **mydriatic** drugs. People with dilated pupils may experience blurred vision for approximately two to four hours. When pupils are dilated, brilliant lights may be bothersome. Dark glasses should be worn until the dilation subsides.

Lubricants restore moisture to a dry eye. Dry eyes may result from exposure to the elements, such as sun or wind; to chemicals, such as chlorine; to allergens; or to some medications.

Originally responding to possible injury or infection, the immune system sends white blood cells and other mediators in the blood to the eye. With more blood, the whites of the eye get redder as blood vessels dilate (open up) to accommodate the influx of blood. Vasoconstrictors or decongestants return blood

when the mediators are no longer needed. Vasoconstriction therapy should be short-term, as a rebound effect will occur with long-term use.

The rebound effect happens after the swelling subsides, and the redness goes away. At that point, the blood vessels become dilated again to counter the vasoconstrictive effect of the medication. This paradoxical overcompensation, or *self-correcting* action, causes the blood vessels to dilate even more, resulting in a tolerance after two to five days. Because the blood vessels have dilated so much, they tend not to constrict well anymore, and the patient needs more drug to counter this residual dilation. The rebound effect will continue with prolonged use of vasoconstricting medications; therefore, the long-term use of vasoconstrictors should be avoided. In fact, some research suggests a connection between long-term use of vasoconstrictors and glaucoma.

❝ Workplace Wisdom **Ophthalmic Medications**

All ophthalmic medication and containers must remain *sterile*. ❞

---

macular degeneration happens when the macula deteriorates.

cycloplegic causing relaxation and paralysis of the intraocular muscles.

mydriatic drugs used to dilate the pupils

Ophthalmic Conversion
Remember: 1 inch = 2.54 cm

■ Procedure 25-2

Applying an Ophthalmic Ointment

In addition to the basic guidelines for applying an ophthalmic medication described in Procedure 25-1, patients should follow these instructions when using an ophthalmic ointment (Figure 25-5). Note that the stream of oil-based ointment is measured by the length of the *ribbon* that comes out of the tube. The measurement can be stated in either centimeters or inches.

1. Hold the tube between your thumb and forefinger. Place it near the eye, but not touching any part of the eye or the eyelid. Tilt your head forward slightly.
2. With the index finger of your other hand, pull the lower eyelid down to form a "V" pocket. Squeeze the tube, and place a ribbon of ointment or gel into the "V" pocket made by the opened lower eyelid. Do not let the tip of the tube touch the eye.
3. Blink the eye gently; do not squeeze lids together. Close the eye for one to two minutes.

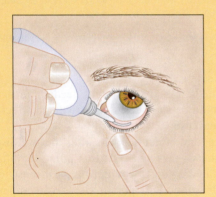

FIGURE 25-5 Applying an ophthalmic ointment.

■ Procedure 25-3

How to Instill an Ophthalmic Solution

Ophthalmic liquid medications must be instilled; otherwise, the medication will immediately drain from the tear duct area. In addition to the basic instructions described in Procedures 25-1 and 25-2, patients should follow these specific instructions for instilling a liquid into the eye (Figure 25-6).

1. Uncap the container, tilt the head back slightly, and look at the ceiling.
2. Use the index finger to gently pull down on the lower eyelid to form a pocket.
3. Position the dropper above the eye. Look up and away from the dropper.
4. Squeeze out the prescribed number of drops and gently close the eye.
5. Apply gentle pressure to the inside corner of the closed eye (near the nose) for about one minute to prevent the liquid from draining down from the tear duct.
6. If using drops in both eyes, repeat the process in the other eye.

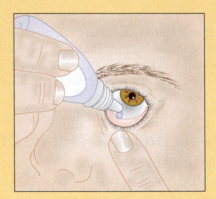

FIGURE 25-6 Instilling ophthalmic drops.

❝ Workplace Wisdom Ophthalmic Suspensions

Ophthalmic suspensions must be mixed properly before administration. Shake the bottle gently or roll it in your hand before administering the medication.

Tables 25-5 through 25-7 list prescription treatments for allergy, inflammation, and infection.

The Ear

Hearing starts at the outer ear, as sound waves or vibrations travel down the external auditory canal and strike the eardrum. When the eardrum vibrates, the vibrations are passed to three tiny bones in the middle ear. These bones amplify the sound and send the sound waves to the inner ear and into the fluid-filled hearing organ, the *cochlea*. The cochlea is lined with

---

PROFILES IN PRACTICE

A customer requests a refill of a Tobradex ophthalmic suspension, which was prescribed for bacterial conjunctivitis. The patient explains that although the medication was used as prescribed, the infection has returned.

▶ *What are some possible reasons for the return of the customer's infection?*

▶ *If no refills are available on the prescription, what should the pharmacy do?*

TABLE 25-5 Prescription Treatments for Allergy

Generic Name	Brand Name	Dosage Forms and Availability	Route of Administration	Common Adult Dosage
emedastine	Emadine	5-mL DROP-TAINER dispensers	Ophthalmic	1–2 gtts bid-qid
lodoxamide	Alomide	10-mL DROP-TAINER dispenser	Ophthalmic	1–2 gtts bid-qid
nedocromil	Alocril	5 mL in 10-mL bottle	Ophthalmic	1–2 gtts bid

TABLE 25-6 Prescription Treatments for Inflammation

Generic Name	Brand Name	Dosage Forms and Availability	Route of Administration	Common Adult Dosage
dexamethasone	Decadron phosphate (solution and ointment), Maxidex (suspension)	0.75-mg, 0.5-mg tablets	Ophthalmic	1–2 gtts hourly during the daytime and every two hours at night until inflammation decreases; then decrease to usually every four hours
diclofenac 1% solution	Voltaren	20-gm tube (physician's sample), 100-gm tube NDC; three pack (three tubes containing 100 gm each); five pack (five tubes containing 100 gm each)	Ophthalmic	1 gtt qid
flurbipofen	Ocufen	2.5 mL in 6-mL bottle	Ophthalmic	1 gtt every 30 minutes beginning two hours before surgery for a total of 4 gtts
ketoprofen ophthalmic	Acular	3 mL in 5-mL bottle, 5 mL in 10-mL bottle, 10 mL in 10-mL bottle	Ophthalmic	1 gtt qid
prednisolone	Pred Forte	1 mL in 5-mL bottle, 5 mL in 10-mL bottle, 10 mL in 15-mL bottle, 15 mL in 15-mL bottle	Ophthalmic	1–2 gtts bid-qid

TABLE 25-7 Prescription Treatments for Infection

Generic Name	Brand Name	Dosage Forms and Availability	Route of Administration	Common Adult Dosage
fluorometholone/ sulfacetamide sodium	FML-S suspension	10 mL in 15-mL bottle, 5 mL in 10-mL bottle, 15 mL in 15-mL bottle	Ophthalmic	1–2 gtts bid-qid
gentamicin, prednisolone acetate	Pred-G	5 mL in 10-mL bottle, 10 mL in 15-mL bottle	Ophthalmic	1–2 gtts bid-qid
loteprednol etabonate, tobramycin	Zylet	2.5 mL in 7.5-mL bottle, 5 mL in 7.5-mL bottle, 10 mL in 10-mL bottle	Ophthalmic	1–2 gtts q4–6h

TABLE 25-7 Prescription Treatments for Infection (*Continued*)

Generic Name	Brand Name	Dosage Forms and Availability	Route of Administration	Common Adult Dosage
Neomycin/polymyxin B/bacitracin zinc	Neocidin	Ointment	Ophthalmic	Apply as directed
Sulfacetamide sodium/prednisone acetate	Blephamide	10%/0.2% ointment	Ophthalmic	Apply as directed
Tobramycin/ dexamethasone	TobraDex suspension	2.5-mL, 5-mL, 10-mL suspension container	Ophthalmic	1 gtt q4–6h

cells that have thousands of tiny hairs (*cilia*) on their surfaces. The sound vibrations make the tiny hairs move. By their movement, the hairs translate the sound vibrations into nerve signals, so that your brain can interpret the sound. The signals travel to the brain along special nerves. After the sound waves reach the inner ear, they are converted into electrical impulses, which the auditory nerve sends to the brain. The brain recognizes these electrical impulses as sound.

Anatomy and Physiology of the Ear

The ear has three major areas: the outer, middle, and inner ear (see Figure 25-7). The outer ear structures, commonly called the *flaps* and *ear lobes*, are the cartilaginous portion known technically as the *pinna* or *auricle*. The pinna acts as a preamplifier that enhances the sensitivity of hearing.

The *tympanic membrane* or *eardrum* receives the vibrations that travel up through the auditory canal. These vibrations

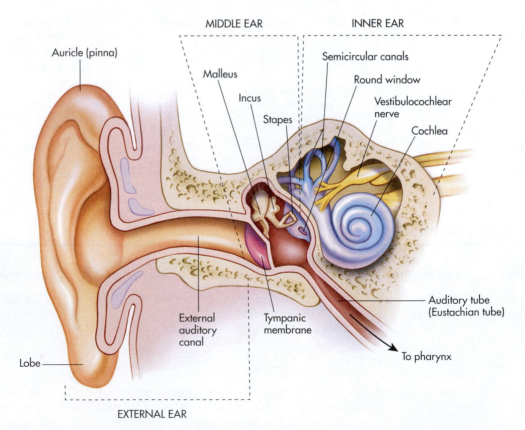

FIGURE 25-7 Anatomy of the ear.

are transferred to three of the smallest bones in the body, the *ossicles*, and then to the oval opening into the inner ear. The *malleus* or hammer, the *incus* or anvil, and the *stapes* or stirrup form the connection between the vibration of the eardrum and the forces exerted on the oval opening of the inner ear. The eardrum provides amplification of about 15 times more than the aural opening. The auditory canal acts as a closed-tube resonator, which boosts and improves sounds in the 2–5 kHz range. At the eardrum, sound energy (air pressure changes) is converted into the mechanical energy of eardrum movement.

External Ear

Without the ears, we would not be able to have the wonderful gift of hearing. The outside part of the ear consists of the pinna, concha, and the external auditory meatus. The outer workings of the ear gain sound and center it on the tympanic membranes. External parts of the ear boost sound pressure. Careful consideration should be taken with the ear in that sounds at high levels can cause hearing loss and/or damage.

Middle Ear

The middle ear is the space between the eardrum and inside of the ear that has three auditory ossicles that produce vibrations within the oval window to the cochlea area, which is also called the tympanum. The middle ear is often host to painful ear infections, which require immediate attention, as pain is unbearable and infection can also lead to hearing loss or other problems if untreated.

Eustachian Tube

The *eustachian tube* connects the middle ear with the nasopharynx of the throat. When a person swallows or coughs, this tube acts to equalize the pressure between the middle ear and the outer ear. Proper transfer of sound waves occurs when the pressure is the same. The eustachian tube is shorter in children and is often oriented more horizontally. It is, therefore, less likely to open and more likely to become blocked by enlarged adenoids. Fluid may collect within the middle-ear area of young children, causing temporary hearing loss and/or a feeling of fullness and pain. This condition is called *serous otitis media* (SOM). SOM may occur shortly after or during an upper respiratory infection when the child has nasal congestion. Allergy-induced congestion or SOM may require antihistamines to dry out the congestion and stop the allergic response that is causing it. SOM is most common among children younger than five years old.

Sometimes a person with SOM needs a *myringotomy*—the surgical relief of fluid pressure—or the surgical insertion of ventilation tubes into the middle ear. A patient with these tubes should avoid swimming, as water may contaminate the surgical site and cause a potentially serious infection.

The middle ear serves as an equalizer, matching the impedance of air in the ear canal to the impedance of the *perilymph* of the inner ear. Perilymph has the same makeup as cerebrospinal fluid, with a low potassium (K^+) concentration and a high sodium (Na^+) concentration. The scala tympani also contain perilymph.

Inner Ear

The inner ear, or the labyrinth of the ear, is the part of the ear located inside the temporal bone that is associated with both hearing and balance—it is also associated with the semicircular canals of the ear, vestibule, and cochlea part of the ear. The inner ear is also prone to infection along with the middle part of the ear. Infections should be taken care of as soon as they are noticed, as further problems or hearing loss can occur if left untreated.

Cochlea

The snail-shaped *cochlea* is the sensory organ of hearing, as it contains the auditory nerves. The wave-like patterns initiated by vibration of the stapes footplate causes a shearing of the cilia of the outer and inner hair cells. This process causes hair cell depolarization, which occurs in the organ of Corti within the scala media of the cochlea. This changes the vibrational energy into neural energy that is transmitted along the eighth cranial nerve to the brain, which interprets these impulses as sound.

Vestibular Labyrinth

The *vestibular labyrinth* is composed of the *saccule* and *utricle*, which are the sense organs for balance. The vestibular labyrinth contains the receptors for balance and notifies the brain about an individual's linear and rotational orientation and movement in space.

Disorders and Diseases of the Ear

This section discusses some common disorders and diseases of the ear.

Complications of Earwax Buildup

The skin of the outer part of the ear canal contains the ceruminous and sebaceous gland that produces earwax (*cerumen*). The purposes of earwax are to:

- Trap dust, dirt, insects, sand, and other particles, preventing them from getting into the eardrum
- Keep the eardrum moist
- Act as a water repellent
- Inhibit the growth of bacteria in the eardrum

In most cases, earwax accumulates in small quantities for a short period of time, carrying particles along with it as it dries and comes out of the ear. Earwax can migrate to the pinna, where it is easily wiped off. Earwax does not form in the deep part of the ear canal near the tympanic membrane. Normal amounts of earwax are healthy.

Dry, itchy ears may be a result of wax deficiency. The homeostasis of self-cleaning—that is, the process of producing earwax, which then dries, flakes, and falls out of the ear canal—is slow and constant. Sometimes, homeostasis is interrupted when the wax builds up against the eardrum. Using cotton swabs or other objects to "clean out" the ear serves only to push the earwax further inside. Continuous scratching of the ear canal, which is very thin skin and can be easily injured, can lead to pain and infection. Hearing aids can prevent the migration of earwax out of the canal.

Annual ear exams can prevent some temporary hearing loss. The audiologist may wash the ear out, vacuum it, or physically remove the wax with special instruments. OTC eardrops may be used to soften the earwax before the wash or suctioning.

Table 25-8 lists prescription treatments for cerumen buildup.

Workplace Wisdom Perforated Eardrums

If the eardrum has been punctured or perforated, infection may result from the use of water or presoftening eardrops. Examples of earwax softeners are Debrox and Murine Ear Drops (carbamide peroxide).

Types of Hearing Loss

Hearing loss may be caused by a number of factors. The most typical hearing losses, and the ones discussed in this section, are conductive, sensory, drug-induced, neural, and presbycusis.

Conductive Hearing Loss

Conductive hearing loss occurs when a problem exists with a part of the outer or middle ear. Usually this is a mild and temporary hearing loss, because, in most cases, medical treatment can help. Causes may include a blow to the head or ear, birth defects, malformation of parts of the outer or middle ear, a tiny hole or perforation in the eardrum, wax buildup in the ear canal, and middle-ear infections.

Sensory Hearing Loss

Sensory hearing loss occurs when the cochlea is not working correctly, because cilia have been damaged or destroyed. This

---

tinnitus

otitis media

problem can affect one or both of the ears. Depending on the extent of loss, sound may be muffled (mild loss), some sounds might become slightly inaudible (moderate loss), or no sounds at all may be heard (severe/profound loss). Speech may also be affected. Sensory hearing impairment is almost always permanent. It may be due to heredity factors or may occur during fetal developmental stages if the pregnant mother gets certain kinds of diseases, such as rubella (German measles). Other possible causes are certain medications, severe injury to the head, frequent listening to extremely loud music, and exposure to other loud noises (factory machinery, race cars, airplane engines).

Workplace Wisdom Hearing Impairments

According to the National Institute on Deafness and Other Communication Disorders, approximately 28 million Americans have some type of hearing impairment, and two to three out of every 1,000 infants born in the United States are deaf or hearing-impaired.

Drug-Induced Hearing Loss

Drug-induced hearing loss can occur with the use of some ototoxic drugs that impair hearing and balance. Hearing loss can be reversible (temporary) or irreversible (permanent). Drugs that may cause hearing loss (see Table 25-9) are found in several classifications, such as:

- IV aminoglycosides
- Loop diuretics
- Antineoplastic agents (anticancer drugs)
- Quinine-containing drugs

In addition, large doses of aspirin can cause ringing in the ears, or **tinnitus**.

Neural Hearing Loss

Neural hearing loss occurs when there is a problem with the connection from the cochlea to the brain. For example, when the nerve that carries the messages from the cochlea to the brain is damaged, neural hearing loss may result. This type of hearing loss is permanent.

TABLE 25-8 Prescription Treatments for Cerumen Buildup

Generic Name	Brand Name	Dosage Forms and Availability	Route of Administration	Common Adult Dosage
carbamide peroxide	Debrox	0.5 fl oz. bottle	Otic	Apply proper amount of eardrops into ear canal; leave for at least five minutes; may use cotton to plug ear
triethanolamine polypeptide oleate	Cerumenex	6-mL, 12-mL bottle	Otic	Fill ear canal with solution; allow the patient to sit for 15 to 30 minutes covering the ear with cotton ball; remove cotton, place tip of syringe into ear, and gently squeeze to allow wax and liquid to drain

TABLE 25-9 Drugs That May Cause Sensory Hearing Loss

Trade Name	Generic Name
Antibiotics	
Amikin	amikacin iv
Garamycin	gentamicin iv
Nebcin	tobramycin iv
Loop Diuretics	
Bumex	bumetanide
Demadex	torsemide
Edecrin	ethacrynic acid
Lasix	furosemide
Antineoplastic Agents	
Paraplatin	carboplatin
Platinol	cisplatin
Quinine Products (Selected)	
Aralen	chloroquine
Quinaglute Dura-tabs, Quinidex Extentab	quinidine
Quinine	quinine sulfate
Tonic water	

Presbycusis

Presbycusis is the permanent loss of hearing due to damaged hearing nerves. When hearing deteriorates with age, sensitivity to high-pitched sounds fades first. This is why people often say that they can hear sounds but cannot understand what is being said. Presbycusis develops slowly and gradually. *Recruitment*, a progression of presbycusis, is a loss of sensitivity to soft sounds and a decreased ability to tolerate loud sounds.

Otitis Media

One of the most common causes of conductive hearing loss is **otitis media**, an inflammation and infection of the middle ear that usually presents in one out of three children. Acute otitis media is an infection that produces pus, fluid, and inflammation within the middle ear; it is usually quite painful. Older children may complain of ear pain, a feeling of fullness in the ear, or hearing loss. Younger children may present with irritability; fussiness; or difficulty in sleeping, feeding, or hearing. Fever is usually present.

These symptoms are frequently associated with signs of upper respiratory infection, such as a runny or stuffy nose or a cough. Otitis media, the most common childhood illness, usually appears four to seven days after the respiratory infection. Severe ear infections may cause the eardrum to rupture. Immediate medical treatment is then necessary. More than 80% of all children will have at least one middle-ear infection before they are three years old. Usually, otitis is easily treatable; however, a temporary hearing loss may result. This conductive hearing loss may cause delays in speech and language development and lead to learning difficulties. If left untreated, permanent hearing loss, rupture of the tympanic membrane, and/or meningitis may develop (see Tables 25-10 and 25-11).

TABLE 25-10 Prescription Treatments for Otitis Media

Generic Name	Brand Name	Dosage Forms and Availability	Route of Administration	Common Adult Dosage
amoxicillin	Amoxil, Amoxil pediatric suspension	250-mg, 500-mg capsule; 500-mg, 875-mg tablets	Oral	Adult dose: 500 mg every 12 hours; pediatric: older than three months, 90 mg/kg daily divided doses every 12 hours
ciprofloxacin/dexamethasone otic suspension	Ciprodex	7.5-mL fill DROP-TAINER	Otic	4 gtts bid for seven days
ciprofloxacin/hydrocortisone otic suspension	Cipro HC	0.3% solution	Otic	3 gtts bid for seven days
sulfamethoxazole/trimethoprim suspension	Bactrim, Septra	80/400-mg, 160/800-mg tablets	Oral	Adult dose: 20 mL every 12 hours for 10 to 14 days; pediatric: two months and older children, dosage is based on weight

TABLE 25-11 Antibiotic Treatment for Otitis Media in Children

Trade Name	Generic Name	Trade Name	Generic Name
Prophylaxis		Biaxin	clarithromycin
Amoxil, Trimox, Wymox	amoxicillin	Cedax	ceftibuten
	sulfisoxazole (DOC)	Ceftin	cefuroxime axetil
First-Line Therapy		Cefzil	cefprozil
Bactrim	trimethoprim-sulfamethoxazole (TMP-SMX)	Lorabid	loracarbef
		Vantin	cefpodoxime proxetil
Septra (used for patients with penicillin allergy)	amoxicillin	Zithromax	azithromycin
Amoxil, Trimox, Wymox	amoxicillin	**Third-Line Therapy**	
Second-Line Therapy		Cleocin (used for resistant pneumococci)	clindamycin
Augmentin	amoxicillin and clavulanate potassium	Rocephin	ceftriaxone sodium

Summary

The most basic of all of our senses is sight. The anatomy and physiology of the eye are discussed extensively in this chapter.

The eyes are prone to many diseases, but eye infections are usually self-limiting and treatable; only on rare occasions do they lead to vision problems. More serious diseases, such as glaucoma, can cause irreversible vision problems.

A wide variety of treatment modalities is available to treat eye disorders. However, it is important that ophthalmic products be used safely and properly. One of your most important responsibilities as a pharmacy technician is to thoroughly understand the basics of safe use of ophthalmic remedies, so that you can properly handle these medications and help educate patients about their use.

The ear consists of three major areas: the outer, middle, and inner ear. The functions of the ear include hearing and the maintenance of equilibrium or balance. Like the eye, the ear is susceptible to a variety of disorders; most can normally be prevented, controlled, or reversed with treatment. Although easily treatable, common problems such as otitis media (a middle-ear infection) can lead to permanent hearing loss if left untreated. It is estimated that more than 80% of children will be affected with this disorder before they reach the age of three years.

Chapter Review Questions

1. _____ is an inflammation of the eyelid margins accompanied by redness.
   a. Conjunctivitis
   b. Blepharitis
   c. Retinopathy
   d. Glaucoma

2. Which part of the eye is composed of light-sensitive nerve endings that take visual impulses to the optic nerve?
   a. macula
   b. vitreous humor
   c. choroid
   d. retina

3. Inflammation of the thin lining that covers the white of the eyeball and inner surface of the eyelid is known as _____.
   a. conjunctivitis
   b. blepharitis
   c. retinopathy
   d. glaucoma

4. Treatment options for open-angle glaucoma include all of the below, *except* _____.
   a. laser surgery
   b. medication
   c. filtration surgery
   d. iridotomy

5. The most common childhood illness is _____.
   a. conjunctivitis
   b. glaucoma
   c. otitis media
   d. pink eye

6. The first line of therapy for otitis media includes which of the following drugs?
   a. clindamycin
   b. azithromycin
   c. clarithromycin
   d. amoxicillin

7. Ototoxicity caused by medications can lead to _____.
   a. conjunctivitis
   b. balance impairment
   c. infection
   d. otitis media

8. Otitis media is _____.
   a. a blockage in the tear ducts
   b. the first sign of the onset of glaucoma
   c. not curable
   d. an inflammation and infection of the middle ear

9. The pinna and lobe are part of the _____ ear.
   a. inner
   b. middle
   c. external
   d. none of the above

10. Which of the following drugs is not indicated for glaucoma?
    a. betaxolol
    b. latanoprost
    c. carbamide peroxide
    d. brinzolamide

Critical Thinking Questions

1. State which sense, eyesight or hearing, is more important to you, and explain why you would rather lose the other sense.

2. Explain why the eye is considered the body's camera.

3. Why do doctors often tell their patients not to "stick anything smaller than an elbow" in the ear?

Web Challenge

1. Visit http://www.glaucoma.org/ and find out what researchers are doing to find a cure for glaucoma. Write a one-page summary of your findings.

2. Go to http://visionsimulations.com to see how various eye diseases actually affect a person's vision. Select one disease and write a one-page description of its effects on vision along with treatment options.

3. Go to http://www.nidcd.nih.gov/ to learn more about diseases and conditions affecting the ear.

References and Resources

Adams, M.P., D.L. Josephson, and L.N. Holland, Jr. *Pharmacology for Nurses: A Pathophysiologic Approach.* (4th edition.) Upper Saddle River, NJ: Pearson, 2013.

"Anatomy, Physiology and Pathology of the Human Eye." http://www.tedmontgomery.com/the_eye/. 23 June 2007. Web.

"Beltone Interactive Internet Site for the Anatomy of the Ear." http://www.beltone.com/ear_anatomy/ear_anatomy.asp#. 24 June 2007. Web.

"Eye Anatomy." http://www.stlukeseye.com. 24 June 2007. Web.

Holland, N. and M.P. Adams. *Core Concepts in Pharmacology.* (3rd edition.) Upper Saddle River, NJ: Pearson, 2010.

"Lumigan® Package Insert." http://www.lumigan.com/pdfs/PI.pdf. 25 June 2007. Web.

"Review of Anatomy: The Ear and Temporal Bone." http://www.bcm.tmc.edu/oto/studs/anat/tbone.html#EAR. 25 June 2007. Web.

"Statistics About Hearing Disorders, Ear Infections, and Deafness." http://www.nidcd.nih.gov/. 25 June 2007. Web.

"Timolol®." http://www.rxlist.com/cgi/generic/timolol_cp.htm. 25 June 2007. Web.

"The Merck Manual of Diagnosis and Therapy." http://www.merck.com/mrkshared/mmanual/section8/chapter94/94c.jsp. 10 August 2013. Web.

"Web MD Reports." *Age-Related Macular Degeneration Treatment.* 4 December 2012. Web.

"What Is Glaucoma?" http://www.glaucoma.org. 25 June 2007. Web.

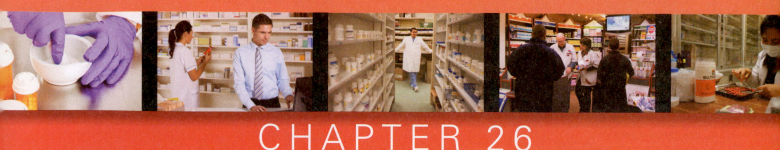

CHAPTER 26

The Gastrointestinal System

LEARNING OBJECTIVES

After completing this chapter, you should be able to:

- Identify the basic anatomical and structural parts of the digestive system.

- Describe the physiology of the digestive system.

- List and define common diseases affecting the gastrointestinal system and understand the causes, symptoms, and pharmaceutical treatments associated with each disease.

- List and describe the three main categories of nutrients.

- Identify the functions and AMDR of the macronutrients.

- State the difference between essential and nonessential amino acids.

- Identify the functions, symptoms of deficiencies, and reference daily intakes (RDIs) of the micronutrients.

- Understand the importance of water to the body.

KEY TERMS

acceptable macronutrient distribution range (AMDR), p. 410

antioxidant, p. 414

chyme, p. 398

dietary reference intake (DRI), p. 409

diverticulitis, p. 409

exogenous, p. 414

fortified, p. 412

high-density lipoprotein (HDL), p. 411

hypermetabolic, p. 413

hypersensitivity, p. 405

kilocalories (kcal), p. 410

lipid, p. 398

low-density lipoprotein (LDL), p. 411

malabsorption, p. 412

mastication, p. 397

monosaccharide, p. 398

pepsin, p. 398

pepsinogen, p. 398

protease, p. 398

mcg, p. 412

INTRODUCTION

The digestive system is responsible for adequate nourishment and hydration of the body. Without proper nourishment and hydration, body cells would die and, eventually, the body itself would die. The main purpose of the digestive system is to fuel the body so that it can continue to survive and function properly.

Lack of proper nutrition and digestion can lead to numerous disease states. The body needs the right amounts of macronutrients, micronutrients, and water to function properly. Nutrition guidelines and recommendations have been

---

mastication chewing.

established to help educate the public and make sure that people receive the correct amount of nutrients.

Anatomy and Physiology of the Digestive System

The digestive system, which extends from the mouth to the anus, is a long tube that twists and turns with a series of hollow organs along its length (see Figure 26-1). This tube is lined with protective mucosa that prevents acid from causing sores or ulcers. In the mouth, stomach, and small intestine, the mucosa also contains tiny glands that produce the liquid digestive juices that help digest food. These liquids contain enzymes and acids.

The liver and pancreas produce digestive juices that are sent to the intestine through small ducts. The liver produces *bile*, which is stored in the gallbladder, and the pancreas produces enzymes. In addition, accessory organs, nerves, and blood play a major role in the digestive system.

Rings of smooth muscle along the digestive tract produce a wave of synchronized contractions, called *peristalsis*, that help propel the food down the tube. The six main parts or organs of the digestive system are the following:

- Mouth
- Esophagus
- Pharynx
- Stomach
- Small intestine
- Large intestine

The six accessory organs of the digestive system are the following:

- Teeth
- Tongue
- Salivary glands
- Liver
- Gallbladder
- Pancreas

Digestion

The body performs digestion to accomplish the following functions:

- Break up food particles into smaller pieces.
- Break down food substances into nutrients that the body can use in body processes as energy or building materials.
- Transfer what it cannot use out of the body as waste; this elimination process is known as *excretion*.
- Reabsorb water into the body's tissues to prevent dehydration.

Digestion involves many different body organs and structures. This section takes you through the digestive process one step at a time.

The Mouth

Digestion begins in the opening of the alimentary tract, or *mouth*, where the teeth, tongue, and saliva aid in physical digestion (see Figure 26-2). **Mastication** occurs as the teeth break up the food pieces into smaller particles. Saliva moistens the food to ease swallowing and adds predigestive enzymes to the mix. The

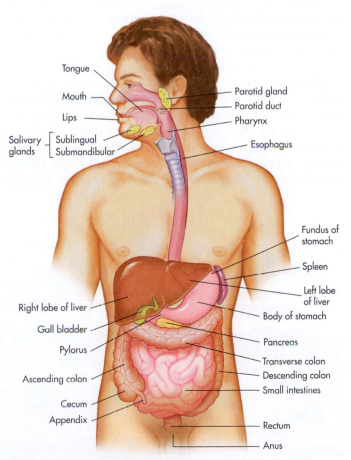

FIGURE 26-1 The digestive system.

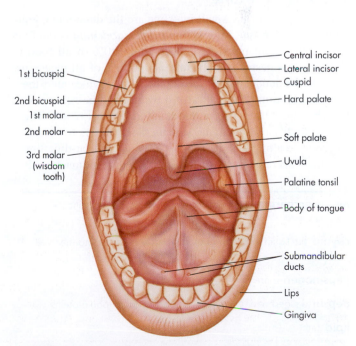

FIGURE 26-2 The mouth.

tongue moves the ball of chewed food, or *bolus*, to the uvula, and both assist in swallowing. Food then passes through the throat (*pharynx*) into the esophagus, as the windpipe or *trachea* is closed off by the epiglottis. Before the food is swallowed, the carbohydrate content of the food is chemically broken down by an enzyme into simple sugars or **monosaccharides**. This enzyme is an amylase known as *ptyalin*.

Monosaccharides are the building blocks of carbohydrates. Because food is usually swallowed before being completely chewed or moistened with enzymes, physical and chemical digestion have not been completed. The bolus passes through the approximately 10-inch-long esophagus, which runs behind the heart before meeting the stomach. Before entering the stomach, the bolus must pass through the cardiac sphincter, also referred to as the *lower esophageal sphincter (LES)*.

The Stomach

The three parts of the stomach are the fundus, body, and pylorus (see Figure 26-3). The smooth muscles of the stomach continue peristalsis, which moves the foodstuff, now called **chyme**, along the digestive tract to break up the food into even smaller pieces. Chyme has the consistency of a thick, soupy liquid. Chemical digestion in the stomach occurs when the walls of the stomach sense the weight or presence of the food and get stretched out. In response, the parietal cells make and secrete hydrochloric acid, which converts **pepsinogen** into the enzyme **pepsin**. The proteolytic enzyme pepsin chemically breaks down protein into amino acids. Amino acids are the building blocks of all proteins. About four hours later, peristalsis continues to move the chyme, consisting of carbohydrates, monosaccharides, proteins, and amino acids, through the pyloric sphincter.

The Small Intestine

The three parts of the small intestine are the duodenum, jejunum, and ileum (see Figure 26-4). The *duodenum* is the first part of the small intestine, where about 80% of all food is chemically digested. As a result, about 80% of all ulcers are found in the duodenum. As the highly acidic chyme enters the duodenum, it must be neutralized by an alkaline substance, bicarbonate. Otherwise, a duodenal ulcer will result. The strong acidity of the chyme signals the pancreas to secrete bicarbonate along with its starch-, protein-, and fat-digesting enzymes. Secreted bicarbonate neutralizes the stomach acids

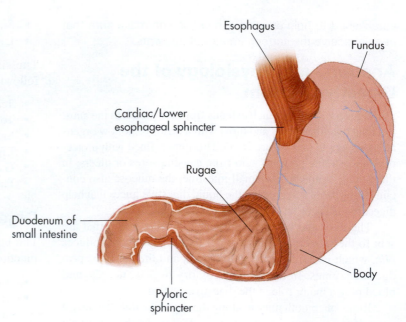

FIGURE 26-3 The stomach.

and raises the pH in the small intestine to slightly acidic (about 5.5); this is the chemical environment in which the pancreatic enzymes work best.

The small intestine calls upon the liver to make and secrete bile to help in digesting **lipids**. Stored bile from the gallbladder is sent to the small intestine to break up large molecules of fats into smaller ones, a process called *emulsification*. Emulsification occurs so that fat and fat-soluble vitamins can be absorbed in the intestine after enzymes break down the smaller globules into absorbable nutrients.

While food is in the small intestine, the pancreas sends out all three of its enzymes in a juice or secretion. Trypsin, a **protease**, further breaks down any remaining proteins or amino acids into the simplest of amino acids. Amylopsin, an amylase, breaks down any remaining carbohydrates and simple sugars into the simplest of sugars (monosaccharides). Finally, a lipase called steapsin, not produced elsewhere in the digestive tract, breaks down the smaller molecules of fat into fatty acids and glycerol

---

monosaccharide simplest form of carbohydrate (e.g., glucose, fructose).

chyme the liquid that food turns into before it passes into the small intestine.

pepsinogen a precursor to pepsin.

pepsin a digestive enzyme needed to break down food proteins.

lipid fat.

protease an enzyme that begins protein breakdown.

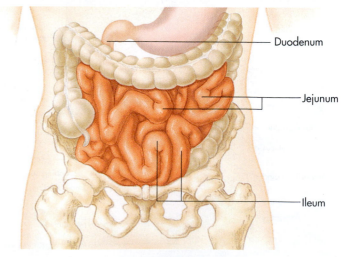

FIGURE 26-4 The small intestine.

(the building blocks of fats). At this point, all food sources—carbohydrates, proteins, and fats (lipids)—have been broken down into their simplest constituent nutrient substances and are ready to enter the bloodstream, so the body can use them as energy to power other body processes. The four nutrients—monosaccharides, amino acids, fatty acids, and glycerol—are then absorbed into the capillaries of the blood system and small lymph vessels by finger-like projections in the small intestine, called *villi* and *microvilli*. Whatever is not absorbed there is then passed out of the small intestine into the large intestine and out of the body as waste.

The small intestine is where the majority of absorption occurs. The nutrients are absorbed into tiny lymph vessels called *lacteals* and are passed through a large portal vein to the liver. The liver breaks down any toxins that may be present and prepares the nutrients for release into the bloodstream. The bloodstream carries the nutrients to every cell in the body, where they are used for energy and for tissue building and repair.

Table 26-1 shows the chemical breakdown of specific foods in a typical sandwich and the function of the nutrient building blocks produced during digestion.

The Large Intestine

The large intestine, or *colon*, is divided into the following seven sections (in order) (see Figure 26-5):

1. Cecum
2. Ascending colon
3. Transverse colon
4. Descending colon
5. Sigmoid colon
6. Rectum
7. Anus

Waste (material or residue that is not absorbed) is moved through the ileocecal valve that connects the lower ileum of the

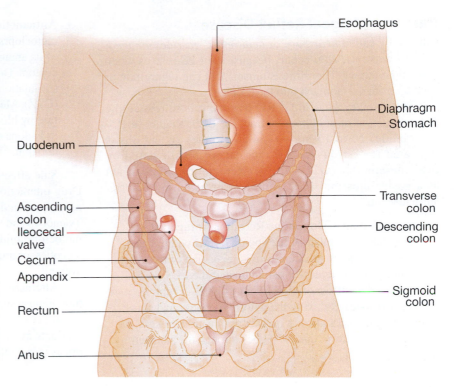

FIGURE 26-5 The large intestine.

small intestine to the cecum. The large intestine utilizes smooth muscle to mix the waste and allows the water to be reabsorbed. The motility of the colon is considered to be unsynchronized or nonperistaltic. A second and very important type of motility that occurs in the large intestine is the high-amplitude propagating contraction. These extremely strong contractions occur about six to eight times per day in healthy people, are longitudinal, and sweep from the cecum to stop just above the rectum. They move the waste down the large intestine and trigger bowel movements. Food waste, along with bacteria, remains in the large intestine for about 30 hours.

Disorders of the Digestive System

The following section discusses some common disorders of the digestive system.

TABLE 26-1 Comparison of Nutrient Functions within the Body

Food Source	Chemical Base of Food Source	Building Block (Nutrient Present at the End of Digestion or Hydrolysis)	Function of the Building Block or Nutrient
Bread or bun	Complex carbohydrates	Simple sugars or monosaccharides	Quick energy
Hamburger patty	Protein	Amino acids	Growth and repair of all cells, tissues, organs, structure (especially muscle)
Mayonnaise	Lipids (fats)	Fatty acids and glycerol	Stored energy, lubrication, protection/padding, insulation

Gastroesophageal Reflux Disease

Commonly called *heartburn* or *acid reflux*, *gastroesophageal reflux disease (GERD)* occurs because the LES relaxes when it should contract. Therefore, stomach acid can regurgitate or back up from the stomach into the esophagus.

The primary goal in GERD treatment is to reduce the overproduction of acid and contract the LES. Reglan (metoclopramide) 10 to 15 mg po qid 30 minutes ac and qhs is indicated for serious GERD that cannot be alleviated by over-the-counter (OTC) drugs. Metoclopramide can act as a gastrointestinal (GI) stimulant or as an antiemetic/antinauseant.

- **GI Stimulant—Dopamine Receptor Antagonist.** It stimulates peristalsis of the upper GI tract without causing more acid production; causes relaxation of the pyloric sphincter and increased resting tone of the LES (i.e., it helps the muscle of the LES stay tighter even in its relaxed state). Relaxing the pyloric sphincter and contracting the LES allow a quicker elimination process, or emptying time, so that food goes through the stomach faster.

- **Antiemetic or Antinauseant.** The antiemetic action of metoclopramide is unknown but is believed to be a result of its antagonism of central and peripheral dopamine receptors. Dopamine causes nausea and vomiting (N/V) by stimulation of the medullary chemoreceptor trigger zone (CTZ). Metoclopramide promotes proper sphincter function by blocking stimulation of the CTZ by agents, such as L-dopa or apomorphine, which are known to increase dopamine levels and to have dopamine-like effects.

Side effects include drowsiness and urinary incontinence. Drug interactions may occur with anticholinergic drugs, such as atropine and scopolamine, and narcotic analgesics, such as Tylenol #3 and Vicodin. Additive sedative effects can occur when metoclopramide is given with alcohol, sedatives, hypnotics, narcotics, or tranquilizers such as Valium, Dalmane, Percocet, or Tofranil.

Alternative therapies used to treat GERD include acupuncture, dietary supplements, herbal medicine, meditation, guided and relaxation therapy. Patients can choose from many OTC products available on pharmacy shelves for fairly reasonable prices (see Table 26-2).

TABLE 26-2 Prescription and OTC Treatments for GERD

Generic Name	Brand Name	Dosage Forms and Availability	Route of Administration	Common Adult Dosage
cimetidine	Tagamet, Tagamet HB	Rx: 300 mg, 400 mg, 800 mg; injection SDV OTC: 100 mg , 200 mg	Oral, IV	Oral dosage Rx, GERD, 400 mg qid or 800 mg bid
dexiansoprazole	Dexilant	30 mg, 60 mg	Oral	Dosage varies depending on the severity of the condition; a common dose is 60 mg qd for initial treatment
esomeprazole magnesium	Nexium	10 mg, 20 mg, 40 mg	Oral	Dosage varies depending on the severity of the condition; a common dose is 20 mg qd
famotidine	Pepcid Pepcid AC	Rx: 20 mg, 40 mg OTC: 10 mg, 20 mg	Oral, IV	Oral dosage Rx, GERD, 20 mg bid
lansoprazole	Prevacid	Rx: 15 mg, 30 mg OTC: 15 mg	Oral, IV	Dosage varies depending on the severity of the condition; a common dose is 20 mg qd; OTC: 15−30 mg qd
nizatidine	Axid, Axid AR	Rx: 150 mg capsule, 300 mg capsule; OTC: 75 mg	Oral	Oral dosage Rx, GERD, 150 mg bid
omeprazole	Prilosec	Rx: 10 mg, 20 mg, 40 mg OTC: 20 mg tablets	Oral	Dosage varies depending on the severity of the condition; a common dose is 20 mg qd; OTC: 20 mg daily for up to 14 days

TABLE 26-2 Prescription and OTC Treatments for GERD (*Continued*)

Generic Name	Brand Name	Dosage Forms and Availability	Route of Administration	Common Adult Dosage
pantoprazole	Protonix	20 mg, 40 mg	Oral, IV	Dosage varies depending on the severity of the condition; a common dose is 40 mg qd
raberprazole sodium	AcipHex	10 mg, 20 mg	Oral	Dosage varies depending on the severity of the condition; a common dose is 20 mg qd
ranitidine	Zantac, Zantac 75, Zantac 150	Rx: Oral: 150 mg, 300 mg tablets; 150 mg, 300 mg capsules; Injection: 20 mg/mL solution; OTC: 75 mg, 150 mg; 15 mg/mL syrup	Oral, IV	Oral dosage Rx, GERD, 150 mg bid

❛❛ Workplace Wisdom Digestive Disorders

An estimated 70 million Americans are said to have one or more digestive disorders, which account for 13% of all hospitalizations. ❜❜

Nausea and/or Vomiting

Nausea precedes vomiting and is a feeling of awareness that something is stimulating the vomit center and that vomiting is going to occur. Vomiting, or *emesis*, is produced by involuntary contraction of the abdominal muscles when the fundus and LES are relaxed, causing a strong ejection of gastric contents. If left untreated, chronic vomiting can cause malnutrition, dehydration, potassium chloride (KCl) electrolyte deficiency, heart problems, and arrhythmias. N/V occur when the vomiting center in the brain is activated by any of the following causes:

- Migraines
- Gallstones
- Intestinal obstructions
- Irritation of the stomach
- Overeating
- Food poisoning
- Overconsumption of alcohol
- Food allergies
- Reactions to medications such as NSAIDs and chemotherapy drugs
- Illness
- Various conditions of the body or disease states
- Pyloric stenosis—a blockage at the stomach outlet that produces projectile vomiting in infants and must be treated immediately.

See Tables 26-3 and 26-4.

- Anesthesia—postoperative vomiting is generally caused by the decreased amount of narcotic or opium derivative in the body after surgery (see Table 26-2).

- Pregnancy—no drugs have been approved for "morning sickness," but vitamin B6 may help to reduce the emotional stress that may accompany it. No nutritional deficiencies are associated with N/V during pregnancy.
- Bacterial or viral gastroenteritis—acute-onset gastroenteritis is most commonly caused by some type of bacteria or virus. This could result from eating contaminated food or catching influenza. Gastroenteritis usually causes a one-time attack of sudden projectile vomiting that does not require medication. The patient generally feels much better after the attack.
- Psychogenic vomiting—some nausea/vomiting is due to depression, anxiety, and emotional stress.
- Motion sickness (*vertigo*)—occurs when the body is subjected to accelerations of movement in different directions or under conditions where visual contact with an actual outside horizon is lost. The balance center of the inner ear then sends information to the brain that conflicts with the visual clues of being still; the resulting confusion causes nausea.

Treatment to relieve N/V is typically through medication. Which medication is to be prescribed depends on the particular patient's problem (see Table 26-3).

Antihistamines work by competitive inhibition or by blocking H1 receptor sites, which slows the response to the stimuli causing the N/V (see Table 26-5). Antihistamines are thought to block excitatory labyrinthine impulses at cholinergic synapses in the region of the vestibular nuclei. Side effects include drowsiness and dry mouth. Listed warnings advise patients with glaucoma or urinary disturbances not to take antihistamines.

N/V may occur as a side effect of chemotherapy, either during or after administration of chemotherapeutic drugs. Serotonin receptors of the 5-HT$_3$ type are located peripherally on vagal nerve terminals and centrally in the CTZ of the area postrema of the brain. During chemotherapy that induces

TABLE 26-3 Prescription and OTC Treatments for Nausea/Vomiting

Generic Name	Brand Name	Dosage Forms and Availability	Route of Administration	Common Adult Dosage
alosetron	Lotronex	0.5 mg, 1 mg tablets	Oral	0.5 mg bid
dimenhyrdinate	Dramamine	50 mg tablets	Oral	Oral: 50–100 mg q4–6h
dolasetron	Anzemet	50 mg, 100 mg tablets; 12.5 mg, 100 mg SDV; 12.5 mg pre-filled syringe; 500 mg/25 mL multi-dose vial	Oral, IV	Oral: 100 mg prior to chemotherapy treatment; IV: 1.8 mg/kg 30 minutes before chemotherapy treatment
granisetron	Kytril	1 mg tablets; 2 mg/10 mL solution; 0.1 mg/mL, 1 mg/mL vial	Oral, IM	Oral: 2 mg daily; IM: 10 mcg/kg 30 minutes before chemotherapy treatment
meclizine	Antivert (Rx), Bonine (OTC)	Rx: 12.5 mg, 25 mg, 50 mg; OTC: 25 mg	Oral	Oral: 12.5–25 mg one hour before exposure to stimulus
metoclopramide	Reglan	5 mg, 10 mg tablets	Oral	Nonchemotherapeutic dosage: 5–10 mg before meals and at bedtime as needed; chemotherapeutic adult dosage: 10 mg in 50 mL of normal saline over 30 minutes, given once before chemotherapy treatment, may repeat every 2 hours × 2 doses or every 3 hours × 3 doses
ondansetron	Zofran	4 mg, 8 mg tablets; 4 mg, 8 mg disintegrating tablets; 4 mg/5 mL solution; 2 mg/mL SDV/MDV	Oral, IV	Oral: 8 mg 30 minutes before chemotherapy treatment, then 8 mg eight hours after dose followed by 8 mg every 12 hours for several days
palonosetron	Aloxi	0.5 mg capsule; 0.25 mg/5 mL SDV	Oral, IV	Oral: 0.5 mg 1 hour before chemotherapy treatment; IV: 0.25 mg 30 minutes before chemotherapy treatment
prochlorperazine	Compro, Compazine	5 mg, 10 mg tablets; 10 mg, 15 mg capsule; 5 mg/mL vials; 2.5 mg, 5 mg, 25 mg suppository	Oral, IM, rectally	5–10 mg tid or qid
scopolamine	Transderm Scöp	1 mg patch	Transdermal skin patch	Apply one patch behind ear four hours before event; change patch every three days, alternating side of application
trimethobenazmide	Tigan	300 mg capsule; 100 mg/mL vial	Oral, IM	Oral: 300 mg tid or qid; IM: 200 mg tid or qid

vomiting, mucosal enterochromaffin cells release serotonin that stimulates 5-HT$_3$ receptors. This evokes vagal afferent discharge, or firing, which induces vomiting.

Drugs used for postemetogenic nausea are called 5-HT$_3$ antagonists. These drugs block serotonin from binding with and stimulating the 5-HT$_3$ receptors, and thus prevent N/V. There are no listed drug interactions for 5-HT$_3$ antagonists.

Side effects are minimal but may include headache, diarrhea, or constipation (see Table 26-6).

❝ Workplace Wisdom Herbal Remedy

Ginger root is an herb that is known to aid in combating N/V. A minor side effect of ginger root is a burning stomach. **❞**

TABLE 26-4 Postoperative Vomiting Drugs

Trade Name	Generic Name	Available Strength and Dosage Forms	Dosage
Compazine	prochlorperazine	5 mg, 10 mg, 25 mg tablets 2.5 mg, 5 mg, 25 mg suppository 5 mg/mL injection	5–10 mg po tid or qid 50 mg pr bid Not to exceed (NTE) 40 mg/day IV
Phenergan	promethazine	12.5 mg, 25 mg, 50 mg tablets 12.5 mg, 25 mg, 50 mg suppository 25 mg/mL, 50 mg/mL injections	12.5–25 mg q4–6h
Tigan	trimethobenzamide	300 mg capsule 100 mg, 200 mg suppository 100 mg/mL injection	300 mg po tid or quid 100–200 mg pr tid or qid 200 mg IM tid or qid

TABLE 26-5 Antihistamines Used as Antiemetics

Trade Name	Generic Name	Dosage
Antivert	meclizine	25–50 mg 1 hour prior to travel
		25–100 mg daily in divided doses (for vertigo)
Dramamine	dimenhydrinate	50 mg tablets: 1–2 tablets q4–6h, NTE 300 mg/6 tablets in 24 hours
Transderm-scop	scopolamine	One patch q3d

TABLE 26-6 Drugs Used for Postemetogenic Nausea

Trade Name	Generic Name	Dosage	
5-HT$_3$ Antagonists			
Aloxi	palonosetron HCl	0.25 mg/5 mL injection	0.25 mg as a single dose 30 minutes before administration of chemotherapy
Anzemet	dolasetron mesylate	50 mg, 100 mg tablets; 20 mg/mL injection	100 mg po within one hour before chemotherapy 1.8 mg/kg as a single dose 30 minutes before chemotherapy
Kytril	granisetron HCl	1 mg tablet; 1 mg/5 mL liquid; 1 mg/mL injection	2 mg po daily or 1 mg po bid 10 mcg/kg IV within 30 minutes before chemotherapy
Zofran	ondansetron HCl	4 mg, 8 mg, 24 mg tablets 2 mg/mL injection 32 mg/50 mL premix IV	8 mg po bid 0.15 mg/kg IV × 3 doses *or* 32 mg IV × 1 dose

Ulcers

Ulcers are sores on the inside *flesh* wall of the stomach or intestines caused by overproduction and secretion of the parietal cells. A *peptic ulcer* is a sore that forms in the lining of the stomach or the duodenum. Ulcer symptoms can include burning pain in the upper abdomen, nausea, vomiting, loss of appetite, weight loss, fatigue, deep recurring ache relieved with food or antacids, gastric pain aggravated by general irritants, and nocturnal (nighttime) pain.

> **❝ Workplace Wisdom** **Peptic Ulcers**
>
> More than 400,000 new cases of peptic ulcers are diagnosed each year, and ulcers are the reason for nearly 40,000 surgeries annually. **❞**

Peptic ulcer disease can affect all age groups, but it is less common in children. In the past, it was believed that men were at twice the risk for ulcers as women due to unhealthy diets and high stress levels. However, it is now known that most ulcers are caused by bacterial infections or medications. Therefore, women and men are at equal risk of developing ulcers. The risk of duodenal ulcers tends to begin around the age of 25 and continues until the age of 75. Gastric ulcers peak in people between the ages of 55 and 65. There is an 80% incidence of duodenal ulcers (see Figure 26-6).

Nonsteroidal Anti-Inflammatory Drugs

Some peptic ulcers can be caused by the extended use of nonsteroidal anti-inflammatory drugs (NSAIDs), such as ibuprofen and naproxen sodium. Many NSAID medications can be found in most stores and are available OTC. Other NSAIDs, such as Celebrex, require a prescription.

NSAIDs are prescribed to reduce inflammation and fever but are also effective for analgesia (pain reduction). However, use of NSAIDs does increase the risk of stomach ulcers. NSAIDs work by blocking the effect of the enzyme cyclooxygenase (COX). Prostaglandins are produced within the body's cells by one of two COX enzymes, COX-1 and COX-2. Prostaglandins promote inflammation, pain, and fever. However, they also protect the lining of the stomach from the damaging effects of acid by stimulating the *gastric mucosa* to secrete a protective fluid. Only COX-1 produces prostaglandins that support platelets and protect the stomach. NSAIDs block all COX enzymes and thus reduce prostaglandin production throughout the body. This can reduce the stomach's natural defenses and promote ulcer development.

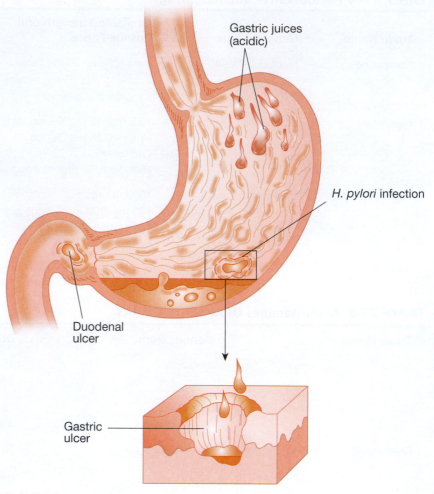

FIGURE 26-6 An ulcer.

> **❝ Workplace Wisdom** **NSAIDs**
>
> Nearly 4% of regular NSAID users develop serious GI conditions. Patients are advised always to take NSAID medications with food to help prevent stomach problems. NSAID-induced ulcers usually heal once the person stops taking the medication. **❞**

Other Causes of Ulcers

Other factors that can induce the overproduction of acid and cause ulcers include the following:

Infection A major cause of peptic ulcers is infection with the bacterium *Helicobacter pylori (H. pylori),* a spiral-shaped bacterium found in the gastric mucous layer or adhering to the epithelial lining of the stomach. It can multiply readily in the right conditions. A by-product of its cell division is an acid that leads to overacidification of the stomach and intestines. *H. pylori* is responsible for about 90% of duodenal ulcers and 80% of gastric ulcers. Many people have *H. pylori* infections, but not everyone with an infection develops a peptic ulcer.

Smoking Ulcers are more likely to occur, less likely to heal, and more likely to cause death in smokers than in nonsmokers. Some studies show that smoking reduces the bicarbonate

---

Hypersensitivities allergy.

produced by the pancreas, interfering with the neutralization of acid in the duodenum. Other research shows that smoking lessens the power of the immune system to fight the *H. pylori* bacteria. The best advice is to discontinue smoking.

Alcohol Research reports are mixed, but some results show that alcohol may aggravate *H. pylori* infections and cause more bleeding. The advice is to decrease alcohol consumption or discontinue consumption completely in severe cases.

Excessive peristalsis. Motility stimulates the parietal cells to secrete more acid, and some researchers believe that the peristalsis that accompanies stress can lead to this. Diarrhea may be caused by an increase in motility and peristalsis, or "spasms of the colon," so antidiarrheals may help in alleviating the overproduction of acid by reducing motility. Antispasmodics, also known as *muscarinic receptor antagonists*, that have a direct effect on smooth muscle are usually prescribed. An example is Donnatal, which contains belladonna alkaloids.

Anticholinergics These medications inhibit the actions of acetylcholine at the postganglionic parasympathetic neuroeffector sites. Large doses block nicotinic sites, inhibit gastric acid secretion, and decrease GI and urinary tract motility. Moderate doses dilate the pupils and increase heart rate; small doses inhibit salivary and bronchial secretions. Drugs prescribed for this include prostaglandin replacement. An example is Cytotec (misoprostol). Available in 100 and 200 mg tablets, a common dosage is 100–200 mcg qid with food. Dose can be reduced to 100 mcg, if the larger dose cannot be tolerated. Because misoprostol is a prostaglandin-like substance or agonist, it stimulates production of prostaglandins by the mucosal lining. By increasing the viscosity of the gastric mucosa, it offers greater protection from the acid when the patient takes an NSAID that blocks prostaglandins. Adverse reactions include diarrhea, cramping, miscarriage, premature labor, and birth defects.

Food hypersensitivities Hypersensitivities to foods, such as peanut butter, shrimp, and milk, can cause the mast cells to release histamine2 (H2). H2 binds to the H2 receptor site of the parietal cells that line the stomach wall, thus triggering the production and release of acid. As the lock-and-key theory suggests, H2 antagonists enter the H2 receptors in the parietal cells, thus preventing H2 from binding there. This blocks both acid production and secretion. This is called *competitive inhibition* (see Table 26-5).

Ulcer Therapy

Therapy for *H. pylori* infection consists of 10 to 14 days of one or two antibiotics, such as amoxicillin, tetracycline (not to be used for children under 12 years old), metronidazole, clarithromycin, plus ranitidine bismuth citrate or bismuth subsalicylate, or a proton pump inhibitor (PPI). Acid suppression by the H2 blocker or PPI, in conjunction with the antibiotics, helps alleviate ulcer-related symptoms, heal gastric mucosal inflammation, and may enhance efficacy of the antibiotics against *H. pylori* (see Tables 26-7 and 26-8).

Adverse reactions to H2 antagonist drugs include fatigue, hypertension, muscle pain, bronchiospasm, grand mal seizures, impotence, and *gynecomastia* (development of breasts in males).

PPIs block the enzyme that turns on the H+−ATPase enzyme system. When this enzyme is blocked, the parietal cells will not secrete hydrogen, which is the last step in making HCl. Side effects include headache, nausea, and vomiting. Drugs with adverse interactions include digoxin (PPIs can cause an increase in plasma levels of digoxin) and ketoconazole (PPIs can cause a decrease in plasma levels of ketoconazole) (see Table 26-9).

Diarrhea

Diarrhea is defined as many lose bowel movements that take place usually in a short period of time. It can last a few hours to a few days. The problem with constant diarrhea is that it can be the cause of an underlying condition or infection. Diarrhea that continues for more than a few days should be checked out by a doctor. Diarrhea can sometimes cause N/V. This can make

TABLE 26-7 H2 Antagonist Drugs Used for Ulcer Treatment

Trade name	Generic name	Available Strength and Dosage Form	Dosage
Axid	nizatidine	150 mg, 300 mg tablets	150 mg po bid or 300 mg po qhs
Pepcid	famotidine	20 mg, 40 mg tablets 40 mg/5 mL oral suspension	20−40 mg po daily
Tagamet	cimetidine	200 mg, 300 mg, 400 mg, 800 mg tablets 300 mg/2 mL injection	300 mg po qid or 400 mg po bid or 800 mg po qhs 300 mg IV q6−8 h
Zantac	ranitidine	150 mg, 300 mg tablets; 25 mg, 150 mg effervescent tablets 75 mg/5 mL syrup 25 mg/1 mL premixed injection; 50 mg IVPB	150 mg po bid or 300 mg po qhs 50 mg IM or IV q6−8 h

TABLE 26-8 Multiple Drug Therapy Used for *H. pylori* Infection

Drug Regimens	Non-PPI Drug Regimen
Bismuth subsalicylate	+metronidazole (Flagyl) 250 mg qid
(Pepto-Bismol) 525 mg qid	+tetracycline 500 mg qid × 2 weeks
	+H2 receptor antagonist therapy as directed × 4 weeks
Double-Drug Theory	
Lansoprazole 30 mg tid	+amoxicillin 1 gm tid × 2 weeks
Triple-Drug Theory	
1. omeprazole 20 mg bid + clarithromycin 500 mg bid + amoxicillin 1 gm bid × 10 days	
2. lansoprazole 30 mg bid + clarithromycin 500 mg bid + amoxicillin 1 gm bid × 10 days	

TABLE 26-9 PPI Drugs Used for Ulcer Treatment

Trade Name	Generic Name	Availability	Dosage
Aciphex	rabeprazole sodium	20 mg delayed-release tablets	20–40 mg daily
Nexium	esomeprazole magnesium	20 mg, 40 mg delayed-release capsules	20 or 40 mg daily
Prevacid	lansoprazole	15 mg and 30 mg enteric-coated delayed-release capsules	15 or 30 mg daily
Prilosec	omeprazole	10 mg, 20 mg, and 40 mg delayed-release capsules	20 or 40 mg daily
Protonix	pantoprazole	20 mg, 40 mg delayed-release tablets	40 mg daily

individuals feel worse when suffering from the problem. Certain medications and antibiotics can cause diarrhea, but probiotics can help combat the effects that the antibiotics have on the stomach and reduce symptoms like diarrhea that occur when having to take a course of antibiotics. Various medications can be used to treat diarrhea, and the severity of diarrhea generally depends on the type of medication used to treat the condition and the amount of drugs the patient needs to take to cure the symptoms. It is important to watch out for dehydration in patients who endure a long bout of diarrhea, as this can cause the patient to feel worse and the condition to become more severe. Foods that irritate or make the stomach upset:

- Using too many laxatives
- Particular cancers
- Diabetes
- Using too much alcohol

There are a variety of medications used to treat the common illness. Lomotil and Octreotide are two prescriptions used to treat loose bowel movements. Lomotil is available in liquid (suspension) form, and Octreotide is given in injection form. It is used mainly for short durations of diarrhea.

Common OTC drugs used to cure or treat the symptoms of diarrhea are Imodium (loperamide) and Bismuth. Bismuth is also known in brand-name form as Kaopectate and Pepto-Bismol. Traditionally, medicines that treat symptoms of diarrhea often work quickly, so the patient does not have to suffer with sometimes disabling symptoms. There are no known safe alternative therapies to treat diarrhea (see Table 26-10).

Constipation

Constipation is a GI condition characterized by hard, dry, and small-sized stools that are difficult to pass. People with constipation usually have fewer than three bowel movements per week, along with other symptoms that may include straining, bloating, abdominal pain and distention, or the sensation of incomplete emptying. Constipation is a symptom, not a disease, and in most cases results from a diet that is high in fat and low in fiber. Other causes of constipation are the following:

- Lack of physical activity
- Medications, such as loperamide, codeine, morphine, and iron supplements
- Abuse of laxatives

TABLE 26-10 Prescription and OTC Treatments for Diarrhea

Generic Name	Brand Name	Dosage forms and Availability	Route of Administration	Common Adult Dosage
bismuth subsalicylate	Pepto-Bismol (OTC)	Tablets; solution	Oral	2 tablets or 30 mL prn, NTE eight doses in a 24-hour period
diphenoxylate/ atropine	Lomotil	2.5/0.025 mg tablets	Oral	2.5–5 mg qid, then bid or tid prn; NTE 20 mg in a 24-hour period.
loperamide	Imodium (Rx); Imodium AD (OTC)	2 mg capsule (Rx)	Oral	2 mg following each loose stool (maximum 16 mg/day × 2 days)

- Suppression of defecation
- Milk
- Diseases such as multiple sclerosis, stroke, and diabetes
- Changes in lifestyle, such as aging, pregnancy, and travel
  See Table 26-11.

Laxatives are drugs that are used to treat constipation or evacuate the colon for medical examinations (see Table 26-12). They include the following types:

- *Bulk-forming*—work in the intestine by absorbing water to make the stool softer. They are considered the most common and safest type of laxative.

- *Emollients*—work by stopping the colon from absorbing fecal water and thereby softening the stool.
- *Evacuants*—used for bowel cleansing before medical exams.
- *Fecal softeners/surfactants*—work in the intestines and help mix fat and water to soften stool.
- *Hyperosmotics*—cause colon fluid retention and thereby increase peristalsis.
- *Saline*—draws water into the colon, making it easier to pass stools.
- *Stimulants/irritants*—work by causing rhythmic intestinal contractions.

TABLE 26-11 Prescription and OTC Treatments for Constipation

Generic Name	Brand Name	Dosage Forms and Availability	Route of Administration	Common Adult Dosage
bisacodyl	Dulcolax	5 mg tablets; 10 mg suppository	Oral, rectal	10 mg orally or rectally qd as needed
docusate calcium	Kaopectate stool softener (formerly Surfak)	240 mg capsules	Oral	240 mg daily
docusate sodium	Colace	50 mg, 100 mg, 250 mg capsules; 100, 250 mg tablets; 20 mg/5 mL syrup	Oral	50–300 mg daily, NTE 300 mg daily
glycerin	Colace Glycerin, Fleet Babylax	Suppository	Rectal	One suppository rectally once daily as needed
lubiprostone	Amitiza	8 mcg, 24 mcg capsules	Oral	Chronic idiopathic constipation dosage: 24 mcg bid; irritable bowel syndrome: 8 mcg bid
psyllium	Metamucil		Oral	1 Tbsp. daily in 8 oz. of water or juice
senna	Senokot	Tablets	Oral	8.5–28 mg daily

TABLE 26-12 Types of Laxatives

Type	Onset of Action	Trade Name	Generic Name
Bulk-forming	12–72 hours		psyllium
		Metamucil	polycarbophil
		FiberCon	methylcellulose
Emollient	6–8 hours	Citrucel	mineral oil
Evacuant	1 hour		polyethylene glycol-electrolyte solution (peg-es)
		CoLyte	polyethylene glycol (peg) solution
		GoLYTELY	
Fecal softener/surfactant	Raise 12–72 hours	GlycoLaxMiraLax	docusate sodium
		Colace	docusate calcium
Hyperosmotic	15 minutes–1 hour	Surfak Liquigels	glycerin suppository
	24–48 hours	Sani-Supp	lactulose
		Colace	
Saline	30 minutes–3 hours	Cephulac	magnesium sulfate
		Enulose	epsom salt
			milk of magnesia
			monobasic sodium phosphate/dibasic sodium phosphate
Stimulant/irritant	6–8 hours	Fleets Phospho-Soda	cascara sagrada
	6–10 hours		sennosides
	Suppository: 15 minutes–1 hour	Ex-lax	bisacodyl
	Tablet: 6–10 hours	Senokot	
		Dulcolax	
		Correctol	

Flatulence

Flatulence, also known as gas or passing gas, is a common problem for most people. Flatulence is combination of gases in the stomach and intestine. Socially, it can be a bit embarrassing, but there are drugs designed to cut down on the amount of gas the body produces. It is quite normal to pass gas several times a day, as it is a regular process of the body. OTC medicines used to combat gas are OTC products such as Gas-X, Mylanta Gas Oral, and Bicarsim Oral; they are inexpensive and work fairly quickly to relieve the pressure, bloating, and the need to expel built-up substances either orally or rectally. The antibiotic Rifaximin can be given to make the symptoms of gas less uncomfortable and reduce bloating as well. Most commonly, flatulence is treated with OTC medications. OTC medications seem to provide significant relief of gas, but many prescriptions do exist and are often covered by insurance as OTC medicines are not.

---

diverticulitis a condition in which the diverticula form in the walls of the colon and portion of the large intestine and become inflamed.

dietary reference intakes (DRIs) nutritional guidelines that include both recommended intakes and tolerable upper intake levels.

Irritable Bowel Syndrome

The cause of irritable bowel syndrome (IBS) is unknown, but all the symptoms are manageable and treatable. IBS is a long-term illness that involves the large and small bowel/intestine. Discomfort of the abdomen and pain in that area are the main characteristics of IBS. Some things that trigger IBS are certain foods, stress, and hormones. IBS can also include symptoms of anxiety and depression, and those who suffer from GI illnesses, such as Crohn's disease and ulcerative colitis (UC), may also have IBS. Some prescription medications used to manage IBS are antidepressants, antidiarrheals, antispasmodics, benzodiazepines, antibiotics, and probiotics. Two types of antidepressants are given to treat anxiety and depression—selective serotonin reuptake inhibitors (SSRIs) and tricyclic antidepressants (TCAs) (see Table 26-13). Alternative therapies can range from yoga and relaxation techniques to managing stress to basic herbal remedies to treat the constant *upset stomach* aspect of IBS. There are no known OTC or alternative remedies to treat IBS approved by the Food and Drug Administration (FDA).

Crohn's Disease

Crohn's disease is a very serious and painful condition that lasts a lifetime and inflames the bowels. It is unknown what causes Crohn's disease, but there are quite a few drugs that are used to treat the illness. Swelling, deep sores, diarrhea, and belly pain are present with the inflammatory disease. Cyclosporine and IV corticosteroids are used in patients who are very ill from Crohn's disease. Biologics, drugs that suppress the immune system, corticosteroids, antibiotics, and aminosalicylates are also used to keep the illness in check. There are no known approved OTC drugs or alternative therapies used to treat Crohn's disease except for reducing stress levels and avoiding foods that will make the illness worse.

Ulcerative Colitis

UC is a part of the family of inflammatory bowel diseases. The two parts of the body it affects are the lining of the large intestine (or colon) and the rectum. Causes of UC are unknown; however, most individuals have a compromised immune system. Some of the medications given to patients to treat the condition are aminosalicylates, corticosteroids, immunomodulators, antibiotics, and biologic therapies. UC is a life-long manageable condition but not curable. There are no known OTC drugs or approved alternative therapies that are used to treat UC. However, it is recommended for patients to watch their diet and not eat foods that upset their condition. Reducing stress is also very important in managing the condition.

Diverticulitis

Diverticulitis is a condition in which the diverticula form in the walls of the colon and portion of the large intestine and become inflamed. The cause of this condition is not known. Some symptoms of diverticulitis are abdominal pain and cramping, nausea, fever, chills, constipation, loose stools, diarrhea, and in some cases, rectal bleeding. Treatment includes prescribing antibiotics, pain relievers, emptying the stomach via a tube, surgery, and changes in diet.

See Table 26-14.

Nutrition

Modern daily food intake recommendations are based on *Nutrition and Your Health: Dietary Guidelines for Americans*. This publication was first developed in 1980 by the U.S. Department of Agriculture (USDA) and the Department of Health and Human Services (DHHS) for use in consumer nutrition education efforts with healthy Americans aged two years and older. The guidelines are revised every five years to include analysis of the most recent research of the Dietary Guidelines Advisory Committee.

The recommended dietary allowances (RDAs) were established to define the nutritional needs of healthy persons living in the United States. The Food and Nutrition Board of the National Academy of Sciences sets the values for the RDAs on the basis of human and animal research.

The RDAs have been revised and are now being replaced by the **dietary reference intake (DRI)**. The DRIs include both recommended intakes and tolerable upper intake levels (ULs). The National Information Resource Center states that the DRIs are based on the evaluation of the following four categories:

1. Estimated average requirement—the nutrient value that is estimated to meet the needs of 50% of the population.
2. RDA—the nutrient value that prevents deficiencies in 98% of the population.

TABLE 26-13 Prescription Treatments for Irritable Bowel Syndrome

Generic Name	Brand Name	Dosage Forms and Availability	Route of Administration	Common Adult Dosage
alosetron	Lotronex	0.5 mg tablets	Oral	0.5 mg bid
dicyclomine	Bentyl	10 mg capsules; 20 mg tablets; 10 mg/5 mL syrup; 20 mg/2 mL injection	Oral, IV	20 mg qid
hyoscyamine sulfate	Levsin SL	0.125 mg tablets	Oral	1–tablets q4h or as needed. Do not exceed 12 tablets in 24 hours.

TABLE 26-14 Prescription Treatments for Crohn's Disease/Ulcerative Colitis

Generic Name	Brand Name	Dosage Forms and Availability	Route of Administration	Common Adult Dosage
adalimumab	Humira	20 mg, 40 mg PFS	SC	160 mg initial dose, then reduced to 40 mg every other week for maintenance
azathioprine	Azathioprine, Imuran	50 mg tablets	Oral	50–100 mg daily
infliximab	Remicade	100 mg SDV	IV	5 mg/kg infused IV and then two and six weeks later; followed by maintenance regimen of 5 mg/kg every eight weeks thereafter
mesalamine	Canasa, Lialda, Pentassa	250 mg capsules; 1.2 gm tablets; 1,000 mg suppository;	Oral, rectal	Oral: 1–1.2 gm daily with a meal; Rectal: 1000 mg HS
prednisone	Deltasone	2.5 mg, 2 mg, 10 mg, 20 mg, 50 mg tablets	Oral	Varies
sulfasalazine	Azulfadine EN	500 mg tablets	Oral	2 gm daily
tacrolimus	Prograf	0.5 mg, 1 mg, 5 mg capsules; 5 mg/mL ampicillin	Oral, IV	Varies

3. Adequate intake—the value set for nutrients that do not have an RDA.
4. Tolerable UL—the highest value of a nutrient that is not likely to pose adverse effects in 98% of the population.

The nutrients needed by the body fall into one of three categories: macronutrients, micronutrients, and water.

Macronutrients

Macronutrients are nutrients that the body requires in relatively large quantities; the three types of macronutrients are carbohydrates, proteins, and fats. **Kilocalories (kcal)** are the units of measure of the energy needed to digest and utilize food and the energy expended with exercise. Fats are the most concentrated source of food energy. One gram of fat supplies about 9 kcal, as compared to the 4 kcal supplied by carbohydrates and protein.

---

kilocalories (kcal) a unit of measurement for food energy.

acceptable macronutrient distribution range (AMDR) the range of intake levels that provide an adequate amount of a nutrient and is associated with a reduced risk of disease.

low-density lipoprotein (LDL) bad cholesterol.

high-density lipoprotein (HDL) good cholesterol.

The micronutrients—vitamins, minerals, and water—provide no calories or energy.

Carbohydrates

Sources of carbohydrates include fruits, vegetables, whole grains, and legumes, all of which contain fiber, starch, and some vitamins and minerals. Carbohydrates can be classified as either simple or complex. Simple carbohydrates are sugars and contain no energy-yielding calories. They are considered *empty calories*, like candy, for example. Complex carbohydrates are starches, take longer to be broken down in the digestive tract, and have more nutritional value than simple sugars. Whole-grain bread is an example of a complex carbohydrate.

Carbohydrates provide immediate energy and are the most readily available sources of food energy. During digestion and metabolism, carbohydrates are broken down into the simple sugar glucose to be used as the body's principal energy source. Glucose is stored in the liver and muscle tissue as glycogen. A carbohydrate-rich diet is necessary to maintain muscle glycogen, the preferred fuel for most types of exercise. The **acceptable macronutrient distribution range (AMDR)** for carbohydrates is 45% to 65% of daily caloric intake. The AMDR is the range associated with the reduced risk of disease while providing needed nutrients. Of course, most health benefits will be derived from ingestion of more complex carbohydrates and fewer simple carbohydrates.

Fats

Lipids play an important role in the body. The main functions of body fat are to:

- Help to provide lubrication
- Store energy reserves
- Act as an insulator to provide and retain warmth
- Provide a cushion and protect vital organs by acting as a shock absorber
- Help metabolize carbohydrates and proteins more efficiently
- Help absorb and transport fat-soluble vitamins such as vitamins A, D, E, and K

Dietary fats (lipids) are the body's only source of linoleic acid, a fatty acid that is essential for growth and skin maintenance. Fats are divided into two categories: saturated and unsaturated (including monounsaturated and polyunsaturated fatty acids). These fatty acids differ from each other chemically based on the nature of the bond between the carbon and hydrogen atoms.

As a general rule, saturated fat is solid at room temperature; most saturated fat is derived from animal sources. Unsaturated fat, which is liquid at room temperature, is derived primarily from plants. Monounsaturated and polyunsaturated fats should be emphasized in the diet, as they tend to lower the blood cholesterol level. Saturated fats tend to raise the level of blood cholesterol. High blood cholesterol levels are associated with an increased risk of coronary heart disease.

Of the two types of fat, saturated is considered *bad* fat, because the entire lipid chain has hydrogen atoms covering it, which leads to increased **low-density lipoprotein (LDL)** and total cholesterol levels. Saturated fats contain more cholesterol, because they are derived from animal sources such as meat and dairy products. Butter, skin of the animal, and mayonnaise are also saturated fats. Some saturated oils, such as palm oil and coconut oil, may actually cause the body to overmanufacture cholesterol.

Unsaturated fat is considered good or better dietary fat, because it is less hydrogenated. Examples of monounsaturated fat are olive oil and canola oil. Polyunsaturated fats are found in most other vegetable oils and nuts, but deep cold-water fish, such as salmon, mackerel, tuna, and bluefish, are also sources of *good* dietary fat.

❝ Workplace Wisdom   Dietary Risks

Current studies show that the diets containing a higher amount of a certain type of polyunsaturated fatty acid are associated with a decreased risk for heart disease in certain people. ❞

Hydrogenated fats are created when an oil or fat that is largely unsaturated, such as corn oil, has hydrogen added to it. Chemically saturating an unsaturated fat, by adding hydrogen atoms, produces trans-fatty acids, which act like saturated fats in the body and have the same capacity to do harm as saturated fats. Research shows that trans-fatty acids increase LDL cholesterol levels, decrease the levels of **high-density lipoprotein (HDL)**

cholesterol, and thus increase the risk of coronary heart disease. Hydrogenated fat, such as margarine, is solid or semisolid at room temperature; it is used in many processed foods, because it is more stable and goes rancid more slowly than unprocessed, unhydrogenated fats and oils.

In addition, trans-fatty acids, which are chemically altered (processed) fats, are also found in many packaged foods and may be listed on the labels as partially hydrogenated or hydrogenated oil. The more solid and hydrogenated the fat is, the more trans-fatty acids there are in the product. Commercial peanut butter is an example.

Palm and coconut oils are also high in saturated fats, even though they stay liquid at room temperature. They will raise blood levels of bad cholesterol (LDL and *VLDL*, which is very low-density lipoprotein) and lower blood levels of good cholesterol (HDL).

Essential fatty acids, omega-3 and omega-6, are fats that are needed by the body but are not produced internally; they must be taken in from foods. Omega-3 fatty acids, found primarily in fish, help prevent heart disease, arthritis, and cancer growth and development.

The AMDR for fats is 20% to 35% of caloric intake—but not more than 10% of calorie intake should be saturated fat. Saturated fats, hydrogenated or partially hydrogenated fats or oils, trans fats (chemically altered), and palm and coconut oils that raise blood bad cholesterol (LDL and VLDL) should be avoided and replaced with healthier fats such as olive and canola oil.

Protein

Proteins make up almost all cells, tissues, and organs of the body and are considered the body's main building blocks. Hormones, enzymes, and blood plasma transport systems are also composed of proteins. Protein is necessary to make and repair body cells, tissue, and muscle.

Proteins are composed of complex strings of amino acids.

Proteins can be divided into two groups: complete and incomplete. *Complete* or *essential proteins* have the essential amino acids necessary to build other proteins. Complete proteins can be found in animal muscle (e.g., beef, chicken, pork, fish). Incomplete proteins are missing one or more of the amino acids needed to build other proteins. *Incomplete protein* can be found in plant-based foods, such as beans and peanuts.

The body requires 20 different amino acids, both essential and nonessential, to maintain proper nutrition. Essential amino acids are not produced within the body. Therefore, essential amino acids have to be derived from food intake. The remaining 11 nonessential amino acids can be produced by the body (see Table 26-15).

Protein is not normally a significant energy source during either rest or exercise. However, the body will use protein for energy when calorie or carbohydrate intake is inadequate (during fasting or a low-carbohydrate diet). The AMDR for protein is 10% to 35% of total caloric intake.

When a person eats excessive amounts of protein, the body must excrete the extra nitrogen. Therefore, the body produces extra urine, requiring extra fluid. This places many athletes,

TABLE 26-15 Essential and Nonessential Amino Acids

Essential	Nonessential
Histidine	Alanine
Isoleucine	Arginine
Leucine	Asparagines
Lysine	Aspartic acid
Methionine	Cysteine
Phenylalanine	Glutamic acid
Threonine	Glutamine
Tryptophan	Glycine
Valine	Proline
	Serine
	Tyrosine

and others who are less than amply hydrated, at risk of dehydration. In extreme cases, excess protein or amino acid intake can lead to kidney damage. In addition, excessive protein intake can cause urinary calcium loss. However, severe restriction of protein intake often results in decreased iron intake.

Micronutrients

Micronutrients are nutrients that the body requires in only small quantities. Micronutrients include both vitamins and minerals.

Vitamins

Following the DRI suggestions for vitamins may help to prevent diseases and maintain good health. Good food sources are preferred to vitamin supplements, because food also is a good source of fiber and other nutrients. Vitamins are classified as either fat-soluble or water-soluble. The reference daily intakes (RDIs) mentioned in the following sections are for the average adult male and female who are 19 to 70 years old.

Fat-Soluble Vitamins The fat-soluble vitamins, A, D, E, and K, are found in the fat and oily parts of foods. They tend to be stored in the liver and adipose tissue and remain there, rather than being excreted like most water-soluble vitamins. The storage of fat-soluble vitamins in the body makes it possible to

survive long periods of time without having to include them in the diet. However, because they are stored so efficiently in the body, fat-soluble vitamins carry a high risk of toxicity.

Vitamin A. Vitamin A (retinol) is found in orange, yellow-orange, and green leafy vegetable foods, such as carrots, pumpkin, apricot, squash, peaches, and spinach. Vitamin A is also found in beef liver and fish liver oil.

Most of the body's vitamin A is stored in the liver as retinyl palmitate and released into the bloodstream as retinal. It binds to retinol-binding protein and prealbumin (transthyretin). It helps with eyesight and epithelial cells and tissues (skin cells).

Deficiencies in vitamin A may cause night blindness; xerosis (dryness) of the conjunctiva and cornea; xerophthalmia and keratomalacia; keratinization of lung, GI tract, and urinary tract tissues; and increased susceptibility to infection. Follicular hyperkeratosis of the skin (raised pink bumps where hair exits) is common in vitamin A deficiency.

Acute toxicity occurs in children taking vitamin A doses greater than 100,000 micrograms (300,000 International Units), resulting in increased intracranial pressure and vomiting. Death may ensue unless ingestion is discontinued. Women who take 13-*cis*-retinoic acid (isotretinoin) for skin conditions during pregnancy may cause birth defects in infants. Adults may also exhibit *carotenosis*, in which the skin (not including the sclera) becomes deep yellow or orange-yellow, especially on the palms and soles. Early warning signs may include sparse or coarse hair, thinning eyebrows, dry rough skin, and cracked lips. The DRI is 900 micrograms (**mcg**)/day for males and 700 mcg/day for females.

Vitamin D. Sunlight enables the skin to make vitamin D with cholesterol. Milk is often **fortified** with vitamin D, as are canned salmon and tuna. The main function of vitamin D is to improve the absorption of calcium from the intestine to make stronger bones and teeth. Deficiency causes metabolic bone softening called *rickets* in children and *osteomalacia* in adults. The DRI is 5 mcg/day (ages 19–50) and 10 mcg/day (ages 51–70) for both males and females.

Vitamin E. Vitamin E is found in wheat germ oil, sunflower seeds, eggs, butter, nuts, and green leafy vegetables. Vitamin E is a strong antioxidant for lipids.

Deficiency is generally caused by **malabsorption**, not by lack of ingestion. Vitamin E deficiency may cause disorders of the reproductive system; abnormalities of muscle, liver, and bone marrow; hemolysis of red blood cells; defective embryo genesis; brain dysfunction; and disorder of capillary permeability. The DRI is 15 mg/day for both males and females.

Vitamin K. Vitamin K (phytonadione) is found primarily in dark green leafy vegetables. Vitamin K is necessary for blood coagulation; it controls the formation of coagulation factors II (prothrombin), VII (proconvertin), IX (Christmas factor, plasma thromboplastin component), and X (Stuart factor) in the liver. Vitamin K is also needed for calcium uptake in the bones. It is used as an antidote for coumadin overdoses.

Deficiency is rare in adults, because the microbiologic flora of the normal gut synthesize menaquinones (from vitamin K).

---

fortified with an added nutrient for enrichment.

malabsorption an abnormality in digestion that causes nutrients to be absorbed poorly or not at all.

hypermetabolic metabolizing at an increased rate.

Vitamin K Deficiency in Infants

In infants, the liver, where vitamin K is stored, is not fully developed. Thus, vitamin K deficiency in breast-fed infants remains a major worldwide cause of infant morbidity and mortality. One to seven days postpartum, the vitamin-deficient infant may have skin, GI, or chest hemorrhage.

However, the following can contribute to an increased need for vitamin K: trauma, extensive surgery, long-term parenteral nutrition with or without treatment with broad-spectrum antibiotics, and overdoses of coumadin. Drugs that contribute to vitamin K-related hemorrhagic disease are anticonvulsants, anticoagulants, certain antibiotics (particularly cephalosporins), salicylates, and megadoses of vitamin A or E. The DRI is 120 mcg/day for males and 90 mcg/day for females.

Water-Soluble Vitamins Water-soluble vitamins, for the most part, are carried in the bloodstream and excreted in the urine. Although they are required only in small doses, intake is needed on a daily basis. Vitamins B1, B2, B6, B12, and C are water-soluble vitamins. Water-soluble vitamins are unlikely to be toxic, but excess intake of vitamins C and B6 may have serious side effects. These vitamins are easily destroyed during storage or preparation.

Vitamin B1. Vitamin B1 (thiamine) can be found in fortified bread and cereals, sunflower seeds, peanuts, wheat bran, beef liver, pork, seafood, egg yolk, and beans. Vitamin B1 is necessary for carbohydrate metabolism.

Deficiency causes the disease *beriberi,* which affects the peripheral neurologic, cerebral, cardiovascular, and GI systems. Those most at risk are breastfeeding infants whose mothers are thiamine-deficient, adults with high consumption of polished rice, alcoholics, patients on renal dialysis, patients on total parenteral nutrition (TPN) (high concentrations of dextrose infusions or frequent or long-term infusions can lead to increased need for B1, especially if vitamin B1 is not administered), and patients with **hypermetabolic** states in which more carbohydrate is needed or metabolized (e.g., fever, infection, pregnancy, and strenuous exercise). The DRI is 1.2 mg/day for males and 1.1 mg/day for females.

Vitamin B2. Vitamin B2 (riboflavin) is found in liver, kidney, heart, nuts, cheese, eggs, milk, green leafy vegetables, whole grains, and fortified cereals. Vitamin B2 is needed for the health of the mucous membranes in the digestive tract and aids in absorption of iron and vitamin B6.

Deficiency of vitamin B2 leads to oral, eye, skin, and genital lesions; dizziness; hair loss; insomnia; light sensitivity; poor digestion; retarded growth; slow mental responses; and burning feet. The DRI is 1.3 mg/day for males and 1.1 mg/day for females.

Vitamin B3. Vitamin B3 (niacin) is found in lean meats, poultry, fish, liver, and peanuts. Vitamin B3 is very important in oxidation–reduction reactions and is vital in protein metabolism.

Deficiency of niacin and tryptophan, an amino acid that allows the body to synthesize niacin, leads to the disease *pellagra*. Pellagra affects the skin, mucous membranes, GI, and brain/CNS systems, with photosensitive rash, scarlet stomatitis, glossitis, diarrhea, and mental aberrations. Common in India and Central and South America, deficiency is found in diets high in corn. The DRI is 16 mg/day for males and 14 mg/day for females.

Vitamin B5. Vitamin B5 (pantothenic acid) can be found in beef, brewer's yeast, eggs, fresh vegetables, kidney, legumes, liver, mushrooms, nuts, pork, fish, whole rye flour, and whole wheat. Vitamin B5 is important for the secretion of hormones such as cortisone, and for maintenance of healthy skin, muscles, and nerves. Pantothenic acid is used in the release of energy, in the metabolism of fat, protein, and carbohydrates, and in the manufacture of lipids, neurotransmitters, steroid hormones, and hemoglobin.

Although vitamin B5 deficiency is extremely rare, symptoms include insomnia, depression, nausea, headache, and muscle spasm. The DRI is 5 mg/day for both males and females.

❝ Workplace Wisdom Vitamin Abbreviations

It is important for pharmacy technicians to know both the vitamin letter and its corresponding generic name. This is because vitamin names written without the generic name raise the risk of transcription and/or filling errors. ❞

Vitamin B6. Vitamin B6 (pyridoxine) is found in fortified cereals, beans, meat, poultry, fish, and some fruits and vegetables. Vitamin B6 is needed for red blood cell formation, antibody production, and cell respiration and growth, as well as for the conversion of tryptophan to niacin. When caloric intake is low, the body needs B6 to help convert stored carbohydrate or other nutrients to glucose to maintain normal blood sugar levels. Vitamin B6 helps maintain the normal range of blood glucose and the health of lymphoid organs (thymus, spleen, and lymph nodes) that make white blood cells. It is needed for the synthesis of the neurotransmitters required for normal nerve cell communication, such as serotonin and dopamine.

❝ Workplace Wisdom Pyridoxine Supplements

Although a shortage of vitamin B6 will limit the functions discussed here, supplements do not enhance them in well-nourished individuals without vitamin B6 deficiencies. ❞

Vitamin B6 deficiency can result in a form of anemia that is similar to iron-deficiency anemia. B6 deficiency can decrease antibody production and suppress the immune response. Signs and symptoms include dermatitis, glossitis (a sore tongue), depression, confusion, and convulsions.

Toxicity of vitamin B6 may cause sensory ataxia, profound impairment of position and vibration sense in the lower limbs, and nerve damage to the arms and legs. This neuropathy is usually related to high intake of vitamin B6 from supplements and can be reversed by stopping supplementation. Senses of touch, temperature, and pain are only somewhat affected. The RDI is 1.3 mg/day for males and females aged 19 to 50 and 1.7 mg/day for males and 1.5 mg/day for females over the age of 51.

Vitamin B9. Vitamin B9 (folic acid) is found in barley, beef, bran, brewer's yeast, brown rice, cheese, chicken, dates, green leafy vegetables, lamb, legumes, lentils, liver, milk, mushrooms, oranges, split peas, pork, root vegetables, salmon, tuna, wheat germ, whole grains, and whole wheat. Vitamin B9 is important for energy production and the formation of red blood cells. It strengthens immunity, promotes healthy cell division and replication, assists in protein metabolism, and prevents depression and anxiety.

Folic acid deficiency can be serious and may result in sore, red tongue, anemia, apathy, digestive disturbances, fatigue, graying hair, growth impairment, insomnia, labored breathing, memory problems, paranoia, and weakness. Spina bifida can occur in the infant if a pregnant woman does not get enough folic acid, especially in the first trimester. The RDI is 400 mcg/day for both males and females.

Vitamin B12. Vitamin B12 (cyanocobalamin) is found in mollusks, clams, beef liver, rainbow trout, and fortified cereals. Vitamin B12 is needed for healthy nerve cells, to make DNA, and for the formation of red blood cells. Vitamin B12 is bound to the protein in the food, and hydrochloric acid in the stomach releases B12 from the protein during digestion. Once released, B12 combines with a substance called intrinsic factor (IF) before it is absorbed into the bloodstream.

Deficiency is a very serious problem, which ultimately leads to irreversible nerve damage signified by numbness and tingling in the hands and feet. Signs and symptoms include fatigue, weakness, nausea, constipation, flatulence, loss of appetite, weight loss, difficulty in maintaining balance, depression, confusion, poor memory, and soreness of the mouth or tongue. The RDI is 2.4 mcg/day for both males and females.

(info) Vitamin B12

Vitamin B12 binds with IF before it is absorbed and used by the body. An absence of IF prevents normal absorption of B12 and results in *pernicious anemia*. Patients with pernicious anemia need IM injections of B12, as it is a chronic condition requiring monitoring by a physician and lifelong supplementation of vitamin B12.

Vitamin C. Vitamin C (ascorbic acid) is found in citrus fruits, including oranges, lemons, limes, and grapefruits. Vitamin C is an **antioxidant** and is essential for collagen formation and maintaining the integrity of connective tissue, bone, and teeth. Important for wound healing and recovery from burns, vitamin C helps in the absorption of iron. Vitamin C functions as a reduction/oxidation system in the cells of the body. It also activates enzymes that hydroxylate procollagen proline and lysine to procollagen hydroxyproline and hydroxylysine.

Severe deficiency results in *scurvy*, a condition characterized by general weakness, bleeding gums, anemia, and skin bleeding. The DRI for vitamin C is 90 mg/day for males and 75 mg/day for females.

Minerals

Minerals are inorganic compounds that are much smaller than vitamins and occur in much simpler forms. Like vitamins, minerals have no calories and do not provide energy to the body. Dozens of minerals are found in nature, and 21 of them are essential for human nutrition. Minerals also act as helpers in delivering nutrients and aiding in certain functions in the body. They differ from vitamins in that they are indestructible; they act as catalysts in body processes but are not consumed or broken down in these processes. Minerals are not made by the body; therefore, **exogenous** sources must be used.

Some minerals, such as calcium and phosphorus, are used to build bones and teeth. Others are important components of hormones, such as iodine in thyroxine. Sodium and potassium are minerals called *electrolytes* that help regulate muscle contraction, conduction of nerve impulses, and normal heart rhythm.

Minerals are classified into two groups based on the body's need. The *major minerals*, or *macrominerals*, are needed by the body in larger quantities; in general, more than 100 mg/day. Calcium, chlorine, magnesium, phosphorus, potassium, sodium, and sulfur fall into this category. *Minor minerals*, or *trace elements*, are needed in amounts of less than 100 mg/day. Iron, zinc, selenium, copper, and iodine are minor minerals.

Minerals are very important in regulation of numerous body functions. Some common minerals, their main functions, and DRIs are listed in Table 26-16.

Water

Water makes up 60% of an adult's body weight. The average adult male should drink 3 L/day of fluids, while women need 2.2 L/day. Most water should come from liquids and foods. Water is an indispensable component of the body; it actually forms a major portion of every tissue and provides the medium in which most of the body's activities are conducted. It also

---

PROFILE IN PRACTICE

A doctor orders TPN for an inpatient; the solution is to contain 25 gm of lipids 20% (fat), 50 gm of amino acids 10% (protein), and 300 gm of dextrose 70% (carbohydrate) per TPN bag.

▸ *What is the total number of kilocalories provided to the patient by one TPN bag?*

---

antioxidant a molecule that slows or prevents the oxidation of other molecules.

exogenous from outside the organism.

TABLE 26-16 Mineral Functions and DRIs

Mineral	Main Function	DRI (males)	DRI (Females)
Calcium	Bone, muscle, nerve, and blood development	1,000 mg/day (ages 19–50)	1,000 mg/day (ages 19–50)
		1,200 mg/day (ages 51 and up)	1,200 mg/day (ages 51 and up)
Iron	Maintains oxygen levels in blood	8 mg/day	18 mg/day (ages 19–50)
			8 mg/day (ages 51 and up)
Magnesium	Aids in energy metabolism, protein synthesis, maintenance of muscle and nerve function. Needed for more than 300 biochemical reactions in the body.	400 mg/day (ages 19–30)	310 mg/day (ages 19–30)
		420 mg/day (ages 31 and up)	320 mg/day (ages 31 and up)
Potassium	Maintains proper muscle memory function	4.7 gm/day	4.7 gm/day
Selenium	Supports immune system and thyroid and helps make antioxidants	55 mcg/day	55 mcg/day
Sodium	Regulates body fluids	1.5 gm/day (ages 19–30)	1.5 gm/day (ages 19–30)
		1.3 gm/day (ages 31–70)	1.3 gm/day (ages 31–70)
Zinc	Aids in the healing process	11 mg/day	8 mg/day

Daily Water Intake Requirements

Use the following formula to determine your water requirements:

Body weight × 0.6 ÷ 12

Example

200 lb. × 0.6 ÷ 12 = 10 (8-0z. glasses of water a day)

Regular intake helps maintain normal functions of the body. Thirst is a signal to drink water. Lack of water can lead to dehydration.

facilitates many metabolic reactions that occur in the body and helps transport vital materials to the cells. One highly important function of water is to serve as the vehicle in which glycogen is transported into muscle cells. *Glycogen* is often referred to as muscle fuel, because it powers muscle contractions.

USDA MyPlate Food Guidance System

The traditional food guide was developed by the USDA with support from the DHHS (see Figure 26-7). With the understanding that "one size does not fit all," the guide was recently revised to reflect more individuals' dietary needs. Now called MyPlate, the USDA guidance system is designed to help people to:

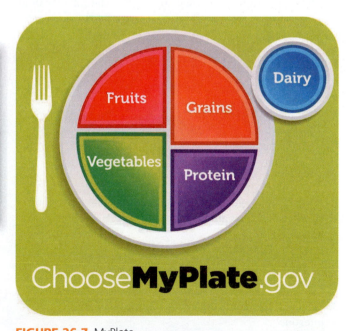

FIGURE 26-7 MyPlate.
Source: USDA

- Make healthy food choices
- Find balance between food and exercise
- Stay within the recommended caloric intake
- Get the most nutrition from their caloric intake

Food Allergies

People develop allergies to all different kinds of foods. Approximately 2% of American adults and 5% of infants and children have a food allergy, and 90% of all food-related allergic reactions are caused by one of the following eight foods: milk, eggs, fish, shellfish, tree nuts, peanuts, wheat, and soybeans. Food allergies involve the immune system and can be quite troublesome for those who experience common symptoms, such as swelling, hives, rashes, nasal congestion, asthma, nausea, diarrhea, and gas. Symptoms can be immediate or delayed up to 48 hours after ingestion of the offending food. Allergic reactions can be severe and life-threatening, causing anaphylactic shock and even death.

Food *intolerances* cause the same symptoms as food allergies but without involving the immune system. For example, a lactose intolerance can cause symptoms similar to mild allergy, such as gas and diarrhea. However, lactose intolerance may also cause thinning of the GI mucous lining, cramping, and bleeding during defecation; an allergy to milk would not produce these effects. All unexpected food reactions should be evaluated by an expert.

Summary

The GI system is the system whereby food travels through the body, and digestion is accomplished. Food is broken down, absorbed, or chemically modified into substances that are required by the cells to survive and function properly. Waste products that the body cannot use are eliminated. The GI system extends from the mouth to the anus. Its six main parts are the mouth, esophagus, pharynx, stomach, and small and large intestines. Various supportive structures, accessory glands, and accessory organs are also parts of the complete digestive system. The main purpose of the digestive system is to fuel the body.

An estimated 70 million Americans suffer from one or more digestive disorders; these disorders account for 13% of all hospitalizations. More than 400,000 new cases of peptic ulcer are diagnosed each year, resulting in nearly 40,000 surgeries annually. As a pharmacy technician, you should be aware of the important digestive disorders discussed throughout this chapter.

Many OTC remedies are available to treat the *milder* forms of digestive disease. More serious GI diseases often require more aggressive therapies, including surgery.

As with any disease, the primary goal is prevention. Pharmacy technicians need to be prepared to assist the pharmacist in providing information to clients about proper nutrition and should have an understanding of USDA recommendations and the current DRIs.

Chapter Review Questions

1. Most ulcers are found in the _____.
   a. stomach
   b. duodenum
   c. jejunum
   d. ileum

2. The waves of synchronized contractions that move food along the GI tract are known as _____.
   a. villi
   b. emulsification
   c. motility
   d. peristalsis

3. Which of the following is not a part of the large intestine?
   a. cecum
   b. transverse colon
   c. duodenum
   d. sigmoid colon

4. All of the following are antihistamines that can be used as antiemetics, *except* _____.
   a. ondanestron
   b. meclizine
   c. scopolamine
   d. dimenhydrinate

5. The three parts of the small intestine are _____.
   a. esophagus, stomach, and duodenum
   b. jejunum, duodenum, and ileum
   c. duodenum, diaphragm, and ileum
   d. stomach, esophagus, and jejunum

6. Which of the following promotes inflammation, pain, and fever?
   a. cyclooxygenase
   b. NSAIDs
   c. 5-HT3 antagonists
   d. prostaglandins

7. Which of the following is an essential amino acid?
   a. alanine
   b. cysteine
   c. lysine
   d. serine

8. Which of the following is classified as a bulk-forming laxative?
   a. Metamucil
   b. Colace
   c. Senekot
   d. Citrucel

9. Carbohydrates should make up what percentage of a person's dietary intake?
   a. 10−35
   b. 20−35
   c. 45–65
   d. 50−75

10. Saturated fat intake should not exceed _____ of a person's total fat intake.
    a. 2%
    b. 5%
    c. 10%
    d. none of the above

Critical Thinking Questions

1. Why are many vitamin deficiencies more prevalent in underdeveloped countries than in the United States?

2. No-/low-carbohydrate and high-protein diets are very popular. Do you think these types of diets are nutritionally sound?

3. What can people do to help reduce their risk of developing ulcers?

Web Challenge

1. Go to http://www.choosemyplate.gov to assess your dietary intake and physical activity levels.

2. Visit http://www.nlm.nih.gov/medlineplus/gerd.html to learn more about GERD.

References and Resources

Adams, M.P., D.L. Josephson, and L.N. Holland, Jr. *Pharmacology for Nurses: A Pathophysiologic Approach.* (4th edition.) Upper Saddle River, NJ: Pearson, 2013.

"Arthritis Today 2004 Drug Guide DMARDs." http://www.arthritis.org/conditions/DrugGuide/about_dmards.asp. 15 July 2007. Web.

"Carbohydrates, Proteins, and Fats." http://www.merck.com/mmhe/sec12/ch152/ch152b.html. 27 July 2007. Web.

"Diverticulitis." Web MD. 11 April 2012. Web.

Drug Facts and Comparisons, 2013 ed. St. Louis: Wolters Kluwer Health.

"Food Allergens." www.fda.gov. 27 July 2013. Web.

Holland, N. and M.P. Adams. *Core Concepts in Pharmacology.* (3rd edition.) Upper Saddle River, NJ: Pearson, 2010.

Mayo Clinic. "Water: How Much Should You Drink Every Day?" http://www.mayoclinic.com/health/water/NU00283. 30 July 2013. Web.

"MOA of APAP News on APAP." http://www.pharmweb.net/pwmirror/pwy/paracetamol/pharmwebpicmechs.html. 15 July 2007. Web.

"National Digestive Diseases Information Clearinghouse (NDDIC)." http://digestive.niddk.nih.gov. 5 August 2013. Web.

"National Institutes of Health Office of Dietary Supplements." http://ods.od.nih.gov/index.aspx. 26 June 2007. Web.

National Library of Medicine. "A Review of SERMs and National Surgical Adjuvant Breast and Bowel Project Clinical Trials." http://www.ncbi.nlm.nih.gov/entrez/query.fcgi?cmd=Retrieve&db=PubMed&listuids=14613021&dopt=Abstract. 15 July 2007. Web.

"The Merck Manual of Diagnosis and Therapy." http://www.merck.com/mrkshared/mmanual/section5/chapter57/57a.jsp. 15 July 2007. Web.

"United States Department of Agriculture." http://myplate.gov. 6 August 2013. Web.

"United States Department of Agriculture." http://www.mypyramid.com. 30 June 2007. Web.

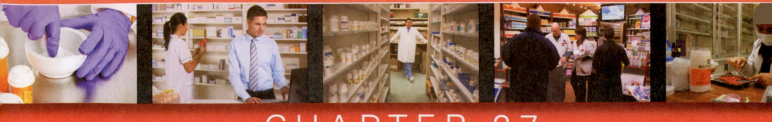

CHAPTER 27

The Musculoskeletal System

LEARNING OBJECTIVES

After completing this chapter, you should be able to:

- List, identify, and diagram the basic anatomical structure and parts of the muscles and bones.

- Describe the functions and physiology of the muscles and bones.

- List and define common diseases affecting the muscles and bones, and understand the causes, symptoms, and pharmaceutical treatments associated with each disease.

- Describe the mechanisms and the complications of the following musculoskeletal diseases and comprehend how each class of drugs works: osteomyelitis, osteoporosis, osteoarthritis, gout, inflammation, multiple sclerosis, and cerebral palsy.

- List the indications for use and mechanisms of action of ASA, NSAIDs, COX-2 inhibitors, antigout agents, calcitonin, bisphosphonates, SERMs, and skeletal muscle relaxants.

KEY TERMS
. . . .

bone marrow, p. 420
bones, p. 419
cartilage, p. 419
joints, p. 425
ligaments, p. 425
muscle, p. 419
myocyte, p. 419
sarcomere, p. 419
synovial fluid, p. 425
tendons, p. 425

INTRODUCTION

The musculoskeletal system is extremely important, as it provides the framework of the human body for both support and movement. All body movement is coordinated between the nervous system and the bones, joints, muscles, ligaments, cartilage, and tendons. Whether you are eating, riding a bike, eliminating waste, or simply breathing, the musculoskeletal system underlies that action.

Anatomy of the Muscles

Skeletal **muscles** are attached to bones and enable body movement (*kinetics*). Skeletal muscles are voluntary, striated in shape, and contain multiple peripheral nuclei.

The heart is made up of cardiac muscle known as the *myocardium*. This muscle contracts rhythmically, and its action is coordinated by the transmission of electrical impulses from nerve to muscle fibers. The cadence and rhythm of the heart, as well as the force of contraction, are dependent on this muscle.

Smooth muscle, or *visceral muscle*, is attached to, or lines, organs such as the stomach, intestines, lungs, and blood vessels. Figure 27-1 shows the three types of muscle.

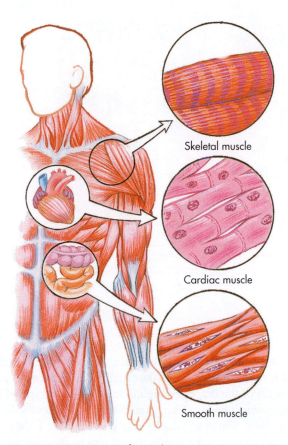

Skeletal muscle

Cardiac muscle

Smooth muscle

FIGURE 27-1 Types of muscle.

---

muscle a specialized tissue that contracts when stimulated.

sarcomere one of the segments into which a fibril of striated muscle is divided.

myocyte a muscle cell.

bones specialized form of dense connective tissue consisting of calcified intercellular substance that provides the shape and support for the body. Bones are made of calcium and phosphate. Injuries can result in fractures.

cartilage soft tissues that line every joint and give shape to the ears and nose. Injuries can result in tears or degeneration of the cartilage and arthritis.

Muscle Action

A muscle's thick and thin filaments do the actual work of the muscle. The thick filaments are made of a protein called *myosin*, formed as a shaft of myosin molecules arranged in the shape of a cylinder. There are about 300 molecules of myosin per thick filament. The enzyme ATPase hydrolyzes adenosine triphosphate, which is required for myosin and actin cross-bridge formation. The thin filaments are composed of three different proteins—actin, tropomyosin, and troponin—and look like two strands of pearls twisted around each other. Together, these are termed the *regulatory protein complex*.

The thick myosin filaments grab onto the thin actin filaments by forming cross-bridges during contraction of the muscle. The thick filaments grab and pull the thin filaments past them, which shortens the **sarcomere**. The signal for contraction in a muscle fiber is synchronized over the entire fiber so that all the myofibrils that make up the sarcomere shorten at the same time. Two proteins in the grooves of each thin filament enable the thin filaments to slide along the thick ones. These proteins are *tropomyosin*, a long rod-like protein, and *troponin*, a shorter bead-like protein complex. Troponin and tropomyosin are the molecular chemicals or *switches* that control the interaction of actin and myosin during muscle contraction.

Chemical and physical interactions between actin and myosin cause the sarcomere length to shorten, and therefore the **myocyte** (muscle cell) to contract, during the process of excitation-contraction coupling.

The Functions of Muscles

The main functions of the muscles include the following:

- Providing movement of and within the body through contraction. This includes large movement, such as running or walking, and finer movement such as smiling or wincing.
- Stabilizing the joints.
- Maintaining body posture.
- Producing heat within the body to maintain body temperature. About 85% of the heat produced inside the body occurs as a result of muscle contraction.

The Bones

A newborn has about 300 *soft* **bones**, which eventually grow together, or *fuse*, to form 206 adult bones. Some baby bones are made of **cartilage**, which is a soft and flexible cushion. During childhood, the cartilage grows and slowly hardens into a bone, as calcium is deposited. At about the age of 25, the cartilage will have finished hardening into a bone. After the cartilage has hardened, there can be no more bone growth. Bones are classified into one of the following five categories:

1. *Flat* bones are generally more flat than round. Examples are the cranial bones and the rib bones.
2. *Irregular* bones have no defined shape. Examples are the scapula and the vertebrae.
3. *Sesamoid* bones often have cartilage and fibrous tissue mixed in. These bones are found in the joints and help to

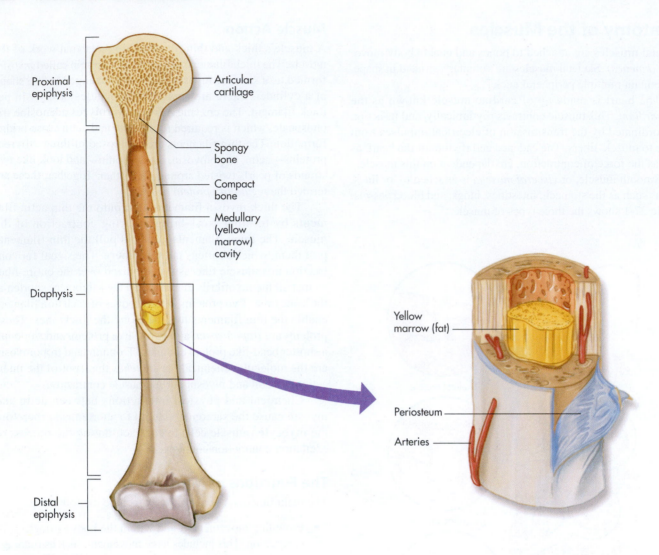

FIGURE 27-2 • The long bone.

lower friction and enhance joint movement. One example is the patella (kneecap).

4. *Short* bones are more cube-shaped. Examples are the carpals of the hand.

5. *Long* bones are the most common (see Figure 27-2). One example is the femur of the leg. The inside of a long bone is divided into two areas: the *epiphysis* (the rounded end of the bone) and the *diaphysis* (the main shaft or central part of the bone).

The epiphysis is covered with smooth, slippery articular cartilage, which helps bones move against each other at the joints. The inside of the epiphysis is made up of spongy or *cancellous* bone, which is made from criss-crossed strands of bone; the spaces between these strands are filled with bone marrow.

---

bone marrow the spongy type of tissue found inside most bones; responsible for the manufacture of red blood cells, some white blood cells, and platelets. Also acts as a storage area for fat.

The diaphysis has a hollow core, the *medullary cavity*, that is filled with red marrow in children and yellow marrow in adults. The walls of the diaphysis are made of a second type of bone called *compact bone*, which is much harder and more solid than spongy bone. The outermost layer of the long bone is the *periosteum*, which covers the diaphysis and part of the epiphysis, but does not cover the articular cartilage. This layer contains cells called *osteoblasts*, which make new bone to replace older bone cells (*osteoclasts*) and also provide nourishment for the bone.

Bone Marrow

Bone marrow is the gelatinous substance inside bones (see Figure 27-3) and occurs in two types: red and yellow. Red marrow is a red, jelly-like substance that contains blood cells and is usually found only in the sternum, vertebrae, ribs, hips, clavicles, and cranial bones. Red bone marrow produces red blood cells, white blood cells, and blood platelets. In infants, red marrow is found in the bone cavities.

Yellow marrow is a fatty yellow substance that replaces red marrow in the long bones of adults; it does not produce blood cells. Yellow bone marrow has fewer pluripotential

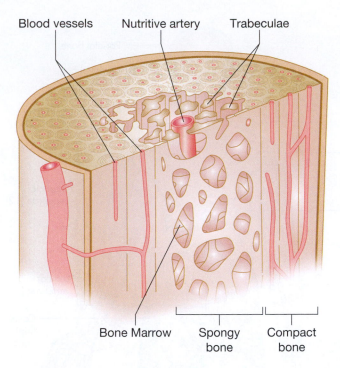

Blood vessels   Nutritive artery   Trabeculae

Bone Marrow   Spongy bone   Compact bone

FIGURE 27-3 Bone marrow.

hematopoietics (stem cells), and what stem cells it does contain are inactive. As one ages, red marrow converts to yellow, containing more fat and less erythrocytes.

The Functions of Bones

The main functions of the bones include the following:

- Providing the framework or foundation of the body.
- Supporting the body against the pull of gravity to keep it in an upright position (see Figure 27-4).
- Protecting the internal organs—heart, lungs, brain, liver—by enveloping them in a *cage*.
- Allowing the exchange of nutrients and waste products via the tunnels within the bone's living tissue.
- Acting as the components of a mechanical lever system that works with the muscular system to allow movement.
- Storing nutrients, such as calcium and phosphorus, in bone marrow. When calcium levels in the blood decrease below normal, the bones release calcium so that there will be an adequate supply for metabolic needs. When blood calcium levels increase, the excess calcium is stored in the bone matrix. The dynamic process of releasing and storing calcium goes on almost continuously to maintain homeostasis.

Musculoskeletal Disorders

Diseases and disorders of the muscles and bones range from minor discomfort to debilitating conditions. This section discusses several of the most common diseases and disorders of the musculoskeletal system.

Osteomyelitis

Osteomyelitis is a bacterial infection inside the bone that destroys bone tissue. Often the original site of infection is in another part of the body, but the infection spreads to the bone via the blood.

Pharmacokinetics plays an important role in selecting anti-infective agents to combat osteomyelitis. The physician generally chooses the drug that exhibits the highest bactericidal or fungicidal activity with the least toxicity at the lowest cost. A penicillinase-resistant semisynthetic penicillin (PCN), such as nafcillin or oxacillin, and an aminoglycoside should ameliorate osteomyelitic infections, at least until culture results and sensitivities are determined.

Staphylococcus aureus is the usual culprit behind spinal osteomyelitis; it responds well to IV clindamycin in PCN-allergic patients. Antimicrobial IV therapy may last six weeks or longer. Surgical debridement of infected, devitalized bone and tissue must be performed in addition to the IV therapy. Occasionally, hyperbaric oxygen therapy (HBO) is required. HBO therapy is a medical treatment in which patients breathe pure oxygen inside a pressurized chamber. The hyperbaric chamber is pressurized to 2.5 times the normal atmospheric pressure and delivers 100% oxygen. This increases the amount of oxygen being carried by the blood, which results in more oxygen being delivered to the organs and tissues in the body. This extra oxygen improves the action of certain antibiotics, activates white blood cells to fight infection, and promotes the healing process in chronic wounds.

Osteoporosis

Osteoporosis is bone brittleness due to lack of calcium. Estrogen helps to keep calcium in the bone and blood; parathyroid hormone (PTH) and calcitonin contribute to the homeostasis of calcium; and vitamin D is required for the absorption of calcium. Osteoporosis is prevalent in postmenopausal women because of their low levels of estrogen. Figure 27-5 compares a normal bone to one affected by osteoporosis.

> **Workplace Wisdom** Osteoporosis
>
> Osteoporosis, which is the most common bone disorder in the United States, is 400% more prevalent in women than in men.

Paget's Disease

Normally, bone continually breaks down and rebuilds itself, but Paget's disease changes the normal process of bone growth: Bone breaks down more quickly and then grows back softer than the normal bone. The softer, weakened bones bend or break more easily and may grow larger than before. Although this disease can affect any bone, it is more common in the skull, vertebra, hip, pelvis, and leg bones.

Treatment of Weak, Fragile, or Soft Bones

As discussed previously, osteoporosis is a major cause of bone fractures, affecting 20 million Americans. Women over the age of 45 commonly suffer fractures of the hip, wrist, or spine due to loss of bone mass from osteoporosis. Think of bone remodeling

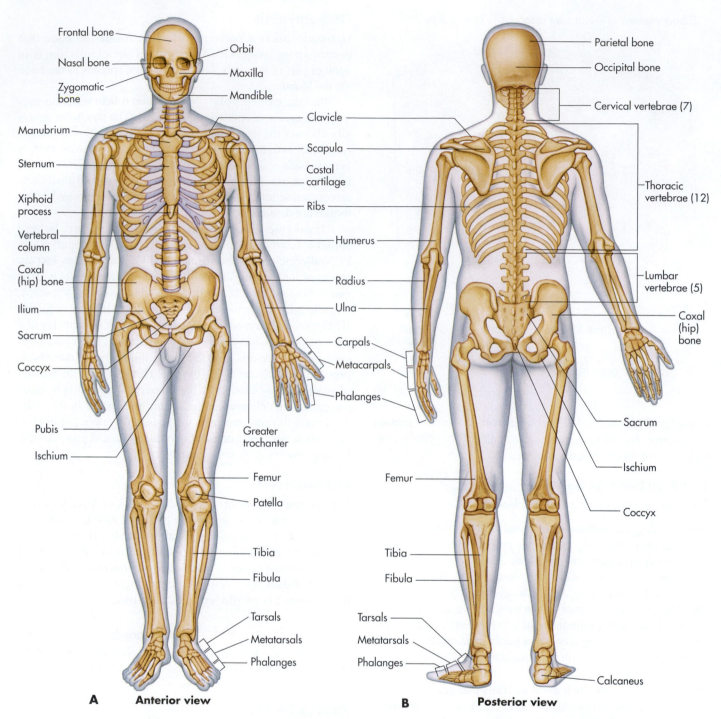

FIGURE 27-4 The skeleton.

as a ditch digger digging a ditch and another person right beside him filling up the ditch. As old bone is worn away or removed, new bone is made. As calcium removal leaves a hole in the bone, new calcium is laid to fill in the holes, making new bone. PTH and calcitonin hormones from the parathyroid gland and thyroid gland, respectively, contribute to this homeostasis.

In addition to vitamin D and mineral calcium replacement therapy, weak, fragile, and soft bones may respond to hormonal therapy (estrogen, calcitonin) and bisphosphonates. Estrogen hormonal therapy (estrogen replacement therapy, hormone

replacement therapy) is used for osteoporosis, while bisphosphonates and calcitonin are used for both Paget's disease and osteoporosis (also see Tables 27-1 and 27-2).

Cholesterol in the skin, along with sunlight, generates an inactive form of vitamin D that becomes cholecalciferol. This is released into the blood system, where it becomes calcifediol. Finally it is sent to the kidneys, where it is changed by enzymes to an active form of vitamin D called *calcitriol*.

The parathyroid gland and the thyroid gland work together to ensure that the bone-building and bone-demineralization

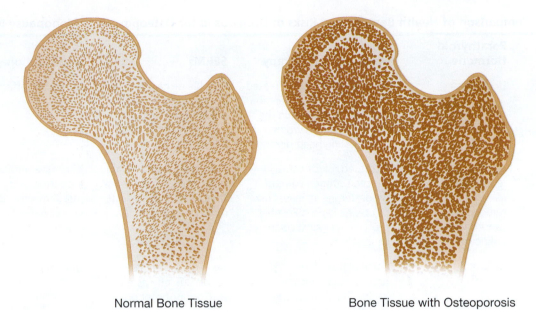

Normal Bone Tissue   Bone Tissue with Osteoporosis

FIGURE 27-5 Bone density.

TABLE 27-1 Bone Resorption Inhibitors

Bone Resorption Inhibitor	Trade and Generic Names	Notes
Nitrogen side-chain bisphosphonates	Actonel (risedronate) Aredia (pamidronate) Boniva (ibandronate) Fosamax (alendronate) Zometa (zoledronic acid)	The newer, more potent bisphosphonates are also called third-generation bisphosphonates Hypercalcemia with metastases, menopausal osteoporosis
Nonnitrogen side-chain bisphosphonates, calcitonin—polypeptide hormone	Didronel (etidronate) Skelid (tiludronate) Miacalcin Nasal Spray	First- and second-generation Paget's disease reduces the risk of vertebral fracture, but not hip or wrist, in postmenopausal women with osteoporosis

TABLE 27-2 Comparison of Health Benefits and Risks of Drugs Used for Osteoporosis in Menopause

	Parathyroid Hormone	Hormone Replacement Therapy	SERMs	Bisphosphonates
Selected examples	Forteo (teriparatide, rDNA origin)	Premarin, Climara	Evista (raloxifene), the only SERM approved for osteoporosis. Others in the investigational pipeline as of 2007	Oral agents: Fosamax (alendronate), Actonel (risedronate)
				Injected agents: Aredia (pamidronate), Zometa (zoledronic acid)
Osteoporosis and fracture	Increases bone mineral density; reduces risk of fracture	Increases bone density; reduces risk of fracture, although not significantly in women over the age of 60. Not currently recommended for prevention of osteoporosis in most women	Increases bone density; reduces risk of spinal fractures. Does not appear to prevent hip fractures as bisphosphonates do	Drug of choice (DOC) for most women. Proven to increase bone mass and prevent fractures, including hip, spine, and wrist

TABLE 27-2 Comparison of Health Benefits and Risks of Drugs Used for Osteoporosis in Menopause (*Continued*)

	Parathyroid Hormone	Hormone Replacement Therapy	SERMs	Bisphosphonates
Heart disease	Unknown	No overall benefit; increased risk of myocardial infarction (MI) and stroke within the first two years in women with existing heart disease	Possible protection, according to a 2002 study, in women with existing heart disease	No known effects
Cancer	Animal studies report higher risk of bone tumors; human cancer risk unknown	Increased risk of breast cancer. Estrogen without progesterone increases risk of uterine cancer. Possible protection against colon cancer	Tamoxifen and raloxifene reduce breast cancer risk. Tamoxifen increases risk of uterine cancer	May have antitumor properties. May slow metastasis to the bone in cancer patients
Other positive effects	Unknown	Possible protection against urinary tract infections with vaginal application *only*, incontinence, glaucoma, macular degeneration	No vaginal bleeding. Fewer side effects than HRT or bisphosphonates	Unknown
Other negative effects	Injectable only (pain)	Increases risk of blood clots, vaginal bleeding, breast pain, asthma, endometriosis, fibroids, temporomandibular joint disorders, varicose veins, and gallstones. Mixed studies on Alzheimer's, osteoarthritis, migraines, and cataracts	Increases risk of blood clots. Side effects include menopausal symptoms of hot flashes and leg cramps. Swelling in the legs	Increases risk of GERD. Possible long-term risk of ulcers, especially in combination with NSAIDs or ASA. Administration of some requires empty stomach and 30 minutes of sitting up

(dissolution) processes maintain homeostasis. *Osteoclasts*, bone cells that arise from marrow stroma cells and found on the surfaces where bone is being formed, are generally regarded as bone-forming cells. Osteoclasts, enriched with identifier acid phosphatase, are large, multinucleated cells that play an active role in bone resorption or breakdown. PTH from the parathyroid gland and calcitonin from the thyroid gland work in tandem to accomplish this. When PTH is released, it stimulates bone demineralization or the breakdown of bone. This process is called *bone resorption* (not to be confused with absorption or reabsorption) in which the smaller minerals enter the bloodstream. One of the minerals that enters the blood system is calcium. Calcium is necessary for proper nerve and muscle function. PTH allows the kidneys to change the calcifediol to calcitriol.

Too much calcitriol released from the kidneys back into the bloodstream would cause hypercalcemia. When this happens, the thyroid gland (if functioning normally) will secrete calcitonin to counter the increase of calcium ions (Ca^{++}) in the blood. While calcium is coming out of the bone into the blood, the bone is left with *holes* in it that may contribute to osteoporosis if the calcium is not replaced—that is, if the bone is not rebuilt.

Bisphosphonates Bisphosphonates are a very common treatment for osteoporosis, as they mimic the natural organic bisphosphonate salts found in the body, inhibiting bone resorption and osteoclast activity and restoring bone mass and density. There are two types of bisphosphonates: nonnitrogen side-chain and nitrogen side-chain bisphosphonates. The nitrogen side-chain type is preferred, because they are more potent. Bisphosphonates irreversibly bind and inactivate osteoclasts and induce apoptosis of the osteoclast. In addition, they decrease osteoclast action. Bisphosphonates work by inhibition of the mevolonate pathway, the pathway responsible for cholesterol synthesis. The inactivated osteoclast is then incorporated into the bone matrix.

---

ligaments strong fibrous bands of connective tissue that hold bones together. Injuries can result in sprains.

tendons cords of connective tissue that attach muscle to bone. Injuries can result in strains, ruptures, or inflammation.

joint the location or position where bones are connected to each other. A joint contains synovial fluid and cartilage.

synovial fluid a liquid that fills the space between the cartilage of each bone; provides smooth movement by lubricating the cartilage.

Calcitonin Calcitonin inhibits bone resorption, and decreases the number of bone fractures from low bone density, by increasing bone growth and the number and action of osteoblasts. It blocks the bone-mineral-absorbing activity of the osteoclasts (bone cells), increases calcium excretion by the kidneys, and slows bone resorption—the speed at which a bone is broken down before it is replaced.

Calcitonin is a polypeptide hormone that is a potent inhibitor of osteoclastic bone resorption, but its effects are only temporary. It acts directly on osteoclasts (via receptors on the cell surface for calcitonin). The calcitonin receptor is specific for osteoclasts and causes rapid shrinkage of the osteoclasts with initial exposure. Osteoclasts avoid the inhibitory effects of calcitonin following continued exposure.

Calcitonin is available in a nasal spray or injection. Often, calcitonin from eel or salmon is used, as it is many times stronger and longer-lasting than the human form. Calcitonin produces small, incremental increases in the bone mass of the spine with a modest reduction of bone turnover in women with osteoporosis. Although calcitonin reduces the risk of vertebral fracture in postmenopausal women with osteoporosis, it does not show much sign of helping nonvertebral fractures, such as in the hip or wrist. Calcitonin may also have an analgesic benefit. Miacalcin Nasal Spray has a new delivery system via the nose, as opposed to injection. Inhalation of 200 units/day may cause the minor side effect of nasal irritation.

Selective Estrogen Receptor Modulators Another option for postmenopausal women is the class of drugs called selective estrogen receptor modulators (SERMs). SERMs have a protective effect on the bones and heart; however, they do not control the hot flashes associated with menopause. Early studies report a significant reduction in the number of cases of breast cancer detected in women using SERMs. Because SERMs do not stimulate the uterus, there is no increased risk of endometrial cancer and no vaginal bleeding. The most common side effects are leg cramps and hot flashes that are worse than without the drug. Contraindications include a history of breast cancer, liver problems, or blood clots or if the patient is on hormone replacement therapy.

Nonpharmacologic Treatments of Osteoporosis Nonpharmacologic treatments for osteoporosis include weight-bearing exercise, such as daily walking. Lifestyle changes include smoking cessation and reduced intake of caffeinated and alcoholic beverages. Calcium intake from diet and supplements should total about 1,500 mg/day for a postmenopausal woman or 1,000 mg/day if she is receiving HRT.

Bursitis

Bursitis is an inflammation of the *bursae,* which are the small, fluid-filled pouches between bones and **ligaments**, or between bones and muscles, that serve as cushions.

Tendonitis

Tendonitis is an inflammation of the **tendons**, which are cords of connective tissue that attach muscle to bone.

Myalgia

Myalgia is muscle pain. It can be caused by many things and range from very minor to severe and acute to chronic.

Bone Marrow Disorders

Any disease or condition that affects blood cell production is considered a bone marrow disorder. This section briefly describes a few of the most common ones.

Anemia

Anemia is failure of the bone marrow to produce the components of the red blood cells. The most common cause is a lack of iron, which causes a lack of oxygen inside the erythrocyte and leads to fatigue. However, blood loss or hemolysis (red blood cell destruction) can also cause a variety of anemias, such as microcytic and normocytic.

Leukemia

Leukemia begins when one or more white blood cells experience deoxyribonucleic acid (DNA) loss or damage. The damaged DNA is then copied and passed on to subsequent generations of cells. These abnormal cells do not die off like normal cells, but instead multiply and accumulate within the body. No one really knows why such changes occur, but some factors that increase the risk of this disorder include genetics, age, environment, and lifestyle. All cancers, including leukemia, begin as a mutation in the genetic material—the DNA within certain cells.

Arthritis

Arthritis is the inflammation of a **joint**. There are several different types of arthritis, which vary in onset, action, and treatment possibilities.

Rheumatoid Arthritis

Rheumatoid arthritis (RA) is a progressive form of arthritis that has devastating effects on the joints, body organs, and general health. It is classified as an *autoimmune* disease, because the disease is caused by the immune system attacking the body itself. Symptoms include painful, stiff, and swollen joints, fever, and fatigue. RA is characterized by an inflammation of the cartilage around the joints that leads to a thickening and hardening of the **synovial fluid**. Eventually, RA attacks the visceral organs, which can cause lung or heart fibrosis, renal amyloidosis, and inflammatory conditions such as endocarditis and pericarditis.

> **❝ Workplace Wisdom** Osteoarthritis
>
> Reports indicate that as many as 40 million Americans are affected by osteoarthritis. **❞**

Osteoarthritis

Osteoarthritis is a progressive disease characterized by the breakdown of joint cartilage. Weight-bearing activities, such as marching, running, and jogging, are the main cause of the wear-and-tear breakdown of joints. Such joint erosion may cause the body to identify particles of the worn bone as foreign material in the joint; an immune reaction sends phagocytes to the site, resulting in irritation and inflammation.

Knee joint pain is the most common musculoskeletal complaint that sends people to their doctors. With today's increasingly active society, the number of knee problems is increasing. See Figure 27-6 for an illustration of the knee joint.   "

Gout

Gout is a painful joint inflammatory disease that was first described in the days of Hippocrates, 400 BCE to 300 BCE. Gout is caused by the deposit of uric acid in the joint synovial fluid of the big toes, knees, and elbows, and some soft tissues. Not necessarily localized to the joints, gout is a systemic disease.

Gout is caused by an excess or overproduction of uric acid or by the inability of the kidneys to adequately excrete uric acid from the body. Uric acid is formed every day from the metabolism of nucleic acids. Because humans cannot use uric acid, it is normally secreted into the urine by renal tubules. The condition of having too much uric acid in the blood is called *hyperuricemia.*

An increase in the amount of uric acid in the blood leads to the formation of needle-like uric acid crystals in the joints, which act as an irritant and cause an arthritis-like pain and inflammation that imitates osteoarthritis. When phagocytes (leukocytes) enter the area and attack the uric acid crystals, leading to a decrease in the pH (acidity) of the joint fluid, more uric acid accumulates in the joint, and the destructive cycle begins again if the uric acid levels in the blood remain high.

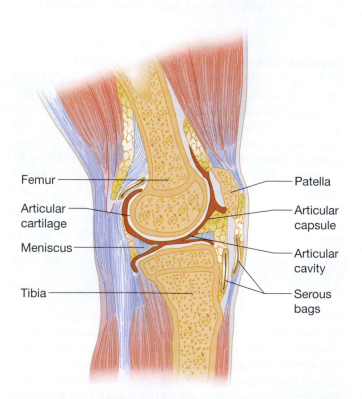

Femur
Articular cartilage
Meniscus
Tibia
Patella
Articular capsule
Articular cavity
Serous bags

FIGURE 27-6 The knee joint.

This occurs when uric acid is not filtered or cleared via the glomerulus of the nephrons in the kidneys.

Acute gout is the vicious cycle of inflammation that produces edema, redness, and severe pain. Chronic gout is characterized by uric acid slowly depositing in soft tissues, causing *tophi* (the bulging, deformed joints characteristic of gout). Uric acid may also collect in the urinary tract as kidney stones. Calcium pyrophosphate deposits, rather than uric acid crystals, cause *pseudoarthritis,* which is sometimes mistaken for gout.

As much as 3% of the U.S. population is affected by gout.   "

An excess of certain fermented alcoholic beverages (wine and beer) and certain foods that are aged and/or contain a high purine content (e.g., legumes [peas, lentils, beans]; cheeses; anchovies and sardines; scallops, mussels, and other shellfish; organ meats [liver, kidneys, heart]; and red meats) increase the uric acid level of the blood. This may precipitate a gout attack. Medications, including hydrochlorothiazide (a diuretic) and some transplant immunosuppressant medications, such as cyclosporine and tacrolimus, can also increase uric acid levels.

Certain disease states and genetic factors can predispose a person to gout. A high incidence has been noted in New Zealanders, Pacific Islanders, and postmenopausal women. However, gout affects men more than women by a ratio of 20:1. Obesity, high blood pressure, kidney disease, and genetics are all risk factors for gout.

Arthritis Treatment

This section describes some common treatments for arthritis.

Disease-Modifying Antirheumatic Drugs If taken early in the course of the disease, disease-modifying antirheumatic drugs (DMARDs) can help prevent the progression of the disease. DMARDs usually take up to six to eight months to evoke a response and thus are considered slow-acting drugs (remittive). DMARDs are now regarded as a long-term solution to symptom control. Generally, DMARDs are used for RA, but some can also be used for juvenile RA, ankylosing spondylitis, psoriatic arthritis, and lupus. DMARDs are immunosuppressants, and a major adverse reaction is an acquired illness due to the mechanism of action that lowers immune system response. Therefore, the patient must watch for such signs of infection as sore throat, cough, fever, or chills. Furthermore, vaccinations may pose a problem for those taking DMARDs, as DMARDs suppress or lower the immune system enough to make a vaccine a source of infection rather than protection. Table 27-3 lists some commonly prescribed antirheumatic agents.

Gold Compounds Gold compounds were discovered accidentally by a French physician, Jacques Forrestier, after he injected gold salts into a tuberculosis patient, who coincidentally had arthritis; the arthritis improved. Gold has been used to treat arthritis ever since. The exact mechanism of action is

TABLE 27-3 Antirheumatic Agents

Trade Name	Generic Name	Available Strength and Dosage Form(s)	Dosage
Arava	leflunomide	10 mg, 20 mg, 100 mg tablets	100 mg daily × 3 days, then 20 mg daily
Aurolate Myochrysine	gold sodium thiomalate (~50% gold)	50 mg/mL injectable solution	Weekly doses: 10 mg IM week 1 25 mg IM weeks 2 and 3 50 mg IM subsequent weeks
Azulfidine	sulfasalazine	500 mg tablets	1 gm bid
Cuprimine	penicillamine	125 mg, 250 mg capsules	125–250 mg daily, up to 750 mg daily
Depen	penicillamine	250 mg titratable tablets	125–250 mg daily, up to 750 mg daily
Plaquenil	hydroxychloroquine sulfate	200 mg tablets	400–600 mg daily
Ridaura	auranofin (29% gold)	3 mg capsule	6 mg daily or 3 mg bid
Solganal	aurothioglucose (~50% gold)	50 mg/mL injectable suspension	Weekly doses:
			10 mg IM week 1
			25 mg IM weeks 2 and 3
			50 mg IM subsequent weeks

not known, but it is believed that the gold interferes with the functions of the white blood cells that are responsible for joint damage and inflammation. Gold slows destruction, but it cannot cure existing joint deformities. Side effects include an itchy rash on the lower extremities and mouth ulcers, which disappear when the medicine is discontinued, and transitory diarrhea or loose bowel movements. Fifty percent of users discontinue this medication because of the side effects.

Penicillamine Penicillamine is related to the antibiotic PCN. However, patients who are allergic to PCN can take penicillamine. Known as a *chelator*, penicillamine binds to heavy metals in the body. It may become more active or potent if combined with copper, which is present naturally in the body. Used since the 1970s for RA, the exact mechanism or mode of action (MOA) of penicillamine is unknown, but it is believed to act like gold, interfering with the functions of the white blood cells that are responsible for joint damage and inflammation. Side effects include skin rashes, mouth sores, loss of taste, and gastrointestinal (GI) upset. Kidney damage may also occur; therefore, the patient must be monitored for protein in the urine.

Sulfasalazines A combination of salicylate and an antibiotic, originally used to treat inflammatory bowel disease, sulfasalazines

have been on the scene since the 1940s. Because sulfasalazine is not as toxic as gold or penicillamine, a renewed interest in its usage for RA has developed. Side effects include loss of appetite, nausea and vomiting (N/V), diarrhea, renal problems, and blood dyscrasias. In addition, it may cause severe allergic reactions or anaphylactic shock in those allergic to sulfa drugs.

Hydroxychloroquine Originally used to treat malaria and recently lupus, this medication has been around for many years. Hydroxychloroquine is indicated for patients with RA who have not responded well to nonsteroidal anti-inflammatory drugs (NSAIDs). It has few side effects and blood test monitoring is not required. Once-a-day dosing is usual with one rare toxic effect: The drug may deposit in the retina and cause visual impairment. Therefore, an ophthalmologic exam is recommended every six months.

Leflunomide Leflunomide helps to slow the progression of joint damage caused by RA. Although there is no cure for RA, leflunomide may keep the disease from progressing. It has been shown to inhibit structural damage (as evidenced by X-rays of erosions and joint space narrowing) and improve physical function. Leflunomide is an isoxazole immunomodulatory agent that inhibits an enzyme involved in pyrimidine synthesis. By blocking this enzyme, leflunomide prevents T-cell actions and proliferation that lead to the disabling inflammation of RA. Side effects include dry mouth, insomnia, hair loss, nausea, diarrhea, tiredness, and acne. Signs of toxicity include dark yellow urine, difficulty breathing or shortness of breath, increase in blood pressure, and yellowing of the skin or eyes. Leflunomide has the potential to cause liver damage; therefore, patients must be monitored. Rash, swelling, and difficulty breathing may be signs of a possible allergic reaction and should be reported immediately.

Secondary Lines of Therapy NSAIDs and other steroidal anti-inflammatory drugs are commonly used for the symptoms of RA, but they do not prevent progression of the disease. There is also some research showing that NSAIDs interfere with the bone-rebuilding process.

Treatment of Gout

Colchicine is mainly used only during the first 48 hours of an acute gout attack, as it will cause N/V when taken for longer periods. Colchicine alters the ability of the phagocytes to attack the uric acid crystals, which prevents the pH of the joint or synovial fluid from decreasing. Thus, the cycle of deposition of uric acid crystals and acid is broken and the gout attack

subsides. If a patient is taking *blood thinners*, such as aspirin, dipyridamole, or warfarin, or is prone to ulcers caused by NSAIDs or acetylsalicylic acid (ASA), colchicines may be the DOC (see Table 27-4).

Anti-inflammatory analgesics, such as aspirin and ibuprofen, can be used to reduce the pain and inflammation of acute gout attacks. Indomethacin is most often prescribed for gout inflammation.

Preventive Treatment *Prophylactic therapy* is the long-term use of drugs to prevent the reoccurrence of gout attacks and tophi. Two major types of drugs are used for preventive treatment: hypouricemic agents and uricosuric agents.

Hypouricemic agents decrease production of uric acid in the blood. The enzyme xanthine oxidase is necessary to convert hypoxanthine into uric acid. The MOA is inhibition of the enzyme xanthine oxidase so that hypoxanthine is not made. Therefore, uric acid is not formed, and hypoxanthine is then excreted in the urine. Over a period of time, the amount of uric acid in the blood decreases, preventing the future formation of tophi and urate stones in the kidney.

Uricosuric agents increase the excretion of uric acid through urination rather than altering the formation of uric acid. Uricosuric drugs promote the excretion of uric acid via the kidney,

TABLE 27-4 Comparison of Drugs Used to Treat Gout

Indication	Classification	Trade Name	Generic Name	Purpose	MOA
Acute gout attack	Antigout agent	No trade name	colchicine	To stop the cycle of deposition of uric acid crystals and lower pH during an immediate acute attack within the first 48 hours	Alters phagocytes' ability to attack uric acid crystals, prevents decrease in the pH of the joint or synovial fluid; stops the cycle of uric acid crystal formation and high pH.
Acute or chronic gout	NSAID	Indocin	indomethacin	Anti-inflammatory analgesics; reduce pain and swelling	Inhibits/blocks the enzyme COX-2, which starts the reaction of inflammation; prevents prostaglandin synthesis
Chronic	Hypouricemic agent	Zyloprim	allopurinol	Prophylactic therapy: decreases production of uric acid in the blood	Inhibition of the enzyme xanthine oxidase, stopping production of hypoxanthine and thus preventing formation of uric acid
	Uricosuric agent	Anturane Benemid	sulfinpyrazone probenecid	Prophylactic therapy: increases the excretion of uric acid	Blocks renal reabsorption of uric acid so that uric acid passes into the urine
	Combination drug	Colbene-mid	probenecid + colchicine	Reduces urate blood levels and prevents further gout attacks	MOA is same as for the individual drugs in combination

which leads to a rapid clearance of uric acid from the blood. These drugs block reabsorption of uric acid in the renal tubules of the kidney so that uric acid passes into the urine. Uricosuric drugs frequently cause GI distress. It is recommended that these drugs be taken with meals, milk, or antacids.

Some drugs for gout combine prophylactic and maintenance drugs. Often, probenecid is administered in combination with colchicine as Colbenemid, which reduces urate blood levels and prevents further gout attacks. To reduce the likelihood of developing renal urate stones, it is also recommended that the patient drink plenty of water daily.

Inflammation

Inflammation is a symptom common to bursitis, tendonitis, muscle pain, dysmenorrhea, arthritis, and gout. Inflammation, along with pain, is the most common symptom of all the previously discussed inflammatory diseases. The inflammatory process is a normal response to injury: When tissues are damaged, substances such as histamine, prostaglandins, and serotonin are released. These substances produce vasodilation and increase permeability of the capillary walls. As inflammation increases, the inflamed tissue hits nerves, which causes pain because the pain receptors are stimulated. This occurs while proteins and fluids leak out of the damaged cells. As blood flow to the damaged area increases, leukocytes migrate to the area to destroy harmful substances introduced by the injury. All of this results in the development of the following cardinal signs of inflammation:

- Redness
- Edema
- Warmth
- Pain
- Loss of function or immobilization

Treatment of Inflammation

There are basically three choices of anti-inflammatory agents to treat inflammation: salicylates, topical corticosteroids, and NSAIDs.

Salicylates Salicylates relieve inflammation by inhibiting the synthesis of prostaglandin. Along with their anti-inflammatory properties, salicylates are also used as analgesics and antipyretics. Side effects of salicylates include the following:

- *Nausea and vomiting*—Salicylates directly irritate the stomach mucosal lining and stimulate the chemoreceptor trigger zone in the medulla oblongata located in the brain stem, which directly excites the vomiting center.

info

Prolonged Inflammation

In some instances, the inflammatory process becomes chronic and repeats over a long period of time, often with little or no provocation. When exaggerated or prolonged, it results in further tissue damage. The inflammation itself becomes a disease.

- *Hemorrhagic (antiplatelet) effect*—Platelets are the sticky element in the blood necessary for clot formation. The anticoagulant effect of ASA inhibits the aggregation of platelets and thins out the blood, increasing the risk of hemorrhage and GI ulcer. Therefore, patients can bleed excessively if cut, undergo surgery, or have dental work while taking ASA and salicylamides.
- *Tinnitus*—In low doses, salicylates relieve pain, aches, and fever. Unfortunately, to relieve the pain of arthritis, gout, and RA, they must be used in large doses for extensive periods of time. Megadose therapy with ASA or NSAIDs is frequently associated with toxic effects and may also cause tinnitus by their effect on the inner ear, cochlea, and spiral ganglion.

The dangerous and often fatal reactions to acute salicylate poisoning are respiratory depression and acidosis. Reye's syndrome, a fatal disease affecting the brain and liver in children who take aspirin after or during a viral infection, has been the main reason for the decrease in the use of ASA in children.

Very good documentation supports the fact that ASA blocks the enzyme cyclooxygenase II (COX-2), thereby blocking the first step in the inflammatory process and further blocking prostaglandins from being made. In addition, the platelet-aggregating substance, thromboxane A2, is also blocked when ASA blocks the production of prostaglandin, thereby preventing further stroke or MI. This is why salicylates are also used for their antiplatelet or anticoagulant effect. If ulcers are not present, continual administration of aspirin may be beneficial to prevent the formation of thromboemboli. Usually, a child's dose of 81 mg is given. In layman's terms, this *thins out* the blood. Although too much aspirin or other salicylates may cause hemorrhage, a small amount on a daily basis for the patient with a potential for stroke or MI will be beneficial. Table 27-5 lists some salicylate drugs.

Corticosteroids Topical corticosteroids are also used to treat inflammation and most of its causes, including chemical, mechanical, microbiological, and immunological agents. When applied to inflammation, corticosteroids inhibit the movement of macrophages and white blood cells into the area, resulting in a decrease in swelling, redness, and itching.

Nonsteroidal Anti-Inflammatory Drugs NSAIDs relieve inflammation and pain (see Table 27-6). Some of the many types of arthritis are also associated with infection. An NSAID will reduce the fever, as well as any pain associated with the fever, but will not affect the infection. Therefore, antibiotics are needed to combat the infection directly.

Long-term use of NSAIDs may have a damaging effect on chondrocyte (cartilage) function, which leads to more arthritic symptoms and disease. With chronic use, all anti-inflammatory and salicylate drugs may produce nausea, GI distress, and ulceration. However, ibuprofen has been reported to produce less gastric distress. Toxic effects of NSAIDs include bone marrow suppression that leads to blood disorders. Therefore, NSAIDs are used more for their anti-inflammatory effect

TABLE 27-5 Salicylate Drugs

Trade Name	Generic Name	Strength and Dosage Form Available	Dosage
Various trade names	acetylsalicylic acid (ASA); aspirin	Various strength tablets	3.2–6 gm/day for RA
			325–650 mg q4h for minor aches/pain
Arthropan	choline salicylate	870 mg/5 mL	870–1740 mg up to qid for RA
Dolobid	diflunisal	250 mg, 500 mg tablets	1 gm first dose, then 500 mg q8–12h for mild/moderate pain
			250–500 mg bid for osteoarthritis and RA
	salsalate (salicylsalicylic acid)	500 mg, 750 mg tablets	3,000 mg/day in divided doses
	sodium salicylate	325 mg, 650 mg tablets	325–650 mg q4h

TABLE 27-6 Examples of NSAIDs

Trade Name	Generic Name	Strength and Dosage Form Available	Usual Adult Dose
Ansaid	flurbiprofen	50 mg, 100 mg tablets	200–300 mg in divided doses bid, tid, or qid
Cataflam	diclofenac	50 mg tablets	100–200 mg/day in divided doses
Voltaren Voltaren-XR		25 mg, 50 mg, 75 mg, 100 mg extended-release (ER) tablets	
Celebrex	celecoxib	100 mg, 200 mg, 400 mg capsules	100 mg bid or 200 mg daily
Clinoril	sulindac	150 mg, 200 mg tablets	300–400 mg/day in two divided doses
Daypro	oxaprozin	600 mg capsules	1,200 mg daily
Daypro ALTA		678 mg oxaprozin potassium (equivalent to 600 mg oxaprozin)	Maximum dose: 1,800 mg/day or 26 mg/kg (whichever is lower) in divided doses
Feldene	piroxicam	10 mg, 20 mg capsules	10 mg bid or 20 mg daily
Indocin	indomethacin	25 mg, 50 mg capsules; 75 mg SA capsules; 50 mg suppository	Taper up to 150–200 mg/day in divided doses
		25 mg/5 mL suspension	
Lodine	etodolac	400 mg, 500 mg tablets; 200 mg, 300 mg capsules	300 mg bid–tid or 400–500 mg bid
		400 mg, 500 mg, 600 mg ER tablets	400–1,000 mg/day (ER tablets)
Meclomen	meclofenamate	50 mg, 100 mg capsules	50–100 mg q4–6h, NTE 400 mg/day

TABLE 27-6 **Examples of NSAIDs** (*Continued*)

Trade Name	Generic Name	Strength and Dosage Form Available	Usual Adult Dose
Motrin IB (OTC)	ibuprofen	OTC: 50 mg, 100 mg, 200 mg tablets	1.2−3.2 gm/day in divided doses tid−qid, NTE 3.2 gm/day
Motrin		200 mg capsules	
		40 mg/mL gtts	
		100 mg/5 mL, 100 mg/2.5 mL suspension	
		Rx: 400 mg, 600 mg, 800 mg tablets	
Nalfon	fenoprofen	200 mg, 300 mg capsules; 600 mg tablets	300−600 mg tid−qid
Naprosyn	naproxen sodium	250 mg, 375 mg, 500 mg tablets	250−500 mg bid
		375 mg, 500 mg delayed-release tablets	
Anaprox		250 mg, 500 mg tablets	
Naprelan		375 mg, 500 mg continuous-release tablets	
Orudis	ketoprofen	12.5 mg tablets; 50 mg, 75 mg capsules	50 mg qid or 75 mg tid
Oruvail		100 mg, 150 mg, 200 mg ER capsules	200 mg daily (ER)
Relafen	nabumetone	500 mg, 750 mg tablets	1,000 mg daily to start, increasing to 1,500−2,000 mg daily. Can divide doses
Tolectin	tolmetin	200 mg, 600 mg tablets	400−600 mg tid
		400 mg capsules	
Toradol	ketorolac tromethamine	10 mg tablets; 15 mg/mL injection	10 mg q4−6h, NTE 40 mg/day
		30 mg/mL injection	15−30 mg q6h, NTE 120 mg/day

than for their analgesic (pain-relieving) or antipyretic (fever-reducing) effects. If another pain reliever or fever reducer with fewer adverse reactions can be used, it is often preferred over an NSAID.

NSAIDs work by inhibiting or blocking the enzyme that starts the reaction of inflammation by making prostaglandin. This enzyme, called COX-2, catalyzes arachidonic acid to prostaglandins and leukotrienes. Further, NSAIDs block the action of the synthesis of prostaglandin that promotes inflammation.

The enzyme cyclooxygenase I (COX-1) produces the prostaglandins that cause the building and thickening of the mucosal lining of the stomach, thereby protecting the stomach against acid. The enzyme COX-2 produces the prostaglandins that contribute to inflammation.

When NSAIDs block *all* prostaglandin synthesis by blocking both COX-1 and COX-2, although the mucosal lining of the GI tract thins out and inflammation is reduced, a patient can then get a GI ulcer. Therefore, COX-2 inhibitors, which block only the COX-2 that makes PGE-2, contribute less to ulcers while still treating inflammation. With COX-2 inhibitors, only the inflammation process is inhibited; the viscosity of the gastric mucosal lining is not affected.

The COX-2 inhibitors have been successfully marketed on the basis of the belief that the main mechanism by which nonselective NSAIDs cause GI ulcers is inhibition of COX-1. According to this hypothesis, selective COX-2 inhibitors will have similar anti-inflammatory activity with less GI toxicity. Short-term clinical studies (CLASS and VIGOR), in which all patients underwent endoscopy, showed fewer cumulative gastroduodenal erosions and ulcers with the COX-2 inhibitors (9–15%) than with nonselective NSAIDs (41–46%). The FDA authorities judged this outcome as insufficient to prove that selective COX-2 inhibitors were better than nonselective NSAIDs in terms of the life-threatening complications of NSAIDs (namely, ulcers complicated by GI bleeds, perforations, and obstructions). Therefore, the monographs and package inserts of celecoxib (Celecoxib) and meloxicam (Mobic) include the same warnings and patient precautions about GI toxicity as all other NSAIDs.

According to the VIGOR and CLASS studies, COX-2 selective inhibitors are associated with an increased incidence of serious adverse events as compared with nonselective NSAIDs. Therefore, more studies are being done to prove or disprove this hypothesis.

A study in Germany shows that the use of leeches in knee arthritis yields a great reduction in swelling and pain. Acetaminophen (trade name, Tylenol), also known as paracetamol or N-Acetyl P-Aminophenol (APAP), is now thought to selectively block the newly discovered enzyme COX-3 in the brain and spinal cord, thereby reducing pain and fever without unwanted GI side effects. Still, APAP has very little or no anti-inflammatory effect.

It is important to emphasize the adverse reactions of NSAIDs. Long-term use of NSAIDs may have a damaging effect on chondrocyte (cartilage) function, which will lead to

PROFILE IN PRACTICE

A customer informs Rachel, a pharmacy technician, that he has been experiencing stomach upset over the past few days. The customer's profile shows that a prescription for piroxicam 10 mg po bid was filled two days earlier.

more arthritic symptoms and disease. Therefore, in the long run, use of NSAIDs may exacerbate any arthritis-related disease.

- Is it possible that the patient's new prescription is causing the stomach upset?
- How can it be alleviated?
- What is Rachel's role in this situation, and what is the role of the pharmacist?

Skeletal Muscle Relaxants

Skeletal muscle relaxants (SMRs) are used to relax specific muscles in the body and relieve the pain, stiffness, and discomfort associated with strains, sprains, or other muscle injuries (see Table 27-7). SMRs may also be used in spastic diseases, such as multiple sclerosis and cerebral palsy,

TABLE 27-7 Skeletal Muscle Relaxants

Trade Name	Generic Name		
Direct-Acting Skeletal Muscle Relaxants			
Dantrium	dantrolene	25 mg, 50 mg, 100 mg capsules	25 mg daily to start, increase to 25 mg bid–qid, then increase up to 100 mg bid–qid; NTE 400 mg/day
		20 mg/vial (0.32 mg after reconstitution)	2.5 mg/kg IV; about one hour before anesthesia, infused over one hour
Central-Acting Skeletal Muscle Relaxants			
Lioresal	baclofen	10 mg, 20 mg tablets	Titrate to 40–80 mg/day
Soma	carisoprodol	350 mg tablets	350 mg tid–qid
Parafon Forte DSC	chlorzoxazone	250 mg, 500 mg tablets	250–750 mg tid–qid
		250 mg capsules	
		500 mg caplet	
Flexeril	cyclobenzaprine	5 mg, 10 mg tablets	20–40 mg/day in divided doses
Valium	diazepam	2 mg, 5 mg, 10 mg tablets	2 mg–10 mg tid;qid
		5 mg/5 mL oral solution	
		5 mg/mL concentration	2–5 mg tid–qid IM/IV
		5 mg/mL injection	

TABLE 27-7 Skeletal Muscle Relaxants (*Continued*)

Trade Name	Generic Name		
Skelaxin	metaxalone	800 mg tablets	800 mg tid–qid
Robaxin	methocarbamol	500 mg, 750 mg tablets	Initial: 1.5 gm qid
			Maintenance: 1 gm qid, 750 mg q4h or 1.5 gm tid
		100 mg/mL injection	IV/IM: NTE 3 gm for longer than three consecutive days
Norflex	orphenadrine citrate	100 mg, 100 mg SR tablets	100 mg qam and qpm
		30 mg/mL injection	60 mg IV/IM; may repeat q12h
Zanaflex	tizanidine HCl	2 mg, 4 mg tablets	Initial: 4 mg q6–8h
		2 mg, 4 mg, 6 mg capsules	Titrate in 2–4 mg steps, maximum 3 doses/day; NTE 36 mg/day

as well as to help relax the patient or a specific part of the body prior to surgery. Drug therapy does not take the place of recommended rest or exercise, nor does it alleviate muscle problems caused by tetanus. SMRs act either in the central nervous system (CNS) or directly on the muscle to produce their relaxant effects.

The use of SMRs can also facilitate surgical and orthopedic procedures and intubations (see Tables 27-7 and 27-8). They may also be used to treat overexertion of the muscles and injuries accompanied by aches and the pain of sore, stiff, and swollen joints. Other drugs used to treat the soreness associated with overworked muscles are analgesics and anti-inflammatory agents.

TABLE 27-8 Agents for Surgical Procedures That Provide Temporary Muscle Paralysis

Trade Name	Generic Name
Nondepolarizing Agents	
Mivacron	mivacurium chloride
Nimbex	cisatracurium besylate
Norcuron	vecuronium bromide
Pavulon	pancuronium bromide
Tracrium	atracurium besylate
Zemuron	rocuronium bromide
Depolarizing Agents	
Quelicin, Anectine, Sucostrin	succinylcholine chloride

SMRs that inhibit neuromuscular function are either peripheral acting or central acting. Direct-acting SMRs are a subtype of peripheral-acting SMRs. The peripheral-acting SMRs block muscle contraction at the neuromuscular junction within the contractile process. The contractile process begins with an electrical impulse originating in the CNS that is conducted via the spinal cord to the somatic, or voluntary, motor neurons. These motor neurons connect to skeletal muscle fibers, creating the neuromuscular junction. Acetylcholine (ACH) forms in the endings of the somatic motor fibers and then travels to the neuromuscular synapse, an area between two neurons. When the ACH attaches to the nicotinic–II (NII) receptors, depolarization occurs, causing the contractile substances of myosin and actin to produce a muscle contraction.

Peripheral-acting SMRs inhibit contraction in two ways: as nondepolarizing agents and as depolarizing agents. Nondepolarizing SMRs block NII receptors, thereby inhibiting depolarization and stopping nerve transmission and muscle contraction. Depolarizing SMRs attach to the NII receptors, stimulating them to cause depolarization and consequent contraction; this changes the NII receptors so that they do not respond to the natural ACH neurotransmitter in the future. This one-two punch is called the *neuromuscular blockade*.

The adverse actions of SMRs vary from mild to major. It is well documented that, to fall asleep, the body and muscles as well as the brain's thoughts and impulses must relax. Therefore, side effects include drowsiness, dizziness, N/V, fatigue, and weakness. An overdose will produce toxic effects with possible paralysis of the respiratory muscles; respiratory failure and death may result. The main problem is potentiation of the neuromuscular blocker by any CNS depressant or other muscle relaxant, which can lead to an increased and faster approach to death by respiratory depression. Table 27-9 gives some examples of drugs that interact with muscle relaxants.

TABLE 27-9 Examples of Drugs That Interact with Muscle Relaxants

Classification	Trade Name	Generic Name
Alcohol	Various	various (even if in another medication preparation)
Antibiotics	Cleocin	clindamycin
	Pipracil	piperacillin
		neomycin
	Achromycin V, Tetracyn, Sumycin	tetracycline (TCN)
Benzodiazepines and other tranquilizers or sedatives	Halcion	triazolam
	Valium	diazepam
	Dalmane	flurazepam
	Xanax	alprazolam
Antiarrhythmics	Xylocaine	lidocaine
General anesthetics	Amidate	etomidate
	Brevital	methohexital
	Diprivan	propofol
	Ethrane	enflurane
	Fluothane	halothane
	Forane	isoflurane
	Ketalar	ketamine
	Penthrane	methoxyflurane
	Pentothal	thiopental sodium

info

From Arrow Poison to Surgical Aide

Curare is a natural product produced by South American plants such as *Strychnos toxifera* and *Strychnos castelnaei* and was originally used as an arrow poison. When prepared and used properly, curare assists in temporary muscle paralysis for surgery.

Spastic Diseases

Spastic diseases are motor diseases characterized by tonic spasms (continued muscular tension) and involuntary, exaggerated muscle contractions coupled with abnormal and automatic reflexes, lack of dexterity, and fatigability. This section briefly discusses two of the most common spastic diseases.

Multiple Sclerosis

More commonly known as MS, multiple sclerosis is characterized by multiple areas of inflammation and scarring of the myelin in the brain and spinal cord. MS is an autoimmune disease in which, for unknown reasons, the body's immune system begins to attack normal body tissues. In the case of MS, the body attacks the cells that make myelin, the tissue that covers and protects the nerve fibers. Nerve communication is thereby disrupted. A person with MS experiences varying degrees of neurological impairment, depending on the location and extent of the scarring. Although there is as yet no known cure for MS, much can be done to make the patient's life easier.

Symptoms of MS may include fatigue, weakness, spasticity, balance problems, bladder and bowel control problems, numbness, vision loss, tremor, and vertigo. Not all symptoms affect all MS patients. Symptoms and signs may be persistent, or the patient may experience periods of remission. Treatment of MS includes the use of steroidal anti-inflammatory agents (synthetic adrenal glucocorticoids) and corticosteroids such as betamethasone, dexamethasone, methylprednisolone, prednisone, and prednisolone.

Cerebral Palsy

Cerebral palsy is a condition in which the affected person has poor control of the brain, muscles, and joints. Cerebral palsy is caused by an injury to the brain before, during, or shortly after birth. Because body movements and muscle coordination are affected, children with cerebral palsy may not be able to walk, talk, eat, or play in the same ways as most other children.

Cerebral palsy is characterized by an inability to fully control motor function, particularly muscle control and coordination, and is manifested by the following symptoms:

- Muscle tightness or spasm
- Lack of muscle coordination
- Disturbance in gait and mobility
- Abnormal sensation and perception
- Impairment of sight, hearing, or speech
- Seizures

Depending on the individual child's needs, physical therapy, occupational therapy, and speech-language therapy are employed to improve posture and movement. Pharmaceutical therapy includes drugs to prevent seizures and spasticity (see Tables 27-10 and 27-11).

TABLE 27-10 Drugs Used to Treat Seizures Associated with Cerebral Palsy

Trade Name	Generic Name
Dilantin	phenytoin
Luminal	phenobarbital
Tegretol	carbamazepine

TABLE 27-11 Drugs Used to Treat Spasticity Associated with Cerebral Palsy

Trade Name	Generic Name
Dantrium	dantrolene—peripheral direct-acting SMR
Lioresal	baclofen—muscle relaxant; acts to decrease activity of nerves, blocking nerves within the reticular formation
Valium	diazepam—benzodiazepine SMR

Summary

The musculoskeletal system, which consists of the bones and skeletal muscles, provides the body with both form and the ability to move. The musculoskeletal system has four main functions: to provide a framework or shape for the body, to protect the internal organs, to allow body movement, and to provide storage for essential minerals. There are 206 bones in the human body. The five classes of bones are long, short, flat, irregular, and sesamoid. Muscles are classified as skeletal (voluntary muscles attached to the bone to provide body movement), cardiac (involuntary muscle attached to the heart), or smooth (involuntary muscles attached to or lining the internal organs).

The musculoskeletal system is affected by numerous disorders, some of which cause only discomfort and pain, and some of which can completely disable the individual. Osteoporosis, the most prevalent bone disorder in the United States, affects approximately 20 million Americans and is a major cause of bone fractures. Osteoarthritis, a progressive disease of the joints, affects up to 40 million Americans.

Chapter Review Questions

1. Which type of muscle enables kinetics?
   a. skeletal muscle
   b. smooth muscle
   c. cardiac muscle
   d. heart muscle

2. A _____ is a specialized dense connective tissue that provides the shape and support for the body.
   a. joint
   b. cartilage
   c. ligament
   d. bone

3. An infection inside the bone is known as _____.
   a. osteoarthritis
   b. osteoporosis
   c. osteoclast
   d. osteomyelitis

4. Which type of muscle is also known as visceral muscle and is considered an involuntary muscle?
   a. skeletal muscle
   b. smooth muscle
   c. cardiac muscle
   d. heart muscle

5. A _____ is a connective tissue that holds bones together.
   a. joint
   b. bone marrow
   c. tendon
   d. ligament

6. A _____ is a connective tissue that attaches muscle to bone.
   a. joint
   b. bone marrow
   c. tendon
   d. ligament

7. Which of the following refers to muscle pain?
   a. bursitis
   b. tendonitis
   c. myalgia
   d. anemia

8. Which of the following is *not* an inflammatory disease?
   a. gout
   b. tendonitis
   c. anemia
   d. bursitis

9. What type of drug is currently considered a long-term solution to controlling arthritis symptoms?
   a. NSAIDs
   b. DMARDs
   c. SMRs
   d. SERMs

10. Which of the following drugs is an NSAID?
    a. phenytoin
    b. phenobarbital
    c. naproxen sodium
    d. carbamazepine

Critical Thinking Questions

1. What are the advantages and disadvantages of using salicylates rather than NSAIDs to treat inflammation?

2. If you had to choose a course of therapy for osteoporosis in menopause, which therapy would you choose and why?

3. Explain why a doctor might choose a drug that only blocks COX-2 over a drug that blocks both COX-2 and COX-1.

Web Challenge

1. Go to http://www.niams.nih.gov/bone/optool/index.asp, and complete the survey to determine the health of your bones.

2. Go to http://www.gwc.maricopa.edu/class/bio201/muscle/mustut.htm for a tutorial and to learn more about muscles.

References and Resources

Adams, M.P., D.L. Josephson, and L.N. Holland, Jr. *Pharmacology for Nurses: A Pathophysiologic Approach.* 4th ed. Upper Saddle River, NJ: Pearson, 2013.

"Arthritis Today, Drug Guide. http://www.arthritis.org/today.org/arthritis-treatment/medications/drug-guide/index.php. 6 August 2013. Web.

Colbert, B., J. Ankney, and K. Lee. *Anatomy and Physiology for Health Professionals: An Interactive Journey.* (2nd edition.) Upper Saddle River, NJ: Pearson, 2010.

DeNoia, V. "Bisphosphonates for Osteoporosis: A Closer Look at Efficacy and Safety." http://www.arthritispractitioner.com/article/7413. 12 April 2008. Web.

Drug Facts and Comparisons, 2012 ed. St. Louis, MO: Wolters Kluwer Health.

"Functions of the Muscular System." http://training.seer.cancer.gov/module_anatomy/unit4_1_muscle_functions.html. 8 April 2008. Web.

Holland, N. and M.P. Adams. *Core Concepts in Pharmacology.* (3rd edition.) Upper Saddle River, NJ: Pearson, 2010.

"MOA of APAP, News on APAP." http://www.pharmweb.net/pwmirror/pwy/paracetamol/pharmwebpicmechs.html. 8 April 2008. Web.

National Institute of Arthritis and Musculoskeletal and Bone Diseases. "Osteoporosis and Medicine: Medications to Treat and Prevent Osteoporosis." http://www.niams.nih.gov/Health_Info/Bone/Osteoporosis/Medicine/default.asp. 7 April 2008. Web.

National Library of Medicine. "A Review of SERMs and National Surgical Adjuvant Breast and Bowel Project Clinical Trials." http://www.ncbi.nlm.nih.gov/entrez/query.fcgi?cmd=Retrieve&db=PubMed&listuids=14613021&dopt=Abstract. 15 July 2007. Web.

"The Merck Manual of Diagnosis and Therapy." http://www.merck.com/mrkshared/mmanual/s`ection5/chapter57/57a.jsp 15 July 2007. Web.

The Virtual Anesthesia Textbook. "Non-Opioid Analgesics." http://www.virtual-anaesthesia-textbook.com/vat/non_narcotics.html#intro. 15 July 2007. Web.

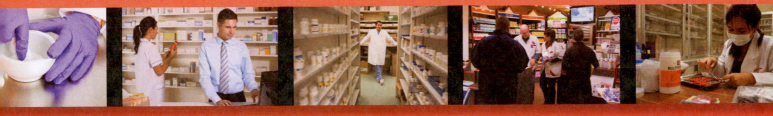

CHAPTER 28

The Respiratory System

LEARNING OBJECTIVES

After completing this chapter, you should be able to:

- Identify and list the basic anatomical and structural parts of the respiratory tract.

- Describe the function or physiology of the individual parts of the respiratory system and the external exchange of oxygen and waste.

- List and define common diseases affecting the respiratory tract and understand the causes, symptoms, and pharmaceutical treatments associated with each disease.

- List the trade and generic names and identify the classification of various drugs used in the treatment of diseases and conditions of the respiratory tract.

KEY TERMS

allergen, p. 448

allergy, p. 448

cilia, p. 439

chronic obstructive pulmonary disease (COPD), p. 452

epiglottis, p. 440

larynx, p. 440

pharynx, p. 438

rhinitis, p. 441

rhinorrhea, p. 441

trachea, p. 440

INTRODUCTION

Children commonly hold their breath to find out what it feels like. Adults do so while swimming. It is hard to consciously *not* breathe for very long without giving up. Oxygen is crucial to sustain life, and humans take in oxygen by the act of breathing.

Some people can survive for weeks (50–80 days) without food, for several days (3–14) without water, and for a few hours without adequate warmth in cold conditions. But after several minutes without air, the brain begins to suffer, major organs shut down, and eventually the person dies. The longer the body goes without air, the more damage is done. The respiratory system is what performs the essential action of receiving and exchanging gases, through the lungs, by the process known as breathing or *respiration*.

Function of the Respiratory System

The respiratory system has the following two purposes:

1. Transport of air (gases) to and from the lungs
2. Exchange of oxygen for carbon dioxide

The primary function of the respiratory system is to supply oxygen to the blood. The blood, in turn, carries the oxygen to all parts of the body, via the "freeways" of the circulatory system (veins, arteries, and capillaries). The heart is the pump that propels blood to and from the lungs.

Respiration is the mechanism through which gases are exchanged. During breathing, one inhales air containing oxygen and exhales carbon dioxide, a by-product after the use of oxygen in the body. During its journey into the lungs, the air is humidified, warmed, and purified (suspended particles are removed). It is through this exchange of gases that the respiratory system gets oxygen into the blood. When blood stops moving, oxygen does not get to the body tissues. If a sufficient supply of oxygen does not get to a specific part of the body, that part will eventually die. Without sufficient oxygen, the whole body will eventually die. The respiratory and circulatory systems work in tandem to accomplish their mutual function of sustaining life.

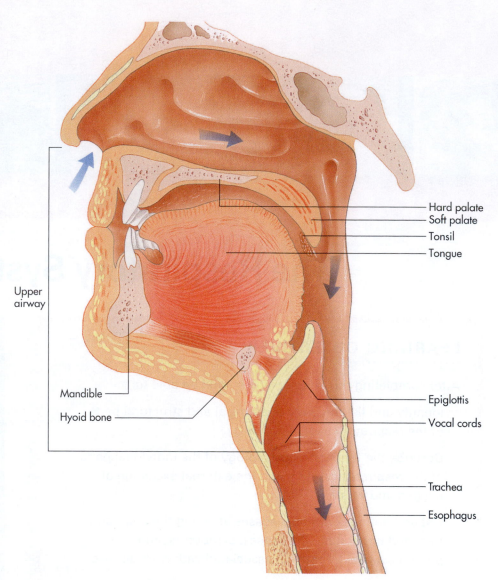

FIGURE 28-1 The upper respiratory tract.

The lymphatic system also supports respiration by maintaining fluids, providing immunity, and removing inhaled solid materials and microorganisms. For example, the flow of lymph from lung-tissue interstitial spaces into the blood helps to eliminate excess fluid, and the lymphoid tissue of the tonsils protects against infection at the entrance to the respiratory tract.

Anatomy of the Respiratory System

The respiratory system is divided into two parts, the upper respiratory tract and the lower respiratory tract. The upper respiratory tract consists of the nose or nasal cavity, paranasal sinuses, **pharynx**, and larynx (see Figure 28-1). The larynx acts in conjunction with the epiglottis to guard the entrance to the trachea and lower airways. The lower respiratory tract consists of the trachea, two lungs, and two main bronchi—the bronchi then branch into bronchioles, alveolar ducts, and alveoli (see Figure 28-2).

The Diaphragm

The dome-shaped *diaphragm* is a layer or sheet of muscle that lies across the bottom of the chest cavity. Breathing occurs as the diaphragm contracts and relaxes. It pushes carbon dioxide out of the lungs during relaxation and pulls oxygen-containing air into the lungs during contraction.

The Upper Respiratory System

The upper respiratory system is comprised of the nose, cavities of the nose, voice box, and throat. The upper respiratory system can become host to infection and illness, which can be serious if not treated properly or at the onset of symptoms. Upper respiratory infections are generally viral infections, but a bacterial

---

pharynx   the part of the throat from the back of the nasal cavity to the larynx.

cilia   the tiny hair-like organelles found in the nose and bronchial passageways.

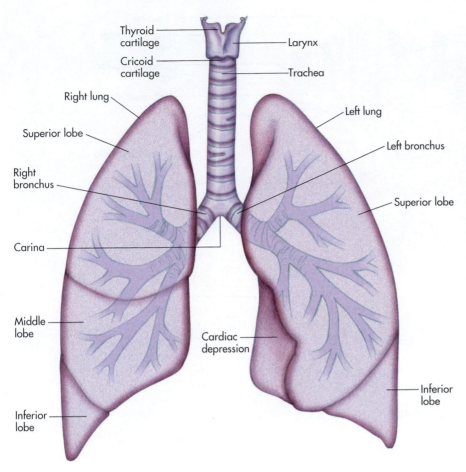

Thyroid cartilage
Cricoid cartilage
Right lung
Superior lobe
Right bronchus
Carina
Middle lobe
Inferior lobe

Larynx
Trachea
Left lung
Left bronchus
Superior lobe
Cardiac depression
Inferior lobe

FIGURE 28-2 The lower respiratory tract.

infection can also be present. These viral infections are contagious and can be passed on to another person if contact is made with someone who already has an upper respiratory infection. The most well-known types of illness of the upper respiratory tract are rhinitis, sinus infection, common cold, and laryngitis. A variety of treatments can be used to treat upper respiratory

viral infections. Some remedies include antibiotics, acetaminophen, nonsteroidal anti-inflammatory medications, antihistamines, nasal ipratropium, cough medications, steroids, decongestants, and nasal solutions. Combination drugs and over-the-counter (OTC) medications can also help alleviate the symptoms of upper respiratory illness. An alternative therapy of using honey can assist in quieting an annoying cough. Respiratory infections require more potent remedies such as antibiotics to clear up infections caused by possibly resistant pathogens. Duration of treatment depends on how serious the illness is and how well an individual responds to various treatment options.

The Lower Respiratory System

The lower respiratory system includes the windpipe, bronchial tree, and lungs. Lower respiratory systems are prone to infection just as the upper respiratory system. Illnesses of the lower respiratory system include infections, bronchitis, bronchiolitis, and pneumonia. Treatment can include antibiotics, antibacterials, bronchodilators, steroids, and combination drugs. Some of the symptoms of lower respiratory illnesses can include cough, chest pain, heavy mucus production, headache, confusion, myalgia, abdominal pain, nausea, diarrhea, and vomiting.

The Lungs

Only about 10% of the lungs is solid tissue (see Figure 28-3). The remainder is filled with air and blood. The functional structure of the lungs can be divided into two parts:

1. The conducting airways (bronchi and bronchioles), which are tubes lined by **cilia** and respiratory mucosa containing varying amounts of muscle and hyaline cartilage in their walls. The conducting airways provide "dead air space" for ventilation and gas-exchange areas for perfusion. They move approximately 10,000 L of inspired (inhaled) air per day.
2. Cartilage, which is a form of protection and cushioning for the bronchi. The bronchi contain hyaline cartilage rings in their walls to keep the airways open. The bronchioles, however, contains little cartilage; instead, they have a thick layer of smooth muscle.

info

What is a hiccup?

A hiccup, technically known as a *singultus*, is a diaphragmatic spasm. The diaphragm usually works without a hitch, but sometimes it can become irritated and jerk, causing the breath to be exhaled differently. An irritation or stimulation of the glossopharyngeal area causes this irregular breath. During the jerking motion, the diaphragm contracts involuntarily, causing the person to take a quick breath of air into the lungs. This irregular breath hits the voice box, and the sound it makes is called the *hiccup*. Things that can irritate the diaphragm are eating or swallowing too quickly, eating too much, an irritation in the stomach or the throat, or nervousness or excitement. Most cases of hiccups last for only a few minutes. However, some cases of hiccups can last beyond a few days, which usually indicate that there is another medical problem. The longest attack of hiccups ever recorded was experienced by an American pig farmer whose hiccups lasted from 1922 to 1987.

info

What is a yawn?

Although it is not completely understood, most medical schools teach that a yawn is caused by a lack of oxygen in the alveoli, which makes the lungs stiffen and react to bring in more oxygen.

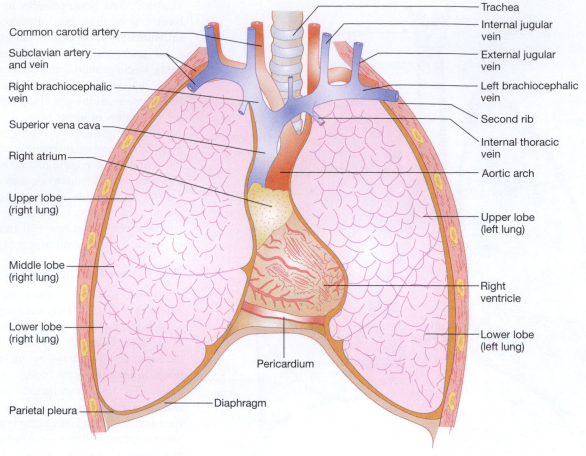

FIGURE 28-3 The lungs.

Respiration

Respiration is achieved through the mouth, nose, trachea, lungs, and diaphragm. Inspiration of air occurs when the pressure inside the lung, known as *intrapulmonary pressure*, becomes lower than the outside or *atmospheric* pressure. This change in pressure allows air to flow into the alveoli of the lungs. During inspiration, the intrapulmonary pressure is less than the atmospheric pressure of 760 mm Hg, which is the average sea-level pressure. Oxygen enters the upper respiratory system through the mouth and the nose, where it is warmed and filtered by cilia.

The oxygen then passes through the **larynx** and the **trachea**, and then into two smaller tubes called the *bronchi*. Each bronchus splits off into the bronchial tubes, which lead into the lungs and in turn branch off into many *bronchioles*, which connect to alveoli.

Alveoli are often described as grape-like clusters of air sacs; the average adult lungs contain about 600 million of them. Oxygenated air passes into the alveoli and then diffuses

larynx the voice box.

trachea the windpipe.

epiglottis the small, leaf-shaped cartilage attached to the tongue that prevents substances other than air from entering the trachea.

rhinitis inflammation of the nasal passages.

rhinorrhea runny nose.

info Do we breathe when we swallow?

The esophagus is located at the back of the throat, and the windpipe for air is located at the front. When we swallow during ingestion, a flap called the **epiglottis** swings down to cover the windpipe, so that food cannot go down the "wrong pipe." This flap blocks the air coming in for just a second, so for that short moment we do not breathe. Therefore, we do not breathe when we swallow. In addition, because smell and breathing are crucial in tasting food, we do not taste our food as we swallow; that has already been done by our taste buds prior to swallowing!

through the membranes into the surrounding capillaries. As oxygen travels into the arterial blood, the waste product carried in the blood, carbon dioxide, is released into the alveoli. Carbon dioxide leaves the lungs during exhalation. If this waste gas is not exhaled, the carbon dioxide will accumulate in the blood, causing all body parts to suffocate.

Diseases and Conditions of the Respiratory Tract

Many diseases and conditions of the respiratory tract can be treated with OTC medications. However, infections and cancer must be treated with specific anti-infectives, antibiotics, and chemotherapeutic drugs. This section explores the common cold, allergies, anaphylactic shock, and chronic obstructive diseases such as emphysema and asthma.

Colds

Colds, caused by viral infections, lead to more absences at work or school each year than any other medical condition. The virus that is responsible for a cold inflames the membranes in the lining of the nose and throat, causing **rhinitis** and sore throat. More than 200 different viruses can cause the common cold. Among the most common are *rhinoviruses*, which thrive in the nasal mucosa, and *coronaviruses*, which cause respiratory, neurological, and enteric infections.

One reason for the increased incidence of colds during the fall and winter months is that people are more often indoors, in heated buildings, and in closer proximity to each other. Also, the lower humidity during colder months makes the nasal passages drier and more vulnerable to infection. Colds usually start two to three days after the virus enters the body, and symptoms last from several days to several weeks. Common cold symptoms are:

- Stuffy nose or congestion
- Difficulty breathing
- Runny nose (**rhinorrhea**), with either a watery discharge from the nose or a discharge that thickens and turns yellow or green
- Sneezing
- Sore or scratchy throat
- Cough
- Headache
- Low-grade fever and/or chills
- Achy muscles and bones
- Fatigue

Coronaviruses are named for their corona-like or halo-like appearance in electron spectrographs, which is due to various projections on the surface of the viral envelope. One of these projections is the E2 glycoprotein, the viral attachment protein—the target of neutralizing antibodies. These viruses primarily affect adults and are difficult to culture in a laboratory.

Colds can be prevented by avoiding contact with others who have colds and doing frequent hand washing. Avoid touching your eyes, nose, or mouth when in contact with others who

are infected with a virus. Using humidifiers and occasionally rinsing the nasal passages with a saline solution may help nasal membranes from becoming overly dry and vulnerable.

How a Cold Virus Causes a Disease

The exact mechanism by which a virus causes a cold is not fully known or understood. The following is the most probable explanation of the sequence of events by which a cold virus causes a disease. Viruses cause infection by overpowering the immune system. The first line of immunity defense is mucus produced in the nose and throat. Mucus captures inhaled material, such as pollen, dust, pollutants, bacteria, and viruses. After a virus contacts a mucous membrane in the nose, ear, eye, or skin, it then enters a cell and takes over protein synthesis in that cell to manufacture new viruses, which, in turn, attack surrounding body cells.

Cold symptoms are most likely a result of the immune response to viral attack. Virus-infected nose cells emit signals that summon white blood cells to the site of the infection. In turn, these cells send out immune system chemicals such as kinins. Kinins lead to the symptoms of the common cold by causing swelling and inflammation of the nasal membranes, leakage of proteins and fluid from capillaries and lymph vessels, and increased production of mucus. Researchers are examining whether drugs to block kinins and other immune system substances, or the receptors on cells to which they bind, might benefit people with colds.

Table 28-1 compares some common symptoms of colds and viral flu.

TABLE 28-1 Comparison of Cold and Flu Symptoms

Cold Symptoms	Flu Symptoms
Low or no fever	High fever
Sometimes a headache	Usually a headache
Stuffy or runny nose	Clear nasal passages
Sneezing	Sometimes sneezing
Mild, hacking cough	Productive cough; may become severe
Slight aches and pains	Often severe aches and pains
Mild fatigue	Severe fatigue; may last for weeks
Sore throat	Usually a sore throat
Normal energy level	Extreme exhaustion
Colds occasionally lead to secondary bacterial infections of the middle ear or sinuses, requiring treatment with antibiotics	Influenzas occasionally lead to secondary bacterial infections of the lungs (bronchi and bronchioles) or to pneumonia

Treating the Common Cold with Medication

The treatment of colds is considered symptomatic treatment. OTC drugs and commonsense therapies are available for uncomplicated cases of the common cold. Among them, bed rest, keeping warm, drinking plenty of fluids, gargling with warm salt water, and using petroleum jelly for a rubbed-raw nose are the most accepted. Treatment of colds is done with medications (whether OTC or prescription) from the following classifications:

- Antihistamines
- Decongestants
- Cough suppressants, expectorants, and mucolytics
- Analgesics
- Antipyretics
- NSAIDs

Coughs

A cough may be a symptom of a cold, flu, other respiratory problems, or even nonrespiratory tract diseases. Most experts agree that a cough most likely begins with an irritation of nerves in the respiratory tract. The irritation may come from a clump of mucus in the airway, exposure to an airborne offender (such as a chemical aerosol like paint fumes), or postnasal drip (PND). PND usually occurs in the patient who has recently had a cold or flu or suffers from allergic rhinitis or acute or chronic sinusitis.

There are, of course, many other causes of coughs. Disease states such as asthma, bronchitis, congestive heart failure, and GERD, as well as side effects of certain drugs (such as ACE inhibitors), can also contribute to cough. A psychogenic or "nervous" cough is emotional or psychological in origin. Cystic fibrosis, an idiopathic pulmonary fibrotic disease, can cause thick mucus to build up that must be expelled or expectorated. Asthma, sinusitis, and GERD are the most frequent causes of chronic cough in children. Serious respiratory complications of GERD include cough, chronic bronchitis, progressively worsening bronchial asthma, and other pulmonary diseases.

Although it goes away in time, postinfectious cough may persist for three or more weeks, usually as the only remaining symptom of an upper respiratory tract viral infection due to persistent inflammation. A persistent acute cough that lasts for three or fewer weeks is usually caused by the common cold, but may be symptomatic of a more serious illness, such as pneumonia or congestive heart failure.

A *chronic cough* is a recurring cough that lasts for three or more weeks at a time. It is sometimes caused by more than one condition. It is most common among tobacco smokers, but also occurs in nonsmokers with postnasal drip syndrome (PNDS), gastroesophageal asthma, and GERD. "Smokers' cough" can mask a more serious condition such as pneumonia or congestive heart failure.

If *pertussis* or whooping cough exists, antibiotic treatment is warranted to fight the bacterial infection, in the patient and possibly in all persons who were exposed to pertussis. Children usually get pertussis. During this disease, it is difficult for the child to stop coughing and get air. Patients experience coughing spasms with a typical "whooping" sound that follows the cough. This sound indicates that the child is trying to catch his or her breath before the next bout of whooping. Complications that may set in are pneumonia, seizures, brain damage, and death. Children under seven years of age need to be vaccinated with a series of five injections of DPT (diphtheria/pertussis/tetanus) vaccine.

An effective, purposeful cough requires normal nerve pathways in the respiratory tract so that cough can occur when needed. Normal muscle tone of the diaphragm and abdomen (respiratory muscles) is required to create a strong push to the lungs for expiration with normal mucus stickiness and viscosity. Excessive coughing can affect normal muscle tone, hampering the ability of the cough to dislodge mucus or phlegm from bronchial airways.

Mucus is brought up out of the lungs by a productive cough; a nonproductive cough is a dry, hacking cough. A productive cough is purposeful, although sometimes drugs are required to promote the removal of mucus, and may help some patients cough up and expel abnormally thick mucus by thinning it out. It is important to keep the airways free of mucus, to prevent invasion by bacteria that can cause serious disease to the respiratory tract.

A nonproductive cough is usually not purposeful and may persist, becoming as problematic as it is annoying. A nonproductive cough can be exhausting depending on the duration and forcefulness of the cough. Intercostal tissue of the rib cage may tear if the cough persists. Drugs can be given to stop the cough; however, some nonproductive coughs result as a side effect of a medication that is being taken for a different condition or disease.

Cough Medications

There are two types of coughs and two types of treatments (see Tables 28-2 and 28-3). Nonproductive cough is treated with a cough *suppressant* or *antitussive* to quiet the cough; these

TABLE 28-2 Prescription and OTC Antitussives

Generic Name	Brand Name	Dosage Forms and Availability	Route of Administration	Common Adult Dosage
dextromethorphan	Delsym	Syrup	Oral	10 mL every 12 hours, not to exceed two doses in a 24-hour period
guaifenesin, dextromethorphan	Robitussin DM, Mucinex DM	Syrup—various strengths; 600-mg, 1,200-mg tablets	Oral	Robutussin DM: 10 mL every four hours, not to exceed six doses in a 24-hour period; Mucinex DM: 600–1,200 mg every 12 hours, not to exceed two doses in a 24-hour period
hydrocodone, guaifenesin	Hycotuss	Syrup	Oral	5 mL every four to six hours, not to exceed six doses in a 24-hour period
phenylpropanolamine, hydrocodone	Hycomine (C-III)	25 mg/5 mg/5 mL	Oral	5 mL every four hours, not to exceed six doses in a 24-hour period
promethazine, codeine	Phenergan with Codeine	Syrup	Oral	5 mL every four to six hours

TABLE 28-3 Comparison of Cough Formula for Nonproductive Versus Productive Coughs

Indications—Nonproductive Cough	Indications—Productive Cough
Symptoms—dry, hacking cough that does not produce mucus or phlegm.	Symptoms—a cough in which there is production and removal of phlegm or mucus; sometimes called a "wet" cough.
Purpose—suppressants (antitussives) are used to suppress the cough centers in the brain and to moisten and lubricate the throat to relieve irritation and quiet the cough.	Purpose—expectorants are drugs that loosen and clear mucus and phlegm from the respiratory tract, and also moisten and lubricate the throat to relieve irritation.
Generic ingredient, nonnarcotic cough suppressants—dextromethorphan.	Generic ingredient, nonnarcotic expectorant—guaifenesin.
Narcotic cough suppressants—codeine and hydrocodone.	
Trade names of nonnarcotic antitussives—Dimetapp, Robitussin-DM, Delsym, Pertussin, Drixoral, Vicks Formula 44, Triaminic, Coricidin.	Trade names of nonnarcotic expectorants—Robitussin, Humibid, Humibid LA, Mucinex, Organidin NR, Fenesin.
Trade names of narcotic antitussives—Hycodan, Mycodone, Tussigon, Tussionex.	
Mechanism of action of dextromethorphan—works on the CNS to suppress cough centers in the brain (in the medulla oblongata). When coughing is suppressed, the throat does not lose moisture.	Mechanism of action of guaifenesin—thins mucus and lubricates the irritated respiratory tract.

(Continued)

TABLE 28-3 Comparison of Cough Formula for Nonproductive Versus Productive Coughs *(Continued)*

Indications—Nonproductive Cough	Indications—Productive Cough
Mechanism of action of codeine—codeine is a centrally acting agent that elevates the threshold for cough in the medulla oblongata. As a result, dry, unproductive coughs become more productive and less frequent. Codeine may be combined with an expectorant.	
Side effects—drowsiness or tranquilization, constipation, overdrying of respiratory secretions, upset stomach. At high doses, can cause nausea, itchy skin, visual and auditory hallucinations, loss of motor control, and a feeling of being "stoned" and "out of it."	Side effects—rare, but may include vomiting, diarrhea, stomach upset, headache, skin rash, and hives.
Contraindications—patients with hypertension, kidney problems, diabetes, or glaucoma must seek approval from their doctor; increases the effects of those conditions. Pregnancy; patients with persistent lingering cough; excessive phlegm; or chronic cough due to bronchitis, smoking, asthma, or emphysema.	Contraindications—pregnancy; patients with persistent lingering cough; excessive phlegm; chronic cough due to bronchitis, smoking, asthma, or emphysema.

allow the upper respiratory tract to stay moistened (coughing dries it out and further irritates the respiratory tract). *Expectorants* are used to increase the moisture content and decrease the viscosity of mucus, to ease removal of mucus during coughing.

Decongestants

Decongestants thin out the mucus in an inflamed, stuffy nose and clear the nasal passages, allowing easier breathing. Indications for use are nasal and bronchial congestion.

Oral pseudoephedrine and phenylephrine are alpha-adrenergic agonists, which act on alpha-adrenergic receptors in the blood vessels of the nasal mucosa to produce vasoconstriction, resulting in decreased blood flow and shrinkage of tissue in the nasal passages. This effect reduces the vascular inflammation and edema that are associated with congestion.

Pseudoephedrine, like ephedra, creates its effect indirectly by releasing norepinephrine from storage sites in the nerve endings. However, pseudoephedrine can also relax the bronchial smooth muscles by acting directly on beta-2 adrenergic receptors in the mucosa of the respiratory tract. This stimulation produces vasoconstriction, which shrinks swollen nasal mucus membranes; reduces tissue hyperemia (excessive blood), edema, and nasal congestion; and increases the patency (openness) of the nasal airway passages. In addition, it promotes an increase in the drainage of sinus secretions. Obstructed eustachian tubes may also be opened.

Side effects of oral decongestants include irregular heartbeat, palpitations, hypertension, and shortness of breath. CNS toxic effects include convulsions, hallucinations, and stimulation. Those with sulfite sensitivities may have allergic reactions and asthmatic attacks.

❝ Workplace Wisdom Oral Decongestants and MAOIs

Patients must not use pseudoephedrine or phenylephrine if they are currently taking a prescription monoamine oxidase inhibitor (MAOI) or for two weeks after stopping the MAOI drug. MAOIs are used in the treatment of depression, psychiatric or emotional conditions, and Parkinson's disease. MAOIs potentiate the cardiovascular effects of oral decongestants. ❞

Benefits and disadvantages of oral decongestants, compared with topical nasal inhalation decongestants, are as follows:

- Oral drugs have prolonged decongestant effects, but delayed onset; topicals usually work quickly within five minutes.
- Oral drugs do not cause rebound congestion; topical has a rebound effect. The *rebound effect* occurs with topical decongestants only when more and more product is needed to produce the same effect. This will increase side effects as well. This happens with prolonged use (more than three to five days) when nasal decongestants lose effectiveness and even cause swelling in the nasal passages. The patient then increases the frequency of the dose. Congestion worsens, and the patient responds by increasing the doses or frequency of doses to as often as every hour. Patients can become dependent on the use of topical decongestants. This effect may occur with ophthalmic decongestants as well. Oral drugs are less potent than topicals; topicals have a more direct effect and less systemic effect.

Pseudoephedrine and Meth

Pseudoephedrine is an essential chemical used in the production of methamphetamine—"meth," an illegal, highly addictive street stimulant. The Combat Methamphetamine Epidemic Act of 2005 requires that any product containing pseudoephedrine, ephedrine, or phenylpropanolamine be sold from a locked cabinet or from behind the pharmacy counter. The seller must ensure that consumers do not have access to the products prior to sale, and must keep an electronic record ("log") of each sale. The act also puts limits on how much of the drug a person can purchase at one time. In addition, pharmacy customers must present a driver's license or state identification card at the time of purchase as well.

PPA and Bleeding

After much debate, public hearings that began in 1985, and a controlled case study that began in 1994, phenylpropanolamine (PPA) was removed from the market in November 2000 because it increased the risk of intracranial bleeding associated with hemorrhagic stroke. PPA was used in OTC cough and cold remedies as a decongestant, as well as an appetite suppressant in weight-loss formulas. This bleeding risk was found to be higher in women than in men, mainly because the incidence of stroke occurred more with diet aids than with cold medications, and diet aids are used more by women than men.

Topical nasal decongestants act as vasoconstrictors, sending edema-causing fluids and blood back to the vessels from which they originally leaked, thereby shrinking the dilated blood vessels. Topical decongestants are used for the temporary relief of nasal congestion or stuffiness caused by hay fever or other allergies, colds, or sinusitis.

Side effects of topical decongestants include burning, dryness, or stinging inside the nose; increase in nasal discharge; and sneezing. Toxic effects of topical decongestants include blurred vision; fast, irregular, or pounding heartbeat; headache; dizziness; drowsiness or lightheadedness; high blood pressure; nervousness; trembling; trouble sleeping, and weakness. One might think that a topical agent is safe for all patients; its simple route of administration fools many people. In fact, there is a long list of contraindications for this simple dosage form of topical (and) nasal sprays and drops. Do not use on patients with the following conditions:

- Diabetes mellitus
- Excessively dry nasal membranes
- Enlarged prostate (difficulty in urinating may worsen)
- Glaucoma (mydriasis may worsen)
- Heart or blood vessel disease such as CHF or coronary artery disease
- High blood pressure (oxymetazoline, in particular, may make the condition worse)
- Overactive thyroid gland (decongestants may increase tachycardia)

Table 28-4 lists prescription and OTC decongestants, Table 28-5 shows some examples of nasal decongestants and Table 28-6 lists examples of prescription allergy treatments.

TABLE 28-4 Prescription and OTC Decongestants

Generic Name	Brand Name	Dosage Forms and Availability	Route of Administration	Common Adult Dosage
oxymetazoline	Afrin Original	Nasal spray, nasal mist	Nasal	Two to three sprays in each nostril every 10–12 hours, not to exceed two doses in a 24-hour period
phenylephrine HCl	Sudafed PE, Neo-Synephrine	10-mg tablets, nasal spray	Oral, nasal	Sudafed PE (oral): 10 mg every four hrs, not to exceed six doses in a 24-hour period. Neo-Synephrine: nasal—two to three sprays in each nostril every 10–12 hours, not to exceed two doses in a 24-hour period
pseudoephedrine HCl	Sudafed	30-mg, 120-mg, 240-mg tablets	Oral	30 mg every four to six hours, not to exceed eight doses in a 24-hour period

TABLE 28-5 Nasal Decongestants

Generic Name	Trade Name
naphazoline HCl	Privine
oxymetazoline HCl	Afrin, Dristan 12-Hr Nasal Spray
phenylephrine HCl	Sudafed PE (oral), Neo-Synephrine 4-Hr, 4-Way Fast Acting, Afrin Children's Pump Mist
phenylephrine HCl + pheniramine maleate	Dristan Fast Acting Formula
pseudoephedrine	Sudafed (oral)
tetrahydrozoline HCl (Rx only)	Tyzine
xylometazoline HCl	Otrivin, Natru-Vent

Note: OTC and topical, unless otherwise indicated.

TABLE 28-6 Prescription Treatments for Allergies

Generic Name	Brand Name	Dosage Forms and Availability	Route of Administration	Common Adult Dosage
acrivastine/ pseudoephedrine	Semprex-D	8-mg/60-mg capsules	Oral	One cap four times daily
azelastine	Optivar	0.05% ophthalmic solution	Ophthalmic	One drop into each affected eye twice daily
beclomethasone	Beconase AQ, QVAR	MDI	Nasal spray, oral inhaler	Beconase AQ: one to two sprays in each nostril twice daily, not to exceed a maximum dose of 336 mcg/day QVAR: 40 mcg to 160 mcg twice daily, not to exceed 320 mcg twice daily.
budesonide	Rhinocort	32-mcg nasal spray	Nasal	One spray per nostril daily
cetirizine	Zyrtec	10-mg tablets, 10-mg capsules	Oral	10 mg, not to exceed a single dose in a 24-hour period
fexofenadine	Allegra	60-mg, 180-mg tablets	Oral	60–180 mg every 12 hours, not to exceed 180 mg in a 24-hour period
fluticasone	Flonase	50-mcg nasal spray	Nasal	One to two sprays in each nostril once daily, not to exceed two sprays per nostril daily.
ketotifen	Zaditor	0.025% ophthalmic solution	Ophthalmic	One drop in affected eye twice daily
loratadine	Claritin RediTabs, Claritin	5-mg, 10-mg tablets; 10-mg capsules	Oral	5–10 mg per dose, not to exceed 10 mg in a 24-hour period

TABLE 28-6 Prescription Treatments for Allergies *(Continued)*

Generic Name	Brand Name	Dosage Forms and Availability	Route of Administration	Common Adult Dosage
loteprednol	Alrex, Lotemax	Alrex—0.2% suspension; Lotemax—0.5% suspension	Ophthalmic	Alrex: use one drop of the 0.2% eye suspension in the affected eye up to four times a day Lotemax: use one or two drops of the 0.5% eye suspension in the affected eye four times a day
mometasone	Nasonex	50-mcg nasal spray	Nasal	Two sprays in each nostril twice daily
olopatadine	Patanol	0.1% ophthalmic solution	Ophthalmic	One drop in each affected eye twice daily
promethazine/ phenylephrine	Phenergen VC	6.25 mg/5 mg/5 mL	Oral	1 tsp. every 4–6 hours
triamcinolone	Nasacort AQ	55-mcg nasal spray	Nasal	Two sprays in each nostril once daily

Influenza

Influenza, or commonly called "the flu," is caused by the influenza virus and is an infection associated with the respiratory tract and system. There are three types of flu—A, B, and C. The flu can become deadly, or recovery can be slowed if not treated properly or right away. Older individuals, those with compromised immune systems, and young children are affected by the flu the hardest. Health professionals recommend obtaining a flu vaccine every year to avoid catching the flu. Antiviral medications and pain medications can be used to treat the flu. Prevention is the best way to avoid catching the flu.

H1N1

The H1N1 virus includes symptoms similar to those of regular flu. This strain first became notable in 2009 and caused many variants of H1N1 to be born. The 2009 Swine Flu Vaccine can help protect against contracting the H1N1 flu, and those who are more susceptible to the flu should get the vaccine. This group includes children, older adults, and those who have compromised immune systems. The annual flu vaccine can also help protect against getting the H1N1 flu. The newest strain of flu is called Swine Flu because the strain parallels between North American pigs and the type of strain humans have contracted in recent years. The Swine Flu can be avoided by getting vaccinated with the appropriate shots and by practicing regular hand washing, keeping the mouth covered when sneezing and coughing, and avoiding continuous touching of the eyes and mouth. Keeping hydrated and getting a lot of rest can also help a person recover from H1N1.

Rhinitis

Rhinitis is a common condition of irritation and inflammation of the mucous membranes of the nose lining. Many things can cause rhinitis such as a cold, flu, allergies, pollution in the air, overpowering odors, perfumes, chemicals, paint, and other irritating factors. Rhinitis can be acute (short-term) or a long-term condition. Symptoms can include runny nose, itchy nose, congestion, sneezing, PND, coughing, headache, and runny and watery eyes. Drug treatment of rhinitis includes nasal spray, steroids, antihistamines, decongestants, and allergy shots. Irrigated salt water, humidifiers, purifiers, limiting exposure to allergens and pollutants, and taking proper care of animals such as bathing and vacuuming pet hair can help cut down on the misery of rhinitis (Table 28-7).

TABLE 28-7 Prescription Treatments for Rhinitis

Generic Name	Brand Name	Dosage Forms and Availability	Route of Administration	Common Adult Dosage
fluticasone	Flonase	50-mcg nasal spray	Nasal	One to two sprays in each nostril once daily, not to exceed two sprays per nostril daily.
triamcinolone	Nasacort AQ	55-mcg nasal spray	Nasal	Two sprays in each nostril once daily.

Treatment of Allergies

The treatment of **allergies** with respiratory responses includes antihistamines and antitussives to alleviate the symptoms and mast cell stabilizers to prevent initial allergic reactions and recurrence.

Antihistamines

Like many drugs, antihistamines have many different uses that are based on their desired effects and side effects. They are used to treat seasonal allergies, to dry up mucous membranes, and as a sleep aid.

If a patient takes an antihistamine before exposure to the **allergen**, such as pollen, the drug will go to the H-1 receptor site. When the person is exposed to the pollen, the mast cells will release histamine-1, which will try to find H-1 receptors. However, because the antihistamine is already bound to the H-1 receptor sites, it blocks or inhibits the histamine from getting in. Thus, no allergic reaction will occur.

If a patient has been exposed to the allergen or pollen first, the receptor sites are already occupied by histamine. If a person takes antihistamines *after* exposure to the allergen, the drug will wait until the histamine, a protein, degrades and exits the receptor site. Since there are histamine and antihistamine molecules waiting to get into open receptor sites while the person is still exposed to the allergen, the antihistamine will race the histamine to get into the receptor site first. Fortunately, antihistamines always win the race! This mechanism of action (MOA) is known as *competitive inhibition*. Once inside of or attached to

---

allergy the result of the immune system's reaction to a foreign substance.

allergen a substance capable of causing a hypersensitivity reaction.

---

the H-1 receptor site, the antihistamine does not fit perfectly, but fits well enough to bind, preventing or blocking the histamine from getting in. This blocking is known as *inhibition*. Because the antihistamine does not fit in the receptor-site "lock" quite as well as the correct histamine "key," the "key" is never "turned," and thus there is no chemical change and no allergic reaction occur. This is somewhat like a jigsaw puzzle piece that looks like it is the right color, right size, and right shape, but just does not fit exactly and so does not snap into place. Individuals with prostate problems or glaucoma should avoid antihistamines, unless they have authorization from their physicians.

Antihistamines have two MOAs to combat colds and one additional MOA to combat allergies. First-generation antihistamines have the anticholinergic effect of drying the mucous membranes of the nose, mouth, and eyes; they do so by attaching to muscarinic or cholinergic receptors, which blocks the effect of acetylcholine (ACH).

> **❝ Workplace Wisdom** **First-Generation Antihistamines**
>
> Only first-generation antihistamines work on cholinergic receptors. This MOA helps to combat both the common cold and allergies. **❞**

First-generation antihistamines are lipophilic; therefore, they cross the blood–brain barrier and enter the central nervous system, causing sedation. This side effect can be desirable for those with a cold, who may need rest and sleep, but is often undesirable for allergy patients. Side effects of antihistamines can include drowsiness, sleepiness, and overly dry mucous membranes. Some antihistamines also stop nausea, vomiting, and motion sickness. Tables 28-8 to 28-12 include some examples of various antihistamines.

TABLE 28-8 Prescription Antihistamines

Generic Name	Brand Name	Dosage Forms and Availability	Route of Administration	Common Adult Dosage
cetirizine	Zyrtec	10-mg tablets; 10-mg capsules	Oral	10 mg, not to exceed a single dose in a 24-hour period
desloratadine	Clarinex	5-mg, 10-mg tablets	Oral	5–10 mg per dose, not to exceed 10 mg in a 24-hour period
diphenhydramine	Oral—Benadryl, topical—Benadryl Itch Stopping Gel, SDV—Benadryl injection	12.5-mg, 25-mg tablets; 12.5-mg, 25-mg capsules; 50 mg/mL SDV	Oral, topical, injection	Oral: 1–2 tablets or capsules every 4–6 hours, not to exceed six doses in a 24-hour period; topical: apply to affected area, not more than four times daily; injection: 10–50 mg intravenously at a rate generally not exceeding 25 mg/min, or deep intramuscularly; 100 mg if required; maximum daily dosage is 400 mg

TABLE 28-8 Prescription Antihistamines *(Continued)*

Generic Name	Brand Name	Dosage Forms and Availability	Route of Administration	Common Adult Dosage
fexofenadine	Allegra	60-mg, 180-mg tablets	Oral	60–180 mg every 12 hours, not to exceed 180 mg in a 24-hour period
loratadine	Claritin	5-mg, 10-mg tablets; 10-mg capsules	Oral	5–10 mg per dose, not to exceed 10 mg in a 24-hour period

TABLE 28-9 Examples of OTC Antihistamines (H-1 Antagonists) Used for Cold and Allergy Symptoms

Generic Name	Trade Name
chlorpheniramine	Chlor-Trimeton
clemastine	Tavist-1
diphenhydramine	Benadryl, Banophen, Diphedryl
loratadine	Alavert, Claritin—does not cause drowsiness
loratadine/pseudoephedrine	Claritin-D—does not cause drowsiness

Note: Formulations cause drowsiness, unless otherwise indicated.

TABLE 28-10 Examples of Prescription Antihistamines (H-1 Antagonists) for Allergy

Generic Name	Trade Name
azelastine	Astelin NS—possible drowsiness
brompheniramine	BroveX CT
cetirizine	Zyrtec—does not cause drowsiness
cyproheptadine	Periactin
desloratadine	Clarinex
fexofenadine	Allegra—does not cause drowsiness
hydroxyzine HCl	Atarax—also used as an antiemetic
hydroxyzine pamoate	Vistaril—also used as an antiemetic
phenyltoloxamine citrate, pyrilamine maleate, pheniramine maleate	Poly-Histine (antihistamine combination)
promethazine HCl	Phenergan—also used as an antiemetic

Note: Formulations cause drowsiness, unless otherwise indicated.

TABLE 28-11 Examples of Prescription Ophthalmic Antihistamines (H-1 Antagonists)

Generic Name	Trade Name
azelastine HCl	Optivar
emedastine difumarate	Emadine
epinastine HCl	Elestat
ketotifen fumarate	Zaditen
olopatadine HCl	Patanol

TABLE 25-12 Comparison of Degree of Sedation of Various Types of Antihistamines

Ethanolamines		Ethylenediamines		Alkylamines
clemastine	Greater sedation than ⟶	pyrilamine	Greater sedation than ⟶	pheniramine
diphenhydramine		thonzylamine		brompheniramine
doxylamine				
				chlorpheniramine
				triprolidine

Mast Cell Stabilizers

The use of antihistamines is one way to treat allergies, as these drugs stop histamine from entering or binding to cells in the nose, eye, skin, or other body area and thus causing an allergic reaction. *Mast cell stabilizers* prevent the allergen from attaching to the mast cell, thereby preventing the mast cell from releasing histamine. If histamine is not released from the mast cell, it cannot be free to seek the new binding receptor site of a body cell. For example, if no histamine is available to bind to the nose receptor site, the nose will not become itchy, have congestion, or become runny. In other words, mast cell stabilizers act prophylactically to prevent allergic responses. They are considered anti-inflammatory agents. The benefits of mast cell stabilizers are that they:

- Stop the allergic response before it begins, without causing drowsiness, irritability, or a decreased ability to think or focus.
- Do not reverse allergy symptoms that are already present, but do prevent exposure to new allergens, thus preventing allergic symptoms.
- Can be used for weeks or months at a time without the fear of rebound effects or threat of addiction that decongestants may pose.

Mast cell stabilizers are used most often to prevent asthma attacks, but can also be used to prevent allergic rhinitis. Mast cell stabilizers are available for use in the nose, lungs, and GI tract. Other names for mast cell stabilizers are *mast cell inhibitors* and *mediator-release inhibitors* (see Table 28-13).

Side effects are so few, and the drug is so gentle that cromolyn sodium, the drug of choice, has been used successfully on infants and children and is now an OTC remedy known as Nasalcrom. A new mast cell stabilizer, Tilade (nedocromil sodium), has also been effective, and has a longer duration. Nedocromil may have more anti-inflammatory properties than cromolyn sodium.

Mast cell stabilizers may reduce renal and hepatic function; therefore, the dosage should be decreased in patients with kidney and liver problems. Due to the presence of propellants, inhalant canisters should be used with caution in patients who have coronary artery disease or a history of cardiac arrhythmias. If a patient develops eosinophilic pneumonia (where white blood cells called eosinophils accumulate in the lungs), this particular treatment should be discontinued.

Cromolyn sodium and nedocromil inhibit mast cell degranulation and activation by creating a protective barrier around the cells in the nose and respiratory tract, so that pollen, mold, dust, and animal dander cannot bind or attach to them. The exact MOA is not fully understood, but it is believed that cromolyn indirectly inhibits calcium ions from entering the mast cell and triggering the release of cellular contents. The mast cell stabilizers inhibit both the early and late phases of bronchoconstriction induced by inhaled antigens. In clinical trials, they have also been shown to be effective in mitigating the response induced by cold air, environmental air pollutants, exercise, sulfur dioxide, and other triggers. It is important to note the following:

- Mast cell stabilizers do not have bronchodilation, anticholinergic, antihistaminic, or glucocorticoid effects.
- Mast cell stabilizers are not used in any acute phase of severe bronchoconstriction.

TABLE 28-13 Mast Cell Stabilizers

Generic Name	Trade Name	Dosage Forms
cromolyn sodium	Intal	Inhalation solution
	Nasalcrom	Aerosol
	Gastrocrom	Oral concentrate
	Crolom	Ophthalmic solution
iodoxamide tromethamine	Alomide	Ophthalmic solution
nedocromil sodium	Tilade	Aerosol
	Alocril	Ophthalmic solution
pemirolast potassium	Alamast	Ophthalmic solution

Cystic Fibrosis

Cystic fibrosis (CF) is a genetic disease in which a defective gene causes the body to produce abnormally thick, sticky mucus. This disease affects approximately 30,000 children and adults in the United States. The abnormally viscous mucus clogs the lungs, and leads to life-threatening lung infections, breathing difficulty, and digestive problems. These thick secretions also block the pancreas, preventing digestive enzymes from entering the intestines; this in turn prevents the metabolism (the chemical breakdown and absorption) of food nutrients. According to the CF Foundation's National Patient Registry, the median age of survival for a person with CF is 33.4 years, and 95% of men with CF are sterile.

CF symptoms include very salty-tasting skin; persistent coughing with or without phlegm; wheezing or shortness of breath; excessive appetite with poor weight gain; and greasy, bulky stools. Symptoms may vary partly because more than 1,000 mutations of the CF gene exist. Treatments include:

- Chest percussion physical therapy, a form of airway clearance performed on a routine daily basis that involves vigorous clapping on the back and chest to dislodge the thick mucus from the lungs
- Antibiotics to treat infections
- Bronchodilator and corticosteroid inhalers
- Nutritional supplements
- Mucolytic treatment

Mucolytics thin out the sticky, viscous mucus that causes the breathing and digestive problems associated with CF. The viscosity of the mucus depends on the amount of mucoprotein produced. The more mucoprotein, the greater the number of disulfide bonds, making the mucus thicker. N-acetylcysteine (the generic name of the active drug in Mucomyst and Airbron) breaks the disulfide bonds in mucin, which thins the mucus and makes it more easily dislodged from the lungs by the mucociliary elevator (MCE).

N-acetylcysteine is also used as an antidote in acetaminophen overdose, to prevent or mitigate hepatic injury (damage to the liver). Toxic effects of acetaminophen poisoning are inevitable if not treated in time. These effects include hepatic necrosis, renal tubular necrosis, hypoglycemic coma, and thrombocytopenia, but the potential for severe, irreversible hepatic failure, damage, and necrosis is usually the main concern. Results of hepatic toxicity may not be measurable, clinically or by laboratory tests, until 48 to 72 hours after administration of the initial oral overdose. Signs and symptoms of acute APAP overdose are dose-related, but may include nausea, vomiting, diaphoresis, and general malaise.

Possible adverse effects of acetylcysteine include hemoptysis, stomatitis, nausea, vomiting, and severe rhinorrhea. Interestingly, bronchoconstriction has also been reported with acetylcysteine therapy. The recommended dose of acetylcysteine is 3 mL to 5 mL of a 20% solution diluted with an equal volume of water or saline, or 6 mL to 10 mL of a 10% solution, administered three to four times daily.

Another agent, Pulmozyme (recombinant human deoxyribonuclease I, rhDNase, or dornase alpha) is an enzyme that cleaves DNA left behind by neutrophils in the lungs. When a neutrophil dies, its DNA leaks out, which then comes into contact with mucus, making it very thick. A patient with cystic fibrosis is affected greatly by this natural process. The MOA is one of hydrolysis; when this recombinant human DNA enzyme is inhaled, it hydrolyzes or cuts the neutrophil DNA apart and subsequently thins out the mucus for an easier removal by the MCE. This agent is delivered by inhalation.

Side effects may include chest pain or discomfort, hoarseness, and sore throat. Less common are difficulty breathing; fever; redness, itching, pain, swelling, or other irritation of eyes; runny or stuffy nose; upset stomach; hives or welts; itching; redness of skin; and skin rash.

Asthma

Asthma is a chronic respiratory disease characterized by inflammation of the airways and tightening of the muscles around the airways. *Bronchoconstriction* occurs when the smooth muscles encircling the airways or tubes tighten, causing the airways to spasm. The actual interior wall constricts because the tissue becomes inflamed, and the inflammation further constricts airflow. The narrowing of the bronchi during an asthmatic attack may be fatal if the person cannot get the passageways opened quickly. In addition, more mucus is made, further narrowing the airways. As a result, the patient may feel weak; exhibit wheezing, coughing, and chest tightness or pain; and be short of breath. Albuterol and other bronchodilators are often the drug of choice for quick relief and restoration of airflow (Table 28-14).

The exact cause of asthma is unknown, but if a family member has it, others in the family are more likely to develop it. Research suggests that allergic triggers (allergens and irritants), as well as viral infections and exercise, play a large role in triggering airway inflammation and asthma symptoms. If a child has allergies, he or she is more likely to develop asthma. Approximately 17 million people (mostly children) have asthma attacks caused by allergies to airborne pollutants such as dust, mold, mites, pollen, and animal dander.

There are many substances, called *biochemical mediators*, inside each mast cell. These mediators can be released during exposure to allergens. Two of the most common mediators released from the mast cells that cause allergies are leukotrienes and histamine. *Leukotrienes* are potent mediators that are released by mast cells, eosinophils, and basophils. They work to contract airway smooth muscle, increase vascular permeability, increase mucus secretion, and attract and activate inflammatory cells in the air passageways of patients with asthma. Among the many other mediators that are released during respiratory inflammation are eosinophilic chemotactic factor of anaphylaxis (ECF-A), various prostaglandins, cytokines such as tumor necrosis factor (TNF), and interleukins.

One of the most important prostaglandin mediators involved in asthma is the slow-reacting substance of anaphylaxis known as SRS-A. Leukotrienes B, C, D, and E are also released; C, D, and E help to make SRS-A. The effects of SRS-A last longer than those of histamine, creating mucosal edema and leukocyte infiltration and causing major bronchoconstriction.

TABLE 28-14 Prescription Treatments for Asthma

Generic Name	Brand Name	Dosage Forms and Availability	Route of Administration	Common Adult Dosage
alubuterol	Proventil HFA, Ventolin HFA, Ventolin, AccuNeb	90-mcg inhalant aerosol; 0.5% inhalant solution	Inhalant, liquid for nebulizer	MDI: two puffs every four to six hours or as needed for rescue of acute attack; neb: 2.5 mg three to four times daily by nebulization
beclomethasone	Beclovent, Beconase AQ	42-mcg nasal spray	Nasal	One spray into each nostril three to four times daily
cromolyn	Nasalcrom	40-mg/mL nasal spray	Nasal	One spray into each nostril three to four times daily
flunisolide	AeroBid, Nasalide	Oral inhaler; 0.025% nasal spray	Inhalation—oral and nasal	Two puffs up to two times daily
fluticasone propionate	Flovent, Flonase	44-mcg, 110-mcg, 220-mcg inhalant aerosol; 50-mcg nasal spray	Inhalation—oral and nasal; topical	Flovent: two to four puffs bid Flonase: two sprays per nostril up to two times daily
fluticasone propionate/ salmeterol	Advair Diskus; Advair HFA	100/50-mcg, 250/50-mcg, 500/50-mcg inhalant powder; 45/21-mcg, 115/21-mcg, 130/21-mcg inhalant powder	Oral inhalation	One blister dose as prescribed every 12 hours
montelukast	Singulair	10-mg tablets; 4-mg, 5-mg chew tablets; 4-mg oral granules	Oral	10 mg once daily in the evening; 4-mg and 5-mg forms for pediatric use
salmeterol	Serevent	50-mcg inhalant powder	Oral inhalation	Two puffs bid (not meant for acute attacks); should not use more than once every 12 hours
triamcinolone acetonide	Azmacort	60-mg inhalant aerosol	Inhalation	Two to three puffs up to four times daily
zafirlukast	Accolate	10-mg, 20-mg tablets	Oral	20 mg two times daily

❝ Workplace Wisdom Asthma Statistics

Asthma affects more than 15 million people and is responsible for as many as 1.5 million emergency room visits and 500,000 hospitalizations each year.

Diagnosis of asthma may include chest X-ray to rule out other diseases, blood tests, sputum studies, physical exam in which the examiner listens to the sounds and notes symptoms, and spirometry tests. A spirometry breathing test measures the amount of air intake and the rate at which air can pass through the patient's airways. Less air will pass through the airways, and at a lower speed, if the airways are narrowed because of inflammation. This results in abnormal spirometry values. ❞

---

chronic obstructive pulmonary disease (COPD) a condition resulting from continual blockage of external exchange of oxygen in the lungs; an umbrella term for emphysema and chronic bronchitis.

Chronic Obstructive Pulmonary Disease

Chronic obstructive pulmonary disease (COPD) is an umbrella term for emphysema and chronic bronchitis. It is a serious respiratory condition that causes breathing difficulty for those affected. COPD is characterized by partially blocked bronchi and bronchioles, which make it very difficult to get air into and out of the lungs and consequently cause shortness of breath. COPD is the fourth leading cause of death in the United States; more than 120,000 people die of it every year. About 80% to 90% of all COPD is related to cigarette smoking (Table 28-15).

Emphysema

Emphysema affects approximately 3.8 million Americans and is ranked (with COPD) as the fourth leading cause of death in the United States. Forty percent more men than women are affected by emphysema.

Individuals suffering from emphysema progressively become characterized with tachypnea (or rapid respiration), which can occur after limited physical activity (such as walking a very short distance). Emphysema involves destruction of the alveoli. The external exchange of gases is interrupted when these thin, fragile air sacs become permanently and irreversibly damaged, as a protein called *elastin* is destroyed. The alveoli become less able to transfer oxygen to the blood system. In addition, bronchioles are less able to dilate and often collapse due to a lack of elastin.

A major symptom is shortness of breath. As alveoli are destroyed, the lungs lose the elasticity needed to keep the airways open. The alveoli stay full of air and carbon dioxide, but are unable to exhale the waste and inhale the much-needed air from which to extract oxygen. Another symptom is great difficulty in exhaling, which leads to the characteristic fully expanded chest, known as a "barrel" chest.

Other symptoms include the inability to perform normal daily activities or exercise. Chronic breathing problems, such as bronchitis and asthma, may also develop before emphysema is diagnosed. The main cause of emphysema is long-term exposure to pollutants that irritate the alveoli, such as tobacco smoke, asbestos, pollution, coal dust, and chemical fumes. Also, it is believed that more than 100,000 Americans have been born with a protein deficiency that can lead to an inherited form of emphysema called alpha 1-antitrypsin (AAT)–deficiency-related emphysema.

Chronic Bronchitis

Chronic bronchitis is characterized by inflammation of the airways that lasts for long periods of time or keeps returning. The main cause is exposure to cigarette smoke, both firsthand and secondhand. A person who smokes is more likely to get chronic bronchitis, and the condition will continue to worsen if the person does not quit. Symptoms of chronic bronchitis include shortness of breath, wheezing, fatigue, headaches, lower extremity swelling that affects both sides, and a cough that produces large amounts of mucus (which may contain blood).

Treatment of Asthma and COPD

The autonomic nervous system plays an important role in COPD and especially in asthma. Stimulation of the sympathetic nervous system's beta-2 receptors by epinephrine creates bronchodilation, whereas stimulation of the parasympathetic nervous system, specifically the activation of the vagus nerve by irritants, causes bronchoconstriction. Bronchodilators act to either open airway passages immediately, prevent attachment of the allergen to mast cells, or stop prostaglandin synthesis. Bronchodilators administered orally include ephedrine, albuterol, and terbutaline. Oral epinephrine is unavailable because it is broken down in the digestive system before it can reach the lungs.

TABLE 25-15 Prescription Treatments for COPD

Generic Name	Brand Name	Dosage Forms and Availability	Route of Administration	Common Adult Dosage
fluticasone/ salmeterol	Advair HFA	45/21-mcg, 115/ 21-mcg, 130/21-mcg inhalant powder	Oral inhalation	Two puffs twice daily
formoterol/ budesonide	Symbicort	80/4.5-mcg, 160/ 4.5-mcg inhalant powder	Oral inhalation	Two puffs twice daily
ipratropium bromide	Atrovent	17-mcg inhalant, 0.03% nasal spray	Oral inhalation, nasal	Oral inhalant: two puffs qid Nasal inhalant: two sprays into each nostril two to three times daily
ipratropium/ albuterol	Combivent, DuoNeb	18/90-mcg inhalant aerosol, 20/120-mcg nasal spray, 0.5/3-mg inhalant solution	Oral inhalation, nasal	Oral inhalant: two puffs qid; one vial four times daily via nebulization; Nasal inhalant: two sprays into each nostril two to three times daily
theophyline	Uniphyl	400-mg, 600-mg tablets	Oral, inhalant, injection, rectal	400–600 mg daily

Treatments that open up the air passageways usually include stimulant inhalers; treatments for the prevention of inflammation usually include anti-inflammatory corticosteroids. The aim of treatment is to reduce inflammation and prevent further injury to the airway. There are also oral medications that can prevent inflammation. There is mounting evidence that, if left untreated, asthma can cause a long-term decline in lung function.

Oral and nasal inhalers used in the treatment of asthma are divided into two groups:

- Treatments used for quick relief, to immediately open the airway passages
- Treatments used for prophylactic maintenance, to decrease and prevent swelling, irritation, and inflammation on a daily basis, and treatments used to prevent the release of histamines and leukotrienes so that asthma attacks will not occur

Bronchodilators

Beta-adrenergic inhalers act within approximately 15 minutes. One exception is salmeterol, which is a long-acting bronchodilator that is not designed to give an immediate effect. The MOA of these *sympathomimetic* drugs is to mimic or simulate epinephrine stimulation of the beta-2 receptors of the respiratory tract, directly relaxing smooth muscles and causing immediate bronchodilation (see Table 28-16).

Xanthines

The exact MOA of xanthines, which are respiratory smooth muscle relaxants, is unknown. However, some of the ways in which xanthines are believed to work are the following:

- Xanthines increase levels of energy-producing cyclic adenosine monophosphate (cAMP).
- They competitively inhibit phosphodiesterase (PDE), an enzyme that chemically breaks down cAMP.
- Inhibition of PDE results in increased cAMP levels, smooth muscle relaxation, bronchodilation, and airflow through air passages.

The result of these actions is increased CNS and cardiovascular stimulation, force of contraction, kidney secretion, and diuretic effect. Side effects include nausea, vomiting, anorexia, gastroesophageal reflux during sleep, sinus tachycardia, extrasystole, palpitations, ventricular dysrhythmias, and

TABLE 28-16 Beta-Adrenergic Bronchodilators

Generic Name	Trade Name	Strength/Dosage Form(s) Available	Average Adult Dosage
albuterol	Ventolin, Proventil	Tablet: 2 mg, 4 mg	2–4 mg tid–qid
		Syrup: 2 mg/5 mL	
		ER tablet: 2 mg, 4 mg	8 mg q12h
		90-mcg inhaler	Two puffs q4–6h
		Inhalant solution: 0.083%, 0.5%, 0.021%, 0.42%	2.5 mg tid–qid via nebulizer
albuterol + ipratropium bromide	Combivent	Aerosol	Two puffs qid
	DuoNeb	Inhalant solution	3 mL qid with two additional doses per day prn
bitolterol	Tornalate	Inhalant solution: 0.2%	
epinephrine	Adrenalin	Inhalant solution:10 mg/mL	0.5 mL no more than q3h
		Aerosol: 0.22 mg	
		Injection: 1 mg/mL, 0.1 mg/mL	
fluticasone + salmeterol combination	Advair Diskus	100 mcg/50 mcg	One inhalation bid
		250 mcg/50 mcg	
		500 mcg/50 mcg	
formoterol	Foradil	12-mcg inhaled powder in capsule	12 mcg q12h via aerolizer inhaler

TABLE 28-16 Beta-Adrenergic Bronchodilators (*Continued*)

Generic Name	Trade Name	Strength/Dosage Form(s) Available	Average Adult Dosage
isoproterenol	Isuprel	Injection: 0.2 mg/mL, 0.02 mg/mL	0.2 mg IV; repeat prn
levalbuterol	Xopenex	Inhalant solution: 0.31 mg/3 mL, 0.63 mg/3 mL, 1.25 mg/3 mL	0.63 mg tid (q6–8h) via nebulizer
metaproterenol	Alupent, Metaprel	0.65-mg inhaler	Two to three puffs tid–qid; NTE q4h
		Inhalant solution: 0.4%, 0.6%, 5%	
pirbuterol	Maxair	0.2-mg inhaler	Two puffs (q6–8h)
salmeterol	Serevent		
salmeterol zinafoate	Serevent Diskus	50 mcg	50 mcg bid
terbutaline	Bricanyl, Brethine (also SQ and po)	Tablet: 2.5 mg, 5 mg Inhalant: 1 mg/mL	5 mg q6h
			0.25 mg sq; repeat dose in 15–30 minutes

transient tonic/clonic convulsions. Some xanthines, such as theophylline, may cause increased nervousness when used with herbs such as St. John's Wort, ma huang, or ephedra.

Anticholinergics

Anticholinergics block the effects of acetylcholine by competing for the ACH receptor site. Bronchoconstriction is prevented, and airway passage dilation is assisted. Possible side effects include dry mouth or throat, gastrointestinal distress, headache, coughing, and anxiety (see Table 28-17).

Anti-Inflammatory Agents

Corticosteroids are not quick acting, so they are used prophylactically. The result of corticosteroid action is decreased

TABLE 28-17 Various Treatments for Asthma

Generic Name	Trade Name	Dosage Form	Adult Dosage
natural xanthines	Caffeine, tea, cocoa, chocolate	po	100 mg = 1 cup coffee
Methyl Xanthines and Derivatives			
aminophylline (79% theophylline)		Tablet: 100 mg, 200 mg	Individualized dosing
		Injection: 250 mg/10 mL	
		Suppository: 250 mg, 500 mg	
oxtriphylline (64% theophylline)		Tablet: 100 mg, 200 mg; 400–mg, 800-mg SR tablets, elixir and pediatric syrup	4.7 mg/kg q8h
theophylline	Theodur, Bronkodyl, Slo-Bid	Tablet/capsule: 100 mg, 125 mg, 200 mg, 300 mg; 100 mg, 200 mg, 300 mg, 400 mg, 450 mg, 600 mg extended- and timed-release tablets/capsules	Individualized dosing
		Syrup: 150 mg/15 mL	
		Elixir: 80 mg/15 mL	

(Continued)

TABLE 28-17 Various Treatments for Asthma (*Continued*)

Generic Name	Trade Name	Dosage Form	Adult Dosage
Anticholinergics			
albuterol + ipratropium combination	Combivent	Aerosol	Two puffs qid
	DuoNeb	Inhalant solution	2 mL qid with two additional doses per day prn
ipratropium bromide	Atrovent	Inhaler	Two puffs qid
tiotropium bromide	Spiriva	Powder for inhalation capsules	One capsule daily in the HandiHaler device

inflammation of the airway passages, which allows the patient to breathe more easily. The MOA is one of inhibition: Glucocorticoids exert their effects by binding to the glucocorticoid receptor (GR), which then inhibits or increases gene transcription through processes known as *transrepression* and *transactivation*, respectively. In this manner they also reduce the immune response (see Table 28-18).

Oral thrush, or *thrush mouth*, is the common term for a yeast infection by *Candida albicans* that occurs in the back of the throat of patients who use corticosteroid inhalers. The main symptom is a white film located at the back of the throat, tongue, and tonsil area. Antifungal mouthwash may be used to treat this infection (all yeast are fungi, but not all fungi are yeast). This common side effect occurs because steroids alter the local bacterial and fungal population of the mouth, enhancing fungal growth. Using a space inhaler or rinsing the mouth very thoroughly after each corticosteroid use will help to prevent it.

Mast Cell Inhibitors

As discussed in the preceding section on allergies, mast cell inhibitors are also known as mast cell stabilizers, mediator-release inhibitors, or prophylactic drugs. Benefits of Intal (cromolyn sodium) and Tilade (nedocromil) include reduction in asthma symptoms, improved peak expiratory flow rates, and decreased need for short-acting beta-2 agonists.

Antileukotriene Drugs

There are two types of antileukotriene drugs: leukotriene receptor antagonists and leukotriene inhibitors. This is the first new class of asthma-fighting drugs to appear in more than 30 years. Leukotriene inhibitors may be used to reduce the need for low-dose corticosteroid inhaler regimens. The long-term effects of leukotriene inhibitors therapy have yet to be determined. It is speculated that, in the future, IV formulations of these agents may be useful in emergency situations. Table 28-19 lists some of the mast cell stabilizers and antileukotrienes.

Leukotrienes are substances released when a trigger, such as animal dander, mold, or dust, starts a series of chemical reactions in the body. Histamine is also released. Leukotrienes attach to the allergen and then to the mast cell, causing

inflammation, increased mucus production, and bronchoconstriction. The patient will experience coughing, wheezing, and shortness of breath.

Antileukotriene agents block or inhibit the leukotrienes from attaching to the receptors on the mast cells in the lungs and the basophils in blood circulation. The result is a decrease in neutrophil and leukocyte infiltration to the lungs that decreases inflammation in the lungs, thus mitigating and preventing asthma symptoms. The specific MOAs of these new drugs are further explained in Table 28-19.

Unfortunately, antileukotriene agents do have toxic effects. They may cause liver dysfunction; therefore, liver assessments must continue during therapy with these agents. Side effects of Accolate and Zyflo may include headache, dyspepsia, diarrhea, dizziness, and insomnia. The toxic effect is liver dysfunction. Montelukast has fewer side effects and no toxic effects on the liver.

Other Treatments

Another drug, atropine, may also be used to fight allergic reactions and anaphylactic shock, because it has antisecretory properties. It decreases the amount of nasal and respiratory secretions in the body.

There are many medications in many different dosage forms and routes of administration for respiratory diseases.

PROFILES IN PRACTICE

Mr. Rodriguez, an older adult patient, currently uses albuterol (two inhalations 15 minutes prior to exercise) and theophylline (100 mg po bid), for the treatment of his asthma. While checking out, he asks the pharmacist which of his breathing medications he should take first, as he takes both drugs before going to the gym.

▸ *Is there any difference based on the order in which Mr. Rodriguez takes his medications? If so, why?*

TABLE 28-18 **Corticosteroids**

Trade Name	Generic Name	Dosage Form	Adult Dose
Inhalers			
Advair Diskus	fluticasone + salmeterol combination	100 mcg/50 mcg	One inhalation bid
		250 mcg/50 mcg	
		500 mcg/50 mcg	
Aerobid	flunisolide	MDI, intranasal form for rhinitis	Two to three puffs bid to tid, NTE 12 puffs per day
Azmacort	triamcinolone	MDI, po, TOP, SC, ID, IM	Two puffs tid–qid, NTE 16 puffs per day
Flovent	fluticasone	MDI	Two puffs bid (44 mcg each), NTE 10 puffs per day (440 mcg/day)
Pulmicort	budesonide	Dry powder inhaler (DPI)	One to two puffs qd (200 mcg/inhalation), NTE four puffs per day (800 mcg/day)
QVar, Beclovent	beclomethasone	MDI, intranasal form for rhinitis	One to two puffs tid–qid
Oral			
Deltasone, Meticorten	prednisone	po only	5–10 mg/day; reduction in dose should be gradual to decrease the risk of adrenal insufficiency
Dexone, Decadron	dexamethasone	Tablet: 0.5 mg, 0.75 mg, 1.5 mg, 4 mg	0.75–9 mg/day
Medrol, Medrol DosePak	methylprednisolone	po: 2 mg, 4 mg, 6 mg, 8 mg, 16 mg, 24 mg, 32 mg tablets; also available IM, SC for neoplasia and adrenal insufficiency	4–48 qd; reduction in dose should be gradual to decrease the risk of adrenal insufficiency
Injectable			
Decadron	dexamethasone sodium phosphate	Injection: 4 mg dexamethasone phosphate in 1 mL ampoule	For anaphylactic shock: 10–100 mg IV (1 mg/kg) slow IV bolus
SoluCortef	hydrocortisone	IV, IM, infusion sterile powder: 100-mg, 250-mg, 500-mg, 1,000-mg Act-O Vial	100–500 mg for 48–72 hours, over 30 seconds to 10 minutes, q2, 4, or 6h, then decreased gradually to a maintenance dose
SoluMedrol	methylprednisolone	IV, IM, and infusion sterile powder: 40-mg, 125-mg, 500-mg, 1-gm Act-O Vial	30 mg/kg over 30 minutes, MR q4–6h × 48 hours at least 30 minutes. Dosage must be discontinued gradually

TABLE 28-19 Mast Cell Stabilizers and Antileukotrienes

Trade Name	Generic Name	Dosage/Mechanism of Action
Mast Cell Stabilizers		
Intal, Nasalcrom (OTC)	cromolyn sodium	MDI; two puffs of 1 mg each qid; takes two to four weeks before results are seen. NTE 8 mg/day
Tilade	nedocromil	MDI; two puffs of 2 mg each qid; NTE 16 mg/day
Leukotriene-Receptor-Blocking Drugs (LTRAs)		
Accolate	zafirlukast	Selectively blocks receptors of leukotrienes D_4 and E_4. LTD_4 and LTE_4 are components of SRS-A
Singulair	montelukast	Binds with high affinity and selectivity to the $CysLT_1$ receptor rather than prostanoid, cholinergic, or beta-adrenegic receptors, and inhibits the actions of LTD_4 at the $CysLT_1$ receptor without any agonist activity
Leukotriene-Formation Inhibitors		
Zyflo	zileuton	Blocks the synthesis of leukotrienes by specifically inhibiting the enzyme that enables the formation of specific leukotrienes from arachidonic acid

Medications taken orally almost always have a much higher *systemic concentration* (concentration in the entire body and blood system) than inhaled medications. Therefore, an inhaled route is preferred whenever possible. The idea behind an inhaler is that the full dose is delivered to the lungs, where it is immediately absorbed by the lung tissue and can take local effect. Excess drug that may be absorbed by the bloodstream is then distributed to the rest of the body. The lungs receive an immediate, high concentration of the drug, while the rest of the body receives very little drug. One advantage of oral medications is that some are available as timed-release formulations, so that the patient takes a tablet only once every 12 hours, whereas the inhaled medication may require dosing every 4 to 6 hours. Keeping track of the number of doses used on an inhaler compared with the number it can deliver is the surest way of telling whether the inhaler is empty. One way to do this is to mark both the beginning date and the date on which the inhaler should be empty if all doses are given.

Products that once relied on chlorinated fluorocarbons (CFCs), such as air-conditioning units, refrigerators, and most aerosol products, have been either totally banned or modified to use alternative chemicals that do not damage the ozone layer. However, metered-dose inhalers (MDIs) have been granted an "essential use" exemption from this ban. This allows the drug manufacturers a few more years to develop new, alternative propellants and devices. The FDA has approved a new non-CFC inhaler, Proventil HFA (albuterol), which uses hydrofluoroalkane instead of CFC propellant.

Pneumonia

Pneumonia is characterized by lung inflammation, which can be caused by an infection. Symptoms can include chills, fever, fatigue, chest pain, coughing, and sore throat. Pneumonia is generally a serious illness that requires immediate attention. Antibiotics, antivirals, bronchodilators, and corticosteroids are used to treat the infection along with much rest and keeping hydrated.

Tuberculosis

Tuberculosis, or TB, is a bacterial infection most commonly found in the lungs, although it can spread to any part of the body. Some patients who develop TB never have any symptoms, and the bacteria can live inactive in the body. When an individual's immune system becomes compromised, the bacteria can become active and cause tissue death, depending on the organs affected. TB is a fatal disease if left untreated. People who are exposed to large groups of people, usually who live within close quarters of each other, can contract the disease. For example, dorm rooms, student apartments, and prisons can be a breeding ground for the possibly deadly disease. There are no alternative therapies or OTC medications; all treatment for TB are prescription medications. (Table 28-20)

TABLE 28-20 Prescription Treatments for Tuberculosis

Generic Name	Brand Name	Dosage Forms and Availability	Route of Administration	Common Adult Dosage
ethambutol	Myambutol	100-mg, 400-mg tablets	Oral	800 mg to 1.2 gm once daily
pyrazinamide	n/a	500-mg tablets	Oral	2,000 mg once daily for two months
rifampin	Rifadin	150-mg, 300-mg capsules	Oral	600 mg once daily one to two hours before or after meals

Summary

The respiratory system is crucial to sustaining life because it is responsible for providing all cells of the body with the oxygen necessary to perform their specific functions. It is the system that performs the intake of oxygen through inhalation, and the excretion of carbon monoxide through exhalation. The respiratory system is divided into two parts, the upper and lower respiratory tracts. The upper respiratory tract consists of the nasal cavity, paranasal sinuses, pharynx, and larynx. The lower respiratory tract is made up of the trachea, two lungs, two main bronchi, secondary and tertiary bronchi, bronchioles, alveolar ducts, and alveoli.

The most common disease of the respiratory system is the common cold. Uncomplicated common colds are generally treated with OTC medications, including antihistamines, decongestants, cough suppressants, analgesics, antipyretics, and anti-inflammatories. The aim of treatment is to provide relief from symptoms. The pharmacy technician should also be familiar with commonsense treatment measures, such as increased fluid intake, bed rest, gargling with warm salt water, and so on, and be able to assist the pharmacist in advising patients suffering from common colds.

Of course, there are many more serious diseases of the respiratory system, one of which is asthma. Asthma affects more than 15 million people and is responsible for as many as 1.5 million ER visits and 500,000 hospitalizations every year. If left uncontrolled, asthma can cause a long-term decline in lung function.

This chapter also discussed other respiratory diseases, ranging from allergies to life-threatening COPD, and their treatments. Because many respiratory diseases are treated with some form of inhalation therapy, it is important for pharmacy technicians to be able to assist the pharmacist in educating clients in the proper, safe use of inhalation products and devices.

Chapter Review Questions

1. Which of the following is *not* available as an inhaler?
   a. Azmacort
   b. Alamast
   c. Atrovent
   d. Aerobid

2. The tiny air sacs of the lungs are known as _____.
   a. bronchial tubes
   b. capillaries
   c. lobes
   d. alveoli

3. A genetic disease in which a defective gene causes the body to produce abnormally thick and sticky mucus is known as _____.
   a. pneumonia
   b. cystic fibrosis
   c. bronchitis
   d. emphysema

4. Mucomyst is indicated for cystic fibrosis and _____.
   a. emphysema
   b. COPD
   c. aspirin overdose
   d. acetaminophen overdose

5. Singulair belongs to which of the following classifications?
   a. nasal decongestant
   b. leukotriene-receptor-blocking drug
   c. expectorant
   d. antihistamine

6. Which of the following antihistamines is also indicated for nausea and vomiting?
   a. azelastine
   b. diphenhydramine
   c. promethazine
   d. loratadine

7. Zyrtec is to _____ as _____ is to fexofenadine.
   a. azelastine; Vistaril
   b. brompheniramine; Clarinex
   c. cetirizine; Tavist-1
   d. cetirizine; Allegra

8. Ventolin is classified as what type of drug?
   a. mucolytic
   b. bronchodilator
   c. antileukotriene
   d. antihistamine

9. Anticholinergic drugs block _____.
   a. norepinephrine
   b. epinephrine
   c. acetylcholine
   d. mast cells

10. Which of the following antihistamines is prescribed for ophthalmic use?
   a. brompheniramine
   b. cetirizine
   d. hydroxyzine
   d. olopatadine

Critical Thinking Questions

1. Discuss the advantages and disadvantages of the different types of treatment for asthma.

2. Which would be a better choice for a person with severe bronchitis, a narcotic or nonnarcotic cough suppressant? Explain your answer.

Web Challenge

1. Go to the American Lung Association's website at http://www.lungusa.org to learn more about asthma and allergies.

2. A "Methacholine Challenge" test may be given to determine if someone has asthma. See http://asthmallergy.com/methacholine.htm for a brief description of this test.

References and Resources

"About Air." http://www.engineeringtoolbox.com. Web. 8 April 2008.

Adams, M.P., D.L. Josephson, and L.N. Holland, Jr. *Pharmacology for Nurses—A Pathophysiologic Approach.* (4th edition.) Upper Saddle River, NJ: Pearson Education, 2013. Print.

American Academy of Allergy, Asthma, and Immunology. http://www.aaaai.org/ Web. 8 April 2008.

"Chronic Obstructive Pulmonary Disease (COPD), Includes Chronic Bronchitis and Emphysema." http://www.cdc.gov. Web. 10 August 2013.

"Cure for the Common Cold?" http://www.quantumhealth.com/news/articlecold.html. Web. 8 April 2008.

"Diaphragm Development." http://www.breathing.com/articles/diaphragm-development.htm. Web. 8 April 2008.

Drug Facts and Comparisons, 2012 ed. St. Louis: Wolters Kluwer. 2011. Print.

"Emphysema." http://www.wrongdiagnosis.com/e/emphysema/intro.htm. Web. 6 April 2008.

"End Allergy and Asthma Misery." http://www.acaai.org/powerpoint/online/slide1.html. Web. 8 April 2008.

"Exchange." http://www.mrothery.co.uk/exchange/exchange.htm. Web. 4 April 2008.

"Hiccup." http://www.tipsofallsorts.com/hiccup.html#facts. Web. 1 April 2008.

Holland, N. and M.P. Adams. *Core Concepts in Pharmacology.* (3rd edition.) Upper Saddle River, NJ: Pearson Education, 2010. Print.

"Into the Thorax." http://www.saburchill.com/chapters/chap0020.html. Web. 8 April 2008.

"Legal Requirement for the Sale and Purchase of Drug Products Containing Pseudoephedrine, Ephedrine, and Phenylpropanolamine." http://www.fda.gov. Web. 15 July 2007.

"Little Mystery: Why Do We Yawn?" http://www.msnbc .com/news/205574.asp?cp1=1. Web. 8 April 2008.

"Molecular Mechanism of Action of Theophylline: Induction of Histone Deacetylase Activity to Decrease Inflammatory Gene Expression." http://www .pubmedcentral.nih.gov/articlerender.fcgi?artid= 124399. Web. 8 April 2008.

National Emphysema Foundation. http://www.emphysema foundation.org. Web. 10 October 2012.

National Institute of Allergy and Infectious Diseases. "Common Cold." http://www.niaid.nih.gov/factsheets /cold.htm. Web. 8 April 2013.

"Respiratory System—Basic Function." http://www.ama-assn .org/ama/pub/category/7165.html. Web. 8 April 2008.

"Respiratory Tract." http://www.radiation-scott.org /deposition/respiratory.htm. Web. 8 April 2008.

"What Allergies Do You Suffer From?" http://allergies.about .com/. Web. 8 April 2008.

"What Is Alpha-1 Antitrypsin Deficiency Emphysema?" http://www.lungusa.org. Web. 10 October 2007.

"What Is COPD?" http://www.nhlbi.nih.gov. Web. 13 August 2013.

"What Kind of Inhalers Are There?" http://www.radix .net/~mwg/inhalers.html. Web. 8 April 2008.

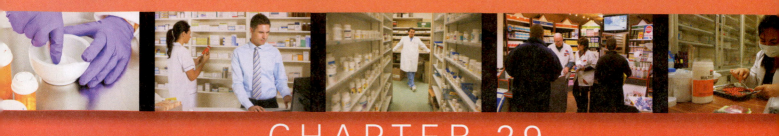

CHAPTER 29

The Cardiovascular, Circulatory, and Lymph Systems

LEARNING OBJECTIVES

After completing this chapter, you should be able to:

- List, identify, and diagram basic anatomical structure and parts of the heart.

- Explain the function of the heart and the circulation of the blood within the body.

- List and define common diseases affecting the heart, including the causes, symptoms, and pharmaceutical treatment associated with each disease.

- Explain how each class of drugs works to mitigate symptoms of heart diseases.

- Describe the mechanism of action of anticoagulants, indications for use, and antidotes for overdose.

- List a variety of drugs intended to affect the cardiovascular system, their classifications, and the average adult dose.

- List the total cholesterol, LDL, HDL, and triglyceride ranges for an average adult, and describe the differences between HDL, LDL, and triglycerides.

- Describe the structure and main functions of the lymphatic system, and explain its relationship to the cardiovascular system.

INTRODUCTION

The heart is both an organ and a muscle. Its main purpose is to send oxygenated blood throughout the body by a pumping mechanism. The heart, which is about the size of a fist, is located just to the left of the sternum in the mediastinum between the two lungs. This unique muscle pumps about 1,900 gal./day of blood, even though the human body contains only about 5.6 L of blood.

Coronary artery disease (CAD), congestive heart failure (CHF), hypertension (HTN), and high cholesterol are serious cardiovascular diseases that affect millions of Americans. This chapter discusses the current classifications of cardiovascular drugs and average adult dosages used for treatment of cardiovascular diseases.

Anatomy of the Heart

The *circulatory system* is composed of organs and blood vessels that transport oxygenated blood to all parts of the body. Specifically, the circulatory system is made up of the heart, lungs, veins, arteries, and capillaries.

The *pericardium* is a double layer of serous and fibrous tissue, a fluid-filled sac that surrounds and protects the heart. It also permits free movement of the heart during contraction. The heart sits inside the pericardial cavity. The *endocardium* is the innermost wall layer that covers the inside surface of the heart. The *myocardium* surrounds the heart and causes chamber contractions.

The heart is composed of four chambers. The *septum* divides the heart into the right and left sides (see Figure 29-1). The top two chambers are the *atria* and the bottom two chambers are the *ventricles*. The right atrium (RA) receives deoxygenated blood from the body, and the left atrium receives oxygenated blood from the lungs. The right ventricle (RV) pumps deoxygenated blood to the lungs to pick up oxygen and drop off waste. The left ventricle, the strongest chamber, pumps oxygenated blood to the rest of the body and back to the heart.

Functionality of the heart can be determined by listening to the *lup-dup, lup-dup* sounds of the opening and closing valves. The four heart valves, which direct blood flow forward in a single direction and prevent the backflow of blood, are the following:

- Tricuspid valve—located between the RA and the RV.
- Pulmonary valve—located between the RV and the pulmonary artery.

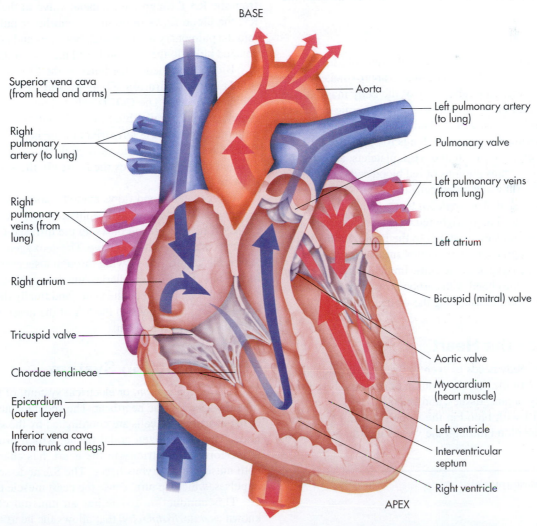

BASE

Superior vena cava (from head and arms)

Aorta

Left pulmonary artery (to lung)

Right pulmonary artery (to lung)

Pulmonary valve

Left pulmonary veins (from lung)

Right pulmonary veins (from lung)

Left atrium

Right atrium

Bicuspid (mitral) valve

Tricuspid valve

Aortic valve

Chordae tendineae

Myocardium (heart muscle)

Epicardium (outer layer)

Left ventricle

Inferior vena cava (from trunk and legs)

Interventricular septum

Right ventricle

APEX

FIGURE 29-1 The heart.

- Mitral or bicuspid valve—located between the left atrium and the left ventricle.
- Aortic valve—located between the left ventricle and the aorta.

Arteries are blood vessels or tubes through which oxygenated blood travels. The largest artery is the *aorta*, which branches off the heart, divides into many smaller arteries, and then divides into the smallest called **arterioles**. *Veins* carry the deoxygenated blood. Veins take deoxygenated blood back to the heart and then to the lungs to pick up more oxygen. *Capillaries* form a network of tiny blood vessels connecting arterioles and carrying oxygenated blood and nutrients to **venules** (the smallest veins) that carry deoxygenated blood and metabolic waste. During its passage through the many capillaries of the body, blood deposits the materials necessary for growth and nourishment into the tissues; at the same time, it receives from the tissues the waste products resulting from metabolism.

Although blood pulses through the chambers at all times, the heart does not receive its needed oxygen and nutrients from this blood. Instead, it receives its own fresh blood supply via the *coronary arteries*, which branch directly off of the aorta. These arteries feed blood deep into the thick heart muscle. Carbon dioxide and waste are removed through the *coronary veins*.

Blood

Blood is a liquid tissue and is considered the fluid of life, growth, and health. The average adult body contains approximately 5.6 L of blood, which constitutes about 7% of the body mass. Blood carries oxygen, nutrients, hormones, disease-fighting cells, and other substances to all parts of the body and transports waste to the kidneys for filtration and to the lungs for expiration. Blood is composed of erythrocytes, **leukocytes**, platelets, and plasma. A drop of blood contains millions of red blood cells (RBCs) but only 7,000 to 25,000 white blood cells (WBCs). RBCs contain a protein chemical called *hemoglobin* that contains the element iron, which makes the blood bright red. As blood passes through the lungs, oxygen molecules attach to the hemoglobin. As the blood passes through the body's tissues and organs, the hemoglobin releases the oxygen to the cells. Immediately, the empty hemoglobin molecules bond with carbon dioxide or other waste gases from the tissues, transporting the waste away.

Function of the Heart

Every cell in the body needs oxygen to live and function properly. The purpose of the heart is to pump or deliver oxygen-rich blood to all body organs, tissues, and cells.

The atria fill with blood at the same time and then contract, pushing the blood through the valves into the ventricles.

arterioles the smallest arteries.

venules the smallest veins.

leukocyte white blood cell.

While relaxed, the ventricles fill with blood; then, they contract simultaneously to push the blood out of the heart through the pulmonary valve and aortic valve into the lungs and the rest of the body, respectively. Therefore, the heart beats top to bottom, not right to left or diagonally, with two pumping actions from left to right within one pumping system.

It is important to know the pattern of blood flow to understand the normal circulation of blood within the body (see Figure 29-2). There are two kinds of blood, venous and arterial. *Venous blood* contains waste, primarily carbon dioxide (CO_2), and is dark red and deoxygenated. Veins carry deoxygenated blood to the heart to be sent to the lungs, where the external exchange of gases occurs. Arterial blood contains nutrients and oxygen (O_2) and is bright red and oxygenated. Arteries carry oxygenated blood to the body to feed and nourish all the body tissues. There is, however, one exception to this rule. The pulmonary artery carries deoxygenated blood from the heart to the lungs, and the pulmonary vein carries oxygenated blood from the lungs back into the heart.

Venous, deoxygenated blood leaving the lower part of the body enters the RA of the heart via the inferior vena cava; the deoxygenated blood from the upper part of the body enters the RA via the superior vena cava. The blood then flows from the RA through the tricuspid valve to the RV. From the RV, the blood flows through the semilunar pulmonary valve into the pulmonary artery, which branches and takes the deoxygenated blood to the right and left lungs (see Figure 29-3).

Blood is cleaned in the lungs as the CO_2 waste is dropped off. During respiration, O_2 is picked up and the external exchange occurs. The CO_2 is exhaled out of the body, while the clean, oxygenated blood travels out of the lungs via the pulmonary vein to the left atrium of the heart. The blood then flows through the bicuspid valve to the left ventricle. The oxygenated blood then leaves the heart via the semilunar aortic valve to the aorta.

Oxygenated blood flows from the aortic arch to the arteries, then to the arterioles and capillaries. The oxygenated blood drops off its oxygen and picks up the diffused CO_2 waste in a process called *internal exchange*. The deoxygenated blood then leaves the capillaries, flowing through a succession of widening vessels. From the capillaries, the deoxygenated blood flows through the venules, then the veins, and finally the superior and inferior vena cavas back to the RA of the heart to start the circulation process over again.

The Conduction System

The *conduction system*, or electrical system, of the heart controls the speed of the heartbeat. The spontaneous contractions of the heart muscle cells are coordinated by the sinoatrial (SA) node. This specialized nodal tissue, which provides energy in the form of electricity to the heart, has characteristics of both muscle and nervous tissue. The SA node sends electrical impulses, which, in turn, cause the heart muscle to contract.

This conduction tissue has an unusual characteristic, known as *autorhythmicity*, that allows the heart to generate its own electrical stimulation. The electrical impulse generated

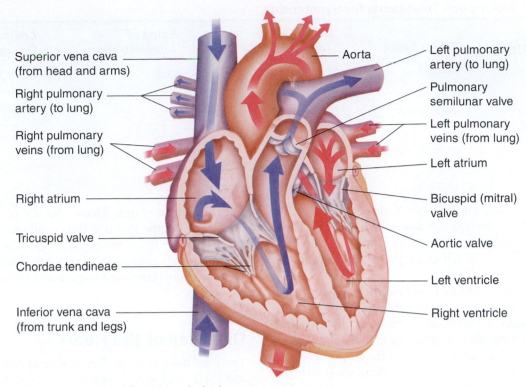

FIGURE 29-2 Blood flow through the heart.

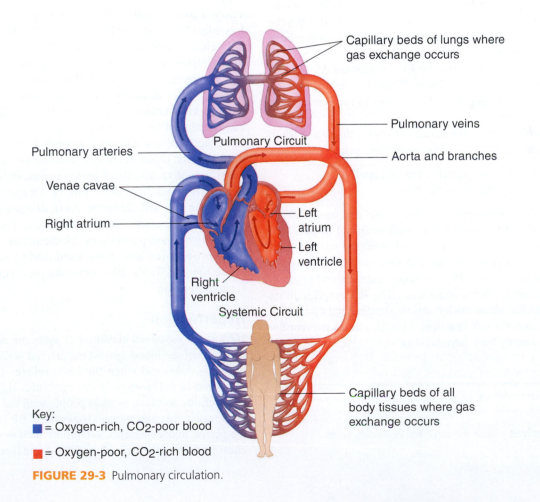

FIGURE 29-3 Pulmonary circulation.

TABLE 29-1 Prescription Treatments for Hypotension

Generic Name	Brand Name	Dosage Forms and Availability	Route of Administration	Common Adult Dosage
fludrocortisone	Florinef	0.1-mg tablets	Oral	0.1–0.2 mg qd* unlabeled use
midodrine	ProAmatine	2.5-mg, 5-mg, 10-mg tablets	Oral	10 mg tid

*Lidocaine PFS dosage forms and availability.

within the SA node is known as the *natural pacemaker*. The impulse continues through the atrioventricular (AV) node, known as the *electrical bridge*, into the common bundle of His (AV bundle) through the left and right bundle branches and Purkinje fibers.

This conduction pathway for an electrical impulse results in contraction of the atria immediately followed by contraction of the ventricles. Therefore, coordination of the contractions of the heart chambers depends on both the SA node and autorhythmicity. In a healthy human, as the electrical impulse moves through the heart, the heart contracts about 60 to 100 times a minute. Known as the *heart rate*, each contraction represents one heartbeat. The atria contract about 1/10 of a second before the ventricles so that the atrial blood empties into the ventricles before the ventricles contract. This delay occurs when impulses reach the AV node and are then sent down the *AV bundle*, a bundle of fibers that branches off into two bundles. From there, the impulses are carried down the center of the heart to the left ventricles and RVs, where the AV bundles divide further into Purkinje fibers. When the impulses reach these fibers, they trigger the muscle fibers in the ventricles to contract.

The *cardiac cycle* is the pattern of events that occur when the heart beats. There are two phases of this cycle:

1. Diastole—when the ventricles are relaxed.
2. Systole—when the ventricles contract.

During the diastole phase, both the atria and ventricles are relaxed and the **AV valves** open to allow blood to pass into both ventricles. Deoxygenated blood from the superior and inferior vena cava flows into the RA and from the pulmonary vein into the left atrium. The SA node contracts and prompts the atria to contract at the same time. The RA empties all its blood into the RV, while the left atrium simultaneously empties its contents into the left ventricle. The AV valves prevent the blood from flowing back into the atria.

During the systole phase, the RV receives electrical impulses from the Purkinje fibers and contracts simultaneously with the left ventricle. The AV valves close and the **semilunar valves** open. Deoxygenated blood is pumped into the pulmonary artery, and oxygenated blood is pumped into the aorta.

Diseases of the Heart

There are three common forms of heart disease: HTN, CHF, and CAD. This section explores the complications that can occur and the pharmaceutical treatment for each.

Hypotension

When a patient suffers from hypotension, they suffer from low blood pressure (BP), specifically BP below 90/60. A BP below 120/80 is considered ideal, and low BP without any symptoms is often not of concern in healthy individuals. Hypotension should still be taken seriously, particularly in older patients, as it can cause inadequate blood flow to vital organs, such as the brain and heart. Low BP can be caused by a number of factors. Prescription drugs, OTC medications, and other everyday stimulants can affect blood levels. Other causes of lowered BP are advanced diabetes, anaphylaxis, heart arrhythmias, dehydration, fainting, heart attack, and heart failure. Drugs can also have an impact on low BP. Some of these drugs are alcohol, anti-anxiety medications, antidepressants, diuretics, high BP medications, and painkillers. Medications used during surgical procedures and those used during surgery can also cause low BP. Table 29-1 presents prescription treatments for hypotension.

Hypertension

HTN is the sustained elevation of systemic arterial BP. *BP* is the force of the blood against the arterial walls when the heart beats (systole) and when the heart relaxes (diastole). BP is measured in millimeters of mercury (mm Hg). HTN can be a very serious problem, as most people with the condition do not even realize that they have it. However, if BP is extremely high, the person may experience symptoms such as severe headache, chest pain, irregular heartbeat, and fatigue (see Table 29-2).

---

atrioventricular valves include the tricuspid and mitral valves of the heart.

semilunar valves include the aortic and pulmonary valves of the heart.

TABLE 29-2 Prescription Treatments for Hypertension

Generic Name	Brand Name	Dosage Forms and Availability	Route of Administration	Common Adult Dosage
benazepril	Lotensin	5-mg, 10-mg, 20-mg, 40-mg tablets	Oral	20–40 mg qd or divided bid; maximum of 80 mg/day
lisinopril	Prinivil, Zestril	5-mg, 10-mg, 20-mg tablets	Oral	10–40 mg qd
captopril	Capoten	12.5-mg, 25-mg, 50-mg, 100-mg tablets	Oral	25–50 mg bid or tid; maximum of 450 mg/day
ramipril	Altace	1.25-mg, 2.5-mg, 5-mg, 10-mg tablets	Oral	2.5–20 mg qd
fosinopril	Monopril	10-mg, 20-mg, 40-mg tablets	Oral	10–40 mg qd
moexipril	Univasc	7.5-mg, 15-mg tablets	Oral	7.5–30 mg daily
nadolol	Corgard	20-mg, 40-mg, 80-mg tablets	Oral	40–80 mg daily
metoprolol	Lopressor	50/25-mg, 100/25-mg, 100/50-mg tablets Metoprolol/hydrochlorothiazide	Oral	50/25: two tablets daily, 100/25: one to two tablets daily, 100/50: one tablet daily
pindolol	Visken	5-mg, 10-mg tablets	Oral	Should be individualized
bisoprolol	Zebeta	5-mg, 10-mg tablets	Oral	Must be individualized
acebutolol	Sectral	200-mg, 400-mg capsules	Oral	400–800 mg qd
verapamil	Calan, Isoptin, Verelan, Calan SR, Ispotin SR	40-mg, 80-mg, 120-mg tablets	Oral, injection (intravenous)	Oral immediate-release dosage form (Calan, Isoptin, Verelan): 40–120 mg tid; Verelan: 240–280 mg qd; Verelan PM: 200 mg qd at bedtime; long-acting dosage forms (Calan SR, Isoptin SR): 120 mg qd to 240 mg q12h
captopril/HCTZ	Capoten, Capozide	12.5-mg, 25-mg, 50-mg, 100-mg tablets	Oral	25–50 mg qd
benazepril/HCTZ	Lotensin	5-mg, 10-mg, 20-mg, 40-mg tablets	Oral	10 mg qd to start, 20–40 mg qd daily maintenance dosage
telmisartan/HCTZ	Micardis	20-mg, 40-mg, 80-mg tablets	Oral	Must be individualized
lisinopril/HCTZ	Prinivil, Zestril	5-mg, 10-mg, 20-mg tablets	Oral	10–40 mg qd
moexipril/HCTZ	Univasc	7.5-mg, 15-mg tablets	Oral	7.5–30 mg qd
fosinopril/HCTZ	Monopril HCT	10-mg, 20-mg, 40-mg tablets	Oral	10 mg qd to start, 20–40 mg qd maintenance dosage

(Continued)

TABLE 29-2 Prescription Treatments for Hypertension (*Continued*)

Generic Name	Brand Name	Dosage Forms and Availability	Route of Administration	Common Adult Dosage
losartan/HCTZ	Cozaar, Hyzaar	15-mg, 50-mg, 100-mg tablets	Oral	25–100 mg daily
valsartan/HCTZ	Diovan HCT	40-mg, 80-mg, 160-mg, 320-mg tablets	Oral	80–320 mg qd
candesartan/HCTZ	Atacand HCT	16–12.5 mg, 32–12.5 mg, tablets	Oral	8–32 mg qd or bid
enalapril/HCTZ	Vaseretic	10–25 mg tablets Enalapril maleate/ hydrochlorothiazide	Oral	10–40 mg qd
atenolol/HCTZ	Tenormin, Tenoretic	50/25-mg, 100/25-mg tablets Atenolol/ chlorthalidone	Oral, injection (intravenous)	25–50 mg qd. Up to 100 mg/day
propranolol/HCTZ	Inderide, Inderide LA	40/25-mg, 80/25-mg tablets Propranolol hydrochloride/ hydrochlorothiazide	Oral, injection (intravenous)	Oral (immediate release) 40–80 mg tid; Inderide LA; 80–160 mg qd
atenolol/ chlorothalidone	Tenoretic, Tenormin, Cozaar	50/25-mg, 100/25-mg tablets Atenolol/ chlorthalidone	Oral	Must be individualized
bisoprolol fumarate/HCTZ	Zebeta, Ziac	5-mg, 10-mg tablets	Oral	Must be individualized
metoprolol/HCTZ	Lopressor HCT, Toprol XL	50/25-mg, 100/25-mg, 100/50-mg tablets Metoprolol/ hydrochlorothiazide	Oral, injection (intravenous)	Oral (immediate release): initially, 12.5–25 mg bid. Up to 450 mg/day in divided does. 50–100 mg bid following MI. Toprol XL: 50–100 mg/day up to 400 mg/day
amldipine/ benzaepril	Norvasc	2.5-mg, 5-mg, 10-mg tablets	Oral	5–10 mg qd
amlodipine/ valsartan	Exforge	5/160-mg, 10/160-mg, 5/320-mg, 10/320-mg tablets	Oral	2.5–10 mg/ 80–320 mg qd
amlodipine/ olmesaran	Azor	5/20-mg, 5/40-mg, 10/20-mg, 10/40-mg tablets Amlodipine equivalent/ olmesartan medoxomil	Oral	5/20 mg–10/40 mg qd
diltiazem/enalapril	Cardizem CD, Cardiazem LA, Cardiazem SR, Dilacor XR, Tiazac	120-mg, 180-mg, 240-mg, 300-mg, 360-mg capsules	Oral, injection (intravenous)	For extended-release products: 180–240 mg qd up to 360–420 mg/day
trandolapril/ verapamil	Tarka, Mavik	2/180-mg, 1/240-mg, 2/240-mg, 4/240-mg tablets Trandolapril/ verapamil hydrochloride	Oral	1/120–4/480 mg qd

(*Continued*)

contractility the ability to contract; also, the degree of contraction.

TABLE 29.2 Prescription Treatments for Hypertension *(Continued)*

Generic Name	Brand Name	Dosage Forms and Availability	Route of Administration	Common Adult Dosage
enalapril/felodpine	Lexxel, Plendial	5/5-mg tablets Enalapril maleate/ felodipine	Oral	2.5–10 mg qd
amlodipine/ valsartan/HCTZ	Exforge HCT	5/160-mg, 10/160-mg, 5/320-mg, 10/320-mg tablets Amlodipine besylate equivalent/ amlodipine free-base with valsartan	Oral	2.5–10/80–320 mg qd
amlodipine/ atorvastatin	Caduet	2.5/10-mg, 2.5/20-mg, 2.5/40-mg, 5/10-mg, 5/20-mg, 5/40-mg, 5/80-mg, 10/10-mg, 10/20-mg, 10/40-mg, 10/80-mg tablets Amlodipine besylate, atorvastatin calcium	Oral	Must be individualized
traimterene/HCTZ	Dyazide	25-mg hydrochlorothiazide and 37.5-mg triamterene capsules	Oral	One capsule daily
amiloride/HCTZ	Midamor, Moduretic, Dyazide, Inspra	5-mg tablets	Oral	One tablet daily

Risk factors for high BP include the following:

- Obesity
- High-sodium diets
- Lack of physical activity
- Stress
- Excessive alcohol consumption
- Genetics
- Age (most HTN occurs in those who are over 35 years of age)
- Race (African-Americans are at higher risk of high BP than other racial groups)

People with HTN are at highly increased risk of heart disease, liver failure, heart attack, and stroke. Reducing stress and getting the right amount of exercise can help individuals with high BP (see Table 29-3).

❝ Workplace Wisdom Heart Failure

Heart failure is responsible for 40,000 deaths each year as well as 2.9 million doctor visits and 875,000 hospitalizations. ❞

Congestive Heart Failure

In *CHF*, the heart fails to cycle all the blood it receives. CHF is caused by a decreased **contractility** of the myocardium. In other words, the heart receives more blood than it can pump out, because the myocardium is not strong enough to push the blood out of the atria through the valves into the ventricles. This causes a backup of blood in the atria, resulting in congestion as blood accumulates inside the atria, stretching and enlarging the heart. This enlargement weakens the heart muscle, which is trying to move ever-increasing amounts of blood each time it contracts. There are no known alternative therapies or OTC drugs used to treat CHF (see Table 29-4). With less blood leaving the atria, less blood is available to be sent to the lungs and the rest of the body. Therefore, less CO_2 leaves the lungs, and less O_2 enters the blood during external exchange. Less blood throughout the body means less oxygen available to feed the organs and body parts; because of the lack of oxygen, *necrosis* (tissue death) may occur.

Symptoms of CHF include upright posture or leaning forward, anxiety and restlessness, cyanotic (bluish), clammy skin, persistent cough, rapid breathing, fast heart rate, and edema (swelling) of the lower limbs.

Ischemia

Ischemia is a condition in which the oxygen-rich blood is stopped, blocked, or restricted to a specific part of the body. *Cardiac ischemia* refers to the lack of blood flow and oxygen to the myocardium. If ischemia is sustained, it can cause a

TABLE 29-3 American Heart Association Classes of Blood Pressure Levels

BP Category	Systolic (mm Hg)		Diastolic (mm Hg)
Normal	>120	and	>80
Prehypertension	120–139	or	80–89
Stage 1 hypertension	140–159	or	90–99
Stage 2 hypertension	160 or higher	or	100 or higher

myocardial infarction (MI) and can lead to heart tissue damage or death. In most cases, a temporary blood shortage (oxygen deprivation) to the heart causes *angina pectoris* (pain in the chest and heart area).

Myocardial Infarction

The result of ischemia is damage to or death of the tissue that did not receive enough oxygen. If this necrotic tissue is in the heart or cardiac muscle, the necrosis is called an *infarction*. If the tissue within the heart dies, it is an MI. This tissue death or damage can be fatal if the area of the infarct is large enough, as in a massive MI. Some people can survive two or three MIs, if they are small and do not overlap to create a large area of damage. Tissue that has undergone an MI will never heal or return to the status of a functional cardiac muscle. Therefore, the functionality of the heart muscle is reduced with each MI. There are no known drugs or alternative therapies used to treat MI.

Crash Cart Medications

Pharmacy technicians should be aware of medications stocked on a crash cart, if they are a hospital pharmacy technician.

TABLE 29-4 Prescription Treatments for Congestive Heart Failure

Generic Name	Brand Name	Dosage Forms and Availability	Route of Administration	Common Adult Dosage
digoxin	Lanoxin	Injection: 500 mcg (0.5 mg) in 2 mL (250 mcg [0.25 mg] per mL); tablets: 125 mcg (0.125 mg) 250 mcg (0.25mg)	Oral, injection (intravenous [preferred], intramuscular	0.125–0.25 mg qd (the dosage and frequency of dosing must be adjusted for body weight and renal function of the patient)
hydrochlorothiazide	Microzide, Ezide, Accuretic	12.5-mg tablets	Oral	25–50 mg daily as single dose or two divided doses
metolazone	Zaroxolyn, Mykrox	0.5-mg tablets	Oral	2.5–20 mg qd
furosemide	Lasix	20-mg, 40-mg, 80-mg tablets	Oral, injection (intravenous, intramuscular)	20–80 mg qd or in divided doses.
bumetanide	Bumex	0.5-mg, 1-mg, 2-mg tablets	Oral, injection (intravenous, intramuscular)	0.5–2 mg qd
spironolactone	Aldactone	25-mg, 50-mg, 100-mg tablets	Oral	Range: 50–200 mg daily in single or divided doses; usual dose for CHF initially is 50 mg bid
acetazolamide	Diamox	500-mg capsules; 500-mg vials	Oral, intravenous	250–375 mg every other day in the morning or for two days followed by one day of rest; one day of rest in the regimen allows kidney recovery to maintain effectiveness against edema

Some of the most common medications stocked for cardiac issues are the following:

- Atropine (1 mg/10 mL)
- Bretylium tosylate (Bretylol, 500 mg/10 mL)
- Calcium chloride (10%, 1 g/10 mL)
- Dextrose (50%, 25 g/50 mL)
- Diazepam (Valium, 10 mg/2 mL)
- Dipenhydramine (Benadryl, 50 mg/vial)
- Dopamine in D5W (400 mg/250 mL)
- Epinephrine (1 mg/10 mL)
- Furosemide (Lasix, 100 mg/10 mL)
- Hetastarch (Hespan, 500 mL/Bas)
- Isoproterenol (Isuprel, 1 mg/5 mL)
- Lidocaine (100 mg/5 mL)
- Lidocaine in D5W (2 g/500 mL)
- Magnesium sulfate (50% in 5 mL)
- Midazolam (Versed 2 mg/2 mL)

Angina Pectoris

Angina Pectoris is a short-term blood shortage to the heart. This shortage of blood causes angina, commonly known as chest pain. As a result of myocardial ischemia, angina pectoris will occur. Both of these conditions are usually because a patient has developed CAD. The three most common types of medications used to treat angina pectoris are nitrates, B-adrenergic blockers, and calcium channel blockers. Nitrates work by relaxing smooth muscle (vascular) and reduce the work of the heart's left ventricle. Nitrates dilate the blood vessels and work to end the attacks of chest pain. B-adrenergic blockers work to reverse heart action (sympathetic) endured because of physical exertion, stress, and exercise. The third medication used to treat angina are calcium channel blockers. These drugs were developed for the care and treatment of angina in the stable form. They work to keep calcium out of smooth muscle cells and myocytes to make arterial vasodilatation and decrease arterial BP. In addition, they decrease myocardial contractility. This results in less myocardial oxygen consumption. There are no known OTC or herbal treatments available to treat angina pectoris (see Table 29-5).

Arrhythmias

Arrhythmias are irregular patterns in the beating of the heart or a change in the force or speed of the heart's contraction. They can occur in the atrium, the ventricle, or both, at one time or at irregular intervals. Arrhythmias can be due to cardiac diseases, such as CHF, CAD, HTN, or MI, or due to the side effects of some medications. The most serious arrhythmia is *ventricular fibrillation*, which constitutes a medical emergency because the ventricles cannot contract efficiently to maintain adequate blood circulation; this results in MI or death. Slow heartbeats are known as *bradycardia*, and fast heartbeats are known as *tachycardia*.

Antiarrhythmic drugs restore normal rhythm patterns but do not cure the cause of the irregular heartbeat. These drugs are grouped into four classes according to their effect on the cardiac cycle (see Tables 29-6 and 29-7).

Class I Antiarrhythmic Agents

Class I antiarrhythmic drugs cause local anesthetic effects, slow down the heart rate, slow conduction velocity, prolong the refractory period, and decrease automaticity of the heart. This is accomplished by blocking the influx of sodium ions to excitatory membranes during depolarization and excitation.

Class II Antiarrhythmic Agents

Beta-adrenergic blockers (class II antiarrhythmic agents) slow down the heart rate, slow conduction velocity, prolong the refractory period, and decrease automaticity by blocking both the release of sympathetic neurotransmitters and their activity. Because they antagonize the effects of norepinephrine (NE) at beta-1 cardiac receptors, these drugs work particularly well on ventricular myocardium.

Class III Antiarrhythmic Agents

Class III antiarrhythmics block the efflux of potassium (K^+) ions during repolarization phases $1-3$, thus prolonging the refractory period and decreasing the frequency of arrhythmias (see Table 29-6).

Class IV Antiarrhythmic Agents

Calcium channel blockers or antagonists (class IV antiarrhythmic drugs) block the pathways for calcium entry to excitable membranes of the heart and blood vessels that develop action potentials. This action decreases SA node activity, slowing down the heart rate and conduction velocity of the AV node. Supraventricular tachycardia often responds to class IV antiarrhythmic agents.

> **❝ Workplace Wisdom** Quinidine
>
> Quinidine is derived from cinchona bark and is also used in the treatment of malaria. Quinidine may cause cinchonism (poisoning). Overdose causes tinnitus, headache, dizziness, excessive salivation, and hallucinations. ❞

Treatment for Heart Disease

Pharmaceutical treatment of CHF involves the administration of drugs from various drug classifications. The following drug classes are discussed in this section:

- Cardiac glycosides
- Diuretics
- Vasodilators
- ACE inhibitors
- Beta-adrenergic blockers
- Phosphodiesterase inhibitors

Cardiac Glycosides

Cardiac glycosides are used to increase the force of myocardial contraction without causing an increase in the consumption of

TABLE 29-5 Prescription Treatments for Heart Conditions

Generic Name	Brand Name	Dosage Forms and Availability	Route of Administration	Common Adult Dosage
lisinopril	Prinivil, Zestril	5-mg, 10-mg, 20-mg tablets	Oral	10–40 mg qd
benazepril	Lotensin	5-mg, 10-mg, 20-mg, 40-mg tablets	Oral	20–40 mg qd
captopril	Capoten	12.5-mg, 25-mg, 50-mg, 100-mg tablets	Oral	25–50 mg bid or tid; maximum 450 mg/day
fosinopril	Monopril	10-mg, 20-mg, 40-mg tablets	Oral	10–40 mg qd
losartan	Cozaar	25-mg, 50-mg, 100-mg tablets	Oral	25–100 mg qd or divided twice daily
valsartan	Diovan	40-mg, 80-mg, 160-mg, 320-mg tablets	Oral	80–320 mg qd
atenolol	Tenormin	25-mg, 50-mg, 100-mg tablets	Oral	25–50 mg qd; up to 100 mg daily
propranolol	Inderal, Inderal LA	40/25-mg, 80-mg, 25-mg tablets Propranolol hydro-chloride/ hydrochloro-thiazide; 1 mL ampuls	Oral, injection (intravenous)	40–80 mg tid; Inderal LA: 80–160 mg qd
metoprolol	Lopressor, Toprol XL	50-mg, 100-mg tablets; 5 mL ampuls	Oral, injection (intravenous)	Oral (immediate release): initially 12.5–25 mg bid. Up to 450 mg daily in divided doses for HTN. 50–100 mg bid following MI. Topprol XL: 50–100 mg daily up to 400 mg daily for HTN
diltiazem	Cardizem CD, Cardiazem LA, Cardiazem SR, Dilacor XR, Tiazac	120-mg, 180-mg, 240-mg, 300-mg, 360-mg capsules	Oral, injection (intravenous)	For extended-release products: 180–240 mg qd up to 260–420 mg/day for HTN
nifedipine	Procardia XL, Adalat CC	30-mg, 60-mg, 90-mg tablets	Oral	Procardia XL: for hypertension, 30–60 mg qd; Adalat CC: 30 mg qd, Maximum: 90 mg/day for HTN
verapamil	Calan, Isoptin, Verelan, Calan SR	40-mg, 80-mg, 120-mg tablets	Oral, injection (intravenous)	Oral immediate-release dosage form (Calan, Isoptin, Verelan); 40–120 mg tid; Verelan: 240–480 mg qd; Verelan PM: 200 mg qd at bedtime; long-acting dosage forms: 120 mg qd to 240 mg q12h
almodipine	Norvasc	2.5-mg, 5-mg, 10-mg tablets	Oral	For hypertension, 5–10 mg qd
felodipine	Plendil	2.5-mg, 5-mg, 10-mg tablets	Oral	2.5–10 mg qd

TABLE 29-6 Prescription Treatments for Arrythmias

Generic Name	Brand Name	Dosage Forms and Availability	Route of Administration	Common Adult Dosage
quinidine sulfate	Quinalan		Intravenous	Quinidine gluconate ER oral: initially, 324 mg bid or tid; then adjusted to patient's response and drug levels
quinidine gluconate	Quinidex	300-mg tablets	Oral	Dosing regimens for the use of quinidine sulfate tablet, film coated, extended release in suppressing life-threatening ventricular arrhythmias have not been adequately studied
procainamide	Procanbid extended-release; Pronestyl, Pronestyl SR	250-mg, 375-mg, 500-mg tablets	Oral	Procanbid oral: 50 mg/kg daily; procainamide determined by weight and age of patient
sotalol	Betapace, Betapace AF	80-mg, 120-mg, 150-mg tablets	Oral	Ventricular arrhythmias: initially 80 mg bid, then 120–160 mg bid; for a-fib, initially 80 mg bid up to 160 mg bid
propafenone	Rythmol, Rythmol SR	150-mg, 225-mg, 300-mg tablets	Oral	Rythmol: 150–255 mg q8h; Rythmol SR: 225–425 mg q12h
amiodarone	Cordarone, Pacerone	200-mg tablets	Oral, injectable (in hospital only)	Dependent on type of arrhythmia; usual maintenance doses range from 200 to 600 mg qd
disopyramide	Norpace, Norpace CR	100-mg, 150-mg capsules	Oral	150 mg q6h; CR: 300 mg q12h
generic name	Brand Name	Dosage Forms and Availability	Route of Administration	Common Adult Dosage
lidocaine PFS	Xylocaine	*See table below	Injection or intravenous drip	50–100 mg IV bolus, then followed by IV infusion at a rate of 1–4 mg/minute (or approximately 20–25 mcg/kg/minute adjustments guided by patient response and drug levels; convert to other antiarrhythmic therapy as soon as possible to avoid drug toxicity with prolonged use

*Lidocaine PFS dosage forms and availability

Xylocaine—How Supplied in Vials

Xylocaine (lidocaine HCl) Concentration (%)	Epinephrine Dilution (if present)	Xylocaine								
		Single-Dose Vials (mL)						Multiple-Dose Vials (mL)		
		2	5	10	20	30	50	10	20	50
0.5							X			X
0.5	1:200,000									X

(Continued)

Xylocaine—How Supplied in Vials (Continued)

Xylocaine (lidocaine HCl) Concentration (%)	Epinephrine Dilution (if present)	Xylocaine								
		Single-Dose Vials (mL)						Multiple-Dose Vials (mL)		
		2	5	10	20	30	50	10	20	50
1		X	X			X		X	X	X
1	1:100,000							X	X	X
1	1:200,000			X		X				
1.5			X							
1.5	1:200,000			X		X		X	X	X
2		X	X						X	X
2	1:100,000									
2	1:200,000			X	X					

TABLE 29-7 Antiarrhythmic Agents

Generic Name	Trade Name	Available Dosage Form(s)/ Strength	Average Adult Dose
Class I Antiarrhythmic Agents			
disopyramide	Norpace	100-mg, 150-mg capsules 100-mg, 150-mg extended-release (ER) capsules	400–800 mg/day in divided doses (q6h for immediate-release forms and q12h for ER)
flecainide	Tambocor	50-mg, 100-mg, 150-mg tablets	50–150 mg q12h; not to exceed (NTE) 400 mg/day
mexiletine	Mexitil	150-mg, 200-mg, 250-mg capsules	200–400 mg q8h
procainamide	Procanbid	250-mg, 500-mg, 750-mg ER tablets 250-mg, 375-mg, 500-mg capsules	50 mg/kg in divided doses
propafenone	Rhythmol	150-mg, 225-mg, 300-mg tablets 225-mg, 325-mg, 425-mg ER capsules	150–300 mg q8h 225–425 mg q12h (ER)
quinidine	Quinaglute Quinadex	200-mg, 300-mg tablets 300-mg, 324-mg SR tablet	200–400 mg tid–qid 300–600 mg q8–12h
Class II Antiarrhythmic Agents			
esmolol	Brevibloc	10 mg/mL, 20 mg/mL, 250 mg/mL injection	50–200 mcg/minute IV
propranolol	Inderal	10-mg, 20-mg, 40-mg, 60-mg, 80-mg, 90-mg tablets 60-mg, 80-mg, 120-mg, 160-mg ER capsules	HTN: 120–240 mg /day po in two to three divided doses 80–160 mg po daily (ER)

(Continued)

TABLE 29.7 **Antiarrhythmic Agents** (*Continued*)

Generic Name	Trade Name	Available Dosage Form(s)/ Strength	Average Adult Dose
		4 mg/mL, 8 mg/mL solution 80 mg/mL conc. solution 1 mg/mL injection	1—3 mg IV q4h
Class III Antiarrhythmic Agents			
amiodarone	Cordarone	100-mg, 200-mg, 400-mg tablets	Loading dose: 800—1,600 mg/day
			Maintenance: 400—600 mg/day
bretylium tosylate		2 mg/mL, 4 mg/mL, 50 mg/mL injection	5—10 mg/kg IV q6h
sotalol	Betapace	80-mg, 120-mg, 160-mg, 240-mg tablets	160–640 mg/day in two or three divided doses
Class IV Antiarrhythmic Agents—Calcium Channel Blockers			
amlodipine	Norvasc	2.5-mg, 5-mg, 10-mg tablets	5–10 mg qd
bepridil	Vascor	200-mg, 300-mg tablets	200–400 mg qd
diltiazem	Cardizem	30-mg, 60-mg, 90-mg, 120-mg tablets	120–360 mg qid
	Dilacor XR	120-mg, 180-mg, 240-mg, 300-mg, 360-mg, 420-mg ER tablets	180–540 mg qd (ER tablets)
		60-mg, 80-mg, 120-mg, 180-mg, 240-mg, 300-mg, 360-mg, 420-mg ER capsules	180–540 mg qd or in two divided doses (ER capsules)
felodipine	Plendil	2.5-mg, 5-mg, 10-mg ER tablets	2.5–10 mg qd
isradipine	DynaCirc	5-mg, 10-mg continuous-release (CR) tablets	5–10 mg qd (CR)
		2.5-mg, 5-mg capsules	2.5–10 mg bid
nicardipine	Cardene	20-mg, 30-mg capsules	20–40 mg tid
		30-mg, 45-mg, 60-mg ER capsules	30–60 mg bid (ER)
nifedipine	Procardia, Adalat	10-mg, 20-mg capsules	10–20 mg tid
		30-mg, 60-mg, 90-mg ER tablets	30–90 mg qd (ER)
nimodipine	Nimotop	30-mg capsules	60 mg q4 × 21 days
nisoldipine	Sular	10-mg, 20-mg, 30-mg, 40-mg ER tablets	10–60 mg qd
verapamil	Calan, Isoptin	40-mg, 80-mg, 120-mg tablets	240–480 mg/day in three or four divided doses
		120-mg, 180-mg, 240-mg (ER tablets and capsules, SR tablets) 100-mg, 200-mg, 300-mg ER capsules	ER and SR: individualize doses

Note: Calcium channel blockers are also indicated for HTN.

oxygen. Cardiac glycosides, which are derived from the *digitalis purpurea* or *digitalis lanata* plants, have been used for hundreds of years. Cardiac glycosides increase blood flow and kidney filtration, thereby reducing sodium and other electrolytes that cause fluid retention, a main culprit in CHF. The main mechanism of action is acceleration of calcium cations inside the myocardium by blocking the enzyme adenosine triphosphate, which in turn shuts off the Na^+/K^+ pump. This pump would normally remove sodium (Na^+) ions from inside the heart muscle. The sodium ions now being brought into the heart muscle will be exchanged for calcium (Ca^{++}) ions.

" Workplace Wisdom **Cardiac Glycoside or Aminoglycoside?**

Be careful not to confuse cardiac glycosides with *aminoglycosides*, which are potent antibiotics.

Calcium ions in the myocardium increase the synthesis of actinomycin and the force of contraction of the heart muscle. With a greater force of contraction, more blood can be pumped out of the heart.

Hypokalemia (low potassium levels in the serum) increases the toxic effects of the glycosides on the heart. Hypokalemia may increase the potential for arrhythmias, ventricular fibrillation, or sudden death. Hyperkalemia (high potassium serum levels) blocks the therapeutic effects of cardiac glycosides. Hypercalcemia (high calcium serum levels) increases the therapeutic effects of cardiac glycosides and can also increase the force of contraction and speed enough to create arrhythmias. A patient taking cardiac glycosides should never consume grapefruit or grapefruit juice, because it decreases absorption rates of these medications.

The most common cardiac glycoside is digoxin. Digoxin doses are highly individualized. Most patients are started on a high dose of digoxin and then maintained on about one-quarter of the original dose. This process, called *digitalization*,

is used to produce a rapid high blood level, somewhat like a loading dose, and then deliver an average adult maintenance dose of 0.125–0.5 mg po daily. The trade name for digoxin is Lanoxin, which is available in the following strengths/forms: 0.5-mg, 0.1-mg, 0.2-mg capsules; 0.125-mg and 0.25-mg tablets; 0.05 mg/mL pediatric elixir; and 0.1 mg/mL and 0.25 mg/mL injections.

Diuretics

Diuretics, commonly called *water pills*, are used to eliminate excess sodium and water via the urinary tract. Retention of sodium results in the retention of water and a subsequent increase in blood volume, which causes edema. Both lead to and aggravate the congestion and blood circulation problems associated with CHF.

Less sodium means less water in the blood and a lower blood volume, resulting in less need for contraction force from the heart. Diuretics lower BP, because they help to decrease blood volume and the force of the blood against vessel walls.

Because they promote water loss, diuretics are used to treat both HTN and CHF. The layperson's term for a diuretic is a *water pill*. Potassium serum levels must be monitored when a patient is taking diuretics. The four main diuretic categories are the following:

- *Thiazide* diuretics—produce mild-to-moderate diuretic effects and are the type of diuretic most commonly used for CHF. Thiazides are also indicated for the treatment of edema, HTN, and renal impairment (see Table 29-8).
- *Loop* diuretics—work in the loop of Henle within the kidneys. These diuretics have a moderate to potent diuretic effect. Used often for acute CHF, loop diuretics are also indicated for edema, HTN, **pulmonary edema**, and nephrotic syndrome (see Table 29-9).
- *Potassium-sparing* diuretics—allow water loss without loss of the important electrolyte, potassium. Low levels of potassium lead to a weak heart muscle that has less

TABLE 29-8 Thiazide Diuretics

Generic Name	Trade Name	Available Dosage Form(s)/ Strength	Average Adult Dose
chlorothiazide	Diuril	250-mg , 500-mg tablet 250 mg/5 mL suspension 500-mg injection	500–1,000 mg po daily
chlorthalidone	Hygroton	25-mg, 50-mg, 100-mg tablets	Edema: 50–100 mg daily HTN: 25–50 mg daily
hydrochlorothiazide (HCTZ)	Hydro-Diuril	25-mg, 50-mg, 100-mg tablets 12.5-mg capsule 50 mg/5 mL solution	Edema: 25–100 mg daily HTN: 12.5–50 mg daily
metolazone	Zaroxolyn	0.5-mg, 2.5-mg, 5-mg, 10-mg tablets	Edema: 5–20 mg daily HTN: 2.5–5 mg daily

pulmonary edema a condition in which fluid accumulates in the lungs

TABLE 29-9 Loop Diuretics

Generic Name	Trade Name	Available Dosage Form(s)/Strength	Average Adult Dose
bumetanide	Bumex	0.5-mg, 1-mg, 2-mg tablets 0.25 mg/mL injection	0.5–2 mg po daily 0.5–1 mg IM or IV; repeat in two to three hours NTE 10 mg
furosemide	Lasix	20-mg, 40-mg, 80-mg tablets 10 mg/5 mL, 40 mg/5 mL po solution 10 mg/mL injection	Edema: 20–80 mg po daily 20–40 mg IM or IV daily–bid HTN: 40 mg po bid
torsemide	Demadex	5-mg, 10-mg, 20-mg, 100-mg tablets	Average dose: 10–20 mg po daily

ability to contract and pump, thereby exacerbating the CHF condition. Any diuretic that has some amount of a potassium-sparing diuretic added as a combination drug is considered a potassium-sparing drug in total. Potassium-sparing diuretics are often used in conjunction with thiazide and loop diuretics (see Table 29-10).

• *Carbonic anhydrase inhibitors* —inhibit the enzyme carbonic anhydrase, resulting in a reduction of the amount of aqueous humor and a decrease in intraocular pressure. Carbonic anhydrase inhibitors are used in the treatment of glaucoma and for the prevention or mitigation of acute mountain sickness symptoms (see Table 29-11).

Vasodilators

By dilating blood vessels, *vasodilators* allow more blood to exit the heart, thereby preventing or mitigating congestion and increasing cardiac output. They have a stronger effect on arteries than they do on veins but will work on both.

Vasodilators relax the arterioles, causing them to dilate so that more blood can pass from the ventricles to the lungs and from the aorta to the rest of the body. They lower BP which, in turn, decreases the workload and oxygen consumption of the heart, so the heart does not have to pump as hard.

Vasodilators can be used alone or in combination with cardiac glycosides and diuretics to treat CHF. Nitro-Bid relaxes smooth muscle, which causes venous dilation and results in

TABLE 29-10 Potassium-Sparing Diuretics

Generic Name	Trade Name	Available Dosage Form(s)/Strength	Average Adult Dose
spironolactone	Aldactone	25-mg, 50-mg, 100-mg tablets	Edema: 25–200 mg daily HTN: 50–100 mg daily
spironolactone + HCTZ	Aldactazide	25-mg spironolactone and 25-mg HCTZ tablets 50-mg spironolactone and 50-mg HCTZ tablets	One to eight tablets daily One to four tablets daily
triamterene	Dyrenium	50-mg, 100-mg capsules	100 mg bid po, NTE 300 mg/day
triamterene + HCTZ	Dyazide, Maxzide	37.5-mg triamterene and 25-mg HCTZ tablets	One to two capsules daily

TABLE 29-11 Carbonic Anhydrase Inhibitors

Generic Name	Trade Name	Available Dosage Form(s)/Strength	Average Adult Dose
acetazolamide	Diamox	125-mg, 250-mg tablets 500-mg SR capsules 500-mg pwd injection	250–1,000 mg po daily in divided doses
methazolamide	Neptazane	25-mg, 50-mg tablets	50–100 mg bid–tid

TABLE 29-12 Peripheral Vasodilators

Generic Name	Trade Name	Available Dosage Form(s)/Strength	Average Adult Dose
hydralazine	Apresoline	10-mg, 25-mg, 50-mg, 100-mg tablets 20 mg/mL injection	10–50 mg po qid 20–40 mg IV/IM prn
isoxsuprine HCl	Vasodilan, Voxsuprine	10-mg, 20-mg tablets	10–20 mg tid–qid
minoxidil	Loniten	2.5-mg, 10-mg tablets	10–40 mg/day; can divide doses
papaverine HCl	Pavabid	150-mg timed-release (TR) capsule	150 mg q12h

a decreased workload for the heart. It also dilates the arteries leading to the heart, which helps improve oxygen supply.

Peripheral vasodilators (see Table 29-12) work directly on the blood vessels in the arms and legs to treat moderate to severe HTN; they are often used in conjunction with diuretics and/or other antihypertensive drugs. Coronary vasodilators are used in the treatment of acute angina to stop the pain and promote immediate dilation of the coronary artery, which allows oxygen to the heart muscle; they can be used prophylactically to manage chronic angina. Nitrates, beta blockers, and calcium channel blockers are all coronary vasodilators (see Table 29-8).

ACE Inhibitors

Angiotensin-converting enzyme (ACE) inhibitors are now thought to be one of the best treatments for CHF (see Table 29-12). ACE inhibitors are considered the **drug of choice (DOC)**

PROFILE IN PRACTICE

Mr. Lopez presents a new prescription for nitroglycerin 0.2 mg/hour transdermal patch—apply one patch every 24 hours—for angina.

▶ *What information should be included in the pharmacist's consultation with Mr. Lopez, particularly if he has never used a patch before?*

TABLE 29-13 Coronary Vasodilators

Generic Name	Trade Name	Available Dosage Form(s)/Strength	Average Adult Dose
isosorbide dinitrate	Isordil, Titradose, Isordil	5-mg, 10-mg, 20-mg, 40-mg tablets 2.5-mg, 5-mg, 10-mg SL and chewable tablets	10–40 mg po q6h 2.5–5 mg SL chewable: 5 mg–titrate upward until relief
isosorbide mononitrate	Monoket, Imdur	10-mg, 20-mg tablets 30-mg, 60-mg, 120-mg ER tablets	20 mg bid given seven hours apart 30–120 mg po daily (ER tablet)
nitroglycerin	Nitrostat, Nitro-Bid, Nitro-Dur	0.3-mg, 0.4-mg, 0.6-mg tablets 2.5-mg, 6.5-mg, 9-mg SR capsules 2% topical ointment 0.2 mg/hour, 0.4 mg/hour, 0.6 mg/hour transdermal patches	1 tablet SL q5min; NTE three tablets in 15 minutes 2.5 mg qid up to 26 mg qid; give smallest effective dose 1–2 inches q8h up to 4–5 inches q4h 0.2–0.8 mg/hour q24h

---

drug of choice (DOC) the drug preferred for treatment of a particular condition or disease.

TABLE 29-14 Angiotensin-Converting Enzyme Inhibitors

Generic Name	Trade Name	Available Dosage Form(s)/ Strength	Average Adult Dose
benazepril	Lotensin	5-mg, 10-mg, 20-mg, 40-mg tablets	10−40 mg daily or divided in two doses; NTE 80 mg/day
benazepril + amlodipine	Lotrel	10-mg/2.5-mg tablets 10 mg/5 mg tablets 20 mg/5 mg tablets 20 mg/10 mg tablets	NTE 80 mg benazepril and 20 mg amlodipine/day
captopril	Capoten	12.5-mg, 25-mg, 50-mg, 100-mg tablets	25−150 mg bid–tid; NTE 450 mg/day
captopril + HCTZ	Capozide	50 mg/25 mg tablets 50 mg/15 mg tablets 25 mg/25 mg tablets 25 mg/15 mg tablets	NTE 150 mg captopril and 50 mg HCTZ daily
enalapril	Vasotec	2.5-mg, 5-mg, 10-mg, 20-mg tablets	10−40 mg daily or in two divided doses
enalapril + diltiazem	Teczem	5 mg/180 mg tablets	NTE 40 mg enalapril and 360 mg diltiazem daily
enalapril + felodipine	Lexxel	5 mg/2.5 mg tablets 5 mg/5 mg tablets	NTE 40 mg enalapril and 10 mg felodipine daily
enalapril + HCTZ	Vaseretic	10 mg/25 mg tablets 5 mg/12.5 mg tablets	
fosinopril	Monopril	10-mg, 20-mg, 40-mg tablets	20−40 mg/day
lisinopril	Prinivil, Zestril	2.5-mg, 5-mg, 10-mg, 20-mg, 30-mg, 40-mg tablets	20−40 mg daily
lisinopril + HCTZ	Prinizide, Zestoretic	20 mg/25 mg tablets 20 mg/12.5 mg tablets 10 mg/12.5 mg tablets	NTE 80 mg lisinopril and 50 mg HCTZ daily
moexipril	Univasc	7.5 mg, 15 mg tablets	3.75−30 mg/day in one or two divided doses
moexipril + HCTZ	Uniretic	15 mg/25 mg tablets 15 mg/12.5 mg tablets 7.5 mg/12.5 mg tablets	
perindopril	Aceon	2-mg, 4-mg, 8-mg tablets	4 mg/day titrated to a maximum of 16 mg/day
quinapril	Accupril	5-mg, 10-mg, 20-mg, 40-mg tablets	10−80 mg/day in one or two divided doses
ramipril	Altace	1.25-mg, 2.5-mg, 5-mg, 10-mg capsules	2.5−10 mg/day
trandolapril	Mavik	1-mg, 2-mg, 4-mg tablets	1−4 mg/day

(Continued)

TABLE 29-14 Angiotensin-Converting Enzyme Inhibitors *(Continued)*

Generic Name	Trade Name	Available Dosage Form(s)/ Strength	Average Adult Dose
trandolapril + verapamil	Tarka	1 mg/240 mg tablets	NTE 8 mg trandolapril and 480 mg verapamil daily
		2 mg/180 mg tablets	
		2 mg/240 mg tablets	
		4 mg/240 mg tablets	

for CHF. They lower high BP and are thought to shrink an enlarged heart, while increasing the vital signs.

The kidneys make renin, which helps to make angiotensin I (AI) in the blood vessels. AI has no effect on BP but is converted to angiotensin II (AII) by ACE. AII is a natural vasoconstrictor that commences the synthesis and release of aldosterone, cardiac stimulation, and renal reabsorption of sodium.

When AII binds to the angiotensin I (AI) receptors in the blood vessels, vasoconstriction occurs, leading to high BP. ACE inhibitors block the conversion of AI to AII by combining with ACE. Because AI is not converted to AII, there is no AII to bind to the AI receptors in the blood vessels; therefore, the blood vessels do not constrict and BP does not increase.

Side effects include dizziness, fainting, or lightheadedness and a very annoying dry cough. Many ACE inhibitors have the suffix of *pril* (such as benazepril or captopril) in the generic name.

Angiotensin II Receptor Blockers

As discussed earlier, once AI is converted to AII by ACE, it binds to AI receptors in the blood vessels, causing vasoconstriction and high BP. AII receptor blockers (angiotensin receptor antagonists) block AII from getting into the AI receptors in the blood vessels (see Table 29-15) by competitive inhibition (competing with AII to get into the AI receptors first). In most cases, angiotensin receptor blockers get to the receptor first, but they have been found to increase blood levels of potassium. Rifampin reduces the blood levels of losartan, and fluconazole reduces the conversion of losartan to its active form, thus decreasing its effects.

Beta-Adrenergic Blockers

Beta-adrenergic blockers are used to block beta-1 and beta-2 receptors from receiving the sympathetic neurotransmitters NE and epinephrine (EPI) (see Tables 29-16 through 29-19). Beta-1 receptors are found in the heart and are stimulated by both NE and EPI. Beta-2 receptors are found in the lungs and are stimulated by EPI but not by NE. When the heart beta-1 receptor is stimulated, the following changes occur first in the heart and then in the lungs:

- Heart rate increases
- Pulse rate increases
- Vasoconstriction increases

TABLE 29-15 Angiotensin II Receptor Blockers (Angiotensin II Antagonists)

Generic Name	Trade Name	Available Dosage Form(s)/ Strength	Average Adult Dose
candesartan	Atacand	4-mg, 8-mg, 16-mg, 32-mg tablets	2–32 mg/day in one or two divided doses
eprosartan	Tevetan	600-mg tablets	400–800 mg/day in one or two divided doses
irbesartan	Avapro	75-mg, 150-mg, 300-mg tablets	150–300 mg daily; NTE 300 mg/day
losartan	Cozaar	25-mg, 50-mg, 100-mg tablets	25–100 mg daily
losartan + HCTZ	Hyzaar	50 mg/12.5 mg, 100 mg/ 12.5 mg, 100 mg/25 mg tablets	25–10 mg losartan daily
olmesartan	Benicar	5-mg, 20-mg, 40-mg tablets	20–40 mg daily
telmisartan	Micardis	20-mg, 40-mg, 80-mg tablets	20–80 mg/day
valsartan	Diovan	40-mg, 80-mg, 160-mg, 320-mg tablets	80–320 mg daily

TABLE 29-16 Nonselective Beta-Adrenergic Blocking Agents

Generic Name	Trade Name	Available Dosage Form(s)/Strength	Average Adult Dose
labetolol	Normodyne	100-mg, 200-mg, 300-mg tablets	100−400 mg bid
nadolol	Corgard	20-mg, 40-mg, 80-mg, 120-mg, 160-mg tablets	80−240 mg daily
pindolol	Visken	5-mg, 10-mg tablets	10−60 mg daily in two divided doses
propranolol	Inderal	10-mg, 20-mg, 40-mg, 60-mg, 80-mg, 90-mg tablets	HTN: 120−240 mg/day po in two to three divided doses
		4 mg/mL, 8 mg/mL solution	
		80 mg/mL conc. solution	
		60-mg, 80-mg, 120-mg, 160-mg ER capsules	80−160 mg po daily (ER)
		1 mg/mL injection	1−3 mg IV q4h
timolol	Blocadren	5-mg, 10-mg, 20-mg tablets	20−40 mg daily in divided doses

TABLE 29-17 Selective Beta-Adrenergic Blocking Agents

Generic Name	Trade Name	Available Dosage Form(s)/Strength	Average Adult Dose
acebutolol	Sectral	200-mg, 400-mg capsules	200−1,200 mg daily in two divided doses
atenolol	Tenormin	25-mg, 50-mg, 100-mg tablets	50−100 mg qd
bisoprolol	Zebeta	5-mg, 10-mg tablets	2.5−20 mg qd
esmolol	Brevibloc	10 mg/mL, 20 mg/mL, 250 mg/mL injection	50−200 mcg/kg/minute IV
metoprolol	Lopressor	25-mg, 50-mg, 100-mg tablets	100−450 mg daily
		25-mg, 50-mg, 100-mg, 200-mg XL tablets	50−400 mg qd (XL)

TABLE 29-18 Antiadrenergic Agents

Generic Name	Trade Name	Available Dosage Form(s)/Strength	Average Adult Dose
clonidine	Catapres	0.1-mg, 0.2-mg, 0.3-mg tablets	100−600 mcg daily in divided doses
		0.1 mg/24 hour, 0.2 mg/24 hour, 0.3 mg/24 hour transdermal patches	One patch every seven days
guanabenz acetate	Wytensin	4-mg, 8-mg tablets	4−32 mg bid
guanadrel	Hylorel	10-mg tablets	10−75 mg daily in two divided doses
guanethidine	Ismelin	10-mg, 25-mg tablets	10−50 mg qd
guanfacine	Tenex	1-mg, 2-mg tablets	1−2 mg daily at bedtime
methyldopa	Aldomet	250-mg, 500-mg tablets	250−2,000 mg daily in two to three divided doses
reserpine		0.1-mg, 0.25-mg tablets	0.5 mg daily for one to two weeks, then decrease to 0.1−0.25 mg daily

- BP increases
- Force and contraction rate of the heart increase
- Breathing rate increases
- Bronchodilation increases
- Oxygen consumption increases

Likewise, when beta-2 receptors in the lungs are stimulated by EPI, the following changes occur, first in the lungs and then in the heart:

- Bronchodilation increases
- Breathing rate increases
- Heart rate increases
- Pulse rate increases
- Vasoconstriction increases
- BP increases
- Force and contraction rate of the heart increase
- Oxygen consumption increases

When the sympathetic neurotransmitters are blocked from the beta-1 and/or beta-2 receptors, the following changes occur:

- Heart rate decreases
- Pulse rate decreases
- Vasoconstriction decreases
- BP decreases
- Force and contraction rate of the heart decrease
- Oxygen consumption decreases (prevents ischemia and angina)
- Breathing rate decreases
- Bronchodilation decreases

If a patient has HTN, angina, or cardiac arrhythmias, beta-1 blockers will mitigate these conditions. Selective beta blockers that block only beta-1 receptors in the heart are used primarily for HTN. Beta blockers may affect insulin and glucose levels. Inderal is also indicated in the treatment of migraine headaches, glaucoma, cardiac arrhythmias, and post-MI.

Antiadrenergic Agents

An *antiadrenergic agent* is a centrally or peripherally acting antihypertensive agent. This drug interferes with the manufacture of NE at nerve endings. Because less NE is being made, the antiadrenergic agents are stored as a false transmitter and are released like natural NE when needed. Drowsiness may occur upon initial therapy.

---

plaque a fatty deposit that is high in cholesterol.

thrombi blood clots (singular, *thrombus*).

hematuria blood in the urine.

dyscrasia an abnormal condition of the body, especially a blood imbalance.

deep venous thrombosis (DVT) a blood clot in one of the veins of the legs or other deep veins.

thrombophlebitis an inflammation of a vein with a thrombus.

Coronary Artery Disease

CAD occurs when there is insufficient blood flow to the heart via the right or left coronary artery. The reduced blood flow is usually due to arteriosclerosis and/or atherosclerosis. Over time, CAD can lead to angina, heart attack, arrhythmias, stroke, pulmonary embolism, and heart failure. CAD is the most common form of heart disease; the National Heart, Lung, and Blood Institute ranks CAD as the leading cause of death in the United States.

Arteriosclerosis, often referred to as "hardening of the arteries," is the actual stiffening of the arteries themselves. It occurs over a period of many years, during which the arteries thicken and lose elasticity, and develop areas that become hard and brittle. This occurs because of the deposition of calcium in the vessel walls. During exercise the arteries should constrict, and during rest they should dilate. With arteriosclerosis, the arteries will become inflexible and will not constrict or dilate as they should, when they should. A *stenosis*, or narrowing of the lumen, may also occur. A person can have both a hardening and a narrowing of the arteries or one condition without the other. Arteriosclerosis can lead to HTN, MI, and stroke. All the organs that are fed by the sclerotic (hardened) arteries can suffer damage and fail to function properly. Causes include genetics, diet, and normal aging.

Atherosclerosis, a specific form of arteriosclerosis, is a condition in which **plaque** builds up on the walls of the coronary arteries and hardens them. Atherosclerosis is believed to be initiated by an injury to the artery wall; the injury may have been caused by a diet high in cholesterol, smoking, high BP, or diabetes. Plaque adheres more easily to a damaged wall and, as it builds up (*accretes*), the lumen soon becomes occluded. Blood clots (**thrombi**) can also form, because the arterial wall is no longer smooth. Instead, the wall has an irregular surface that platelets stick to easily. This will further impede blood flow and lead to ischemia, which may in turn cause angina, MI, stroke, or pulmonary embolism. The terms *arteriosclerosis* and *atherosclerosis* are often used interchangeably. It should be noted that there are no OTC drugs or alternative therapies used to treat CAD.

Treatment of Coronary Artery Disease

CAD, especially atherosclerosis, creates a condition in which blood clots form easily. Normal blood contains platelets that help the blood to clot when necessary. As more blood with more sticky platelets runs through the narrowed tunnels of coronary arteries with atherosclerosis, the platelets aggregate (clump together). Blood clots *snowball*, getting larger and larger, until the lumen is eventually occluded, causing ischemia and angina. To prevent blood clots from forming or getting bigger, antiplatelet drugs are given to reduce the number of platelets and anticoagulants are given to reduce the stickiness of the platelets. Think of a platelet as a piece of adhesive tape. The more tape there is, the more stickiness there will be. To reduce stickiness, you can either reduce the number of tape pieces or reduce the amount of adhesive on each piece of tape.

Doing both achieves the best results, reducing both the number of platelets and their stickiness—and hence reducing blood's ability to clot.

Antiplatelets

Also called *platelet aggregation inhibitors*, antiplatelet drugs (see Tables 29-19 and 29-21) reduce and prevent platelet aggregation by interfering with the extrinsic and intrinsic pathways. Because antiplatelets reduce the ability of the blood to coagulate, the chance of internal and external hemorrhage exists. Side effects include **hematuria**, blood in the feces or tarry stools, and/or heavy menstrual bleeding.

The patient's blood-clotting ability, urine, and stools should be monitored. Gastrointestinal (GI) upset and bleeding may also lead to GI ulcers. Therefore, platelet inhibitors should be taken on a full stomach and at least two hours apart from antacids. Ticlid has been known to cause blood **dyscrasias** such as thrombotic thrombocytopenia, neutropenia/agranulocytosis, and thrombotic thrombocytopenic purpura.

Anticoagulants

Sometimes erroneously called *blood thinners*, anticoagulants do not thin out the blood (see Table 29-16). Instead, they prevent clots from forming or existing clots from getting bigger. However, they *cannot* dissolve existing blood clots. Warfarin is the oral DOC, and heparin is the parenteral DOC.

Warfarin is used in the long-term prevention or management of venous thromboembolic disorders, including **deep venous thrombosis (DVT)**, pulmonary embolism, and clotting associated with atrial fibrillation and prosthetic heart valves. It is also used after MI to prevent reinfarction, venous thromboembolism, and death. It works by preventing the synthesis of clotting factors II, VII, IX, and X. Warfarin dosages are monitored by prothrombin time (PT) values. Signs of bleeding are usual indications for treatment with vitamin K. Warfarin takes several days for onset with a long duration of two to five days after it is discontinued.

Heparin is a parenterally administered anticoagulant used prophylactically to prevent and treat DVT and pulmonary embolism, to treat **thrombophlebitis**, and to prevent clotting during cardiac and vascular surgery, extracorporeal circulation, hemodialysis, blood transfusions, and in blood samples for laboratory tests. Heparin is a mucopolysaccharide found in bovine (cattle) and porcine (pig) lung and intestinal tissue. Heparin combines with antithrombin III to inactivate clotting factors IX, X, XI, and XII. This inhibits the conversion of prothrombin to thrombin, thus preventing the formation of fibrin, one of the main clotting ingredients of blood, and thereby inhibiting the formation of a clot. Heparin also interferes with platelet aggregation and inhibits thromboplastin so that more thrombin cannot be manufactured. Heparin must be administered parenterally by IV or subcutaneous injection or by IV infusion. It is destroyed by gastric juices and cannot be given orally. The onset of action of

TABLE 29-19 Prescription Treatments for Antiplatelets

Generic name	Brand name	Dosage Forms and Availability	Route of Administration	Common Adult Dosage
aspirin	Bayer aspirin, others	81-mg, 325-mg tabletss	Oral	81–325 mg daily
dipyridamole	Persantine	25-mg, 50-mg, 75-mg tablets	Oral	75–100 mg daily
ticlopidine	Ticlid	250-mg tablets	Oral	250 mg bid
clopidogrel	Plavix	75-mg, 300-mg tablets	Oral	75 mg daily
prasugrel	Effient	5-mg, 10-mg tabs	Oral	5–10 mg daily

TABLE 29-20 Antiplatelet Agents

Generic name	Trade Name	Available Dosage Form(s)/ Strength	Average Adult Dose
anagrelide hcl	Agrylin	0.5-mg, 1-mg capsules	0.5 mg qid or 1 mg bid
cilostazol	Pletal	50-mg, 100-mg tablets	100 mg bid
clopidogrel	Plavix	75-mg tablet	75 mg daily
dipyridamole	Persantine	25-mg, 50-mg, 75-mg tablets	75–100 mg qid with warfarin therapy
dipyridamole + ASA	Aggrenox	200 mg SR dipyridamole/25 mg ASA capsules	One capsule bid
ticlopidine	Ticlid	250-mg tablet	250 mg bid with food

TABLE 29-21 Comparison of Antiplatelet Agents

First-Generation Subclassification: Platelet Inhibitors	Second-Generation Subclassification: Thienopyridines	Third-Generation Subclassification: Parenteral Glycoprotein II/IIIA Platelet Inhibitors (Antagonists)
Aspirin (acetylsalicylic acid or ASA)	Ticlid (ticlopidine)	ReoPro (abciximab)
	Not used as much as Plavix, because it causes blood disorders such as thrombocytopenia	
Persantine (dipyridamole)	Plavix (clopidogrel)	Centocor (abciximab)
		Aggrastat (tirofiban)
		Integrilin (eptifibatide)
Mechanism of Action		
The MOA of ASA is the inhibition of cyclooxygenase, which prevents prostaglandin G2 from forming, which, in turn, prevents the formation of thrombaxane A2, a potent platelet aggregator and vasoconstrictor		Glycoprotein II/IIIa receptor inhibitors/antagonists block certain receptors on the platelets responsible for clumping and, therefore, block platelet activity
Side Effects		
Bleeding gums, poor healing of scratches or sores, bruises, hematuria or heavy menstrual bleeding, GI upset with external or internal bleeding	Bleeding gums, poor healing of scratches or sores, bruises, hematuria or heavy menstrual bleeding, GI upset with external or internal bleeding	Bleeding gums, poor healing of scratches or sores, bruises, hematuria or heavy menstrual bleeding, GI upset with external or internal bleeding
Toxic Effects		
Anemia	Rare but serious blood disorders or dyscrasias, thrombocytopenic purpura, anemia, neurological changes, acute onset of altered mental status, renal failure	Anemia
Special Considerations and Warnings		
Blood must be monitored to dose patients properly and to avoid anemia or blood disorders	Blood must be monitored to dose patients properly and to avoid anemia or blood disorders (especially with Ticlid)	Blood must be monitored to dose patients properly and to avoid anemia or blood disorders

heparin is immediate when given IV and within 20–30 minutes when given subcutaneously. However, it has a short duration and must be given continuously while needed.

Bioequivalence is still a disputed issue among different manufacturers of warfarin and unfractionated heparin (UFH). It is still considered sound judgment not to switch manufacturers of products during therapy for an individual patient once therapy has begun. Low-molecular-weight heparins (LMWHs) are also not interchangeable. Both UFH and LMWHs inactivate factor Xa by interacting with antithrombin. UFH inactivates factors IIa and Xa, whereas LMWHs inhibit factor Xa but only minimally affect thrombin (factor IIa).

Some advantages of LMWHs over UFH are the following:

• Longer half-life of LMWHs allows less frequent dosing and yields more predictable response.

• Reduce hospital stay times and therefore are cost-efficient.
• UFH has less bioavailability, because it binds to more blood components; there is greater variability in patient response to each dose.
• Lower incidence of heparin-induced thrombocytopenia with LMWHs than with UFH.
• LMWHs are smaller molecules, because some mucopolysaccharides have been removed; thus, subcutaneous absorption is better.

The disadvantage of LMWHs is that there is *no* specific antidote, as there is for UFH. Protamine sulfate reverses only about 60% of the antifactor Xa activity of LMWH.

Tables 29-22 and 29-23 list the anticoagulants and prescription treatments for anticoagulants.

TABLE 29-22 Prescription Treatments for Anticoagulants

Generic Name	Brand Name	Dosage Forms and Availability	Route of Administration	Common Adult Dosage
heparin	Heparin	5-mL, 10-mL vials	Injection	Ranges from 5,000 to 10,000 units subcutaneously q8h for DVT prevention to weight-based IV infusions given as 18 units/kg/hour IV and adjusted to lab values
warfarin	Coumadin, Jantoven	1-mg, 2-mg, 2.5 mg, 3-mg, 4-mg, 5-mg, 6-mg, 7.5-mg, or 10-mg tablets	Oral	Based on PT/INR response to drug

TABLE 29-23 Anticoagulants

Generic Name	Trade Name	Available Dosage Form(s)/Strength	Overdose Antidote
heparin sodium (Na)		1,000 units/mL, 2,000 units/mL, 5,000 units/mL, 10,000 units/mL, 20,000 units/mL, 40,000 units/mL injection	Protamine sulfate
warfarin Na	Coumadin	1-mg, 2-mg, 2.5-mg, 3-mg, 4-mg, 5-mg, 6-mg, 7.5-mg, 10-mg tablets	Vitamin K
LMWHs			
dalteparin Na	Fragmin	2,500 units/mL, 5,000 unit/mL, 7,500 units/mL, 10,000 units/mL, 25,000 units/mL injection	
enoxaparin Na	Lovenox	30 mg/0.3 mL, 40 mg/0.4 mL, 60 mg/0.6 mL, 80 mg/0.8 mL, 100 mg/1 mL, 120 mg/0.8 mL, 150 mg/1 mL, 300 mg/3 mL injection	
tinzaparin Na	Innohep	20,000 units/mL	

Note: Doses vary with blood monitoring results.

Tissue Plasminogen Activators

Tissue plasminogen activators (t-PAs) and other thrombolytic enzymes chemically break down blood clots by reversing the clotting order and interfering with the synthesis of various clotting factors (see Table 29-24). The main indication for use of these *clot-busting* drugs is in the management of acute, severe thrombolytic diseases such as MI, pulmonary embolism, and iliofemoral thrombosis.

t-PAs must be administered by parenteral infusion within a *window of opportunity* to avoid intracranial hemorrhage. This window is usually less than three hours from the onset of symptoms; however, some thrombolytics may be used within six hours of the onset of symptoms. A fatal error occurs if a thrombolytic is given for an MI caused by a stenosis instead of

a clot. Therefore, because of their potency and possible adverse reactions, t-PAs are used only in emergency cases for acute MIs, acute ischemic stroke, and pulmonary embolism caused by blood clots. Quick, expensive blood testing and electrocardiography must be performed before a thrombolytic can be administered. This takes precious time in the window of opportunity, but it is well worth it. Thrombolytics stimulate the synthesis of fibrinolysin, which breaks down a clot into soluble products (see Table 29-24).

These drugs are extremely expensive: thousands of dollars just for the product alone, not including diagnosis, the ER personnel who order and administer the drug, and pharmacy preparation of the drug. A recently compounded thrombolytic usually has an expiration time of 8 to 24 hours. Because of the

TABLE 29-24 Thrombolytics and Tissue Plasminogen Activators

Generic Name	Trade Name	Type	Average Adult Dose
alteplase recombinant	Activase	t-PA, thrombolytic	15-mg IV bolus, then 50 mg over 30 minutes, then 35 mg over 60 minutes
anistreplase	Eminase	Thrombolytic	30 units IV over two to five minutes
retiplase recombinant	Retivase	r-PA, thrombolytic	10 units IV bolus over two minutes, repeated 30 minutes later
streptokinase	Strepase	Thrombolytic	1.5 million units IV over 60 minutes
tenecteplase	Metalyse	TNKase	30–50 mg IV bolus over five seconds (based on patient's weight)
urokinase	Abbokinase	Thrombolytic	4,400 units/kg at 90 mL/hour over 10 minutes, then 4,400 units/kg at 15 mL/hour for 12 hours

expense and short shelf life of the compounded drug, thrombolytics are usually prepared by the pharmacy just prior to administration.

Contraindications include previous stroke, major surgery, head injury, and history of stomach ulcers or abnormal bleeding problems. Patients who have previously had an injection of streptokinase should not receive a further dose of streptokinase at any time, unless it is within four days of the first dose. Streptokinase stimulates the formation of antibodies that will reduce the effectiveness of a second dose. A second heart attack or clot treatment will require administration of an alternative thrombolytic drug.

Thrombolytics should not be given if the ECG wave pattern shows no ST segment elevation. Possible side effects include nausea and vomiting; bleeding at the injection site, gums, or other areas; and large bruises.

Thrombin Inhibitors

Traditionally, anticoagulant therapy has been used to prevent the production of thrombin or its activity (see Table 29-25). However, new direct thrombin inhibitors inactivate bound thrombin by binding to the enzyme and blocking its interaction with its fibrin substrates. There are two receptor sites on thrombin IIa.

The active site-directed thrombin inhibitor, argatroban, binds to the thrombin without displacing the fibrin, which inactivates the thrombin so that it cannot form a clot. Bivalent direct thrombin inhibitors, such as hirudin and bivalirudin, displace thrombin from fibrin during binding and the inactivation process.

These new agents may have potential advantage over heparin because thrombin inhibitors produce a more predictable anticoagulant response, as they do not bind to plasma proteins like heparin does. Therefore, there is greater capability for maintained and accurate dosing and response with thrombin inhibitors.

Antidotes for Overdose of Antiplatelets or Anticoagulants

Should overdose of antiplatelet or anticoagulant drugs occur, a number of antidotes exist.

Warfarin Overdose

Vitamin K is a natural precursor to the synthesis of some clotting factors. Vitamin K is found in cabbage, cauliflower, spinach, other green leafy vegetables, cereals, soybeans, and egg yolks. It is also made by the bacteria that line the GI tract. Vitamin K may reduce the effectiveness of the oral anticoagulant

TABLE 29-25 Thrombin Inhibitors

Generic Name	Trade Name	Available Dosage Form(s)/ Strength	Average Adult Dose
argatroban	Novastin	100 mg/mL injection	2 mcg/kg/minute IV
bivalirudin	Angiomax	250-mg pwd for injection	1 mg/kg IV bolus, followed by a four-hour infusion of 2.5 mg/kg/hour
desirudin	Iprivask	15-mg pwd for injection	15 mg SC q12h
lepirudin	Refludan	50-mg pwd for injection	0.4 mg/kg for patients up to 110 kg

warfarin. Because of this, vitamin K may also be used as an antidote to stop hemorrhage when too much warfarin has been given and is causing excessive bleeding. Bleeding may be internal or external. Note the locations and clotting factors on the coagulation pathway where vitamin K is required, particularly factors VII and IX and prothrombin (see Table 29-25).

Information

Here is a note about factor VIII that has little to do with diseases of the heart but pertains to the subject of clotting factors. Hemophilia A is the most common hereditary disorder affecting blood coagulation; (*heme* = blood, *philia* = loving). It is caused by a lack of plasma protein factor VIII.

The disorder is caused by an inherited, sex-linked recessive trait. The defective gene is located on the X chromosome. Because females have two copies of the X chromosome, there is a good chance that there will not be a defective gene on both chromosomes. Males, however, carry only one X chromosome, so if the factor VIII gene on that chromosome is defective, male offspring will be born with the disease. Hemophilia A affects about 1 out of 5,000 men. Females with one defective factor VIII gene are carriers of this trait. All female children of a male hemophiliac are carriers of the trait.

Although some cases of hemophilia go unnoticed until later in life, when trauma, surgery, or injury occurs, many cases show the classic symptoms of severe bleeding. Hemorrhage may be internal or external.

Heparin Overdose

The only antidote for heparin overdose is protamine sulfate, which is used for the emergency reversal of heparin-induced bleeding. Heparin's clotting ability centers around the clotting factor called factor IXa. Activated partial thromboplastin time of more than 100 seconds may require administration of protamine sulfate.

Thrombolytic Enzyme Overdose

Aminocaproic acid and tranexamic acid can be used to counter a thrombolytic enzyme overdose. The fibrinolysis inhibitory effects of aminocaproic acid are exerted principally via inhibition of plasminogen activators and to a lesser degree through antiplasmin activity. Tranexamic acid competitively inhibits the activation of plasminogen to plasmin (see Table 29-26).

TABLE 29-26 Prescription Treatments for Thrombolytics

Generic Name	Brand Name	Dosage Forms and Availability	Route of Administration	Common Adult Dosage
streptokinase	Streptase, Kabikinase	50-mL, 6.5-mL vials	Intravenous, intracoronary infusion	Acute MI: 1,500,000 units within 60 minutes of event; within seven days: PE: LD 250,000 units over 30 minutes, then 100,000 units over 24 hours; arterial thrombosis: LD 250,000 units over 24–72 hours; DVT: LD 250,000 units over 30 minutes, then 100,000 units/hour for 72 hour; embolism: LD 250,000 units over 30 minutes, then 100,000 units/hour for 24–72 hours
urokinase	Kinlytic	250,000 international units urokinase activity, 25-mg mannitol, 250-mg albumin (human), and 50-mg sodium chloride vials	Urokinase injection	Acute MI: LD 440 units/kg to run at 90 mL/hour X 10 minutes, then 15 mL X 12 hours; PE: Both LD and continuous infusion are based on weight (kg) of patient; dose ranges between 2,250,000 and 6,250,00 units/kg
alteplase	Activase (t-PA)	50-mg vials containing vacuum and 100-mg vials without vacuum.	Intravenous	Acute MI: 15-mg IV bolus, then 0.75 mg/kg IV (maximum: 50 mg) infused over 30 minutes, and then 0.5 mg/kg IV (maximum 35 mg) over next 60 minutes. PE: 100 mg over 2 hours X 1 dose; ischemic stroke: 0.9 mg/kg maximum 90 mg over 60 minutes X 1 dose

(Continued)

TABLE 29-26 Prescription Treatments for Thrombolytics (*Continued*)

Generic Name	Brand Name	Dosage Forms and Availability	Route of Administration	Common Adult Dosage
reteplase	Retavase	Lyophilized powder in 10.4 units (equivalent to 18.1 mg Retavase (reteplase)) vials without a vacuum; Kit: two single-use Retavase (reteplase) vials 10.4 units (18.1 mg), two single-use diluent vials for reconstitution (10 mL sterile water for injection, USP), two sterile 10-mL syringes, two sterile dispensing pins, four sterile needles, two alcohol swabs, and a package insert; Half-Kit: 1 single-use Retavase (reteplase) vial 10.4 units (18.1 mg), one single-use diluent vial for reconstitution (10 mL sterile water for injection, USP), a sterile dispensing pin, and a package insert.	Intravenous	Acute MI: first bolus given over two minutes, second bolus given 30 minutes after first bolus
tenecteplase	TNKase	Lyophilized powder in a 50-mg vial under partial vacuum	Intravenous	Acute MI: dose is based on weight, NTE 50 mg
anistreplase	Eminase		Intravenous	Acute MI: 30 units over two to five minutes

Cholesterol

Cholesterol is a waxy fat-like substance that is found in all cells and is needed to make hormones, vitamin D, and digestive substances. The liver may synthesize cholesterol or may take up all the cholesterol the body needs from circulating lipoproteins or from what is absorbed in the small intestines. However, because it is found in many foods, many people have more cholesterol than the body needs. When there is excess cholesterol and other fats in the blood, the condition is called **hyperlipidemia**. These fats are transported in the blood via larger molecules called *lipoproteins*. The five categories of lipoproteins are the following:

- Chylomicrons
- Very-low-density lipoproteins (VLDLs)
- Intermediate-density lipoproteins (IDLs)
- Low-density lipoproteins (LDLs)—*bad* cholesterol
- High-density lipoproteins (HDLs)—*good* cholesterol

Regular screenings for hyperlipidemia are needed, because high cholesterol is asymptomatic. The first line of defense in the fight against high cholesterol is diet and exercise. When this fails to bring the LDL and VLDL levels down to normal, or if the amount of HDL decreases, a prescription medication must be employed. Normally, HDL carries LDL and VLDL away from artery walls. Hyperlipidemia occurs when there is a higher than normal amount of LDL.

---

hyperlipidemia high concentrations of lipids in the blood.

Triglycerides

Triglycerides are a form of energy stored in adipose and muscle tissues. They are gradually released and metabolized between meals as the body's energy needs fluctuate. Lipids are also found in the adipose tissue, the liver, and the blood. Immediately after a meal, triglycerides can be found in the blood. Triglycerides are often measured to depict fat ingestion and metabolism, and the measurements can be used to assess CAD risk factors.

Chylomicrons, which are produced in the intestines, deliver dietary cholesterol and triglycerides. Usually, the fatty acids are removed from the triglycerides, found in the center of the chylomicrons, as they pass through various tissues, particularly adipose and skeletal muscle. The remainder of chylomicron is then delivered to the liver and disappears from the blood within two or three hours. The remaining triglycerides, plus any triglycerides synthesized by the liver, are then secreted into the blood by the liver as VLDL (see Tables 29-27 through 29-30).

Antihyperlipidemics

Antihyperlipidemics are drugs that help prevent the progression of CAD by lowering plasma lipid levels (see Table 29-31). Some are also useful in treating diabetes insipidis and in prevention of

TABLE 29-27 Total Cholesterol Levels

Cholesterol Levels	Ranges for Most Adults
Optimal cholesterol level—*Good*	200 mg/dL or lower
Borderline high cholesterol	200–239 mg/dL
High cholesterol—*At Risk*	240 mg/dL or higher

TABLE 29-28 High-Density Lipid (HDL) Levels (Good Cholesterol)

	Ranges for Most Adults
High HDL/low HDL—*Good*	60 mg/dL or higher
Borderline low HDL	40–59 mg/dL
Low HDL—*At Risk*	Less than 40 mg/dL

TABLE 29-29 Low-Density Lipid (LDL) Levels (Bad Cholesterol)

	Ranges for Most Adults
Optimal LDL—*Good*	Less than 100 mg/dL
Near or above optimal LDL	100–129 mg/dL
Borderline high LDL—*At Risk*	130–159 mg/dL
High LDL—*At Risk*	160 mg/dL or higher

TABLE 29-30 Triglycerides

	Ranges for Most Adults
Normal triglycerides—*Good*	Less than 150 mg/dL
Borderline high triglycerides	150–199 mg/dL
High triglycerides	200–499 mg/dL
Very high triglycerides—*At Risk*	500 mg/dL or higher

TABLE 29-31 Prescription Treatments for Hyperlipidemia

Generic Name	Brand Name	Dosage Forms and Availability	Route of Administration	Common Adult Dosage
cholestyramine	Questran, Arava	210 gm, 378 gm cans	Oral	4 gm qd or bid; maximum 24 gm daily
colestipol	Colestid, Niacor	1 gm tablets	Oral	Initially 5 gm qd or bid; maximum 30 gm daily
lovastatin	Altoprev, Mevacor	20-mg, 40-mg tablets	Oral	10–80 mg qd; Altoprev 10–mg qd
simvastatin	Zocor	5-mg, 10-mg, 20-mg, 40-mg, 80-mg tablets	Oral	5–80 mg qd
pravastatin	Pravachol, Pravigard	10-mg, 20-mg, 40-mg, 80-mg tablets	Oral	10–80 mg qd
atorvastatin	Lipitor	10-mg, 20-mg, 40-mg, 80-mg tablets	Oral	10–80 mg qd
pitavastatin	Livalo	1-mg, 2-mg, 4-mg tablets	Oral	1–4 mg qd
rosuvastatin	Crestor	5-mg, 10-mg, 20-mg, 40-mg tablets	Oral	5–40 mg qd
fluvastatin	Lescol	20-mg, 40-mg, 80-mg capsules	Oral	20–80 mg daily
gemfibrozil	Lopid	600-mg tablets	Oral	600 mg bid
ezetimibe	Zetia	10-mg capsules	Oral	10 mg qd
nicotinic acid	Niaspan, Niacor	Niaspan: 500-mg, 750-mg, 1000-mg tablets Niacor: 500-mg tablets	Oral	Niacor: 1–2 gm tid; Niaspan: 500 mg at bedtime, then 1–2 gm/day at bedtime after titration

stroke and MI. Patients with CAD and high cholesterol are most likely to benefit from treatment with long-term antihyperlipidemic drug therapy.

There are various steps in the synthesis of cholesterol. Therefore, drugs with various mechanisms of action are needed to lower or reverse cholesterol synthesis. The most frequently prescribed drugs, called *statins*, have been found to be highly effective in lowering LDL cholesterol. The statins are a group of drugs that suppress cholesterol synthesis by inhibiting the enzyme HMG CoA reductase (see Tables 29-31 and 29-32).

Statins decrease the synthesis of cholesterol by the liver, which has two important effects: (1) the upregulation of LDL receptors by hepatocytes and consequent increased removal of certain lipoproteins from blood circulation and (2) a reduction in the synthesis and secretion of lipoproteins by the liver. The net effect of statin therapy is to lower plasma concentrations of cholesterol-carrying lipoproteins, the most prominent of which is LDL.

Statins also increase the removal of and reduce the secretion of remnant particles, specifically VLDL and IDL. For patients with elevated LDLs and triglycerides, a statin is one of the therapies of choice because of its ability to effectively lower LDL and non-high-density lipoprotein cholesterol (non-HDL-C) levels.

A newer antihyperlipidemic drug, ezetimibe, also enables patients to reach their lipid goals but works in the digestive tract rather than the liver. However, it does not affect fat absorption. Ezetimibe selectively inhibits cholesterol absorption by intestinal microvilli and villi. This prevents cholesterol from entering the blood system, which in turn decreases hepatic storage of cholesterol, and increases clearance from the blood. The cholesterol moves right through the intestinal tract, leaving the body essentially unchanged and without affecting bowel function or the absorption of fat-soluble vitamins. This distinct mechanism is complementary to that of HMG-CoA reductase inhibitors.

Another alternative is vitamin B3 (niacin), which works indirectly to reduce total cholesterol by reducing the production of building blocks for LDL and increasing production of HDL.

TABLE 29-32 Antihyperlipidemics

Generic Name	Trade Name	Available Dosage Form(s)/Strength	Average Adult Dose
atorvastatin calcium	Lipitor	10-mg, 20-mg, 40-mg, 80-mg tablets	10–80 mg qd
atorvastatin + amlodipine	Caduet	Antihyperlipidemic/HTN combination—various strengths	Individualized dosing
cholestyramine	Questran	Powder for suspension	4 gm daily or bid
colesevelam	WelChol	625-mg tablet	Three tablets bid or six tablets daily
colestipol	Colestid	1 gm tablet	5–30 gm daily or in divided doses
		5 gm/dose granules	
ezetimibe	Zetia	10-mg tablets	10 mg qd
ezetimibe + simvastatin	Vytorin	10 mg/10 mg, 10 mg/20 mg, 10 mg/40 mg, 10 mg/80 mg tablets	One tablet daily
fenofibrate	Tricor	48-mg, 145-mg tablets	48–145 mg/day
fluvastatin sodium	Lescol	20-mg, 40-mg tablets	20–80 mg/day
	Lescol XL	80-mg XL tablets	80 mg qd (XL)
gemfibrozil	Lopid	600-mg tablets	600 mg 30 minutes before the morning and evening meal
lovastatin	Mevacor	10-mg, 20-mg, 40-mg tablets	10–80 mg daily or in two divided doses
	Altoprev	10-mg, 20-mg, 40-mg, 60-mg ER tablets	10–60 mg qd (ER)
niacin		500-mg tablets	1–2 gm bid–tid

(Continued)

TABLE 29-32   Antihyperlipidemics (*Continued*)

Generic Name	Trade Name	Available Dosage Form(s)/Strength	Average Adult Dose
		500-mg, 750-mg, 1,000-mg ER tablets	500–2,000 mg daily (ER)
pravastatin sodium	Pravachol	10-mg, 20-mg, 40-mg, 80-mg tablets	Initial dose: 40 mg/day, may increase to 80 mg/day
rosuvastatin calcium	Crestor	5-mg, 10-mg, 20-mg, 40-mg tablets	5–40 mg qd
simvastatin	Zocor	5-mg, 10-mg, 20-mg, 40-mg, 80-mg tablets	55–80 mg/day qd or in divided doses

The Lymphatic System

The lymphatic system is a complex system of lymph organs, nodes, ducts, tissues, vessels, and capillaries that transport lymph fluid to the circulatory system. The cardiovascular and lymphatic systems work in tandem and are joined by a capillary system through which lymph and blood move (see Figure 29-4). Blood circulates in the closed, revolving circulatory system; in contrast, lymph fluid moves in one direction to eliminate waste such as bacteria, old blood cells, debris, and cancer cells.

Some medical experts consider the lymphatic system to be a part of the blood circulatory system, because lymph fluid comes from blood and returns to blood and because the lymphatic ducts are very similar to the blood vessels. Others consider it the main component of the immune system. Throughout the body, wherever blood vessels are located there are also lymph vessels, and the two systems work together.

Lymph fluid is not pumped, as the heart pumps blood. The lymphatic system uses the contraction of skeletal muscles to move the fluid through the lymph vessels. Bone marrow produces certain cells called **lymphocytes**, **monocytes**, and leukocytes. *Lymph nodes* are areas where lymphocytes concentrate along the lymphatic veins. The lymphatic system supports the immune system by:

- Filtering out organisms that cause disease
- Producing specific WBCs
- Manufacturing antibodies
- Distributing fluids and nutrients throughout the body
- Draining excess fluids and protein so that tissues do not swell or become inflamed

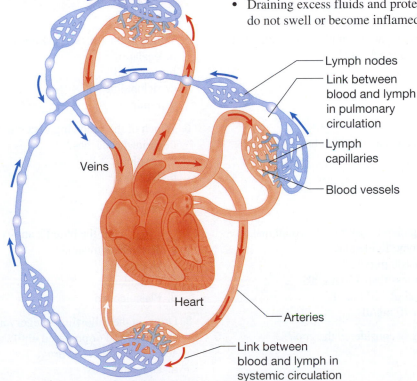

FIGURE 29-4 The lymphatic system and the circulatory system.

---

lymphocyte a type of white blood cell.

monocyte a type of white blood cell.

Summary

The cardiovascular system, often referred to as the circulatory system, is responsible for transporting blood to all parts of the body. It consists of the heart, arteries, arterioles, veins, venules, and capillaries. The arteries are responsible for carrying oxygen-rich blood to the cells; the veins carry deoxygenated blood back to the heart and lungs. The lungs and respiratory system work in tandem with the cardiovascular system to sustain life.

To accomplish its primary purpose of pumping blood to all parts of the body, the heart relies on a conduction system comprised of nodes and nodal tissues that regulate the various aspects of the heartbeat. In addition, the nervous system plays a vital role in regulating heart rate.

The two most common diseases affecting the cardiovascular system are CHF and CAD. CHF occurs when the heart pumps out less blood than it receives, resulting in a weakened and enlarged heart and in less blood being pumped out to feed the body. Complications of CHF include ischemia, MI, and cardiac arrhythmias. CHF is responsible for 40,000 deaths each year as well as for 2.9 million doctor visits and 875,000 hospitalizations.

CAD is characterized by insufficient blood flow to the heart. CAD is the result of atherosclerosis or arteriosclerosis; however, many factors can contribute to CAD, including diet, stress, smoking, normal aging, and genetics. As a pharmacy technician, you need to be aware of lifestyle factors that can lead to the development of CAD.

HTN and hyperlipidemia are two additional conditions that affect the cardiovascular system. HTN is high BP, for which many pharmaceutical treatments exist, including diuretics, vasodilators, ACE inhibitors, beta blockers, and calcium channel blockers. Hyperlipidemia is high blood cholesterol. Both HTN and hyperlipidemia often go undetected, as these conditions do not have substantial symptoms.

The lymphatic system and circulatory system work closely together, as blood and lymph fluid move through the same capillary system. Lymph fluid removes wastes and debris from the body and supports the immune system by filtering out pathogens and draining excess fluid from the body.

This chapter contains a thorough discussion of the available treatments for diseases of the cardiovascular system. Keep in mind that although great strides have been made in the ability to treat CHF and CAD, cardiovascular disease remains the leading cause of death in the United States.

Chapter Review Questions

1. Approximately how many gallons of blood are estimated to be pumped by the heart each day?
   a. 1,900
   b. 3,300
   c. 2,300
   d. 1,300

2. How much blood does the average adult body contain?
   a. 7.6 L
   b. 6 L
   c. 5.6 L
   d. 5 L

3. Which of the following cholesterol ranges would make the patient *at risk* for hyperlipidemia?
   a. LDL level less than 100 mg/dL
   b. triglyceride level of less than 150 mg/dL
   c. total cholesterol level of 220 mg/dL
   d. HDL level less than 40 mg/dL

4. Which of the following is considered the *good* cholesterol?
   a. VLDL
   b. HDL
   c. LDL
   d. both a and c

5. Which of the following drugs is an antiplatelet agent?
   a. enalapril
   b. captopril
   c. ticlopidine
   d. ramipril

6. Which of the following beta blockers is also used to treat migraine headaches?
   a. timolol
   b. labetalol
   c. esmolol
   d. propranolol

7. _____ is the blood's ability to clot.
   a. Thrombocytopenia
   b. Hematuria
   c. Coagulation
   d. Plasminogen

8. Drugs in the following category are very expensive and are not mixed or prepared until the patient is ready for the administration of the drug.
   a. anticoagulants
   b. antiplatelet agents
   c. diuretics
   d. tissue plasminogen activators

9. Which of the following is used as an antidote for heparin overdose?
   a. warfarin
   b. aminocaproic acid
   c. protamine sulfate
   d. tranexamic acid

10. Which of the following drugs is not an antihyperlipidemic drug?
    a. atorvastatin
    b. lovastatin
    c. colestipol
    d. verapamil

Critical Thinking Questions

1. Diagram the flow of the blood through the body.

2. Explain the process of blood oxygenation and carbon dioxide exchange.

3. Why might a doctor prescribe a diuretic along with an antihypertensive drug for a patient with hypertension?

Web Challenge

1. To view an animation of how the heart works, go to http://www.smm.org/heart/

2. Find out how much you know about heart disease. Go to http://www.webmd.com/content/tools/1/quiz_heart_disease and take the heart disease quiz.

References and Resources

Adams, M.P., D.L. Josephson, and L.N. Holland Jr. *Pharmacology for Nurses: A Pathophysiologic Approach.* (4th edition.) Upper Saddle River, NJ: Pearson, 2013.

"Arteriosclerosis/Atherosclerosis." http://www.mayoclinic.com/health/arteriosclerosis-atherosclerosis/DS00525. 10 July 2007. Web.

"Atherosclerosis." http://www.americanheart.org/presenter.jhtml?identifier=4440. 10 July 2007. Web.

"Cholesterol." http://www.americanheart.org. 15 October 2007. Web.

"Endocardium and Periocardium." http://www.medterms.com/script/main/art.asp?articlekey=3236. 8 April 2008. Web.

"Geriatic Drug Review: Nitrobid." http://agenet.agenet.com/?Url=link.asp?DOC/1339. 6 April 2008. Web.

Holland, N. and M.P. Adams. *Core Concepts in Pharmacology.* (3rd edition.) Upper Saddle River, NJ: Pearson, 2010.

"Hypertension: Symptoms of High Blood Pressure." www.webmd.com. 9 July 2007. Web.

"Lymphatic System." http://www.innerbody.com/image/lympov.html. 8 April 2008. Web.

Maybaum, S. *Medical Treatments for Congestive Heart.* Columbia, NY: New York Presbyterian Hospital and Ainat Beniaminovitz.

"Myofilaments, Sarcoplasmic Reticulum (SR)." www.biology.eku.edu/RITCHISO/301notes3.htm. 1 April 2008. Web.

"Spleen Disorders." http://www.merck.com/mrkshared/mmanual_home2/sec14/ch179/ch179a.jsp. 1 April 2008. Web.

"The Cardiac Cycle." http://www.jdaross.cwc.net/cardiac_cycle.htm. 8 April 2008. Web.

"The Heart." http://www.leeds.ac.uk/chb/HUMB2040/prac3thor.pdf. 8 April 2008. Web.

"Thrombophlebitis." http://www.nlm.nih.gov/medlineplus/thrombophlebitis.html. 8 April 2013. Web.

"What is Coronary Heart Disease?" http://www.nhlbi.nih.gov/health/dci/Diseases/Cad/CAD_WhatIs.html. 9 July 2013. Web.

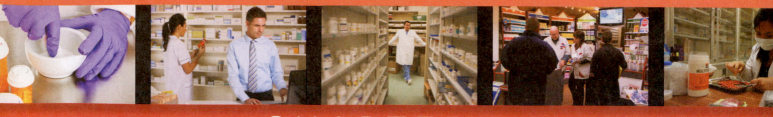

CHAPTER 30

The Immune System

LEARNING OBJECTIVES

After completing this chapter, you should be able to:

- Explain how the body's nonspecific and specific defense mechanisms work to keep the body safe from disease-causing microorganisms.

- Understand the basic relationships between the immune system and the various body systems.

- List and describe the different types of infectious organisms.

- List the five stages of progression of HIV to AIDS.

- Explain how the different classes of HIV drugs work.

- Describe autoimmune disease, and identify various types.

- Understand how drug resistance develops, and what steps can be taken to stop it.

- List and define common anti-infective drug classifications, their mechanisms of action, and their side effects.

- Describe both tuberculosis and malaria and their causes, treatments, and prevention.

- Identify the different types and uses of vaccines, and how they work in the body.

KEY TERMS

aerobic, p. 498

anaerobic, p. 498

antibodies, p. 495

antigens, p. 497

complement, p. 497

DNA, p. 498

epitope, p. 495

genome, p. 501

hematopoietic, p. 497

lysis, p. 518

macrophage, p. 495

pathogen, p. 497

phagocyte, p. 495

RNA, p. 498

INTRODUCTION

The immune system protects the body from foreign invaders that would otherwise destroy it, or parts of it, via infection or cancer. The immune system uses numerous kinds of responses to fend off attacks from these foreign invaders and is amazingly effective most of the time. Its defensive barriers and mechanisms include the skin, mucus, and cilia in the linings of the respiratory and digestive passageways, the blood clotting process, white blood cells and other infection-fighting substances, the thymus gland, and the lymph nodes.

Many different classes of medications affect the immune system. These include drugs for the treatment of human immunodeficiency virus (HIV)/acquired immune deficiency syndrome (AIDS), tuberculosis (TB), and malaria, as well as for many other immune-related conditions and diseases. It is important for pharmacy technicians to have a clear understanding of what these drugs are, and how they work to protect the body.

The Body's Defense Mechanisms

A human body protects itself with nonspecific defense mechanisms, which are considered the first line of defense against disease and infection. Specific defense mechanisms are the body's second line of defense. When these mechanisms fail or are destroyed and leave a person susceptible to infection, the person is said to be *immunosuppressed* or *immunocompromised*.

Nonspecific Defense Mechanisms

Nonspecific defense mechanisms include physical barriers, natural deterrents (fluids or chemicals and immune cells that prevent or attack invaders), and the inflammatory process. These mechanisms effectively reduce the workload of the immune system by preventing the entry and spread of microorganisms in the body. The body's physical and anatomical barriers against disease and infection include the following:

- Mucus in the respiratory tract—traps particles and microbes before they can infect the lungs.
- Vertebral column, spinal cord fluid, and the meninges—protect the central nervous system from injury or infection.
- Skin—protects the inside of the body from attack with its hard, dry, dead skin cell layer and its salty and somewhat acidic pH. These qualities of skin work together to prevent microorganisms from reproducing and growing.

phagocyte a specialized cell that engulfs and ingests other cells.

macrophage a white blood cell, found primarily in connective tissue and the bloodstream.

antibodies proteins that specifically seek and bind to the surface of pathogens or antigens.

epitope a region on the surface of an antigen that is capable of producing an immune response.

Natural physiological deterrents to pathogens include the following:

- Acidic secretions of the vagina—create an environment that prevents the growth of many pathogens.
- Tears—continually flush irritants and microorganisms out of the eyes.
- Lysozyme—an enzyme that breaks down bacterial cell walls and aids in the prevention of microorganism growth. Lysozyme is present in tears, saliva, mucus, blood, sweat, and many other tissue fluids.
- Nonspecific immune system cells, such as **phagocytes** and **macrophages**, can detect, target, track, engulf, and kill invading microorganisms, host cells, and debris.

Blood components act as defense mechanisms in the following ways:

- Clotting factors found in blood cause clotting at the site of injury (scabbing), which can prevent pathogens from entering or invading. This is a type of *perimeter* effect.
- Proteins aid in inflammation and release of phagocytes. Proteins bind to the surface of bacterial or viral host cells and destroy (*lyse*) them. Inflammation can aid in prevention or recognition of invasion; however, uncontrolled inflammation may lead to more tissue damage and even death.

The *normal flora* consists of a group of microorganisms that occur naturally in the mouth, skin, and gastrointestinal (GI) tract. These flora do not usually cause disease unless they move outside of their natural environment. Instead, they prevent infection by exogenous microorganisms by competing with them so that the foreign pathogens cannot penetrate, invade, or grow in the human host tissues.

Suppression of the natural endogenous microorganisms of the normal flora (*good* microorganisms) allows opportunistic exogenous (*bad*) microorganisms to infect and cause disease. The natural flora may become suppressed during antibiotic treatment, in some females, or in some cancer patients during chemotherapy.

Specific Defense Mechanisms

When the nonspecific mechanisms of defense fail, the body initiates a second, specific, line of defense—the immune system (see Table 30-1). The immune system can create specialized protein molecules and cells that function to fight foreign invaders. Two types of these specialized protein molecules are called *antibodies* and *complement*. In simple terms, antibodies mark an invading substance as a target; complement destroys the invader.

Antibodies, sometimes called *immunoglobulins,* have a concave area on the surface called a *combining site*. The **epitopes** of antigens fit perfectly into the combining sites of antibodies. When the two combine with or bind to each other, the antigen is inactivated and unable to harm the body. This process makes a toxin nonpoisonous or makes harmful substances stick together (*agglutinate*). Macrophages or phagocytes then consume the disabled foreign invaders. The ability of antibodies to disable or inactivate foreign invaders is called *humoral immunity*.

TABLE 30-1 Relationships between Body Systems and the Immune System

System	The System's Role in and Effect on the Immune System	The Immune System's Effects on and Role in the System
Integumentary	• Provides a physical barrier to microorganisms. • Utilizes inflammation as a caution signal. • Aids in reduction and prevention of further inflammation.	• Provides antibodies found in skin (IgA, IgG, etc.) to assist in immune function of protection.
Digestive	• Provides important nutrients to the lymph tissues. • Digestive acids/enzymes destroy microorganisms.	• The tonsils destroy infective bacteria and viruses of the mouth and throat. • Lymph vessels carry absorbed lipids to the bloodstream.
Musculoskeletal	• Muscles protect and cushion lymph nodes and vessels. • Muscles contract to help push lymphatic fluid through vessels, into the circulatory system, and to elimination. • Lymphocytes and other immune cells are produced and stored in bone marrow.	• Assists in repair after injuries. • Assists in repair of bone. • Macrophages (phagocytes) fuse to make bone cells.
Respiratory	• Lung cells present antigens to trigger the immune defense response. • Provides essential oxygen and eliminates carbon dioxide, both necessary for optimum immune cell function.	• Tonsils, which are lymphoid tissue, protect against infection at the entrance to the respiratory tract. • Lungs remove inhaled and deposited solid material and microorganisms. • Plays a supportive role in maintaining and eliminating fluids.
Circulatory	• Distributes white blood cells and antibodies. • Clotting factors in blood make thrombi to assist as barriers to microorganisms.	• Fights circulatory and blood vessel infections. • Returns interstitial tissue fluid to circulation via veins.
Renal	• Eliminates waste produced by immune cells as a by-product of reproduction, phagocytosis, and attack. • Acidic pH of urine kills microorganisms.	• Fights bladder and kidney infections.
Endocrine	• Adrenal gland corticosteroid hormones have an anti-inflammatory effect. • Thymus hormone, *thymosin*, stimulates the development and maturation of lymphocytes.	• Thymus gland secretes thymosin.
Reproductive	• Certain enzymes (*lysozymes*) and chemicals in vaginal and other body secretions kill bacterial microorganisms. • Reproductive hormones have been shown to regulate the immune system. Estrogen has been shown to regulate the expression, distribution, and activity of immune chemicals called *cytokines*.	• Produces antibodies to assist in immune system function. • Through cytokine- and interleukin-mediated pathways, regulates the reproductive system by inducing the release of gonadotropins (luteinizing hormone and follicle-stimulating hormone).
Nervous	• Neurons have antigens that stimulate specific immune defense responses—the second line of defense.	• Produces *cytokines*, immune hormones that affect the production of other hormones by the hypothalamus.

Complement is a group of normally inactive enzymes that is activated by the antibodies and **antigen** attachment. The antibody-antigen binding changes the shape of the antigen, exposing two complement binding sites. This activates two different complement enzymes, each of which binds to one of the sites. Thus, the antibody *holds* the antigen and makes it vulnerable while the complement enzymes bind to it. The function of complement is to kill invading cells by *drilling* a hole in the cell membrane wall, which allows body fluid to fill the inside of the invading cell and burst it open. There are about 30 different complement enzymes in the plasma.

The specific immune response empowers the body to seek and target specific **pathogens** and the body's own infected cells for destruction. It depends on specialized white blood cells called *lymphocytes*, which include *T cells* (produced from lymphocytes that matured in the thymus gland) and *B cells* (produced from lymphocytes that matured in the bone marrow). There are two complementary parts of the specific immune response: the cell-mediated response and the antibody-mediated response.

The *cell-mediated response* involves T cells and is responsible for the following:

- Destroying body cells that are infected with a virus.
- Destroying cancerous cells (mutated cells that grow rapidly).
- Activating other immune cells to be more efficient pathogen killers.

The *antibody-mediated response* involves both T cells and B cells and is necessary for the destruction of invading pathogens and for the elimination of toxins. After a macrophage engulfs a pathogen, both the cell-mediated and antibody-mediated responses commence. Macrophages digest the pathogen and then exhibit antigens from the pathogen on their surfaces. By this *flagging* or targeting of pathogenic proteins, the macrophages stimulate specific helper T cells to release signal molecules called *lymphokines*. The lymphokines, in turn, stimulate both the cell-mediated and antibody-mediated responses.

In the cell-mediated response, the lymphokines released from the helper T cells stimulate killer T cells and phagocytic cells to help destroy the pathogen-infected cells. These natural killer T cells attach themselves to the pathogen-infected cells and destroy them; phagocytic cells produce toxin molecules that directly kill the pathogen.

In the antibody-mediated response, the lymphokines activate specific B cells to produce antibodies that act like a *flag* or signal to the phagocytic cells. Other B cells go on to become *memory B cells*, which respond by quickly producing more antibodies upon future infection by the same pathogen—even if the reinfection is years later. The memory of healthy B cells lasts for the person's lifetime. The memory B cell response is very quick, so the pathogen does not have time to reproduce enough to cause disease before the host's body destroys it. The effectiveness of vaccination is explained by the mechanism of the memory response, which prevents many diseases even at the first encounter.

Lymphocytes

Immune system cells are *on the lookout* for invading cells and other foreign substances that may have entered the body. *Lymphocytes* circulate within the body fluids, especially the blood and lymph, and may reside in the lymph nodes, lymphatic tissue, thymus gland, spleen, or liver. Lymphocytes are made in the bone marrow from primitive cells called **hematopoietic** stem cells. Lymphocytes may be either B cells or T cells.

B cells are produced and matured in the bone marrow. After entering the bloodstream, they are carried to the lymph nodes (see Figure 30-1), where they multiply and divide. If the B cell attaches to an antigen that fits into its receptor site, it becomes an activated B cell. These activated B cells transform into either *plasma cells* or *memory B cells*. Plasma cells immediately make and secrete hundreds of thousands of antibodies

---

complement a large group of proteins that are activated in sequence when cells are exposed to a foreign substance; activation eventually results in the death or destruction of the substance. In general, complements amplify or enhance the effects of antibodies and inflammation.

antigens specific molecules that trigger an immune response.

pathogen a disease-causing organism.

hematopoietic blood-forming.

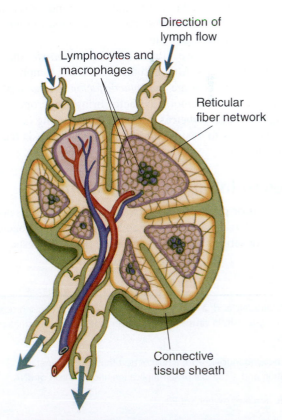

FIGURE 30-1 Lymph node and structure.

Direction of lymph flow

Lymphocytes and macrophages

Reticular fiber network

Connective tissue sheath

Common Cell Structures

All cells have at least three common structures:

- **Cell membrane**—a selectively permeable phospholipid membrane that allows some material to pass into or out of the cell while preventing other material from doing so.
- **Cytoplasm**—a fluid where cell respiration takes place; usually contains **RNA** (a nucleic acid that enables protein synthesis).
- **DNA**—the genetic code of an organism, floating freely in the cytoplasm of some cells or isolated inside the nucleus of other cells.

into the blood to attack the antigen, but they have a short life span. The B cells that are not converted to plasma cells transform into memory cells. These memory cells, which *remember* that particular invader, have a much longer life span; therefore, they quickly secrete the appropriate antibodies when the body comes into subsequent contact with the same antigen.

T cells are first produced by stem cells in the liver, just before and after birth. The T cells are then carried to the thymus gland, where they undergo the first stage of development; hence the name *T cell*. A T cell undergoes a second change when it moves to the lymph node, where it will reside. There, it develops a binding site, shaped for a specific protein, that will attach to a specific kind of antigen. This binding sensitizes the T cell and allows it to produce cell-mediated immunity or resistance to disease organisms.

Some T cells release a toxin, called *lymphotoxin,* that kills foreign invading cells. Although there are many lymphotoxins, two of the primary ones are *chemotactic factor* and *macrophage-activating factor*. Chemotactic factor brings macrophages to invading substances, whereas macrophage-activating factor tells the macrophages to destroy the cells by phagocytosis (eating/engulfing them).

Types of Infectious Organisms

Any animal or plant microorganism that causes a disease is called a *pathogen*. Animal pathogens are parasites, bacteria, rickettsia, or viruses. Plant pathogens are fungi or yeasts.

RNA ribonucleic acid; a nucleic acid needed for the metabolic processes of protein synthesis. In viruses, RNA may carry the genetic information of the virus.

DNA deoxyribonucleic acid; a nucleic acid that carries genetic information and is capable of self-replication and synthesis of RNA.

aerobic requires oxygen for life.

anaerobic does not require oxygen for life.

Animal Microorganisms

The differences in pathogens can be observed under a microscope. They vary in shape, size, motility, and other characteristics.

Parasites

Parasites may be bacterial, protozoal, or helminthes. The most common parasites in the United States are pinworms, roundworms, and tapeworms. Transmission usually occurs via ingestion of contaminated food or soil. Some types are large enough to see with the naked eye. Infecting worms can perforate the intestines by burrowing. They can also do this to the muscles, lungs, and liver.

Parasites can damage or block organs by clumping together in balls. These balls are often mistaken for cancer tumors, as they travel into the brain, heart, or lungs. These worms rob the host of the crucial vitamins, minerals, and amino acids needed for human digestion and nutrition, leaving some people anemic or drowsy after meals. Some worms give off metabolic waste products that are poisonous to their human hosts (*verminous intoxification*). The toxins are not easily eliminated and usually are reabsorbed through the intestines. Because it must work harder to counteract these toxins, the immune system becomes overtaxed and suppressed, which leads to further fatigue and leaves the host vulnerable to other illnesses. Symptoms of parasitic infestation are diarrhea, loss of appetite, intense anal itching (worms lay eggs there), and abdominal cramping.

Protozoa

Protozoa are single-celled eukaryotes that play a vital role in controlling the numbers of bacteria. (Note, though, that bacteria are necessary for maintaining soil, plant, and animal and human life.) An example is the protozoan that lives in the mosquito and is transmitted via a mosquito bite, causing malaria. There are four types of protozoa, distinguished by their methods of obtaining food:

- *Ameboids* are protozoa that most often consume algae, bacteria, or other protozoans.
- *Ciliates* have a specialized opening in the outer edge to capture their prey.
- *Zooflagellates* exist in symbiotic relationships, meaning that their coexistence in another living creature has mutual benefits.
- *Sporozoans* are parasites that live inside a host and often cause disease by robbing the host of vital nutrients.

Bacteria

Most bacteria are round (*coccus/cocci*), rod-shaped (*bacillus/bacilli*), or spiral-shaped. These organisms can be **aerobic** or **anaerobic**. Bacteria are unicellular, prokaryotic microorganisms that multiply by dividing or splitting into two parts in a process called *binary fission. Bacteria* is plural and *bacterium* is singular.

A *coccus* bacterium is spherical, oval, elongated, or flattened on one side and has an approximate measurement of about 0.5 μm in diameter. After cell replication, division in one plane produces the following:

- *Coccus*—one bacterium.
- *Diplococcus*—two bacteria connected side by side.
- *Streptococcus*—several bacteria aligned in a row or a chain (which may be straight or curved).

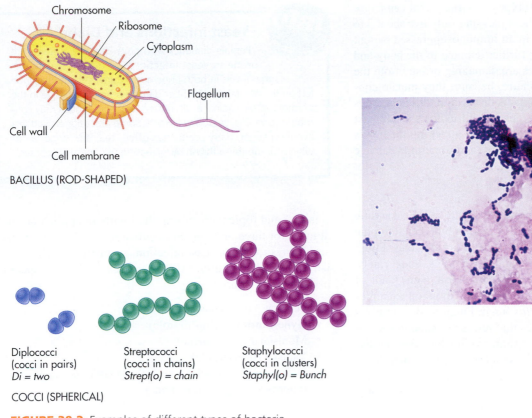

FIGURE 30-2 Examples of different types of bacteria.

Division in two planes produces a *tetrad* arrangement of four bacteria in a square. Division in three planes produces a *sarcina* arrangement, an *eight-pack* cube. Division in random planes produces a *staphylococcus* arrangement, which looks like a bunch of grapes (see Figure 30-2). Examples of the latter are *Staphylococcus aureus*, which causes skin, respiratory, and wound infections and *Clostridium tetani,* which produces a toxin that can be lethal to humans.

A *bacillus*, or rod-shaped, bacterium has an approximate measurement of 0.5 to 1 μm in width and from 1 to 4 μm in length. Bacillus bacteria are found in three possible arrangements:

- *Bacillus*—a single bacterium.
- *Streptobacillus*—a chain or a string of bacilli.
- *Coccobacillus*—an oval bacillus similar to oval cocci.

Spiral or wave-shaped bacteria appear in one of the following arrangements:

- *Vibrio*—a comma-shaped or resembling part of a wave.
- *Spirillium*—a rigid spiral wave.
- *Spirochete*—a thin and flexible spiral wave.

Rickettsia

Rickettsia is the genus of several parasitic microorganisms, made up of small rod-shaped coccoids, that live in the gut of arthropods such as lice, fleas, ticks, and mites. These bacteria are transmitted to humans and other animals via a bite. The diseases they cause in humans have flu-like symptoms and include typhus, scrub typhus, Q fever, and Rocky Mountain spotted fever.

Viruses

A *virus* is an ultramicroscopic infectious pathogen that can replicate only within cells of a living host by using the DNA and RNA of the host. Viruses consist of nucleic acid covered by protein, although some animal viruses are surrounded by a membrane. Viruses are both nonliving pathogens and intracellular parasites. Very tiny and surrounded by a capsid or protein coating, a basic virus contains only a few genes (DNA and RNA) with which it replicates itself by commandeering the *machinery* inside the host cell. Although most viruses are host-specific, some can cross, or *jump*, species. It is thought that HIV, the retrovirus that causes AIDS, jumped species from monkeys to humans. Figure 30-3 shows an illustration of a virus.

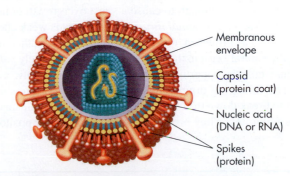

FIGURE 30-3 An illustration of a virus.

There are more than 200 types of viruses that can cause the common cold. Although these parasites only live about 3 to 10 days in a healthy human, in an immunosuppressed patient they can live longer, causing further damage to the body and immune system. Some viruses are damaging or fatal from the start. Viruses are difficult to cure, because they mutate constantly and develop different strains that require different drugs for treatment. In addition, because the virus lives inside host cells, attacking the virus usually means attacking the host's own cells. This leads to suppression of (and sometimes damage to) whatever system is affected.

Plant Microorganisms

Fungus is a plant-like, filamentous, or single-celled eukaryotic organism characterized by a lack of chlorophyll, heterotrophic growth, and the production of extracellular enzymes. Fungi include yeasts, molds, mildews, and mushrooms. Fungi can be parasitic or saprobic. Canker sores, ringworm, some kinds of molds, and mildews are fungal diseases. Common examples are the *Candida* and *Aspergillus* fungi. Fungi feed themselves by secreting digestive enzymes that release organic molecules from the tree, soil, or organism (human) in which they are living. The fungus then absorbs those released organic molecules. Fungal infections flourish in moisture, heat, and darkness; tropical conditions allow fungi to grow easily. Athlete's foot is an example of growth of fungus in a moist, hot, dark environment—the sneaker. Fungal infections of the blood are the hardest to cure. Many drugs used to fight fungal and yeast infection end in *azole*. Examples are ketoconazole (which has many drug interactions), sulfamethoxazole, fluconazole, and itraconazole. Another antifungal drug is amphotericin B, which can have many side effects.

Yeast is a microscopic, dehydrated, hydrophilic single-celled organism of the fungus family, which eats sugar and produces alcohol and carbon dioxide as it grows and ferments. *Candida albicans* is a yeast-like fungus that causes vaginal yeast infections (*candidiasis*). *Candida glabrata* is a more resistant yeast that also causes thrush and vaginal yeast infections.

Antibiotics taken to kill pathogenic bacteria may also kill friendly bacteria that are part of the normal flora. These bacteria, such as lactobacilli, help to keep yeast in the vagina under control. Without lactobacilli, the balance of yeast in the vagina is disrupted and *Candida* can take over. Antibiotics have no effect on yeast itself; however, they can change the environment in the vagina just enough to cause a yeast overgrowth or infection (also known as *vaginal thrush*). If the body is weak after an illness such as influenza, or too busy fighting off another infection, the natural yeast in the body may not be adequately *policed* and may take the opportunity to multiply uncontrollably.

The following drugs are antifungals that work in similar ways to break down the cell wall of the *Candida* organism until it disintegrates. They are available as vaginal suppositories

Yeast Infections and Diabetes

Female diabetics with poor immune systems are prone to yeast infections, as diabetes increases sugar levels in both urine and vaginal secretions. Urine left on the genital area, tight or damp clothing, a change in the normally acidic vaginal environment, and some foods may contribute to vaginal yeast overgrowth. Some practitioners suggest avoiding sugar, dairy products, coffee, tea, and wine, all of which contribute to thrush by increasing urinary sugar content.

(inserts) and topical creams applied with an applicator once at night for three or seven consecutive nights. It takes at least seven days to cure a yeast infection, no matter which administration method is used. All the applications in the specific package must be used.

- Femstat 3 (butoconazole nitrate)
- Gyne-Lotrimin (clotrimazole)
- Monistat 7 (miconazole)
- Vagistat (tioconazole)
- Diflucan (fluconazole), one 150-mg tablet po×1 dose (approved for yeast infections)

HIV/AIDS

HIV can be categorized as either HIV-1 or HIV-2. Unless specified otherwise, most references here are to HIV-1, the most common worldwide. Both types are transmitted by sexual contact; through blood, semen, and vaginal fluid; and from mother to child. Both types of HIV cause clinically indistinguishable AIDS. AIDS is the eventual outcome of HIV infection, as the body's immune system becomes severely suppressed and cannot fight opportunistic infections. People with AIDS often suffer lung, brain, skin, eye, and other organ diseases along with diarrhea, debilitating weight loss, candidiasis and other fungal infections, toxoplasmosis, dementia, and Kaposi's sarcoma. The presence of HIV antibodies in the blood confirms that an individual has been infected. On March 19, 2004, the FDA approved the first oral fluid-based rapid HIV test kit (Ora-Quick), which provides results in 20 minutes with more than 99% accuracy.

Five-Stage Progression of HIV to AIDS to Death

- Stage 1—initial transmission and infection with HIV
- Stage 2—infection without presentation of signs or symptoms (may last 10 or more years)
- Stage 3—signs and symptoms of HIV begin to appear
- Stage 4—AIDS opportunistic infections begin; CD4 cell count or level at or below 200 per cubic millimeter of blood
- Stage 5—final stage of wasting and infections; ends in death

genome the complete hereditary material or code of an organism.

HIV/AIDS Drugs

Reverse transcriptase inhibitors block the conversion of the HIV single-strand viral RNA to double-strand viral DNA, thus preventing the synthesis of copies of the viral RNA. There are two types of reverse transcriptase:

- *Nucleoside analogs,* often called *nukes*, mimic the building blocks used by reverse transcriptase to make copies of the HIV genetic material. The fake building blocks interrupt or interfere with viral replication.
- *Nonnucleoside* reverse transcriptase inhibitors (NNRTIs) prevent the reverse transcriptase enzyme from working.

Once the new double-strand hybrid DNA is transcribed to a viral RNA, the RNA serves as a **genome** for new HIV viruses. *Protease inhibitors (PIs)* block the protease enzyme, which blocks translation. This means that the HIV makes copies of itself that cannot infect new cells. Studies have proven that PIs can reduce the amount of virus in the blood and increase CD4 cell counts.

Currently, the best way to avoid drug resistance is to stop or reduce production of HIV virus in the body. The less HIV there is in the body, the less chance there will be of creating a virus that is resistant to anti-HIV drugs. It is recommended that PIs be taken in combination with at least two other anti-HIV drugs (see Table 30-2). This treatment protocol is known as *highly active anti-retroviral therapy (HAART).* The implementation of HAART increases the anti-HIV effect and prevents or overcomes resistance; this is sometimes referred to as *protease boosting.* Drug resistance tests are ordered to determine which combination of drugs to use. The following is an example of one such combination, or *cocktail*, given to HIV/AIDS patients:

Zidovudine	+	Lamivudine	+	Efavirenz
600 mg/day		300 mg/day		600 mg/day

TABLE 30-2 Antiretroviral Agents

Anti-AIDS Drug Classification	Trade/Generic Name	Possible Side Effects
Vaccine	In research	—
Attachment inhibitors	In research	—
Fusion (fusion inhibitors)	Fuzeon (enfuvirtide)	Itching, swelling, redness, pain, tenderness, hardened skin and bumps near the injection sites, asthenia, insomnia, depression, myalgia, constipation, pancreas problems, numbness of feet and legs, dyspnea, fever, uremia, peripheral edema (feet)
Reverse Transcriptase Inhibitors		
Nucleoside reverse transcriptase	Combivir (zidovudine + lamivudine) (AZT + 3TC)	Headache, nausea
	Emtriva (emtricitabine) (FTC)	Skin rash and skin discoloration on palms and soles
	Epivir (lamivudine) (3TC)	Lactic acidosis
	Epzicom (abacavir + lamivudine) (ABC + 3TC)	Severe hepatomegaly with steatosis Possible redistribution of body fat, peripheral wasting, facial wasting, breast enlargement, and cushingoid appearance
	Hivid (zalcitabine) (ddC)	
	Retrovir (zidovudine) (AZT or ZDV)	
	Trizivir (abacavir + zidovudine + lamivudine) (ABC + AZT + 3TC)	
	Truvada (tenofovir disoproxil fumarate + emtricitabine) (TDF + FTC)	
	Videx (didanosine, buffered versions); Videx EC (didanosine, delayed-release capsules)	

(Continued)

TABLE 30-2 Antiretroviral Agents (*Continued*)

Anti-AIDS Drug Classification	Trade/Generic Name	Possible Side Effects
	Viread (tenofovir disoproxil fumarate) (TDF or Bis(POC) PMPA)	
	Zerit (stavudine) (d4T)	
	Ziagen (abacavir) (ABC)	
Nonnucleoside reverse transcriptase (NNRTIs)	Viramune (nevirapine)	Headache
	Rescriptor (delavirdine mesylate)	Dizziness
	Sustiva (efavirenz)	Fatigue
		Nausea, vomiting, diarrhea
		Rash (may be severe)
		Liver problems that can be severe and life-threatening. Regular blood tests may be needed to monitor for liver problems.
		Insomnia
		Drowsiness (sedation)
Protease inhibitors	Agenerase (amprenavir)	Increased blood pressure
	Lexiva (fosamprenavir)	Diabetes
	Crixivan (indinavir)	Lipodystrophy—inability to absorb fat
	Kaletra (lopinavir/ritonavir)	Liver toxicity may worsen hepatitis
	Norvir (ritonavir)	
	Invirase and Fortovase (saquinavir)	
	Viracept (nelfinavir)	
	Zrivada (atazanavir)	

Autoimmune Diseases

A person with an autoimmune disease has an immune system that mistakenly targets and attacks the cells, tissues, and organs of its own body. The immune system cells and molecules accumulate at a target site in a gathering broadly referred to as *inflammation*. Approximately 75% of autoimmune diseases affect women.

Some autoimmune diseases are prevalent in specific populations. For example, lupus is more common in Hispanic and African-American women than in Caucasian women of European ancestry. Rheumatoid arthritis and scleroderma affect more residents of some Native American communities than the general population of the United States.

Autoimmune diseases are not contagious and are not related to AIDS or cancer (see Table 30-3). Many are inherited, some are triggered by sunlight (lupus), others are caused by dormant viruses that are reactivated and mistakenly *protected*

by the immune system, while the original antibody is attacked (such as in the case of rheumatoid arthritis). Most autoimmune diseases are not curable but are treatable with appropriate drug therapy to manage daily living.

Therapeutic agents that slow or suppress immune system response, in an attempt to stop the inflammation during an autoimmune attack, are called *immunosuppressive medications*. These drugs include corticosteroids, azathioprine, cyclosporin, cyclophosphamide, and methotrexate (MTX). Unfortunately, these medications also suppress the ability of the immune system to fight true infections, and they cause potentially serious adverse reactions. The common pharmacotherapeutic goal in the care of patients with autoimmune diseases is to discover treatments that produce remissions with few side effects. New research for agents that have therapeutic antibodies against specific T cell molecules may produce drugs with fewer long-term side effects than the chemotherapies currently being used.

TABLE 30-3 Common Autoimmune Diseases

Disease	Notes
Autoimmune Oophoritis and Orchitis	
Site of action: the gonads.	Endocrine system
Treatment includes: no known treatment or cure; hormone replacement therapy is used, but it cannot return fertility.	Patients with oopheritis may have premature menopause before 40 years of age, or the ovaries are destroyed before the first menstruation (no treatment available).
	Orchitis is an enlargement of the testis in which infertility antisperm antibody can be detected.
Crohn's Disease	
Site of action: the gut or intestine.	Gastrointestinal system
Treatment includes: Remicade (infliximab), a monoclonal antibody engineered as an inhibitor of tumor necrosis factor alpha, a protein that promotes inflammation in the body.	Inflammation of the bowel, both in the ileum (lower small intestine) and in the colon (large intestine), possibly caused by a reaction to a virus.
Entocort EC (budesonide), which uses the high affinity of budesonide for glucocorticosteroid receptors; potent anti-inflammatory effect about 200 times that of cortisol and 15 times that of prednisolone.	
Graves' Disease	
Site of action: the thyroid.	Endocrine system
Treatment includes: propylthiouracil iodine (radioactive).	Immune cells attack both the eye muscles and the thyroid, leading to dysfunction of both. This may cause hyperthyroidism and increased thyrotoxicosis that produces intolerance of heat and weight loss.
	May have exophthalmy in which the eyes appear protruded or unusually popped out
Lupus or Systemic Lupus Erythematosus	
Site of action: affects various tissues and organs; also varies among individuals with the same disease.	Multiple organs, including the musculoskeletal system
Treatment includes: corticosteroids, NSAIDs, immunosuppressant COX-2 inhibitors.	Ultimate damage to specific tissues may be permanent. Example is destruction of insulin-producing cells of the pancreas, resulting in Type 1 diabetes mellitus. Immune cell complexes and inflammatory molecules can block blood flow and ultimately destroy organs such as the kidney.
	Lupus may be worsened or triggered by sunlight.
Multiple Sclerosis	
Site of action: the brain.	Nervous system
Treatment includes: glatiramer acetate, interferon beta 1-a, interferon beta 1-b.	Patients with MS produce antibodies that attack the white matter in the brain and spinal cord, causing the myelin sheath, or coating of nerve fibers, to become inflamed in the brain and spinal cord, which results in an inability to transmit signals along the nerves.
Myasthenia Gravis	
Site of action: the muscles.	Nervous system

(Continued)

TABLE 30-3 Common Autoimmune Diseases *(Continued)*

Disease	Notes
Treatment includes: thymectomy (removal of thymus gland) to improve immune system function.	Autoantibodies attack a part of the nerve that stimulates muscle movement.
Plasmapheresis—abnormal antibodies are removed from the blood.	
High-dose intravenous immune globulin, which temporarily provides the body with normal antibodies from donated blood.	
Pernicious Anemia	
Site of action: the blood.	Circulatory system
Treatment includes: restorative vitamin B12 shots, folic acid.	Pernicious anemia is caused by the inability of the body to absorb vitamin B12 from the digestive tract into the bloodstream; the supply of this vital nutrient to organs and bone marrow is compromised and eventually results in immune attack on organs such as the liver, spleen, kidneys, heart, and brain.
Psoriasis	
Site of action: the skin. Treatment includes: corticosteroids such as Dovonex (calcipotriene). Coal tars, Anthra-Derm (anthralin). Topical receptor-selective retinoid—tazarotene (thought to normalize the proliferation of keratinocytes as well as to decrease cutaneous inflammation). Immunosuppressive dimeric fusion protein—Amevive (alefacept) primarily blocks the activation of immune system T cells.	Integumentary system Very small areas of skin or the entire body may be covered with a buildup of red and silvery scales called *plaques*; may be painful and unattractive. Epidermal cell kinetics with abnormal activation of immune mechanisms are thought to be the major contributors.
Rheumatoid Arthritis	
Site of action: the joints and other tissues and organs.	Multiple organs including the musculoskeletal system
Treatment includes: DMARDs, which slow down the disease process by modifying the immune system in some way other than by inhibition of prostaglandin.	In rheumatoid arthritis, reactive oxygen intermediate molecules and other toxic molecules are made by overproductive macrophages and neutrophils that invade the joints. The toxic molecules contribute to inflammation, which is observed as warmth and swelling, and participate in damaging the joint.
Scleroderma	
Site of action: the skin and blood vessels. Treatment includes: pallative only; no cure. Immunosuppressants—cyclophosphamide. Nifedipine and calcium channel blockers. Antibiotics.	*Cytokines*, proteins that may cause surrounding immune system cells to become activated, grow, or die; may also influence nonimmune system tissues. Some cytokines may contribute to the thickening of the skin and blood vessels that is symptomatic of scleroderma. Systemic sclerosis (scleroderma) is characterized by fibrosis of the skin, vasculature (blood vessels), and internal organs.
Ulcerative Colitis	
Site of action: the large intestine. Treatment includes: anti-inflammatories—aka 5-ASA (mesalamine), Azulfidine (sulfasalazine), Asacol (sulfur-free), Pentasa, Colazal (balsalazide), Rowasa enema, corticosteroids. Immunosuppressants—Imuran, 6-MP, cyclosporin. Immune modulators—Remicade (infliximab).	Gastrointestinal system An irritable bowel disease; inflammation due to ulcers of a part of the large intestine, or the entire colon and rectum, possibly resulting from a weakened immune response to bacteria.

(Continued)

TABLE 30-3 Common Autoimmune Diseases *(Continued)*

Disease	Notes
Vitiligo	
Site of action: the skin.	Integumentary system
Treatment includes: pallative with cosmetics and self-tanning products.	The body makes antibodies to its own pigment cells or melanocytes, creating patches of lighter skin.
	Cycles of pigment loss, followed by remission during which the pigment does not change, may continue indefinitely.

Gram Staining

The *Gram stain* is a method of identifying and separating two main types of bacteria. This important technique is named after Hans Christian Gram, a Danish bacteriologist who devised the test in 1844. It is almost always the first test performed for the identification of bacteria in culture and sensitivity (C&S) laboratory tests. The main stain used in Gram staining is crystal violet, although methylene blue is sometimes substituted. The microorganisms that retain the crystal violet–iodine complex appear purple/brown or blue when examined under a microscope. The microorganisms that stain blue or purple are commonly classified as gram-positive (or gram-nonnegative). Other bacteria, not stained by crystal violet but appearing red, are referred to as gram-negative. The theory of Gram staining is based on the ability of the bacterial cell wall to retain the violet dye during a solvent treatment. The cell walls of gram-positive microorganisms have a higher peptidoglycan (a protein) and lower lipid content than gram-negative bacteria and thus retain the dye.

Methods of Transmission of Pathogens

Pathogens are transmitted by three main routes: ingestion, inhalation, and physical contact. Sexually transmitted diseases (STDs) are transmitted via physical contact. The most common form of transmission of pathogens is via unwashed hands. Microorganisms can survive on inanimate objects, such as desks, pencils, and doorknobs, for a very long time. Thus, handwashing is the number one method for preventing the transmission of pathogens and the most important way in which you can prevent pathogens from contaminating a drug being prepared.

Anti-Infectives

Anti-infective is an umbrella name under which various types of drugs are subclassified (see Table 30-4). Some anti-infectives treat bacteria only (antibacterials), whereas others treat viruses only (antivirals) or fungi only (antifungals). Other anti-infectives treat more than one type of pathogen. Another word for anti-infective is *antimicrobial* (against the growth of a microorganism or microbe).

Antibacterials

This section describes the various types of antibacterials.

Penicillins

Penicillins (PCNs) are divided into four groups of varying spectrum of activity: natural PCNs, penicillinase-resistant PCNs, amino PCNs, and extended-spectrum PCNs (see Tables 30-5). There are four *generations* of PCNs; each newer generation covers a broader spectrum of pathogens. PCNs work by binding to the proteins in the cell wall of a pathogen, inhibiting them from making the cell wall or continuing to grow. However, the cytoplasm continues to grow and eventually bursts out of the cell along with the nucleus, destroying the bacterial cell.

There are more allergies to PCNs than to any other drug classification. The usual reaction is a rash or GI disturbance. The worst case is a severe allergy that results in anaphylactic shock; epinephrine must be administered within 5 to 20 minutes or the person may die. In an anaphylactic reaction, there is swelling in the airway passages, such as the mouth, tongue, throat, nose/nasal tissue, or in the respiratory bronchi, bronchioles, or air sacs. When this happens, oxygen supply is cut off, and death may result if the patient is not treated appropriately and very quickly.

Cephalosporins are chemical cousins to PCNs, because they have a similar chemical structure. For this reason, any patient who has a known reaction to PCN must be monitored if given a cephalosporin, as there is a 5% to 20% chance that this patient may also be allergic to these anti-infectives (*cross-sensitivity*). A better choice for the PCN-allergic patient is macrolides, such as erythromycin, tetracyclines (TCNs), or quinalones.

The best antibacterial to use depends on the culprit pathogen. C&S tests are employed to identify the infecting bacterium so that drug and pathogen can be matched. Carbapenems may be used on stronger bacteria, but only when PCN is not effective or safe, due to cross-sensitivity to PCN and the potential for the adverse reactions of pseudomembranous colitis, heart failure, arrhythmias, and kidney or hepatic failure.

Certain enzymes produced by some bacteria provide resistance to specific antibiotics. These enzymes are produced by both gram-positive and gram-negative bacteria and are found on both chromosomes and plasmids. These enzymes counter

TABLE 30-4 Comparison of Various Anti-Infectives

Anti-infective Classification	Common Side Effects	Toxic Effects	Drug, Food, and Herb Interactions	Special Notes and Cross-Hypersensitivity
Antibacterials	Rash GI disturbances Nausea/vomiting/diarrhea (N/V/D) Stomach pain Vaginal itching or discharge	Anaphylactic shock	1. Reduces effect of birth control pills. 2. Avoid taking with hot drinks; the heat from the drink may stop the medicine from working or make it work too fast. 3. Cross-hypersensitivity to a similar drug/classification.	1. Patient who has been taking an antibiotic (AB) must tell doctor or dentist before having surgery with a general anesthetic. 2. ABs may cause incorrect results with some urine sugar tests used by patients with diabetes.
Penicillins (PCNs)	Most common side effects, plus allergic reactions	Anaphylactic shock	1. Drugs that reduce the effect of PCNs: chloramphenicol, erythromycin ethylsuccinate (EES), sulfonamides, TCNs, methotrexate (MTX). These drugs also increase chances of side effects.	1. Take PCNs with a full glass of water on an empty stomach (either one hour before or two hours after meals). 2. May be taken with food or milk to avoid GI upset. PCNs are high in sodium content.
Cephalosporins	Most common side effects, plus joint aches and pain	Anaphylactic shock for PCN cross-hypersensitive patients Severe or bloody diarrhea and/or black, tarry stools Chest pain Chills, cough, fever Painful or difficult urination Shortness of breath Sore throat, sores, ulcers, or white spots on lips or in mouth	1. Drugs that increase chance of bleeding: anticoagulants, dipyridamole sulfinpyrazone, ticarcillin, valproic acid, heparin, thrombolytic agents, furosemide. These drugs may increase blood levels of cefuroxime. 2. Avoid acidic fruit juices/drinks (e.g., grapefruit juice or orange juice) within one hour of taking this medication.	1. Hypersensitivity to PCN.
Tetracyclines (TCNs)	Most common side effects, plus may cause the teeth to become discolored and/or mottled.	Photosensitivity, which may cause a skin rash, itching, redness, or other discoloration of the skin, or a severe sunburn and thinning of skin, which could lead to skin cancer Slows down the growth of bones, especially in children	1. Drugs that reduce TCN effects: antacids or calcium supplements, cholestyramine, medicines containing iron and magnesium 2. Antagonistic effect: PCNs decrease TCN effect.	1. Patient who is taking TCN must tell doctor or dentist before having surgery with a general anesthetic. 2. Do not give to children under eight years of age.
Macrolides	Most common side effects, plus: Stomach upset or cramps Sore mouth or tongue Fever Loss of appetite	Anaphylactic shock (rare)	1. PCN may decrease the effect of EES. 2. May increase blood levels of theophyllin, warfarin, digoxin, dilantin, and tegretol.	1. Abnormal liver tests or liver dysfunction can also occur with erythromycin.

(Continued)

TABLE 30-4 Comparison of Various Anti-Infectives *(Continued)*

Anti-infective Classification	Common Side Effects	Toxic Effects	Drug, Food, and Herb Interactions	Special Notes and Cross-Hypersensitivity
Quinolones (fluoroquinolones)	Most common side effects, plus: Headache Restlessness	1. Status epilepticus and coma (rare) 2. Anaphylactic shock 3. Loss of consciousness 4. Photosensitivity	1. Do not take with food or drink that contains a lot of calcium, such as milk, yogurt, or cheese. 2. Caffeine or stimulant drugs will increase gamma-aminobutyric acid (GABA) inhibitory effect.	1. Take with a full glass of water on an empty stomach (either one hour before or two hours after meals). 2. If food must be eaten, avoid calcium. 3. Avoid antacids—take four hours before or after when taking Cipro; others two hours before or after. 4. Also a GABA inhibitor: contraindicated for patients with preexisting neurological problems or seizures.
Sulfur-containing antibiotics (e.g., trimethoprim-sulfamethoxazole)	Most common side effects, plus: Tiredness Headache Dizziness	1. Depression 2. Weakness 3. Eye light sensitivity 4. Yellowing of eyes/skin, dark urine 5. Abdominal pain 6. Ringing in the ears 7. Gastrointestinal problems, damage to kidneys, and anemia (rare)	1. Some diuretics and anticoagulants	Anything containing sulfur: 1. Cross-hypersensitivity to furosemide, birth control pills, acetazolamide, thiazide diuretics, oral antidiabetics, antiglaucoma agents, phenazopyridine (e.g., Pyridium). 2. Foods with preservatives or dyes. 3. Take with plenty of fluids; due to side effect crystalluria.

TABLE 30-5 Types of Penicillins

Groups of Penicillins	Examples	Spectrum	Specific Infections	Important Notes
Natural PCNs: first-generation PCNs	pen G benzathine (Bicillin IM) pen G potassium IM, IV/IM, IV pen G sodium pen V potassium (Pen V K, V-Cillin K, Pen-Vee K), po	Gram + streptococci pneumococci	Ear, throat, gonorrhea, syphilis	The least effective, though still used.
Penicillinase-resistant penicillins	cloxacillin (Tegopen), po dicloxacillin (Dynapen), po methocillin (Staphcillin), IM, IV nafcillin (UniPen, Nafcil), IM, IV oxacillin (Prostaphlin), po, IM, IV	Staph (resistant), *Staphylococcus aureus*	Endocarditis, abscesses, difficult-to-treat pneumonia	Effective against PCNase-producing organisms that are difficult to treat and do not respond to other-generation PCNs.

(Continued)

TABLE 30-5 Types of Penicillins (*Continued*)

Groups of Penicillins	Examples	Spectrum	Specific Infections	Important Notes
Aminopenicillins: second-generation PCNs	ampicillin (Omnipen), po, IM, IV amoxicillin (Amoxil), po bacampicillin (Spectrobid), po	Gram + and gram – organisms: *E. coli, Proteus mirabilis, Haemophilus influenzae*	Ear, urinary, and respiratory tract infections	Amoxicillin is well absorbed and causes less or no GI disturbance or diarrhea. Second-generation PCNs are not effective against PCNase-producing organisms.
Extended-Spectrum Penicillins				
Third-generation PCNs	carbenicillin (Geocillin) ticarcillin (Ticar)	Broader spectrum than second-generation PCNs, with gram + and gram – coverage: *Pseudomonas aeruginosa, Proteus vulgaris*	Difficult-to-treat respiratory and urinary tract infections	May require additional combination therapy with antibiotics such as aminoglycosides. Not resistant to PCNase.
Fourth-generation PCNs	mezlocillin (Mezlin), IM, IV piperacillin (Pipracil), IM, IV	Broader than third-generation PCNS, with gram + and gram– coverage: *Klebsiella pneumoniae, Bacterioides fragilis* (anaerobe), *Pseudomonas aeruginosa, Proteus vulgaris*	Serious infections of skin, urinary tract, and respiratory tract	Made with mono-sodium salts; reduce sodium intake. Great for CHF, HTN, or diabetic patients. To date, require IV therapy. May require combination therapy.

the antibacterial activity of the drugs, so the bacteria survive while the drug is altered and rendered inactive; meanwhile, the patient's infection gets worse.

Scientists were challenged to make a drug that would be impervious to (not affected by) these beta-lactamase enzymes, which are also called *penicillinases*. A drug or agent that destroys or interferes with the action of penicillinase or beta-lactamase is known as a *beta-lactamase inhibitor*.

Beta-lactamases work by hydrolysis of the beta-lactam ring of the basic PCN structure, which adds a molecule of water (H_2O) to the carbon-nitrogen bond and opens up the ring, thus making the PCN drug ineffective. Most extended-spectrum beta-lactamase (ESBL) enzymes remain susceptible to beta-lactamase inhibitors. Currently, there is no oral, broad-spectrum, penicillinase-resistant PCN; therefore, in some cases, combination therapy is required.

Table 30-6 shows some additional antibacterials that are related to PCNs.

Cephalosporins

Discovered in 1948, *cephalosporins* are grouped into four *generations* according to their antimicrobial properties (see Table 30-7). Each newer generation of cephalosporins has

significantly greater gram-negative antimicrobial properties than the preceding (earlier) generation. Likewise, older generations have better gram-positive coverage than the newer generations. The first generation is the oldest. The frequency of dosing decreases with increasing generation(s) as does palatability. Cephalosporins are chemical cousins to PCNs, and, like PCNs, bind to the proteins in the cell wall of the pathogen, inhibiting them from making the cell wall or growing. The cell wall collapses after the cell contents burst out. The body's natural defenses also continue to fight infection.

Tetracyclines

TCNs are used as systemic agents against acne, bacteria, protozoans, and as antirheumatic agents (see Table 30-8). Some unusual uses are as a diuretic, for the syndrome of inappropriate antidiuretic hormone, and as an intrapleural sclerosing agent. Use of TCNs by patients with diabetes, renal disease, or hepatic disease may make the condition worse. Use of this substance when it is outdated, warm, or changed in taste or appearance may cause *serious side effects*. TCN may be used to treat various systemic diseases, such as Lyme disease, malaria, shigellosis, and pneumothorax.

TABLE 30-6 Other Antibacterials Related to Penicillins

Classification	MOA	Examples	Spectrum and Specific Indications	Important Notes
Beta-lactamase inhibitors:	Block and inactivate the beta-lactamase enzyme, thereby not allowing the molecule to hydrolyze the basic PCN beta-lactam ring.	clavulanic acid+ amoxicillin (Augmentin)	Otitis media and acute otitis media caused by PCNase- or beta-lactamase-producing bacteria—strains of *H. influenzae*, *Streptococcus pneumoniae*, *M. catarrhalis*, *Klebsiella pneumoniae*, *E. coli*, *Enterobacter* sp., *S. aureus*, etc.	Used for suspected resistance to PCNase.
clavulanic acid,		clavulanic acid + ticarcillin (Timentin)		Mainly active against rapidly dividing bacteria.
sulbactam,		sulbactam+ ampicillin (Unasyn)		
tazobactam		tazobactam+ piperacillin (Zosyn)		
Carbapenems	Similar to PCNs: Interfere with synthesis of cell wall by binding to penicillin protein-binding targets.	meropenem (Merrem), IV	Complicated intra-abdominal infections due to clostridum, *E. coli*, *Peptostreptococcus*, *Bacterioides fragilis* (anaerobe)	Structurally related to PCNs. Can be used against PCNase-resistant organisms.
		imipenem-cilastatin (Primaxin), IM, IV	Bacterial meningitis due to *S. pneumonaiae*, *N. meningitides, H. influenzae*	
		ertapenem (Invanz), IM, IV		
Monobactams	Similar to PCNs: Interfere with synthesis of cell wall by binding specifically to protein 3 (PBP 3).	aztreonam (Azactam)	Skin, urinary, respiratory tract, gynecological, and intra-abdominal infections. Enterococcus and gram–bacteria.	Structurally related to PCNs. Can be used against PCNase-resistant organisms. Unlabeled use for PCNase-resistant gonorrhea as an alternative to spectinomycin.

TABLE 30-7 Cephalosporins

Drug	Route and Adult Dose
First Generation	
cefadroxil (Duricef, Ultracef)	po; 500 mg–1 gm qd–bid (maximum 2 gm/day)
cefazolin sodium (Ancef, Kefzol)	IM, IV; 250 mg–2 gm tid (maximum 12 gm/day).
cephalexin (Keflex)	po; 250–500 mg qid
Second Generation	
cefaclor (Ceclor)	po; 250–500 mg tid
cefamandole naftate	IM; 500 mg–1 gm tid–qid (maximum 12 gm/day)
cefonicid sodium (Monocid)	IM; 1 gm qd (maximum 2 gm/day)
cefprozil (Cefzil)	po; 250–500 mg qd–bid
cefuroxime sodium (Ceftin, Kefurox, Zinacef)	po; 250–500 mg bid Can be given via IV route as well.
Third Generation	
cefdinir (Omnicef)	po; 300 mg bid
cefixime (Suprax)	po; 400 mg qd or 200 mg bid
cefotaxime sodium (Claforan)	IM; 1–2 gm bid–tid (maximum 12 gm/day)
ceftriaxone sodium (Rocephin)	IM; 1–2 gm qd–bid (maximum 4 gm/day)
Fourth Generation	
cefepeime (Maximpime)	IM; 0.5–1 gm bid (maximum 3 gm/day)

TABLE 30-8 Tetracyclines

Drug	Route and Adult Dose
tetracycline hydrochloride (Achromycin, Panmycin, Sumycin)	po; 250–500 mg bid–qid (maximum 2 gm/day)
demeclocycline hydrochloride (Declomycin)	po; 150–300 mg bid–qid (maximum 2.4 gm/day)
doxycycline hyclate (Doryx, Doxy, Monodox, Vibramycin)	po, IV; 100 mg on day 1, then 100 mg qd (maximum 200 mg/day)
minocycline hydro-chloride (Dynacin, Minocin, Vectrin)	po; 200 mg as one dose, followed by 100 mg bid
oxytetracycline (Terramycin)	po; 250–500 mg bid–qid

TABLE 30-9 Macrolides

Drug	Route and Adult Dose
azithromycin (Zithromax)	po; 500 mg for one dose, then 250 mg qd for four days
clarithromycin (Biaxin)	po; 250–500 mg bid
dirithromycin (Dynabac)	po; 500 mg qd
erythromycin (E-mycin, Erythrocin)	po; 250–500 mg qid or 333 mg tid

TCNs are bacteriostatic and therefore slow down the growth and reproduction of bacteria. TCNs enter the bacterial cell, utilize energy, and bind to a subunit of the ribosome, which blocks protein synthesis of the cell membrane wall. The growth of the cell slows down and replication is hindered. The body's immune system then takes over to kill the bacteria.

Macrolides

The antibacterial agents known as macrolides are active against both aerobic and anaerobic gram-positive cocci, with the exception of enterococci (see Table 30-9). They are also active against some gram-negative anaerobes. Macrolides are mainly bacteriostatic. Erythromycin can be bacteriostatic at low doses and bactericidal at high doses; it works by inhibiting the protein synthesis that depends on RNA. Erythromycin has been used orally in combination with an oral aminoglycoside to prepare the bowel before bowel or GI tract surgery.

Aminoglycosides

Aminoglycosides are potent bactericidal antibiotics that act by creating fissures in the outer membrane of the bacterial cell (see Table 30-10). The mechanism of action (MOA) is to interrupt protein synthesis. They are active against aerobic, gram-negative bacteria and act synergistically against certain gram-positive organisms. Because of their antibacterial activity, spectrum, and toxic effects, they are usually reserved for the treatment of severe infections of the abdomen and urinary tract, endocarditis, and bacteremia. They are given IV only for systemic conditions and topically for ocular infections.

Toxic effects include nephrotoxicity and ototoxicity. Toxic effects result, because the body does not metabolize

TABLE 30-10 Aminoglycosides

Drug	Route
amikacin sulfate (Amikin)	IM/IV
gentamicin sulfate (Garamycin, G-mycin, Jenamicin)	IM, topical, ophthalmic
kanamycin (Kantrex)	IM/IV/po
neomycin sulfate (Mycifradin)	po
netilmicin sulfate (Netromycin)	IM
paromomycin sulfate (Humatin)	po
streptomycin sulfate	IM
tobramycin sulfate (Nebcin)	IM, IV, ophthalmic route

TABLE 30-11 Fluoroquinolones

Drug	Route and Adult Dose
ciprofloxacin (Cipro)	po; 250–750 mg bid
levofloxacin (Levaquin)	po; 250–500 mg/day
ofloxacin (Floxin)	po; 200–400 mg bid
sparfloxacin (Zagam) moxifloxacin (Avelox, Vigamox)	po; 400 mg on day 1, then 200 mg daily

aminoglycosides due to inhibition of certain metabolic enzymes. Renal toxicity is most often documented and is usually reversible by stopping aminoglycoside treatment. Nephrotoxicity results from renal cortical cumulation that causes tubular cell degeneration and sloughing. Ototoxicity is usually irreversible. Studies in animals have shown that aminoglycoside accumulation in the ear is dose-dependent but can reach a saturation point at low serum levels. Therefore, toxicity to the cochlear organ of Corti and inner ear is dose-dependent.

Aminoglycosides are associated with postantibiotic effect. It is believed that after exposure to higher doses of aminoglycosides, leukocytes have enhanced phagocytosis and ability to kill; these effects last for relatively long periods of time after the dose is given. The once-standard dosing of gentamicin 80 mg q8–12h is no longer recommended. Correct multiple daily dosing of aminoglycosides often requires pharmacokinetics expertise and close monitoring of drug serum levels and renal function and is both labor- and lab-intensive. It is now recommended that single daily dosing be used. This method, with high concentrations of aminoglycosides and long dosing intervals of q24–48h, is called *pulse dosing.*

Fluoroquinolones

Fluoroquinolones are used to treat severe infections, such as infections of the bone and joints, skin, urinary tract, serious ear infections, bronchitis, pneumonia, TB, inflammation of the prostate, some STDs or sexually transmitted infections (STIs), and some infections that affect people with AIDS (see Table 30-11). Some fluoroquinolones may weaken the tendons in the shoulder, hand, or heel, making the tendons more likely to tear. Some people feel drowsy, dizzy, lightheaded, or less alert when taking quinolones. Special attention should be paid to patients with renal, hepatic, or CNS disease, or sclerotic cranial arteries, epilepsy, and other seizure disorders.

Fluoroquinolones, which are bactericidal, act by inhibiting gyrase, an important enzyme for replication of DNA, during bacterial replication. Because the affected bacteria cannot reproduce, they die off.

Sulfonamides

Antibiotics containing sulfur are called *sulfa drugs* or *sulfonamides.* Sulfonamides (see Table 30-12) are used to treat urinary tract infections, bronchitis, middle ear infections, and traveler's diarrhea. They are also used for the prevention and treatment of *Pneumocystis carinii* pneumonia. Sulfonamides competitively inhibit both para aminobenzoic acid and the enzymatic substrate dihydropteroate to block the essential synthesis of folic acid of the bacterial cell.

Antifungals

The MOA of an antifungal depends on its subclass (see Table 30-13). Imidazoles, such as ketoconazole, interfere with synthesis of ergosterol, the vital, major component of the cell wall membranes of fungi and yeast. The reduced availability of ergosterol increases the permeability of the cell wall, allowing outside material to enter the cell and encouraging leakage of cytoplasm and nucleus to the outside of the fungal cell. This ultimately causes the collapse of the fungal cell and inhibits cell growth.

Triazole antifungals, such as ketoconazole, fluconazole, itraconazole, and voriconazole, also inhibit or interfere with the fungal cell's ability to synthesize ergosterol. Though each drug has a slightly different action, all promote increased

PROFILE IN PRACTICE

A patient mentions to the pharmacy technician that every time she takes an antibiotic for the full course of therapy, she ends ups with diarrhea and vaginitis and therefore does not normally complete the full prescription.

▶ *What could the pharmacist suggest to help alleviate this recurring problem?*

TABLE 30-12 Sulfonamides

Drug	Route and Adult Dose	Notes
Gantanol (sulfamethoxazole)	500-mg tablets: four tablets (2 gm) initially, then two tablets (1 gm) tid	Must take with plenty of water to prevent crystallization in the kidneys.
Gantrisin (sulfisoxazole)	500-mg tablets, 4−8 gm in four to six divided doses	Must take with plenty of water to prevent crystallization in the kidneys.
Septra, Bactrim, Bactrim DS (sulfamethoxazole+trimethoprim)	Bactrim and Septra—400 mg/80 mg Dose: one tablet q6h Bactrim DS and Septra DS—800 mg/160 mg Dose: one tablet q12h	Must take with plenty of water to prevent crystallization in the kidneys. May cause photosensitivity.
Sulfadiazine (various generics)	500-mg tablets: 2−4 gm in three to six divided doses	Must take with plenty of water to prevent crystallization in the kidneys.

Note: All may require a loading dose.

TABLE 30-13 Antifungal Agents

Generic (Trade) Name	Strength and Dosage Form(s) Available	Usual Adult Dose	Notes
amphotericin B, desoxycholate (Fungizone)	Powder for injection: 50-mg vials	Depends on weight and diagnosis; 0.25−1.5 mg/kg/day 4 gm maximum daily dose, given 4−12 weeks	Only used for life-threatening systemic fungal infections because of drug interactions and toxic effects. Monitor renal patients. May cause respiratory reactions and nephrotoxicity.
amphotericin B, lipid-based (Amphotec)	Powder for injection: 50-mg single-dose vials. Vials should be stored in the pharmacy refrigerator.	Depends on weight and diagnosis; 3−6 mg/kg/day	Reserved for life-threatening systemic fungal infections. May cause N/V/D, headache, anxiety, asthma, convulsions, MI, anemia, leukemia, and more.
fluconazole (Diflucan)	Tablets: 50 mg, 100 mg, 150 mg, 200 mg Powder for po suspension: 10 mg/mL and 40 mg/mL when reconstituted Injectable: 2 mg/mL	200 mg on day 1, then 100 mg qd For vaginal candidiasis, one 150-mg tablet qd×7 days	Double the daily dose on day 1 for a loading dose. Caution with renally or hepatically impaired patients. May cause hepatoxicity. Has 26% incidence of adverse reactions associated with 150 mg qd for vaginal candidiasis.
flucytosine (Ancobon)	Capsule: 250 mg, 500 mg	50−150 mg/kg in four divided doses, q6h	Warning: monitor renally impaired patients. Usually given with amphotericin B to increase therapeutic action, but combination may also increase toxicity. May cause bone marrow depression.

(Continued)

TABLE 30-13 Antifungal Agents *(Continued)*

Generic (Trade) Name	Strength and Dosage Form(s) Available	Usual Adult Dose	Notes
griseofulvin (Fulvicin)	Tablet: 250 mg, 500 mg	Depends on weight and diagnosis. One tablet daily.	Photosensitivity and lupus-like syndrome.
griseofulvin, ultramicrosize (Fulvicin PG and Gris-Peg)	Tablet: 125 mg, 165 mg, 250 mg, 330 mg		Possible PCN cross-sensitivity.
itraconazole (Sporanox)	Tablet: 100 mg Suspension po: 10 mg/mL Pwd for injection: 10 mg/mL	100–200 mg qd Take whole capsules with food to increase absorption.	Do not give to CHF patients; may increase CHF symptoms.
ketoconazole (Nizoral)	Tablet: 200 mg 1% OTC and 2% Rx strength and cream	200–400 mg qd	Side effects: headache, dizziness.
			Toxic effects: May cause anaphylaxis on first dose, hepatoxicity, gastric acidity.
			Contraindicated with triazolam (may cause CNS depression and psychomotor impairment or suicidal tendencies).
			Contraindicated with antacids, which may reduce the effect of ketoconazole; delay administration by two hours.
terbinafine (Lamisil)	Tablet: 250 mg OTC cream	250 mg qd × 6 or 12 weeks	Do not give to patients with liver damage or transplants. May cause renal or hepatic function impairment and Stevens–Johnson syndrome. Inhibits CYP450 enzyme. Caution in use with drugs that also interact with CYP450: MAOIs, TCA, SSRIs, beta blockers.
voriconazole (V-fend)	Tablet: 50 mg, 200 mg (take one hour before or one hour after meal/empty stomach) Pwd for injection: 200 mg SDV	po: 50–300 mg q12h UAD 200 mg q12h	Increase dosage of voriconazole if coadministered with phenytoin.

permeability, leakage of the cell's inner contents, and collapse of the cell wall, resulting in death of the fungal cell.

In contrast, flucytosine competitively inhibits the cell's production of purine and pyrimadine. Biosynthesis of purine and pyrimadine nucleotides is an essential process in all growing cells, because these molecules are the direct precursors of DNA and RNA. Therefore, by blocking the cell's own production of purine and pyrimadine, flucytosine also blocks production of DNA and RNA. In addition, flucytosine metabolizes to 5-fluorouracil (5-FU), which is then incorporated into the RNA of the fungal cell, where it blocks the synthesis of both DNA and RNA, leading to fungal cell death.

Amebicides/Antiprotozoals

Metronidazole is amebicidal, bactericidal, and trichomonacidal. Its selectivity for anaerobic bacteria is a result of these organisms' ability to reduce metronidazole to its active form intracellularly; it then disrupts the helical structure of DNA, inhibiting nucleic acid synthesis by the bacterial cell. This eventually results in bacterial cell death. Metronidazole is equally effective against dividing and nondividing cells. The electron transport proteins necessary for this reaction are found only in anaerobic bacteria. Metronidazole's spectrum of activity includes protozoa and obligate anaerobes, including *Bacteroides* group (including *B. fragilis*), *Fusobacterium*, *Veillonella*, the *Clostridium* group (including *C. difficile* and *C. perfringens*), *Eubacterium*, *Peptococcus*, and *Peptostreptococcus*. Its protozoan coverage includes *Entamoeba histolytica*, *Giardia lamblia*, and *Trichomonas vaginalis*. It is not effective against the common aerobes, but it combats *Gardnerella (Haemophilus) vaginalis*.

Tables 30-14 and 30-15 list some common antifungal and antiprotozoal agents.

TABLE 30-14 Common Antifungal Agents

Drug	Uses	Basic Mechanism of Action
Amphotericin B	Systemic fungal infections	Alters permeability of cell membrane
Azoles such as clotrimazole, miconazole, and fluconazole	Local candidiasis and dermatological infections. Systemic fungal infections	Inhibit sterol synthesis
Flucytosine	Serious fungal infections	Competes with uracil

TABLE 30-15 Common Antiprotozoal Agents

Drug	Uses	Mechanism of Action
Chloroquine, quinine	Malaria	Inhibits nucleic acid synthesis
Imidazoles such as metronidazole and tinidazole	Entamoeba, giardia, trichomoniasis	Interferes with several metabolic pathways, disrupts DNA's helical structure
Pentamidine	*Pneumonia carinii, Trypanosoma rhodesiense/ gambiense*	Inhibits aerobic glycolysis
Pyrimethamine	Malaria, toxoplasmosis	Inhibits folic acid reduction

> ### ❝ Workplace Wisdom Metronidazole and Alcohol
>
> If patients who are taking metronidazole drink alcoholic beverages, they may experience disulfiram-like side effects, which include nausea and vomiting, headache, flushing, and abdominal cramps. It is possible for these effects to last two to three weeks after the last dose of metronidazole has been taken. Disulfiram (the generic name for Antabuse) is used as an anti-alcoholic treatment. Disulfiram also causes cramping with the slightest amount of alcohol, such as that in mouthwash. ❞

Tuberculosis

TB is caused by a bacterium called *Mycobacterium tuberculosis*, which is very common in Latin America, the Caribbean, Africa, Asia, Eastern Europe, and Russia. These bacteria may attack any part of the body but usually attack the lungs. Once a leading cause of death in the United States, it was almost eradicated in the 1940s when scientists discovered the drug treatments that are still used today. However, due to complacency and a decrease in funding for TB programs, there has been a resurgence of the illness, and drug-resistant types are appearing.

Despite new programs to combat TB, tens of thousands of cases are still reported in the United States each year. The bacteria are spread by breathing the air that infected people cough or sneeze into. Usually, TB is spread among people in close proximity, who see each other on a day-to-day basis. It is found most commonly in homeless shelters, migrant farm camps, prisons, jails, and some nursing homes in the United States. TB can become active in a person whose immune system is weak and cannot fight it off, or it can be the latent type of TB that stays dormant, alive but inactive, in the body (especially in a person with a strong immune system). Symptoms are different for the two states of TB.

Symptoms include weakness, weight loss, fever, lack of appetite, chills, and sweating at night. Other symptoms of TB disease depend on where the bacteria are growing in the body. If the infection is in the lungs (pulmonary TB), the symptoms may include a bad cough, pain in the chest, and coughing up blood (*hemoptysis*). Those most at risk for developing active TB are patients with the following conditions:

- Substance abuse
- Diabetes mellitus
- Silicosis
- Cancer of the head or neck
- Leukemia or Hodgkin's disease
- Severe kidney disease
- Low body weight
- Certain medical treatments, such as corticosteroid treatment or organ transplants

Latent TB infection is characterized by having dormant bacteria in the lungs or other parts of the body. Though the dormant pathogens cause no symptoms, the bacteria can become active again whenever the immune system is stressed or weakened. Infected persons in whom the disease is latent can still spread TB to others and will develop the active form of the disease later in life, if they do not receive treatment for the latent infection.

Diagnosis of TB disease usually begins with a positive skin test reaction. This indicates the presence of TB but does not necessarily indicate infection. Further diagnostic tests usually include a chest X-ray and sputum test. Because TB bacteria may be found somewhere besides the lungs, blood or urine may also be tested.

The drug of choice for treatment is isoniazid (INH) (see Table 30-16). INH is taken for at least six to nine months and longer, if the patient has a weakened immune system. Compliance is a major problem in the treatment of TB, as many low-income or transient patients do not complete the full course; incomplete treatment builds drug resistance and creates a public health hazard.

A toxic effect is the development of hepatitis. This effect is age-related with a higher incidence in persons aged 50 to 64 years. The use of alcohol during treatment can be dangerous and can increase the chances of hepatitis. Precaution statements on the label placed by the pharmacy technician should include a warning that the patient is not to drink alcoholic beverages (wine, beer, or liquor) while taking INH. Side effects should be reported immediately; they may include the following:

- Lack of appetite
- Nausea
- Vomiting
- Jaundice (yellowish skin or eyes)
- Fever for three or more days

- Abdominal pain
- Tingling in the fingers and toes

❝ Workplace Wisdom TB Resistance

Because resistance to TB can develop rapidly, both mycobactericidal or tubercularcidal and tubercularstatic drugs should be given—rifampin and INH/ethambutol, respectively. ❞

Antivirals

The common cold and influenza are discussed in Chapter 28. This chapter investigates antiretrovirals for HIV/AIDS and vaccinations for influenza. Some oral antivirals can be used to prevent the onset of influenza if used within 24 to 48 hours after the onset of signs and symptoms. Amantadine should be continued for 24 to 48 hours after the disappearance of signs and symptoms.

Antivirals change or metabolize to acyclovir triphosphate; acyclovir inhibits the virus-specific DNA polymerase, an enzyme important for viral growth, multiplication, and replication. Replication is interrupted and the viruses die (see Table 30-17).

❝ Workplace Wisdom Viruses

Because viruses use the host cell's machinery to replicate, they are very difficult to target. The viruses can mutate quickly enough to elude some antiviral drugs. ❞

TABLE 30-16 Common Antituberculosis Regimens

Regimen 1	Regimen 2	Regimen 3
Daily INH, rifampin, and pyrazinamide for eight weeks. Subsequent administration of INH and rifampin daily or two to three times weekly for 16 weeks. Ethambutol or streptomycin should be added to the initial regimen until sensitivity to INH and rifampin is demonstrated. In addition, a fourth drug is optional if the relative prevalence of isoniazid-resistant *Mycobacterium tuberculosis* isolates is present.	Daily INH, rifampin, pyrazinamide, and streptomycin or ethambutol for two weeks. Subsequent administration of same drugs twice weekly for six weeks. Subsequently twice weekly INH and rifampin for 16 more weeks.	Three times weekly with INH, rifampin, pyrazinamide, and ethambutol or streptomycin for six months.

Antituberculin Drugs	Usual Maximum Daily Dose	Maximum Twice Weekly Dose
ethambutol	2.5 gm	50 mg/kg
isoniazid	300 mg	900 mg
pyrazinamide	2 gm	50–70 mg/kg
rifampin	600 mg	600 mg
streptomycin	1 gm (> 60 years old, 750 mg)	20–30 mg/kg

TABLE 30-17 Common Antiviral Drugs

Drug	Uses	Mechanism of Action
acyclovir, famciclovir, valacyclovir	Herpes viruses	Nucleoside analogue
amantadine, rimantadine	Influenza A	Inhibit virus uncoating and assembly
ganciclovir	Cytomegalovirus (group of herpetoviruses that inhabit the salivary glands, causing immunocompromised individuals, such as AIDS and transplant patients, to develop retinitis, pneumonia, colitis, and/or encephalitis)	Nucleoside analogue
ribavirin	Respiratory syncytial (RS) virus (common cause of acute bronchitis in small children)	Nucleoside analogue
Antiretrovirals—Used Specifically for HIV		
azidothymidine	HIV	Nucleoside analogue
nevirapine	HIV	Protease inhibitor

Drug Resistance

Resistance is a microorganism's ability to live and grow despite the presence of an anti-infective or antimicrobial drug. Resistance is a result of genetic mutation during the replication or cell division process that causes the pathogen to evade or avoid the mechanism by which a drug destroys the pathogen. A pathogen, such as a bacteria, fungus, or virus, becomes resistant to a drug; a person does not become resistant to a drug or a pathogen. The ability of the bacterium or pathogen to survive the mechanism of destruction of the antibiotic, or resistance, is promoted by several factors. Basically, though, the process is Darwinian *survival of the fittest* on a small and rapid scale, any pathogens that happen to survive after a patient is treated with a particular drug will reproduce similarly hardy (resistant) cells.

This is one reason it is so important for patients to finish a course of antibiotics. Some patients, who are prescribed antibiotics, do not take the full dosing regimen; they quit taking the drug when they start to feel better. This often kills off only some of the weaker, nonresistant bacteria, and enhances the resistance ability of the remaining pathogens, which multiply and become stronger. Soon the prescribed antibiotic will no longer work and a stronger antibiotic will be needed. If the patient again breaks off treatment with the prescribed drug, a stronger antibiotic may not be available or may not be effective upon a subsequent infection.

Contributing to the problem is the fact that bacteria and other pathogens are remarkably resilient and can develop ways to evade drugs meant to kill or weaken them. The increasing use of antibiotics contributes to this action and is called *antibiotic resistance, antimicrobial resistance,* or *drug resistance.* Research has shown that antibiotics are given to patients more often than recommended by federal guidelines. For example, many patients ask their doctors for antibiotics to treat a cold, cough, or the flu, all of which are viral in etiology and do not respond to antibacterials. Food-producing animals given antibiotic drugs for therapeutic, disease-prevention, or production-enhancement reasons can harbor microbes that become resistant to drugs used to treat human illness. This results in harder-to-treat human infections.

According to the FDA, about 70% of *nosocomial* bacteria, which cause infections in hospitals, are resistant to at least one of the most commonly prescribed antibiotics. Some organisms are resistant to all FDA-approved antibiotics and can be treated with only experimental and potentially toxic drugs.

Antibiotic resistance problems must be detected as soon as they emerge, and actions must be taken to contain them; otherwise, the world will be faced with previously treatable diseases that have once again become untreatable. It will be as it was in the days before antibiotics were first discovered and used.

Antibiotic resistance results when bacteria acquire genes conferring resistance in any of the following three ways:

- In spontaneous DNA mutation, bacterial genetic material may change spontaneously to a form that serendipitously resists the action of a drug or drugs. Drug-resistant TB occurs this way.
- In a type of microbial sex called *transformation*, one bacterium may take up DNA from another bacterium. PCN-resistant gonorrhea results from microbial transformation.
- Most powerful is the resistance acquired from a small circle of DNA (a plasmid) that can *hop* from one type of bacterium to another. A single plasmid can provide a great number of different resistances. In 1968, 12,500 people in Guatemala died in an epidemic of *shigella* diarrhea, because a pathogen harbored a plasmid-carrying resistances to four antibiotics.

Timeline of PCN-resistant Pathogens

Only four years after drug companies began mass-producing PCN in 1943, PCN-resistant pathogens began to appear.

1943—The first bug to battle PCN was *S. aureus,* which caused pneumonia or toxic shock syndrome from infected wounds.

1967—American military personnel in Southeast Asia were acquiring PCN-resistant gonorrhea from prostitutes.

1967—*Streptococcus pneumoniae*, called pneumococcus, surfaced in a village in Papua New Guinea, causing PCN-resistant pneumonia.

1979 to 1987—According to the Centers for Disease Control and Prevention (CDC), only 0.02% of pneumococcus strains are PCN-resistant.

1983—A hospital-acquired intestinal infection caused by the bacterium *Enterococcus faecium* appears.

1987—First vancomycin-resistant enterococcus is reported in England and France.

1989—Vancomycin-resistant enterococcus is discovered in a New York hospital.

1994—A full 6.6% of pneumococcus strains are resistant.

2002—The CDC reports a Michigan patient with diabetes, vascular disease, and chronic kidney failure who developed the first *S. aureus* infection completely resistant to vancomycin.

2003—Epidemiologists report in the *New England Journal of Medicine* that 5% to 10% of hospital patients acquire an infection during their stay.

2003—Study in the *New England Journal of Medicine* found that the incidence of sepsis (blood and tissue infections) almost tripled from 1979 to 2000.

Solutions to Resistance

Pathogens exist in huge numbers. They have short generation times and the ability to swap genes, which make them flexible and dangerous. Although there may be no ultimate cure for resistance, it can be slowed down.

- Avoid using antibiotics unnecessarily. Use only when bacterial infections warrant such treatment. Do not use for viral or fungal infections.
- Complete any antibacterial regimen; do not have leftover doses.
- Use the most specific antibiotic possible with the most precise target or narrowest *spectrum*. This kills the offending bug without triggering resistance among other bacteria that live in the patient, as broader-spectrum drugs do.

- Use the common antibiotics first; if they work, do not use second line of defense drugs. Reserve these latter drugs for infections on which the first-generation drugs do not work.
- Reduce hospital-transmitted infections by improving infection control in hospitals. This will kill the bugs before they get inside patients.
- Invent new antibiotic drugs that use new mechanisms to kill microbes, and find new drugs that improve the action of existing antibiotics.
- Invent vaccines against common viral diseases to prevent initial infections.
- Reduce the widespread use of antibiotics in animal feeds.

> **Workplace Wisdom** **Your Role in Reducing Drug Resistance**
>
> It is important that pharmacists educate patients regarding medications. To reduce resistance, patients must understand how important it is to complete their prescribed anti-infective therapy, even if they begin to feel better.

Vaccines

Vaccines were first used by the Chinese who called it *variolation*. They were observed by Lady Mary Wortley Montagu, wife of the British ambassador to Turkey, who brought them back to England in the early 1700s. In the late 1700s, Edward Jenner experienced variolation as a child, survived, and later became a doctor who was told by a milkmaid that she could not catch smallpox, because she had already contracted cowpox. In 1796, Jenner infected a boy with cowpox. After the boy's recovery, Jenner injected the pus from a smallpox lesion directly under the boy's skin. The boy never contracted smallpox. Thus, the first inoculation was born.

Most of today's immunizations are either inactivated, acellular, or attenuated vaccines (see Table 30-18). *Inactivated* vaccines are composed of killed disease-causing microorganisms. *Acellular* vaccines are taken from the antigenic part of the disease-causing organism, such as the capsule or flagella. These types of vaccines cannot cause disease and therefore can be used in immunocompromised patients. With these vaccine types, booster shots are required every few years. *Attenuated* vaccine contains a live microorganism that has been weakened by aging or altering the viral growth conditions. They are lifelong and do not require booster shots. Although these are the most successful vaccines, they carry a high risk of mutation to virulent strains. Therefore, these types of vaccines should not be used in immunocompromised patients.

Another type of vaccine, called a *toxoid*, is made from viral toxins that have been treated with aluminum salts. Yet another vaccine uses a part of the organism to stimulate a strong immune system response; these are called *subunit* vaccines. They are made from bacterial or yeast host cells that have had the genome of the infectious agent inserted into them.

TABLE 30-18 Types of Vaccines

Type of Vaccine	Examples	Notes
Acellular vaccines	Haemophilus influenzae B (HIB)	Requires booster shots
Attenuated vaccines	Measles, mumps, and rubella	Highest risk of mutation
		Lifelong immunization
		Does not require booster shots
Biotechnology and genetic engineering techniques	Hepatitis B vaccine	Safe for immunocompromised patients
Inactivated or killed vaccines	Typhoid vaccine	Organism is killed using formalin
	Salk poliomyelitis vaccine	
Toxoid vaccines	Diphtheria	Administered with an adjuvant—an agent that increases or enhances the immune response
	Tetanus	
	Diphtheria/pertussis (whooping cough)/tetanus (DPT) vaccine	
Use of an organism similar to a lethal organism	BCG vaccine against *Mycobacterium tuberculosis*	

The national goal to fully vaccinate 90% of 2-year-old children depends on the support of private healthcare providers. The 12 diseases that the Vaccines for Children program currently provides protection against are the following:

- Diphtheria
- Haemophilus influenzae type B
- Hepatitis A
- Hepatitis B
- Measles
- Mumps
- Pertussis
- Pneumococcal disease
- Poliomyelitis
- Rubella
- Tetanus
- Varicella (chicken pox)

Various Infectious Disease States

In addition to varying in appearance, microorganisms vary in the specific disease(s) they cause. Table 30-19 displays some of the most common diseases and their origins.

Malaria

Malaria is a disease transmitted by parasites found in malaria-infected mosquitoes. Malaria is common in large areas of Central and South America, Haiti and the Dominican Republic,

Africa, the Indian subcontinent, Southeast Asia, the Middle East, and Oceania. In these areas of risk, about 1 million deaths per year are caused by malaria. The United States sees only a few cases each year.

Malaria can be cured with prescription drugs (see Table 30-20). The type of drugs used and duration of the treatment depend on which type of malaria is diagnosed, where the patient was infected, the patient's age, and the progression of the disease state at the start of treatment. Antimalarial drugs should be taken before, during, and after travel to the high-risk areas. One drug, in particular, is reserved for travelers who cannot take other drugs: Primaquine can cause **lysis** (bursting and destruction) of red blood cells. This occurs in persons who are deficient in glucose-6-phosphate dehydrogenase (G6PD) and can be fatal. Travelers *must* be tested for G6PD deficiency and have a documented G6PD level in the normal range before primaquine is used.

The main focus of treatment is prevention:

- Vaccinations are given four to six weeks before foreign travel, and an antimalarial drug is prescribed. This antimalarial drug must be taken exactly on schedule without missing doses.
- Prevent mosquito and other insect bites by using DEET insect repellent on exposed skin and flying insect spray in the room where you sleep.
- Protective clothing: Wear long pants and long-sleeved shirts, especially from dusk to dawn, the time when mosquitoes that spread malaria bite.
- Bed nets dipped in permethrin insecticide should be employed, if screened or air-conditioned housing is not available.

lysis the destruction of cells.

TABLE 30-19 Origin of Various Human Infectious Diseases

Bacterial Origin	Viral Origin	Fungal Origin	Yeast Origin	Parasitic Origin
Anthrax	Childhood diseases: mumps, measles, German measles (rubella), chicken pox	Athlete's foot (*Tinea pedis*)	Vaginal yeast infections (*Candida albicans*, candidiasis, moniliasis)	Malaria
Cholera	Common cold	Cryptococcal meningitis	*Cryptococcus neoformans* (opportunistic infection that occurs as a complication of AIDS or use of immunosuppressant drugs)	Pediculosis
Diphtheria	Hepatitis	Histoplasmosis (found in bird or bat droppings; when inhaled, causes severe eye disease or blindness)		Scabies
Dysentery	HIV (progresses to AIDS)	Jock itch, thigh area (*Tinea cruris, Trichophyton rubrum*)	Jock itch, inclusive of penis and scrotum (*Candida albicans*)	
Meningitis (bacterial, not all)	Influenza	Ringworm		
Pneumonia (bacterial, not all)	Meningitis (viral, not all)	Sporotrichosis (caused by *Sporothrix schenckii*, found in thorny plants such as roses, hay, and sphag num moss; causes boils and open lesions)		
Rocky Mountain spotted fever (*Rickettsia rickettsii*; bacteria spread by ixodid (hard) ticks)	Polio (poliomyelitis)	Thrush (caused by a yeast-like fungus)		
Scarlet fever	Pneumonia (viral, not all)	Toxoplasmosis		
Some STDs: syphilis, gonorrhea, chlamydia	Rabies			
Tetanus	Shingles			
Toxic shock syndrome	Smallpox			
Tuberculosis	Warts and genital warts			
Typhoid fever (*Salmonella typhi*)				
Whooping cough	Yellow fever (spread by mosquitoes)			

TABLE 30-20 Antimalarial Drug Regimens

Travel to Africa, South America, the Indian Subcontinent, Asia, and the South Pacific		Travel to Mexico, Haiti, Dominican Republic, and Certain Countries in Central America, the Middle East, and Eastern Europe (their antimalarial drug is available as an alternative)	
Antimalarial Drug	**Antimalarial Drug Regimen**	**Antimalarial Drug**	**Antimalarial Drug Regimen**
Malarone—a combination of Mepron (atovaquone) 250 mg and proguanil 100 mg	Usual adult dose (UAD): one tablet qd, with food or milk, same time each day. First dose: one to two days before travel to the malaria-risk area. Last dose: once a day for seven days after leaving the malaria-risk area.	chloroquine (Aralen)	UAD: 500 mg once a week on the same day of the week. Take on a full stomach to lessen the risk of nausea and stomach upset. First dose: one week before arrival in the malaria-risk area. Last dose: four weeks after leaving the malaria-risk area.
doxycycline (a type of TCN, various trade names)	UAD: 100 mg qd, same time each day. First dose: one or two days before arrival in the malaria-risk area. Last dose: four weeks after leaving the risk area.	hydroxychloroquine sulfate (Plaquenil)	UAD: 400 mg once a week on the same day of the week. Take on a full stomach to lessen nausea and stomach upset. First dose: one week before arrival in the malaria-risk area. Last dose: four weeks after leaving the risk area.
mefloquine (Lariam)	UAD: 250 mg tablet once a week on a full stomach with a full glass of liquid.		
	First dose: one week before arrival in the malaria-risk area; once a week on same day of week thereafter.		
	Last dose: four weeks after leaving the risk area.		
primaquine (in special circumstances)	UAD: two tablets (30 mg base primaquine) once a day.		
	Take the first dose one to two days before travel and last dose seven days after leaving the high-risk area.		

Cancer

According to the American Cancer Society, *cancer* is a group of diseases characterized by the uncontrolled growth and spread of abnormal cells. If the spread is not controlled, it can result in death. It is important to note that increased growth rate alone is not cancer; the cells must be mutated or abnormal to the extent that normal cell function is altered or impaired. As some cells stop functioning normally, they no longer serve a useful or purposeful function, and thus they become cancerous cells.

Normal cells reproduce in a regulated and systematic manner. However, after injury, the cell division and reproduction of normal cells is speeded up until the injury is healed. In comparison, cancer cells divide in a haphazard process. The typical result is that they pile up into a nonstructured mass or *tumor*. When the cancer cells become invasive, they destroy the part of the body where they originated and then spread to other parts of the body. When the cancer spreads, or *metastasizes*, the disease can become life-threatening. Benign growths, in contrast, stay localized and are not cancer, even though the cells may grow or divide fast. The most common types of metastatic cancers include the following:

- Bladder
- Breast
- Colon and rectal
- Endometrial
- Kidney (renal cell)
- Leukemia
- Lung
- Melanoma
- Non-Hodgkin's lymphoma
- Ovarian
- Pancreatic
- Prostate
- Skin (nonmelanoma)

Cancer Treatments

Cancer is treated with a variety of methods. Treatment may include only one method, or a combination of methods, depending on the type and severity of the cancer.

Surgery is usually the first line of treatment for solid tumors. In early-stage cancer, it may be sufficient to cure the patient by removing all cancerous cells. Benign growths may also be removed by surgery.

Radiation may be used in conjunction with surgery and/or drug treatments. The goal of radiation is to kill the cancer cells by damaging them with direct high-energy beams.

Chemotherapy uses cytotoxic agents—a wide array of drugs—to kill cancer cells. Chemotherapy damages the dividing cancer cells and prevents their further reproduction.

Hormonal treatments prevent cancer cells from receiving the signals necessary for Continued growth and division.

Specific inhibitors are a relatively new class of drugs that work by targeting specific proteins and processes used by cancer cells. Inhibition of these proteins and processes prevents cancer cell growth and division.

- *Antibodies* are used to target cancer cells, depriving the cancer cells of necessary growth signals or causing the direct death of the cells. Antibodies may also be called *specific inhibitors.*
- *Biological response modifiers (BRMs)* are naturally occurring, normal proteins that stimulate the body's own defenses against cancer.
- *Vaccines* for cancer also stimulate the body's defenses against cancer, increasing the body's response against the abnormal cancer cells.

Drugs Used to Treat Cancer

Alkylating antineoplastic agents cause the disruption of DNA function and cell death by three methods. Alkylating agents:

- Bind or latch alkyl groups to DNA bases, preventing DNA synthesis and RNA transcription from the affected DNA.
- Cause a formation of cross-bridges that link two bases together, thus preventing DNA from being separated for synthesis or transcription.

- Induce the mispairing of nucleotides, leading to mutations of the cancer cell. (Nucleotide *A* always pairs with *T*, and *G* always pairs with *C*. Alkylated G bases may erroneously pair with T bases. If this altered pairing is not corrected, it may lead to a permanent mutation—in this case, a fatal mutation is desired).

Antimetabolites inhibit ribonucleotide reductase and DNA polymerase to decrease DNA synthesis. They primarily kill cells undergoing DNA synthesis (S phase) and, under certain conditions, block the progression of cells from the G1 phase to the S phase. Although the MOA is not completely understood, it appears that antimetabolites act through the inhibition of DNA.

Sometimes body misregulation causes overproduction of hormones, such as too much estrogen or testosterone. Prostate cancer is caused by too much testosterone, activating cell growth in the prostate. Breast cancer can be caused by too much estrogen, activating cell growth in the breast. In some cases, the opposite androgenic hormone is given to suppress the overproduced hormone. For example, estrogen may be given to prostate cancer patients.

BRMs are substances that help to fight infections; they are found naturally in small amounts in the body. BRMs are produced in the laboratory in large amounts and then injected into the body to treat cancer. BRMs are sometimes combined with chemotherapy drugs to help improve the effect of the cytotoxic agents. Unfortunately, BRMs are not effective against most cancers. The following are general types of BRMs: cytokines, monoclonal antibodies, tumor vaccines, and other immunotherapy.

- *Cytokines,* such as interferon, travel into the cells that are affected by a virus or a cancer and stop the virus or cancer from multiplying. Interferon has been used to treat viral infections, such as hepatitis A, B, C, and D, and cancers such as chronic myelocytic leukemia, melanoma, and breast cancer. Special classes of cytokines are called *colony-stimulating factors.*.These agents are used to stimulate the bone marrow to recover after chemotherapy.
- *Monoclonal antibodies* are designed to cause the body to attack a cancerous tumor in the same way that it responds to a viral infection. The antibody can be attached to a medication used in chemotherapy and targeted against a specific cancer or tumor. When the antibody attacks the tumor, the chemotherapy medication is then delivered directly to the tumor.
- *Tumor vaccines* are mostly experimental medications made from bits of tumors. It is hoped and expected that, when the tumor vaccine is administered, the body will attack the tumor—and any similar tumorous tissues— and keep them from growing.
- *Other immunotherapy* includes a bacterium called bacillus Calmette-Guerin (BCG), which is injected into the body to treat certain types of bladder and melanoma cancers. BCG causes the body to mount a general immune response, in the course of which the body also attacks the cancer.

The side effects of most BRMs are similar to flu symptoms. These symptoms include high fever, chills, fatigue, nausea, vomiting, and loss of appetite.

Antitumor *antibiotics* work by binding with DNA to prevent RNA synthesis, thus preventing DNA replication and cell growth. Antitumor antibiotics may also prevent the DNA from mending or reattaching itself, thus again causing cell death. Antibiotics, which are given IV, are used to treat a wide variety of cancers, including testicular cancer and leukemia.

Plant (vinca) alkaloids prevent cell division by binding to tubulin, which prevents the formation of mitotic spindles. During metaphase, mitotic spindles hold the two sets of DNA that the cell needs to divide. Cancer cells cannot divide without mitotic spindles. These drugs, which are derived from plants, are used to treat cancers of the lung, breast, and testes.

Table Table 30-21 lists some common anticancer drugs.

TABLE 30-21 Anticancer Agents

Trade/Generic Name	Cancers or Disorders Treated	Classification or Type of Antineoplastic Agents
Adriamycin PFS	Variety of cancers	Antibiotic
Adriamycin RDF, Rubex (doxorubicin)	In combination with other cytotoxic agents	
Adrucil, Carac, Efudex, Fluoroplex (fluorouracil)	Variety of cancers	Antimetabolite
Arimidex (anastrozole)	Breast cancer in postmenopausal females	
Busulfex, Myleran (busulfan)	Primary brain cancers, leukemias, and bone marrow disorders	Alkylating agent
Casodex (bicalutamide)	Prostate cancer	Androgen
Cytosar-U (cytarabine)	Variety of cancers	Antimetabolite
Cytoxan, Neosar (cyclophosphamide)	Variety of cancers	Alkylating agent
	Prevent rejection after organ transplants	
	Treat autoimmune diseases	
Ellence (epirubicin)	Breast cancer	Anthracycline
Femara (letrozole)	Breast cancer in postmenopausal women	Aromatase inhibitor, antiestrogenic agent
Gleevec (imatinib)	Chronic myelocytic leukemia	Tyrosine kinase inhibitor
	Specific gastrointestinal cancers	
Hexalen (altertamine)	Ovarian cancer	Antineoplastic agent, miscellaneous
Imuran (azathioprine)	Prevents rejection of solid organ transplants and autoimmune diseases	Immunosuppressant agent
Megace (megestrol acetate)	Endometrial cancer	Progestin
	Breast cancers that have spread	
	Appetite stimulant	
Mylotarg (gemtuzumab ozogamicin)	Acute myeloid leukemia (AML)	Natural source (plant)
		Derivative antineoplastic agent

(Continued)

TABLE 30-21 Anticancer Agents *(Continued)*

Trade/Generic Name	Cancers or Disorders Treated	Classification or Type of Antineoplastic Agents
Nolvadex (tamoxifen)	Breast cancer in women and men	Miscellaneous antineoplastic agent
	Prevention of breast cancer in women at increased risk	
	Induce ovulation	
Navelbine (vinorelbine)	Variety of cancers	Natural source plant (vinca alkaloids) derivative antineoplastic agent
Oncovin [DSC], Vincasar PFS (vincristine)	Variety of cancers	Natural source plant (vinca alkaloids) derivative antineoplastic agent
Onxol Taxol (paclitaxel)	Variety of cancers	Natural source plant (vinca alkaloids) derivative antineoplastic agent
Platinol, Platinol-AQ (cisplatin)	Variety of cancers	Alkylating agent
Propecia, Proscar (finasteride)	Symptoms of benign prostatic hypertrophy (BPH)	Antiandrogen
Avodart (dutasteride)		
Rheumatrex, Trexall (methotrexate)	Variety of cancers	Antimetabolite
	Psoriasis	
	Arthritis	
Rituxan (rituximab)	Non-Hodgkin's lymphoma	Monoclonal antibody
Toposar, VePesid (etoposide)	Variety of cancers	Podophyllotoxin derivative
Trelstar Depot (triptorelin)	Prostate cancer	Luteinizing hormone-releasing hormone analog
		Antineoplastic agent
Xeloda (capecitabine)	Breast cancer	Antimetabolite

Summary

The immune system is the body's defense system. Its function is to protect the body from foreign invaders that might otherwise destroy the body or parts of it. These foreign invaders, called pathogens, include parasites, bacteria, viruses, rickettsia, and fungi or yeast. Pharmacotherapeutic treatment of pathogens (with antibacterials, anti-infectives, antifungals, etc.) is an important part of a pharmacy technician's knowledge base.

The body's defense mechanisms are either nonspecific or specific. The nonspecific defense mechanisms include physical barriers, such as the skin and the linings of the respiratory and digestive systems. They also include the lining of the spinal column, clotting factors in the blood, and normal flora (microorganisms) in the digestive tract that compete with invading pathogens so that they cannot penetrate host tissues. Specific defense mechanisms are defined by specialized protein molecules and cells. These include antibodies and their complements, and lymphocytes (B cells and T cells).

Sometimes, the immune system malfunctions. A person with an autoimmune disease, such as lupus erythematosus or rheumatoid arthritis, has an immune system that mistakenly attacks itself and the body itself. The end result of this misplaced defense reaction is often inflammation. Autoimmune diseases are treated both pharmacologically and nonpharmacologically. The pharmacotherapeutic goal of treatment is to reduce inflammation or to stop or suppress the inflammatory process.

Many viral diseases are difficult to treat because of the nature of viral infection. Hence, vaccines play an important part in protecting people from many preventable diseases.

Most vaccines are either inactivated, acellular, or attenuated. Some vaccinations last for the lifetime of the person; others require booster shots.

Cancer is the uncontrolled growth of abnormal or mutated cells. Cancer can be treated in a variety of ways, including radiation, surgery, and chemotherapy. Treatments can be given alone or in combination with other treatments. It is important for pharmacy technicians to understand chemotherapy and cancer drug therapy, as well as how to prepare the drugs safely.

Chapter Review Questions

1. Immune system molecules are composed of two types of protein called _____.
   a. mucus and cilia.
   b. antibodies and antigens.
   c. immunoglobulins and enzymes.
   d. antibodies and complement.

2. The main stain used in Gram staining is _____.
   a. green
   b. orange
   c. red
   d. violet

3. _____ are two bacteria connected side by side.
   a. Coccus
   b. Diplococcus
   c. Streptococcus
   d. Staphylococcus

4. In the progression of HIV to AIDS, in which stage do AIDS opportunistic infections begin?
   a. stage 1
   b. stage 2
   c. stage 3
   d. stage 4

5. Tetanus is an example of which type of vaccine?
   a. inactivated
   b. attenuated
   c. toxoid
   d. acellular

6. Which of the following is an aminoglycoside?
   a. penicillin
   b. cleocin
   c. erythromycin
   d. tobramycin

7. Which of the following is a second-generation cephalosporin?
   a. cefazolin
   b. cefepime
   c. ceftriaxone
   d. cefaclor

8. If a person is allergic to a penicillin drug, what is the chance that he or she will also have cross-sensitivity to cephalosporins?
   a. 1% to 5%
   b. 5% to 10%
   c. 5% to 20%
   d. 10% to 20%

9. Which of the following drugs is commonly used to treat the herpes virus?
   a. amantadine
   b. ribivirin
   c. penicillin
   d. acyclovir

10. INH is the drug of choice for the treatment of _____.
    a. HIV
    b. TB
    c. malaria
    d. otitis media

Critical Thinking Questions

1. Why do you think some cancer treatments include only one type of therapy, while other treatments combine several different therapies?

2. Why do you think a vaccine for HIV/AIDS has not yet been discovered or developed?

3. Why is the national goal to fully vaccinate 2-year-old children only at 90% rather than 100%?

Web Challenge

1. Go to http://www.aids.org to learn more about the disease AIDS and the new treatments that are available.

2. Search the website of the National Institute of Allergies and Infectious Diseases at http://www.niaid.nih.gov/ to learn more about the immune system, infectious diseases, and vaccines.

References and Resources

"About cells." http://staff.jccc.net/pdecell/cells/basiccell.html#introduction. Web. 8 April 2008.

Adams, M.P., D.L. Josephson, and L.N. Holland, Jr. *Pharmacology for Nurses: A Pathophysiologic Approach.* (4th edition.) Upper Saddle River, NJ: Pearson, 2013. Print.

"HIV and AIDS Treatments." http://www.hivandhepatitis.com/hiv_and_aids/emtriva.html.Web. 8 April 2008.

"HIV and Hepatitis.com. http://www.hivandhepatitis.com. Web. 16 August 2013.

Holland, N. and M.P. Adams. *Core Concepts in Pharmacology.* (3rd edition.) Upper Saddle River, NJ: Pearson, 2010. Print.

"Introduction to Microorganisms." http://www.sparknotes.com/biology/microorganisms/intro/summary.html. Web. 5 April 2013.

McLaughlin Centre, Institute of Population Health, University of Ottawa Health Systems Concerns. "Immune System Fact Sheet."http://www.emcom.ca/health/immune.shtml. Web. 8 April 2008.

"The Body: An AIDS and HIV Information Resource." http://www.thebody.com/treat/protinh.html. Web. 8 April 2013.

"The Body's Defenses." http://www.langara.bc.ca/biology/mario/Biol1215notes/biol1215chap43.html. Web. 8 April 2008.

"The Immune System—In More Detail." www.nobelprize.org Web. 11 August 2013.*(Continued)(Continued)(Continued)(Continued)(Continued)(Continued)***(Continued)**

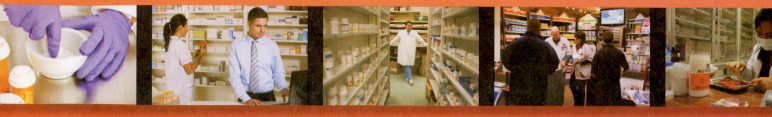

CHAPTER 31

The Renal System

LEARNING OBJECTIVES

After completing this chapter, you should be able to:

- List, identify, and diagram the basic parts of the renal system.

- Explain the functions of the nephron, kidney, and bladder.

- List and define common diseases and conditions affecting the renal system, and explain the mechanisms of action of each class of drugs used to treat each disease.

- Explain how homeostasis of fluid and electrolytes affects the body.

KEY TERMS

acidosis, p. 528

bilirubin, p. 529

dialysis, p. 535

Kegel exercises, p. 530

ketone, p. 529

palliative, p. 534

pH, p. 528

specific gravity, p. 529

urobilinogen, p. 529

void, p. 528

INTRODUCTION

The renal system or urinary system is a fairly simple system with few components; however, its condition has a grave impact on many parts of the body. Genitourinary tract infections, poor kidney filtration, and water imbalance can indicate or cause diabetes, high blood pressure, or dehydration. The proper functioning of the kidneys is essential to maintain life. The drugs most commonly used to treat diseases of the renal system are anti-infectives and diuretics. The use of strong diuretics to remove excess water may also lead to a loss of potassium, which can cause muscle and heart problems. A delicate balance of electrolytes, kidney function, filtration, and waste removal must be maintained at all times, especially during illness and while taking medications that affect or treat the urinary tract.

Anatomy and Physiology of the Renal System

The renal system includes two kidneys, two ureters, one bladder, and the urethra (see Figure 31-1). The filtering system of the kidneys is composed of millions of microscopic kidney cells called *nephrons*. The by-products created as food and drugs are continually metabolized and filtered through the nephrons of the kidneys. The wastes then

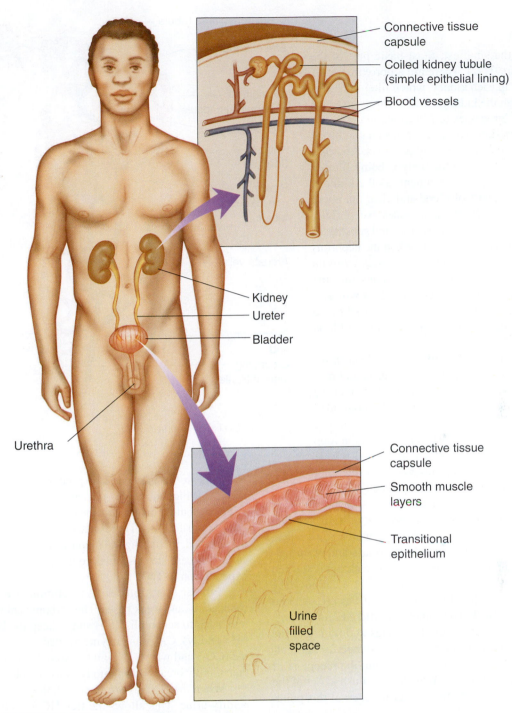

FIGURE 31-1 The renal system.

exit the kidneys as urine via the ureters. The *ureters* are tubes that allow urine to flow into the bladder, where it is stored until it is released. The kidneys, each of which is about the size of a fist, are located in the posterior abdomen just above the waist. The right kidney is slightly lower than the left because of the location of the liver. The kidneys are protected by adipose tissue and the ribcage.

The organs of the renal system are responsible for the following life-sustaining processes:

- Filtration of waste from the blood
- Removal of urine from the body
- Maintenance of water balance
- Maintenance of electrolyte balance
- Maintenance of acid–base balance

The Kidney

The human body contains two pairs of kidneys. Their function is to filter blood and remove waste, control body fluid balance, and regulate the body's balance of electrolytes. When the kidneys filter blood, they also make urine. The urine collects in the kidney's pelvis area, which is funnel shaped, and drains to ureters to the bladder. The kidney loses about 90% function when the body experiences various problems, diseases, or conditions.

The Nephron

The *nephron* is the smallest, most basic part of the kidney (see Figure 31-2). There are a pproximately 1 million nephrons in each kidney, which filter the blood that passes through the kidneys. The nephrons produce urine through the processes of filtration, tubular reabsorption, and secretion. These functions enable blood to reabsorb water, electrolytes, and nutrients. Approximately 25% of the blood in the body is being filtered by the kidneys at any given moment, as the kidneys process about 200 quarts of blood and clear out about 2 quarts of waste per day. Waste includes excess fluid, minerals, toxic substances such as urea, and substances that cannot be utilized by the body. When the nephrons fail to filter correctly, harmful toxic wastes build up in the body. The waste may then flow back into the bloodstream, causing blood infections. This will also result in the retention of excess fluid, increased blood pressure, and a reduction in the number of red blood cells produced.

The filter station of the kidney, the *glomerulus*, is located inside the nephrons and is housed and protected by the glomerulus capsule. The tubule that the filtrates flow into from the glomerulus is subdivided into three major parts: the proximal convoluted tubule (PCT), the loop of Henle (LOH) (also called the loop of the nephron), and the distal convoluted tubule (DCT). The urine then flows into the collecting duct and finally out of the kidney via the ureters.

Tubular reabsorption is the means of transporting ions back into the blood. Facilitating the process of transportation and reabsorption is *tubular secretion*, in which ions, acids, and bases are secreted to maintain homeostasis and water balance. Ions are reabsorbed when positively charged sodium (Na^+) cations are exchanged for hydrogen (H^+) cations. The Na^+ cations returns to the blood; the H^+ cations are secreted in the PCT and the DCT. The mineralocorticoid *aldosterone*, produced by the adrenal cortex, facilitates and regulates the secretion of potassium (K^+) cations in exchange for Na^+ cations in the DCT. When aldosterone gets into the receptors of the distal tubule, it releases K^+ ions that are flushed out of the tubule along with urine into the collecting duct; at this point,

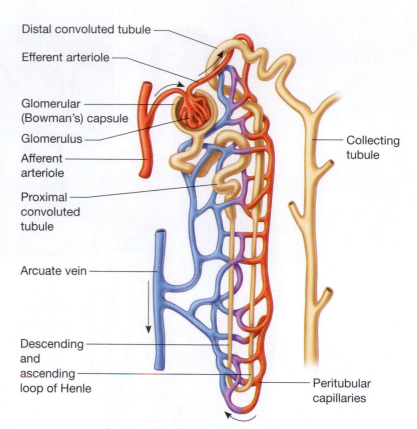

Labels: Distal convoluted tubule, Efferent arteriole, Glomerular (Bowman's) capsule, Glomerulus, Afferent arteriole, Proximal convoluted tubule, Arcuate vein, Descending and ascending loop of Henle, Collecting tubule, Peritubular capillaries

FIGURE 31-2 The nephron.

Na^+ ions are reabsorbed. This process creates an *osmotic gradient*, in which more Na^+ ions are in the blood than are in the urine or tubule. This follows the principle that wherever sodium goes, water follows. Therefore, water will follow the Na^+ ions in the blood, increasing the blood volume. This may exacerbate certain disease states such as congestive heart failure (CHF) or hypertension (HTN).

Tubular secretion serves to eliminate K^+ ions, H^+ ions, weak acids, and weak bases. The carbonic anhydrase (CA) system helps to accomplish this and to keep the blood at a proper **pH** (acidity). CA is an enzyme needed to convert carbon dioxide (CO_2) and water (H_2O) into carbonic acid (H_2CO_3), which then rapidly breaks down into H^+ ions and bicarbonate (HCO_3).

When the H^+ ions are liberated, they become available to acidify urine. This allows the free HCO_3 to be transported or reabsorbed back into the blood, reducing blood acidity by neutralizing the metabolic and toxic wastes. This process raises the blood pH to normal values. Metabolic **acidosis** can occur when CA is blocked. Table 31-1 displays some of the substances found in the nephron and their mechanisms of action.

The Bladder and Urine

The capacity of the average adult bladder is approximately 350 mL to 550 mL of urine; about 250 mL triggers a sensation of needing to **void**. Increased volume in the urinary bladder stretches the bladder wall and activates the micturition reflex. After voiding, it is normal to have about 50 mL left in the bladder. The micturition reflex is the relaxation of the

---

pH the measure of acidity or alkalinity of a solution.

acidosis the excessive acid in the body fluids.

void emptying the bladder.

specific gravity a measure of the density of a substance as compared to water; the specific gravity of water is 1.

ketone a by-product of fat metabolism.

urobilinogen a substance produced by the breakdown of bilirubin.

bilirubin a substance produced by the breakdown of hemoglobin.

TABLE 31-1 Actions of Selected Substances in the Nephron

Substance	Mechanism	Comments
Water	Reabsorbed by PCT and collecting ducts	Creates osmotic gradient
Sodium ions (Na^+)	Reabsorbed by PCT and DCT	Cation exchange for H^+
Hydrogen ions (H^+)	Secreted by PCT and DCT	Na^+ and HCO_3 go back into the blood; acidifies urine to a pH less than 7
Potassium ions (K^+)	Secreted by DCT	Cation exchange for Na^+, when aldosterone receptors are filled with aldosterone
Chloride ions (Cl^-)	Reabsorbed by loop of Henle	Na^+ ions follow Cl^- ions
Antidiuretic hormone	Released by pituitary gland; opens the pores of the collecting ducts. Water immediately flows toward sodium and is reabsorbed	Decreases the amount of water in urine

urethral sphincter in response to the increased pressure in the bladder.

Normal urine may vary in color from colorless to dark yellow. Some foods and medications can produce great variations in urine color:

- Red—produced by beets, blackberries, rifampin, and some anticoagulants
- Orange—produced by phenazopyridine
- Green or blue-green—produced by amitriptyline and vitamin B complex
- Brown/black—produced by levodopa and iron products

The **specific gravity** of urine ranges between 1.006 and 1.03. The higher the specific gravity, the higher the concentration of the urine. The specific gravity value will vary, depending on the time of day, amount of food and liquids consumed, and the amount of recent exercise.

The pH of urine is influenced by a number of factors. Generally, a normal urine pH range is from 4.6 to 8, with an average of 6. Usually, there is no detectable urine glucose, urine **ketones**, or urine protein, unless various disease states—notably diabetes—exist. Usually, no red blood cells, white blood cells, hemoglobin, or nitrites are present in urine. Although there may be a trace of **urobilinogen** in the urine, **bilirubin** is normally not detected in the urine.

Diseases, Conditions, and Treatments of the Urinary System

The urge to urinate varies depending on how much liquid has been consumed and the capacity of the bladder. The first signal occurs when the bladder is about half full. The average person should empty the bladder every three to six hours or four to six times a day. Frequency of urination will vary as a person ages. Usually, the first signal/urge will subside, if urination is postponed. As the bladder gets fuller and urination is further delayed, the signal or sensation becomes stronger.

Renal Failure

Renal failure means complete kidney failure. The kidneys are an important part of the body, because they help remove waste products and balance sodium, water, and vital electrolytes in the body. Kidney failure is a deadly build up of these products and requires immediate treatment (see Table 31-2). Patients sometimes do not know that they are suffering from renal failure until they incur a hospital stay or a visit to a clinic.

Prostatitis

Prostatitis, a common condition in males, can cause many uncomfortable symptoms. They can include urges to urinate, urination pain, fever, chills, sexual problems, and pelvic pain. Treatment for this illness can include surgery or medication. Some of the drugs used to treat prostatitis are antibiotics, anti-inflammatory drugs, and alpha-blocker medications.

Urinary Incontinence

Certain conditions may cause a person not to be able to hold even half of the bladder's capacity or not hold the urine long enough to reach a toilet. The inability to hold urine is called *incontinence*; the majority of incontinence occurs in females. There are seven types of incontinence:

- *Stress incontinence*—leakage occurs during exercise, coughing, or laughing.
- *Urge incontinence*—also known as *overactive bladder*; the person has little bladder control, especially when hearing running water, drinking, or sleeping.
- *Overflow incontinence*—occurs when a person cannot completely empty the bladder and there is a constant leakage.
- *Functional incontinence*—occurs when a person is not able to get to the toilet in time because of mobility limitations. Functional incontinence is the most common form of incontinence in older patients.
- *Mixed incontinence*—when a person has more than one form of incontinence, which may or may not be related.

TABLE 31-2 Pharmaceutical Treatments for Renal Failure

Generic Name	Brand Name	Dosage forms and Availability	Route of Administration	Common Adult Dosage
calcitrol	Rocaltrol	0.25-mcg, 0.5-mcg capsules; 15 mL solution	Oral	Dialysis patients: 0.25–1 mcg daily; based on serum calcium levels, other parameters
calcium acetate	Phoslo	667-mg tablets	Oral	1334 mg tid
calcium carbonate	TUMS, Actonel w/calcium, Renacidin, Tequin	35-mg tablets, 1,250-mg calcium carbonate tablets	Oral	500–2,000 mg tid
darbepoetin alfa	Aranesp	25 mcg, 40 mcg, 60 mcg, 100 mcg, 200 mcg, 300 mcg, and 500 mcg Aranesp/1 mL, and 150 mcg Aranesp/0.75 mL SDV; Single-dose prefilled syringes: 25 mcg Aranesp/ 0.42 mL, 40 mcg Aranesp/ 0.4 mL, 60 mcg Aranesp/ 0.3 mL, 100 mcg Aranesp/ 0.5 mL, and 150 mcg Aranesp/0.3 mL, 200 mcg Aranesp/0.4 mL, 300 mcg Aranesp/0.6 mL, and 500 mcg Aranesp/1 mL PFS	SC, IV	Dialysis patients: 0.45 mcg/kg once weekly; doses adjusted for hemoglobin levels
epoetin alfa (erythropoietin)	Epogen, Procrit	2,000 units, 3,000 units, 4,000 units, 10,000 units, and 40,000 units Epogen/1 mL SDV; 20,000 units Epogen/2 mL and 20,000 units Epogen/1 mL MDV	SC, IV	Dialysis patients: 75 units/kg three times weekly; doses adjusted for hemoglobin levels
ferrous sulfate	Feosol	45-mg, 65-mg caplets	Oral	325 mg qd or tid
sevelamer	Renagel, Renvela	400-mg, 800-mg tablets	Oral	800–1,000 mg tid

- *Anatomic incontinence*—occurs when a person has a physical abnormality.
- *Temporary incontinence*—may be due to urinary infection or severe constipation or occur as a side effect of certain medications.

Common causes of incontinence include the following:

- Childbirth, if supportive muscles and nerves of the urethra are damaged
- Obesity
- Hysterectomy (increases risk of incontinence by 30% to 40%)
- Recurrent bladder infections

- Medical condition or illness, such as diabetes, lung disease, or stroke
- Drugs that can relax the bladder too much and permit involuntary urine flow (e.g., first-generation, drowsy-formula antihistamines, such as diphenhydramine and chlorpheniramine, as well as some older antidepressants)

Treatment for incontinence will depend on the cause. **Kegel exercises** may be beneficial in controlling urine leakage. Kegel exercises strengthen the muscles of the pelvic floor, thereby improving the urethral sphincter tone and function. Surgery is also available. Medications used to treat stress incontinence are aimed at increasing the contractility of the urethral sphincter muscle.

Treatment with medications tends to be most successful in patients with mild-to-moderate stress incontinence (see Table 31-3). Alpha-adrenergic agonist drugs, such as pseudoephedrine, found in common over-the-counter (OTC)

Kegel exercises pelvic muscle training and toning exercises.

TABLE 31-3 Pharmaceutical Treatments for Urinary Incontinence

Generic Name	Brand Name	Dosage Forms and Availability	Route of Administration	Common Adult Dosage
darifenacin hydrobromide	Enablex	7.5-mg, 15-mg tablets	Oral	7.5–15 mg qd
flavoxate HCl	Urispas	100-mg tablet	Oral	100–200 mg tid–qid
oxybutynin	Ditropan, Oxytrol, Gelnique	5-mg, 10-mg, 15-mg tablets; 5 mg/5 mL syrup. 3.9-mg patch	Oral, transdermal	5 mg bid–tid; transdermal path: apply patch every three to four days; transdermal gel: apply one packet topically qd
solifenacin succinate	Vesicare	5-mg, 10-mg tablets	Oral	5–10 mg qd
tolterodine tartate	Detrol, Detrol LA, Detrol XL	1-mg, 2-mg tablets; 2-mg, 4-mg capsules	Oral	Detrol: 1–2 mg bid; Detrol LA: 2–4 mg qd
trospium chloride	Sanctura, Sanctura XR	20-mg tablets	Oral	Sanctura: 20 mg bid; Sanctura XR: 60 mg every a.m.

decongestants, may be used to treat stress incontinence. They work by increasing the strength of the urethral sphincter; in about 50% of patients, symptoms improve with this treatment. The tricyclic antidepressant imipramine has similar properties, so it too may be used to treat stress incontinence. Estrogen replacement therapy (ERT) can decrease urinary frequency, urgency, and burning in postmenopausal women. ERT has also been shown to increase the tone of and blood supply to the urethral sphincter muscles. However, the use of estrogen as a treatment for stress incontinence is controversial.

Urinary Retention

An inability to urinate is more common in men than in women. When approximately 200 to 300 mL of urine has collected in the bladder, a signal is sent via nerves in the spinal cord to the brain. The brain then returns a signal that starts contractions or spasms in the bladder wall. At this same moment, the internal sphincter muscle relaxes. With urinary retention, the bladder is not able to release the urine, even though the urge exists. Common causes of urinary retention include the following:

- Blockage or obstruction of the urethra. The most common cause of urethral blockage in men is the enlargement of the prostate gland, called *benign prostatic hypertrophy (BPH)*. The enlarged prostate gland presses against the urethra, blocking the outflow or passage of urine.
- Disruption or damage to the delicate and complex system of nerves that connects the urinary tract with the brain. Common causes include spinal cord injury, spinal cord tumor, herniated disk in the back, or an infection or blood clot that places pressure on the spinal cord.
- Infection in the pelvic area, such as herpes, chlamydia, or pelvic inflammatory disease. The inflammation and swelling that accompany infection can interfere with nerves in the area and/or compress the urethra. Infections of the spinal cord place pressure on the cord, leading to retention, because nerve signal transmission is hampered.
- Anesthetic effects during or after surgery. This is a relatively common and temporary cause.
- Other drugs that act to tighten the ureters and block or restrict the flow of urine. These drugs include the ephedrine and pseudoephedrine found in nasal decongestants.

PROFILE IN PRACTICE

Mrs. Lange arrives at the window of an independent retail pharmacy and explains to the pharmacist that her urine has recently taken on a brownish color, but she has not gotten any new prescriptions filled. When asked what OTC medicines she might be on, Mrs. Lange states that she takes 81 mg of aspirin, a psyllium laxative, and a multivitamin every day, but also says that she has been taking these medications for quite some time with no problems. However, she recently changed the brand of her multivitamin.

▸ *Could this change in the brand of her multivitamin cause the discoloration? Why or why not?*

Functional urinary retention is treated with the insertion of a Foley catheter and possibly antibiotics to avoid or treat urinary tract infection (UTI). Urinary cholinergics (bethanechol and neostigmine methylsufate) can be used to treat nonfunctional incontinence in postoperative and postpartum patients.

Urinary Tract Infections

UTIs are bacterial infections of the urinary system. UTIs are most common among women, because the distance from the urethra to the anus is shorter in women, thus bacteria do not need to travel as far. UTI symptoms include a frequent urge to void, a burning sensation during voiding, cloudy or strong-smelling urine, and blood in the urine. Two of the most common UTIs are cystitis and pyelonephritis.

Cystitis is an inflammation of the bladder caused in most cases by *E. coli* and staphylococcus bacteria.

Pyelonephritis is an inflammation of the kidney and upper urinary tract that is usually caused by a bacterial infection of the bladder or cystitis. The backflow of infected urine from the bladder goes up into the ureters and then into the kidney and nephrons.

Pyelonephritis may occur when urine becomes stagnant. In most cases, urine stagnates because of an obstruction of urinary flow caused by a blockage, such as kidney stones, tumors, congenital deformities, or loss of bladder function from nerve disease. When no obstruction is present, the *E. coli* bacterium, normally found in the feces, is the cause of about 80% to 90% of acute bladder and kidney infections. Other bacteria that may cause both cystitis and pyelonephritis are *Klebsiella, Enterobacter, Proteus, Pseudomonas*, and *Mycoplasma*.

Symptoms of acute pyelonephritis include sudden onset of fever and chills, burning or frequent urination, aching pain on one or both sides of the lower back or abdomen, nausea and vomiting, cloudy or bloody urine, and fatigue. The flank pain may be extreme. The symptoms of chronic pyelonephritis include HTN, anemia, and protein and blood in the urine.

If left untreated, both cystitis and pyelonephritis can progress to a chronic condition that lasts for months or years and may lead to scarring and possible loss of kidney function. In one study, researchers found that a substance in cranberry juice keeps infection-causing bacteria from attaching to the walls of the urethra. Cranberry juice also makes the urine more acidic.

In addition to treating the infection, phenazopyridine (200 mg po tid) can be used to manage the symptoms of a burning and itching urethra. Treatment of a UTI with phenazopyridine should not exceed two days, because there is little or no evidence that the coadministration of phenazopyridine HCl and an antibacterial provides greater benefit than administration of the antibacterial alone after two days. Table 31-4 shows some anti-infectives used to treat UTIs.

info
UTIs in Women and Men
Approximately 30% of all women will experience a UTI in their lifetimes, as compared with 3% of all males. The most common causes of UTI in the male are prostatic enlargement and diabetes. The incidence of UTI in men nears the incidence of UTI in women only in men over 60 years of age. There is evidence that circumcised male neonates have more UTIs than noncircumcised (intact) male neonates.

❝ Workplace Wisdom Common Abbreviations
The abbreviation for sulfamethoxazole is SMZ, and the abbreviation for trimethoprim is TMP. ❞

TABLE 31-4 **Pharmaceutical Treatments for Urinary Tract Infections**

Generic Name	Brand Name	Dosage Forms and Availability	Route of Administration	Common Adult Dosage
amoxicillin	Amoxil, Trimox	250-mg, 500-mg capsules; 500-mg, 875-mg tablets; 125 mg/5 mL, 150 mg/5 mL, 400 mg/5 mL suspension	Oral	500 mg q12h
amoxicillin/clavulanate	Augmentin	150-mg, 500-mg, 875-mg tablets; 125 mg/5 mL suspension	Oral	500 mg q12h
cefaclor	Ceclor	250-mg, 500-mg pulvules; 125 mg/5 mL, 187 mg/5 mL, 250 mg/5 mL, 375 mg/5 mL suspension	Oral	150–500 mg q8h
cefadroxil	Duricef	500-mg capsules; 50 mL, 75 mL, 100 mL suspension	Oral	For cystitis: 1–2 gm daily; for all other UTIs, 1 gm bid

(Continued)

TABLE 31-4 Pharmaceutical Treatments for Urinary Tract Infections (*Continued*)

Generic Name	Brand Name	Dosage Forms and Availability	Route of Administration	Common Adult Dosage
cefpodoxime	Vantin	100 mg, 200 mg tablets; 50 mL, 75 mL, 100 mL suspension	Oral	100 mg q12h, Acute; 200 mg × 1 dose
ceftriaxone	Rocephin	500 mg, 1 gm crystalline power	Intravenous	500 mg–1 gm bid (IV or IM only)
cefuroxime	Ceftin	250-mg tablets; 50 mL, 100 mL suspension	Oral	250 mg bid
cephalexin	Kelfex	250-mg, 333-mg, 500-mg, 750-mg capsules	Oral	250 mg q6h or 500 mg q12h
demeclocycline	Declomycin	150 mg, 300 mg tablets	Oral	150 mg qid or 300 mg bid
doxycycline	Vibramycin	100 mg of doxycycline with 480 mg of ascorbic acid; packages of 5 mg powder; 100-mg capsules	Oral, intravenous	100 mg q12h for one day, then 100 mg daily
flavoxate	Uripas	100-mg tablets	Oral	100 mg tid–qid
fosfomycin	Monurol	3-gm SD sachet	Oral granules	3-gm packet in 90–120 mL cold water, given as a single dose
fosfomycin	Monurol	3-gm sachet	Oral	3 gm (dissolve one sachet) × 1 dose
methenamine	Urised, Urex	1-gm tablets	Oral	Two tablets qid
minocycline	Minocin	5 mL suspension; 50-mg, 100-mg capsules	Oral	100 mg q12h
nitrofurantoin	Macrobid, Macrodantin	100-mg capsules	Oral	Macrobid: 100 mg bid; Macrodantin: 50–100 mg qid
nitrofurantoin	Macrodantin, Macrobid	100-mg capsules	Oral	Macrodantin: 50–100 mg q6h; Macrobid: 100 mg q12h
norfloxacin	Noroxin	400-mg tablets	Oral	400 mg q12h
ofloxacin	Floxin	200-mg, 300-mg, 400-mg tablets	Oral	200 mg q12h
phenazopyridine	Pyridium	100-mg, 200-mg tablets	Oral	200 mg tid
sulfamethoxazole/ trimethoprim	Septra, Bactrim	80/400-mg, 160/800-mg tablets; 473 mL oral suspension	Oral, intravenous	One DS tablet q12h TMP IV divided q6–12h; Info: dose, duration varies w/infection type, severity
tetracycline	Sumycin	250-mg, 500-mg tablets	Oral	500 mg q 6h, qid
trimethoprim/ sulfamethoxazole	Bactrim, Bactrim DS, Septra	80 mg/400 mg tablets; 160 mg/800 mg DS tablets	Oral	160 mg TMP/800 mg SMZ po q12h × 10–14 days

Other Signs and Symptoms of Renal System Conditions

A person may have many indicators that he or she has a renal system problem; signs and symptoms may include the following:

- *Anuria*—production or excretion of less than 100 mL of urine per day. If wastes are not eliminated from the body, the person may die from toxemia or septicemia.
- *Dysuria*—difficult or painful urination.
- *Hematuria*—blood in the urine, possibly from an injured kidney or infection.
- *Nephritis*—inflammation of the nephron that causes the tissue of the whole kidney to become inflamed; usually due to infection.
- *Oliguria*—decreased urine production (100–400 mL/day).
- *Pyuria*—pus or bacteria in the urine.
- *Uremia*—urine in the blood.

Kidney Stones

Kidney stones (*urolithiasis*) is a common and painful urinary tract disorder in which solid mineral deposits accumulate in the urinary tract. In addition to possibly obstructing urinary flow, urolithiasis may also lead to UTIs. The pain of *passing* such a blockage or stone is considered excruciating. The mineral masses develop when waste is not completely dissolved in the urine. A microscopic, hard crystal that remains in the kidney is called a *calculus*. The waste substances most commonly found in kidney stones are calcium, oxalate, phosphate, and uric acid. (see Table 31-5)

It is also possible to have solids in the urine, because the body does not produce enough water in the urine to dissolve them. In addition, there may be a deficiency of certain chemicals that are normally present in the urine that help break down and dissolve the waste solids. These *helpers* are citrate, magnesium, and pyrophosphate. If calculi obstruct one of the ureters, they can cause the urinary tract to go into a spasm, causing great pain. Large calculi can cause organ damage and even renal failure.

---

palliative reducing the severity of symptoms.

dialysis a medical procedure that removes waste from the blood of patients with renal failure.

Caucasian males between 30 and 60 years are the most prone to urolithiasis. Diet plays an important role, as diets high in animal protein increase uric acid levels in the body and can lead to gout and kidney stones. The routine intake of rhubarb, spinach, pepper, cocoa, nuts, or tea can result in excess oxalate in people who have a high level of risk. Dehydration and diarrhea contribute to a lack of water available to dissolve the stones. The following chemical imbalances can contribute to the formation of kidney stones: hypercalcemia, hypernatremia, and hypocitraturia. Also, people who have been diagnosed with hyperthyroidism or hyperparathyroidism are at higher risk, because both conditions allow excess calcium to combine with phosphate or oxalate in the kidneys, resulting in the formation of calculi.

Treatment of urolithiasis is **palliative**, with pain management, and preventive, with diet consisting of mineral and vitamin supplements and increased fluid intake. Most calculi measure less than $\frac{1}{4}$ inch (4 mm) and spontaneously pass in the urine without need for any treatment. Stones that measure 5 to 7 mm can be passed without intervention in about 50% of cases. When a stone exceeds 7 mm in diameter, however, some form of intervention is usually required.

Pain management depends on the degree of pain. Oral analgesics for mild-to-moderate pain include diclofenac and acetaminophen with codeine. Severe pain requires injections of narcotics such as morphine or meperidine. Because narcotics can cause nausea, vomiting, and constipation, it is important not to let the patient get dehydrated if this side effect should occur.

Collection and analysis of the stones can allow the physician to make specific diet and medication recommendations, such as avoiding high-protein and high-fat foods, taking the antigout drug allopurinol, increasing fluid intake, and using calcium citrate, magnesium, and cholestyramine to reduce oxalate levels. Taking a potassium citrate supplement or eating citrus fruits increases citrate levels and helps dissolve waste. Taking vitamin B6 supplements helps fight high levels of oxalate. Taking thiazide diuretics may reduce high urinary calcium levels. The patient should avoid increasing calcium in the diet, as this may lead to the formation of calcium calculi.

Edema and Hypertension

Kidney damage can lead to HTN, which can then lead to kidney failure. Consistently elevated blood pressure levels can lead to the damage of the arteries, in particular, the kidney

---

TABLE 31-5 Pharmaceutical Treatments for Kidney Stones

Generic Name	Brand Name	Dosage Forms and Availability	Route of Administration	Common Adult Dosage
allopurinol	Zyloprim	100-mg tablets 300-mg tablets	Oral	200–300 mg qd
potassium citrate	Urocrit-K	5 mEq, 10 mEq, 15 mEq tablets	Oral	10–20 mEq tid; maximum dosage of 100 mEq/day

arteries, which become thickened and narrowed with prolonged high blood pressure. When this happens, less blood gets to the kidneys, resulting in a reduced oxygen supply. Kidney failure can lead to an excess of fluid in the body, peripheral edema, and ascites. (see Table 31-6) This excess fluid places an excessive workload on the heart, raising blood pressure and possibly leading to heart failure or myocardial infarction. Diuretics play an important role in reducing high blood pressure, because they reduce the volume of fluid in the body and in the blood. Certain disease states, such as CHF, also require less blood volume.

Diabetes Mellitus and the Kidneys

Diabetes affects many organs of the body, including the eyes, kidneys, and blood vessels. Kidney damage, bladder problems, and UTIs are long-term complications affecting people with diabetes and can lead to renal failure. Diabetic kidney disease (*diabetic nephropathy*) and *end-stage renal disease (ESRD)* require the diabetic person to have either **dialysis** or a kidney transplant. Native Americans and African-Americans are at even higher risk for developing ESRD than diabetics. The warning sign of protein in the urine can trigger early diagnosis and treatment. Familial ESRD, diet, high blood pressure, high blood glucose, and noncompliance are a few of the factors that lead to diabetic nephropathy.

Health goals for the diabetic patient include the following:

- Blood sugar less than 126 mg/dL
- Hemoglobin A1C less than 7%
- Blood pressure less than 130/80 mm Hg
- Yearly microalbumin tests to check for protein in the urine

TABLE 31-6 Pharmaceutical Treatments for Edema

Generic Name	Brand Name	Dosage Forms and Availability	Route of Administration	Common Adult Dosage
acetazolamide	Diamox	250-mg capsules 500-mg capsules	Oral, intravenous	250–375 mg every other day for two days followed by one day of rest
amiloride	Moduretic	5-mg, 50-mg tablets	Oral	1–2 tablets daily
amiloride/ hydrochlorothiazide (HCTZ)	Midamor	5-mg tablets	Oral	5–10 mg daily
bumetanide	Bumex	0.5-mg, 1-mg, 2-mg tablets	Oral, intravenous	0.5–2 mg qd or bid
chlorothiazide	Diuril	250 mg oral suspension 500-mg capsules	Oral, intravenous	Oral: 0.5–1 gm daily in one to two divided doses
furosemide	Lasix	20-mg, 40-mg, 80-mg tablets	Oral, intravenous	20–80 mg qd
hydrochlorothiazide	Ezride, Microzide	12.5-mg, 25-mg, 50-mg capsules	Oral	12.5–50 mg daily or intermittently
indapamide	Lozol	1.25-mg tablets	Oral	2.5 mg po qd
metolazone	Mykrox	0.5-mg tablets	Oral	5–20 mg qd
spironolactone	Aldactazide	25-mg, 50-mg tablets	Oral	One to two tablets daily
spironolactone/ HCTZ	Aldactone	15-mg, 50-mg, 100-mg tablets	Oral	25–200 mg daily
torsemide	Demadex	5-mg, 10-mg, 20-mg, 100-mg tablets	Oral, intravenous	10–20 mg qd
triamterene	Dyazide	25-mg, 37.5-mg capsules; 25-mg, 37.5-mg, 50-mg, 75-mg tablets	Oral	One to two tablets daily
triamterene/HCTZ	Dyrenium	50-mg, 100-mg capsules	Oral	100 mg bid

When the glucose in the blood becomes high, the body tries to get rid of the excess sugar by trying to eliminate it in urine. This leads to dehydration and is the reason why diabetics are usually excessively thirsty and urinate frequently. The effects of dehydration depend on the degree of water loss:

- 2% body weight loss reduces performance significantly.
- 5% body weight loss causes heat exhaustion.
- 7% to 10% body weight loss results in heat stroke or death.

Diuretics

Diuretics increase urine output in various ways. Most diuretics inhibit or block sodium absorption by the blood system in the nephron, thus promoting the secretion of sodium. Recall that wherever sodium goes, water follows. Chloride also follows the sodium. The diuresis increases as sodium levels in the tubule increase.

Diuretics play a significant role in the renal system as well as the cardiovascular system. See Chapter 29 for a more in-depth look at diuretics.

Summary

The renal system is fairly simple, yet its proper functioning is essential to maintain life. The renal system consists of two kidneys, two ureters, the bladder, and the urethra. The functions of the renal system are to filter waste from the blood and remove it from the body, maintain water and electrolyte balance, and maintain acid–base balance. Any dysfunction of the renal system can have grave impacts on many parts of the body. Kidney damage can lead to HTN, muscle problems, and serious cardiac disorders.

Common diseases of the renal system include urinary retention or urinary incontinence, kidney stones, and UTIs. Approximately 30% of all women will experience a UTI in their lifetimes.

The two drugs most commonly used to treat diseases of the renal system are anti-infectives and diuretics. This chapter contains a thorough discussion of the importance of the renal system in maintaining homeostasis, the incidence of diseases of the urinary tract, and the drug therapies available to treat these conditions.

Chapter Review Questions

1. Which of the following is *not* a function of the urinary system?
   a. remove urine from the body
   b. filter waste from the body
   c. produce hormones
   d. maintain water balance

2. The filter station of the kidney is the _____.
   a. nephrons
   b. glomerulus
   c. loop of Henle
   d. distal convoluted tubule

3. The generic name for Duricef, which can be used to treat UTIs, is _____.
   a. cefadroxil
   b. sulfamethoxazole and trimethoprim
   c. fosfomycin
   d. demeclocycline

4. An inflammation of the kidney is _____.
   a. nephritis
   b. pyelonephritis
   c. cystitis
   d. urolithiasis

5. _____ is a condition of blood in the urine.
   a. Uremia
   b. Pyuria
   c. Dysuria
   d. Hematuria

6. An inflammation of the bladder is _____.
   a. nephritis
   b. pyelonephritis
   c. cystitis
   d. urolithiasis

7. The development of kidney stones is known as _____.
   a. phlebitis
   b. pyelonephritis
   c. cystitis
   d. urolithiasis

8. _____ is a condition of urine in the blood.
   a. Uremia
   b. Pyuria
   c. Dysuria
   d. Hematuria

9. The medical term for decreased urine production is
   _____.
   a. oliguria
   b. urolithiasis
   c. nephritis
   d. incontinence

10. Which of the following is used to treat urinary incontinence?
    a. furosemide
    b. chlorthalidone
    c. tolterodine
    d. bumetanide

Critical Thinking Questions

1. Explain why women are much more likely than men to develop urinary tract infections.

2. Explain why it is so important to the body that the kidneys work properly. What can happen if the kidneys are not working properly?

3. What causes (other than those listed in this chapter) can contribute to incontinence?

Web Challenge

1. Go to http://kidney.niddk.nih.gov/kudiseases/pubs/yoururinary/index.htm to learn more about how the kidneys work.

2. Choose one of the conditions discussed in this chapter. Go online and research alternative methods of treatment for the condition.

References and Resources

Adams, M.P., D.L. Josephson, and L.N. Holland, Jr. *Pharmacology for Nurses: A Pathophysiologic Approach.* (4th edition.) Upper Saddle River, NJ: Pearson, 2013.

"Circumcision and Urinary Tract Infection." http://www.cirp.org/library/disease/UTI. Web. 8 April 2008.

"Control of the Hydrogen Ion Activity (pH) in the Body." http://www.usyd.edu.au/su/anaes/lectures/acidbase_mjb/control.html. Web. 8 April 2008.

Drug Facts and Comparisons, 2013 ed. St. Louis: Wolters Kluwer. 2012. Print.

"Health Ask the Doctor BBC." http://www.bbc.co.uk/health/ask_doctor/cystitis_cranberry.shtml. Web. 8 April 2008.

Holland, N. and M.P. Adams. *Core Concepts in Pharmacology.* (3rd edition.) Upper Saddle River, NJ: Pearson, 2010.

"Micturition Reflex." The Free Dictionary. Web. 13 December 2012.

National Institute of Diabetes and Digestive and Kidney Diseases (NIDDK), NIH. http://diabetes.niddk.nih.gov/ Web. 13 December 2012.

"Types of Urinary Incontinence." www.mayoclinic.org. Web. 24 July 2013.

Whorton, J.C. *Nature Cures: The History of Alternative Medicine in America*. New York: Oxford University Press, 2004.

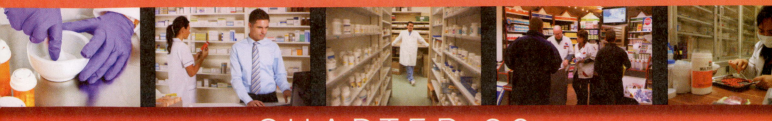

CHAPTER 32

The Endocrine System

LEARNING OBJECTIVES

After completing this chapter, you should be able to:

- Identify and describe the glands of the endocrine system.

- Describe the functions of the hypothalamus and pituitary gland, and list other body parts that are affected by these glands.

- List and define the hormones of the endocrine system and know which gland or organ secretes each hormone.

- Describe male and female hormones and some products used for replacement in cases of deficiency of these hormones.

- Identify and describe the major diseases and conditions that affect the endocrine system.

- Compare and contrast diabetes mellitus and diabetes insipidus.

- Understand the effects of anabolic steroid use.

KEY TERMS

corticosteroid, p. 542

gonads, p. 542

homeostasis, p. 540

hormone, p. 540

isotonic, p. 542

negative feedback, p. 540

polydipsia, p. 550

polyphagia, p. 550

polyuria, p. 550

priapism, p. 548

INTRODUCTION

The endocrine system is a collection of glands that produce hormones to help regulate the body's growth, metabolism, and sexual development and function. In fact, hormones, which are transported to tissues and organs throughout the body, influence every cell in some way. Because the glands of the endocrine system are ductless, the hormones they secrete are released directly into the bloodstream and travel through the circulatory system to reach the specific target organs where they exert their primary effects.

The nervous system is considered the mass communicator of the human body, and hormones are the chemicals that do the communicating. *Endocrinology* is the study of the chemical communication system that controls a large number of physiologic processes. It is also the study of hormones, their receptors, and the intracellular signaling pathways that they follow and call upon. As mentioned, all cell types, organs, and processes are influenced by hormone signaling, though some more strongly than others. Growth from birth to adulthood involves the endocrine system, critical GHs, and other contributing hormones.

Anatomy of the Endocrine System

The endocrine system (see Figure 32-1) is an internal *communication* system that consists of the hypothalamus, pituitary gland, other hormone-producing cells and glands, hormones, and receptors. The major driving forces of the endocrine system are the hypothalamus and the pituitary gland. The pituitary gland controls the thyroid, parathyroid, pancreas, adrenal glands, and gonads. During pregnancy, the placenta also acts as an endocrine gland.

The *hypothalamus*, part of the brain stem, controls the activity of the pituitary gland. Also known as the *hypophysis*, the *pituitary gland* is only about the size of a large pea, but it is called the *master gland* because it controls many of the other glands. Attached to the base of the hypothalamus in the brain, the pituitary gland is composed of an anterior lobe and a posterior lobe. Each lobe contains a number of hormones, which may be released into the general blood circulation.

Some parts of the endocrine system also secrete substances other than hormones. The pancreas, for example, secretes digestive enzymes. The testes and ovaries secrete ova and sperm. Organs such as the stomach, heart, and intestines

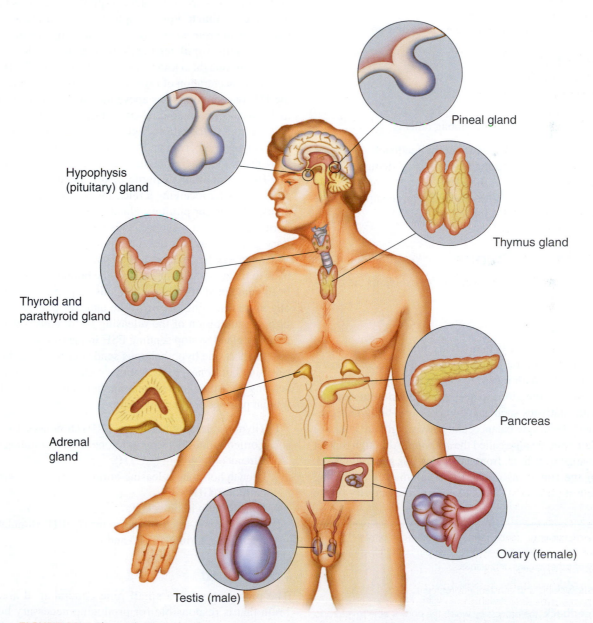

Hypophysis
(pituitary) gland

Pineal gland

Thymus gland

Thyroid and
parathyroid gland

Pancreas

Adrenal
gland

Testis (male)

Ovary (female)

FIGURE 32-1 The endocrine glands.

are involved in hormone production, too, but this is not their primary function.

Hormones

Hormones are the chemicals that take *messages* to the cells through the bloodstream. Hormones transfer information and instructions from one set of cells to another. Each hormone affects only the cells that are genetically programmed to receive and respond to its message. Many factors can affect the level of hormones in the body at any given time. Age, stress, infection, and changes in the balance of fluid and minerals in blood are only a few examples.

Hormones are divided into two groups according to their structure:

1. Steroids
   - Slow-acting
   - Long-lasting
   - Names usually end in *rone* (e.g., testosterone, progesterone)
2. Peptides and amines
   - Made of proteins
   - Fast-acting
   - Short-lived
   - Include insulin and ADH, among others

Hormone production is controlled by feedback. *Feedback control* depends on a monitoring of supply and demand. When the level of hormone is low, the gland secretes the hormone until the level rises again. When there is a large supply of the hormone, the gland stops making it.

The Endocrine Glands

This section briefly describes each of the glands in the endocrine system.

Hypothalamus

The *hypothalamus* controls many body functions, especially a number important to the female menstrual cycle, pregnancy, birth, and lactation. With regard to the nervous system, the hypothalamus mainly functions to keep the body in **homeostasis**. Dynamic vital statistics such as blood pressure, body temperature, fluid and electrolyte balance, and body weight are held to a given, predetermined value called the *set point*. Although this set point can change over time, from day to day it is generally fixed.

One of the functions of the hypothalamus in achieving and maintaining homeostasis is to control the activity of the

---

hormone a chemical substance, produced by an organ or gland, that travels through the bloodstream to regulate certain bodily functions and/or the activity of other organs and glands.

homeostasis a stable and constant environment.

negative feedback the process by which the body is able to return to homeostasis.

---

pituitary gland. The hypothalamus produces hormones known as *releasing factors*. These are sent to the pituitary gland via small blood vessels, which connect the hypothalamus to the anterior lobe of the pituitary gland. The releasing factors stimulate the release of hormones that are produced in the anterior lobe.

The hormones of the anterior lobe are known as *tropic hormones*. *Tropic* means *growth*. The tropic hormones are released into the general blood circulation to control the activities of the other endocrine glands. Sometimes these hormones are called *stimulating hormones,* because they stimulate other glands either to produce other hormones or to perform an activity.

The hypothalamus also produces oxytocin and antidiuretic hormone (ADH), two hormones that are stored in the posterior lobe of the pituitary gland. The posterior lobe, also known as the *neurohypophysis*, sits behind the anterior lobe and is actually a continuation of the hypothalamus.

The mechanism that controls the release of tropic or stimulating hormones from the anterior pituitary gland is known as **negative feedback**. For example, the thyroid-releasing factor stimulates the release of thyroid-stimulating hormone (TSH), which in turn stimulates the thyroid gland to release the hormone thyroxine (also known as thyroid hormone [TH]). As a result, the concentration of thyroxine in the blood increases. When the TH concentration rises above normal, this signals the hypothalamus to stop sending releasing factor. Because no releasing factor is sent to the pituitary gland, the pituitary gland does not send out any more TSH and the thyroid gland does not produce more thyroxine. Therefore, these mechanisms are *inhibited*.

Here is another example of the mechanism of negative feedback: After receiving a releasing factor from the hypothalamus, the anterior pituitary gland releases follicle-stimulating hormone (FSH) in response. This FSH from the anterior pituitary gland stimulates the maturation of an egg in the ovary. When the egg has matured, the ovary releases negative feedback to the hypothalamus, telling the brain that the activity has been completed. The hypothalamus responds by *not* sending any more releasing factor to the anterior pituitary gland. In turn, the inhibition of the releasing factor causes the anterior pituitary gland to stop sending FSH to the ovary.

In short, the hypothalamus sends out releasing factors, or releasing hormones, to the pituitary gland, which responds by sending out tropic, or stimulating, hormones. Some of the important pairings are the following:

1. Thyroid-releasing hormone (TRH) stimulates TSH.
2. Corticotropin-releasing hormone (CRH) stimulates adrenocorticotropin (ACTH).
3. Growth hormone-releasing hormone stimulates growth hormone (GH).
4. Somatostatin inhibits GH.
5. Gonadotropin-releasing hormone (GnRH) stimulates both luteinizing hormone (LH) and FSH.

Pineal Gland

The pineal gland is a small pine cone-shaped area in the brain that is responsible for producing necessary hormones and is part of the diencephalon of the brain. One of the many important hormones the pineal gland produces is melatonin, a hormone that is responsible for sleep and wake cycles. Melatonin can be taken in supplement form to help with insomnia and sleep problems. As individuals get older, melatonin levels drop off or can become nonexistent. Light is a big player in determining just how much melatonin the body produces.

Pituitary Gland

The anterior pituitary gland secretes hormones that regulate the activities of the other endocrine glands (see Figure 32-2). All the hormones stimulate a specific endocrine gland, except the GH or *somatotropin,* which regulates the growth and maintenance of all body tissues. An excess of GH in a child results in gigantism; a lack or deficiency results in pituitary dwarfism. *Acromegaly* results when the increase in GH occurs in an adult. If this happens, parts of the body, such as the head, hands, feet, jaw, arms, and legs, grow to be unusually large.

The pituitary gland sends a signal to the respective gland or body part to initiate its glandular functions:

1. TSH stimulates the thyroid gland (TH production).
2. FSH/LH stimulates the gonads (gametogenesis and steroid production).

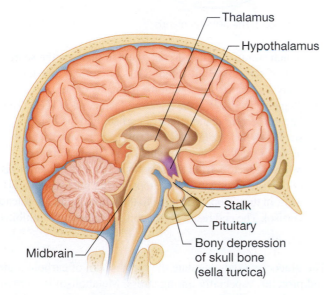

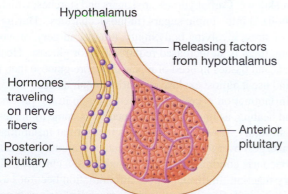

FIGURE 32-2 The pituitary gland.

3. GH is sent to all body parts for linear growth and intermediate metabolism.
4. ACTH is sent to the adrenal glands to cause growth of the adrenal cortex and synthesis and secretion of cortisol.
5. Prolactin stimulates the mammary glands to produce milk during and after pregnancy.

Classes of pituitary hormones and their other, more technical names are as follows:

1. Somatomammotrophs
   a. Somatotrophs—GH or somatotropin
   b. Mammotrophs—also called lactotrophs or PRL

2. Glycoproteins
   a. Thyrotrophs—TSH or thyrotropin
   b. Gonadotrophs—LH and FSH
   c. Corticotrophs—ACTH or corticotropin
   d. Pro-opiomelanocortin - ACTH, LPH, endorphins (not described in this book)

Thyroid and Parathyroid

The *thyroid* is a small gland, weighing less than 1 oz., located in the front of the neck. It is made up of two lobes that lie along the windpipe and are joined together by a narrow band of tissue called the *isthmus.* The thyroid is directly regulated by the anterior pituitary gland and indirectly regulated by the hypothalamus.

Two types of cells make up the thyroid tissue: follicular cells and parafollicular cells. The majority of the thyroid tissue consists of the *follicular cells,* which secrete iodine-containing hormones called thyroxine (T4) and triiodothyronine (T3). The *parafollicular cells* secrete the hormone calcitonin.

The normal thyroid gland produces about 80% T4 and about 20% T3; however, T3 possesses about four times the hormone *strength* of T4. When the level of THs drops too low, the pituitary gland produces TSH, which stimulates the thyroid gland to produce more hormones.

The thyroid gland needs iodine to produce these hormones. Thyroid cells are the only cells in the body that can absorb iodine. The richest sources of iodine are seafood and seaweed (especially kelp). In the United States, the primary source of iodine is iodized salt. Thyroid cells combine iodine and the amino acid tyrosine to make T3 and T4. T3 and T4 are then released into the bloodstream and are transported throughout the body, where they control metabolism. Every cell in the body depends on THs for regulation of metabolism. The thyroid gland is also responsible for the enhancement of growth and development and for nervous system maturation in children.

The thyroid is a very important gland that affects parts of the body and functions that regulate growth, such as:

- Thermogenesis—T4 and T3 produce heat by increasing the body's oxidative metabolism. This is accomplished by the synthesis of Na^+/K^+ ATPase.
- Growth and development—T4 and T3 are essential for growth in childhood. T4 and T3 stimulate growth by exerting a direct effect on tissue and a permissive effect on GH action.

- Nervous system—in childhood, T4 and T3 are essential for normal myelination and development of the nervous system. Thyroid deficiency in childhood causes mental retardation. In adults, T4 and T3 deficiency causes lethargy and blunting of intellect. T4 and T3 excess causes restlessness and hypersensitivity.
- Heart—excess T4 and T3 can increase heart stroke volume and heart rate by increasing the heart's sensitivity to catecholamines. A deficiency of T4 and T3 has the opposite effect.

Parathyroid Gland

The parathyroid glands are located behind the thyroid gland in the neck. These glands help control the amount of blood calcium in the body and how much calcium the body produces. Parathyroid glands can be the cause of disease and tumors, as many other glands in the body are susceptible to falling victim to problems and diseases.

> **Workplace Wisdom** **Thyroid Cancer Statistics**
>
> Every year, approximately 15,000 new cases of thyroid cancer are diagnosed.

Adrenal Glands

Adrenal glands are located on the upper part of each kidney (see Figure 32-3). These glands have an inner or center part known as the *adrenal medulla* and an outer part known as the *adrenal cortex*. The adrenal medulla, which is part of the sympathetic nervous system, secretes epinephrine (EPI) during sympathetic activation. EPI is a catecholamine.

The adrenal cortex secretes two types of **corticosteroids** or hormones: *glucocorticoids* and *mineralocorticoids*. The hormones of the adrenal cortex, the adrenocorticosteroids, are generally referred to as *corticosteroids* or simply *steroids*. As a pharmacological agent, the glucocorticoids, or glucocorticosteroids, are used frequently in the treatment of inflammatory or allergic conditions such as arthritis or bee sting.

The following three factors induce the hypothalamus to secrete the releasing factor called *ACTH*:

- Sleep-wake cycle—larger amounts of ACTH (from the anterior pituitary gland) and cortisol (a glucocorticoid from the adrenal gland) are secreted while a person is awake. Smaller amounts of these hormones are present during sleep. During the wake period, cortisol requires body metabolism to meet the requirements of this active period. Cortisol is a natural anti-inflammatory substance.
- Stress—occurs when the body is subjected to increased demands of physical or mental exertion. Stress may be induced by cold weather, exercise, infections, burns, surgery, and anxiety. Stress produces an increase in ACTH,

---

corticosteroid steroidal hormones produced in the adrenal cortex.

isotonic having the same salt concentration as that of blood.

gonads testes and ovaries.

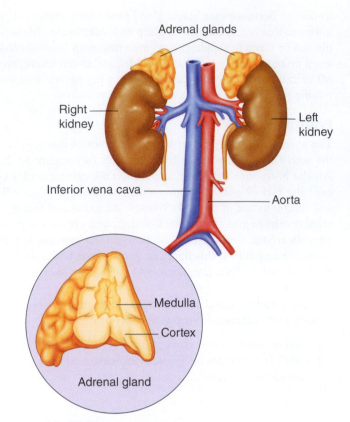

FIGURE 32-3 The adrenal glands.

which stimulates the adrenal gland to increase the secretion of cortisol. High amounts of cortisol increase the body's ability to cope with the demands of stress.
- Negative feedback—the releasing factor and ACTH stimulate the secretion and return of cortisol into the bloodstream. When the level of cortisol rises above normal, negative feedback begins, which stops the secretion of releasing factors from the hypothalamus to the anterior pituitary gland, which in turn stops further release of ACTH. This, in turn, stops the signal to the adrenal gland to release cortisol. The end result is that cortisol secretion is inhibited.

Glucocorticoids

The glucocorticoids regulate the metabolism of carbohydrates and proteins, especially during stress. Metabolism is a chemical breakdown. Carbohydrates are sugars and starches, which are metabolized into simple sugars (monosaccharides). During periods of stress involving body injury, trauma, surgery, or wound healing, there is an increased requirement for glucose. Healing wounds and tissues in need of repair use more glucose than normal and use it almost exclusively during repair stages.

Inflammation is considered the first step in the process of wound healing, as immune system mediators come to the rescue after an injury. However, sometimes the normal inflammatory response gets overworked, as in an acute inflammatory reaction, or it becomes continual or is prolonged, as in a chronic inflammatory reaction. In this situation, inflammation becomes a disease in itself. Inflammation is also present in various types of allergic reactions, asthma, and anaphylactic shock. Therefore, the glucocorticoids are useful in treating these conditions. The glucocorticoids have potent anti-inflammatory effects. The synthetic glucocorticoids are frequently used to treat inflammatory and allergic conditions, because they have a longer duration of action than naturally occurring adrenocorticosteroids.

Although some topical steroids are available over the counter, the higher strengths (all po forms) are available by prescription only. The topical preparations are specifically labeled for temporary relief. They can be used for relief of minor skin irritations, itching, dermatitis, rashes, eczema, insect bites, poison ivy, reactions to cosmetics (perfumes) and detergents, and itching in the anal and genital regions. Glucocorticoids are also given via the IM and IV routes.

Mineralocorticoids

The main function and purpose of mineralocorticoids is to regulate the *electrolyte*, or salt and fluid, balance of the body. Mineralocorticoids are essential for life. Therefore, a deficiency requires replacement therapy so that the patient will not dehydrate, to maintain pH balance in the body, and to assist the electrical functions and processes in the body.

The most important mineralocorticoid is *aldosterone*. The site of action of aldosterone is in the distal tubules of the nephrons in the kidneys (refer to Figure 31-2 for an illustration of the nephron). Nephrons are the smallest working unit (cell) of the kidneys. The hormone aldosterone increases the reabsorption of sodium ions. *Reabsorption* means that the sodium leaves the tubule and returns to the blood supply. During this process, there is an exchange of potassium ions for sodium ions. The potassium cations are led into the nephron tubule and transported into the urine.

Water is also reabsorbed with sodium. Consequently, normal sodium and water levels are maintained in the blood and other body tissues, which are **isotonic**.

Table 32-1 gives examples of glucocorticoids and mineralocorticoids.

TABLE 32-1 Examples of Glucocorticoids and Mineralocorticoids

Trade Name	Generic Name
Glucocorticoids	
Aristocort, Kenalog	triamcinolone
Celestone	betamethasone
Cortef, Hydrocortone, Corticaine	hydrocortisone
Decadron, Hexadrol	dexamethasone
Deltasone, Destasone, Orasone	prednisone
Medrol, Solu-Medrol (injection)	methylprednisolone
Mineralocorticoids	
Florinef	fludrocortisone

Pancreas

The pancreas is both an endocrine gland and a digestive organ. As an endocrine gland, it produces many important hormones that include insulin, glucagon, and finally somatostatin. The pancreas also acts as a digestive organ that secretes pancreatic juice that contains digestive enzymes, which help in the absorption of nutrients and digestion in the part of the small intestine. These enzymes help to further break down the carbohydrates, proteins, and lipids. The pancreas is an organ that is no stranger to contracting cancer and other digestive illnesses. Depending on the severity of the cancer and when it is diagnosed, patients can recover and find that they are cancer free after proper treatment. Early detection is the key, as with any cancer.

Gonads

GnRH is the hormone released by the hypothalamus that precipitates the onset of sexual maturity in both males and females. GnRH is needed for both sexual maturity and normal reproduction. It acts by stimulating the release of LH and FSH from the anterior pituitary. LH and FSH act by stimulating the production of sex hormones in the **gonads**, known as *testes* in males and *ovaries* in females.

Both LH and FSH are responsible for the development and secretion of sex hormones and the development of sex organs and secondary sex characteristics. *Secondary sex characteristics* are physical features that start to develop at puberty and serve to distinguish males from females. The primary sex characteristics are the genitals.

Female Sex Hormones

The sex hormones of the female are estrogen and progesterone. *Estrogen* is responsible for the development of secondary sex characteristics as well as the formation of osteoblasts, inhibition of osteoclasts, and bone loss. *Progesterone* prepares the lining of the uterus for the implantation of a fertilized egg (ovum).

Two additional pituitary hormones are involved in childbirth. *Oxytocin*, secreted by the posterior pituitary gland, but made by the hypothalamus, stimulates the uterus to start contracting at the beginning of labor. *Prolactin* signals the mammary glands to start producing milk.

Male Sex Hormones

Male sex hormones, or *androgens*, are also known as the *masculinizing hormones*. The main sex hormone of the male, *testosterone*, is produced in the testes. The major functions of testosterone are to stimulate the development of male sex organs and to maintain the secondary sex characteristics of the male.

Men also require *progesterone* that is produced in the adrenal gland and testes. This hormone plays an integral part in maintaining a healthy prostate.

Table 32-2 is a list of the endocrine glands, the hormones each gland secretes, and the main function of each hormone.

TABLE 32-2 Endocrine Glands and Secreted Hormones

Endocrine Gland	Hormone Secreted	Hormone Function
Adrenal (cortex)		
	Aldosterone	Maintains sodium and water balance
	Cortisol	Increases blood glucose levels
	Gonadocorticoids (androgens and estrogens)	Develops gender characteristics
Adrenal (medulla)		
	Epinephrine, Norepinephrine	Prepares body for action in emergencies
Ovaries		
	Estrogen	Develops female sex/reproductive characteristics
	Progesterone	Prepares uterine lining for pregnancy
Pancreas		
	Glucagon	Raises blood sugar level
	Insulin	Lowers blood sugar level
Parathyroid		
	Parathyroid hormone	Increases blood calcium levels
Pineal		
	Melatonin	Affects daily physiologic cycles and reproductive development
Pituitary (anterior lobe)		
	Growth hormone	Stimulates the growth of muscles, bones, and organs; influences height
	Thyroid stimulating hormone (TSH)	Stimulates thyroid to secrete thyroid hormones
	Adrenocorticotropic hormone (ACTH, corticotropin)	Stimulates secretion of cortical hormones of the adrenal gland
	Gonadotropic hormones	Regulate the development of the gonads
	Prolactin	Initiates and maintains milk production
	Follicle-stimulating hormone (FSH)	Stimulates the growth of ovary follicles
	Luteinizing hormone (LH)	Stimulates ovulation
Pituitary (posterior lobe)		
	Antidiuretic hormone (ADH)	Promotes reabsorption of water in kidneys
	Oxytocin	Stimulates contraction of uterus and release of breast milk
Testes		
	Testosterone	Develops male sex/reproductive characteristics
Thyroid		
	Thyroid hormone	Affects growth, maturation, and metabolism
	Calcitonin	Reduces blood calcium levels

(Continued)

TABLE 32-2 Endocrine Glands and Secreted Hormones *(Continued)*

Endocrine Gland	Hormone Secreted	Hormone Function
Other Organs with Hormone Secretion		
Gastric Mucosa		
	Gastrin	Stimulates the production of gastrin and hydrochloric acid
Heart		
	Atriopeptin	Involved in homeostasis of body water, sodium, and fat
Placenta		
	Human chorionic gonadotropin	Signals ovaries to secrete hormones to maintain uterine lining
Small Intestine Mucosa		
	Secretin	Regulates pH levels
	Cholecystokinin	Stimulates contraction of gallbladder
Thymus Gland		
	Thymosin	Involved in immune system development

Estrogen Replacement Therapy and Menopause

After menopause, estrone is the most active circulating estrogen; at that point, it is made in the adrenal glands only. Estrogen replacement therapy is, literally, the replacement of estrogen for postmenopausal women (see Table 32-3). It is prescribed for the symptomatic treatment of the common symptoms associated with menopause, such as hot flashes and vaginal dryness, the prevention of bone fractures associated with osteoporosis, reduction of the risk of heart attacks and strokes, and to treat excessive and painful uterine bleeding. Topical or vaginal estrogen creams are prescribed for vaginal or vulvar atrophy associated with menopause.

Estrogens reduce LDL cholesterol and increase HDL cholesterol in the blood. When taken alone or in combination with a progestin (synthetic progesterone), estrogens have been shown to reduce the risk of myocardial infarction (MI) and stroke by 40% to 50%. In addition, they have bone-promoting effects, which means that they reduce the risk for hip and knee fracture from osteoporosis by 20% to 30%.

However, estrogens used in replacement therapy have also been associated with an increased risk of liver disease, through an unknown mechanism, in patients receiving dantrolene. Women over 35 years of age and those with a history of liver disease are especially at risk. Estrogens increase the liver's ability to manufacture clotting factors, and those taking warfarin must have their blood monitored for reduction of the blood-thinning effect. Blood clots are occasional, but serious, side effects of estrogen therapy and are dose-related; that is, they occur more frequently in patients taking higher doses. Cigarette smokers are at higher risk than nonsmokers. Therefore, patients requiring estrogen therapy are *strongly* encouraged to quit smoking.

Estrogens can cause a buildup of the uterine lining (*endometrial hyperplasia*) and increase the risk of endometrial carcinoma. The addition of a progestin to estrogen therapy has been shown to prevent endometrial cancer from developing. There is conflicting data regarding an association between estrogen and breast cancer. It is not known at this time if the addition of a progestin to ERT reduces the risk of breast cancer as it does for uterine cancer. There is no evidence that estrogens are effective for nervous symptoms or depression that might occur during menopause. Estrogens increase the incidence of gallbladder disease and abnormal blood clotting. Indications for estrogen include the following:

- Moderate to severe vasomotor symptoms associated with menopause
- Atrophic vaginitis
- Kraurosis vulvae—atrophy and shrinkage of the skin of the vagina and vulva
- Female hypogonadism
- Hysterectomy
- Primary ovarian failure
- Breast cancer, for palliative therapy only in appropriately selected women and men with metastatic disease
- Prostatic carcinoma (palliative therapy of advanced disease)

Estrogen is contraindicated in women with:

- Undiagnosed abnormal genital bleeding
- Known, suspected, or history of the breast cancer, except in appropriately selected patients being treated for metastatic disease
- Known or suspected estrogen-dependent neoplasia
- History of deep vein thrombosis or pulmonary embolism

TABLE 32-3 Estrogen Replacement Therapy Choices

	Trade Name	Dosage	Comments
From Natural Sources			
Animal-derived estrogen replacements have been considered more natural than plant-derived estrogens.	Premarin (conjugated animal estrogen)	0.3-mg, 0.625-mg, 1.25-mg, and 2.5-mg tablets qd; NTE 2.4 mg/day	Extracted from pregnant mares' urine; contains a mixture of different estrogens
		Vaginal cream: 1 app of 0.5–1 gm/day	Cream for short-term use for atrophic vaginitis or kraurosis vulvae
		Injection: 25 mg q6h prn hemorrhage	Injection for abnormal interuterine bleeding
From Plant Sources			
Plant-derived estrogens are chemically identical to animal estrogen made by the ovaries.	Estrace	1–2 mg daily	Estradiol is the most potent form of estrogen in premenopausal women
	Estrasorb	Apply two 1.74-mg packets to calf or thigh/day	Topical estradiol emulsion
	Estrogel	Apply once daily on one arm from wrist to shoulder	Estradiol gel avoids first-pass metabolism in the liver and minimizes application-site skin irritation; gel dries in as little as two to five minutes
	Estring (estradiol)	Soft, flexible vaginal ring with 2-mg estradiol delivery system; placed in the upper third of the vagina by the physician or the patient; worn continuously for 90 days, then removed and replaced if therapy is to be continued	Discontinue during treatment for vaginal infection with vaginal antimicrobial therapy
	Alora (estradiol transdermal system)	Apply 0.025 mg/day twice a week to hips, abdomen, or thigh, NTE 1 mg/day twice a week	May not be suitable for women with narrow, short, or stenosed (constricted) vaginas, and prolapse (who are more prone to irritation from a tight-fitting ring), or those with symptoms of vaginal irritation
	Climara TDP (transdermal patch)	Apply one TDP once a week to abdomen, buttocks, inner thigh, upper arm, or hips as directed	Continuous delivery for twice-weekly dosing; applied to abdomen, hips, and thigh—6.5 cm^2, 12.5 cm^2, 18.75 cm^2, and 25.0 cm^2

(Continued)

TABLE 32-3 Estrogen Replacement Therapy Choices *(Continued)*

	Trade Name	Dosage	Comments
Plant-derived progesterones are chemically identical to animal progestins made by the ovaries.	Prometrium (progesterone)	Dosage varies	
Lab-Modified Estrogens			
Plant-derived estrogens that have been chemically modified in a laboratory and are therefore not truly *natural*.	Cenestin	0.625-mg tablets, NTE 1.25 mg qd	Conjugated plant estrogens Treatment of vasomotor symptoms due to menopause. Dosages for other conditions may vary
	Ogen	One 0.625-mg (0.75-mg estropipate) tablet to two 2.5-mg tablets daily	Estrone estropipate
	Ortho-est	Avail: 0.3–1.25 mg tablets, one tablet qd, NTE 1.25 mg/day	Esterified estrogens
	Estratab	Dosage varies per patient and condition/indication	
	Menest	Dosage varies	Given cyclically for short-term use only
Synthetic progesterones are known as progestins.	Aygestin (norethindrone acetate)	5-mg tablet Dosing varies per indication: amenorrhea, uterine cancer, endometriosis	Lab-created progestins
	Provera, Depo-Provera (medroxyprogesterone acetate [MPA])	2.5-mg, 5-mg, 10-mg tablets Contraceptive injection: 1 mL × 150 mg/90 days	Contraceptive injection
	Cycrin (MPA)	2.5-mg, 5-mg, 10-mg tablets	
Combination synthetic progesterone and animal estrogens	Prempro	One tablet qd	Combines norethindrone acetate or MPA with Premarin
	Premphase	One maroon tablet qd for days 1–14, then one blue tablet for days 15–28	Dosage varies with indications: postmenopausal vasomotor symptoms, prevention of osteoporosis
Combination synthetic progesterone and plant estrogens	Activella (estradiol/norethindrone acetate)	One tablet daily (1 mg/ 0.5 mg)	Prevention of osteoporosis, vasomotor menopausal symptoms

- Active or recent (within the past year) arterial thrombo-embolic disease, such as stroke or MI
- Liver dysfunction or disease
- Known hypersensitivity to ingredients of the particular estrogenic formula
- Known or suspected pregnancy

Testosterone Hormonal Replacement

Testosterone also produces an anabolic effect that promotes the synthesis and retention of proteins, for muscle and bone, in the body. The more testosterone there is, the easier it is for the body to build muscle, and the more muscle can be built. In some diseases, muscle will atrophy or become weak. Pharmaceutical anabolic steroids can help the patient with such a disease to rebuild muscle tissue; in addition, they promote weight gain after surgery, trauma, or serious infection (see Table 32-4). Unfortunately, overuse of the steroids (as evidenced by illegal use for athletic performance enhancement) can cause some irreversible effects.

The FDA has approved pharmaceutical steroids for the following uses:

- Weight gain for chronic nutritional deficiencies or wasting syndromes, such as those in cancer or AIDS patients
- Relief of bone pain associated with osteoporosis
- Corticosteroid-induced catabolism
- Hereditary angioedema
- Severe antimetastatic breast cancer in women
- Hypogonadism (hormonal replacement for hormonal deficiency states in males)
- To stimulate the beginning of puberty in certain boys who are late starting puberty naturally
- Cryptorchidism (failure of one or both testicles to descend)

Angioedema is an autosomal dominant disorder characterized by recurring episodes of swelling of the face, extremities, genitalia, bowel wall, and upper respiratory tract. It is caused by deficient or nonfunctional C1 esterase inhibitor (C1 INH).

TABLE 32-4 Androgens

Trade Name	Generic Name
Androderm, Testoderm TTS	testosterone; transdermal patches (abdomen, back, thigh, and arm)
Androgel, Testim	testosterone; topical gel applied to shoulders, upper arms, and/or abdomen
Delatestryl	testosterone (parenteral) for testosterone replacement therapy
Halotestin	fluoxymesterone (oral tablets)
Oreton	methyltestosterone (oral capsules)
Oxandrin	oxandrolone for AIDS wasting syndrome (oral tablets); for bone pain, weight gain, postsurgery/trauma, corticosteroid-induced protein catabolism
Testoderm	testosterone; transdermal patches (scrotal)
Winstrol	stanozolol (oral tablets); anabolic androgen for angioedema

Stanozolol cannot stop, but can prevent, slow the frequency of, and control the severity of attacks of angioedema and can increase blood serum levels of C1 INH and C4.

Anemia caused by the administration of myelotoxic drugs, as well as acquired aplastic anemia, congenital aplastic anemia, and myelofibrosis, may respond to androgens. Oxymetholone enhances the production and excretion of erythropoietin in patients with anemias caused by bone marrow failure and often stimulates erythropoiesis in anemias stemming from deficient red cell production.

Oral testosterone or testosterone derivatives are contraindicated in male patients who have prostate or breast cancer and in females with hypercalcemia or breast cancer.

❝ Workplace Wisdom AndroGel Warning

AndroGel can be passed to another person through unwashed clothing or skin-to-skin contact. Any persons who come in direct contact with clothing or skin that has had the drug applied to it should immediately wash the area of contact with soap and water. ❞

Side Effects of Anabolic Steroids

Too much testosterone or anabolic steroid signals the pituitary gland to stop producing the hormone *gonadotropin*. This fact is the basis for research into a male contraceptive, as gonadotropin is necessary for spermatogenesis. When excessive amounts of anabolic steroids are used, a domino effect occurs, causing testicular atrophy, decreased size and function of the testicles and testes, lowered sperm count, reversible sterility, **priapism**, prostate enlargement, and frequent or continuing erections. Upon cessation of steroid use,

---

info — Risks and Benefits of HRT

In conjunction with their physician, each patient must weigh the risks and benefits before starting hormone replacement therapy.

- Risks: Estrogen increases the risk of blood clots, gallbladder disease, uterine cancers, and breast cancer.
- Benefits: Relief from frequent hot flashes is achieved with estrogen hormonal treatment. *Hot flashes* are sudden episodes of increased uncomfortable warmth, skin flushing, and sweating, which occur in about 70% of women during menopause. These hot flashes are sometimes severe enough to cause insomnia, fatigue, and irritability.

---

priapism a painful, extended-duration erection.

the natural ability to produce testosterone may remain completely shut down, possibly leading to a permanent imbalance of the hormone.

Side effects of anabolic steroids in both men and women include the following:

- Edema and weight gain due to sodium and water retention
- Jaundice due to an increased concentration of bilirubin in the liver
- Hepatic carcinoma after prolonged steroid use
- High cholesterol and associated diseases
- Increased or decreased libido
- Chills
- Decreased glucose tolerance
- Increased serum levels of LDLs and decreased levels of HDLs
- Increased excretion of creatine and creatinine

In women, the following effects of masculinization are reversible if the drug is discontinued in time, except as noted:

- Acne
- Hirsutism (growth of facial hair)
- Increases in body hair (permanent)
- Deepening of the voice (permanent)
- Amenorrhea or other menstrual irregularities
- Enlargement of the clitoris (permanent)
- Uterine atrophy
- Shrinkage of breast size
- Masculinization of female fetuses in pregnant women

In men, the following side effects have been documented:

- Infertility
- Impotence (after as little as 25 mg of testosterone a day for six weeks; spermatogenesis declines; androgens will cause the same effect even after drug withdrawal)
- Increased frequency of erections
- Prepuberty penis enlargement
- Testicular atrophy (shrinkage)
- Decline in testicular function and decrease in spermatogenesis
- Decrease in seminal volume
- Chronic priapism
- Epididymitis
- Bladder irritability and decrease in seminal fluid volume
- Gynecomastia (enlarged breast) and nipple tenderness

> ❝ **Workplace Wisdom** **Federal Regulation of Anabolic Steroids**
>
> Because of the widespread abuse, the Anabolic Steroids Control Act of 1990 was passed, making anabolic steroids a Schedule III controlled substance. This means that the drugs may be kept under lock and key in the pharmacy. ❞

Androgen Precautions

Although the newer topical testosterone gels have fewer side effects than oral or injectable testosterone, without protection and contact precautions these drugs may contaminate other partners and family members and cause severe side effects. For example, anabolic steroids may cause suppression of clotting factors II, V, VII, and X, and an increase in prothrombin time.

Glandular Disease States

Some cancers, especially those involving the breast, uterus, and prostate gland, are dependent on the presence of sex hormones. The use of sex hormones opposing those found in the cancerous tissue receptors most often appears to antagonize or inhibit tumor growth. Endocrine therapy is palliative (soothing) only.

The following are examples of conditions that benefit from endocrine therapy:

- *Breast cancer*—Breast tissue has estrogen receptors. In breast cancer, estrogen *feeds* the cancer cells. Therefore, adding more estrogen exogenously causes more breast cancer or enhances the growth of cancer that is already present. Obese men have higher levels of estrogen in their bodies, because fat cells produce estrogen from other hormones; these patients may also produce fewer androgens. Taking an androgen as an antiestrogenic therapy will lower the amount of endogenous estrogen; this sort of therapy is used in females, although (as noted) there may be significant side effects. Androgens (and possibly progesterone) exert a protective influence, are used to treat breast cancer in males, and include the drugs tamoxifen (Nolvadex) and megestrol (Megace). Tamoxifen, an antiestrogen, works by blocking estrogen in the breast, thus slowing the growth and reproduction of breast cancer cells that depend on estrogen for survival. Megestrol, an antiandrogen, blocks the effect of androgen (a male hormone) on breast cancer cells. Researchers do not know for certain why blocking androgen in the breast helps treat male breast cancer.
- *Polycystic ovary syndrome (PCOS)*—PCOS involves enlarged ovaries containing many fluid-filled sacs. Female PCOS patients exhibit high levels of male hormones (androgens, testosterone). More testosterone would only exacerbate the problem. Therefore, giving these female patients estrogen increases their estrogen levels and helps lower the levels of male hormones.
- *Prostate cancer*—Researchers have found that small amounts of estrogen help reduce the amount of bone loss caused by a common prostate cancer treatment. If the estrogen level in the body is high, the body does not make as much testosterone, so the cancer cannot feed on it. Estrogens actually block prostate cancer growth but only to a point.
- *Endometrial cancer*—This cancer is dependent on estrogen. Certain stages may be treated with estrogen antagonists such as aromatase inhibitors.

Endocrine System Disorders

Following are some of the abnormalities caused by defects of the endocrine system.

Pituitary Gigantism

Gigantism results from excessive secretion of GH in childhood and is usually caused by a nonmalignant tumor of the pituitary gland. The affected child grows excessively and is bigger in all areas of the body: height, weight, and size. The size is, however, proportionate. Treatment may include surgical removal or radiation therapy of the pituitary tumor. Medications include somatostatin analogs, such as octreotide or long-acting lanreotide, which reduce secretion of GH. Also used, but less effective, are dopamine agonists such as bromocriptine mesylate and cabergoline.

Pituitary Dwarfism

Pituitary dwarfism results from a lack of GH. The affected individual may be somewhat short at birth, but in most cases the child's growth in height and weight is normal from birth up to 6 to 12 months of age. At that point, it may become apparent that the child is not growing normally; large amounts of exogenous GH are needed.

The person may have hypoglycemia or low blood sugar, because GH is not present to counter insulin. Patients with pituitary dwarfism may have an exaggerated *puppet* or *baby-doll* face and may be proportionately short, with a chubby body build, because both the height and the growth of all other structures are decreased. Each case differs: There may be an unusually high deficiency of GH, or the person may produce no GH at all. It has been shown that patients with the form of isolated GH deficiency develop anti-GH antibodies when GH replacement therapy is administered (using exogenous GH). Thus, treatment may not be possible or effective for some patients.

The parents' stature may or may not be relevant to the child's dwarfism. Some syndromes are caused by genetic mutations at the moment of conception. Other syndromes are caused by the random combination of two recessive genes that may have been dormant for generations. (The child must receive one recessive gene from each parent to show the trait.) The main course of therapy is GH replacement therapy, with GH (somatotropin), when there is lack of GH in the body. Somatrem, Protropin, and Humatrope, among others, may be used.

A pediatric endocrinologist usually administers this type of therapy before a child's growth plates have fused (joined together). GH replacement therapy is rarely effective after the growth plates have joined, which usually occurs before the child reaches the age of 17. When therapy is effective, height may increase by as much as 4 to 6 inches (10 to 15 cm) in the first year of treatment. Treatment of pituitary dwarfism involves GH injections given at home, which can be given once or several times a week.

polyuria excessive urination.

polydipsia ingestion of abnormally large amounts of fluids.

polyphagia excessive hunger or eating.

Acromegaly

Acromegaly results from an excessive secretion of GH during the adult years. It is characterized by enlarged bones of the cheek, hands, feet, and jaws; the patient will have a predominant forehead and a large nose. The arms, legs, and hands are disproportionately large compared to the rest of the body, but the person will have slender arms, sometimes exacerbated by atrophy of the muscles. There is often a curvature of the spine associated with a deformity of the chest. The lower part of the sternum may project forward, because the bones of the chest are increased in size. Ultimately, the person with acromegaly will suffer considerable disability, with joint pain, cardiovascular disease, hypertension, insulin resistance, visual impairment, and severe headaches.

The cause is usually a tumor on the pituitary gland, called a *pituitary adenoma*. Too much GH after the age of 17 will lead to acromegaly, but seldom to gigantism, because the long bones of the limbs have fused and cannot grow any more. Treatment includes surgical removal of the tumor. Medications that may decrease the secretion of GH and reduce the size of the tumor include the following:

- Somatostatin—a brain hormone that inhibits GH release
- Octreotide (Sandostatin)—a synthetic form of somatostatin
- Lanreotide (Somatuline LA)—a synthetic, long-acting form of somatostatin

Table 32-5 shows a list of treatments.

Diabetes

It is estimated that approximately 6.6% of the U.S. population has diabetes, with about one-third of that number unaware of their serious medical condition. Diabetes mellitus (DM) is a disease in which the body does not produce or properly use insulin, a hormone that is needed to convert sugar, starches, and other food into the energy necessary for daily life. The cause of diabetes is not certain, but both genetics and environmental factors, such as obesity and lack of exercise, appear to play roles. Some cases appear to be caused by autoimmune reactions.

Diabetes can be categorized as:

- *Type 1*—results from the body's failure to produce insulin. It is estimated that 5% to 10% of Americans who are diagnosed with diabetes have type 1 diabetes (see Table 32-6).
- *Type 2*—results from *insulin resistance* (a condition in which the body fails to properly use insulin) combined with relative insulin deficiency (see Table 32-7). Most Americans who are diagnosed with diabetes have type 2 diabetes.
- *Gestational*—affects about 4% of all pregnant women (135,000 cases) in the United States each year.
- *Prediabetes*—a condition in which a person's blood glucose levels are higher than normal but not high enough for a diagnosis of type 2 diabetes.

Many people remain undiagnosed, because many of the diabetes symptoms seem harmless. Studies indicate that the early detection of diabetes symptoms and treatment can decrease the chances of developing the complications of diabetes.

TABLE 32-5 Prescription Treatments for Pituitary Gigantism and Acromegaly

Classification	Generic Name	Brand Name	Availability	Route of Administration	Common Adult Dosage
Somatostatin analogs	lanreotide	Somatuline Depot	60-mg, 90-mg, 120-mg PFS	SC injection	90 mg every four weeks for three months (initial); 60–120 mg every four weeks (maintenance)
	octreotide acetate	Sandostatin	50-mcg, 100-mcg, 500-mcg amps; 200 mcg/mL, 1,000 mcg/mL MDV	SC or IV injection	50 mcg bid or tid
Dopamine agonists	bromocriptine mesylate	Palodel Cycloset	2.5-mg tablets; 5-mg capsules 0.8-mg tablets	Oral Oral	2.5–15 mg daily 1.6–4.8 mg daily
	cabergoline	Dostinex	0.5-mg tablets	Oral	0.25–1 mg twice a week
Growth hormone receptor blockers	pegvisomant	Somavert	10-mg, 15-mg, 20-mg SDV	SC injection	40 mg (initial); 10–30 mg daily (maintenance)

Diabetes symptoms include the following:

- Frequent urination (**polyuria**)
- Excessive thirst (**polydipsia**)
- Extreme hunger (**polyphagia**)
- Unusual weight loss
- Increased fatigue
- Irritability
- Blurry vision

Type 2 diabetes may be delayed, or even prevented from developing, through diet and exercise. Most people with diabetes have high risk factors for other conditions, such as high blood pressure and cholesterol, which increase their risk for heart disease and stroke. It is estimated that more than 65% of people with diabetes die from heart disease or stroke. With diabetes, heart attacks occur earlier in life and often result in death.

Diabetes should not be taken lightly. Anyone can assess their individual risk through prediabetes screening. Diabetes is a major chronic disease that causes significant morbidity and mortality from heart and circulatory conditions, renal failure, and blindness. By managing diabetes, high blood pressure, and cholesterol, people with diabetes can greatly reduce their risk of complications. Treatment may include proper diet and exercise, oral hypoglycemics, insulin, or a combination of therapies. Many of the oral hypoglycemics listed in Table 32-8 are available as combination drugs.

Insulin

For some diabetic patients who are insulin dependent (type 1), an array of injectable insulins is available (see Table 32-6). Which insulin is best for which patient is assessed by the health care provider. Available insulins include the following:

- *Lente (L)*—Humulin L, Novolin L
- *NPH*—Humulin N, Novolin N
- *Peakless/Basal Action*—Lantus (glargine)
- *Premixed*—Humulin 70/30, Novolin 70/30, Humulin 50/50
- *Rapid-acting*—Humalog (lispro), Novolog (aspart)
- *Regular*—Novolin R, Velosulin BR, Humulin R
- *Ultralente*—Humulin U

As with the oral medications, some combination insulins are now available and others are being developed. Research continues on insulin with the following considerations:

- Rapid-acting insulins
- Short-acting insulins
- Intermediate-acting insulins
- Long-acting insulins
- Ultra-long-acting insulins
- Insulin mixtures

TABLE 32-6 Insulin Treatments for Diabetes Mellitus

Classification	Generic Name	Brand Name	Onset	Duration
Rapid-acting	insulin lispro	Humalog Humalog Cartridge Humalog KwikPen Humalog Pen	5–15 minutes	3–4 hours
	insulin aspart	NovoLog NovoLog FlexPen NovoLog PenFill		
Short-acting	insulin regular	Humulin R Novolin R ReliOn Novolin R	30–60 minutes	6–8 hours
Intermediate-acting	isophane insulin	Humulin N Humulin N Pen Novolin N ReliOn Novolin N	1–2 hours	14–20 hours
	insulin zinc	Humulin L		
Long-acting	insulin glargine insulin determir	Lantus Levemir	2 hours	Up to 24 hours
Mixed	isophane and regular insulin	Humulin 50/50 Humulin 70/30 Humulin 70/30 Pen Novolin 70/30 ReliOn Novolin 70/30	Biphasic	Up to 24 hours
	lispro and lispro protamine	Humalog 50/50 Humalog 50/50 Pen Humalog 50/50 KwikPen Humalog 75/25 Humalog 75/25 Pen Humalog 75/25 KwikPen	Biphasic	Up to 24 hours

Insulin delivery technology has developed the following innovations:

- Insulin injection
- Insulin pens (injectors that are about the size and shape of a fountain pen)
- Insulin jet injectors
- External insulin pumps
- Implantable insulin pumps
- Transdermal insulin
- Oral spray insulin
- Inhaled insulin

Diabetes Insipidus

Diabetes insipidus (DI) is a condition that results from a decrease in or hyposecretion of ADH. The primary symptom of DI is the same as for DM—high amount of sugar in the blood. Other symptoms include the following:

- Polyuria
- Polydipsia
- Polyphagia

The lack of ADH in patients with DI is caused by kidneys that do not concentrate urine well. Because the urine is more

TABLE 32-7 Prescription Treatments for Type 2 Diabetes Mellitus

Classification	Generic Name	Brand Name	Availability	Route of Administration	Common Adult Dosage
Alpha-glucosidase inhibitors	acarbose	Precose	25-mg, 50-mg, 100-mg tablets	Oral	25 mg tid (initial); 50–100 mg tid (maintenance)
	miglitol	Glyset	25-mg, 50-mg, 100-mg tablets	Oral	25 mg tid (initial); 50–100 mg tid (maintenance)
Amylinomimetics	pramlintide	Symlin	60 pen injector of 15-mcg, 30-mcg, 45-mcg, and 60-mcg doses 120 pen injector of 60-mcg and 120-mcg doses 600 mcg/mL MDV	SC	15 mcg tidww(initial); 30–60 mcg tid (maintenance)
Biguanides	metformin	Fortamet Glucophage	500-mg, 850-mg, 1,000-mg tablets	Oral	500 mg bid to 2,000 mg daily, in divided doses
		Glucophage XR	500-mg, 750-mg tablets	Oral	
Meglitinides	nateglinide	Starlix	60-mg, 120-mg tablets	Oral	60–120mg tid
	repaglinide	Prandin	0.5-mg, 1-mg, 2-mg tablets	Oral	0.5–4 mg tid
Sulfonylureas	chlorpropamide	Diabinese	100-mg, 250-mg tablets	Oral	100–500 mg daily
	glimepiride	Amaryl	1-mg, 2-mg, 4-mg tablets	Oral	1–8 mg daily
	glipizide	Glucotrol	5-mg, 10-mg tablets	Oral	5–40 mg daily in divided doses if >15 kg
		Glucotrol XL	2.5-mg, 5-mg, 10-mg tablets	Oral	5–20 mg daily
	glyburide	DiaBeta Micronase	1.25-mg, 2.5-mg, 5-mg tablets	Oral	1.25–20 mg daily
	tolazamide	Tolinase	100-mg, 250-mg, 500-mg tablets	Oral	100–1,000 mg daily
	tolbutamide	Orinase			
Thiazolidinediones	pioglitazone	Actos	15-mg, 30-mg, 45-mg tablets	Oral	15–45 mg daily
	rosiglitazone	Avandia	2-mg, 4-mg, 8-mg tablets	Oral	4–8 mg daily
Misc.	exenatide	Byetta	5-mcg, 10-mcg PFS	SC	5 mcg bid
	sitagliptin	Januvia	25-mg, 50-mg, 100-mg tablets	Oral	100 mg daily

(Continued)

TABLE 32-7 Prescription Treatments for Type 2 Diabetes Mellitus *(Continued)*

Classification	Generic Name	Brand Name	Availability	Route of Administration	Common Adult Dosage
Combination drugs	glipizide/ metformin	Metaglip	2.5/250-mg, 2.5/500-mg, 5/500-mg tabs	Oral	varies, NTE 20/2,000 mg daily
	glyburide/ metformin	Glucovance	1.25/250-mg, 2.5/500-mg, 5/500-mg tablets	Oral	1.25/250–5/500 mg qd or bid
	pioglitazone/ glimepride	Duetact	30/2-mg, 30/4-mg tablets	Oral	30/2–30/4 mg daily
	pioglitazone/ metformin	Actoplus Met	15/500-mg, 15/850-mg tablets	Oral	15/500– 45/2,550 mg daily
	repaglinide/ metformin	PrandiMet	1/500-mg, 2/500-mg tablets	Oral	varies, NTE 10/2,500 mg daily
	rosiglitazone/ glimepride	Avandryl	4/1-mg, 4/2-mg, 4/4-mg, 8/2-mg, 8/4-mg tablets	Oral	4/1–8/4 mg daily
	rosiglitazone/ metformin	Avandamet	2/500-mg, 4/500-mg, 2/1,000-mg, 4/1,000-mg tablets	Oral	up to 8/2,000 mg total, taken in two doses
	sitagliptin/ metformin	Janumet	50/500-mg, 50/1000-mg tablets	Oral	50/500– 100/2,000 mg daily

TABLE 32-8 Oral Hypoglycemic Agents

Class	Example(s)	Primary Site of Action	Mechanism of Action
Alpha-glucosidase inhibitors	Precose (acarbose) Glyset (miglitol)	Intestine	Slow digestion of carbohydrates
Biguanides	Glucophage (metformin)	Liver	Reduce glucose release
Meglitinides	Prandin (repaglinide) Starlix (nateglinide)	Pancreas	Increase insulin release
Sulfonylureas	Glucotrol (glipizide) Amaryl (glimeprimide) Diabeta, Micronase (glyburide)	Pancreas	Increase insulin release
Thiazolidinediones	Avandia (rosiglitazone) Actos (pioglitazone)	Muscle	Increase insulin sensitivity

diluted, the patient must urinate more often, frequently getting up two or three times in the night. People with DI are thirsty all the time and may often want to drink liquids every hour. Excessive urination may cause DI patients to become dehydrated, making them feel lethargic and thirsty. When people feel tired or lethargic, they sometimes interpret the feeling as meaning that they need to eat; weight gain and poor metabolism of food just exacerbate the problem.

Two things are known to cause DI. In the first case, the hypothalamus does not make enough ADH. In the second case, the kidneys do not respond to ADH the way they should. Most people with DI acquire it after a head injury or after a brain surgery, or it may be caused by a brain tumor. DI can also be congenital and run in families. DI can be drug-induced, such as by lithium, which is used to treat bipolar disorder. About 25% of the time, however, the cause is unknown. Treatment for pituitary DI is with DDAVP nasal spray, which contains a substance much like the body's natural ADH, *vasopressin*. If a person taking DDAVP takes in too much liquid, the body will get overloaded with fluids, making the patient feel weak, dizzy, or generally bad all over (see Table 32-9).

Table 32-10 compares DI with DM.

TABLE 32-9 Prescription Treatments for Diabetes Insipidus

Generic Name	Brand Name	Availability	Route of Administration	Common Adult Dosage
chlorpropamide	Diabinese	100-mg, 250-mg tablets	Oral	100–500 mg daily
desmopressin acetate	DDAVP	0.1-mg, 0.2-mg tablets; 4 mcg/mL MDV and amps	Oral SC	0.1–0.8 mg daily; 2–4 mcg daily
vasopressin	n/a	10 units, 20 units, 200 units MDV	IM or SC	5–10 units bid or tid as needed

TABLE 32-10 Comparison of Diabetes Insipidus and Diabetes Mellitus

Factors	Diabetes Insipidus	Diabetes Mellitus Type 1	Diabetes Mellitus Type 2
Onset	Birth	Birth; may show up in childhood or adolescence; currently also being seen in older adults.	Adult onset, usually after 40 years of age; current trend of development in younger, overweight children.
Mechanism of the disease	Lack of ADH or vasopressin secreted by posterior pituitary gland	Beta cells of islets of Langerhans do not manufacture insulin; patient is unable to transport sugar from the bloodstream into cells.	Beta cells of islets of Langerhans do not manufacture enough insulin, or the muscles do not utilize insulin properly; creates inability to transport sugar from the bloodstream into cells.
Other names	Neurogenic, hypothalamic, pituitary, water diabetes	DM type 1, insulin-dependent diabetes, IDDM, juvenile-onset diabetes, sugar diabetes	DM type 2, noninsulin-dependent diabetes, NIDDM, adult-onset diabetes, sugar diabetes
Subtypes	Gestational Dipsogenic	—	—
Causes	Destruction of posterior pituitary; tumors, infections, head injuries, infiltrations; various inheritable defects	Familial, congenital, acquired	Familial, acquired
Symptoms	Polydipsia, polyuria, polyphagia	Polydipsia, polyuria, polyphagia, weight loss, tiredness/fatigue	Polydipsia, polyuria, polyphagia, weight gain; sometimes asymptomatic

(Continued)

TABLE 32-10 Comparison of Diabetes Insipidus and Diabetes Mellitus *(Continued)*

Factors	Diabetes Insipidus	Diabetes Mellitus Type 1	Diabetes Mellitus Type 2
Notes	Rare	Accounts for 10% of DM	Most common; 90% of all DM
Danger	Dehydration, rapid heart rate, fatigue, headache, muscle pain, dry mucous membranes	Too much glucose in the bloodstream and not enough glucose within the cells themselves. Result: Cells attempt to derive energy from fat breakdown. Excessive breakdown causes production of harmful by-products called *ketones*. The accumulation of ketones causes the body's pH to become acidic (*ketoacidosis*), which makes the cellular environment inhospitable for normal metabolic functions. This condition can ultimately become life-threatening; requires aggressive medical therapy.	Too much glucose in the bloodstream and not enough glucose within the cells themselves. Result: Cells attempt to derive energy from fat breakdown. Excessive breakdown causes production of harmful by-products called *ketones*. The accumulation of ketones causes the body's pH to become acidic (*ketoacidosis*), which makes the cellular environment inhospitable for normal metabolic functions. This condition can ultimately become life-threatening; requires aggressive medical therapy.
Treatment	DDVAP (desmopressin) Pitressin (vasopressin) Diapid (lypressin)	Insulin injections	Diet, exercise, oral hypoglycemics; insulin injections as a last resort
Complications	Dehydration, electrolyte imbalance, rapid heart rate, high blood pressure, weight loss, dry skin, muscle pain	Diabetic retinopathy, glaucoma, HTN, renal impairment, neuropathy, heart disease	Diabetic retinopathy, glaucoma, HTN, renal impairment, neuropathy, heart disease

Hyperthyroidism

Hyperthyroidism is a common misfunction of the thyroid gland. It is due to an oversecretion of hormones that are produced by the thyroid gland and is mainly caused by three common conditions. These conditions are Graves' disease, goiter, and postpartum thyroiditis. Graves' disease is the body attacking itself. The cause of the attack is unknown, but antithyroid drugs can be given to treat the disease. Another condition that affects the thyroid is goiter. Goiter is the enlargement of the large neck that is caused by a noncancerous tumor or nodules present on the thyroid gland that are due to the overproduction of a certain TH. Surgery and medications can be given to reduce the size of the noncancerous tumor. The third type of thyroid condition is thyroiditis and affects children after birth. This condition is generally temporary and can be resolved after the onset of the condition. The illness can however cause ongoing hypothyroidism (see Table 32-11).

TABLE 32-11 Prescription Treatments for Hyperthyroidism

Generic Name	Brand Name	Availability	Route of Administration	Common Adult Dosage
methimazole	Tapazole	5-mg, 10-mg tablets	Oral	15–60 mg (initial); 5–15 mg (maintenance); divided into three equal doses
propylthiouracil (PTU)	n/a	50-mg tablets	Oral	300 mg (initial); 100–150 mg (maintenance); divided into three equal doses

TABLE 32-12 Prescription Treatments for Hypothyroidism

Generic Name	Brand Name	Availability	Route of Administration	Common Adult Dosage
levothyroxine sodium	Synthroid Levothroid Levoxyl Levo-T Unithroid	25-mcg, 50-mcg, 75-mcg, 88-mcg, 100-mcg, 112-mcg, 125-mcg, 137-mcg, 150-mcg, 175-mcg, 200-mcg, 300-mg tablets	Oral	1.7 mcg/kg/day
liothyronine sodium	Cytomel Tirostat	5-mcg, 25-mcg, 50-mcg tablets	Oral	5–25 mcg daily (initial); 25–100 mcg daily (maintenance)
liotrix	Thyrolar	3.1/12.5-mcg, 6.25/25-mcg, 12.5/50-mcg, 25/100-mcg, 37.5/150-mcg tablets	Oral	12.5/50–25/100 mcg daily
thyroid	Amrour Thyroid Westhroid	15-mg, 30-mg, 60-mg, 90-mg, 120-mg, 180-mg, 240-mg, 300-mg tabs (also listed as grains)	Oral	60–120 mg daily

Hyperparathyroidism

Hyperparathyroidism is a condition that includes an increased amount of parathyroid hormone (PTH), which can be gained by one of the body's four parathyroid glands. The reason for the condition can be benign tumors. Treatment can range from removing tumors and glands to more simple remedies such as decreasing calcium levels. Calcium levels can be increased because of the higher PTH levels. Because of this process, calcium is released into the bloodstream that leads to bone weakening, an increased possibility of fractures, and kidney stones. Replacement therapy includes calcium and vitamin D supplements.

Hypothyroidism

Hypothyroidism is a condition in which the thyroid gland does not produce a sufficient amount of certain hormones, such as thyroxine (T4) and triiodothyronine (T3). The leading cause of hypothyroidism is iodine deficiency. There are numerous prescription treatments available for hypothyroidism (see Table 32-12).

Hypoparathyroidism

Hypoparathyroidism is the nonfunctioning of the parathyroid gland. When the nonfunctioning happens, it is often necessary to have the parathyroid gland removed. However, when the gland is removed, it can lead to hypocalcemia. This condition is a decrease in the vitamin D volumes in the human body, which can cause muscle spasms, irregular heart contractions, and problems with nerve conduction. To help with these illnesses, replacement therapy is given. Additional supplements of vitamin D and calcium may be used as well.

Osteoporosis

Osteoporosis is the lack of calcium in the body where bones are brittle and break more easily. Treatment for osteoporosis includes exercise, drug therapy, and changes in a patient's diet. Early prevention of osteoporosis helps tremendously to reduce symptoms and problems in the later years of life. Vitamin D and multivitamins containing vitamin D can be taken along with drugs, such as Boniva, Fosamax, and Actonel, to fight the battle against osteoporosis (see Table 32-13).

Abnormalities of the Adrenal Gland

The following are common disorders that can occur with abnormalities of the adrenal gland. Table 32-14 provides a summary of endocrine disorders and conditions.

Cushing's Syndrome

Also known as *hypercortisolism* or *hyperadrenocortism*, *Cushing's syndrome* occurs when the body is exposed to high levels of the hormone cortisol for long periods of time. This may occur during long-term or high-stress situations; long-term therapy with glucocorticoid hormones, such as prednisone, for asthma, rheumatoid arthritis, lupus, and other inflammatory diseases; or from immunosuppression after transplantation and overproduction of natural cortisol. Cortisol performs vital tasks in the body by maintaining blood pressure and cardiovascular function, reducing the immune system's inflammatory response, balancing the effects of insulin in breaking down sugar for energy, and regulating the metabolism of proteins,

TABLE 32-13 Prescription Treatments for Osteoporosis

Generic Name	Brand Name	Availability	Route of Administration	Common Adult Dosage
alendronate	Fosamax	5-mg, 10-mg, 35-mg, 40-mg, 70-mg tablets; 70-mg oral solution	Oral	5–10 mg daily or 35–70 mg weekly
calcitonin-salmon	Fortical, Miacalcin	Nasal spray	Nasal	One spray daily
ibandronate	Boniva	2.5-mg, 150-mg tablets; 3-mg PFS	Oral; IV	150 mg monthly; or 2.5 mg daily; 3 mg every three months
raloxifene	Evista	60-mg tablets	Oral	60 mg daily
risedronate	Actonel	5-mg, 20-mg, 25-mg, 75-mg, 150-mg tablets	Oral	5 mg daily; 35 mg weekly; or 150 mg monthly
teriparatide	Forteo	MD PFS	SC	20 mcg daily
zoledronic acid	Reclast	5-mg SDV	IV	5 mg annually

TABLE 32-14 Endocrine System Disorders

Disorder	Hormonal Change	Characteristics	Treatment
Acromegaly	Increased GH in adults	Enlargement of extremities and certain parts of the body such as hands, feet, legs, arms, chin, and head	Somatostatin analogs such as Somatuline LA (long-acting lanreotide) or Auto-gel SC Octreotide (synthetic somatostatin) Sandostatin (octreotide) LAR IM injection (a long-acting, slow-release form of octreotide)
Addison's disease	Decreased cortisol or decreased aldosterone	Weight loss, muscle weakness, fatigue, low blood pressure	Synthetic cortisol replacement: oral hydrocortisone tablets, qd or bid Aldosterone replacement with an oral mineralocorticoid qd: Florinef (fludrocortisone)
Cushing's disease	Increased ACTH	May have a moon face, buffalo hump, obese torso	Surgical removal of pituitary tumor; possibly cortisol inhibitors such as mitotane, aminoglutethimide, metyrapone, trilostane, and ketoconazole
Cushing's syndrome	Increased ACTH	May have a moon face, buffalo hump, obese torso	Treatment varies by cause: Synthetic cortisol; cortisol inhibitors such as mitotane, aminoglutethimide, metyrapone, trilostane, and ketoconazole

(Continued)

TABLE 32-14 Endocrine System Disorders *(Continued)*

Disorder	Hormonal Change	Characteristics	Treatment
Diabetes insipidus	Decreased ADH	HTN, high blood glucose, polydipsia, polyphagia, polyuria	DDVAP (desmopressin), Pitressin (vasopressin), Diapid (lypressin)
Diabetes mellitus	Decreased insulin	High blood glucose, polydipsia, polyuria, polyphagia; may have HTN	Type 1—insulin injections Type 2—diet modification, weight control, regular exercise, oral hypoglycemic agents Sulfonylureas stimulate the beta cells to secrete more insulin: Orinase (tolbutamide), Diabinese (chlorpropamide) Meglitinides: Prandin (repaglinide) Biguanides decrease hepatic glucose output, reducing insulin resistance and lowering blood glucose—Glucophage (metformin) Thiazolidinediones reduce insulin resistance and improve insulin sensitivity Alpha-glucosidase inhibitors block the breakdown of complex carbohydrates and delay the absorption of monosaccharides from the GI tract: Precose (acarbose), Glyset (miglitol)
Gigantism	Increased GH in child	Large stature, proportional	Somatostatin analogs such as Sandostatin (octreotide) or Somatuline LA (long-acting lanreotide) Auto-gel SC reduces growth hormone secretion Also treated, less effectively, with dopamine agonists, such as bromocriptine mesylate and cabergoline
Goiter	Decreased iodine	Enlargement of the thyroid gland in neck	Add iodine to diet
Graves' disease	Increased TH in adult	Weight loss, feels hot or warm	Propacil (propylthiouracil [PTU])
Hirsutism	Increased androgens or increased testosterone	Facial hair on females, unrelated to menopause	Vaniqa (eflornithine cream applied five minutes after hair removal)
Hypothyroidism/ cretinism	Decreased TH in child; also caused by decreased iodine in the fetus	Small stature, not proportional; short limbs, may be overweight; dry skin, thick tongue, and large nose	Post-birth: Immediate treatment with synthetic thyroid hormone is imperative. Treat child with synthetic thyroid hormone or iodine replacement.
Myxedema	Decreased TH in adult	Weight gain, cold	Treat with synthetic thyroid hormones: Synthroid, Levoxyl (T4, L-thyroxine, levothroid, levothyroxine)

(Continued)

TABLE 32-14 Endocrine System Disorders (*Continued*)

Disorder	Hormonal Change	Characteristics	Treatment
			Cytomel (triiodothyronine, liothyronine)
			Armour Thyroid (synthetic desiccated animal thyroid hormones)
Peripheral edema	Increased ADH	Water and sodium retention, bloating	Exercise, elevate legs and ankles, mild potassium-sparing diuretics such as spironolactone
Pituitary dwarfism	Decreased GH in child	Small stature, proportional	Growth hormone such as Protopin (somatrem) or Humatrope (somatropin)

carbohydrates, and fats. One of cortisol's most important jobs is to help the body respond to stress of all kinds.

Considered rare, Cushing's syndrome most commonly affects adults aged 20 to 50 but only affects 10 to 15 people out of every 1 million people each year. People at risk are those suffering from depression, alcoholism, malnutrition, and panic disorders who have increased cortisol levels. Symptoms vary but may include upper body obesity, rounded face, increased fat around the neck, and thinning of arms and legs. Children with this syndrome tend to be obese with slow growth rates. Purplish-pink stretch marks may appear on the abdomen, thighs, buttocks, arms, and breasts. There may be weakened bones that fracture easily, fatigue, weak muscles, high blood pressure, and high blood sugar. Irritability, anxiety, and depression are common. Women may experience excess hair growth on the face and body

and have irregular menstrual cycles or absence of menstruation. Men have decreased fertility with diminished or absent libido.

Treatment of Cushing's syndrome varies, depending on the cause, and ranges from surgery to the use of synthetic cortisol to maintain and balance the amount needed in the body. Cortisol inhibitors, such as mitotane, aminoglutethimide, metyrapone, trilostane, and ketoconazole, are also used (see Table 32-15).

Addison's Disease

Also called *hypocortisolism*, *Addison's disease* occurs in 1 out of 100,000 people. In this disease, the adrenal glands do not produce enough of the hormone cortisol and, in some cases, also underproduce the hormone aldosterone. For this reason, the disease is sometimes called *chronic adrenal insufficiency*. The disease is characterized by weight loss, muscle weakness, fatigue, low blood pressure, and sometimes darkening of the skin. Causes of cortisol deficiency are a lack of ACTH due to gradual destruction of the adrenal cortex (the outer layer of the adrenal glands) by the body's own immune system as seen with an autoimmune disease. This, in turn, may cause polyendocrine deficiency syndrome in which many glands are affected. A secondary cause may be the long-term use or overuse of glucocorticoids, such as prednisone for asthma, ulcerative colitis, and rheumatoid arthritis.

The addition of exogenous cortisol sends negative feedback to the hypothalamus, causing it to stop making CRH; because there is no releasing factor, ACTH is not sent to the adrenal glands. This can happen when someone suddenly stops taking glucocorticoids or abruptly interrupts long-term therapy. Another cause is removal of a tumor of, or injury to, the pituitary gland. Symptoms may include darkening of the skin, penetrating

---

PROFILE IN PRACTICE

Mr. Reynolds has diabetes and is a regular customer at the pharmacy. He brings in a new prescription for a loop diuretic.

▶ *What important information should be provided to Mr. Reynolds regarding his preexisting condition and his new medication?*

▶ *What is the role of the pharmacy technician in this situation?*

TABLE 32-15 Prescription Treatments for Cushing's Syndrome

Generic Name	Brand Name	Availability	Route of Administration	Common Adult Dosage
aminoglutethimide	Cytadren	250-mg tablets	Oral	250 mg qid
mitotane	Lysodren	500-mg tablets	Oral	2–6 gm/day in divided doses;

TABLE 32-16 Prescription Treatments for Addison's Disease

Classification	Generic Name	Brand Name	Availability	Route of Administration	Common Adult Dosage
Mineralocorticoids	fludrocortisone acetate	Florinef	0.1-mg tablets	Oral	0.1 mg daily
Glucocorticoids	hydrocortisone	Cortef	5-mg, 10-mg, 20-mg tablets	Oral	Varies
	methylpred-nisolone	Medrol	2-mg, 4-mg, 6-mg, 8-mg, 16-mg, 32-mg tablets	Oral	Varies
	methylprednis-olone acetate	Depo-Medrol	20-mg, 40-mg, 80 mg MDV	IM	Varies
	methylprednis-olone sodium succinate	Solu-Medrol	40-mg, 125-mg, 500-mg, 1-gm, and 2-gm vials	IV	Varies
	prednisolone	Prelone, Pedi-pred, Oraped	5-mg tablets; 15 mg/5 mL syringe	Oral	Varies
	prednisone	Deltasone Predone	2.5-mg, 5-mg, 10-mg, 20-mg, 50-mg tablets; Dosepak	Oral	Varies
	dexamethasone	Decadron	0.75-mg, 0.5-mg tablets	Oral	Varies

pain in the lower back, abdomen, or legs, severe vomiting and diarrhea followed by dehydration, low blood pressure, and loss of consciousness. Left untreated, an Addison's disease crisis can be fatal. Treatment is by synthetic cortisol replacement with oral hydrocortisone tablets, taken once or twice a day (see Table 32-16). If aldosterone is also deficient, it is replaced with oral doses of the mineralocorticoid fludrocortisone acetate.

Cretinism

An underactive thyroid gland, or *congenital hypothyroidism*, is caused by a lack of fetal or childhood TH secretion. *Cretinism* may also be due to lack of iodine in the diet of the expectant mother, and therefore in the fetus. The result is babies who are born with, or children who later develop, mental retardation and a type of dwarfism. Other symptoms include coarse, dry skin and a slightly swollen tongue. Immediate treatment with synthetic TH is imperative. Prescription treatments include those available for hypothyroidism (see Table 32-12).

Myxedema (Secondary Hypothyroidism)

Myxedema may also be caused by a deficiency of TH, due to a lack of secretion of TSH by the pituitary gland, or lack of TRH from the hypothalamus in an adult. It is common among women. Usual symptoms are a coarse thickening of the skin and roughness that may be open with sores. Treatment is with synthetic TH. Prescription treatments include those available for hypothyroidism (see Table 32-12).

Graves' Disease

Graves' disease is also known as *thyroid eye disease* or *thyroid orbi-topathy*. Characterized by *proptosis* (protruding eye) and swollen and congested eye muscles, it makes the affected eye appear larger than the other eye (see Figure 32-4). The cause is *not* an overactive thyroid gland, as is commonly believed; those with Graves' disease often do have an overactive thyroid gland, but not always. Rather, Graves' disease is an autoimmune disorder in which immune cells attack

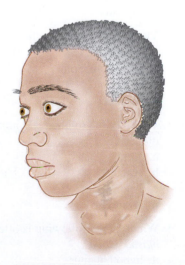

FIGURE 32-4 Eye characteristics of Graves' disease.

both the eye muscles and the thyroid, leading to dysfunction of both. Treatment of Graves' disease depends on the severity of signs and symptoms. Dry eye due to exposure requires the use of nonpreserved, lubricating eye drops. Acute episodes of inflammation result in double vision and optic nerve compression, and corticosteroids such as prednisone are used in these instances.

Radiation therapy is also used to treat optic nerve compression to preserve vision, but unfortunately it may result in radiation retinopathy. Only when the disease is under control, surgical orbital decompression should be employed to decrease proptosis or strabismus surgery be used to realign the eyes. Of course, the complication of hyperactive thyroid should be addressed with propylthiouracil (PTU), marketed under the trade name Propacil.

Summary

The endocrine system is a collection of glands that secrete hormones directly into the bloodstream to be distributed to specific target cells. This very complex system interacts with many other body systems via the release of hormones, which act as *messengers* between sets of cells. Some of the main functions of the endocrine system are regulation of the body's growth, metabolism, and sexual development and function.

The primary drivers of the endocrine system are the hypothalamus, located in the brain stem, and the pituitary gland, which is attached to the base of the hypothalamus. The hypothalamus directs the pituitary gland which, in turn, controls the thyroid, parathyroid, pancreas, adrenal glands, and gonads. A complete review of these glands, their secretions, and their effects on body systems illustrates how important the endocrine system is to the proper functioning of the body. For

example, every cell in the body depends on TH for regulating metabolism.

For the most part, the release of hormones is a self-regulating feedback mechanism that acts according to a simple *supply and demand* model. However, many outside factors can influence the amount of hormones in the body at any given time. Such factors include age, stress, infection, and changes in fluid or mineral balance in the blood, to name a few.

Many of the diseases, disorders, and conditions of the endocrine system discussed in this chapter are very common and familiar to most people (e.g., menopause and diabetes). This chapter also discussed less common disorders, such as Graves' disease, Cushing's syndrome, and Addison's disease, along with the various treatment modalities used to treat disorders of the endocrine system.

Chapter Review Questions

1. The enlargement of extremities, hands, feet, and head is known as _____.
   a. pituitary dwarfism
   b. diabetes insipidus
   c. acromegaly
   d. gigantism

2. The _____ secretes the hormone atriopeptin.
   a. adrenal cortex
   b. adrenal medulla
   c. heart
   d. placenta

3. Which of the following is *not* used in the treatment of diabetes?
   a. Actos
   b. Amaryl
   c. Androderm
   d. Avandia

4. Which of the following is often considered the body's *master gland*?
   a. hypothalamus
   b. thyroid
   c. thymus
   d. pituitary

5. Which of the following hormones is not produced in the pituitary gland?
   a. insulin
   b. GH
   c. TSH
   d. LH

6. Which of the following glands is located in the front of the neck?
   a. pituitary
   b. hypothalamus
   c. thymus
   d. thyroid

7. A decreased amount of GH in a child can result in which of the following conditions?
   a. acromegaly
   b. gigantism
   c. pituitary dwarfism
   d. peripheral edema

8. FSH and LH stimulate which of the following?
   a. gonads
   b. pituitary gland
   c. adrenal gland
   d. mammary glands

9. Which of the following is *not* a symptom of diabetes?
   a. polycoria
   b. polydipsia
   c. polyphagia
   d. polyuria

10. Which of the following diseases is characterized by protruding eyes and swollen/congested eye muscles?
   a. cretinism
   b. myxedema
   c. Graves' disease
   d. Cushing's syndrome

Critical Thinking Questions

1. Why do you think anabolic steroids are now classified as a controlled substance (C-III)?

2. Why is the pituitary gland considered the *master gland*?

3. Why do you think most people with diabetes do not know that they have the disease?

Web Challenge

1. Go to www.youtube.com, conduct a search for the endocrine system, and watch videos on how the system works.

2. Go to http://www.vivo.colostate.edu/hbooks/pathphys/endocrine/index.html to learn more about the endocrine system. Describe what you learn about the *diffuse endocrine system* and some of the hormones that these organs secrete.

References and Resources

"Acromegaly and Gigantism: A Historical Portrait of a Disease." http://www.cladonia.co.uk/acromegaly/ampc.html. Web. 8 April 2008.

Adams, M.P., D.L. Josephson, and L.N. Holland,Jr. *Pharmacology for Nurses: A Pathophysiologic Approach.* (4th edition.) Upper Saddle River, NJ: Pearson, 2013. Print.

"Carbohydrates: Fuel for Your Brain and Body." http://www.iemily.com/Article.cfm?ArtID=274. Web. 8 April 2008.

"Endocrine Glands and Their Hormones." http://training.seer.cancer.gov. Web. 17 October 2007.

"Endometrial Cancer Hormonal Therapy: Prolactin." 2003 (January 3). http://sharedjourney.com/define/prolactin.html. Web. 8 April 2008.

Hitner, N. *Pharmacology: An Introduction.* 6th ed. New York: McGraw-Hill, 2011. Print.

Holland, N. and M.P. Adams. *Core Concepts in Pharmacology.* (3rd ed.) Upper Saddle River, NJ: Pearson, 2010. Print.

Rolf, C., U. Knie, G. Lemmintz, and E. Nieschlaq. "Interpersonal Testosterone Transfer after Topical Application of a Newly Developed Testosterone Gel Preparation." *Clinical Endocrinology.* 56 (2002): 637–641. http://www.fsdinfo.org/pdf/Interpersonal_testosterone_transfer.pdf

"Medical Supervision of Individuals Using Anabolic-Androgenic Steroid (AAS) for Muscle Growth." http://www.mesomorphosis.com/articles/haycock/medically-supervised-steroid-use-02.htm. Web. 8 April 2008.

Medline Pulse. "Diabetes Insipidus" http://www.nlm.nih.gov/medlineplus/ency/article/000377.htm. Web. 5 April 2013.

"Pituitary Dwarfism." http://www.ecureme.com/emyhealth/Pediatrics/Pituitary_Dwarfism.asp. Web. 8 April 2013.

"Unimed Package Insert Online." http://www.unimed.com/pdfs/Anadrol.pdf. Web. 2 April 2008.

Zaccardi, N. *Anabolic Steroids.* Amherst, MA: University of Massachusetts. http://www.wellnessmd.com/anabolics.html. Web. 8 April 2008.(*Continued*)

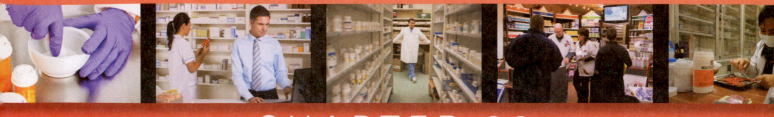

CHAPTER 33

The Reproductive System

LEARNING OBJECTIVES

After completing this chapter, you should be able to:

- List, identify, and diagram the basic anatomical structures and parts of the male and female reproductive systems.

- Describe the functions and physiology of the male and female reproductive systems and the hormones that govern them.

- List and define common diseases affecting the male and female reproductive systems, and understand the causes, symptoms, and pharmaceutical treatments associated with each disease or condition.

- Describe the indications for use and mechanisms of action of various contraceptives.

INTRODUCTION

At the onset of sexual maturity, in both males and females, the hypothalamus secretes gonadotropin-releasing hormone (GnRH). It is needed for both sexual maturation and normal reproduction and acts by stimulating the release of luteinizing hormone (LH) and follicle-stimulating hormone (FSH) from the anterior pituitary. LH and FSH act by stimulating the production of sex hormones in the gonads (the testes and ovaries).

This chapter discusses both the female and male reproductive systems as well as conditions that affect these systems, such as sexually transmitted diseases (STDs) and infertility. Different methods of contraception are also introduced, including oral and topical contraceptives and intrauterine devices (IUDs) and barrier devices.

The Female Reproductive System

The female reproductive system includes the organs and hormones that allow females to reproduce and give them their gender characteristics. This section discusses female reproductive anatomy, contraception, and conditions and diseases (including infertility and STDs).

Anatomy

The female reproductive system is composed of internal organs and external genitals. The internal reproductive organs are two **ovaries**, two fallopian tubes, the uterus, and the vagina (see Figure 33-1). The external genitals are known together as the *vulva*. The vulva consists of the labia minora, labia majora, and clitoris.

Reproductive Cycle

The menstrual cycle consists of two stages: ovulation and menstruation. Females are born with about 2 million **oocytes**. By the time of puberty, only about 400,000 oocytes remain. At the beginning of each monthly cycle, FSH causes one of the many underdeveloped ovarian follicles to fully develop and mature. Within an ovary, an **ovum** (egg) matures about 11 to 17 days before the woman's next menstrual period, or approximately once every 28 to 30 days. As the follicle gets larger, cells that are dedicated to producing the estrogenic hormones estriol, estrone, and estradiol become active.

Estradiol is the most abundant and active of the estrogens. Its main function is to stimulate the development of the uterine lining and the mammary glands to ready the body for pregnancy. The estrogens are known as *feminizing hormones,* because they are responsible for the female secondary sex characteristics, such as a higher voice, breast development, curvaceous body shape, and less bulky muscle. Estradiol is the most potent form of estrogen in premenopausal women. Estrone, which accounts for most estrogen in postmenopausal women, is made only in very small quantities by the ovaries; the majority is converted from another hormone, androstenedione, in fat and other body tissues. Estriol, a weaker estrogen, is formed when estradiol and estrone are metabolized.

Progesterone, the second major type of female sex hormone made in the ovaries, develops the **endometrium** and the mammary ducts for lactation. Progesterone also maintains the

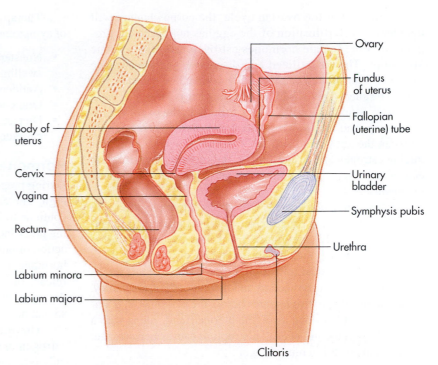

Body of uterus
Cervix
Vagina
Rectum
Labium minora
Labium majora
Ovary
Fundus of uterus
Fallopian (uterine) tube
Urinary bladder
Symphysis pubis
Urethra
Clitoris

FIGURE 33-1 The female reproductive system.

uterine lining if egg implantation occurs. Progesterone literally means *hormone for life.*

If the female reproductive cycle is considered on average a 28-day cycle, during the first 12 days, estrogen has little effect. After that, it has a positive effect on the production of gonadotropins, causing a large increase in LH and a small increase in FSH. Midway through the cycle, after approximately 14 days of development, the sudden increase in LH causes the mature follicle to rupture, releasing the ovum. This generally occurs 12 to 14 days before a woman's next period. The mature egg is released from the ovary, passes into a fallopian tube, and is swept by tiny cilia and smooth muscle action into the uterus. It takes about five days before the egg reaches the uterus. This *trip* is known as **ovulation**. If a woman has a cycle shorter or longer than 28 days, ovulation may occur on a different day (day 7 or day 20), but generally takes place 12 to 14 days before she has a menstrual period.

After ovulation, the ruptured ovarian follicle (which remained in the ovary) undergoes a change. LH transforms the follicle into a corpus luteum, which continues to produce estrogen and begins to produce progesterone to prepare the uterine lining for possible implantation. A woman is most fertile around the time she is ovulating. Some women can tell when they are ovulating by watching for changes in vaginal discharge or body temperature. Some women feel pain when the egg is released.

If implantation of the egg does occur, the high levels of estrogen and progesterone will be maintained; these exert a negative feedback effect on the secretion of gonadotropins by the anterior pituitary gland, and pregnancy continues. If implantation does not occur, there is no need for progesterone, so production of that hormone stops.

---

ovaries the female reproductive organs that produce eggs.

oocyte an immature egg.

ovum a mature egg.

endometrium the lining of the uterus.

ovulation the process in which the ovarian follicle ruptures and releases the egg.

At the end of the ovarian cycle, the corpus luteum will disintegrate if fertilization of the egg has not occurred; production of the female hormones estrogen and progesterone also stops. The unfertilized egg dissolves, and the absence of the two hormones causes the endometrium (uterine lining) to be shed. This shedding begins what is known as *menstruation*. Simultaneously, a new follicle in the ovary begins to develop, and the cycle repeats again. Somewhere roughly between the ages of 40 and 55, a woman's ovaries stop producing estrogen and progesterone and monthly menstruation ceases. One year from the last menstrual cycle is known as *menopause*.

If pregnancy does occur, the corpus luteum continues to produce estrogen and progesterone until the placenta is developed around day 12 (see Figure 33-2). The placenta, acting as an endocrine gland, then assumes the role of producing these hormones. The critical transitional time usually occurs and is completed between the second and third month of pregnancy. If the corpus luteum disintegrates before the placenta can maintain the correct hormone level, the uterine lining, along with a fetus, will rupture and shed. This rupture causes hemorrhage, and the end result is a miscarriage.

About 75% of postpubescent women experience a mild-to-moderate condition called *premenstrual syndrome (PMS)*, which occurs during the phase before menstruation begins. Some women have both PMS and uncomfortable periods. Symptoms of PMS include the following:

- Pain or cramping before and during periods
- Weight gain before and during periods due to water retention
- Moody or irritable feeling before or during periods
- Breakout of acne or pimples before period is due
- Diarrhea, constipation, or upset stomach during periods

About 8% of menstruating women experience a more severe form of PMS called *premenstrual dysphoric disorder (PMDD)*. In addition to PMS symptoms, women experiencing PMDD may also experience the following:

- Fatigue
- Depression
- Anxiety
- Anger or irritability
- Changes in sleep patterns
- Changes in appetite

Therapy for PMDD focuses on prevention and mitigation of symptoms. Treatments may include the following:

- Nonsteroidal anti-inflammatory drugs for pain and swelling
- Antidepressants
- Oral **contraception** to help even out hormone levels
- Diet and lifestyle changes, such as exercise, reductions in caffeine intake, and eating more carbohydrates

Hormone Contraception

During pregnancy, the levels of estrogen and progesterone are high. The constant high levels of estrogen and progesterone continue to inhibit the release of FSH and LH. Therefore, during pregnancy, no other follicle can develop. The mechanism of action of hormone contraception is to maintain a high level of hormone in the blood. A hormonal contraceptive prevents the release of FSH by imitating what happens during pregnancy, thus preventing the development of another follicle or follicles so that no egg is available for fertilization.

There are several types of hormone contraceptives: estrogen and progesterone combinations, and progesterone only (see Table 33-1). Prefertilization and postfertilization are two main mechanisms of action of contraceptives.

- *Prefertilization* mechanisms of action include: (1) prevention of ovulation and (2) thickening of cervical mucus to act as a barrier to sperm, reducing the likelihood of implantation.
- *Postfertilization* mechanisms of action include changing the lining of the uterus to block implantation of the embryo.

Although most people define *conception* as the conjoining of an egg and sperm, the blocking of implantation after the conjoining of the egg and sperm is considered an interference with conception. The low-dose progestins or progestin-only pills (POPs) used to prevent pregnancy are also called *minipills*. Progestins can prevent fertilization by preventing the egg from fully developing and by thickening the cervical mucus so that it slows down the flagellation of the sperm (tail movement), preventing the sperm from entering the uterus. Simply put, the sperm cannot *swim* through the thick mucus, so they cannot reach the uterus or fallopian tubes to fertilize the egg. Birth control pills (BCPs) also lower the midcycle LH and FSH peaks. Progestin-only pills are about 93% effective; that is, 7 out of 100 women taking a POP will become pregnant each year.

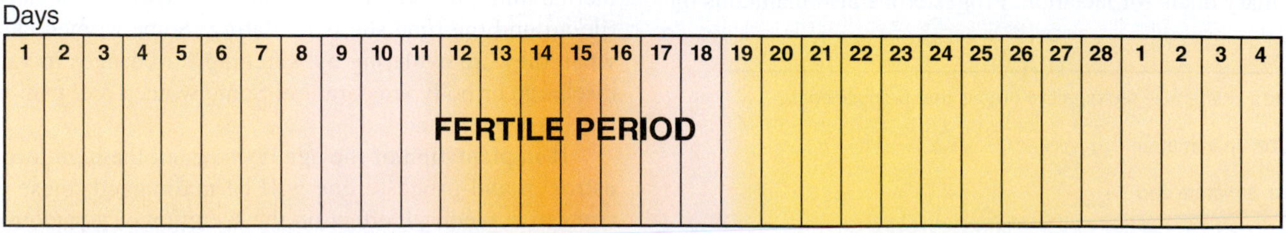

Days

| 1 | 2 | 3 | 4 | 5 | 6 | 7 | 8 | 9 | 10 | 11 | 12 | 13 | 14 | 15 | 16 | 17 | 18 | 19 | 20 | 21 | 22 | 23 | 24 | 25 | 26 | 27 | 28 | 1 | 2 | 3 | 4 |

FERTILE PERIOD

FIGURE 33-2 Fertility and the menstrual cycle.

contraception birth control.

TABLE 33-1 Examples of Hormone Contraception

Type of Contraceptive	Trade Name	Special Notes
Progestin-Only		
estradiol cypionate/ medroxyprogesterone acetate injection	Lunelle	Given monthly, injected into the arm, thigh, or buttock.
levonorgestrel subdermal implant	Norplant	
medroxyprogesterone injection	Depo-Provera	Given every 13 weeks (3 months).
norethindrone tablets	Ortho-Micronor	Can be given during lactation.
norgestrel tablets	Ovrette	Used normally as birth control pills (BCPs). As an emergency contraceptive, 20 tablets are given within 72 hours and repeated within 12 hours.
Emergency Pregnancy Prevention		
levonorgestrel tablets	Plan B	Used following unprotected intercourse or a suspected contraceptive failure.
levonorgestrel/ethynyl estradiol	Preven	The first tablet should be taken as soon as possible within 72 hours of intercourse. The second tablet must be taken 12 hours later.
Combination Progestin and Estrogen		
estrogen and progestin (varying strengths of each)	Alesse, Levlen, Lo/Ovral, Nordette, OrthoCyclen, Ortho-Novum 7/7/7, OrthoTri-Cyclen Lo, Seasonale, Triphasil-28, Trivora, Yasmin	Seasonale, a new type of BCP, changes the menstrual cycle to only four periods per year. The active pills are taken 84 days in a row, followed by seven days of non-hormonal pills. The woman has her period while taking the nonhormonal pills.
etonogestrel 120-mcg and ethinyl estradiol 15-mcg vaginal ring	NuvaRing	A small (about 2 inches in diameter), flexible, colorless ring, inserted at home by patient. Releases a continuous low dose of hormones to prevent pregnancy for that month. Used for three weeks per month for continuous contraception. The ring is removed in the fourth week so that the woman can have a menstrual period. The exact position of the ring in the vagina is not critical for it to work.
norelgestromin 150-mcg and ethinyl estradiol 20-mcg transdermal patch	Ortho Evra Patch	Each small adhesive patch lasts seven days.

❝ **Workplace Wisdom** **Patient Package Inserts**

Federal law requires that all drugs containing estrogen *must* be dispensed with a patient package insert. Therefore, a pharmacy technician must know which drugs contain estrogen. These drugs are usually birth control and hormone replacement therapy (HRT) agents. Examples are Lo/Ovral, Ortho Evra Patch, NuvaRing, PremPro, and Premarin. ❞

Drug–Drug and Drug–Herb Interactions with Hormone Contraception

Antibiotic, antifungal, antiepileptic, and anticonvulsant drugs may interfere with the active ingredients of birth control agents. The drugs and herbs in Table 33-2 prevent birth control drugs from working well, and the patient may become pregnant.

❝ **Workplace Wisdom** **Contraception Interactions**

If a woman must take drugs or herbs that interact with chemical contraception, another method of birth control should be used along with the birth control pills. Condoms with spermicide are a good alternative. If the drugs or herbs are to be used over the long term, she should consult a physician. ❞

TABLE 33-2 Drugs and Herbs That Interact with Oral Birth Control

Classification	Examples
Antibiotics	nitrofurantoin (Macrodantin)
	penicillins (PCNs)
	rifampin
	sulfa drugs
	tetracyclines (TCNs)
Anticonvulsants	carbamazepine (Tegretol)
	ethosuximide (Zarontin)
	phenobarbital
	phenytoin (Dilantin)
	primidone (Mysoline)
Antifungals	fluconazole (Diflucan)
Herbs	St. John's wort (some studies suggest that St. John's wort may reduce the effectiveness of birth control)

Side Effects of Hormone Contraceptives

Side effects may include the following:

- Weight gain
- Mild headaches
- Breast tenderness
- Nausea and vomiting
- Hypertension
- Decrease of libido
- Vaginitis, vaginal skin irritation, and vaginal discharge

Toxic effects can include the following:

- Shortness of breath (SOB)
- Chest pain
- Stomach or intestinal pain
- Severe lingering headache
- Changes in vision (blurred, flashing lights, or diminished vision)
- Infertility for 3–12 months after discontinuation
- Blood clots (lung, brain/stroke)
- Liver tumors
- Gallbladder disease

Contraindications apply to women who:

- Are over the age of 35 and who smoke
- Are pregnant or suspect pregnancy
- Are breastfeeding
- Experience unexplained vaginal bleeding
- Experience migraine headaches
- Have active liver disease (hepatitis) or a history of liver tumors
- Have breast cancer or a history of breast cancer or of cancer of any reproductive organs
- Have a history of heart disease, stroke, or high blood pressure; blood clotting problems; or diabetes

Topical Contraceptives

Spermicides are topical forms of contraception that are available in various dosage forms, including creams, foams, gels, suppositories, and vaginal films. The active ingredient in most spermicides is nonoxynol-9. Nonoxynol-9 has been reported to cause the lining of the vaginal wall to thin or erode faster, and when used often may actually help bacteria and viruses to enter the flesh faster. Apply and reapply spermicides before sexual intercourse, no earlier than the time stated in the directions, which varies from 20 minutes to 1 hour. It is important for the female to prevent the spermicide from dripping out of the vagina after intercourse so that it can be effective. Although the use of a panty liner may help, lying down for four to eight hours will better enhance the effectiveness of such products. Also, women should not douche for at least eight hours after intercourse, because douching may interfere with the effectiveness of the spermicide.

❝ Workplace Wisdom Nonoxynol-9

Studies indicate that nonoxynol-9 spermicides irritate vaginal and rectal linings, increasing the recipient's exposure risk to human immunodeficiency virus (HIV) or a sexually transmitted infection (STI). Anyone using a product containing nonoxynol-9 who notices any genital irritation should discontinue use. ❞

Spermicidal foam, the most effective spermicide, helps prevent pregnancy in two ways:

1. By forming a physical barrier to the entry of sperm into the cervix.
2. By immobilizing and killing the sperm.

Simple skin irritations and allergies to ingredients other than the active ingredient can deter use. Gels must be reapplied if not used within 20 minutes before intercourse. Vaginal filmstrips are good for one hour after insertion.

Contraceptive Devices

Oral contraception, in tablet form, is not the only birth control option. Many alternatives are available, such as barrier devices, diaphragms, cervical caps, and IUDs.

Barrier Devices—Male Condoms Lamb intestine condoms do not provide protection from STDs or STIs. Latex condoms are the most effective protection against transmission of bacterial and viral infections. The main drawback of these is allergic

PROFILE IN PRACTICE

Stephen, a pharmacy technician, is entering demographic data into the computer system for Mrs. Abbott, a new customer. During the conversation, Mrs. Abbott reveals to Stephen that she is 10 weeks pregnant.

▶ *Why is it important for Stephen to include Mrs. Abbott's pregnancy in her patient profile?*

reactions by either the female or the male. Polyurethane condoms should be used if either partner is allergic to latex. Some condoms also contain a spermicide.

Condoms should never be used with greasy or oily substances, such as Vaseline, because these substances will cause the condom to weaken and burst. Personal water-based lubricants, such as K-Y Jelly, are made for this purpose.

Barrier Devices—Female Condoms A polyurethane tube or sheath approximately 6.5 inches long, with an inner ring at the closed end that loosely lines the vagina, provides protection from unintended pregnancy and the transmission of STDs. This material does not cause allergies and need not be removed immediately after ejaculation, though it should be taken out before the woman stands up to avoid the semen spilling out. Upon removal, the outer ring should be twisted to seal the condom so that no semen leaks out. Current standard directions indicate that a female condom should be used only once. However, it can be used with either oil- or water-based lubricants. The simultaneous use of both a male and a female condom is contraindicated, because the condoms may create friction, resulting in either or both condoms slipping or tearing and/or the outer ring of the female condom being pushed inside the vagina. Table 33-3 compares male and female condoms.

Diaphragms and Cervical Caps A *diaphragm* is a latex or silicon cervical barrier form of birth control. When properly inserted, the diaphragm forms a seal against the vaginal wall that prevents sperm from entering. Only a trained health care provider can fit a woman for these devices. The size of the diaphragm must match the distance from the pubic bone to the posterior fornix of the vagina (or the largest size that is comfortable for the client).

A *cervical cap* is similar to a diaphragm except that it fits over the cervix to prevent sperm from entering the uterus. Cervical caps come in four sizes. A cap that is too small can injure the cervix; one that is too large can slip off during intercourse. A woman may need to have these devices refit if she undergoes any of the following changes:

- Gains or loses weight
- Has a baby
- Has a second- or third-trimester abortion

Both the diaphragm and the cervical cap should be used with spermicides. Diaphragms must be worn for at least six hours after intercourse. Because rubber deteriorates, the devices should be periodically checked for small holes and replaced as needed.

TABLE 33-3 Male and Female Condom Comparison

Male Condom	Female Condom
Brands: Durex, Lifestyles, Magnum, Trojan	Brands: Dominique, Femidom, Femy, Myfemy, Reality
Nickname: rubber	Nickname: FC
Rolled on the man's penis, fits snugly on the penis	Inserted into the woman's vagina, loosely lines the vagina
Lubricant	**Lubricant**
• Can include spermicide	• Can include spermicide
• Can be water-based only; cannot be oil-based	• Can be water-based or oil-based
• Located on the outside of the condom	• Located on both the inside and the outside of the condom
Specifications	**Specifications**
Requires erect penis	Can be inserted prior to sexual intercourse; not dependent on erect penis
Must be removed immediately after ejaculation	Need not be removed immediately after ejaculation; must be removed before the female stands
Covers most of the penis and protects the woman's internal genitalia	Provides broader protection by covering both the internal and external genitalia of the woman and the base of the man's penis
Latex condoms can decay if not stored properly	Polyurethane is not susceptible to deterioration from temperature or humidity
Can be used *only* once; is then discarded	Recommended as one-time-use product
Disadvantage: must interrupt foreplay to use	Can be inserted before foreplay, and intercourse occurs without interrupting foreplay
Easy placement	Disadvantage: Takes a while for the female to learn how to use it confidently. Takes practice. Makes a noise that can be silenced with use of more lubricant.

Intrauterine Devices *IUDs* are small, flexible devices made of metal and/or plastic. These devices are inserted into a woman's uterus through her vagina; the procedure is done by a health care provider during an office visit. Approximately 15% of women of reproductive age currently use IUDs. These devices work to prevent pregnancy by a combination of mechanisms. They inhibit sperm migration in the upper female genital tract, which in turn inhibits ovum transport and stimulates

endometrial changes that will not support implantation. Most are unmedicated, but some IUDs are progestin-releasing (levonorgestrel or progesterone). IUDs are safe for 5 to 10 years but have the drawback of tending to cause heavy menstrual bleeding. IUDs are 97% to 99.6% effective.

Conditions That Affect the Female Reproductive System

The following is a description of common conditions that may affect the female reproductive system. Note that menopause, while not a condition, is included in this discussion.

Menopause

Menopause is a normal process that women of a certain age go through, generally about the age of 51. It is the absolute final menstrual period and is reduced functioning of the ovaries. Hormone levels operate at lower levels and the ability to reproduce stop with the event. Symptoms of menopause include bone loss, hot flashes, insomnia, sleep disturbance, and vaginal dryness. Various medications can be used to treat the annoying symptoms of menopause, including both OTC and prescription drugs. HRT and lifestyle changes are some of the remedies to help ease menopause symptoms (see Tables 33-4 and 33-5).

Pelvic Inflammatory Disease

Pelvic inflammatory disease (PID) is an inflammation of the female reproductive organs that causes a host of serious symptoms. Inflammation occurs within the uterine lining, fallopian tubes, and ovaries. Symptoms of PID are increased vaginal discharge, abdominal discomfort, bleeding in between periods, painful periods, uncomfortable urination, painful bowel movements, painful sex, fever, and upper right abdominal pain.

PROFILE IN PRACTICE

Joan is working at an independent retail pharmacy. A woman comes into the pharmacy for Plan B tablets. The pharmacist has a moral objection to this form of emergency contraception and has clearly communicated this to the pharmacy staff.

▶ *How should the situation be handled? What is Joan's role? What is the pharmacist's role?*

TABLE 33-4 Pharmaceutical Treatments for Menopause

Generic Name	Brand Name	Dosage Forms and Availability	Route of Administration	Common Adult Dosage
conjugated estrogens	Premarin	0.3-mg, 0.45-mg, 0.625-mg, 0.9-mg, 1.25-mg tablets	Oral, injection, vaginal	Oral: 0.3–2.5 qd; vaginal cream: 2–4 gm
conjugated estrogens with medroxyprogesterone	Prempro, Premphase	0.3-mg, 0.45/1.5-mg, 0.625/2.5-mg, 0.625/5-mg tablets	Oral	0.625/2.5–0.625/5 mg qd
esterified estrogen	Menest	0.3-mg, 0.625-mg, 1.25-mg, 2.5-mg tablets	Oral	0.3–1.25 mg qd
estradiol	Estrance, Femtrace, Gynodiol,	0.5-, 1-, 2-mg tablets	Oral, transdermal	Oral: 0.5–2 mg qd; transdermal: vary with brand
estropipate	Ogen, Ortho-Est	0.75/0.625-mg, 1.5/1.25-mg, 3/2.5-mg tablets	Oral	0.75–3 mg qd

TABLE 33-5 Comparison of Progestins

Generic Name	Brand Name	Dosage Forms and Availability	Route of Administration	Common Adult Dosage
medroxyprogesterone	Provera (oral), Depo-Provera (injection)	150 mg/mL SD syringe	Oral, injection	Oral: 2–10 mg qd for 5–10 days; Injection: 150 mg deep IM every three months
norethidrone	Aygestin (hormone replacement), Ortho Micronor (contraceptive)	5-mg tablets	Oral	2.5–10 mg in cycles for amenorrhea; 0.35 mg qd for contraception; 5 mg for prevention of endometrial hyperplasia given cyclically with estrogen HRT
progesterone	Crinone	4% (45 mg), 8% (90 mg), SU applicator	Vaginal	45 mg (4% gel) every other day × 6 doses

Certain antimicrobials, IV antibiotics can be given to treat the condition. Treatment may include an in-hospital stay or outpatient options for the patient to get well.

Female Hypogonadism

Female hypogonadism is defined as inadequate production of the hormone estrogen in the ovaries. Because of this condition, females may lack a menstrual cycle and breast development and have stunted growth. Females with this condition may find that they do not have a period, hot flashes, less interest in sex, and less body hair. Adult females may experience early menopause and infertility. The hormones estrogen and progestin are used to treat this condition and are available in pill, lotion, gel, and patches (see Table 33-6).

Mammary Glands and Childbirth

During the fourth or fifth month of gestation, the pituitary gland secretes prolactin, which causes the mammary glands to produce colostrum—the first suckle does not contain breast milk. Breast milk follows after about three days.

Oxytocin, secreted by the posterior pituitary gland, causes labor contractions. Immediately after the baby leaves the birth canal, oxytocin allows the milk that has been made, according to the prolactin signal, to be secreted. After the birth, sucking also causes oxytocin to be secreted by the posterior pituitary gland; the oxytocin causes the milk ducts in the breast to contract and relax, pushing the milk toward the nipple. Therefore, prolactin causes milk production, while oxytocin enables milk secretion. Many other hormones, such as FSH, LH, and human placental lactogen, also play vital roles in milk production. When dopamine, a prolactin-inhibitory factor, inhibits prolactin, milk is no longer produced or secreted.

Research shows that oxytocin may also be responsible for the *bonding* attraction between mother and child as well as between life partners. Injectable oxytocin is available under the trade name Pitocin. Figure 33-3 shows the relationship between oxytocin and breastfeeding.

TABLE 33-6 Pharmaceutical Treatments for Female Hypogonadism

Generic Name	Brand Name	Dosage Forms and Availability	Route of Administration	Common Adult Dosage
estrogen	Prempro, Premphase	0.3-mg, 0.45/1.5-mg, 0.625/2.5-mg, 0.625/6-mg tablets	Oral	One 0.625-mg Premarin (conjugated estrogens [CE]) tablet daily on day 1–14 and one 0.625-mg CE and 5 mg of medroxyprogesterone acetate (MPA) taken on day 15–28
progestin	Activella	1.0/0.5-mg, 0.5/0.1-mg tablets	Oral	Patients should be started at the lowest dose.

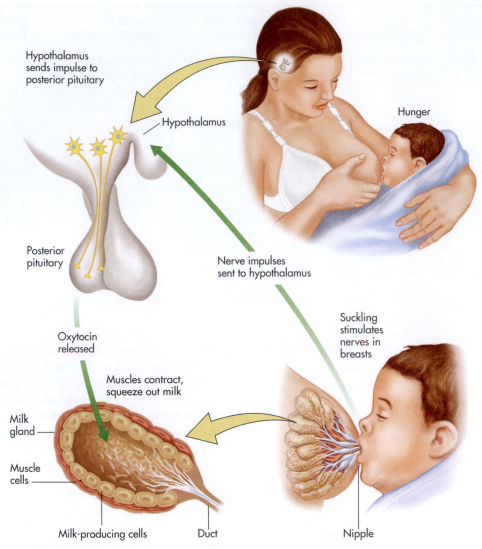

FIGURE 33-3 The relationship between oxytocin and breastfeeding.

Female Infertility

Infertility is defined as the failure to conceive after one year of regular, unprotected intercourse. Infertility may occur as a result of a problem in either partner or because of a combination of problems in both partners.

Causes of Female Infertility

About 35% of all cases of infertility stem from problems in the man's system; another 35% arise from abnormalities in the woman's system; in about 20% of cases, both the man and the woman have fertility problems. In about 10% of cases, no cause can be found. It is known, however, that age often increases the risk of infertility.

- *Age*—a woman's age (more accurately, the age of her eggs) can contribute to infertility. At the age of 25, the chance of getting pregnant within the first six months of trying to conceive is 75%. By the time the woman is 40 years old, her chances are lowered to only 22%. This decrease in fertility appears to be caused by a higher rate of chromosomal abnormalities occurring in the eggs as the woman ages.

- *Weight*—fat cells make 30% of estrogen. However, overweight patients have an overload of estrogen that throws off the reproductive cycle. Conversely, strict vegetarians, athletes, and dancers who lack sufficient body fat may not produce enough estrogen; these women may also have difficulties because of a lack of vitamin B12, zinc, iron, and folic acid. These deficiencies can lead to irregular periods and possibly complete shutdown of the reproductive process.

- *Endometriosis*—a condition in which fragments of the lining of the uterus are found in other parts of the pelvic cavity. These pieces of endometrium still respond to the menstrual hormonal cycle, slowly increasing in number and size. Because the blood cannot escape during menstruation, it builds up and leads to the development of small or large painful cysts, causing scarring and inflammation.

- *Hormonal changes*—about one-third of infertility cases can be traced to ovulation and hormonal problems.
- *Progesterone deficiency*—progesterone keeps the uterine lining ready to accept implantation. Without it, or with decreased progesterone levels, implantation cannot occur, or an implanted embryo may abort.
- *Polycystic ovarian syndrome (PCOS)*—occurs in 6% of women and is the major cause of infertility in American women. PCOS increases androgen production, producing high LH levels and low FSH levels. This prevents the maturation of eggs, so eggs are not released. Inflammation and edema occur in the fallopian tube, hampering passage of any matured ova and creating a cyst (which may create other cysts).
- *Elevated prolactin levels*—in women who are not lactating, increased prolactin levels inhibit ovulation and may also indicate a pituitary tumor. Parlodel is the drug of choice in these cases.
- *Medications*—certain medications can cause temporary infertility. These include prescription antibiotics, antidepressants, hormones and narcotic analgesics, and OTC medications such as ASA and ibuprofen (when taken midcycle). Taking acetaminophen regularly may reduce levels of estrogen and LH. In most cases, once the drugs are discontinued, fertility is restored.
- *Antibodies to sperm*—some women have antibodies to sperm that attack sperm as if they were harmful foreign bodies or substances.

Sometimes a woman is able to conceive, but the fertilized ovum cannot implant or the endometrial lining sheds despite implantation, carrying the ovum with it. *Spontaneous abortion* has been associated with use of an electric blanket during the month of conception.

Pharmaceutical Treatment of Infertility in Women

Persistent infertility, if untreated, often has damaging psychological effects, creating feelings of guilt or depression in either or both partners and breaking down communication between a couple. Having to have intercourse at specific times of the menstrual cycle, and times at which the female has a specific basal temperature, can add more stress. Therefore, persons who wish to conceive often turn to pharmaceutical treatment to help increase fertility. An example of an antiestrogenic drug is the fertility drug clomiphene (Clomid, Serophene). Clomiphene tricks the brain and pituitary gland into *thinking* that there is less estrogen available in the female's body. This stimulates pituitary production of FSH and LH, boosting follicle growth and the release of mature eggs.

Side effects include hot flashes, breast tenderness, mood swings, visual problems, thick cervical mucus, and luteal phase deficiency. The time from ovulation to onset of the next period is known as the *luteal phase*, during which the corpus luteum makes progesterone. Progesterone prepares the uterine lining for embryo implantation. A luteal phase deficiency or a short luteal phase results from a lack of progesterone production by the corpus luteum or poor response of the endometrium to normal progesterone levels. This lack of progesterone or response to it may cause or exacerbate infertility.

Toxic effects of fertility drugs include long-term safety risks. Use for more than a year may increase the risk of ovarian cancer. The risk of multiple births and low birth weight also increases with the use of fertility drugs (see Table 33-7).

TABLE 33-7 Pharmaceutical Treatments for Infertility

Generic Name	Brand Name	Dosage forms and Availability	Route of Administration	Common Adult Dosage
bromocriptine	Parlodel	2.5-mg, 5-mg snap tablets	Oral	Half to one 2.5-mg scored tablet daily
cetrorelix injection	Cetrotide	0.25-mg, 3-mg SDV	Injection	Single dose regimen: 3 mg of Cetrotide (cetrorelix) is administered when the serum estradiol level is indicative of an appropriate stimulation response, usually on stimulation day 7 (range: day 5–9). If hCG has not been administered within four days after injection of Cetrotide (cetrorelix) 3 mg, Cetrotide (cetrorelix) 0.25 mg qd should be administered until the day of hCG administration Multiple dose regimen: 0.25 mg of Cetrotide (cetrorelix) is administered on either stimulation day 5 (morning or evening) or day 6 (morning) and continued daily until the day of hCG administration

(Continued)

TABLE 33-7 Pharmaceutical Treatments for Infertility (*Continued*)

Generic Name	Brand Name	Dosage forms and Availability	Route of Administration	Common Adult Dosage
choriogonadotropin alfa injectable	Ovidrel	250-mcg SDS	Injection	250 mcg should be administered one day following the last dose of the follicle-stimulating agent
clomiphene	Clomid	50-mg tablets	Oral	50 mg qd for five days
danazol	Danocrine	50-mg, 100-mg, 200-mg capsules	Oral	Starting dose of 800 mg given in two divided doses is recommended with a gradual downward titration
folitropin alfa injection	Gonal-f	1 amp/75 IU, 10 amp/75 IU, 100 amp/75 IU, 1 amp/150 IU sterile lyophilized powder	Subcutaneously	Recommended that the initial dose of the first cycle be 75 IU. An incremental adjustment in dose of up to 37.5 IU may be considered after 14 days
folitropin beta injection	Follistim AQ	75 IU/0.5 mL, 150 IU/0.5 mL SDV	Injection	Starting dose of 150–225 IU is recommended for at least the first four days of treatment. After this, the dose may be adjusted for the individual patient based upon her ovarian response
gonadotropins, chorionic intramuscular	Pregnyl, Novarel	Two Vial Pack: 1–10 mL lyophilized, MDV; 1–10 mL vial of solvent containing: water for injection with sodium chloride 0.56% and benzyl alcohol 0.9%	Injection	5,000–10,000 USP units one day following the last dose of menotropins
menotopins injection	Repronex, Menopur	75 IU FSH and 75 IU of LH activity, SDV	Injection	Recommended initial dose is 150 IU daily for the first five days of treatment. Subsequent dosing should be adjusted according to individual patient response
metformin	Glucophage	500-mg, 850-mg, 1,000-mg tablets	Oral	In general, clinically significant responses are not seen at doses below 1,500 mg/day. However, a lower recommended starting dose and gradually increased dosage is advised to minimize gastrointestinal symptoms
progesterone vaginal gel	Crinone, Prochieve	4% (45 mg), 8% (90 mg), SU applicator	Topical	Crinone 8% is administered vaginally at a dose of 90 mg qd

testes the male reproductive organs that produce sperm.

The Male Reproductive System

The male reproductive system includes the organs and hormones that allow males to reproduce and gives them their gender characteristics. This section discusses male anatomy and some conditions and diseases of the male reproductive system, including infertility, erectile dysfunction (ED), benign prostatic hyperplasia (BPH), and STDs.

Anatomy

The prostate gland is situated at the base of the bladder and encircles the urethra. The organ is roughly the size and shape of a large walnut with an average normal weight of 20–30 gm. Secretions produced in the prostatic glands empty into the urethra during ejaculation, via the prostatic ducts, to make up a sizable volume of the ejaculate. Although the function of this fluid is not fully understood, it is speculated that it neutralizes the acidic environment of the vagina and possibly provides nutrition for the spermatids (young sperm cells). Though not absolutely necessary for fertilization, prostate solutions increase the chances of fertilization.

The **testes**, a pair of organs located in the scrotum and surrounded by a thin mesothelial membrane, are responsible for the production of sperm as well as androgens. The testes are made up of thousands of tiny tubules supported by fibrous septae, and the entire gland is surrounded by a thick fibrous capsule called the *tunica albuginea*. Mature sperm are stored in the *epididymis*. During ejaculation, the sperm are propelled along the vas deferens into the urethra (see Figure 33-4).

Conditions That Affect the Male Reproductive System

The following presents a description of common conditions that may affect the male reproductive system.

Male Infertility

Fertility in the male begins with the production of GnRH in the hypothalamus, which instructs the pituitary gland to manufacture FSH and LH. FSH causes sperm production, and LH stimulates production of the male hormone testosterone. Both sperm and testosterone production occur in the testes. The life cycle of sperm is about 70–75 days. The ability of a sperm to move straight forward rapidly is determined by its *flagellum* (tail) and is probably the most important factor that determines male fertility. During sexual excitement, nerves stimulate the muscles in the epididymis to contract, forcing the sperm into the vas deferens and then through the penis. The *seminal vesicles*, clusters of tissue, contribute seminal fluid to the sperm. The vas deferens also collects fluid from the nearby prostate gland. The mixture of the fluids from the seminal vesicles, the secretions from the prostate gland, and the sperm is called *semen*. The two vas deferens join together to form the ejaculatory duct, which conducts the semen through to the urethra. The urethra is the same pathway in the penis through which urine passes. During orgasm in a healthy male, the prostate closes off the bladder so that urine cannot enter the urethra. The semen is forced through the urethra

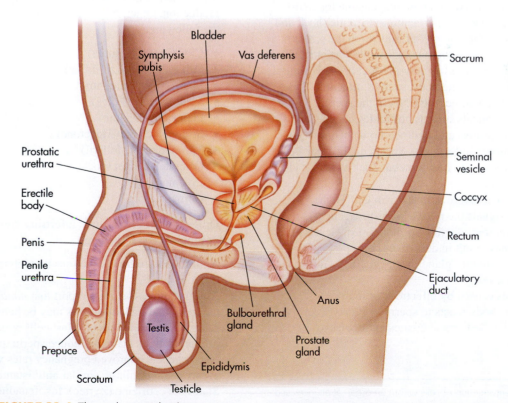

FIGURE 33-4 The male reproductive system.

TABLE 33-8 Categories of Male Infertility

Category	Medical Name	Description/Comment
Low sperm count (most common cause)	Oligospermia	Sperm count is less than 10 million sperm/mL of semen. Numerous and varied causes of temporary and permanent low sperm count.
No sperm	Azoospermia	Complete absence of sperm. Relatively rare, affecting less than 1% of all men and 10% to 15% of infertile men. Causes: Obstruction or production failure of sperm in the testes, which can be caused by mumps, genetic disorders, radiation, or exposure to chemicals.
Low-quality sperm	Dysspermia	Quality is determined by sperm motility (ability to move), which depends on its flagella or its morphology (shape and structure). The quality of the sperm is usually more significant than the number of sperm (count).
No semen production	Aspermia	Ejaculation does not secrete any semen.

during *ejaculation*, the final stage of orgasm. Of the 100 to 300 million sperm that are in the ejaculate, about 400 survive the acidic environment of the vagina, and only about 40 reach the egg.

Activities that increase a male's risk for infertility (see Table 33-8) include the following:

- Smoking, which impairs sperm motility and reduces sperm's lifespan.
- Poor nutrition, especially deficiency of vitamin C, selenium, zinc, and/or folate.
- Bicycling. Pressure from a bike seat may damage the blood vessels and nerves that are responsible for erections. Biking exposes the perineum to extreme shock and vibrations, increasing the risk of injuries to the scrotum.
- Oxygen-free radicals (oxidants). Unstable particles called *free radicals* are released as a by-product of many natural chemical processes in the body, such as infection. These oxidants negatively affect the DNA in the sperm.
- Exposure to chemicals such as pesticides, the phylates used to soften plastics, and hydrocarbons (benzene, ethylbenzene toluene, and xylene). Sperm quality may be affected by exposure to heavy metals such as lead, cadmium, or arsenic.
- Hypogonadism, a severe deficiency in GnRH, the hormone that signals the release of testosterone and other important reproductive hormones. Low levels of testosterone may result in defective sperm production. Tumors of the pituitary gland may also affect GnRH, FSH, or LSH levels.
- Autoantibodies caused by infections or injury. Sometimes the body reacts to sperm as if they were invading foreign bodies and creates antibodies to destroy them.

- Retrograde ejaculation, which occurs when the muscles of the urethra do not propel the semen properly during orgasm. The sperm are forced backward into the bladder instead of forward out of the urethra. Retrograde ejaculation may be caused by several conditions, including diabetes, HTN, MS, spinal cord injury, tranquilizers, and HTN medication.
- Cryptorchidism, associated with mild to severely impaired sperm production, is a failure of the testes to descend from the abdomen into the scrotum during fetal development. The testes are exposed to the higher degree of internal body heat, which kills sperm.
- Medications. Anabolic steroids severely impair sperm production. Other drugs that affect male fertility include the following:

  - Cimetidine (Tagamet)
  - Sulfasalazine (Azulfidine)
  - Methadone (Dolophine)
  - Methotrexate (Folex)
  - Phenytoin (Dilantin)
  - Spironolactone (Aldactone)
  - Thioridazine (Mellaril)
  - Calcium channel blockers
  - Colchicine
  - Corticosteroids

Drugs that can treat male infertility caused by hormonal changes include the following:

- Antibiotics—to treat infections that interfere with infertility.
- Antihistamines—studies report that *nondrowsy* antihistamines that block mast cells may be beneficial in some cases of low sperm count. Mast cells release inflammatory immune factors that may reduce sperm quality. Overseas studies report improved pregnancy rates with two agents, ebastine and tranilast. Similar antihistamines in the United States are cetirizine (Zyrtec), fexofenadine (Allegra), and loratadine (Claritin).

hyperplasia the reproduction of cells within an organ at an increased rate.

- Anti-ED agents—drugs such as sildenafil (Viagra), vardenafil (Levitra), and tadalafil (Cialis) may enhance fertility by increasing sperm motion and *capacitation* (the explosive energy release in the sperm that aids the act of fertilization).
- Bromocriptine (Parlodel)—used to reduce excess prolactin manufactured by the pituitary in some infertile men.
- GnRH—beneficial for men with gonadotropin deficiency and hypogonadism and helps to restore sperm production after chemotherapy.

Erectile Dysfunction

Male sexual *impotence* is defined as the inability to sustain an erection for penetration. Impotence has many causes. A specific sequence of events (such as nerve impulses in the brain, spinal column, and area around the penis, and response in muscles, fibrous tissues, veins, and arteries in and near the corpora cavernosa) must take place, in the proper order, for an erection to occur. It is much like a domino effect and can be interrupted at many different points in the sequence by various factors and agents. Diseases, such as diabetes, kidney disease, chronic alcoholism, multiple sclerosis, atherosclerosis, vascular disease, and neurologic disease, account for about 70% of ED cases. Damage that these conditions cause to nerves, arteries, smooth muscles, and fibrous tissues is the most common cause of *ED*.

Researchers believe that psychological factors such as stress, anxiety, guilt, depression, low self-esteem, and fear of sexual failure cause 10% to 20% of ED cases. Men with an organic physical cause may also experience psychological factors. Smoking, which restricts blood flow in veins and arteries and reduces hormonal (testosterone) secretions, can contribute to ED.

Levitra (vardenafil), Cialis (tadalafil), and Viagra (sildenafil) are used in the treatment of ED (see Table 33-9). Early tests showed that Cialis does not affect blood pressure as much as Viagra. Following sexual stimulation, Cialis works by helping the blood vessels in the penis to relax, allowing the flow of blood into the penis. Cialis will not improve sexual performance if the male does not have ED. Levitra works within 16 minutes with physical stimulation; Viagra takes longer, up to one hour. Levitra is to be taken from 30 minutes to 4.5 hours before desired intercourse. Levitra can be taken with food but Viagra should not.

Levitra and Cialis cause no vision or heart side effects. Viagra helps maintain an erection by blocking the action of an enzyme called phosphodiesterase type 5 in penile tissue. Researchers believe that nonselective blockade of other forms of phosphodiesterase enzymes may trigger some of the drug's adverse side effects, especially facial flushing and visual disturbances (seeing blue).

Benign Prostatic Hyperplasia

Because of their close physical placement, the urethra is susceptible to pressure from hyperplastic enlargement of the prostate. The prostate actually has two anatomical zones: the central zone and the peripheral zone. The central zones are prone to **hyperplasia**; the peripheral zone is much more frequently affected by carcinoma.

As men get older, the prostate gland enlarges. Such an enlargement is called *benign prostatic hyperplasia (BPH)*. This noncancerous growth is the most common benign tumor in men over the age of 50. The enlargement causes the following problems:

- Difficult urination
- Urinary blockage, urinary retention, or the inability to urinate
- Urinary frequency
- A feeling of incomplete voiding (the sensation of incomplete bladder emptying)

Other symptoms include hesitancy or slow initiation of urination (slow start), decreased force of the urinary stream (weak stream), and intermittence (stopping and starting) of the urinary stream. A variety of other symptoms may also occur, including frequent nocturia (nighttime urination) and urgency to urinate.

Changes caused by prostate enlargement are gradual and may often be ignored by the patient. It is thought that from 20% to 30% of men will need medical or surgical treatment of BPH before they reach the age of 80.

TABLE 33-9 Pharmaceutical Treatments for Erectile Dysfunction

Generic Name	Brand Name	Dosage Forms and Availability	Route of Administration	Common Adult Dosage
alprostadil urethral suppositories	Caverject	10-mcg, 20-mcg SD syringe; 10 mcg, 20 mcg, 40 mcg vials	Injection	Inject before sexual activity
sildenafil	Viagra	20-mg, 50-mg, 100-mg tablets	Oral	Take one hour before sexual activity
tadalafil	Muse	1 suppository	Suppository	Insert before sexual activity
vardenafil	Levitra	5-mg,10-mg, 20-mg tablets	Oral	Take one hour before sexual activity
yohimbine	Aphrodyne	5.4-mg capsules	Oral	One capsule tid

Pharmaceutical Treatment of BPH

Drugs such as finasteride (Proscar) and dutasteride (Avodar), which are 5-alpha reductase inhibitors, prevent the conversion of testosterone to the hormone dihydrotestosterone. A treatment period of six months may be necessary before one can tell if the therapy is going to work. Finasteride is available in tablet form, and dutasteride is available as soft gelatin capsules. These are taken orally once a day. Patients should see their physicians regularly to monitor side effects and adjust the dosage, if necessary.

Side effects include reduced libido, impotence, breast tenderness and enlargement, and reduced sperm count. Long-term risks and benefits have not been studied.

Women who are pregnant or may be pregnant must avoid handling dutasteride capsules and broken or crushed finasteride tablets, as exposure to these drugs may cause serious side effects to a male fetus. To prevent pregnant women from being exposed to the drug and causing teratogenic effects through blood transfusion, patients should wait at least six months after treatment with a 5-alpha reductase inhibitor to donate blood (see Tables 33-10 and 33-11).

Alpha-adrenergic blockers relax smooth muscle tissue in the bladder neck and prostate, thereby increasing urinary flow. They typically are taken orally, once or twice a day (see Table 33-11).

TABLE 33-10 Pharmaceutical Treatments for BPH

Generic Name	Brand Name	Dosage Forms and Availability	Route of Administration	Common Adult Dosage
doxazosin	Cardura, Cardura XL	1-mg, 2-mg, 4-mg, 8-mg tablets	Oral	Cardura: 1–8 mg qd; Cardura XL: 4–8 mg qd
dutasteride	Avodart	0.5-mg capsule	Oral	0.5 mg qd
finasteride	Proscar	5-mg tablets	Oral	5 mg qd
tamsulosin	Flomax	0.4-mg capsules	Oral	0.4–0.8 mg qd
terazosin	Hytrin	1-mg, 2-mg, 5-mg, 10-mg tablets	Oral	1 mg initial dose at bedtime, increase to 2-mg, 5-mg and then 10-mg qd

TABLE 33-11 Alpha-Adrenergic Blockers

Generic Name	Trade Name	Strength/Dosage Form Available	Average Adult Dose
alfuzosin	Uroxatral	10-mg extended-release (ER) tablets	BPH: 10 mg qd
doxazosin mesylate	Cardura	1-mg, 2-mg, 4-mg, 8-mg tablets	BPH: 1–8 mg qd HTN: 1–16 mg qd
prazosin	Minipress	1-mg, 2-mg, 5-mg capsules	HTN: 3–20 mg/day in divided doses
tamsulosin	Flomax	0.4-mg ER capsules	BPH: 10 mg qd
terazosin	Hytrin	1-mg, 2-mg, 5-mg, 10-mg tablets and capsules	BPH: 1–10 mg qd HTN: 1–20 mg qd

sexually transmitted disease (STD) a disease caused by a pathogen (virus, bacterium, parasite, or fungus) that is spread from person to person through sexual contact.

sexually transmitted infection (STI) a sexually transmitted disease.

Side effects of alpha-adrenergic blockers include the following:

- Headache
- Dizziness
- Low blood pressure
- Fatigue
- Weakness
- Difficulty breathing

Prostate Cancer

In prostate cancer, cells in the prostate form tumors at an accelerated rate and the blockage of cancer cells inhibits the flow of urine. Prostate cancer is extremely painful for the male and can prove deadly if not treated early on in the disease. This type of cancer causes problems with urination, problems in sexual functioning, and may also spread throughout the body if not treated early. Symptoms of prostate cancer include dysuria, nocturia, blood present in semen and urine, painful ejaculation, and continual pain in the pelvis and/or lower back. Treatment for prostate cancer includes hormone therapy and chemotherapy. Early detection and treatment is the key in curing the disease.

Hypogonadism

Hypogonadism is a condition in which males cannot produce enough of the male hormone testosterone. Symptoms include fatigue, decreased sex drive, trouble concentrating, hot flashes, stress, anxiety, and osteoporosis. Treatment includes HRT and androgen treatment, which may be given as an intramuscular (IM), transdermal patch, topical gel, or buccaly (see Table 33-12).

Sexually Transmitted Diseases

An **STD** is a disease caused by a pathogen (virus, bacterium, parasite, or fungus) that is spread from person to person through sexual contact. STDs may also be referred to as **STIs**. STDs can be painful, irritating, debilitating, and sometimes life-threatening. More than 20 STDs have been identified.

STDs occur most commonly in sexually active teenagers and young adults but are found among men and women of all economic classes. The risk of contracting an STD increases in those who engage in sex with multiple partners. It is estimated that approximately 200 to 400 million people worldwide are infected with a STD. Examples of STDs are the following:

- Bacterial vaginosis (change in the normal bacteria of the vagina)
- *Chlamydia trachomatis* (bacterium that can cause an STI)
- Genital warts (wart-like bumps)
- Gonorrhea (bacterium that can cause an STI)
- Hepatitis B and hepatitis C (liver diseases)
- Herpes (virus)
- HIV/AIDS (acquired immune deficiency syndrome)
- Lice and crabs (parasites)
- Molluscum (viral infection)
- Syphilis (bacterial infection)
- Trichomonas (parasite)
- Vaginal yeast (fungal infection)

Many STDs do not cause much harm or severe symptoms. However, some produce persistent asymptomatic or minimally symptomatic disease. Some people may carry a disease for days, weeks, or even longer. During this time, the infected individual, or *carrier*, can spread disease even if he or she is asymptomatic. Complications of STD infection include the following conditions:

- PID
- Inflammation of the cervix (*cervicitis*) in women

info

Microbicides

Microbicide products are being developed for use either vaginally or rectally to reduce the transmission of HIV and/or other STDs. Microbicides decrease the ability of a microbe to cause an infection. They may become available in many forms, including gels, creams, suppositories, films, sponges, or vaginal rings. Some microbicides will also offer contraceptive benefits. Microbicides are not currently available, but the demand is great, so the public can expect to find them on the market soon.

TABLE 33-12 **Pharmaceutical Treatments for Male Hypogonadism**

Generic Name	Brand Name	Dosage Forms and Availability	Route of Administration	Common Adult Dosage
methyltestosterone	Testred, Android, Methitest	10-mg capsules	Oral	10–50 mg daily
testosterone	Androderm transdermal system	2.5-mg, 5-mg transdermal patch	Topical	5-mg patch qd
testosterone (C-III)	Androgel	2.5-gm, 5-gm packs; two 75-gm pump	Topical	5 gm qd on abdomen, upper arm or shoulder,
testosterone	Striant	Topical	30-mg buccal striant	Apply to gums q12h

- Inflammation of the urethra (*urethritis*)
- Inflammation of the prostate (*prostatitis*) in men
- Fertility and reproductive system problems in both sexes
- Damage to an infant infected while in the womb or during birth; consequences include stillbirth, blindness, and permanent neurological damage

A person infected with an STD is more likely to become infected with HIV, and a person infected with both HIV and another STD is more likely to transmit HIV.

Treatment and Prevention of STDs

The only sure way to avoid becoming infected with an STD is to practice abstinence or practice monogamy with an uninfected partner. The symptoms of viral STDs, such as genital herpes (Herpes simplex virus - HSV) and HIV, can be managed with medication, but the infections cannot be cured. Bacterial STDs, such as gonorrhea and chlamydia, can be cured with antibiotics. Fungal and parasitic diseases can be cured with antifungal and anthelmintic agents, respectively. Early diagnosis and treatment increase the chances for cure.

Summary

The reproductive system is made up of internal reproductive organs, associated ducts, and external genitalia. Its primary function is the reproductive process. Sex hormones are produced in the gonads (in males, the testes; in females, the ovaries).

Although many diseases can affect the reproductive system, a pharmacy technician will most frequently encounter conditions involving contraception, infertility, STDs, and BPH. It is important that a pharmacy technician be well informed regarding the different types of contraceptives, including their side effects and contraindications.

Chapter Review Questions

1. The most fertile time during the female reproductive cycle is _____.
   a. day 1–14
   b. day 20
   c. midcycle, usually day 12–14
   d. end of cycle

2. The main function of estradiol is _____.
   a. to stimulate development of the uterine lining and the mammary glands
   b. to maintain the uterine lining if implantation occurs
   c. to start menstruation
   d. to give feminine features

3. The main function of progesterone is _____.
   a. to stimulate development of the uterine lining and the mammary glands
   b. to maintain the uterine lining if implantation occurs
   c. to start menstruation
   d. to give feminine features

4. Azoospermia is a condition characterized by _____.
   a. low sperm count
   b. low-quality sperm
   c. no sperm production
   d. no semen production

5. Which of the following drugs is *not* indicated for the treatment of infertility?
   a. Avodart
   b. Clomid
   c. Danocrine
   d. Ovidrel

6. BPH can be treated with _____.
   a. cardiac stents
   b. beta blockers
   c. calcium channel blockers
   d. alpha-adrenergic blockers

7. The main risk factor for BPH is _____.
   a. race
   b. HTN
   c. diabetes
   d. age

8. Which of the following is *not* a contraindication for women who are taking oral contraceptives?
   a. over 35 years of age
   b. low blood pressure
   c. history of breast cancer
   d. smoking

9. Which of the following contraceptive agents is a subdermal implant?
   a. Lunelle
   b. Plan B
   c. Ovrette
   d. Norplant

10. Which of the following is *not* a mechanism of action for oral contraceptives?
    a. prevent ovulation
    b. reduce likelihood of implantation
    c. block implantation
    d. prevent sperm from entering vaginal canal

Critical Thinking Questions

1. A pregnant women comes into your pharmacy to pick up her husband's Avodart prescription. What potential complications might arise? What can you do to help to prevent them?

2. Why is a person with an STD more likely to become infected with HIV?

Web Challenge

1. Research current patient information resources on the morning-after pill (emergency contraception), as offered by Planned Parenthood, at http://www.plannedparenthood.org/. Write a one-page summary of your findings.

2. Research microbicide products to find the latest information on their development. Write a one-page summary of your findings. For example, you might discuss safety issues of whether microbicides protect against all STDs.

References and Resources

Adams, M.P., D.L. Josephson, and L.N. Holland, Jr. *Pharmacology for Nurses: A Pathophysiologic Approach.* (4th edition.) Upper Saddle River, NJ: Pearson, 2013. Print.

"CDC Statement on Study Results of Product Containing Nonoxynol-9 (Released at the XIII International AIDS Conference Held in Durban, South Africa, July 9–14, 2000)." http://www.cdc.gov/mmwr/preview/mmwrhtml/mm4931a4.htm Web. 14 April 2008.

Drug Facts and Comparisons, 2013 ed. St. Louis: Wolters Kluwer. 2012. Print.

"FDA Dockets of Noncontraceptive, Estrogen-Containing Drugs." http://www.fda.gov/OHRMS/DOCKETS/98fr/092799d.txt and http://a257.g.akamaitech.net/7/257/2422/14mar20010800/edocket.access.gpo.gov/cfr_2002/aprqtr/pdf/21cfr310.517.pdf. Web. 14 April 2008.

"FindLaw on Estrogen and Package Inserts." http://caselaw.lp.findlaw.com/scripts/getcase.pl?court=ny&vol=i99&invol=0168. Web. 14 April 2008.

Holland, N. and M.P. Adams. *Core Concepts in Pharmacology.* (3rd edition.) Upper Saddle River, NJ: Pearson, 2010.

"Hormone Involved in Reproduction May Have Role in the Maintenance of Relationships." http://www.oxytocin.org/oxytoc/. Web. 14 April 2008.

"Premenstrual Dysphoric Disorder." www.mayoclinic.com. Web. 17 October 2007.

"Shands at the University of Florida." http://www.shands.org/professional/drugs/bulletins/0601.pdf Web. 14 April 2008.

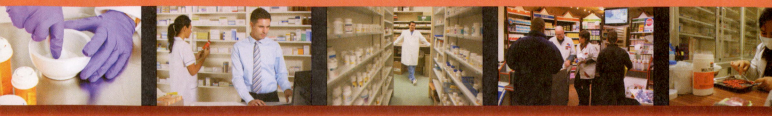

CHAPTER 34

The Nervous System

LEARNING OBJECTIVES

After completing this chapter, you should be able to:

- Explain the functions of the nervous system and its division into the central and peripheral nervous systems.

- Compare and contrast the sympathetic and parasympathetic nervous systems.

- Describe the function or physiology of neurons and nerve transmission and the various neurotransmitters.

- Explain the relationship of the nervous system to the other body systems.

- Explain the functions of the blood–brain barrier, and describe what types of substances will and will not cross it.

- List and define common diseases affecting the nervous system, and discuss the causes, symptoms, and pharmaceutical treatments associated with each disease.

- Identify the common drugs used to treat diseases and conditions of the nervous system.

KEY TERMS

adjuvant, p. 610

afferent, p. 583

anxiety, p. 588

anxiolytic, p. 598

central nervous system (CNS), p. 583

cerebrospinal fluid (CSF), p. 586

efferent, p. 583

electroencephalogram (EEG), p. 602

gray matter, p. 587

narcolepsy, p. 600

peripheral nervous system (PNS), p. 583

white matter, p. 587

INTRODUCTION

The endocrine and nervous systems work together to maintain homeostasis in the body. The endocrine system communicates relatively slowly via hormones secreted by ductless glands into the circulatory system and carried by the blood to muscles, glands, and various other parts of the body. By contrast, the nervous system communicates messages very quickly through nerve impulses conducted from one part of the body to another using the transmission of neurotransmitter chemicals from one nerve cell to another. The nervous system is complex and one of the least understood parts of the body.

At its core, the brain has billions of individual connecting pieces and makes trillions of connections. The specific function of these pieces, known as nerve cells or neurons, is to allow learning, reasoning, and remembering. The brain works on electrochemical energy, allowing you to read this book, smile at a friend, remember a computer password, and decide between eating apples or oranges. The brain also controls emotions, sex drive, heart rate, breathing and respiration, appetite, and sleep.

The brain requires energy in the form of glucose, a sugar. Essential substances, such as vitamins and minerals, as well as sources of dietary carbohydrate energy, help the brain to function properly. The brain cannot turn off like a computer or radio. While you are asleep, your brain is still active, as if on automatic pilot. This is when you digest and metabolize most of your food; you also continue breathing, but at a much slower rate.

The nervous system is tied into every other system in the body. It interacts with every system to ensure homeostasis. Therefore, diseases and disorders of the nervous system may have far-reaching effects and be difficult to diagnose and treat.

Anatomy of the Nervous System

As shown in Figure 34-1, the nervous system is made up of the brain, spinal cord, nerves, and sensory organs (skin, eyes, and ears). The *neuron* is the basic cell of the nervous system. The nervous system is divided into two parts called the **central nervous system (CNS)** and the **peripheral nervous system (PNS)**. Like the central processing unit (CPU) of a computer that controls other devices, the CNS is the main area that controls all othernervous systemfunctions, some directly and others indirectly via the PNS.

The CNS includes the brain and spinal cord; the PNS consists of all other nerves and sensory organs. The PNS is divided into two parts: the somatic nervous system and the autonomic nervous system (ANS).

The *autonomic nervous system* is further divided into two more parts, called the sympathetic and the parasympathetic nervous systems. Many drugs directly affect these two systems, whether beneficially or adversely. Therefore, comparing and contrasting these two subdivisions is critical to understanding how the nervous system works.

Functions of the Nervous System

The nervous system has the following three basic functions (see Table 34-1):

1. *Sensory* or **afferent**—this function sends impulses from muscles and other parts of the body toward the CNS. It senses or recognizes external changes in the environment, such as cold or heat, and internal changes in the body such as a decrease in potassium or calcium.
2. *Integrative*—this function processes perceived information about the sensory changes and interprets or explains them in the external and internal environments.
3. *Motor* or **efferent**—this function sends impulses away from the CNS to muscles and other parts of the body. The efferent system responds to the brain's interpretation of afferent signals and integrates the external and internal environments by making muscles move, groups of muscles interact, and glands secrete hormones or other chemicals into the bloodstream.

The Neuron

About 10 microns in width, the smallest unit of the nervous system is a nerve cell called the *neuron* (see Figure 34-2). The brain is made up of approximately 100 billion neurons. Neurons are similar to other cells, as they are surrounded by a membrane wall; have a nucleus that contains genes; and contain cytoplasm, mitochondria, and other organelles. However, neurons differ from other cells in that they have projections called *dendrites* and *axons*. These projections have the following specialized functions:

- Dendrites bring information to the cell body from the CNS.
- Axons take information away from the cell body to the CNS.

Nervous System cells communicate with each other through an electrochemical process, which can be compared to the way a computer sends electrical signals through its wires. The brain sends electrical signals, but does so through neurons. Neurons transfer information to other neurons to control glands, organs, or muscles. Electrochemical hormones called *neurotransmitters* are produced by neurons and stored in the ends of the nerve cells. These neurotransmitters, such as acetylcholine (ACh), are then released from the end of the neuron and cross the space between neurons, called a *synapse*, to a different neuron. This crossing of the synapse is also a part of transmission of a nerve impulse. The neurotransmitters travel across synapses to reach a receiving neuron, where they attach themselves to special structures called *receptors*.

The attachment results in a small electrical response within the receiving neuron. This response may be the *end* or terminal message, or transmission may be continued by the second, receiving neuron sending out neurotransmitter messengers of its own. However, this small response does not mean that the message will result in an action by the gland, organ, or muscle. Only when the total signal from all the synapses involved exceeds a certain level will a large signal, called an *action potential*, generated, and the message continued.

Neuronal studies can encompass the function of groups of neurons or nerve cells, the role of neurotransmitters, what

---

central nervous system (CNS) the part of the nervous system made up of the brain and spinal cord.

peripheral nervous system (PNS) all parts of the nervous system excluding the brain and spinal cord.

afferent sending an impulse toward the CNS.

efferent sending impulses away from the CNS.

happens at ion channels on a neuronal and cell membrane, reproduction, or the genetic basis of neuronal function. The nervous system uses neuronal circuits throughout the brain to store memory and undergoes continual modification so that a person can learn new things. The brain can actually *rewire* itself when necessary. After some kinds of brain injuries, undamaged brain tissue can take over functions previously performed by the injured area.

The changes in the environment that set off the nerve impulse to communicate with another neuron are called *stimuli*. The action of the impulse that triggers the release of a neurotransmitter to another neuron is called the *firing of neurons* and is both electrical and chemical in nature. There are about 50 different neurotransmitters in the brain. These are made of amino acids by the body, with the help of other proteins called *enzymes,* and are stored in the neuron vesicles. Adding

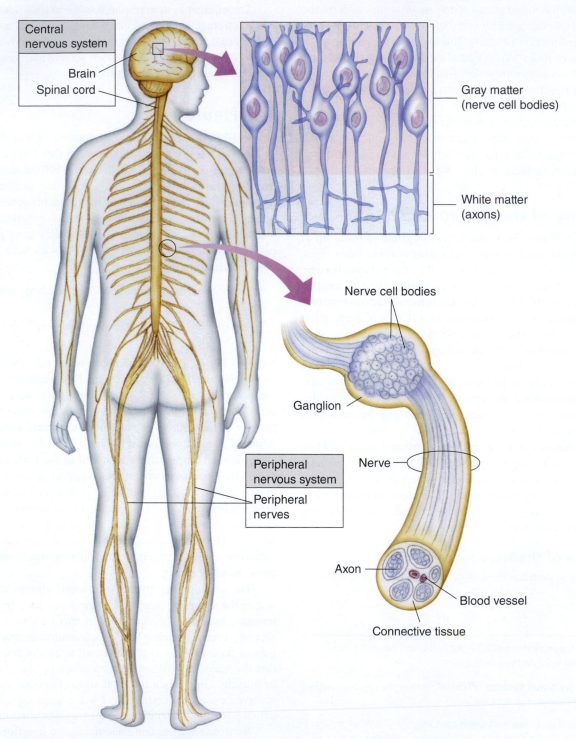

Central nervous system

Brain

Spinal cord

Gray matter (nerve cell bodies)

White matter (axons)

Nerve cell bodies

Ganglion

Nerve

Axon

Blood vessel

Connective tissue

Peripheral nervous system

Peripheral nerves

FIGURE 34-1 The nervous system.

TABLE 34-1 The Nervous System and Its Relationship with the Body

Interactive System	Nervous System
Cardiovascular	Endothelial cells maintain the blood–brain barrier, protecting the brain from harmful substances. Baroreceptors send information to the brain about blood pressure. The brain responds by regulating vasodilation, thereby changing heart rate and blood pressure. Cerebrospinal fluid drains into the venous blood supply, removing harmful waste from the brain.
Digestive	Digestion of food provides the building blocks of the hormones and neurotransmitters. The autonomic nervous system controls the tone of the digestive tract via peristalsis. The nervous system (NS) controls the smooth muscles for peristalsis to allow eating and elimination of food. The nervous system responds to thirst and hunger and controls drinking and eating.
Endocrine	The hypothalamus controls all other endocrine glands by controlling the pituitary gland. Reproductive hormones affect the development of the nervous system. Hormonal feedback to the brain affects the processing and integration of neuronal information.
Integumentary	Receptors in the skin send sensory information to the brain, which then regulates peripheral blood flow and sweat glands. Nerves control muscles that connect to hair follicles (arrector pili).
Lymphatic/immune	The brain stimulates the mechanisms of defense against infection.
Muscular	Muscle receptors send the brain information about body position and movement. The brain controls the contraction of skeletal muscle. The nervous system regulates heart rate (myocardial contractions) and the speed at which food moves through the digestive tract (peristalsis).
Renal or urinary	The bladder sends sensory information to the brain, which controls urination and, therefore, hydration and thirst.
Respiratory	The brain monitors respiratory volume and blood gas levels. The brain responds by regulating the respiratory rate.
Skeletal	Bones provide essential calcium for the proper functioning of the nervous system. The skull and vertebrae protect the brain and spinal cord from injury. Sensory receptors in bone joints send signals about body position to the brain. The brain regulates the position of bones by controlling muscles.

a substance that mimics natural neurotransmitters may help the body, or it may cause certain conditions or disease states. Most addictive drugs change the effect of neurotransmitters on neurons.

Neurotransmission and Receptors

A name for the constant exchange of chemical messages between neurons, or firing of neurons, is *neurotransmission*. It is achieved by three basic steps:

1. Neurons release neurotransmitters—when a neuron is excited, it fires, releasing a neurotransmitter.
2. Neurotransmitters bind to receptors–the released neurotransmitters *swim* across the synapse until they *land*, or meet, the dendrites of the next neuron. This is called *uptake*. The neurotransmitters recognize molecules/sites on the neighboring neuron that are waiting to receive them; these are called *receptors*. Neurotransmitters *dock*,

or attach, to these specific receptors via a chemical reaction in a process called *binding*. The neurotransmitters are then released by the receptors. Several things can happen next:
- Some neurotransmitters may be broken down or destroyed by enzymes.
- Carrying proteins may transport the neurotransmitters back to the axon from which they originally came, a process called *reuptake*.
- Neurotransmitters may be used again in a type of recycling of chemical messengers.
3. Binding passes on or continues (*transduces*) the neurotransmitter's message. The binding itself causes a set of chemical reactions within the receiving neuron. The same kind of impulse that was fired by the sending neuron continues along the nerve pathway from neuron to neuron until it reaches its terminal destination of a muscle, gland, or organ. The result of this can be a change in the way we respond, behave, think, feel, or react physically.

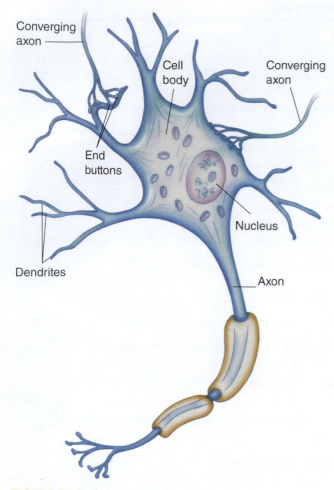

FIGURE 34-2 The neuron.

The Central Nervous System

The CNS includes the brain and spinal cord. The human brain weighs approximately 1.3 to 1.4 kg (2.8 to 3 lb), as compared to the brain of an elephant (6 kg) or the brain of a rhesus monkey (1 kg). The spinal cord is the main pathway for information connecting the brain to the PNS.

Spinal Cord

The spinal cord has 31 paired nerves, which are classified as follows:

- 8 cervical
- 12 thoracic
- 5 lumbar
- 5 sacral
- 1 coccygeal

---

cerebrospinal fluid (CSF) the fluid surrounding the brain and spinal cord.

gray matter a major component of the nervous system, composed of nonmyelinated nerve tissue with a gray-brown color.

white matter a major component of the CNS, composed of myelinated nerve tissue that is white in color.

The spinal cord is considered to be divided into five main regions:

- Skull
- Cervical vertebrae
- Thoracic vertebrae
- Lumbar vertebrae
- Sacral vertebrae (sacrum)

The spinal cord is protected from injury by **cerebrospinal fluid (CSF)**, which is contained within a system of fluid-filled cavities called *ventricles*. Receptors in the skin send information to the spinal cord through the spinal nerves. The following are the main functions of CSF:

- Protection—CSF protects the brain from damage by acting like a cushion to absorb energy and lessen the impact in the event of a blow to the head.
- Excretion of waste products—the one-way flow of CSF into the blood takes harmful metabolites of drugs and other toxic substances away from the brain.
- Endocrine communication—CSF serves as the vehicle to transport hormones to other areas of the brain. Hormones released into the CSF can be carried to remote sites of the brain.

Brain

The head or cephalic region of the body has a bony structure, the *skull*, to protect the brain from injury. Further protection is provided by the three layers of meninges that cover the brain: dura mater, arachnoid, and pia mater (see Figure 34-3). The outermost, hardest layer is the dura mater. The arachnoid has spaces in it that resemble a cobweb and are filled with CSF for further protection.

The brain can be divided down the middle, lengthwise, into two halves called the *cerebral hemispheres*. Each hemisphere (left or right) of the cerebral cortex is divided into the following four lobes:

- Frontal lobe—the frontal lobe is concerned with higher intellect or reasoning, problem solving, parts of speech, movement or motor cortex, and emotion.
- Parietal lobe—the parietal lobe is involved in the stimuli and perception of touch, pressure, temperature, and pain.
- Temporal lobe—the temporal lobe processes perception and recognition of auditory stimuli for hearing and memory (involving the hippocampus).
- Occipital lobe—the occipital lobe is involved with stimuli pertaining to vision.

For the purposes of this overview, we can consider the brain as consisting of three main parts: the cerebellum, the cerebrum, and the brainstem.

Cerebellum

The cerebellum is located behind the brainstem and below the cerebrum. The main purposes of the cerebellum are to coordinate the movement of the body and to maintain equilibrium and balance. Some drugs, such as alcohol, can depress the

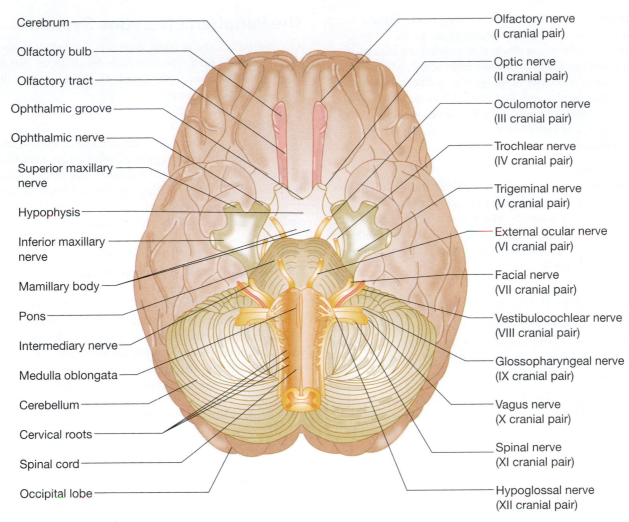

Cerebrum

Olfactory bulb

Olfactory tract

Ophthalmic groove

Ophthalmic nerve

Superior maxillary nerve

Hypophysis

Inferior maxillary nerve

Mamillary body

Pons

Intermediary nerve

Medulla oblongata

Cerebellum

Cervical roots

Spinal cord

Occipital lobe

Olfactory nerve (I cranial pair)

Optic nerve (II cranial pair)

Oculomotor nerve (III cranial pair)

Trochlear nerve (IV cranial pair)

Trigeminal nerve (V cranial pair)

External ocular nerve (VI cranial pair)

Facial nerve (VII cranial pair)

Vestibulocochlear nerve (VIII cranial pair)

Glossopharyngeal nerve (IX cranial pair)

Vagus nerve (X cranial pair)

Spinal nerve (XI cranial pair)

Hypoglossal nerve (XII cranial pair)

FIGURE 34-3 The brain.

cerebellum, resulting in a decrease in body coordination and reaction or response time.

Cerebrum

The cerebrum is divided into two main parts:

- Cerebral cortex—the cerebral cortex contains **gray matter** made up of the neurons that control voluntary action. The cerebral cortex is tied in with the somatic part of the PNS.
- Cerebral Medulla—the cerebra medulla contains **white matter** made up of the myelinated axons of neurons, which conduct nerve impulses to and from different areas of the nervous system. The cerebral medulla also contains more gray matter, known as the *basal ganglia*. The basal ganglia regulate motor activity or movement. Damage to the basal ganglia may result in disorders such as Parkinson's disease.

Brainstem

The brainstem, an extension of the spinal cord, is divided into four main parts:

- Thalamus—sits at the top of the brainstem; regulates and evaluates the sensory impulses of pain, hot, cold, and touch. The thalamus directs the sensory information to the correct part of the cerebral cortex or regulates the response.

- Hypothalamus—located just below the thalamus; controls body functions such as water balance, body temperature, sleep, hunger and appetite, sex drive, the ANS, and some emotional and behavioral responses.
- Pons—located below the hypothalamus; regulates respiration. The pons is considered the *relay* station for nerve fibers that travel to other parts of the brain.
- Medulla oblongata—located at the base of the brainstem and the top of the spine. The medulla oblongata contains the three vital centers that keep the body alive and functioning: cardiac (heart), respiratory (breathing), and vasomotor (blood vessels). Injury to this area of the brain usually results in death. The reflexes for gagging, swallowing, coughing, and vomiting are regulated by the medulla oblongata.

Reticular Formation

Located throughout the brainstem and cerebrum, a network of nerve fibers known as the *reticular formation* affects the degree of alertness. It is made up of two types of fibers:

- Excitatory fibers—when stimulated by external stimuli such as noises, bright lights, or danger, the degree of alertness is increased. Certain stimulant drugs, such as Ritalin and caffeine, can increase the activity in the reticular formation and thus affect the degree of alertness.

- Inhibitory fibers—an absence of external stimuli causes the inhibitory fibers to become more active, which in turn decreases the activity of the excitatory fibers and therefore the degree of alertness. Inhibitory fibers are usually more active during sleep or rest. Certain drugs, such as alcohol, hypnotics, and barbiturates, can decrease the activity of the reticular formation.

Limbic System

One of the least understood areas of the brain is the *limbic system*, a collection of nerve cells in various areas of the brain, especially the hypothalamus, that form a specific neural pathway. The limbic system is associated with such emotional and behavioral responses as sexual behavior, anger, rage, fear, anxiety, reward, and punishment.

Blood–Brain Barrier

The *blood–brain barrier (BBB)* is a semipermeable membrane that allows some substances to cross and reach the brain but prevents others from getting through. The following are the general properties of the BBB:

- Water-soluble or low lipid- and fat-soluble molecules do not penetrate into the brain. High lipid- and fat-soluble molecules, such as barbiturates, rapidly cross the BBB into the brain.
- Large molecules do not easily pass through the BBB.
- Highly electrically charged molecules are slowed down by the BBB.

The functions of the BBB are to:

- Protect the brain from foreign invaders or substances in the blood that could injure the brain.
- Protect the brain from hormones and neurotransmitters in the rest of the body.
- Maintain a constant, homeostatic environment for the brain.

The BBB can be broken down. The following disease states can compromise the barrier:

- Hypertension (high blood pressure) can open up the BBB.
- Infectious agents can open up the BBB.
- Hyperosmolarity—a high concentration of a substance in the blood can cause the BBB to open up.

The following physical changes can also break down the BBB:

- When a particular developmental stage is interrupted, the BBB is not fully formed at birth and thus remains open.
- Exposure to microwaves can open up the BBB.
- Exposure to radiation can open up the BBB.
- Injury to the brain can open up the BBB. Examples include trauma, ischemia, inflammation, and pressure.

---

anxiety an uncomfortable emotional state of apprehension, worry, and fearfulness.

The Peripheral Nervous System

As noted earlier, the nervous system is divided into two parts, the CNS and the PNS. The PNS includes all nerves that are not located in the brain and spinal cord. The PNS is further divided into the somatic and the ANSs.

Autonomic System

The ANS controls the nerves that connect to smooth and cardiac muscles, and thus regulates involuntary movement to perform intricate functions without conscious or voluntary direction. The ANS is further subdivided into two nervous systems called the sympathetic nervous system (SNS) and the parasympathetic nervous system (PSNS).

Sympathetic Nervous System

The SNS is governed by the neurotransmitter norepinephrine (NE); the PSNS is governed by ACh.

The SNS prepares the body for energetic tasks, handles stressful situations, and controls the *fight or flight* response. When NE is inside the receptors of the heart, lungs, and blood vessels, it stimulates or *revs them up*. Heart rate, breathing rate, blood pressure, and vasoconstriction increase; gastrointestinal (GI) and genitourinary functions decrease temporarily.

Parasympathetic Nervous System

The PSNS readies the body for sleep in nonstressful periods and affects the *rest and relaxation* response. When NE is not present inside the receptors of the heart, lungs, or blood vessels, or if ACh is high, the organs are depressed or slowed down. Heart rate, breathing rate, blood pressure, and vasoconstriction decrease; GI and genitourinary functions increase.

> ❝ **Workplace Wisdom** ANS Neurotransmitters
>
> Understanding what each neurotransmitter does to each branch of the ANS is essential to understanding disease states and how they are treated. ❞

Somatic System

The somatic system is the section of the PNS, which is responsible for carrying motor and sensory data both to and from the CNS, for voluntary muscle movements, and for processing sensory information such as hearing, touch, and sight. The somatic nervous system consists of the nerves that connect to the skeletal muscles and control voluntary movement of the whole body.

Neurotransmitters

Neurotransmitters are essential in the proper functioning of the brain and in determining how messages are sent and received. Without neurotransmitters, the brain would not function properly. These chemical messengers act as communication signals between various brain cells. Messengers are molecular substances that can alter mood, appetite, anxiety, sleep, heart rate, body temperature, fear, aggression and other psychological conditions.

Diseases Affecting the Central Nervous System

Mental illness is the most common disorder of the CNS. Mental illness can range from mild and temporary to serious and long-lasting. Pharmacotherapeutics has empowered many people with mental disorders to enhance their lives and reach their fullest potential. The first antipsychotic drug, chlorpromazine, was introduced in the 1950s. Psychotherapy and counseling can be more effective when combined with the use of psychotherapeutic agents. For example, people who were once too depressed to talk to a psychiatrist often begin to respond after a few weeks of treatment with psychotherapeutic drugs.

The following mental disorders may be treated psychotherapeutically: psychosis, depression, anxiety, obsessive–compulsive disorder (OCD), posttraumatic stress disorder, and panic disorder. Some mental illnesses can be fully cured, while others can be managed with medications. Some drugs will help the patient to have a better experience in daily living and to function more effectively. The National Institute of Mental Health established the following four classifications of psychotherapeutic agents: anti-anxiety, antidepressant, antimanic, and antipsychotic medications.

Anxiety

Anxiety is associated with the following risk factors: genetics, brain chemistry, life events, and personality. Less than one-third of all those suffering from anxiety seek medical treatment, yet it is a most treatable condition. There are many forms of anxiety, categorized: generalized anxiety disorder (GAD), obsessive–compulsive disorder (OCD), panic disorder or panic attack, posttraumatic stress disorder (PTSD), social anxiety disorder (SAD), and specific phobias. Anxiety can strike anyone at any time but is usually slowly progressive. Some anxiety occurs as a result of a traumatic or childhood event. Specific symptoms or behaviors interfere with work, social situations, or everyday tasks. Table 34-2 describes different types of anxiety.

> ❝ **Workplace Wisdom** Anxiety Statistics
>
> More than 19 million Americans report experiencing anxiety each year. Among the leading causes are phobia, posttraumatic stress, generalized anxiety, obsessive compulsions, and panic. ❞

A lack of a certain neurotransmitter, *gamma-aminobutyric acid (GABA)*, is associated with anxiety. The more GABA there is, the less anxiety there will be. Conversely, the less GABA there is, the more anxiety there will be. The drug used to treat anxiety depends on the type of anxiety (the cause) and the symptoms. Cognitive and behavioral therapy should be utilized in the treatment of anxiety, along with psychotherapeutic drugs, for the greatest and most beneficial effect.

TABLE 34-2 Types of Anxiety

Type of Anxiety and Cause	Description	Symptoms
GAD—the person has chronic worry about everyday living issues, such as health, money, or work/career.	Uncontrollable worry about things that occur in daily living usually is considered GAD if it persists for six months or longer; focus may shift from issue to issue.	Trembling, muscular aches, insomnia, abdominal upsets, dizziness, irritability, easy fatigability, trouble sleeping.
OCD—the person has continuous and recurring thoughts (*obsessions*) that reflect exaggerated anxiety or fears. Obsessions can lead to performing a ritual or routine (*compulsions*), which may be repeated many times.	Typical obsessions/compulsions: Fear of germs (washes hands) Fear of improper performance or behavior (repeats phrases that are *magical*) Persistent doubts that everything is in order, and thus checks things over and over again (is the iron shut off?)	Symptoms are the compulsions that are manifested to relieve the anxiety: constant cleaning, checking and rechecking if things are all right (doors locked), repeating phrases/words, spending time organizing, hoarding unnecessary items such as junk mail or old bills, unable to part with old, useless items (rooms may get literally filled and dangerous).
Panic attack—an abrupt or sudden onset of fear or discomfort.	Usually accompanied by fear of having a panic attack in the future after experiencing the first one. Usually has at least four symptoms. Most predominant feeling is one of impending doom.	Physical: palpitations, sweating, trembling, nausea or GI disturbances, chest pain or discomfort, tingling sensations, chills or hot flashes, dizziness, and lightheadedness. Emotional: a feeling of imminent danger or doom; a feeling of choking, creating a need to escape; sense of things being unreal or surreal; depersonalization; fear of going crazy; fear of death.

(Continued)

TABLE 34-2 Types of Anxiety *(Continued)*

Type of Anxiety and Cause	Description	Symptoms
PTSD—experience of or witnessing a traumatic event, such as criminal assault, a serious accident, a natural disaster, or a death.	The after effects of exposure to a traumatic experience impede normal functions of everyday living. Is accompanied by intense fear, helplessness, and/or horror.	Relives the trauma; has recurrent dreams or nightmares; loses interest in things/people previously enjoyed; has excessive response to being startled; becomes irritable or angry.
SAD—extreme fear of being judged or ridiculed by others.	Extreme fear of social or performance situations and embarrassment that may potentially occur. Fear that others will think poorly of them. Usually have anxiety in anticipation of a feared event.	Heart palpitations, faintness, blushing, profuse sweating, diarrhea, or panic attack; leads to avoidance behavior.
Specific phobias—usually caused by an event in early childhood.	An extreme fear of, or an intense reaction to, a specific object or situation, such as spiders, heights, being outdoors, being among people.	Fear that may produce panic attacks, which lead to avoidance of everyday situations such as work and intimacy.

Anxiety is normally pharmaceutically treated with benzodiazepines but may also be treated with antidepressant drugs, such as selective serotonin reuptake inhibitors (SSRIs), tricyclic antidepressants (TCAs), monoamine oxidase inhibitors (MAOIs), beta blockers, or any combination of them. Barbiturates are not used as often for anxiety as they once were, because they are highly addictive (C-II) and currently better alternatives are available.

An inability to fall asleep or stay asleep is a common symptom, because the person has obsessive thoughts of anticipated or previously experienced events. Serotonin receptors have long been associated with sleep. One antidepressant, Effexor XR, inhibits the reuptake of both serotonin and NE.

The beta-adrenergic blockers, such as propranolol, reduce the autonomic symptoms of anxiety (including changes in breathing rate, heart palpitations, tremors, sweating, and shaking). Nonbenzodiazepine hypnotics, such as Ambien (zolpidem) and Sonata (zaleplon), selectively bind only to omega-1 or benzodiazepine-1 (BZ-1) receptors affecting the GABA-A receptor, and therefore do not produce an anticonvulsant or muscle relaxant effect. However, an off-label use of these drugs is for anxiety, as they help the person who worries at bedtime and cannot fall asleep. The nonbenzodiazepine Buspar (buspirone) has an antianxiety effect without marked sedation or euphoria. As an antagonist, it binds to the serotonin 5-HT1A receptor at postsynaptic sites. As an agonist, it binds at 5-HT1A presynaptic receptors. It has no direct effect on the GABA system.

Depression

Neurotransmitters are generally monoamines, which can be destroyed in the synaptic cleft by enzymes called *monoamine oxidases* (see Table 34-3). Another cause of depression is the excessive reuptake of neurotransmitters or reabsorption into the proximal nerve. Either event leads to a lack of the neurotransmitters serotonin, NE, and dopamine, and the result is *depression*. Thus, it is hypothesized that clinical depression is related to decreases in concentration of the neurotransmitters. For this reason, pharmaceutical research and current drug therapy are centered around drugs that can either block the reuptake of neurotransmitters (e.g., cyclic antidepressants and newer SSRIs) or interfere with the breakdown of the monoamines within the synaptic cleft (MAOIs).

There are many types of depression, including seasonal major depression (seasonal affective disorder), postpartum depression, bipolar disorder (BD), and dysthymia (mild depression on most days of the year). Depression is very treatable. People with depression have symptoms that include a feeling of a *black curtain* of despair coming down over their lives, lack of energy and inability to concentrate, and feeling irritable for no apparent reason. If the symptoms occur for more than two weeks to six months and are interfering with daily life, the person may be clinically depressed. Depressed patients will show behavior changes including:

- Constant feelings of sadness, worthlessness, hopelessness, or guilt
- Irritability or tension
- Decreased interest or pleasure in usual activities or hobbies
- Changes in appetite (increase or decrease) with significant weight loss or weight gain
- Change in sleeping patterns (increase or decrease) such as difficulty sleeping, early morning awakening, or sleeping too much
- Restlessness, fidgeting, or feeling slowed down
- Decreased ability to make decisions or concentrate
- Thoughts of suicide or death

TABLE 34-3 Pharmaceutical Treatments for Anxiety

Classification	Generic Name	Brand Name	Dosage Forms and Availability	Route of Administration	Common Adult Dosage
Benzodiazepines	alprazolam (C-IV)	Xanax	0.25-mg, 0.5-mg, 1-mg, 2-mg tablets	Oral	0.25–0.5 mg tid up to a maximum of 4 mg daily divided doses
	chlordiazepoxide (C-IV)	Librium	5-mg, 10-mg, 25-mg tablets; 100-mg pwd for injection	Oral IV	Mild anxiety: 5–10 mg tid or qid; severe anxiety: 20–25 mg tid or qid
	clorazepate (C-IV)	Tranxene-T Tranxene-SD Tranxene-SD Half Strength	3.75-mg, 7.5-mg, 15-mg tablets; 22.5-mg tablets; 11.25-mg tablets	Oral	15–60 mg daily in divided doses; Tranxene-SD typically given as a single dose daily
	diazepam (C-IV)	Valium	2-mg, 5-mg, 10-mg tablets; 5 mg/mL injection; 5 mg/5 mL, 5 mg/mL solution	Oral IV, IM Oral	2–10 mg bid, tid, or qid orally; 2–20 mg IV or IM
	lorazepam (C-IV)	Ativan	0.05-mg, 0.25-mg, 1-mg, 2-mg tablets; 2 mg/mL solution; 2-mg, 4-mg PFS	Oral IV	2–6 mg/day given bid or tid
	oxazepam (C-IV)	Serax	10-mg, 15-mg, 20-mg capsules	Oral	10–30 mg daily in divided doses depending upon severity
Nonbenzodiazepines	buspirone	BuSpar	5-mg, 10-mg, 15-mg, 30-mg tablets	Oral	Initial dose: 7.5 mg bid; Maximum dose: 30 mg bid
	zalepon (C-IV)	Sonata	5-mg, 10-mg capsules	Oral	5–20 mg HS
	zolpidem (C-IV)	Ambien	5-mg, 10-mg tablets	Oral	5–10 mg HS

There is no one specific known cause of depression; rather, it results from a combination of factors. Risk factors for becoming depressed include the following:

- Genetics—plays an important part in predisposition to depression.
- Trauma and stress—negative issues such as financial problems, the breakup of a relationship, or the death of a loved one can bring on depression; however, it can also be caused by positive situations or after such life changes as starting a new job, getting married, divorce, moving, or graduating from school.
- Pessimistic personality, low self-esteem, or a negative outlook—can contribute to clinical depression; dysthymia can actually have the same characteristics.
- Physical conditions—serious medical conditions or diseases such as cancer, HIV, heart disease, and infertility can contribute to depression, partly because of the physical weakness and stress they bring on. Depression can worsen medical conditions, because it weakens

the immune system and can make pain more intense. Depression can be induced as a side effect by medications used to treat medical conditions.

- Other psychological disorders—anxiety disorders; schizophrenia; anorexia, bulimia, or compulsive eating disorders; and substance abuse often are masked by or appear with depression.

Depression can make a person feel afraid, alone, and hopeless. It can change how the patient thinks and feels and affect social behavior, as it depletes the sense of physical well-being. Depression can affect anyone, of any age, at any time.

Once the illness is identified, most people diagnosed with depression are successfully treated. Psychotherapy and medication are the two primary treatment approaches. Antidepressant medications can enhance psychotherapy for some people, but they cannot cure depression. Antidepressants are not stimulants, like coffee or amphetamines, but they do remove or reduce the symptoms of depression, helping depressed persons feel the way they did before the onset of depression. Antidepressants are also used for anxiety disorders, mainly to block the physical symptoms of panic: rapid heartbeat, nausea, terror, dizziness, chest pains, and breathing problems. They can also be used to treat some phobias, which are also a type of anxiety (see Table 34-4).

BD, which is discussed in more detail in a later section, is characterized by bouts of oscillating high and low moods. Therefore, the depression phase of BD may require the use of an antidepressant. There are many types of antidepressants, such as SSRIs. TCAs, once the most commonly used antidepressants, have many drug interactions. MAOIs were often used for atypical depressions that have symptoms of oversleeping, anxiety, panic attacks, and phobias. However, they have some major side effects and drug–food interactions. Both TCAs and MAOIs take two to four weeks to begin working. SSRIs have successfully replaced the use of MAOIs, except in some cases.

A major depressive episode is categorized as a DSM-V episode by the American Psychiatric Association's (APA's) *Diagnostic and Statistical Manual for Mental Disorders* (currently in its fifth revision; hence DSM-V). This type of depressive episode is characterized by an observable and relatively persistent dysphoric mood that is present almost every day for at least two weeks, which usually interferes with daily living or functioning, and includes at least five of the following nine symptoms: depressed mood, insomnia or hypersomnia, loss of interest in usual activities, significant change in weight and/or appetite, psychomotor agitation or retardation, increased fatigue, feelings of guilt or worthlessness, slowed thinking or impaired concentration, and a suicide attempt or suicidal ideation.

Bipolar Disorder

Manic-depressive disorder, now called *BD*, is characterized by peaks and valleys of severe highs (*mania*) and lows (*depression*). Episodes referred to as *mood swings* can be spread over hours, days, months, or years. In the manic state, the patient is overactive and overtalkative, displays a great deal of energy, and sleeps less. Manic patients cannot speak fast enough to catch up with their thoughts. They will have unrealistic

thoughts; they may present an angry or irritable state with false ideas about their importance to others or in the world at large. During a manic high, the patient uses poor judgment in business dealings and may plan and carry out careless romantic encounters or *flings*. If left untreated, mania may worsen, developing into a psychotic disorder. As discussed earlier, in the depressive cycle the patient presents with difficulty in concentration, lack of energy, lethargy, slow thinking and moving, and more sleeping and eating. The patient has feelings of hopelessness, helplessness, despair, sadness, worthlessness, and guilt. This may be accompanied by thoughts of suicide.

The biological causes of mania are an excess of the neurotransmitter NE and possibly other neurotransmitters as well; the depression is caused by a deficiency of monoamines (neurotransmitters) such as serotonin, NE, or dopamine. Lithium (Li^+) interferes with sodium ion-potentiated conduction of nerve impulses.

In mania, an excessive amount of lithium ions help the reuptake of NE and dopamine. Lithium also appears to reduce the release of NE and dopamine from the neurons. Someone who does not have enough lithium, or has too much sodium, will exhibit hyperexcitability of the nerves and signs of mania. Therefore, lithium, a mood-stabilizing drug, is given to reduce the hyperexcitability and hyperactivity (see Table 34-5). This allows the patient to form slower and more realistic thoughts. Sometimes, antidepressant drugs are also given to the patient to manage the lows.

Side effects of lithium include drowsiness, weakness, nausea, fatigue, hand tremor, and increased thirst and urination. Too much lithium contributes to complications in the thyroid, kidney, heart, and brain. Lithium increases the risk of congenital malformations in babies. Too much lithium may be toxic, and too little may not be effective. The difference between the two amounts is very small; this is called a *narrow therapeutic index*. Therefore, blood levels must be monitored. Decreased salt intake or increased output may cause a lithium buildup that could lead to toxicity. Dehydration, fever, vomiting, and diuretics (coffee or tea) can contribute to a decrease in sodium and resultant lithium toxicity. Signs of lithium toxicity include drowsiness, mental dullness, slurred speech, blurred vision, confusion, muscle twitching, irregular heartbeat, and seizures. A lithium overdose can be life-threatening. Lorazepam or clonazepam (2 to 4 mg tid IM or po) can be given in conjunction with lithium for acute management. These agents boost the effects of the antipsychotic lithium so that high doses can be reduced, diminishing the possibility of toxicity.

Because of the toxicity associated with lithium, doctors are prescribing alternative anticonvulsant drugs. Anticonvulsants are also prescribed when lithium does not prove effective. Equally effective for nonrapid-cycling BD, and superior to lithium in rapid-cycling BD, is valproic acid (Depakote, divalproex sodium). Adverse side effects include GI symptoms, headache, dizziness, double vision, anxiety, and confusion. Valproic acid has caused liver dysfunction in some cases; therefore, liver function tests should be performed before therapy and at frequent intervals after therapy begins. Research shows

TABLE 34-4 Pharmaceutical Treatments for Depression

Classification	Generic Name	Brand Name	Dosage Forms and Availability	Route of Administration	Common Adult Dosage
SSRIs	citalopram	Celexa	10-mg, 20-mg, 40-mg tablets	Oral	20 mg qd
	paroxetine	Paxil, Paxil CR	10-mg, 20-mg, 30-mg, 40-mg tablets; 10 mg/5 mL oral suspension	Oral	Depression: 20 mg, 25 mg qd; Obsessive–compulsive disorder: 40 mg qd
	fluoxetine	Prozac, Sarafem	10-mg, 20-mg, 40-mg, 90-mg capsules	Oral	60 mg qd maximum; usually 10–20 mg daily
	sertraline	Zoloft	25-mg, 50-mg, 100-mg tablets	Oral	50 mg qd, up to 200 mg qd
SNRIs	duloxetine	Cymbalta	20-mg, 30-mg, 60-mg capsules	Oral	40 or 60 mg qd
	venlafaxine	Effexor	25-mg, 37.5-mg, 50-mg, 75-mg, 100-mg tablets	Oral	75 mg/day, administered in two or three divided doses
TCAs	amitriptyline	Elavil	10-mg, 25-mg, 50-mg, 75-mg, 100-mg, 150-mg tablets	Oral	75 mg daily divided doses, can be increased to 150 mg daily
	doxepin	Sinequan	10-mg, 25-mg, 50-mg, 75-mg, 100-mg, 150-mg capsules	Oral	75 mg daily
	imipramine	Tofranil	10-mg, 25-mg, 50-mg tablets	Oral	In hospital: 100 mg daily divided doses; outpatients: 75 mg daily
	clomipramine	Anafranil	25-mg, 50-mg, 75-mg capsules	Oral	25 mg qd, up to 100 mg daily in divided doses
MAOIs	tranylcypromine	Parnate	10-mg tablets	Oral	30 mg daily, up to 60 mg daily
	phenelzine	Nardil	15-mg tablets	Oral	15 mg tid, up to 60 mg daily
	isocarboxazid	Marplan	10-mg tablets	Oral	10 mg bid
Miscellaneous	trazadone	Desyrel	150-mg, 300-mg tablets	Oral	150–400 mg daily, split into divided doses
	bupropion	Wellbutrin	75-mg, 100-mg tablets	Oral	100–150 mg tid

TABLE 34-5 Pharmaceutical Treatments for Bipolar Disorder

Classification	Generic Name	Brand Name	Dosage Forms and Availability	Route of Administration	Common Adult Dosage
Antimanic	lithium carbonate	Eskalith, Lithobid, Lithotabs	300-mg, 450-mg tablets	Oral	Acute mania: 900–2,400 mg daily
Anticonvulsants	carbamazepine	Tegretol	100-mg tablet and chewable tablet; 200-mg, 400-mg ER tablet; 300-mg ER capsule; 100 mg/5 mL suspension	Oral	400–1,200 mg daily
	clonazepam (C-IV)	Klonopin	0.5-mg, 1-mg, 2-mg tablets	Oral	0.75–20 mg daily
	divalproex sodium, valproic acid	Depakote	125-mg, 250-mg, 500-mg tablets; 500-mg ER tablet; 125-mg capsules	Oral	750 mg initial dose; NTE 60 mg/kg/day
	gabapentin	Neurontin	100-mg, 300-mg, 400-mg capsules; 600-mg, 800-mg tablets; 250 mg/5 mL solution.	Oral	100–1,200 mg daily
	lamotrigine	Lamictal	25-mg, 100-mg, 150-mg, 200-mg tablets; 2-mg, 5-mg, 25-mg chew tablets	Oral	Up to 200 mg daily
	topiramate	Topamax	25-mg, 50-mg, 100-mg, 200-mg tablets; 15-mg, 25-mg capsules	Oral	600–1,600 mg daily

that anticonvulsant therapy is more effective for acute mania than for long-term management of BD. Other anticonvulsants may also be used, although they lack formal FDA approval for treatment of BD (see Table 34-5).

Psychosis

A person who is out of touch with reality is considered *psychotic*. Symptoms of a particular psychosis, schizophrenia, include the following:

- Illogical thoughts or paranoia, such as the certain *knowledge* of being followed by someone all the time
- Hearing someone else's thoughts
- Hearing disembodied voices
- Seeing people, events, and things that are not there (hallucinations)
- Belief that one is someone else, usually of extreme importance or celebrity

Patients with schizophrenia or other psychoses may also have poor hygiene, spend much time alone, and pass the time at night awake, but sleep during the day. The patient may exhibit delusions of grandeur but also a lack of insight and poor judgment.

Early antipsychotic drugs caused muscle stiffness, tremor, and abnormal movements. An irreversible adverse reaction called *tardive dyskinesia* characterized by involuntary movements, affected about 5% of the patients using the older antipsychotics over a long term.

Newer drugs developed in the 1990s, called *atypical antipsychotics*, have lessened the side effects and improved compliance. The most common side effects are drowsiness, rapid heartbeat, dizziness upon moving from one position to another, weight gain, and decreased sexual function or libido.

The degree of effectiveness and the side effects of these drugs vary from patient to patient. In most cases, the drugs take effect within two to six weeks, and improvement can be noticed after a few days, up to several months. Antipsychotic drugs interact with many other drugs, including antihypertensive agents, antiepileptics, anticonvulsants, and anti-Parkinson drugs.

 Workplace Wisdom Psychosis Statistic

More than 2.5 million Americans suffer from psychosis.

Mechanism of Action of Antipsychotic Drugs

One of the well-documented causes of psychosis is an increase in dopamine. Antipsychotic drugs attach to the dopamine D2 receptor, blocking its action and thereby decreasing dopamine activity. Conventional or traditional (typical) antipsychotics do this too, but also induce involuntary movements and elevate serum prolactin.

When given within the accepted clinical effective ranges, atypical antipsychotics do not cause these adverse reactions. To understand how these drugs work, it is important to examine the mechanism of action (MOA) of atypical antipsychotics and how it differs from that of the more typical drugs. The key difference is a physical one: The atypical antipsychotics bind more loosely than dopamine to the dopamine D2 receptor. They also have dissociation constants higher than that of dopamine; in contrast, the conventional antipsychotics bind more tightly than dopamine itself to the dopamine D2 receptor, with dissociation constants that are lower than that of dopamine. (Dissociation measures how easily a molecule is released or unbinds from the receptor.) It is also postulated that atypical drugs block receptors for serotonin, another neurotransmitter, at the same time they block dopamine receptors and that this serotonin–dopamine balance somehow keeps prolactin levels normal, spares cognition, and does not promote involuntary movement.

Clozaril, the first atypical antipsychotic, has helped 25% to 50% of patients who did not respond to conventional antipsychotics. Unfortunately, Clozaril is associated with a 2% risk of agranulocytosis, which is a deficiency of a specific white blood cell. Agranulocytosis is potentially fatal but reversible if diagnosed early. When affected by agranulocytosis, the immune system function is decreased, rendering the patient susceptible to infection. Patients using Clorazil must have their blood checked regularly. Doctors now recommend that Clozaril be used only after at least two other safer antipsychotics have been tried without success. It should be noted that patients who take the drug and those who prescribe the drug must be registered with the Clozaril National Registry (CNR).

Conventional antipsychotics are becoming obsolete because of their serious side effects. Experts usually recommend using a newer, atypical antipsychotic rather than a conventional one unless the patient is already doing well on the older treatment. If the person is noncompliant with multiple daily dosing, the once-a-day dosing of Haldol or Prolixin may be more suitable.

Conventional, traditional, or typical antipsychotic drugs include the following:

- Haldol (haloperidol)
- Stelazine (trifluoperazine)
- Mellaril (thioridazine)
- Thorazine (chlorpromazine)
- Navane (thiothixene)
- Prolixin, Permitil (fluphenazine)

Newer, atypical antipsychotic drugs are being prescribed more often to reduce side effects, thus improving the quality of life for patients with psychosis (see Table 34-6).

TABLE 34-6 Pharmaceutical Treatments for Psychosis

Generic Name	Brand Name	Dosage Forms and Availability	Route of Administration	Common Adult Dosage
aripiprazole	Abilify	2-mg, 5-mg, 10-mg, 15-mg, 20-mg, 30-mg tabs; 1 mg/mL oral solution; 7.5 mg/mL vial	Oral, injection	10–30 mg daily
asenapine	Saphris	5-mg, 10-mg tablets	Oral	10 mg bid
chlorpromazine	Thorazine	10-mg, 25-mg, 50-mg, 100-mg, 200-mg tablets	Oral, injection	25 mg tid, up to 400 mg daily
clozapine	Clozaril	25-mg, 100-mg tablets	Oral	12.5 mg qd or bid with increased increments of 25 mg/50 mg qd. Maximum 300–450 mg/day
fluphenazine	Prolixin	5-mg, 10-mg tablets; 0.5 mg/mL elixir	Oral, injection	10–15 times the normal daily dose given once every month (maximum monthly dose should not exceed 100 mg)

(Continued)

TABLE 34-6 **Pharmaceutical Treatments for Psychosis** (*Continued*)

Generic Name	Brand Name	Dosage Forms and Availability	Route of Administration	Common Adult Dosage
haloperidol	Haldol	Units of 10 × 1 mL ampules	Oral, injection	10–15 times the normal daily dose given once every month (maximum monthly dose should not exceed 100 mg)
iloperidone	Fanapt	1-mg, 2-mg, 4-mg, 6-mg, 8-mg, 10-mg, 12-mg tablets	Oral	6–12 mg bid
loxapine	Loxitane	4 fl oz (120 mL) w/calibrated dropper	Oral	60–100 mg daily
molindone	Moban	5-mg, 10-mg, 25-mg, 50-mg tablets	Oral	50–75 mg daily, increasing to 100 mg daily
olanzapine	Zyprexa	2.5-mg, 5-mg, 7.5-mg, 10-mg tablets; 10-mg vials	Oral, IM	Oral: 5–10 mg qd; 10 mg daily IM
paliperidone	Invega	1.5-mg, 3-mg, 6-mg, 9-mg tablets	Oral	6 mg daily
quetiapine	Seroquel	25-mg, 50-mg, 100-mg, 200-mg, 300-mg, 400-mg tablets	Oral	300–400 mg daily
risperidone	Risperdal	0.25-mg, 0.5-mg, 1-mg, 2-mg, 3-mg, 4-mg tablets	Oral, injection	1 mg bid, up to 8 mg qd–bid
thioridazine	Mellaril	10-mg, 15-mg, 25-mg, 50-mg, 100-mg, 150-mg, 200-mg tablets; 30 mg/mL, 100 mg/mL oral solution	Oral	Maximum of 800 mg daily
thiothixene	Navane	1-mg, 2-mg, 5-mg, 10-mg; 20-mg capsules	Oral	20–30 mg daily
trifluoperazine	Stelazine	1-mg, 2-mg, 5-mg, 10-mg tablets; 10-mL MDV	Oral	1–5 mg qd or bid
ziprasidone	Geodan	20-mg, 40-mg, 60-mg, 80-mg capsules; 20 mg/mL SDV	Oral, injection	Up to 80 mg bid

Insomnia

Each individual's requirement for sleep varies, as do feelings of satisfaction from sleep. *Insomnia* is described as an individual's complaint of inadequate or poor-quality sleep. Insomnia is characterized by one or more of the following complaints:

- Difficulty falling asleep
- Difficulty returning to sleep if awakened during the night
- Waking up frequently during the night
- Waking up too early in the morning
- Poor energy or not feeling refreshed in the morning, as if there had been no sleep at all

Insomnia may cause problematic symptoms such as a lack of energy, tiredness, daytime sleepiness, difficulty in focus or concentration, impaired performance, irritability, and a tendency to feel anger. People most likely to experience insomnia include the following:

- Older people—people over 60 years of age are most likely to have sleep problems. It has been incorrectly stated that the need for sleep decreases with age; in fact, it is the *ability* to sleep that decreases with age.
- Females, especially after menopause.
- People with a history of depression.

Certain risk factors contribute to the increased likelihood of insomnia:

- Anxiety
- Stress
- Medications
- Certain foods and drinks
- Sleep–wake scheduling problems
- Interruptions, such as jet lag or a change in work shift schedules or nighttime activity
- Change in physical surroundings
- Change in the environment, such as noise, light, climate, or temperature alterations

Chronic insomnia is multifaceted and results from a combination of factors. Common causes are physical or mental disorders, especially depression, arthritis, kidney disease, diabetes, hyperthyroidism, congestive heart failure, asthma, restless legs syndrome, sleep apnea, fibromyalgia, and narcolepsy.

To overcome insomnia, patients can make changes to their environment, schedules, medications, and diet (such as eliminating caffeine). Also, playing soft music, reading a book, taking a warm bath, and drinking warm milk are good evening habits. Light exercise, yoga, hypnosis, relaxation techniques, and sleep restriction therapy may all work. In some cases, an over-the-counter (OTC) sleep aid, such as Nytol (diphenhydramine 25 mg), Sominex (diphenhydramine 50 mg), or Unisom (doxylamine 25 mg), which are antihistamines, can help. Recall that the side effects of some OTC antihistamines are drowsiness and sleepiness. The antihistamine ingredient most commonly used is diphenhydramine, although some combination products include analgesics as well. When all else fails, prescription sedatives and hypnotics are available (see Table 34-7).

TABLE 34-7 Pharmaceutical Treatments for Insomnia

Classification	Generic Name	Brand Name	Dosage Forms and Availability	Route of Administration	Common Adult Dosage
Benzodiazepine hypnotics	quazepam	Doral	7.5-mg, 15-mg tablets	Oral	15 mg 30 minutes–1 hour before bedtime
	temazepam	Restoril	7.5-mg, 15-mg, 22.5-mg, 30-mg capsules	Oral	7.5–15 mg at bedtime
Nonbenzodiazepine hypnotics	eszopiclone	Lunesta	1-mg, 2-mg, 3-mg tablets	Oral	2 mg at bedtime only
	ramelteon	Rozerem	8-mg tablets	Oral	8 mg within 30 minutes of bedtime
	zaleplon	Sonata	5-mg, 10-mg capsules	Oral	5–20 mg at bedtime
	zolpidem	Ambien, Ambien CR	5-mg, 10-mg tablets	Oral	IR: 10 mg at bedtime; CR: 12.5 mg at bedtime
Barbituates	butabarbital	Butisol	30-mg, 50-mg tablets	Oral	Sedation: 15–30 mg tid/qid; sleep: 50–100 mg; pre-op: 50–100 mg
	mephobarbital	Mebaral	32-mg, 50-mg, 100-mg tablets	Oral	Sedative: 32–100 mg tid/qid; seizures: 400–600 mg daily
	phenobarbital	Luminal, Nembutal	15-mg, 30-mg, 100-mg tablets; 5-mL oral elixir; 20-mL, 50-mL MDV	Oral, IM	Sedative: 30–120 mg daily; seizures: 60–120 mg daily; sleep. 100–200 mg at bedtime; pre-op: 1–3 mg/kg or 100–200 mg IM
	secobarbital	Seconal	100-mg capsules	Oral	Sleep. 200 mg; pre-op: 200–300 mg

Hypnotics, Sedatives, and Barbiturates

A *hypnotic* is a drug that causes drowsiness, induces sleep onset, and/or maintains sleep. A *sedative* or *tranquilizer* is a drug that calms and relaxes a person. Pharmacologically speaking, a hypnotic and a sedative may have the same active ingredients, varying only in amounts to vary the degree of response. For example, a higher dose of a hypnotic would put patients to sleep very quickly, whereas a smaller dose of the same drug would merely calm them down, reducing nervous tension. Both hypnotics and sedatives decrease mental activity and nervous system function; that is, the nervous system is depressed. By this action, these agents can reduce anxiety, stress, irritability, and excitement. Because relaxation is essential to falling asleep—that is, the muscles and mind must relax—sedatives may cause a person to fall asleep by merely relaxing or calming the mind or loosening the muscles. Because of this, when patients take a sedative close to bedtime to "calm their nerves," they will more than likely fall asleep rather than stay calmly awake.

Barbiturates are very addictive, as they, along with hypnotics and sedatives, are depressants. The pupils become constricted, the vision is blurred, and the breathing is shallow. Large doses of barbiturates can cause respiratory depression, coma, and death.

Barbiturates, hypnotics, and sedatives are used when the cause of insomnia is any emotional disturbance other than depression. Tolerance and addiction can result from long-term use. Therefore, all patients should be counseled to use hypnotics only over a short term (two to four weeks) or episodically (no more than a few times a week). Because depressed patients may be prone to suicide, they should be prescribed small quantities requiring frequent refills, rather than supplying them with large amounts, to reduce the opportunity for suicide attempts.

Benzodiazepines

Because benzodiazepines bind to all three BZ receptors, they can relax the muscles, which can lead to a feeling of total relaxation and sleepiness. They are used as hypnotics and sedatives in higher doses, and in lower doses when used as **anxiolytics**. Proper dosing is important so that antianxiety drugs can be given during the day to prevent anxiety episodes and avoid sleepiness. These drugs are also used as anticonvulsants and antiepilectics.

Benzodiazepines are used to treat many disorders other than anxiety due to their sedative and hypnotic effects. Benzodiazepines can be used for:

- Insomnia
- Epilepsy
- Muscle spasticity
- Anesthesia, as preanesthetic or presurgery medication
- Alcohol withdrawal
- Various psychiatric diagnoses

Side effects are related to dosing and coadministration with drugs or alcohol. High doses taken with alcohol produce lethal effects. Benzodiazepines may cause dependence with long-term use and are therefore classified as Class IV controlled substances. Because of this, it is now recommended that prescriptions for these drugs be only for short-term use. Research is currently underway to make more selective anxiolytic compounds, such as partial agonists at the benzodiazepine receptor.

Mechanism of Action of Benzodiazepines

Benzodiazepine drugs bind to the GABA-A receptors and *potentiate* (increase) the actions of GABA. When there is a lack of GABA, they act like GABA; when GABA cannot cross the synapse, they facilitate the crossing and binding of GABA into the GABA-A receptors.

Management of Benzodiazepine Overdose

The primary use of Romazicon (flumazenil) is as a benzodiazepine antagonist in the event of overdose. Romazicon competitively antagonizes the binding and allosteric effects of benzodiazepines at the BZ GABA-A receptors. An additional use is in the reduction of benzodiazepine effects in general anesthesia or diagnostic procedures. Flumazenil is available for only intravenous administration, because it has a high first-pass effect (hepatic/liver). The physician must be certain of the cause of overdose, because flumazenil may increase the risk of seizures in patients who are comatose because of alcohol intoxication or overdose of TCA agents.

Nonbenzodiazepine Drugs

The characteristics of nonbenzodiazepines, a miscellaneous group of drugs, vary depending on the specific agent. Conventional benzodiazepines, such as triazolam and flurazepam (the treatment of choice for short-term insomnia for many years), are associated with adverse effects such as rebound insomnia, withdrawal, and dependency. The newer *hypnosedatives*, sometimes called the Z drugs, include zolpidem, zaleplon, and zopiclone. These agents are starting to be preferred over conventional benzodiazepines to treat short-term insomnia, because they are considered less likely to cause significant rebound insomnia, or tolerance, and are just as efficacious as the conventional benzodiazepines.

---

info

TCA Dosing

Patients with depression are commonly prescribed a sedating TCA, such as Elavil (amitriptyline), Tofranil (imipramine), or Anafranil (clomipramine), to be taken about one hour before bedtime. In general, these drugs are prescribed at the lowest dose and for the shortest duration needed to relieve the symptoms of insomnia. Some drugs should be tapered off gradually as the medicine is discontinued, because the insomnia may recur if they are stopped abruptly.

---

anxiolytics drug used to treat anxiety.

Ambien (zolpidem), an imidazopyridine, acts by increasing GABA potential but is not useful for anticonvulsant therapy or skeletal muscle relaxation. It is used mainly as a hypnotic for short-term therapy, usually for 7 to 10 days, but extendable up to 28 days. Zolpidem selectively binds to omega-1 BZ receptors and causes little next-morning residual sleepiness or decreased psychomotor function. Sonata (zaleplon) belongs to the pyrazolopyrimidine class of hypnotics and has the same selective binding as zolpidem. Tables 34-8 and 34-9 show some MOAs of sedative and hypnotic drugs.

PROFILE IN PRACTICE

While ringing up Mr. Carson's phenobarbital prescription, the pharmacy technician notices that he is also purchasing OTC diphenhydramine.

▶ *Does the pharmacy technician need to bring Mr. Carson's OTC purchase to the attention of the pharmacist on duty, and if so, why?*

TABLE 34-8 Sedative and Hypnotic Drugs

Classification Type	Site and MOA	Side and Toxic Effects/ Special Notes	Drug Interactions
Barbiturate	SOA: reticular formation and cerebral cortex MOA #1—low doses increase GABA, causing relaxation. MOA #2—high doses cause sleep and depression of CNS.	Dry mouth, lethargy, drowsiness. Overdose: cardiovascular and CNS depression, kidney failure, low blood pressure, death. No known antidote.	Increased effect with other CNS depressants and alcohol.
Nonbarbiturates	SOA and MOA vary. Zolpidem and zaleplon selectively bind to omega-1 BZ receptor, potentiating GABA. Eszopiclone mildly binds to omega-1.	Produce less tolerance and addiction. Exception: Z drugs produce more dependence in patients with preexisting substance-related addictions. Zolpidem: GI and CNS disturbances; rare—delirium, nightmares, hallucinations; may reduce memory or psychomotor function within first two hours after administration of single oral dose. Zaleplon: does not impair memory or psychomotor function but may cause side effect such as headache.	Rifampin induces metabolism of newer hypnosedatives and decreases sedative effects. Ketoconazole, erythromycin, and cimetidine also induce metabolism.
Benzodiazepines	SOA: reticular formation MOA #1—low doses increase GABA, causing relaxation. MOA #2—high doses cause sleep and depression of CNS.	Do not cause REM rebound when discontinued. Less addictive than barbiturates; may be used a few weeks longer before tolerance builds up. Halcion may cause rebound insomnia, nightmares, and daytime anxiety.	Decreased effect with cimetidine. Increased effect with other CNS depressants and alcohol.

TABLE 34-9 Pharmaceutical Treatments for ADD/ADHD

Generic Name	Brand Name	Dosage Forms and Availability	Route of Administration	Common Adult Dosage
amphetamine/ dextroamphetamine	Adderall	5-mg, 7.5-mg, 10-mg, 12.5-mg, 15-mg, 20-mg, 30-mg tablets	Oral	5–60 mg daily
atomoxetine	Strattera	10-mg, 18-mg, 25-mg, 40-mg, 60-mg, 100-mg capsules	Oral	1.2 mg/kg daily
dexmethylphenidate	Focalin	2.5-mg, 5-mg, 10-mg tablets	Oral	Dosage should be individualized according to the needs and responses of the patient
dextroamphetamine	Dexedrine	5-mg, 10-mg, 15-mg capsules	Oral	5–60 mg daily
lisdexamfetamine	Vyvanse	20-mg, 30-mg, 40-mg, 50-mg, 60-mg, 70-mg capsules	Oral	30 mg qd
methylphenidate C-II	Ritalin	5-mg, 10-mg, 20-mg tablets	Oral	20–30 mg in divided doses
methylphenidate LA/SR	Daytrana	27.5-mg, 41.3-mg, 55-mg, 82.5-mg patch	Topical	Applied to the hip area two hours before an effect is needed and should be removed nine hours after application

Stimulants

Stimulants are a class of drugs that enhance brain activity and increase alertness, attention, and energy. They speed up the physiological and metabolic activity of the body. In addition, they elevate blood pressure and increase respiration and heart rate. Therefore, they are used to treat **narcolepsy**, attention deficit hyperactivity disorder (ADHD), attention deficit disorder (ADD), and depression that has not responded to other treatments. They may also be used as appetite suppressants for short-term treatment of obesity and for patients with asthma to increase breathing rate. Because of their potential for abuse and addiction, prescription stimulants are usually classified as controlled substance Schedule II drugs and reserved for treatment of only a few diseases or conditions.

Stimulants have chemical structures similar to the monoamine neurotransmitters found in the brain, including NE and dopamine. Stimulants act like these compounds, increase the amount of them, or promote the synthesis or production of these chemicals in the brain. The results of stimulation of the SNS include:

- Increase in blood pressure and heart rate
- Constriction of the blood vessels
- Increase in blood glucose
- Dilation of the respiratory system pathways for easier breathing

In addition, the increase in dopamine is associated with a sense of euphoria that can accompany the use of these drugs. Cocaine is a stimulant that can produce this euphoric effect. Other C-II stimulants are amphetamines, such as Ritalin (methylphenidate), used for ADD/ADHD and Dexedrine (dextroamphetamine), a synthetically altered amphetamine used for weight loss, narcolepsy, and ADD/ADHD.

Adverse Actions of Stimulants

High doses of some stimulants, taken repeatedly over a short period of time, may lead to feelings of paranoia, anger, or hostility. Other detrimental outcomes are fatally high body temperatures, seizures, arrhythmias, and cardiovascular (CV) failure. Less serious side effects include headache, dizziness, diarrhea or

narcolepsy a condition characterized by frequent and uncontrolled periods of deep sleep.

constipation, restlessness, tremor, nervousness, anxiety, insomnia, dry mouth, unpleasant taste in the mouth, erectile dysfunction, changes in libido, GI disturbances, and weight loss.

Contraindications

Because stimulation of the SNS can exacerbate glaucoma, hypertension, coronary artery disease, or an overactive thyroid gland, patients with these conditions should not take stimulant prescriptions or OTC stimulant products. Stimulants cause a fatally acute rise in blood pressure when taken within two weeks of taking an MAOI antidepressant (such as Nardil or Parnate). Therefore, patients must be warned and counseled on these drug contraindications. Stimulants should not be given to those with agitation or anxiety.

Withdrawal Treatment

Addiction to prescription stimulants may first be treated with a tapering off of the drug. Withdrawal treatment may include antidepressants to help manage the symptoms of depression that occur during the early phase of abstinence from stimulants. Detoxification involves behavioral and cognitive psychotherapy. Recovery support or 12-step groups may also be effectively employed in conjunction with psychotherapy.

ADHD and ADD

ADHD is a condition in which a person (child or adult) has a very short attention span and is easily distracted, excessively active, and possibly overly emotional or highly impulsive. ADD does not present the excessive movement or activity (*hyperkinesia*) associated with ADHD. Treatment should include psychological, educational, and pharmacological approaches.

Stimulants Used in the Treatment of ADHD and ADD

- Ritalin (methylphenidate) is a *mild* CNS stimulant.
- Dexedrine (dextroamphetamine) is a strong CNS stimulant, much more potent than methylphenidate.
- Adderall (dextroamphetamine sulfate, dextroamphetamine saccharate, amphetamine aspartate, amphetamine sulphate) is a combination drug used to treat ADD/ADHD and narcolepsy. Amphetamine is more potent than dextroamphetamine, and amphetamine sulfate is a widely abused street drug. Adderall XR is an extended-release, once-daily dosage form of Adderall. Adderall and Adderall XR may be better choices than methylphenidate or Dexedrine, as they last longer and are more powerful. Because the *speed rush* is brought about more gradually, the patient *comes down* more easily and gradually. Most people on Dexedrine experience a *crash* in which they may sleep for many hours after the drug wears off.
- Concerta (methylphenidate) is the first once-daily treatment for ADD/ADHD with a 12-hour time-release formula. Medical studies have demonstrated that Concerta can help children with ADHD improve focus in the classroom and even perform better on math tests. It has a lower incidence of side effects than the immediate-release form of methylphenidate. Taking immediate-release methylphenidate, dextroamphetamine alone, or dextroamphetamine plus an amphetamine usually produces weight loss in patients. In contrast, only 4% of patients taking Concerta reported any loss of appetite or sleep. Sustained-release methylphenidate can be taken with or without food.

Once-a-day dosing is preferable for convenience and patient compliance. It also allows the parent to do the medication administration from home and eliminates worry about a school nurse or official administering the medication and the stigma to the child associated with being medicated at school.

Nonstimulants Used in the Treatment of ADHD and ADD

Strattera (atomoxetine), a serotonin/NE reuptake inhibitor, is a nonstimulant used in the treatment of ADHD and ADD. It is the first nonstimulant drug that has been approved by FDA for ADD. It is not a controlled substance and is not addictive. Strattera is an oral capsule for once- or twice-a-day dosing. Strattera is the only ADHD medication approved for adults by the FDA.

In addition to those mentioned for stimulants, Strattera has the following side effects:

- Mood swings
- Ear infections
- Influenza

Because this drug has been tested and is also used on adults with ADD and ADHD, sexual side effects in adults have been reported, including:

- Decreased libido
- Difficulty in ejaculation
- Erectile dysfunction
- Urination problems
- Painful menstrual cycles

Although rare, potentially serious allergic reactions (anaphylaxis) may occur with use of Strattera. In addition to having the *same* contraindications as stimulants, Strattera should not be given to patients with epilepsy or seizure disorders, liver disease, or kidney disease.

Convulsions, Seizures, and Epilepsy

Epilepsy is a disorder of the CNS in which the patient may have convulsions or seizures. *Convulsions* are physical/muscular manifestations of the disorder; a *seizure* is irregular electrical activity in the brain, which may cause convulsions. A sudden onset of violent, uncontrollable, and involuntary contractions of the muscles, possible uncontrollable shaking, and twitching of arms or legs, characterize convulsive seizures. The patient may fall on the ground and lose bladder and bowel control.

Seizures occur due to an abnormal electrical discharge of neurons, in which they fire uncontrollably. The nerve cells in this state are said to be *hyperexcitable*. The seizure causes a sudden break in the stream of thought and activity and may include loss of consciousness. Brain seizures may cause a temporary loss of memory or fainting spells. The presence of the two together is more severe than the seizure alone. Causes may be injury to the brain, high fever (possibly due to infection), head trauma, cephalic tumor, stroke, alcohol dependence, or overintoxication. In these cases, the injury is to the neurons. Epilepsy can be diagnosed by the specific wave patterns shown in an **electroencephalogram (EEG)** recording.

Types and Classifications of Seizures

Seizures are classified as either partial and generalized, depending upon where the seizure begins and ends within the nervous system and the body. *Partial seizures* travel short distances on one side of the brain. *Generalized seizures* can travel anywhere throughout the brain, on both sides. Partial seizures are further classified as simple partial seizures and partial complex seizures.

Simple partial seizures affect only one side or portion of the brain and usually occur without loss of consciousness. The patient may experience an intense emotion, such as elation, sorrow, or sadness. The following characteristics are associated with simple partial seizures:

- Muscle contractions of a specific body part
- Abnormal sensations such as numbness and tingling, especially in the hands, feet, arms, or legs
- Nausea, skin flushing, sweating, or pupil dilation
- Hearing noises, seeing things, or having other hallucination-type symptoms
- Loss of awareness of position for a brief time

A patient having a *partial complex seizure* may or may not lose consciousness. All or any of the symptoms of partial simple seizures may occur in addition to any of the following:

- Being on *automatic pilot*—performance of complex behaviors (such as driving) without conscious awareness
- Abnormal sensations
- Changes in personality or alertness
- Loss of consciousness
- Olfactory or gustatory hallucinations or impairments if the epilepsy is focused in the temporal lobe of the brain
- Usually a specific body movement such as smacking the lips or tapping the foot (often referred to as *psychomotor* manifestations)
- Recalled or inappropriate emotions

Generalized seizures involve two sides of the brain and are further subclassified as tonic–clonic, myoclonic, and absence seizures.

- *Tonic–clonic,* also known as grand mal, seizures affect the whole brain. They are considered the most severe, causing the whole body to convulse with rhythmic, sustained contractions alternating with relaxation of the muscles. Infections that cause high fever may induce these seizures, called *febrile seizures*, in small children and infants. Sometimes brought on by a light or sound, the experience can last up to several minutes with possible difficulty breathing and/or loss of bladder/bowel control.
- *Myoclonic seizures* are characterized by convulsive twitching of specific body parts or muscle groups for a brief period of time. Children with infantile spasms may present quick, *jack-knifing* muscular spasms of the head, trunk, and extremities. These seizures may become severe.
- *Absence,* also known as petit mal, seizures affect the whole brain. When a person is having an absence seizure, an onlooker may think that he is merely daydreaming or *zoning out*. These patients look like most people do when bored or distracted, staring blankly into space. This type of seizure typically lasts a few seconds to two minutes. For this reason, absence seizures are difficult to diagnose. They are rare in adults and most common in girls beginning between the ages of 6 and 12. Medication usually helps, and some outgrow this type of seizure.

Status Epilepticus

Any seizures that are generalized, sustained longer than five minutes, or repeated constitute a medical emergency called *status epilepticus.* Irregular heartbeat, lack of oxygen due to difficulty breathing, and hypertension or hypotension can occur, because the muscles of the heart or the diaphragm may also be convulsing. Hyperglycemia, hypoglycemia, lactic acidosis, and rise in body temperature are all due to movement. Immediate administration of IV anticonvulsant/antiepileptic medication is warranted before cerebral cortex damage or death occurs as a result of the catecholamine surge.

Treatment of status epilepticus is usually with a benzodiazepine, administered as follows:

Step 1: Uncontrolled in two minutes
Ativan (lorazepam) IV—0.1 mg/kg, give 1 mg/minute to a maximum of 10 mg over 10 minutes.

Versed (midazolam)—10 mg IM (0.15−0.3 mg/kg IM).

Valium (diazepam)—0.5–1.0 mg/kg rectally, using the IV solution per rectal tube or the diazepam gel preparation.

Step 2: Uncontrolled in 10 minutes
Cerebyx (fosphenytoin)—20 mg/kg IV at a maximum IV rate of 150 mg/minute in the average-sized adult (~3 mg/kg/minute).

Step 3: An additional dose of:

1. Fosphenytoin—10 mg/kg IV over five minutes to a maximum total dose of 30 mg/kg (recommended treatment) or
2. Phenobarbital—20 mg/kg IV at a maximum rate of 50–100 mg/minute in the average-sized adult (~1 mg/kg/minute)

Step 4: An additional dose of phenobarbital 10 mg/kg IV to a maximum total dose of 30 mg/kg or give a fourth drug

---

electroencephalogram (EEG) a graphic record of the electrical activity of the brain.

loading dose IV until the seizure ceases. Pentobarbital is the *traditional* choice when using a fourth drug—15 mg/kg (maximum rate of 25−50 mg/minute).

Treatment of Seizures and Convulsions

Most drugs used to prevent or treat epilepsy or convulsions characteristically treat the alternate relaxation and contraction of muscles and motor centers. Antiepileptic drugs treat the CNS neuronal state of hyperactivity. As noted in the discussion on neurons, ionic concentration affects discharge or firing. Increased neuronal activity is caused by an increase of specific ions traveling into the neuron or nerve cell (*influx*).

Following are three specific MOAs to prevent and treat epilepsy and hyperexcitability of the neuron (also see Table 34-10):

- Drugs that slow down an influx of sodium ions (Na^+, go outside neuron)
- Drugs that slow down an influx of calcium ions (Ca^{++}, stay outside neuron)
- Drugs that speed up the influx of chloride ions (Cl^-, go inside the neuron)

Parkinson's Disease

Parkinson's disease occurs as brain neurons that produce the neurotransmitter dopamine begin to malfunction and progressively die. These neurotransmitters enable the CNS to communicate with the somatic nervous system to translate thought into motion. Because dopamine acts as a chemical messenger that transmits signals to other parts of the brain that control movement and coordination (the cerebral medulla and cerebellum, respectively), a change in body movement is an expected symptom of Parkinson's disease. Other symptoms include tremors, stiff or rigid muscles and joints, and/or difficulty in moving. Too much or too little dopamine can disrupt the normal balance between the dopamine system and the PNS that uses ACh; thus, the imbalance interferes with smooth and continuous movement.

Excess dopamine that does not get bound to the postsynaptic neuron is broken down by a chemical in the synapse called MAO-B. This constant transmission of dopamine to and from neurons, and its subsequent disintegration, creates a homeostasis. The balance of dopamine activity is essential to body coordination and movement. However, as more of the

TABLE 34-10 Three Major Drug Classes Used to Control Seizures

Drugs That Stimulate an Influx of Chloride Ions		
Benzodiazepines	**Barbiturates**	**Miscellaneous**
clonazepam (Klonopin)	amobarbital (Amytal)	gabapentin (Neurontin)
clorazepate (Tranxene)	pentobarbital (Nembutal)	primidone (Mysoline)
diazepam (Valium)	phenobarbital (Luminal)	tiagabine (Gabitril)
lorazepam (Ativan)	secobarbital (Seconal)	topiramate (Topamax)
Drugs That Delay an Influx of Sodium Ions		
	Hydantoins	**Miscellaneous**
	phenytoin (Dilantin)	carbamazepine (Tegretol)
	fosphenytoin (cerebyx)	divalproex (Depakote)
		felbamate (Felbatol)
		lamotrigine (Lamictal)
		valproic acid (Depakene)
		zonisamide (Zonegran)
Drugs That Delay an Influx of Calcium Ions		
	Succinimides	**Miscellaneous**
	ethosuximide (Zarontin)	divalproex (Depakote)
	methsuximide (Celontin)	valproic acid (Depakene)
	phensuximide (Milontin)	zonisamide (Zonegran)

dopamine-producing cells die, less and less dopamine is produced, which causes Parkinson's disease. In addition, MAO-B continues to destroy the little remaining dopamine in the synapse. The balance of dopamine to ACh is thrown off.

Factors contributing to the malfunction that causes the death of neurons that produce dopamine include the following:

- High fevers at a young age, such as those that accompany viral infections
- Infections of the brain
- Injury to the brain, specifically the basal ganglia
- Antipsychotic drugs that act as dopamine antagonists and block dopamine receptors Currently, there is no way to stop the death of the cells that make dopamine. However, certain drugs, such as dopamine agonists, can help the

patient to *manage* the decline in motor function and activity in the early stages of the disease. By mimicking dopamine activity, dopamine agonists help to relieve symptoms such as shaking and slow movement.

Currently, there is no way to stop the death of the cells that make dopamine. However, certain drugs can help manage the decline in motor function and activity as the disease progresses.

Pharmaceutical Treatments

Levodopa is a fat-soluble substance that can cross the BBB and then, with the help of an enzyme, be converted to dopamine in the brain. However, dopamine is a water-soluble substance and cannot cross the BBB. One of the problems with this Parkinson's disease treatment is that the enzyme often converts

TABLE 34-11 Pharmaceutical Treatment for Parkinson's Disease

Drug Trade/ Generic Name	Availability	Dosage and Administration	MOA	Side Effects and Special Notes
Artane (trihexyphenidyl HCl) Cogentin (benztropine mesylate)	Artane: 2-mg, 5-mg tablets; 2 mg/5 mL elixir Cogentin: 0.5-mg, 1-mg, 2-mg tablets	Artane: start low at 1 mg, with 2 mg/ day increments. UAD: 6–10 mg. Maximum: 12–15 mg qd. Daily dose is given in three divided doses, usually with a meal. Cogentin: Cogentin: 0.5–6 mg qd. May be given at bedtime in one dose or in divided doses.	Artane, an antispasmodic drug, inhibits the PSNS. Cogentin is both anticholinergic and antihistaminic. Both drugs restore the dopamine/ ACh balance by reducing the activity of acetylcholine in the brain.	Used in early stages of Parkinson's disease, to be taken in combination with Sinemet (adjunct therapy). Successfully reduce the tremor and muscle stiffness that result from having much more ACh than dopamine. These agents do not correct the problem of too little dopamine. Artane side effects: dryness of the mouth, blurred vision, dizziness, mild nausea, nervousness. Artane toxic effects: delusions, hallucinations, paranoia. Cogentin side effects: tachycardia, constipation, dry mouth. Cogentin toxic effects: psychosis. Contraindications: antipsychotic drugs, antidepressants.
Eldepryl (selegiline hydrochloride)	5-mg tablets	Two 5-mg tablets; one at breakfast and one at lunch	Selective MAO type B inhibitor. Actually blocks MAO-B, the chemical in the synapse that breaks down dopamine, thus conserving the dopamine already in the brain and keeping it in the synapse so that it can bind to postsynaptic dopamine receptors.	Side effects: nausea/ vomiting, dizziness, abdominal pain, headache. Contraindications: nonselective MAOIs, TCAs, SSRIs, meperidine. Toxic effects of these drug interactions: severe agitation, hallucinations, death.

(Continued)

TABLE 34-11 **Pharmaceutical Treatment for Parkinson's Disease** *(Continued)*

Drug Trade/ Generic Name	Availability	Dosage and Administration	MOA	Side Effects and Special Notes
Parlodel (bromocriptine mesylate), Permax (pergolide mesylate) Parlodel, Permax (*continued*)	Parlodel: 2.5-mg, 5-mg tablets. Permax: 0.05-mg, 0.25-mg, 1-mg tablets	Parlodel: start with half of 2.5-mg tablet qd; increase to safe amount NTE 100 mg/day. Permax: start with 0.05 mg qd; increase to a maximum dose NTE 5 mg/day. UAD 3 mg/day in three divided doses.	Dopaminergics: mimic the action of dopamine by attaching to the dopamine receptor sites on the surface of the receiving neuron (postsynaptic neuron), acting like dopamine. This is a substitution-like action. Parlodel is an ergot with dopamine receptor agonist activity. Permax is an ergot-derivative dopamine receptor agonist at both D1 and D2 receptor sites.	Dyskinesias are less common because dopamine itself is not being increased, only the dopamine-like action. Parlodel side effects: nausea, vomiting, abnormal involuntary movements, hallucinations, confusion, dizziness, drowsiness, fainting, asthenia, abdominal discomfort, visual disturbance, ataxia, insomnia, depression, hypotension, shortness of breath, constipation, vertigo. Contraindications: decreased efficacy when taken with dopamine antagonist, butyrophenones, phenothiazines, haloperidol, metoclopramide, pimozide. Permax side effects: dyskinesia, hallucinations, somnolence, insomnia.
Sinemet, Sinemet CR (carbidopa and levodopa)	10 mg/100 mg, 25 mg/100 mg, 25 mg/250 mg tablets 25 mg/100 mg, 50 mg/200 mg CR tablets	Sinemet: start with one tablet qd; increase to two tablets qid. Sinemet CR: UAD 200 − 300 mg levodopa bid or tid, NTE 1,000 mg levodopa per day in three to four divided doses.	Levodopa is converted to dopamine, and carbidopa slows down the conversion so that levodopa can cross the BBB.	Can be used to control symptoms for several years. As dopamine-producing cells decrease, symptoms continue to worsen, and the dose of Sinemet has to be increased. Ultimately, the side effects of high doses of Sinemet are unacceptable, and the drug may have to be discontinued. Dyskinesias (involuntary muscular movements) result from an overload of Sinemet or dopamine in the brain.
Symmetrel (amantadine hydrochloride)	100-mg gel capsules	Start with 100 mg qd UAD: 100 mg bid NTE 400 mg qd	Allows the dopamine-producing nerve cell storage sites to open more easily and wider to release dopamine from the presynaptic neuron into the synapse.	Used in milder cases of Parkinson's disease. Contraindications: decrease the dose in patients with CHF, peripheral edema, orthostatic hypotension, or impaired renal function.

levodopa before it gets a chance to cross the BBB; the quick conversion to water-soluble dopamine keeps the dopamine away from the brain, where it is needed.

Sinemet is the agent most commonly used in the treatment of Parkinson's disease (also see Table 34-11). Sinemet is a combination of levodopa and carbidopa. The enzyme carbidopa slows down the conversion of levodopa to dopamine. As Parkinson's disease progresses, more Sinemet is required, which means more side effects occur. One way to prevent the need for high doses of Sinemet is by the addition of adjunctive therapy. Two examples of adjunctive therapy are:

- Parlodel—mimics the action of dopamine upon attaching to the postsynaptic dopamine receptor.
- Eldepryl—blocks the MAO-B that destroys dopamine.

Dementia

Dementia is a progressive brain dysfunction with a loss of cognition that leads to gradually increasing restriction of daily activities. Patients with irreversible dementias, such as Alzheimer's disease, eventually become unable to care for themselves and may require around-the-clock care. According to the APA, Alzheimer's disease is the fourth leading cause of death in America. The changes in the brain may occur gradually or quickly and may be caused by disease or trauma, which may determine if the dementia is permanent or temporary.

Dementia may interfere with decision making, judgment, memory, thinking, reasoning, verbal communication, and spatial orientation. Behavioral and personality changes may also result, depending on the areas of the brain affected. It is believed that the changes in the brain cause a lack of ACh, which is thought to be the root of Alzheimer's disease. Treating dementia quickly may result in partial or total reversal of the disease.

Signs and Symptoms of Dementia

Early stages of dementia are characterized by loss of short-term memory. As the disease progresses, the patient has trouble with abstract thinking, which may show up as problems with counting or handling money, paying bills, understanding what was just read, or organizing daily activities. In late stages, the patient becomes disoriented about times and dates, confused, and unable to remember or describe their current residence or a recently visited place. Behavioral and personality changes may include the patient:

- Being unable to dress without help
- Being unable to eat or losing the desire to eat
- Having toileting problems, leading to incontinence
- Being unable to do self-care or grooming
- Abandoning interests and hobbies
- Being unable to perform routine activities such as household tasks
- Displaying personality changes with inappropriate responses, lack of emotional control, apathy, or social withdrawal

As the disease progresses, patients with dementia may become more irritable, agitated, and quarrelsome and less neat in appearance, with diminished attention to grooming habits. In late stages of dementia, the patient stops talking, has erratic mood swings, and becomes uncooperative.

Age is the most commonly accepted contributing factor for dementia. However, according to the APA, only 15% to 25% percent of older people suffer from significant symptoms of mental illness. Untreated infections, metabolic disease, and substance abuse can also lead to dementia. The following disorders are risk factors for dementia: brain tumors, hypertension, coronary artery disease, head injury, renal failure, hepatic disease, and thyroid disease. Dietary deficiencies of vitamin B12 (cyanocobalamin), folic acid, and B1 (thiamine) have also been associated with dementia. Genetic disorders such as Huntington's disease, infections such as HIV/AIDS, amyotrophic lateral sclerosis (also known as Lou Gehrig's disease), and Parkinson's disease have also been associated with dementias. Substances associated with drug-induced dementias include the following:

- Anticholinergics
- Barbiturates
- Benzodiazepines
- Cough suppressants
- Digitalis medications
- MAOIs
- TCAs

Treatment of Dementia

First, the underlying cause of the dementia must be treated. Infections, such as HIV/AIDS, are treated with antiretroviral agents. Antibiotics and antifungals are applied for neurosyphilis dementia and other infections. Antihypertensives and antihyperlipidemics are used for CV disease.

The goals of direct treatment of dementia are to improve the quality of life and maximize physical function. Some objectives include improvement of cognitive skills, mood, and behavior. Realistically, the goal of pharmacotherapy for irreversible conditions is to control symptoms and delay worsening if possible.

Tranquilizers and sedatives can modify personality changes manifested by agitation, anxiety, and aggression. Medications may be used to help manage insomnia, restlessness, and incontinence. Caretakers and family must employ safety precautions to protect the confused and disoriented patient from wandering away from home.

In 1993, the FDA approved tacrine, the first agent specifically designed for the treatment of cognitive symptoms in Alzheimer's disease. Cognex (tacrine) is a reversible cholinesterase inhibitor and is believed to work by increasing the availability of ACh in the synapses between the neurons in the brains of Alzheimer's disease patients (see Table 34-12).

Other approaches to treatment of dementias include:

- *Vitamin E,* an antioxidant, may slow nerve cell damage and death in Alzheimer's disease.
- *Eldepryl (selegiline),* a selective MAO-B inhibitor, is used in the United States for Parkinson's disease. It is used off-label by some doctors to slow the progression of Alzheimer's disease.
- *Ergoloid mesylates (hydergine),* derived from rye, are used for dementias other than Alzheimer's disease and as

TABLE 34-12 Drugs Used to Treat Alzheimer's Disease

Drug Trade/ Generic Name	Availability	Dosage and Administration	MOA	Side Effects and Special Notes
Aricept (donepezil)	5-mg, 10-mg tablet	One tablet qh, NTE 10 mg/day.	Reversible acetylcholinesterase inhibitor; blocks the enzyme that destroys ACh.	Nausea/vomiting/diarrhea (N/V/D), insomnia, muscle cramps, fatigue, anorexia
Cognex (tacrine)	10-mg, 20-mg, 30-mg, 40-mg capsule	Start with 10 mg qid. UAD: 20 mg qid. NTE 120 mg/day and 160 mg/day. Transaminase levels should be monitored every other week from at least week 4–16, then decrease monitoring to every three months.	Parasympathomimetic reversible cholinesterase inhibitor; blocks the enzyme that destroys ACh.	N/V/D, myalgia, ataxia, anorexia; high serum ALT/SGPT or liver damage
Exelon (rivastigmine)	1.5-mg, 3-mg, 4.5-mg, 6-mg capsule	Start with 1.5 mg bid, NTE 6 mg bid (12 mg/day). Take with morning and evening meals.	Reversible acetylcholinesterase inhibitor blocks the enzyme that destroys ACh.	Common: N/V/D, insomnia, UTI, fatigue Rare: abnormal hepatic function
Razadyne (galantamine)	4-gm, 8-gm, 12-gm tablet 4 mg/mL oral solution	4 mg bid, with morning and evening meals, NTE 24 mg bid	Reversible, competitive acetylcholinesterase inhibitor.	If therapy is interrupted, patient should restart at lowest dose; lower dose for hepatically impaired patients

an alternative when cholinesterase inhibitors, vitamin E, or selegiline prove ineffective in the Alzheimer's patient. UAD is 3 mg/day, NTE 9 mg/day. It is thought to enhance mental abilities by improving oxygen supply to the brain because of its ability to act as a mild vasodilator. In addition, it is believed to possess antioxidant properties that protect the brain and heart from free-radical damage, improving the number of brain dendrites and their ability to make connections.

Migraine Headaches

A *migraine* is a very painful headache, usually on one side of the head, that tends to recur. The patient may feel nauseated, feel the urge to vomit, and be very sensitive to light and noise. Body movement can make the headache worse. Although there are many types of migraine headaches, the two major kinds are the classic and the common migraine headaches.

Classic Migraine

The major distinction of a classic migraine headache is the experience of an *aura* 10–30 minutes before the attack. The aura may manifest as flashing lights, zigzag lines in the visual field,

or a temporary vision loss, and may or may not be accompanied by speech difficulty, confusion, weakness of an arm or leg, and tingling of the face or hands. The pain of a classic migraine headache is characterized by an intense throbbing or pounding in the forehead, temple, ear, jaw, or the entire area around the eyes. Beginning on one side of the head, a classic migraine may spread to the other side. It may last one to two days.

Common Migraine

The common migraine is the one that is most frequently observed in the general population. It is not preceded by an aura. A variety of vague symptoms may be experienced before onset of a headache, such as mental fog, mood swings, fatigue, and unusual retention of fluid. During the migraine headache phase, the patient may experience abdominal pain, polyuria, and N/V/D.

Causes and Treatment of Migraines

A classic or common migraine can occur as often as several times a week or as rarely as once every few years. The cause of migraines may be a chemical or electrical problem in certain parts of the brain where blood flow is changed. In response to a trigger, such as stress, a food, a sound, or a smell, spasms occur at the base of the brain, which constricts some of the arteries that supply blood to the brain, thereby restricting blood flow and oxygen to the brain. Platelets clump together, releasing the chemical serotonin, a powerful constrictor of arteries; this process further reduces the blood and oxygen supply to the brain. In response to the reduced blood flow and oxygen supply, certain arteries within the brain dilate to meet the brain's energy needs. Scientists believe that this vasodilation causes the pain of the migraine headache. Some migraines are influenced by hormonal changes, especially in women.

Common known migraine triggers include:

1. Medications:
   - Cimetidine
   - Estrogens/BCPs/HRT
   - Indomethacin
   - Nifedipine
   - Nitroglycerin (NTG)
   - Theophylline

2. Foods:
   - Aged foods, including cheese, beer, wine, and hard liquor
   - Yeast-containing foods, such as doughnuts and fresh breads
   - Caffeine, contained in coffee, tea, colas, and some medicines
   - Citrus fruits, bananas, figs, and raisins
   - Dairy products
   - Monosodium glutamate (MSG) and other seasonings
   - Legumes, such as peas, peanuts, lima beans, and nuts
   - Sulfites, aspartame, and saccharin
   - Fermented foods, such as pickled herring

Nonpharmaceutical treatments of migraine headaches include:

- Stress reduction
- Biofeedback training
- Removal of certain foods from the diet
- Regular exercise to increase endorphins and reduce stress
- Reducing the inflammation of the arteries with cold packs

Table 34-13 shows some drugs used in the treatment of migraines.

Cancer Pain

The International Association for the Study of Pain defines *pain* as "an unpleasant sensory and emotional experience in association with actual or potential tissue damage, or described in terms of such damage." Approximately 30% to 50% of patients with cancer experience pain while undergoing treatment, and 70% to 90% of patients with advanced cancer experience pain.

Pain can be acute or chronic. *Acute pain* starts suddenly; it may be sharp and is often a signal of a quick onset of injury to the body. Sometimes other bodily reactions, such as sweating or elevated blood pressure, occur with pain.

Chronic pain lasts beyond the time expected for an injury to heal or an illness to be resolved. Cancer pain can be chronic, but sometimes a patient will have acute flare-ups of pain that are not completely controlled by the usual medication or therapy. This is called *breakthrough pain*. Cancer pain is most often controlled with morphine and other opioid-like compounds.

Cancer causes pain by the mere pressure of a tumor on an organ, on bone, or on nerves. Surgical treatments and other procedures (biopsies, blood draws, lumbar punctures, and laser treatments) can also cause pain. Chemotherapy may result in the following sources of pain:

- Mouth sores (*mucositis*)
- Peripheral neuropathy (numb and sometimes painful sensations in the feet, legs, fingers, hands, and arms)
- GI upset—constipation, diarrhea, nausea, vomiting, abdominal cramps
- Bone and joint pain

Management of cancer pain can be problematic, because some physicians do not always prescribe the right medications or permit sufficient doses of the medication. These mistakes may be due to underestimation of the degree of pain the cancer patient is experiencing and/or the doctor's concerns about the potential for addiction. The use of a pain assessment scale (e.g., a scale in which *0* means *no pain at all* and *10* means *the worst pain one has ever felt before*) can help the physician determine the appropriate drug and dosage.

Pain itself is both electrical and chemical in nature. When pain receptors are triggered by mechanical, chemical, or thermal stimuli, the pain signal is transmitted through the nerves to the spinal cord and then to the brain. The most common cancer pain is from tumors that metastasize to the bone. Tumors erode the bone, forming large holes that make the bone thin and weak. Nerve endings in and around the bone send pain signals to the brain.

Treatment of Cancer Pain

Analgesics do not cure the cause of the pain and provide only temporary relief. However, they may make both short-term and long-term pain tolerable.

Mild pain may be managed with nonopioid analgesics such as acetaminophen and NSAIDs. About 30% of cancer pain can be treated with this type of OTC medication. Severe pain is treated with opioid analgesics such as Duragesic (fentanyl transdermal system), which provides continuous pain relief for 72 hours. Respiratory failure, hypotension, and hypoventilation may result from an overdose. Repeated administration may result in tolerance and physical and psychological dependence. Other side effects of opioid analgesics include the following:

- Constipation, nausea, vomiting
- Dry mouth, excessive sweating
- Excessive sleepiness (somnolence)
- High blood pressure (hypertension) or low blood pressure (hypotension)
- Confusion

TABLE 34-13 Drugs Used in the Treatment of Migraines

Drug Trade/ Generic Name	Availability	Dosage and Administration	MOA	Side Effects and Special Notes
Amerge (naratriptan)	1-mg, 2.5-mg tablet	2.5-mg single dose; may repeat in 4 hours, NTE 5 mg/24 hour or NTE 2.5 mg/24 hour in hepatically impaired patients	A selective 5-hydroxytryptamine$_1$ receptor subtype agonist that binds with high affinity to 5-HT$_{1D}$ and 5-HT$_{1B}$ receptors, resulting in cranial blood vessel constriction and a decrease in prostaglandin proinflammatory neuropeptide release.	Common: paresthesias, dizziness, drowsiness, malaise/fatigue. Rare: fatal cardiac events, HTN crisis
Axert (almotriptan)	6.25-mg, 12.5-mg tablet	NTE 12.5–25 mg/24 hour	A selective 5-HT$_{1B/1D}$ receptor subtype agonist, resulting in cranial blood vessel constriction and a decrease in prostaglandin proinflammatory neuropeptide release.	Common: paresthesias, dizziness, drowsiness, malaise/fatigue. Rare: fatal cardiac events, HTN crisis
Elavil (amitriptyline) Unlabeled use for pain associated with migraine headaches and to reduce pain perception	10-mg, 25-mg, 50-mg, 75-mg, 100-mg, 150-mg tablet; 10 mg/mL injection	75–300 mg/day	TCA that blocks neuronal reuptake of NE and serotonin. Lowering serotonin lowers pain perception and causes vasodilation.	Common: skin rash, GI upset, edema, MI, hepatic failure, coma, seizures, hallucinations. Drug interactions: Avoid cimetidine and MAOIs
Ergotamine + caffeine	1 mg/100 mg tablet	Start with two tablets. May take one additional tablet every half hour, if needed for full relief. NTE 6 tablets/attack or 10 tablets/week	Partial alpha-adrenergic agonist and antagonist, with direct stimulating effect on smooth muscle of cranial and peripheral blood vessels, causing vasoconstriction. Added caffeine is also vasoconstrictive.	Numbness and tingling of the fingers and toes, weakness in the legs, tachycardia
Frova (frovatriptan)	2.5-mg tablet	2.5-mg tablet; may take a second dose in two hours. NTE 3 tablets/24 hour	A selective 5-HT$_{1B/1D}$ receptor subtype agonist, resulting in cranial blood vessel constriction and a decrease in prostaglandin proinflammatory neuropeptide release.	Common: paresthesias, dizziness, drowsiness, malaise/fatigue. Rare: fatal cardiac events, HTN crisis
Imitrex (sumatriptan)	25-mg, 50-mg, 100-mg tablet; Nasal spray: 20 mg/spray, 5 mg/spray	po: 25–50 mg at onset. May be repeated in 2 hours; NTE 200 mg/day. Nasal: one spray; may repeat once in two hours (maximum 40 mg/day)	A selective 5-HT$_{1D}$ and 5-HT$_{1B}$ agonist, resulting in cranial blood vessel constriction and a decrease in prostaglandin proinflammatory neuropeptide release.	Common: diarrhea, numbness, sinusitis, tinnitus. Rare: fatal cardiac events, HTN crisis.

(Continued)

TABLE 34-13 Drugs Used in the Treatment of Migraines (*Continued*)

Drug Trade/ Generic Name	Availability	Dosage and Administration	MOA	Side Effects and Special Notes
Inderal LA (propranolol) Used for prophylaxis of common migraine headache	60-mg, 80-mg, 120-mg, 160-mg tablet	Dosage varies. Start 80 mg LA UAD 160–240 mg qd	Synthetic nonselective beta-adrenergic receptor-blocking agent causing vasodilation. Used in the treatment of hypertension.	Common: CHF, bradycardia, lightheadedness, insomnia, N/V/D, agranulocytosis. Contraindications: avoid reserpine-containing drugs; may lead to bradycardia and hypotension.
Maxalt (rizatriptan)	5-mg, 10-mg tablet 5-mg, 10-mg oral disintegrating tablet	5 mg or 10 mg in a single dose; may be repeated in 2 hours NTE 30 mg/24 hour	A selective 5-HT$_{1B/1D}$ receptor agonist, resulting in cranial blood vessel constriction and a decrease in prostaglandin proinflammatory neuropeptide release.	Common: chest pain, dry mouth, GI upset, N/V, paresthesia Rare: fatal cardiac events, HTN crisis.
Relpax (eletriptan)	20-mg, 40-mg tablet	UAD 20–40 mg/ 24 hour	A selective 5–HT$_{1B/1D}$ receptor subtype agonist, resulting in cranial blood vessel constriction and a decrease in prostaglandin proinflammatory neuropeptide release.	Common: paresthesias, dizziness, drowsiness, malaise/ fatigue Rare: fatal cardiac events, HTN crisis.
Sansert (methysergide)	2-mg tablet	UAD 4–8 mg qd with meals	Ergot derivative that blocks effects of serotonin, a substance that causes vasoconstriction; also lowers pain threshold. Results in vasodilation along with ability to perceive pain differently.	Rare: May cause retroperitoneal fibrosis, pleuropulmonary fibrosis, and fibrotic thickening of cardiac valves in patients receiving long-term therapy.
Zomig (zolmitriptan)	2.5-mg, 5-mg tablet Nasal spray: 5 mg/ spray	1 mg, 2.5 mg, or 5 mg in a single dose; may be repeated in 2 hours NTE 10 mg/24 hour	A selective 5–HT$_{1B/1D}$ receptor agonist, resulting in cranial blood vessel constriction and a decrease in prostaglandin proinflammatory neuropeptide release.	Monitor hepatically impaired patients.

Oral opioids, the most convenient and least expensive form, have a slower onset of action. Thus, they may remain in the bloodstream longer than necessary, often causing intolerable side effects such as dizziness, sedation, and vomiting.

Oral transmucosal fentanyl citrate (Actiq) is a lozenge attached to a plastic handle, which can take 15 minutes to dissolve. There are six lozenge strengths, ranging from 200 to 1,600 mcg. The patient should not exceed four doses in a 24-hour period.

Adjuvant drugs enhance the pain-relieving actions of opioid analgesics. Antidepressants used in smaller amounts than are prescribed for depression are usual choices for adjuvant drugs. Elavil is an example.

---

adjuvant helping or assisting.

Bone pain associated with bone fracture due to metastasis can be alleviated by bisphosphonates. These bind to the damaged areas of the bone and slow down the destruction caused by cancer cells.

Table 34-14 describes some drugs that are used to relieve pain.

Nonpharmaceutical Pain Relief

A transcutaneous electric nerve stimulation (TENS) unit produces mild electrical currents to stimulate certain nerve endings that, when activated, block pain transmission. It is a proven safe, noninvasive, and effective method for relief of many different types of pain, including neuropathic pain.

TABLE 34-14 Selected Narcotics Used to Treat Pain

Drug Trade/Generic Name	Availability	Dosage and Administration	MOA	Side Effects and Special Notes
Codeine Use as antitussive, prn for mild to severe pain	15-mg, 30-mg, 60-mg tablet 30-mL, 60-mL injection 15 mg/5 mL po oral solution	po, SC, IV, or IM: 15–60 mg q4–6h NTE 360 mg/day	Centrally active analgesic	Common side effects: constipation, dysphoria, drowsiness, N/V, respiratory depression, coma, death
Demerol (meperidine) Post-op and pre-op pain Obstetrical analgesia *Not* for long-term pain management	50-mg, 100-mg tablet 25 mg/1 mL, 50 mg/1 mL, 75 mg/1 mL, 100 mg/1 mL injection 50 mg/5 mL po syrup	50–150 mg IM, SC, or po q3–4h prn	Opioid agonist that binds to the opioid mu receptor sites in the brain, producing analgesia and sedation and increasing tolerance to pain.	Common side effects: constipation, dysphoria, drowsiness, N/V, respiratory depression, coma, death Drug interactions: phenothiazines and many other tranquilizers increase the action of meperidine.
Dilaudid (hydromorphone) May be used prn for pain and breakthrough pain	1-mg, 2-mg, 3-mg, 4-mg tablet 3 mg rectal suppository Single-dose ampules for injection: 1 mg/1 mL, 2 mg/1 mL, 4 mg/1 mL Multiple-dose vials for injection: 2 mg/1 mL–20 mL	po: 2 mg q4–6h prn	Opioid agonist that binds to the opioid mu receptor sites in the brain, producing analgesia and sedation and increasing tolerance to pain.	Common side effects: constipation, dysphoria, drowsiness, N/V, respiratory depression, coma, death
Duragesic (fentanyl transdermal system)	25-mcg, 50-mcg, 75-mcg, 100-mcg patches	One patch q72h	Opioid agonist that binds to the opioid mu receptor sites in the brain, producing analgesia and sedation and increasing tolerance to pain.	Common side effects: constipation, dysphoria, drowsiness, N/V, respiratory depression, coma, death
Numorphan (oxymorphone) Use prn for pain	SD ampule: 1mg/1 mL × 1 mL Injection: 1.5mg/1mL × 5mL MVD vials 5 mg rectal suppository	1–1.5 mg q4–6h prn	Semisynthetic opioid agonist	Common side effects: constipation, dysphoria, drowsiness, N/V, respiratory depression, coma, death

(Continued)

TABLE 34-14 Selected Narcotics Used to Treat Pain *(Continued)*

Drug Trade/ Generic Name	Availability	Dosage and Administration	MOA	Side Effects and Special Notes
Oramorph, MS Contin (morphine sulfate) May be used prn for pain and break-through pain	15-mg, 30-mg, 60-mg, 100-mg, 200-mg tablet (immediate or slow release)	Immediate-release: 5−30 mg q4h prn SR: swallow whole 15−200 mg q12h NTE 400 mg/day	Opioid agonist that binds to the opioid mu receptor sites in the brain, pro-ducing analgesia and sedation and increasing toler-ance to pain.	Common side effects: constipation, dyspho-ria, drowsiness, N/V, respiratory depression, coma, death
Oxycontin (oxycodone) Used for con-tinuous ATC pain, chronic/cancer pain	10-mg, 20-mg, 40-mg, 80-mg, 160-mg CR tablet	CR: 10−160 mg q12h Must be swallowed whole	Opioid agonist that binds to the opioid mu receptor sites in the brain, pro-ducing analgesia and sedation and increasing toler-ance to pain.	Common side effects: constipation, dyspho-ria, drowsiness, N/V, respiratory depression, coma, death
Sublimaze (fentanyl)	0.05 mg/mL	0.05−1 mg IM 30−60 minutes pre-op	Opioid agonist that binds to the opioid mu receptor sites in the brain, pro-ducing analgesia and sedation and increasing toler-ance to pain.	Common side effects: constipation, dysphoria, drowsiness, N/V, respira-tory depression, coma, death

Bell's Palsy

Bell's palsy occurs when the muscles in the face are frozen due to trauma to the body's cranial nerve VII. The frozen state can affect either the right or left side of the face. The condi-tion is not forever, and others cannot catch the paralysis. Preg-nant women in the third trimester and people suffering from diabetes and immunocompromised illness are more prone to Bell's palsy. Drug treatment for the condition is corticosteroids or acyclovir (if the illness is associated with the herpes virus). Pain relief can be given by applying a towel or gel packs to the face and plenty of rest is advised so that the patient can fully recover.

Stroke

A stroke is defined as the disturbance of blood flow or seep-ing out of blood from outer vessel walls. Many strokes can be related to ischemia. Ischemia is the decrease of blood flow to the brain, as blood vessels can be blocked by clots. The ves-sels can also become narrow as well. It is also possible for strokes to be because of a blood vessel hemorrhage. The ves-sels can become damaged or ruptured that causes the tissue to be damaged. Patients who suffer a stroke will need physical and speech therapy along with drug therapy. Some of the drug treatments include antithrombotic medications to reduce dam-age to the brain. Medications used to treat blood blockages and drugs used to lower cholesterol and blood pressure are also given to patients who suffer from a stroke. Antidepressants are also prescribed for depression and insomnia. Aspirin, warfarin, and drugs like Plavix may also be prescribed.

Tourette's Syndrome

Tourette's Syndrome (TS) is a disorder of the brain that is neu-rological. Symptoms include vocal noises called tics, invol-untary movements, jerking, kicking, stomping, strange vocal sounds, rapid blinking, shouting, barking, or clearing the throat often. Repetitive thoughts, compulsions, self-inflicted damage, hitting, and punching of the self can also occur. There are no cures for TS, and the condition is thought to be a disorder in the body's genes that control neurotransmitters within the brain. TS can, however, be controlled by medications. Drugs that may help to cure the symptoms of the condition are Klonopin, Cata-pres patch or tablet, Prolixin, Tenex, Haldol, and Orap.

Summary

The nervous system is a very complex system that interacts with every other system in the body to ensure homeostasis and to regulate the body's responses to internal and external stimuli. The nervous system communicates to all cells in the body through nerve impulses that are conducted from one part of the body to another through the transmission of chemicals called neurotransmitters.

The nervous system is divided into two parts: the CNS and the PNS. The CNS includes the brain, the spinal column, and their nerves. The PNS is likewise divided into two parts: the somatic nervous system, which controls voluntary movement of the body through muscles; and the ANS, which controls involuntary motor functions such as heart rate and digestion.

Diseases and conditions affecting the nervous system include anxiety, depression, BD, Parkinson's disease, alcohol addiction, and seizures. Pain due to injury or cancer also affects the nervous system. This chapter discusses many of these conditions and the most common treatments.

Neuropharmacology (pharmacology related to the nervous system) is one of the most diverse and complicated areas of pharmacology. A pharmacy technician must have a solid understanding of the common diseases affecting the nervous system and the pharmaceutical treatments associated with these diseases.

Chapter Review Questions

1. The smallest functional unit of the nervous system is the
   _____.
   a. spinal cord
   b. nerve
   c. neuron
   d. brain

2. Which of the following is not a part of the central nervous system?
   a. the cerebellum
   b. nerves in the hand
   c. the spinal cord
   d. the cerebrum

3. A person who is out of touch with reality is suffering from
   _____.
   a. depression
   b. dementia
   c. psychosis
   d. mania

4. Which type, or cause, of anxiety often results in a fear of going crazy or fear of death?
   a. general anxiety disorder
   b. panic attack
   c. posttraumatic stress disorder
   d. obsessive–compulsive disorder

5. Which of the following drugs is used to treat hypertension and migraine headache?
   a. Imitrex
   b. Elavil
   c. Sansert
   d. Inderal LA

6. Which of the following is responsible for the body's *fight or flight* reaction?
   a. parasympathetic nervous system
   b. somatic nervous system
   c. central nervous system
   d. sympathetic nervous system

7. Which of the following hypnotics/sedatives is classified as a nonbenzodiazepine?
   a. Amytal
   b. Dalmane
   c. Lunesta
   d. Noctec

8. Which of the following is responsible for the body's *rest and relaxation* response?
   a. parasympathetic nervous system
   b. somatic nervous system
   c. central nervous system
   d. sympathetic nervous system

9. Which of the following medications is *not* known to trigger migraines?
   a. birth control pills
   b. cimetidine
   c. sumatriptan
   d. theophylline

10. Sinemet is indicated in the treatment of _____.
    a. dementia
    b. Parkinson's disease
    c. anxiety
    d. seizures

Critical Thinking Questions

1. How does the body react when the sympathetic nervous system is activated, as compared to when the parasympathetic nervous system is activated?

2. Why can the central nervous system be compared to a computer's CPU?

3. Why use a stimulant in the treatment of patients with ADHD when they are already hyperactive?

Web Challenge

1. Go to http://www.depression.com/understanding_depression.html to learn how depression affects the brain. What did you learn that surprised you?

2. Go to http://faculty.washington.edu/chudler/disorders.html and choose a neurological disorder that you would like to find out more about. Write a one-page summary on this disorder, including an overview of the disorder, signs and symptoms, treatment(s), and prognosis.

References and Resources

Adams, M.P., D.L. Josephson, and L.N. Holland Jr. *Pharmacology for Nurses: A Pathophysiologic Approach.* 4th ed. Upper Saddle River, NJ: Pearson, 2013. Print.

"American Psychiatric Association." http://www.psych.org/public_info/elderly.cfm

"Anxiety Disorders Association of America (ADA)." http://www.adaa.org/

"Atypical Antipsychotics: Mechanism of Action." Web. 15 August 2007. http://www.ncbi.nlm.nih.gov/entrez/query.fcgi?cmd=Retrieve&db=PubMed&list_uids=11873706&dopt=Abstract. Web. 15 August 2007.

"Dementia." http://penta.ufrgs.br/edu/telelab/3/dementia.htm. Web. 15 August 2007.

Drug Facts and Comparisons, 2013 ed. St. Louis: Wolters Kluwer. 2012. Print

"Effexor XR Approved in the U.S. for Anxiety, March 12, 1999." http://www.pslgroup.com/dg/ebe9a.htm. Web. 15 August 2007.

Family Practice Notebook. "Smoking Cessation—Tobacco Cessation." http://www.fpnotebook.com/PSY52.htm. Web. 15 August 2007.

Grieve, M. *A Modern Herbal.* 1931. http://www.botanical.com/botanical/mgmh/g/guaran43.html

Holland, N. and M.P. Adams. *Core Concepts in Pharmacology.* 3rd ed. Upper Saddle River, NJ: Pearson, 2010.

"Internet Mental Health—Monograph for Lamotrigine." http://www.mentalhealth.com/drug/p30-l06.html#Head_1. Web. 1 August 2013.

Mallin, R. "Smoking Cessation: Integration of Behavioral and Drug Therapies." *American Family Physician.* 15 (2002): 1107–1115. Print. http://www.aafp.org/afp/20020315/1107.html. Web. 15 August 2007.

"Mechanism of Action of Atypical Antipsychotic Drugs: Critical Analysis." http://www.ncbi.nlm.nih.gov/entrez/query.fcgi?cmd=Retrieve&db=PubMed&list_uids=8935797&dopt=Abstract. Web. 15 August 2007.

"National Institute of Mental Health." http://www.nimh.nih.gov. Web. 1 August 2013.

"Schizophrenia Information." http://www.schizophrenia.com/newsletter/buckets/hypo.html. Web. 1 August 2013.

"Stimulants." http://www.drugabuse.gov/ResearchReports/Prescription/prescription4.html. Web. 15 August 2007.

The Merck Manual of Diagnosis and Therapy. Section 15. Psychiatric Disorders, Chapter 189. Mood Disorders—Treatment. http://www.merck.com/mrkshared/mmanual/section15/chapter189/189d.jsp Web. 15 August 2007.

Tropical Plant Database. "Guaraná *(Paullinia cupana).*" http://www.rain-tree.com/guarana.htm. Web. 15 August 2007.

Tuen, C. "Neuroland." http://neuroland.com/psy/anxiety.htm. Web. 15 August 2007.

Uchiumi, M., S. Isawa, M. Suzuki, and M. Murasaki. "The Effects of Zolpidem and Zopiclone on Daytime Sleepiness and Psychomotor Performance." http://www.biopsychiatry.com/zolpidemvzopiclone.htm. Web. 15 August 2007.

SECTION V

Special Topics

35. Medication Errors

36. Workplace Safety and Infection Control

37. Special Considerations for Pediatric and Geriatric Patients

38. Biopharmaceuticals

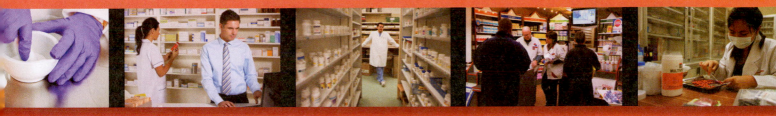

CHAPTER 35

Medication Errors

LEARNING OBJECTIVES

After completing this chapter, you should be able to:

- List and describe the five rights of medication administration.

- Outline and define the various categories of medication errors.

- Discuss key statistics related to medication errors and pharmacy practice.

- Identify look-alike, sound-alike drugs and tall-man lettering.

- Review specific case studies of medication errors, and discuss the causes, outcomes, and recommended preventable solutions.

- Outline and describe best practices for preventing medication errors.

- List various agencies involved in the monitoring and reporting of medication errors and describe their role(s).

KEY TERMS

extra dose error, p. 617

omission error, p. 617

unordered or unauthorized drug error, p. 617

wrong dosage form error, p. 617

wrong dose error, p. 617

wrong route errors, p. 617

wrong time errors, p. 617

INTRODUCTION

Medication errors are a very serious problem in the medical field and, unfortunately, happen quite frequently. For example, suppose that a pharmacy has a 1% prescription error rate. In most professions, this would be considered a very low number and would be acceptable. However, if the pharmacy fills 10,000 prescriptions per year, it would make 100 prescription errors. Although this may seem like a small number of errors, any error can be quite serious and even deadly; thus, *any* error in pharmacy should be considered unacceptable. This section discusses why it is important for a pharmacy technician to know and be able to identify the different types of medication errors, and to learn how to avoid them.

The National Coordinating Council for Medication Error Reporting and Prevention defines a *medication error* as "any preventable event that may cause or lead to inappropriate medication use or patient harm while the medication is in the control of the health care professional, patient, or consumer. Such events may be related to professional practice, health care products, procedures, and systems, including prescribing; order communication; product labeling, packaging, and nomenclature; compounding; dispensing; distribution; administration; education; monitoring; and use." Medication errors can occur at any point in the medication distribution process, from the moment the prescription is written until the medication is ultimately administered to the patient. However, although everyone involved in the process must take precautions to detect and prevent medication errors, the majority of responsibility and blame seems—perhaps too often—to fall on pharmacy staff.

The Five Rights

Let us review the Five Rights of medication administration presented earlier in Chapter 3, as they can greatly decrease the occurrence of medication errors. The Five Rights are the following:

1. Right patient—the drug must always go to the correct patient.
2. Right drug—the right drug must always be chosen.
3. Right route—the drug must be given via the correct route of administration. If the correct drug and dose are given, but via the wrong route, a medication error may occur.
4. Right dose—the patient must receive the right dose. A dose that is too high or too low is considered a medication error.
5. Right time—the patient must receive the medication within the prescribed time frame. Many inpatient institutions have a time window within which the medication can be given; any administration outside that window is considered a medication error. For example, if a dose is due at 9:00 A.M., the nurse may be permitted to give the medication any time between 8:30 A.M. and 9:30 A.M. Medication given outside the set parameters is considered a medication error.

Two new, additional *rights* of medication administration are outside of the five traditional rights. The first is the *right technique*. The correct technique must be used when preparing the drug (e.g., IV products must be made in sterile environments). The second is the *right documentation*. Correct documentation must be completed (whether by the doctor, nurse, pharmacy, etc.), or a medication error may take place.

Types of Errors

According to the National Coordinating Council for Medication Error Reporting Program, a medication error is defined as "[a]ny preventable event that may cause or lead to inappropriate medication use or patient harm while the medication is in the control of the health care professional, patient or consumer. Such events may be related to professional practice, health care products, procedures and systems, including prescribing, order communication, product labeling, packaging and nomenclature, compounding, dispensing, distribution, administration, education, monitoring and use."

The American Hospital Association lists the following as some common types of medication errors:

- Incomplete patient information, such as not knowing about patients' allergies, other medicines they are taking, previous diagnoses, and lab results.

---

info

Little Changes in History of Reasons for Errors

The 1848 Code of Ethics of the Philadelphia College of Pharmacy identified four specific reasons for errors such as illegible handwriting on prescriptions, from which many errors do occur. These still exist some 163 years later. The four reasons for these errors were:

1. Poor handwriting of prescribing physicians.
2. Improper and mistaken use of medical and pharmaceutical abbreviations and selection of wrong drugs with various synonyms.
3. Poor conditions of the environment making it easy to lose concentration while dispensing and selecting the medications correctly.
4. Poor training of pharmacy staff and lack of follow through by the pharmacist in the dispensing process.

---

unordered or unauthorized drug error   the administration or dispensing of a dose of medication that was never ordered for that patient.

extra dose error   the administration or dispensing of a dose given in excess of the total doses ordered by a physician.

omission error   the failure to administer or dispense an ordered dose.

wrong dose error   the administration or dispensing of any dose that contains the wrong number of preformed dosage units of is at least 17% greater or less than the correct dosage.

wrong route errors   the administration of a dosage to a patient using a different route than was ordered.

wrong time errors   the administration of a dosage more than 30 minutes before or after the scheduled administration time, unless there is an acceptable reason for the time difference.

wrong dosage form error   the administration or dispensing of a dose form that is different than that ordered by the physician.

- Unavailable drug information such as lack of up-to-date clinical warnings.
- Miscommunication of drug orders, which can be caused by poor handwriting, confusion between drugs with similar names, misuse of zeroes and decimal points, confusion of metric and other dosing units, and inappropriate abbreviations.
- Lack of appropriate labeling as a drug is prepared and repackaged into smaller units.
- Environmental factors, such as lighting, heat, noise, and interruptions, that can distract health professionals from their medical tasks.

The research-based definition of a medication administration error is any deviation from the prescriber's written order, or as entered into a computer system by the prescriber. Medication errors are typically viewed as being related to drug administration, while dispensing errors refer to mistakes made by pharmacy staff when distributing medications to nursing units or directly to patients in an ambulatory, or outpatient, pharmacy setting. A medication error has been defined to include errors in the process of ordering or delivering a medication, whereas errors by the ordering prescriber have typically been labeled prescribing errors. Error category definitions that have been tested in research studies are described here. Categories may not be mutually exclusive; therefore, the reader is cautioned that rates for different error types cannot always be simply added to obtain an overall error rate.

An **unordered or unauthorized drug error** is defined as the administration of a dose of medication that was never ordered for that patient. This is also called a wrong drug error. An **extra dose error** is counted if a dose is given in excess of the total number of times ordered by the physician, such as a dose given on the basis of an expired order, after a drug has been discontinued, or after a drug has been put on hold. If a patient fails to receive a dose of medication that was ordered, an **omission error** is noted if no attempt was made to administer the dose. Reasons for the omission should be sought, such as doses withheld according to policy (e.g., nothing by mouth before surgery).

A **wrong dose error** occurs when any dose is given that contains the wrong number of preformed dosage units (such as tablets) or was, in the judgment of the observer, more than 17% greater or less than the correct dosage. Some researchers use a narrower definition of wrong dose errors for injectable doses that are measured by the nurse—any dose that is more than 10% different from the correct dosage administration would be in error. Wrong dose errors are counted for ointments, topical solutions, and similar medications only when the dose was quantitatively specified by the physician (e.g., in inches of ointment). **Wrong route errors** are typically defined as those situations where a medication is administered to the patient using a different route than was ordered, an example of which would be the oral administration of a drug ordered for intramuscular use. Also included in this category are doses given in the wrong site, such as the left eye instead of the right eye. **Wrong time errors** are typically defined

as the administration of a dose more than 30 minutes (or 60 minutes depending on the site) before or after the scheduled administration time, unless there is an acceptable reason for this time difference. Acceptable reasons include situations where the physician has ordered that the patient not consume anything by mouth (NPO), or when the patient is off the floor at a diagnostic test or in surgery. The hospital's standardized dose administration schedule should be used to determine the time at which a regularly scheduled dose should be given. The schedule programmed into the pharmacy's computer system can be used to define correct administration times, but input from the nurse and patient preference should be accommodated. A **wrong dosage form error** involves the administration of a dose form that is different from that ordered by the physician, provided the physician specified or implied a particular form. If an extended-release tablet is crushed, a wrong dosage form error is counted, and it is likely that the timing of the release of the drug has been destroyed.

Age-Related Errors

Although medication errors may occur with patients of any age, pediatric patients are especially vulnerable to errors. They more often suffer from incorrect dosing, particularly dosages based on incorrect computations and wrong dosage intervals. Pediatric patients pose a unique challenge to pharmacy staff. Preverbal children cannot say if they have problems such as pain or nausea. The calculations often involve very small quantities, so even a slight error is potentially more serious. Calculations for drugs such as digoxin, epinephrine, theophylline, and narcotics should be checked and rechecked.

EXAMPLE 35.1

Digoxin is available in tablet form as 0.125 mg, 0.25 mg, and 0.5 mg. The recommended doses are as follows:

Infant: 25–35 mcg/kg
Children 1–24 months: 35–60 mcg/kg
Children 2–5 years: 30–40 mcg
Children 5–10 years: 20–35 mcg
Children over 10 years: 10–15 mcg

Many drugs that are used to treat pediatric illnesses are available as over-the-counter (OTC) products but do not contain pediatric dosing indications or dosing guidelines. This greatly increases the risk of errors. As discussed previously, children vary in weight, organ maturity, and physiological differences that affect their metabolism and excretion rates. Medication improvement programs are necessary and should include every member of the health care team, including the family member or caregiver, the pharmacy technician, the pharmacist, and the physician. These improvement programs should also include quality performance activities and drug adverse reaction reporting.

Statistics

More people die each year from medical errors than motor vehicle accidents, breast cancer, or AIDS. Of the estimated 98,000 deaths occurring from medical errors, more than 7,000, or approximately 7%, are a result of medication errors. The average rate for medication errors is 1.8%. That is nearly two prescriptions in every 100 that are dispensed. This translates to 60 million errors in the three billion prescriptions filled annually in the United States.

According to a Harvard study, pharmacy dispensing mistakes account for approximately 12% of all medication errors. The balance of medication errors are a result of transcription (12%), nurse administration (38%), and physician ordering mistakes (39%).

Technology and Errors

Another common cause for pharmacy error is computer problems or errors. Shorthand directions are often mistyped, and then misread, causing more work problems. Sometimes, the computer does not recognize the shorthand abbreviations being used. Even when the directions are typed out fully, a mistake may go unnoticed. For example, when choosing a drug from the database, it is easy to pick the wrong one when several medications start with the same letters. It is just as easy to choose the wrong strength when there are several strengths listed for a particular medication.

Be sure to read what is typed as you are typing it, and then again when you produce the label. Compare the original prescription with the patient record and the printed label. Double check the medication on the label for accuracy. Read the label fully one last time before the pharmacist does the final check. Pharmacists learn the *triple check* process in pharmacy school, and pharmacy technicians should also be trained to follow this procedure.

Look-Alike–Sound-Alike Drugs

Drugs with similar spelling or similar sounding names can result in name confusion. The same is true when working with chemicals with similar names. Table 35-1 provides a brief list of examples of medications with similar sounding names that have been involved in medication errors.

Generic drug manufacturers will typically have a standard design on their label. This can be a problem when the drugs are stored alphabetically, because two different drugs from the same manufacturer may be stored side by side, with the only difference in appearance being the actual name of the drug. When a drug starts with a few of the same letters in the beginning, it is easy to grab the wrong one from the shelf. Likewise, several strengths of a generic medication may all be from the same manufacturer.

The FDA created a solution to this label confusion called *Tall-Man Lettering* to help flag potential problem medications with similar names. When they receive multiple reports for a particular set of drugs, they insist that drug manufacturers change their labels to incorporate the *Tall-Man Lettering*.

Here are just two examples of drugs labeled in this style:

EPINEPHrine and ePHEDrine

PREDnisone and predNISOLONE

Top 10 Drugs that Cause Medication Errors

According to a nationwide study involving every type of practice setting of pharmacy, these are the top 10 drugs associated with medication errors:

1. Insulin
2. Albuterol
3. Morphine
4. Potassium chloride
5. Heparin
6. Cefazolin
7. Warfarin
8. Furosemide
9. Levofloxacin
10. Vancomycin

The top three drug classes for medication errors are the following:

1. Central nervous system medications
   a. Opioid analgesics
   b. Sedatives/hypnotics/anxiolytics
   c. Anticonvulsants
2. Cardiovascular
   a. Beta-blockers
   b. Diuretics
   c. Calcium-channel blockers
3. Hormones/synthetics/modifiers
   a. Insulin
   b. Anti-diabetic agents
   c. Adrenal corticosteroids

TABLE 35-1 Examples of Look-Alike–Sound-Alike Drugs

Zyrtec	Zantac
Flomax	Volmax
Valcyte	Valtrex
Prednisolone	Prednisolone sodium phosphate
Metronidazole	Metronidazole benzoate
Phenobarbital	Phenobarbital sodium

Case Studies

Throughout the textbook, Profile in Practice have been presented to provide opportunities for you to reflect and discuss real-world applications. In this chapter, we have changed the format to include Case Studies—accounts of actual medication errors—for your reflection and discussion. For each of the following Case Studies, consider:

1. What was the cause of the error?
2. What was the impact of the error?
3. What could have been done to prevent the error?

Glynase/Ritalin Mixup

A South Carolina pharmacist dispenses Glynase 6 mg instead of the Ritalin that was prescribed. The patient, a seven-year-old girl, ingests 16 times the recommended adult starting dose. She suffered permanent brain damage and is mentally retarded. The jury awarded 16 million dollars to provide care for the child and as punitive damages for the drugstore chain.

mcg/mg Mixup

A Pittsburgh pharmacist mistranscribes a telephone prescription that calls for two 0.25-mcg Rocatrol pills four times per day. Confusing milligrams and micrograms, she writes down two 0.5-mg pills four times per day. The patient received more than 2,000 times the recommended maximum dose. He is now totally disabled and suffers from complex partial seizures.

Cycrin/Coumadin Mixup

A Florida pharmacist dispenses Cycrin, a female hormone, instead of the Coumadin that was prescribed. The patient took the drug for 11 days before his wife discovered the error. Two days later, he suffered a stroke, followed by a heart attack. Still in a coma, he resides in a constant care facility. The insurance company for the drugstore chain that was responsible agreed to pay six million dollars in order to settle the suit.

Tainted IV Bags in Alabama

Alabama health officials have identified a compounding pharmacy in Birmingham as the source of the *Serratia marcescens* bacteria outbreak that affected 19 patients in six hospitals.

The CDC and the Alabama Department of Health (ADPH) have found that the patients became infected with *S. marcescens* after receiving total parental nutrition (TPN) IV solutions from Meds IV Pharmacy in Birmingham. Nine of the 19 infected patients have died. The earliest reported case occurred in January, according to a statement released by the ADPH on Tuesday, but it was not until March that health officials recognized a pattern.

"Illness with *Serratia marcescens* bacteremia in March occurred in approximately 35% of patients receiving TPN from Meds IV," ADPH reported in a follow-up statement released on Wednesday. "The affected Alabama hospitals are in the process of contacting the patients and their families who received the TPN associated with this outbreak."

Meds IV recalled all its compounded IV products and discontinued production on March 24. The pharmacy's website also is currently offline. According to a statement from Meds IV president William "Tim" Rogers that The Birmingham News published, the pharmacy is cooperating with the investigation.

The family of Mary Ellen Kise, who died at Baptist Health Systems hospital in Prattville, Alabama after receiving the tainted IV bag, filed a lawsuit against Meds IV on Thursday. Health officials at this time cannot determine whether the bacteremia was directly responsible for the patient deaths. All nine patients were seriously ill at the time they received the tainted IV bag. Reuters also reported that a law firm in Birmingham has at least three more cases pending against Meds IV.

Emily Jerry Case Study

At nearly 18 months old, Emily Jerry was diagnosed with a yolk sac tumor. The tumor, which was roughly the size of a grapefruit, was located in her abdomen. Emily's cancer was not only treatable but also curable. After months of surgeries, testing, and harsh chemotherapy sessions, the doctors declared that the tumor was gone.

On her second birthday, Emily went to the hospital to begin her last chemotherapy session as a measure to ensure that no traces of cancer remained in her body. Everything changed on the third day of this final chemotherapy session. Emily awoke from an afternoon nap groggy and moaning that her head hurt. She attempted to take a sip of her mom's Coke but started screaming, "Mommy, my head, my head hurts! MY HEAD HURTS!," while grabbing a hold of the sides of her head. She went limp and began vomiting abundantly. Emily was rushed to the intensive care unit and was on life support within an hour.

Emily suffered massive brain damage and died as a result of a medication error. The pharmacy technician who had prepared Emily's final chemotherapy bag decided to not use a standard bag of sodium chloride solution. She filled a plastic bag concentrated with 23.4% sodium chloride, whereas it was supposed to be less than 1%. The human body is not able to withstand such a high concentration of sodium, and so Emily died a painful, agonizing death caused by salt toxicity.

The pharmacy technician responsible for the error claims that she knew something was not right, but she was not sure. She sought advice from the pharmacist, who was allegedly distracted by a personal phone call. The pharmacist released the toxic solution for administration, which ultimately cost him the loss of his license and incarceration. At that time, pharmacy technicians were not required to be registered with the Ohio State Board of Pharmacy, nor were they required to complete any standardized training, education, or certification. Shortly after this event, the pharmacy technician responsible for the error was employed as a technician supervisor/trainer at one of the largest chain retail pharmacies in the United States. The State Board of Pharmacy had no legal authority to take action against the technician or prevent her from working in another pharmacy. As a result of this tragedy, legislation has since been passed in Ohio, requiring pharmacy technician registration and certification exams.

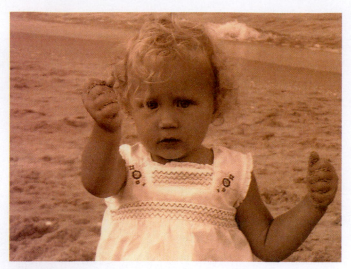

FIGURE 35-1 Emily Jerry

Preventing Medication Errors and the Role of The Pharmacy Technician

Pharmacy technicians are responsible for many of the activities involved in the filling and dispensing of prescription medications. With the evolution of pharmacy technician roles, their duties include more and more of the responsibilities that once were performed only by a pharmacist. With these added expectations, it is imperative that pharmacy technicians accomplish the tasks set before them without error.

Developing technicians to possess and utilize the necessary skills required of them, along with impressing upon them the importance of their role, can provide opportunities to reduce medication errors. Every pharmacy technician should be thoroughly and properly trained and their abilities assessed by the staff educator/trainer. The staffing of pharmacy technicians who have been trained and tested for competency will promote a work environment designed for reducing medication errors.

Pharmacy technicians play an important role in the prevention of medication errors, and the following section discusses some preventive measures they can take. Even though pharmacy technicians work under the direct supervision of a pharmacist, they should always ensure that a medication is correct before a final check takes place. Remember, a team is only as good as its players.

Hospital-Wide Action to Prevent Medication Errors

Within the hospital setting, the following steps can help prevent medication errors:

- Provide adequate staffing.
- Establish a formulary system with therapeutic uses and evaluations for pediatric uses of certain drugs.
- Track medication errors through formal systems and report errors to families.
- Encourage a team environment.

Pharmacy Actions to Prevent Medication Errors

Medication errors exist when breakdowns occur in the systems that have been developed for handling and processing drugs. Whether it is in the prescribing and ordering phase or the distribution and administering phase, teamwork is vital to prevent breaks in the system. Usually, the errors are *multi-factorial*, meaning you cannot take a single incident and blame it on a single factor. No matter the industry, there is always room for improvement.

Pharmacy technicians can use past errors to suggest improvements to their information technology (IT) department or the pharmacy manager to supplement their pharmacy's computer systems with better pharmacy software. Incorporating technology across the entire medication management spectrum should be your organization's target goal. Merely purchasing the latest and greatest software automation systems is not enough. Without sufficient planning and training, system failures can occur across wide spectrums of a health care organization, especially in the pharmacy. There is no room for instrumentation error in a professional health care establishment.

Pharmacists and CPhTs face environmental, physical and emotional stressors in their careers and must accommodate the needs of patients without losing their patience. Patients are usually there for a good reason. They are ill and tired of waiting. They had to wait for their MRI appointment, their doctor appointment, their specialist appointment, and then finally, they have to wait again at pharmacy. They get frustrated, and sometimes they lash out at pharmacy technicians. When pharmacy technicians let this get to them, it can break their concentration, resulting in slips that can subsequently lead to errors in processing prescriptions or oversight of a labeling error. This is especially prevalent at peak times where demand is high on all pharmacy team members. Pharmacy technicians must not let themselves be overcome by stress. When in doubt, take extra cautionary measures during peak pharmacy hours such as reading a prescription more than once (three times or more if necessary). If there is anything unclear about the timing, the drug being prescribed, the dosage, and the number of pills or their ingredients (such as an ingredient that may cause an allergic reaction in the patient), contact the patient's medical provider before filling the prescription to prevent a possible double error (a provider/pharmacy error). Always feel free to ask the pharmacist or pharmacy manager for help at any time regarding a prescription question. It is better to ask questions than make mistakes, because pharmacy technician errors can cause serious harm, illness, or death.

The ultimate tool in preventing medication errors will always be education: education for the pharmacist, education for the pharmacy technician, and education for the patient. Patient education should be encouraged with extensive pamphlets provided by physicians/health care providers at their appointments and Internet information to help them understand their newly diagnosed or chronic medical conditions and the medications used to treat them. To help minimize medication errors, pharmacies and health care providers should urge their pharmacy staff to continue their education through mandatory continuing education courses and training in both automated pharmacy technology and certification training courses (IV, compounding, etc.). Pharmacy technicians can also continue their education on their own by keeping up with news reports, safety advisories, and continuing education programs.

Within the pharmacy, the pharmacy staff can take the following steps to help prevent medication errors:

- Recheck calculations against weight-based dosage ranges.
- Reconfirm confusing orders with physician/pharmacist.
- Check for current allergies and drug compatibilities.
- Prepare drugs in a clean environment, and avoid interruptions during preparation.
- Obtain the original written order before dispensing.
- If possible, use a unit-dose or ready-to-use medication form.
- Do not store sound-alike or look-alike drugs next to each other.

Pharmacy Education and Communication

Establishing best practices for ongoing education and disseminating information among the pharmacy staff can also help prevent medication errors. Steps may include the following:

- Check medication calculations with another team member, especially if unusual in dosage or amount to be given.
- Confirm patient identity and pertinent information before dispensing.
- Educate patients or caregivers about medication before dispensing.
- Implement a tracking system for errors, and communicate with all staff involved on a regular basis to review.
- Answer all questions from caregivers, and listen attentively to them.
- Double-check all orders.
- Always use proper dispensing utensils, such as droppers or medicine cups; do not use inexact utensils, such as household teaspoons, for measurement or dispensing.

Monitoring and Reporting Errors

The Institute of Medicine (IOM) has focused on the identification of a common medication error of illegible handwriting. It firmly believes that with the use of e-prescribing (eRx) a great

number of errors can be eliminated. A
handwriting from a federal perspective
the Medicare Improvements for Patient
2008 authorizes new and separate incer
gible professionals who are electronic
Incentive Program went into effect on
tronic prescribers could earn a 2% incentive payment during the current year. Paying physicians to prescribe electronically on their Medicare Part B claims may encourage them to also prescribe and transmit non-Medicare prescriptions electronically, which should overall reduce a great number of potential medication errors due to handwriting mistakes. eRx participation is now on a voluntary basis, but was with a penalty in the year 2012 for prescribers who do not eRx for Medicare and Medicaid patients. Some doctors do not feel *up to par* when it comes to eRx. They may feel as though they are not fully knowledgeable in eRx or do not have enough updated technology to practice this updated prescribing practice.

The IOM also found that errors can occur through the use of abbreviations and believes that most abbreviations should be avoided. Certain abbreviations are misinterpreted today as easily as they were 150 years ago. The Institute for Safe Medication Practices (ISMP) has identified many easily misinterpreted abbreviations that are directly linked to patient harm. These can be viewed on the ISMP website, www.ismp.org, which will be discussed in the Web Challenge.

The FDA also receives medication error reports on marketed human drugs (including prescription, generic, and OTC drugs) and nonvaccine biological products and devices. Such events may be related to professional practice, health care products, procedures, systems, prescribing, order communication, product labeling, packaging, nomenclature, compounding, dispensing, distribution, administration, education, monitoring, and use.

In 1992, the FDA began monitoring medication error reports that were forwarded to FDA from the United States Pharmacopeia (USP) and ISMP. The agency also reviews MedWatch reports for possible medication errors. Currently, medication errors are reported to the FDA as manufacturer reports (adverse drug events resulting in serious injury and for which a medication error may be a component), direct contact reports (MedWatch), or reports from USP or ISMP. The Division of Medication Errors and Technical Support includes a medication error prevention program staffed with pharmacists and support personnel. Among their many duties are program staff review medication error reports that are sent to the USP Medication Errors Reporting Program (MERP) and MedWatch, which evaluate causality and analyze the data to provide feedback to others at the FDA.

info

More Ways to Prevent Medication Errors

Other ways to prevent errors include using a zero before a decimal whole number (e.g., 0.25 instead of .25), not using abbreviations in names of drugs, and using calibrated syringes or droppers for dosing.

❝ Workplace Wisdom Institute for Safe Medication Practices

One of the leading organizations for monitoring and reporting medication errors, as well as industry education and resources is the ISMP. To learn more, go to **www.ismp.org**. ❞

ummary

Medication error rate continues to rise despite our knowledge, training, and awareness of this situation. Despite awareness of the problem, the problem not only continues to exist, it is increasing.

It is important to learn the areas where medication errors occur. We must understand the problem areas in the practice of filling and dispensing prescription medications and be aware of breakdowns in training or communication in order to avoid mistakes. Making a conscience effort will result in

the reduction of medication errors regardless of which type of pharmacy setting is involved.

It is beneficial for everyone involved in the pharmacy profession to report medication errors to appropriate agencies so that everyone can learn from these mistakes. These reports can be made anonymously or with full detail of the parties involved. Either way the error will be documented, studied, and published if necessary.

Chapter Review Questions

1. A medication administration error is defined as _____.
   a. an incorrect formulation from the pharmaceutical manufacturer
   b. an administered dose of medication that deviates from the physician's order
   c. absence of a medication administration record during drug administration
   d. an incorrect drug or dose compounded by the pharmacy

2. What is the FDA's solution for drugs with similar names?
   a. tall-man lettering
   b. underlining the name of the drug
   c. italicizing the name
   d. highlighting the name

3. Pharmacy dispensing errors account for what percentage of all medication errors?
   a. 38
   b. 12
   c. 19
   d. 7

4. The medication error where a patient has failed to receive a dose is called _____.
   a. unauthorized drug error
   b. extra dose error
   c. wrong time error
   d. omission error

5. MERP is an acronym that stands for _____.
   a. Medication Education Reporting Program
   b. Medication Errors Reporting Program
   c. Management Error Responsibility Program
   d. Magnetic Emergent Resonating Program

6. According to the National Coordinating Council for Medication Error Reporting Program, a medication error is _____.
   a. any error that cannot be prevented
   b. an event that may cause or lead to inappropriate medication use that should not be addressed by or mentioned to the health care professional, patient, or consumer
   c. any preventable event that may cause or lead to inappropriate medication use or patient harm while the medication is in the control of the health care professional, patient, or consumer
   d. unable to be defined

7. A patient receives Claforan 1 gm IV 24 hours after it was discontinued. If this is an error, what type of error is it?
   a. unauthorized drug error
   b. extra dose error
   c. wrong time error
   d. omission error

8. Which of the following drugs is not considered one of the top 10 drugs associated with medication errors?
   a. albuterol
   b. cefadroxyl
   c. furosemide
   d. insulin

9. Why do medication errors occur?
   a. imperfections in automated pharmacy software
   b. distractions
   c. lack of knowledge, communication, and/or training on the part of the person who made the error
   d. all of the above

10. The average error rate for medication errors is _____.
    a. 0.018%
    b. 0.18%
    c. 1.8%
    d. 18%

Critical Thinking Questions

1. If pharmacists are required to provide the final *check* on all prescriptions, in what ways can a pharmacy technician be held liable for contributing to a medication error?

2. What role do ethics play in reporting medication errors?

3. Do you feel that pharmacists or pharmacy technicians should be held liable, criminally, for medication errors that result in death or serious injury? Defend your position.

Web Challenge

1. Visit the ISMP website, www.ismp.org, search for, and print out a copy of the following: (a) ISMP's list of high-alert medications, (b) ISMP's list of error-prone abbreviations, symbols and dose designations, and (c) the ASSESS-ERR medication system worksheet.

2. Search the Internet for news articles on recent, or local, pharmacy or medication errors. Write a summary of the incident, including the classification of the type of error and recommendation(s) on how it could have been prevented on the basis of the material covered in this chapter.

References and Resources

Cohen, M. *Medication Errors*. 2nd ed. Washington, DC: APhA, 2007. Print.

Institute of Medicine. *Preventing Medication Errors*. Eds. P. Aspden, J.A. Wolcott, J.L. Bootman, and L.R. Cronenwett. Washington, DC: National Academies Press, 2007. Print.

"Medication Errors." http://www.fda.gov/drugs/drugsafety/medicationerrors/default.htm. Web. 1 August 2013.

Pavlic, B. "Solutions for Common Medication Errors." *Today's Technician*. 5 (6) (2005). Print.

Tinervia, J. "Medication Errors Update—How Can the Pharmacy Technician Help."
Today's Technician. 11 (4) (2011). Print.

Velgos, B.Z. "Reducing Medication Errors in the Pharmacy." *Today's Technician*. 11 (4) (2010). Print.

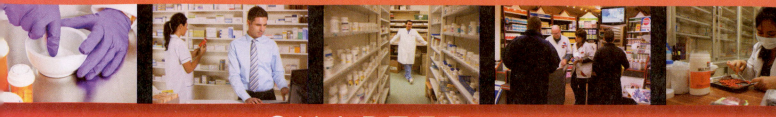

CHAPTER 36

Workplace Safety and Infection Control

LEARNING OBJECTIVES

After completing this chapter, you should be able to:

- Define and describe the importance of workplace safety.

- Explain the difference between an accident and an incident.

- Outline the four key elements of workplace safety.

- Identify specific workplace safety concerns related to pharmacy practice.

- Outline the key requirements as prescribed by OSHA, state regulations, and institutional policies.

- Define and describe infection control.

KEY TERMS

accident p. 625
aseptic isolator p. 626
incident p. 625
infection control, p. 624
workplace safety p. 624

INTRODUCTION

The concerns of **workplace safety** and **infection control** are of great importance for pharmacy technicians. It is critical to understand that workplace safety is a must whether the technician is working in an institutional or community-based pharmacy practice setting. There are a variety of rules and best practices regarding workplace safety and infection control, for pharmacy professionals, based on the specific state, practice setting, and institution, in addition to federal regulations. In this chapter, we will review the major provisions of workplace safety and infection control measures.

---

workplace safety a category of management that includes workplace analysis, hazard prevention and control and safety and health training and education.

infection control policies and procedures designed to monitor and control the transmission of disease.

Workplace Safety

As a technician, you may be wondering what exactly is workplace safety in a pharmacy. Generally speaking, workplace safety refers to the prevention of injury and illness of employees, and volunteers, in the workplace. Two key workplace safety definitions to distinguish are **accident** and **incident**. An accident refers to a specific event that results in unintended harm or damage, whereas an incident is an event that has the potential to result in unintended harm or damage. Workplace safety covers a variety of elements, including:

- Management leadership and employee involvement
- Workplace analysis
- Hazard prevention and control
- Safety and health training and education

Management Leadership and Employee Involvement

Workplace safety must be an integral part of an organization's culture, equal in importance as the organization's finances, efficiency, quality, and security. This requires involvement and communication on both the part of the employer, or corporate headquarters, and the employees. In highly successful and effective organizations, management will involve employees in safety activities and discussions on safety and health issue policies.

Workplace Analysis

In order to ensure optimum workplace safety, an analysis of all workplace conditions should be performed on a regular and timely basis to identify or eliminate existing and potential hazards. In addition to analyzing the workplace for potential hazards, workplace design should also be considered. The primary goal of workplace design is to maximize the productivity potential of employees, while avoiding errors or accidents, over extended periods of time.

Hazard Prevention and Control

Health and safety hazards exist in every work environment, but there are additional hazards affiliated with working in health care environments, such as pharmacies. Hazard prevention and control can include special equipment, maintenance, supplies, personal protective equipment (PPE), policies, procedures, and regular training. Specific areas of hazard prevention and control for pharmacies are covered in more detail later in this chapter.

Safety and Health Training and Education

Pharmacies, like other businesses, should have a safety manual so that pharmacy technicians can review work policies and proper safety procedures. Employees will sometimes be asked

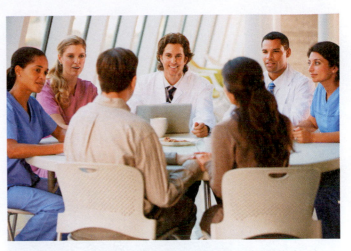

FIGURE 36-1 Safety meetings are used to establish and review work policies and safety procedures.
Source: Monkey Business Images/Shutterstock

to read and sign declarations saying they understand safety procedures and will abide by all the rules. In addition, safety meetings are sometimes held in the workplace to remind and inform technicians of new safety rules and procedures. Meetings like these can also be held as part of new employee orientations as well (see Figure 36-1).

Workplace training sessions must be available to all employees in the pharmacy. The training sessions should always be *at no cost* to employees in the pharmacy. Training should be available at the beginning of employment and throughout the duration of employment as well. Sessions of training are usually provided annually if there is a need for continual initial explanation of procedures. Following proper protocol and following the rules can ensure less mishaps and more productive workflow for all involved in the workplace as well as putting safety first.

The pharmacist and pharmacy technician both play a role in responding to workplace emergencies, such as injury, heart attack, stroke, or other health-related concerns that may affect a customer, co-worker, or other person in the vicinity. The facility should maintain a well-stocked first aid kit and keep the phone numbers for the fire department, police, poison control, local hospital, and emergency medical services in a central location. The pharmacy staff should receive basic first aid training and ideally obtain training and certification in basic life support (BLS) through a program that is accredited by the American Heart Association.

Special Areas for Handling Hazardous Drugs

Pharmacy technicians come in contact with different potentially hazardous chemicals and mixtures when compounding. Special care should be taken when working with these chemicals and drugs. Proper PPE should be worn at all times when working with hazardous materials, chemicals, or body fluids (see Figure 36-2). Hands should be washed before and after applying gloves. Drugs can be absorbed through the skin and be absorbed in the body's system, which can lead to sickness or even death. Protective gear usually consists of latex gloves, a dressing gown, covered mask, and mesh cap to cover the hair.

---

accident a specific event that results in unintended harm or damage

incident a specific event that has the potential to result in unintended harm or damage

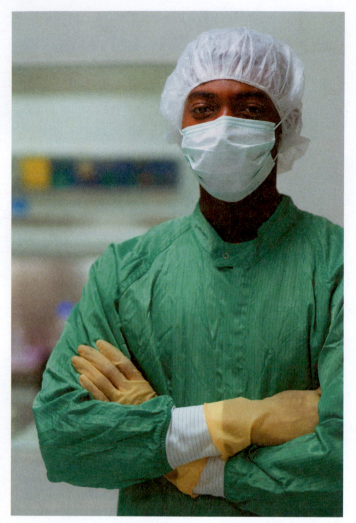

FIGURE 36-2 A pharmacy technician wearing PPE.
Source: Diego Cervo/Shutterstock

Women should pull long hair up under the cap so that no hair is exposed. Keeping fingernails short is also a good idea, as long nails can make tears in latex gloves. Substances and chemicals can get under fingernails, and skin exposure can occur. When working with certain drugs, there is the potential for spraying, splattering, and aerosolization. This can happen in the hospital pharmacy setting when the following occurs:

- When needles are withdrawn from drug vials.
- Transfer of drugs using syringes, needles, or filter straws. The breaking open of drug ampoules and possible explosion of air from a drug-filled syringe can also occur, causing potential harm or hazards.

A restricted area for preparing dangerous chemicals and drugs, such as cytotoxic agents, should be designated along with safety posters and signs, restricting access to only qualified personnel. Activities, such as drinking, smoking, eating, or applying

makeup, should be avoided in these restricted areas. Important labeling practices are vital—all hazardous drugs should be labeled. IV bags and syringes fall under this category and should be labeled as "*Special Handling/Disposal Precautions*," according to occupational health and safety administration (OSHA). Priming of tubing should be run with a nondrug solution prior to the hazardous drug administration, or a backflow closed system should be utilized.

Drug Spills

A pharmacy must have policies and procedures in place to prevent drug spills and manage them if they occur. Per OSHA, the procedures must include who is responsible for cleaning up the spill, and that individual must be properly trained. The American Society of Health-System Pharmacists (ASHP) classifies spills as small or large. A small spill is less than 5 ml, while a large spill is anything that goes beyond that size. A spill kit must also be made available in areas where hazardous drugs are handled on a regular basis. The ASHP recommends the following contents for a hazardous drug spill kit:

1. Sufficient supplies to absorb a spill of about 1000 mL (volume of one i.v. bag or bottle).
2. Appropriate PPE to protect the worker during cleanup, including two pairs of disposable gloves (one outer pair of heavy utility gloves and one pair of inner gloves); nonpermeable, disposable protective garments (coveralls or gown and shoe covers); and face shield.
3. Absorbent, plastic-backed sheets or spill pads.
4. Disposable toweling.
5. At least two sealable, thick plastic hazardous waste disposal bags (prelabeled with an appropriate warning label).
6. One disposable scoop for collecting glass fragments.
7. One puncture-resistant container for glass fragments.

Laminar Airflow Hoods

Laminar airflow hoods are pieces of pharmaceutical equipment that are designed to handle materials when sterile compounding is needed. Two types of laminar airflow hoods exist—vertical and horizontal. Horizontal airflow hoods are used for the compounding of parenteral drugs and products that are sterile. Vertical airflow hoods are often used for chemotherapeutic agents. Laminar airflow hoods need to be serviced (and certified every six months).

Compounding Aseptic Isolator

A compounding **aseptic isolator** is made for compounding drugs, pharmaceutical ingredients, and preparations. These isolators are created to keep an aseptic compounding environment in the isolator through the pharmaceutical compounding environment. In addition, the isolator gives a safe and sterile place where hazardous drugs are prepared and ventilation is taken care of properly. Airflow and many other factors play a role in the safe handling and creation of different pharmaceutical substances and drugs.

---

aseptic isolator a form of isolator specifically designed for compounding pharmaceutical ingredients or preparations.

■ Procedure 36-1

ASHP Recommendations for Hazardous Drug Spill Clean Up

1. Assess the size and scope of the spill. Call for trained help, if necessary.
2. Spills that cannot be contained by two spill kits may require outside assistance.
3. Post signs to limit access to spill area.
4. Obtain spill kit and respirator.
5. Don PPE, including inner and outer gloves and respirator.
6. Once fully garbed, contain spill using spill kit.
7. Carefully remove any broken glass fragments and place them in a puncture-resistant container.
8. Absorb liquids with spill pads.
9. Absorb powder with damp disposable pads or soft toweling.
10. Spill cleanup should proceed progressively from areas of lesser to greater contamination.
11. Completely remove and place all contaminated material in the disposal bags.
12. Rinse the area with water and then clean with detergent, sodium hypochlorite solution, and neutralizer.
13. Rinse the area several times and place all materials used for containment and cleanup in disposal bags. Seal bags and place them in the appropriate final container for disposal as hazardous waste.
14. Carefully remove all PPE using the inner gloves. Place all disposable PPE into disposal bags. Seal bags and place them into the appropriate final container.
15. Remove inner gloves; contain in a small, sealable bag; and then place into the appropriate final container for disposal as hazardous waste.
16. Wash hands thoroughly with soap and water.
17. Once a spill has been initially cleaned, have the area recleaned by housekeeping, janitorial staff, or environmental services.

Eyewash Stations

Pharmacy technicians may come in contact with chemicals or drugs that may be harmful to the eyes. They may also come in contact with blood and body fluids that may splash in the eyes. All properly equipped pharmacies will have eyewash stations where technicians can wash their eyes of any potentially harmful chemicals, body fluids, or blood.

OSHA—Occupational Safety and Health Administration

OSHA is the organization that provides protocols for the safe removal of different hazards and substances, chemicals, needles, body fluids, blood, fire safety and control, and emergency plans in case of a fire. Pharmacy technicians will come in contact with a variety of issues pertaining to materials used on the job, prescriptions, over-the-counter products, compounding substances, body fluids, blood, and needles that will need to be disposed of or safely handled. These substances should always be cleaned up properly and if direct contact occurs, technicians should always wash and disinfect their hands (or area of the body that was affected) immediately. Chemotherapy agents and administration are also an area pharmacy technicians will need to be properly trained in.

OSHA does many things, but listed here are four of the major areas they are mostly well known for:

- Research
- Education
- Information
- Training

OSHA professionals may train pharmacy technicians in proper and safe handling of items found in a hospital or retail pharmacy. In the hospital pharmacy, workers will be exposed to needles that will need safe handling and disposal and chemicals that may be flammable, poisonous, caustic, carcinogenic, or teratogenic. OSHA also performs routine workplace inspections to ensure all safety measures are met and all employees are working in safe conditions. In a community pharmacy (retail setting), OSHA will make sure that pharmacies are kept clean and sanitized, and employees are following the proper procedures for workplace safety. They will also enforce fire safety rules and evacuation in case of a fire. According to OSHA's rules, a pharmacy must have a complete fire safety plan.

The right to inspect health care sites (both private and public) is at OSHA's complete discretion to ensure that the correct guidelines and protocols are followed at all times. Citations are sometimes issued if the proper guidelines and rules that OSHA sets aside are not followed. The employee is not cited, but the workplace can be cited for violations.

Hazard Communication Plan and Exposure Control Plan

Knowing the types of hazards one will encounter in the workplace is of utmost importance. A plan called the hazard communication plan protects the rights of workers and allows them to know what types of hazards will be present in their workplace. It also outlines the types of risks that they will encounter in regards to their health while on the job. Pharmacies are required to have a material safety data sheet (MSDS) (see Figure 36-3). The maker of the hazardous chemical can

info

OSHA Manuals

OSHA offers workplace manuals and training packages. Manuals cover a wide variety of topics such as blood-borne pathogen standards, chemical hazards, exposure to mercury, latex allergies, fire safety standards, recordkeeping requirements, and many other topics pertaining to workplace safety and hazards. To learn more, visit **www.oshamanual.com/medical_OSHA.html**.

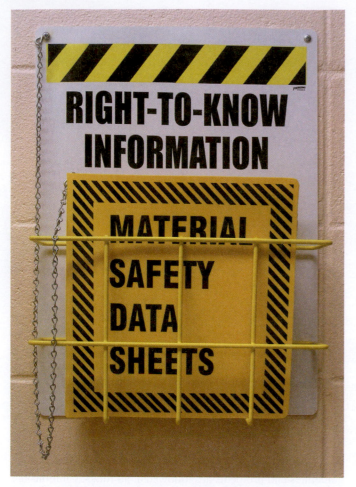

FIGURE 36-3 MSDS sheets are typically stored in a designated binder.
Source: Travis Klein/Shutterstock

Handling Hazardous Materials and Waste

Pharmacy technicians have the potential for coming in contact with various hazardous substances. According to OSHA, workers who are not aware of proper work practices and controls may be exposed to hazardous drugs through the skin, mouth, or breathing the drugs into their lungs.

Technicians may also come in contact with blood, semen, vaginal secretions, cerebrospinal fluid, pleural fluid, synovial fluid, urine, feces, nasal secretions, sputum, breast milk, tears, saliva, and vomit. Technicians are told to follow standard precautions at all times. Standard precautions are a set of guidelines to be followed for infection control and to be assumed that blood and particular body fluids are infectious and the potential to contract the human immunodeficiency virus (HIV) is always there. An OSHA technical manual can issue guidance in regards to health effects that are adverse due to hazardous medications. Some of these adverse effects are nausea, dizziness, or adverse results in birth (better known as birth defects). A Hazard Communication Standard says that drugs that are hazardous and pose a health hazard (exempting pills or tablets) need to be a part of the OSHA Standard Interpretation.

Blood-borne Pathogens

The Occupational Safety and Health Administration (OSHA) implemented the Occupational Exposure to Blood-borne Pathogens Standard. The standard was formed in 1991 and was created to protect 5.6 million health care workers from risky exposure to blood-borne pathogens that may cause HIV and the potential of contracting hepatitis B virus (HBV). In 2010, approximately 4, 690 workers were killed while working.

Pharmacy technicians may come in contact with excreta (urine) and that urine may contain traces of hazardous drugs. Patients given these drugs in a 48-hour time period will have traces of the drugs in their system. Technicians should wear PPE, gloves, and gowns to protect themselves from the possibility of coming in direct contact with the urine.

Institutional policies will somewhat vary from pharmacy to pharmacy. Much will depend on whether the pharmacy technician is working in a hospital or retail pharmacy, as their exposure to substances will be completely different. In a retail setting, there is less chance for the employee to contract blood-borne diseases and conditions. However, it is possible to come in contact with germs and bodily fluids in the retail pharmacy setting (e.g., mucus) if a fellow coworker or customer sneezes or does not have clean and sanitary hands. Pharmacy technicians will also come in contact with kids and adults with colds and flu, so care should be taken to minimize germs with proper hand sanitization through frequent hand washing and sanitization.

Pregnant Women and Workplace Hazards

Pharmacy technicians who are pregnant must be careful with their exposure to certain drugs, as these drugs can affect their unborn fetus. That is why wearing PPE and proper protective gear is even more important for these individuals. Hazardous exposure to chemicals, certain drugs, chemotherapy treatments, preparations, compounding agents, anesthetic gases, radiation,

provide these data sheets, or they can be provided by OSHA. Data sheets contain information about the dangerous chemical or product, and each pharmacy technician should familiarize themselves with the information. Information listed on data sheets contains the following:

1. Chemical name
2. Trade name
3. Synonyms for the chemical
4. Manufacturers name
5. Family of the hazardous chemical
6. Makers name, address, and telephone numbers for emergencies
7. Hazardous contents and information about ingredients
8. Fire and explosion data, health hazard, and protection information

Another type of plan is in order when it comes to safety in the workplace. The exposure control plan minimizes the risks associated with coming in contact with blood-borne diseases and material that has the potential for being hazardous. More can be found out about hazardous materials by visiting **www.sha.gov**.

and exposure to blood-borne substances and infectious disease can potentially harm an unborn child. Workplaces generally have specific rules concerning pregnant workers and exposure to dangerous chemicals and agents.

The Pharmacy and Ergonomics

The potential for pharmacists and pharmacy technicians to suffer from musculoskeletal disorders is always a possibility in the workplace. This can be due to performing repetitive tasks, awkward posture, and performing tasks such as typing and opening and closing prescription bottle lids. Pharmacies should also have proper ergonomically correct keyboards, computer chairs, mouse, and office supplies. Long-term damage to muscles and nerves can cause long-term health issues and pain for the worker.

Workplace Violence in the Pharmacy

The OSH Act passed in 1970 also covers workers and their human safety and protects them from being not only harmed at work, but also from workplace violence. In a pharmacy setting, there is also the potential for being robbed because drugs and money are kept on site. Employers should cover the issue of workplace violence and how to handle such potentially violent issues. OSHA offers some suggestions on how to keep pharmacists and pharmacy technicians out of harm's way and also how to deal with the issue of stealing and robbery. OSHA also advises employees to create a *Violence Prevention Program*. OSHA also suggests these options for keeping workplace violence in check.

Workplace Situation	Possible Solution
Robbery	Installation of Plexiglas in pharmacy payment windows. Better visibility and lighting (inside and outside of the pharmacy). Training for pharmacy staff to recognize strange, hostile, or assertive or assaultive behavior, speech, or mannerisms.

Workers Rights under OSHA

OSHA works to protect workers and pharmacy employees fall under that category. Employees have the right to report unsafe, harmful, or hazardous conditions to their employer and to OSHA. Employees can ask OSHA to inspect their workplace and use employee rights (that are under law) without worry about any type of discrimination or backlash from other workers or bosses. Employees can also receive copies of employee records, which include records of job-associated injuries or sickness. Copies of medical records can also be obtained for interested employees.

State Regulations

All 50 states have their own workplace safety laws. All states have the option of submitting a plan to the U.S.

Secretary of Labor for proper approval. If the U.S. secretary of labor finds the plan acceptable, state laws will stand. These states that fall into this category are called state plan states. This means employees follow the specific state laws, rules, regulations, and standards instead of following the federal OSHA rules and regulations on health and safety. A full list of individual state plans for workplace safety can be found by visiting http://www.osha.gov/dcsp/osp/states.html.

Institutional Policies

Institutional policies will vary from worksite to worksite. Each pharmacy must follow all rules and regulations when it comes to safety in the pharmacy. Posters concerning state safety and rules are to be clearly posted for all employees to view. Posters contain obligations and protections, as they pertain to work safety rules and regulations. Often a policy manual will be on site and also given to new employees when they begin their work as a pharmacy technician. Institutional policies will vary for hospital technicians as well as for retail technicians because of their exposure to different workplace mishaps, hazards, accidents, chemicals, substances, and drugs. Again, each type of institution will have a policy manual covering issues such as fire safety, hazard communication plans, exposure control plans, as well as a record-keeping book to record injuries in.

Record keeping is an important part of injury prevention and control. Pharmacies with more than 10 employees will maintain a log of work-related injuries and illnesses. Employees and employers have full right to review records. Work-related injuries that resulted in the stopping of work, restricted work, loss of consciousness, job transfer, getting fired, death, or medical attention all need to be recorded and reported. Good record keeping of accidents can help prevent issues in the future and help cut down on injuries. Record-keeping forms are available from OSHA. In addition, these records may be kept on paper or on a computer. There are various establishments that are exempted from keeping records and a full list can be viewed by visiting www.osha.gov.

The Joint Commission

In 1951, The Joint Commission was formed to assist health care organizations and health care programs in improving quality health care standards, accreditation, and certification for better, safe, and effective workplaces for health care workers and patients. It both certifies and accredits over 19,000 health care programs and organizations in the global United States. It also gives a disease-specific care certification and a Health Care Staffing Services Certification. The Joint Commission's name was changed in 2007.

Infection Control

Infection control is highly important in any pharmacy technician setting, whether it is in a hospital or retail setting. However, the risk for infection and disease is more of a problem in a hospital setting as pharmacy technicians will be exposed to many different types of pathogens, potentially HIV-causing substances, and

Other Potentially Infectious Materials, also known as OPIM. Because it is important to keep exposure to dangerous pathogens and blood-borne substances at a minimum, employers should have what is called an exposure control plan. The employer's exposure control plan is a written word plan that states the protective measures a particular employer will take to ensure safety on all accounts to get rid of or minimize exposure to human blood and OPIM. The exposure control plan can be thought of as a hazardous materials plan that states tasks, procedures, job classifications, and certain procedures where OPIM would be present in the workplace. The plan will also include the procedures for taking into account an issue of exposure and a schedule of how and when certain provisions of the regular plan and how that plan will be executed. This will include incident record keeping and processes of compliance with the incident. If hazardous waste is not dealt with according to a plan, OSHA has the right to issue citations. Citations are for incidences that breech regulations for handling and exposure to blood-borne pathogens that can potentially cause HIV or HBV. According to an article published in Pharmacy Times magazine, correct infection control needs to be inclusive of education of patients, patient's caretakers, health care workers, and proper instruction concerning impeccable preventive measures in infection control.

The American Society of Health-System Pharmacists (ASHP) encourages and believes the pharmacist's and pharmacy technician's need to possess a direct responsibility in infection control programs in pharmacies and health care facilities worldwide. Further, ASHP believes that the pharmacist's role in issues of infection control and correct use of antimicrobials throughout the pharmacy and health system can help with increased compliance in controlling infections and infectious diseases. The ASHP issued a statement on the Pharmacist's Role in Infection Control stating "these efforts should minimize the misuse of antimicrobials, ultimately resulting in successful therapeutic outcomes for patients with infectious diseases, and reduce the risk of infections for other patients and employees."

The pharmacists as well as the pharmacy technician have a set of responsibilities when it comes to promoting infection quality control and maintenance. The ASHP has officially issued the following points in their statement on *Pharmacist's Role in Infection Control*:

1. Reducing the transmission of infections—educate and inform of the proper use of antiseptics, disinfectants, and sterile products. Promote in-house pharmacy policies, and procedures, and quality control programs and training.
2. Promoting the use of antimicrobial agents—antimicrobial Agents are drugs, chemicals, or other substances that totally kill or slow down the growth of microbes. Antimicrobial agents can be antibacterial medications, antiviral agents, antifungal drugs, and antiphrastic agents.
3. Educational activities (which include educating professionals, patients, and the public) about the use of antimicrobials, immunizations for children and adults, and appropriate infection-control techniques and safeguards.

Sanitation Management

There are certain signs to indicate a biohazard. All containers with the biohazard symbol should be an immediate note to the pharmacy technician that the containers may contain used,

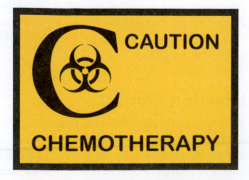

FIGURE 36-4 Biohazard symbols.
Source: Eireann/Shutterstock

contaminated, broken, or altered needles. Red plastic bags with a box that has the biohazard symbol printed on it are used for items such as gloves, paper towels, dressings, and other medical items that are soft. You may have seen rigid red containers with a clear top and the biohazard symbol printed on it going to a doctor's office. These containers are for the disposal of *sharps*. Sharps are needles, glass slides, scalpel blades, and syringes that are disposable. All pharmacy employees are to use these containers to dispose of medical waste in a proper manner (see Figure 36-4).

Hospitals, medical complexes, and doctor's offices should possess these proper waste disposal containers and bags. Pharmacy technicians will need to warn cleaning support staff not to empty these boxes, bags, and containers as they should be left for trained health care staff only to dispose of. Health care workers will need to wear gloves, protective eyewear, and masks to handle biohazard containers and bags and double bag those bags in which there may be any leakage.

Proper Hand Hygiene

According to the CDC, the following considerations and techniques should be followed for proper hand hygiene (see Figure 36-5):

1. When decontaminating hands with an alcohol-based hand rub, apply product to palm of one hand and rub hands together, covering all surfaces of hands and fingers, until hands are dry. Follow the manufacturer's recommendations regarding the volume of product to use.

2. When washing hands with soap and water, wet hands first with water, apply an amount of product recommended by the manufacturer to hands, and rub hands together vigorously for at least 15 seconds, covering all surfaces of the hands and fingers. Rinse hands with water and dry thoroughly with a disposable towel. Use towel to turn off the faucet. Avoid using hot water, because repeated exposure to hot water may increase the risk of dermatitis.

3. Liquid, bar, leaflet, or powdered forms of plain soap are acceptable when washing hands with a nonantimicrobial soap and water. When bar soap is used, soap racks that facilitate drainage and small bars of soap should be used.

4. Multiple-use cloth towels of the hanging or roll type are not recommended for use in health care settings.

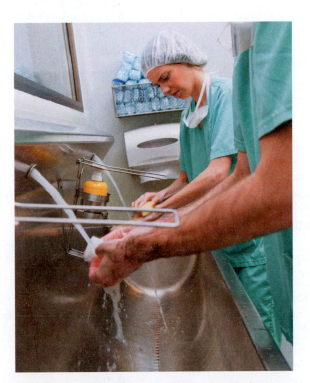

FIGURE 36-5 Proper hand hygiene is a critical component to infection control.
Source: Tyler Olson/Shutterstock

Summary

Workplace safety is shared by the employer and employee. There are noncompliance penalties if the employer does not follow certain safety. The OSHA is a federal agency that enforces work environment rules. All health care employers must post a control plan and a written chemical hygiene plan.

A written exposure control plan tells of the measure of protection to blood-borne pathogen transmission to workers.

A written chemical hygiene plan shows the chemicals present, safe handling, and proper chemical disposal. The training and mandatory compliance in all safety types is of utmost importance for complete workplace safety. Patients are also protected. There are certain processes of disinfection, sterilization, and aseptic technique that are to be followed in the health care workplace.

Chapter Review Questions

1. The Occupational Safety and Health Administration was established in _____.
   a. 1970
   b. 1990
   c. 1961
   d. 1981

2. Which of the following is not required to be provided on a MSDS?
   a. chemical name
   b. fire and explosion data
   c. indication for use
   d. manufacturer's name and address

3. Which of the following is not provided by OSHA?
   a. education
   b. research
   c. training
   d. hazardous waste collection

4. A(n) _____ says that drugs that are hazardous and ones that pose a health hazard need to be part of the OSHA Standard Interpretation.
   a. Joint Commission Communication Protocol
   b. Infection Control Protocol
   c. Hazard Communication Standard
   d. Written Exposure Control Plan

5. Latex gloves, gowns, masks and hair covers are examples of _____.
   a. LAF
   b. OSH
   c. PPE
   d. none of the above

6. Which of the following states does not fall under the U.S. Secretary of Labor "State Plans" for workplace safety?
   a. Alaska
   b. California
   c. Texas
   d. Washington

7. Workplace safety requires the involvement of _____.
   a. management only
   b. employees only
   c. both management and employees
   d. both management and the CDC

8. Sharps containers are to be used for the disposal of _____.
   a. blades
   b. needles
   c. glass slides
   d. all of the above

9. An event that has the potential to result in unintended harm or damage is referred to as a(n) _____.
   a. accident
   b. incident
   c. illness
   d. injury

10. According to the CDC, when washing hands with soap and water, hands should be rubbed together vigorously for at least _____ seconds.
    a. 15
    b. 30
    c. 45
    d. 60

Critical Thinking Questions

1. Explain why workplace violence policies and procedures are important for pharmacy work environments.

2. List two challenges that can occur in implementing a culture of workplace safety, and your recommendation on how to overcome, or solve, those challenges.

3. List and describe the three primary roles of pharmacists in infection control, according to ASHP.

Web Challenge

1. Visit the OSHA website at http://www.osha.gov/dcsp/osp/states.html">http://www.osha.gov/dcsp/osp/states.html, and print out information specific to your state on workplace safety.

2. Using the Internet, search for three MSDS for different pharmaceutical products or chemicals, which contain at least one health hazard and print them out.

References and Resources

"About the Joint Commission." *JCAHO*. Web. 23 May 2012.

"ASHP Statement on the Pharmacist' Role in Infection Control." *American Journal of Health-System Pharmacy*. 55 (1998): 1724–1726. Print.

American Society of Health-System Pharmacists. ASHP guidelines on handling hazardous drugs. American Journal of Health System Pharmacy. 63 (2006):1172–93.

Boyce, J.M. and D. Pittet. "Guidelines for Hand Hygiene in Health-Care Settings." *CDC*. Web. 27 May 2012.

Candow, K. "What Went Wrong: Understanding the Accident/Incident Investigation Process." *Newfoundland & Labrador*. Web. 27 May 2012.

Cross, R.. "Infection Control: Focus on Prevention." *Pharmacy Times*. Web. 23 May 2012.

Johnston, M. *Certification Exam Review for the Pharmacy Technician*. 2nd ed. Upper Saddle River, NJ: Pearson, 2011. Print.

"Occupational Safety & Health Administration." *OSHA*. Web. 19 May 2012.

"OSHA—Common Stats." *OSHA*. Web. 23 May 2012.

"OSHA—Complying Workplace Health Safety Laws." *Nolo*. Web. 19 May 2012.

"OSHA—Ergonomics & Workplace Violence." *OSHA*. Web. 22 May 2012.

"OSHA—Pharmacy." *OSHA*. Web. 21 May 2012.

"OSHA Standards for Blood-borne Pathogens." OSHA. Web. 20 May 2012.

"OSHA Technical Manual (OTM): Section VI: Chapter 2." https://www.osha.gov/dts/osta/otm/otm_vi/otm_vi_2.html Web 2 August 2013.

"OSHA: We Can Help." *OSHA*. Web. 23 May 2012.

"State Occupational Safety and Health Plans." *Nolo*. Web. 19 May 2012.

"State Occupational Safety and Health Plans." *OSHA*. Web. 20 May 2012.

"Workplace Safety Toolkit." *Nonprofit Risk Management Center*. Web. 27 May 2012.

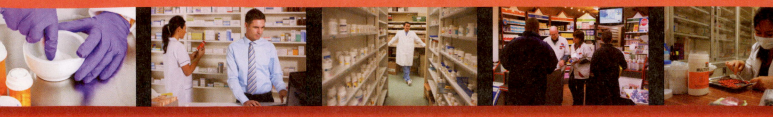

CHAPTER 37

Special Considerations for Pediatric and Geriatric Patients

LEARNING OBJECTIVES

After completing this chapter, you should be able to:

- Discuss the differences between neonatal and pediatric patients.

- Explain how the processes of pharmacokinetics in pediatric patients affect drug dosing.

- Discuss pediatric drug administration and dosage adjustment considerations.

- List two common childhood illnesses or diseases in pediatric patients.

- Discuss the physiological changes that occur in geriatric patients.

- List several factors that affect pharmacokinetic processes in geriatric patients.

- Discuss polypharmacy and noncompliance in geriatric medication therapy.

- Discuss Medicare Part D and its effects on medication dispensing to the geriatric population.

- Explain ways in which geriatric medication dispensing will change in the future, and how extended life expectancy will change pharmacy practice.

KEY TERMS

absorption, p. 635
asthma, p. 640
distribution, p. 636
excretion, p. 636
geriatric, p. 641
half-life, p. 642
infant, p. 635
intramuscular (IM), p. 635
lipid-soluble, p. 636
metabolism, p. 636
neonate, p. 635
noncompliance, p. 643
pH, p. 635
pharmacokinetics, p. 635
polypharmacy, p. 644
side effects, p. 641
toxicity, p. 642
water-soluble, p. 635

INTRODUCTION

Providing medical and pharmaceutical care for the younger set and for older patients is a bit more challenging than caring for adults who need medications. Drug dosing is different for children than adults and carries the same responsibility for accuracy and attention to detail when filling prescriptions for this age group. For older adult patients, there is often more concern about side effects and how well the drug is tolerated by them. These two age groups need extra care and consideration when it comes to pharmaceutical services and care.

Pediatrics

There are many differences between pediatric patients and adults. Pediatric patients are not just small adults, and you must consider a number of factors other than the obvious one of body weight when administering medication. **Neonates** are newborn babies from birth to one month of age; **infants** are between the ages of one month and two years. Finally, a patient is considered a *child* if he or she is between 2 and 12 years of age.

Significant physiological differences also exist between pediatric patients and adults. The **pharmacokinetics** processes known as absorption, distribution, metabolism, and excretion occur quite differently in children, compared to adults, because children's organ systems are not fully developed. Providing medication therapy to pediatric patients can present a challenge if these differences are not considered (see Figure 37-1). This section discusses some of the pharmacological differences in neonatal, infant, and pediatric patients, special medication administration considerations, and some of the common disorders of these special patients.

Pharmacological Differences in Pediatric Patients

Compared to adults, neonates and infants weigh less and usually require a reduction in the dosage of medication. However, there are many other factors to consider when dosing these patients. Drug **absorption** is the process by which a drug enters the bloodstream, whether from the digestive system or

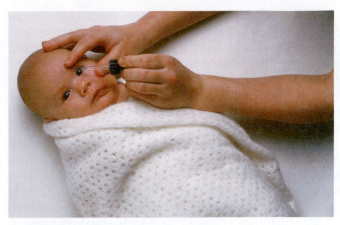

FIGURE 37-1 A baby getting eye drops.
Source: Dave King, Dorling Kindersley

an injection site where it is dissolved into body fluids. Neonates and infants have smaller skeletal structures, and this can affect the absorption of medication just as much as overall weight.

These youngest of patients have limited physical activity, so there is less blood flow to their muscles. Therefore, with an **intramuscular (IM)** injection, medication will be absorbed more slowly and reach the bloodstream later than it would with an adult. The slower absorption increases the risk of muscle and nerve damage with any IM injection.

The neonate's skin is thinner than an adult's skin, so a topical medication, such as an ointment or cream, may be absorbed more completely and rapidly into the systemic circulation. This may cause unexpected or enhanced drug effects not seen in adult patients who receive the same topical medication.

When an oral medication is given, the **pH** of the neonate's digestive system must also be considered; it is less acidic than an adult's digestive system. This can lead to decreased bioavailability and sometimes lower blood levels of the drug.

> ❝ **Workplace Wisdom** **Dosages for Neonates versus Infants**
>
> Remember: A dose that is appropriate for an infant or toddler may not be appropriate for a neonate. For example, digoxin dosage varies:
>
> - For a neonate (one month or younger)—0.03–0.04 mg/kg
> - For an infant (one month to two years)—0.04–0.06 mg/kg ❞

After a medication is absorbed, it enters the bloodstream and is then distributed to the organs and tissues. Several factors, such as blood flow and plasma protein binding, influence how much of a drug reaches the target organ or area of the body. The liver and kidneys have the largest blood supply and receive a greater concentration of a drug than other organs. In addition, the adult brain has a protective barrier, called the blood–brain barrier, which protects it from **water-soluble** substances. Drugs must have a certain degree of lipid or fat solubility to penetrate this barrier and reach the brain.

---

neonate a child from birth to one month of age.

infant a child between the ages of one month and two years.

pharmacokinetics the study of the processes of absorption, distribution, metabolism, and excretion of drugs.

absorption the process by which a drug enters the bloodstream.

intramuscular (IM) within or into a muscle.

pH a scale that measures the alkalinity or acidity of a substance; 7 is the neutral point on this scale (less than 7 is acidic and greater than 7 is alkaline).

water-soluble dissolvable in water; describes drugs that are composed mostly of water and can be excreted by the kidneys.

In pediatric patients, liver function and the blood–brain barrier are still immature. Children usually have a higher percentage of body water and a lower percentage of body fat than adults. If a **lipid-soluble** drug is administered to a pediatric patient, there will be a decreased **distribution** of the drug to the organs and body tissues because of the lower percentage of fat in the child's body. This causes more of the medication to stay in the blood, resulting in higher drug blood levels.

In comparison, water-soluble drugs administered to pediatric patients may cause lower drug concentrations in the blood, because the percentage of water in the child's body is higher and thus results in more peripheral drug distribution. There are fewer plasma proteins in pediatric patients as compared to adults, which allows more of the drug to remain unbound or *free* in the body. Only unbound medications exert a drug effect, so the pediatric patient may have more effective drug in the body, enhancing the drug action and possibly even producing an overdose.

Diarrhea and vomiting are particular concerns in the pediatric patient, as these conditions may cause them to become dehydrated very quickly. When dehydrated, children's bodies retain more of a drug in their organs, and this often leads to amplified drug effects and higher drug concentrations.

Drug Metabolism

Metabolism is the chemical alteration of a drug (or other substance) by the body, and **excretion** is the process by which the body eliminates a drug. The liver and the kidneys are the main organs involved in these processes, and they are not fully developed in pediatric patients. This may result in slower metabolism and excretion in children as compared to adults, so drugs stay in their bodies for a longer period of time. This places pediatric patients at risk of drug accumulation and possible toxicity.

Children (aged 2 to 12 years) also metabolize certain drugs more rapidly than adults; this rate usually continues to increase between 1 and 12 years. Examples of drugs that are metabolized more rapidly in children include valproic acid, which is often given for seizures, and clindamycin, often used for skin and respiratory infections. Medications containing benzyl alcohol, such as bacteriostatic sodium chloride used to dilute powder forms of injectable medications, should not be used in neonates because the alcohol can reach toxic levels. Phenobarbital and some pain medications are rapidly absorbed in some older

infants because of their liver physiology; thus, children often require larger doses or more frequent administration to reach the desired effect. Steroids can stunt pediatric growth; tetracycline can stain permanent teeth and affect bone development.

Pediatric Medication Administration

When administering medications to pediatric patients, dosage adjustments must be considered in addition to the route and dosage forms available because of pediatric physiological differences. Compliance in pediatric

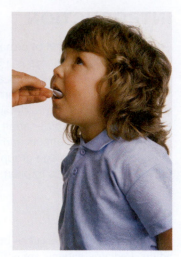

FIGURE 37-2 A child being given the liquid form of an antibiotic.
Source: Dave King, Dorling Kindersley

patients is another important consideration; sometimes, the available dosage form plays a major role in determining which medication to administer. For example, liquids are the dosage form most commonly used, because color and flavors can usually be added to mask bitter or other unpleasant tastes (see Figure 37-2). Tablets and capsules are not easy for small children to swallow and certainly are not appropriate for neonates and infants.

> ### ❝ Workplace Wisdom   Compounding
>
> As a pharmacy technician, you will sometimes need to compound formulations. This involves using a formula (recipe) and special equipment to create a patient-specific product. Sometimes, the medication is not available commercially, or the dosage form available is not appropriate. A pharmacy technician can help ensure that a pediatric patient completes the entire course of therapy by adding flavoring to a bad-tasting medicine to make it more palatable to the child. ❞

Body weight is the basis of the most common method for determining the correct dose for a particular patient. Several formulas are used, including those based on weight, age, body surface area (BSA), or milligrams per body weight per day. Age is considered the least reliable of these, because a pediatric patient may be smaller or larger than the norm for his or her age.

Many over-the-counter (OTC) medications are also available for pediatric patients, but often they are intended for older pediatric patients and contain no dosing instructions for very young children. Parents or caregivers with dosage questions about these OTC medicines should always be referred to a pharmacist.

If the manufacturer does not suggest an exact pediatric dosage for a medication, several methods are available to calculate or estimate the proper dose (see Chapter 14 for a review). The age-based formula that is sometimes used for determining

---

lipid-soluble dissolvable in fats; describes drug that pass readily into cell membranes composed mostly of fatty substances, such as the brain.

distribution the process by which a drug reaches the various organs and tissues of the body.

metabolism the chemical alteration of drugs, food, or foreign compounds in and by the body.

excretion the elimination of a drug from the body; usually occurs through urine, feces, or the respiratory system.

info
OTC Cough & Cold Products
The FDA recommends that OTC cough and cold products should not be used for infants and children under two years of age, because serious and potentially life-threatening side effects can occur.

patient is overweight or underweight for a particular age group, dosages could be off considerably. In addition, the actual appropriate pediatric dose can vary greatly depending on the patient's condition, response, and adverse reactions to the medication. These formulas are not widely used today for this reason.

A method more commonly used to determine dosage is based on weight in kilograms and the normal adult dosage range as stated by the manufacturer.

a pediatric dosage is called *Young's rule*. The other formula, known as *Clark's rule*, uses only the patient's weight.

Young's rule

$$\frac{\text{Age (in years)}}{\text{Age (in years)} + 12 \text{ years}} \times \text{Adult dose} = \text{Pediatric dose}$$

Clark's rule

$$\frac{\text{Weight (in lbs.)}}{150 \text{ lbs.}} \times \text{Adult dose} = \text{Pediatric dose}$$

EXAMPLE 37.1

A child needs to receive a medication that has a suggested adult dose of 650 mg. The child is five years old and weighs 44 lbs. What would the dose be using Young's rule?

$$\frac{5 \text{ yrs old}}{5 \text{ yrs} + 12 \text{ yrs}} \times 650 \text{ mg} = 191.10 \text{ mg}$$

EXAMPLE 37.2

Calculate the dose for the same patient using Clark's rule.

$$\frac{44 \text{ lbs.}}{150 \text{ lbs.}} \times 650 \text{ mg} = 190.45 \text{ mg}$$

Both of these formulas use the usual adult dosage as the basis of the calculation. Clark's rule uses only the weight of the patient; Young's rule uses only the patient's age. If a pediatric

EXAMPLE 37.3

The manufacturer recommends a dosage of 0.5 mg/kg/day. For a child weighing 80 kg, what is the proper dose?

0.5 mg × 80 kg = 40 mg per day

Dosing tables are standard practice today and appear on many OTC packages for products such as acetaminophen and ibuprofen. Table 37-1 shows the recommended dosages for various forms of acetaminophen; these dosages are determined by the manufacturers using both the child's weight and age. For more information on calculating pediatric dosages, refer to Chapter 18

PROFILE IN PRACTICE

Mrs. Richards is the mother of a 2-year-old boy. She has just filled a prescription for Augmentin suspension for her son at your pharmacy. An hour after picking up the prescription, she calls to tell you that her son will not take the Augmentin, because it tastes bad and asks you if there is any way to mask the taste or improve the flavor. You know that if the child does not like the way the medicine tastes, he probably will not take even another dose, let alone the entire course of the antibiotic.

▸ *What options can you offer Mrs. Richards?*
▸ *Where can you find more information on safe ways to flavor Augmentin?*

TABLE 37-1 Recommended Acetaminophen Dosages

Form	Brand Names	Concentration	Dosage
Drops	Tylenol, Liquiprin	80 mg/0.8 mL	6–11 lbs is 0.4 mL
Elixir	Tylenol, Genapap	160 mg/5 mL	12–17 lbs and 4–11 months is 0.5 mL
Suppositories	Uniserts, Feverall	80 mg, 160 mg, 325 mg, 650 mg	Ages 2–3 years, 24–35 lbs is 160 mg
Tablets	Tylenol, Panadol	325 mg, 500 mg, 650 mg	24–35 lbs, 2–3 years is 160 mg
Tablets, chewable	Tylenol, Tempra, Panadol	80 mg	24–35 lbs, 2–3 years is 160 mg

Poisoning

According to the National Poison Data Systems, nearly 2.5 million human exposures to potentially toxic substances were reported, and more than 50% occurred in children under the age of six. Although most of these exposures are unintentional and result in minor or no harm, poisonings do often require emergency care in children.

Among the most common substances of exposure reported in children are cosmetics, analgesics, and household cleaners, representing nearly one-third of all incidents. Other substances commonly encountered include cough/cold medications, toys/ foreign objects, topical preparations, vitamins, antihistamines, pesticides, and plants. Although most toxic exposures result in minimal harm, certain substances can cause severe toxicity in children as a result of very small ingestions, such as a single table or less than a teaspoon. Among these highly toxic substances for children are sulfonylureas, antihistamines, benzocaine gel, beta-andrenergic antagonists, calcium channel blockers, camphorated oil, diphenoxylate/atropine, methyl salicylate, opioids, and tricylcic antidepressants.

Gastric decontamination is often the preferred, if not only, method of intervention available to treat a poisoned patient. Although often used in the past, syrup of ipecac is seldom used for gastric decontamination today, because it is considered to only increase the risk of adverse outcomes in most cases. Both the American Academy of Pediatrics and the American Academy of Clinical Toxicology have issued statements discouraging the use of syrup of ipecac. Other methods of gastric decontamination include gastric lavage, active charcoal, and whole bowel irrigation.

Common Childhood Illnesses

Measures such as immunizations and well-baby checkups can help prevent many childhood illnesses. The CDC has a recommended schedule of vaccinations for persons from 0 to 18 years of age. These include hepatitis, whooping cough, pneumonia, measles, mumps, and rubella, as well as some other common childhood illnesses. Figure 37-3 reproduces the recommended immunization schedules approved by the CDC. In addition, the CDC has developed a *catch-up* immunization schedule for persons 4 months through 18 years old who start late or who are more than one month behind schedule. The *catch-up* immunization schedule can be found on the CDC website.

Conditions such as eye, ear, nose, and throat infections are very common in children. Before the age of three years, a child will probably have at least one ear infection. Earaches are common in the pediatric patient, because the eustachian tube is narrower and shorter than in adults. This tube connects the middle ear to the back of the throat. Normally, this tube allows fluid to drain from the middle ear, but if it gets infected, the tube may become inflamed, swell, and fill with mucus. Bacterial growth causes pressure on the eardrum and pain. If left untreated, this condition, known as *otitis media*, can cause temporary hearing loss and, in acute ongoing cases, even trouble with developing speech and language skills. The most common signs are pain and fever. If the child is too small to communicate pain verbally, he or she may cry or pull on the ear as an indication.

If the doctor thinks the infection is caused by bacteria, an antibiotic will be prescribed. If it is a viral infection, pain relievers and warm compresses are used. If a child has had more than three infections in six months, ear drains are often used to help balance the pressure in the ears and improve drainage. This is accomplished by surgically inserting a plastic tube into the eardrum, which allows air into the middle ear so that fluid can drain out properly. Such drains/tubes are left in for six to nine months on average.

Children who live with smokers, have a predisposing family history, attend day care, or were born prematurely are often at higher risk of infections. Viral infections, such as croup, colds, and flu, are often spread due to the close contact situations found in day care facilities. Bacterial infections, such as chickenpox, strep throat, and whooping cough, are also commonly transmitted in these areas. Bacterial cells can form a protective wall around them, and thus may persist in the environment for some time. Antibiotics can be used to destroy the wall; this kills the cells and therefore rids the body of the infection. In contrast, viruses require a host or living cell to sustain life. Because they invade the host's cells, antibiotics are ineffective against viruses.

Antibiotic medications should be used for only bacterial infections. Each time a person takes an antibiotic, some bacteria are killed. However, others *learn* to defend themselves against the antibiotic and develop drug resistance. To prevent this, make sure the child takes the entire course of antibiotic exactly as prescribed and use antibiotics only when the doctor says they are needed. Proper instructions regarding dosage and storage should be included in the dispensing of medication.

info National Capital Poison Center Hotline

The poison center hotline, which provides free assistance and guidance on exposure to potentially toxic substances, is available 24/7 at 1-800-222-1222, for both parents and health care providers. Nearly two-thirds of poison center calls are able to be treated safely at home. For more information on the National Capital Poison Center or for additional resources, visit **www.poison.org**

info Household Teaspoons

Common household teaspoons are not accurate enough for measuring medication. Provide patients or their caregivers with an oral syringe, measuring dropper, or calibrated cup when dispensing liquid dosage forms.

These recommendations must be read with the footnotes that follow. For those who fall behind or start late, provide catch-up vaccination at the earliest opportunity as indicated by the green bars in Figure 1. To determine minimum intervals between doses, see the catch-up schedule (Figure 2). School entry and adolescent vaccine age groups are in bold.

Vaccines	Birth	1 month	2 months	4 months	6 months	9 months	12 months	15 months	18 months	19–23 months	2–3 years	**4–6 years**	7–10 years	**11–12 years**	13–15 years	16–18 years
Hepatitis B[1] (HepB)	◄1st dose►	◄------2nd dose------►		◄------------------------3rd dose------------------------►												
Rotavirus[2] (RV) RV-1 (2-dose series); RV-5 (3-dose series)			◄1st dose►	◄2nd dose►	See footnote 2											
Diphtheria, tetanus, & acellular pertussis[3] (DTaP: <7 years)			1st dose	◄2nd dose►	◄3rd dose►		◄------------4th dose------------►					5th dose				
Tetanus, diphtheria, & acellular pertussis[4] (Tdap: ≥7 years)														(Tdap)		
Haemophilus influenzae type b[5] (Hib)			◄1st dose►	◄2nd dose►	See footnote 5		3rd or 4th dose, see footnote 5									
Pneumococcal conjugate[6a,c] (PCV13)			◄1st dose►	◄2nd dose►	◄3rd dose►		◄------4th dose------►									
Pneumococcal polysaccharide[6b,c] (PPSV23)																
Inactivated Poliovirus[7] (IPV) (<18 years)			◄1st dose►	2nd dose	◄----------------3rd dose----------------►							◄4th dose►				
Influenza[8] (IIV; LAIV) 2 doses for some: see footnote 8					Annual vaccination (IIV only)						Annual vaccination (IIV or LAIV)					
Measles, mumps, rubella[9] (MMR)							◄------1st dose------►					◄2nd dose►				
Varicella[10] (VAR)							◄------1st dose------►					◄2nd dose►				
Hepatitis A[11] (HepA)							◄------2 dose series, see footnote 11------►									
Human papillomavirus[12] (HPV2: females only; HPV4: males and females)														(3-dose series)		
Meningococcal[13] (Hib-MenCY ≥ 6 weeks; MCV4-D ≥ 9 months; MCV4-CRM ≥ 2 years)				see footnote 13										◄1st dose►		booster

- ■ (red) Range of recommended ages for all children
- ■ (green) Range of recommended ages for catch-up immunization
- ■ (tan) Range of recommended ages for certain high-risk groups
- ■ (olive-green) Range of recommended ages during which catch-up is encouraged and for certain high-risk groups
- □ Not routinely recommended

This schedule includes recommendations in effect as of January 1, 2013. Any dose not administered at the recommended age should be administered at a subsequent visit, when indicated and feasible. The use of a combination vaccine generally is preferred over separate injections of its equivalent component vaccines. Vaccination providers should consult the relevant Advisory Committee on Immunization Practices (ACIP) statement for detailed recommendations, available online at http://www.cdc.gov/vaccines/pubs/acip-list.htm. Clinically significant adverse events that follow vaccination should be reported to the Vaccine Adverse Event Reporting System (VAERS) online (http://www.vaers.hhs.gov) or by telephone (800-822-7967). Suspected cases of vaccine-preventable diseases should be reported to the state or local health department. Additional information, including precautions and contraindications for vaccination, is available from CDC online (http://www.cdc.gov/vaccines) or by telephone (800-CDC-INFO [800-232-4636]).

This schedule is approved by the Advisory Committee on Immunization Practices (http://www.cdc.gov/vaccines/acip/index.html), the American Academy of Pediatrics (http://www.aap.org), the American Academy of Family Physicians (http://www.aafp.org), and the American College of Obstetricians and Gynecologists (http://www.acog.org).

NOTE: The above recommendations must be read along with the footnotes of this schedule.

FIGURE 37-3 Recommended immunization schedules for persons aged 0 through 18 years.
Source: U.S. Department of Health and Human Services

Respiratory Diseases

Asthma is a condition that affects about 7 million children under the age of 18 each year in the United States according to the National Institute of Allergy and Infectious Diseases. It is the most common chronic condition among children and accounts for several million absences from school each year. Hospitalizations from asthma occur at alarming rates and treatment costs are estimated to be in the billions. Allergies are the number one cause of asthma in pediatric patients, followed by the following:

- Upper respiratory infections
- Weather conditions
- Second-hand tobacco smoke inhalation

Early symptoms include coughing or breathing changes, reduced energy, dark circles under the eyes, and trouble sleeping. Symptoms that develop later are tightness in the chest, wheezing, and shortness of breath. Asthma can be life-threatening, because it may cause respiratory failure. Children with asthma have breathing difficulties, because the air passages in their lungs are narrower and do not allow correct air flow. Many triggers can bring on a full-blown asthma attack because of the oversensitivity of lungs and airways. Diagnosis includes spirometry with a device that measures lung function. This may be followed by chest X-rays, blood tests, and peak flow monitoring, which measures how much air a person can blow out of the lungs.

School activities, such as sports and running, may trigger an attack in some children. Inhalers are often prescribed to treat these attacks. Medications known as *bronchodilators* relieve the symptoms of asthma by relaxing the muscles that tighten around the airways (see Figure 37-4). Bronchodilators also help clear mucus from the lungs and open the airways. This allows more air to move in and out of the lungs, improving breathing and allowing coughing to clear mucus out of the lungs more effectively.

Another class of medications known as *anti-inflammatory agents* is also used on an ongoing basis. These can actually prevent attacks, because they reduce swelling and mucus production, making the airways less sensitive and less likely to react to triggers.

Treatment for pediatric patients with asthma often includes a combination of both of these drug types in the form of inhalers, nebulizers, and pills. Quick-acting medications are intended to provide prompt relief during an attack; long-term control medications can be taken to prevent attacks from occurring. In general, treatment focuses on prevention of attacks,

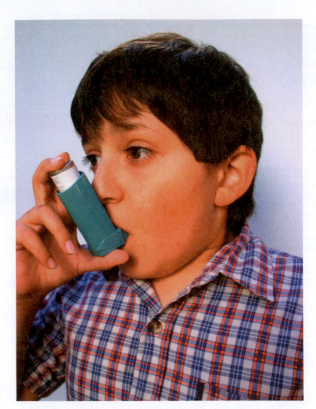

FIGURE 37-4 A child using an asthma bronchodilator.
Source: Peter Elvidge/Shutterstock

through medication and patient or caregiver education, and long-term medications to control and prevent chronic symptoms. Added to these strategies are quick-relief medications and monitoring of daily asthma symptoms.

Other respiratory diseases include whooping cough and pneumonia. Whooping cough, also known as *pertussis*, can be fatal in young children. There is a vaccine, given during childhood, along with diphtheria and tetanus (DPT) immunizations, which can prevent a child from contracting this disease. Treatment usually includes antibiotics such as erythromycin, clear liquids, and fruit juices. Pertussis can last for several weeks or even months and is highly contagious (can be spread easily).

Croup is a viral respiratory disease in which the trachea and larynx become inflamed. It usually occurs in children between six months and three years of age, because the trachea is still very soft and pliable. The airway swells and becomes partially blocked. The child's breathing becomes difficult due to the excess mucus being produced and the partial collapse of the airway. This causes a *barking* sound when the child coughs. Once the child gets a little older, the trachea becomes more rigid, and collapse is less likely to occur. Croup usually goes away over time without treatment, and medication is not prescribed.

Cardiovascular and Blood Disorders

About 50% of newborns will develop *jaundice* in the first two to four days postpartum (after birth). This condition is caused by a buildup of excess bilirubin in the blood and results in the skin and the whites of the eyes appearing yellow. The infant's

---

asthma a respiratory disease characterized by wheezing, shortness of breath, and bronchoconstriction.

geriatric refers to persons over the age of 65.

side effects drug effects other than the intended one; usually undesirable but not harmful.

liver cannot break down bilirubin as fast as the body makes it. It is reabsorbed in the intestines before the infant can eliminate it in the stool. If left untreated, high bilirubin levels can cause deafness, cerebral palsy, and even brain damage.

A simple test for jaundice is to press a fingertip on the tip of a child's nose. If the skin shows a yellowish color, parents should contact a doctor. Jaundice in most infants resolves in a few days during the first week or two of life—without intervention. If this does not occur, phototherapy can be used. In phototherapy, the infant is exposed to a special light that helps break down the bilirubin.

Kawasaki disease is a condition that causes irritation and inflammation of many body tissues, including hands, feet, mouth, lips, and throat. Lymph nodes in the neck may become swollen and often cause heart-related complications. These may be temporary but can turn into long-term problems, especially if related to the coronary artery. Kawasaki disease weakens the wall of the artery and causes it to balloon or bulge out. This, in turn, can cause an aneurysm or blood clot. Treatment includes fever reducers and increased fluid intake. Sometimes aspirin is prescribed to prevent both inflammation from the disease and clot formation.

Rheumatic fever is another pediatric disease that can cause permanent damage to the heart valves. This may occur when the underlying streptococcal infection is not treated properly, or when strep infections occur frequently. The inflammation caused by this disease may damage the heart by scarring the valves, so the heart then has to work harder to pump blood.

Symptoms usually occur about one to five weeks after an infection by Streptococcus bacteria. The infection moves from one joint to another, causing small bumps under the skin. A pink rash follows, as do weight loss, stomach pain, and fatigue. Antibiotic therapy to kill the strep bacteria is the best way to prevent more serious damage and get rid of the infection. If heart valve damage occurs, surgical replacement or repair may be required.

Other common pediatric diseases can also affect the heart and cardiovascular system. In addition, heart problems may be congenital (defects present at birth) or brought on by lifestyle and habits. It is estimated that about 30% of U.S. children aged 6 to 18 are obese. Diet and proper education of family or caregivers is important in the prevention of heart disease in the pediatric population.

Geriatric Patients

Similar to pediatric patients, older adult patients have unique needs that require more specific care and understanding. The number of **geriatric** patients is increasing—and this fact will affect pharmacy practice in very significant ways. There are nearly 40 million Americans who are 65 years of age or older, and this figure is expected to grow to 70 million by 2030. Advances in medical technology, and the resulting extension of life and improvements in quality of life, have increased the number of geriatric patients seeking medical treatment, as well as the number of prescriptions filled each year (see Table 37-2). Currently, geriatric prescriptions account for the

TABLE 37-2 An Aging Society

Year	Median Age (in years)	Life Expectancy at Birth
1800	16	30
1850	19	38.3
1900	22.8	48.2
1950	28	66.1
1975	30.1	67.9
2000	35.5	74.8
2050 (projected)	40.7	82.6

greatest percentage of medication orders filled. Some experts have reported that 50% of all OTC products sold today, and 30% of prescription medications, are consumed by older patients.

Other factors, such as physiological changes, polypharmacy, multiple diseases, and noncompliance, also affect geriatric medication therapy and should be considered when treating this population.

The Physiological Factors

Geriatric patients experience many changes in the body's pharmacokinetic processes as aging occurs. According to Nathan Shock and his colleagues, as a general rule of thumb, most human physiologic systems accrue impairment at a rate of 5% to 10% per decade after the age of 30. These changes affect the way drugs are processed once they enter the body. Cardiac output decreases significantly with age, affecting the amount of blood that the kidneys and liver receive. By the age of 65, a person's liver and kidneys receive significantly less blood flow than they did at age 40. Because the kidneys, liver, and brain are the organs that require the most blood flow to function properly, the metabolism and excretion processes slow as people age. These changes allow certain drugs to stay in the body longer, so the drugs may cause increased **side effects**. Organs also decrease in size as patients age; this further slows the process of metabolism and may intensify any drug effects, whether intended or not.

Drug absorption in the geriatric patient is usually slower due to a decrease in intestinal blood flow, reduced gastric mobility, reduced stomach acid, and smaller intestinal surface area. These factors can delay the onset of action, so it takes longer to get the desired effect. However, these same factors also mean that the drug stays in the system longer, which means that the drug effect can last longer and have unwanted side effects.

Drug distribution is also affected in the aging adult, because the percentage of lean body mass and the total percentage of body water are lower than in younger adults. Drug levels are thus lower, because less water is available to distribute them throughout the body. The amount of body fat increases with age and can cause lipid-soluble drugs, such as general anesthetics, to be widely distributed to the organs that contain the most adipose tissue. This diverts such drugs away from the kidneys and liver, where the metabolism and excretion processes should occur, slowing the elimination of the drug from the body and causing the drug to have a longer **half-life** and possibly greater **toxicity** because of the increased levels of medication in the bloodstream.

As mentioned previously, metabolism and excretion generally decrease during the aging process. The frequent occurrence of kidney and liver disease in older people can also affect these processes. Such diseases as hypertension, coronary artery disease, diabetes, and cancer reduce the blood flow and production of some important microsomal metabolizing enzymes that are necessary for the process of chemically altering a drug so that it can be distributed into the blood and tissues. Excretion is also slower, which allows drugs to stay in the body longer. Because of these changes, geriatric patients are generally more sensitive to medications than younger people and often must take a lower dosage than the usual adult amount. In an older person, the dosage amount taken by a younger adult may produce a greater pharmacological effect. Therefore, drugs such as CNS depressants can actually increase mental depression and the appearance of episodes in older patients.

Although excretion is affected by aging, only the other three traditional components of pharmacokinetics—absorption, distribution, and metabolism—are meaningfully affected by age. Age-related changes in pharmacodynamics, on the other hand, are much more difficult to define.

As people approach their sixties and beyond, health challenges greatly increase. Among the most common health concerns among older people are:

- Muscle and bone loss
- Decreased lung function
- Increased blood pressure and exercise-induced heart rate
- Decreased kidney function
- Overactive bladder function
- Intestinal and colon complications
- Increased thyroid disorders
- Significant changes in sleeping patterns
- Vision impairment
- Declining dental health

Nutrition and the Presence of Disease

Nutritional status is extremely important to the geriatric patient's health (see Figure 37-5). Many older patients live alone and may have inadequate diets because of lack of social contact, tight finances, inability to do grocery shopping, or simple lack of appetite or interest in eating. Proper nutrition is very important to liver function and the ability to metabolize drugs. If protein intake is insufficient, the body has lower amounts of plasma protein, which is necessary for plasma protein drug binding. Many drugs bind to plasma proteins as they are distributed throughout the body, but only unbound (free) drugs cause a pharmacological effect. For example, albumin usually decreases with age. This albumin deficiency allows more unbound drug to remain in the patient's system; thus, the drug effects in the body are intensified. Nutritional deficiencies also make patients more susceptible to infections, other diseases, and drug–disease interactions.

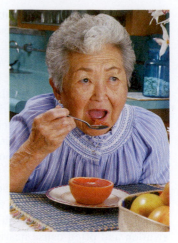

FIGURE 37-5 Maintaining proper nutrition is critical for older people, who often live alone.
Source: Carme Balcells/Shutterstock

The incidence of major chronic diseases, such as diabetes, hypertension, and mental depression, and respiratory illnesses often increases with aging and can have a great impact on medication therapy. General good health and proper nutrition are vital to proper physiological processes.

❝ Workplace Wisdom Immunizations and Older Patients

Numerous vaccine-preventable illnesses affect older people, therefore immunizations are of central importance. Specifically, influenza, pneumococcal disease, herpes zoster and tetanus are among those that are considered most important. In addition, MMR (measles, mumps and rubella) is recommended for patients born after 1957 or in high-risk groups with no documentation of immunization. The hepatitis B vaccine is also recommended for many older patients. ❞

Disease–Drug Interactions

Disease–drug interactions are medication effects that occur because of a preexisting disease or condition. Such interactions often occur because of the decrease in the number of drug receptors caused by aging. These reactions can be extreme; for example, a patient with congestive heart failure who uses drugs such as verapamil may suffer cardiac arrest and a renal disease patient who uses NSAIDs could develop complete renal failure. Patients with a chronic condition, such as anxiety or insomnia, may find that their symptoms grow worse. Drugs such as antianxiety agents or hypnotics may cause excessive *adverse effects* in older patients, because these patients are more sensitive to drugs that depress the central nervous system.

Certain drugs, such as antipsychotics, antidepressants, and antihistamines, can cause excessive side effects known as *anticholinergic effects,* which include urinary retention and

---

half-life the amount of time it takes the body to break down and excrete one-half of a drug dosage.

toxicity drug poisoning; can be life-threatening or extremely harmful.

noncompliance when a patient does not follow a prescribed drug regimen.

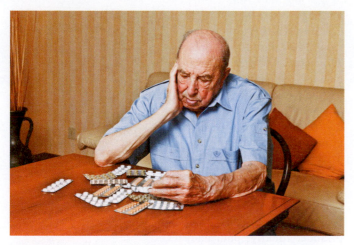

FIGURE 37-6 Overmedication is a growing problem in older people; patients in this population often take numerous prescription and OTC drugs at the same time.
Source: tommaso lizzul/Shutterstock

constipation. Special consideration and attention are required when prescribing for or dispensing to an older patient.

Overmedication is also a growing problem for the geriatric population (see Figure 37-6). Some patients think, "If one pill is good, then two pills should be better." This philosophy can lead to increased drug interactions, increased side effects, and higher medication costs. The more medications a patient takes, the higher the chance that interactions will occur. Common side effects, such as insomnia, dizziness, and dry mouth, occur more often in older people than in younger people and may be more intense in geriatric patients. A greatly increased risk of falls is another major negative effect of over-medication (see Figure 37-7). Falls account for 10% of all emergency room visits, and one out of ten results in a serious injury.

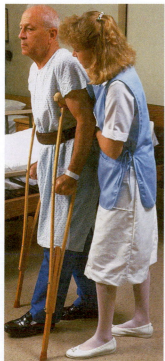

FIGURE 37-7 Older patients often fall because of the dizziness that some medications can cause.
Source: George Dodson/Pearson Education/PH College

Noncompliance

Drug *compliance*, or following a medication regimen, is another factor in geriatric medication. **Noncompliance**, which is defined as a patient's refusal or inability to follow a prescribed drug regimen, is very common in older patients. Those who live alone, have other diseases or conditions, or have problems with memory are at greatest risk of noncompliance.

There are many reasons why a patient may not take medication as prescribed. Sometimes the dosing schedule is confusing, and the patient

has difficulty understanding or remembering what the drug is and exactly why it was prescribed. The more complicated the drug regimen, the more likely it is that an older patient—or any patient, for that matter—will be noncompliant. Some other reasons for noncompliance by older patients include inability to afford the drug, belief that the medication is unnecessary, dislike of the drug's taste or inability to administer the dosage form, not understanding the directions, and not tolerating a drug's side effects. How can pharmacy technicians, as part of the health care team, help improve compliance?

Role of the Pharmacy Technician

The following are some ways in which pharmacy technicians and other health care team members can help ensure medication compliance:

- Greet each patient by name, and mention the name often.
- Keep the directions on the prescription label as simple as possible. Make sure that directions and instructions are legible! Many patients, especially older ones, have trouble reading small type.
- Give clear instructions on the exact treatment regimen, preferably in writing.
- Provide a card listing the medication dose, indication (reason for taking the medication), and time.
- Provide audiovisual aids, written materials, and computerized drug information.
- Ask the patient to repeat the directions on how to take the medication back to you.
- Suggest special reminder containers and calendars.
- Offer to call the patient if a refill is needed.
- Explain consequences of medication noncompliance.
- At each visit, emphasize the importance of adherence to the proper drug schedule.
- At each visit, acknowledge patients' efforts to take their medicines as ordered.
- Involve the patient's family and caregivers (see Figure 37-8).
- Avoid medical jargon when discussing the patient's medication therapy.
- Use short words and short sentences.
- Repeat instructions.
- Make advice as specific and detailed as possible.
- Find out what the patient's worries are; do not confine yourself merely to gathering objective medical information.
- Adopt a friendly demeanor rather than a strictly business-like attitude.
- Spend some time conversing about nonmedical topics.
- Suggest a behavioral contract.
- Ask patients to monitor their drug intake by keeping a log or diary.
- Help the patient link medication administration times to events in the daily routine.
- Ask the patient to recall in detail the medication(s) taken.
- Instruct patients to pay attention to adverse side effects and to inform the physician if they become concerned.
- Increase motivation by enlisting the patient in the decision-making process.
- Request that new patients bring in all medications to you to review, and create a current profile that includes them all.

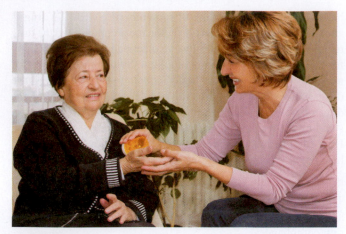

FIGURE 37-8 Involving family members in an older patient's drug routine can often help prevent noncompliance.
Source: Frank Conaway, Getty

 Preventing Overmedication & Adverse Reactions

The following is a list of some ways a pharmacy technician can help prevent overmedication and adverse reactions in older patients:

■ Help the pharmacist create a patient profile that includes all medications.

■ Make a note for the pharmacist to review the profile if you notice a duplication in medication class (e.g., more than one medication in the same class being taken for high cholesterol).

■ Provide nutritional information to patients to assist them in maintaining a proper diet regimen.

■ Identify any OTC products the patient is also taking and include them on the patient's current profile.

Compliance Issues Related to Dosage Forms and Timing

Another important consideration in compliance is the dosage form and administration times. Many older patients have difficulty swallowing, and large capsules or tablets are a problem. This requires evaluating the form to be dispensed and possibly changing to a liquid; depending on the medication, you may suggest crushing a pill into juice. Once-a-day medications are more user friendly and easier for geriatric patients to remember.

Community-based pharmacies and nursing homes also use a packaging technique called *unit dosing*, in which each

---

polypharmacy the administration of more medications than clinically indicated.

package contains a single dose of the drug(s) that should be taken at one time. This makes the drug regimen less confusing and easier for the patient to know what drugs to take and when to take them. If unit dosing is not possible, describing the different drugs as *the big green one* or the *football-shaped one* can help patients identify the correct medication and thus enhance compliance. Ideally, pharmacy instructions would be given to caregivers and family as well as to the patient.

Medication boxes and other reminders can also be very helpful in increasing medication compliance (see Figure 37-9). These devices can be used to help the patient stay on a schedule. Older patients may also find that associating their daily medication schedule with meals or other daily tasks, such as brushing their teeth, can act as reminders to take the medications properly.

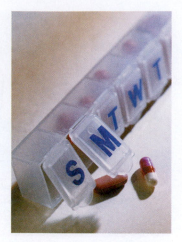

FIGURE 37-9 Encourage older patients to use a medication box to keep track of their daily medications.
Source: Steve Cole/Getty Images

❝ Workplace Wisdom Helping Patients Remember Their Medications

Many tools are available to help seniors better manage the multitude of medications they are often required to take. Pill containers, as well as some new electronic reminders, can be set up initially during a counseling session with the pharmacist.

Another consideration is drug packaging. Lids and caps on medication bottles are sometimes hard to remove, especially if the patient has arthritis. Easy-to-open lids can be substituted. For those with impaired eyesight or who have trouble reading, large print on labels and other direction or instruction sheets are very helpful. ❞

Polypharmacy

Polypharmacy is the administration of more medications than are clinically necessary or multiple drug prescriptions. Studies show that this occurs with 55% to 59% of the geriatric population. Due to the aging process and the incidence of multiple diseases, older patients often end up taking many medications (see Figure 37-10). Conditions such as diabetes, osteoporosis, Alzheimer's disease, dementia, and depression are very common in the older population and often require complicated and multiple drug regimens frequently prescribed by several different physicians. Polypharmacy is a significant cause of noncompliance, adverse effects, and drug interactions. Good pharmacy practitioners will help patients coordinate administration of these multiple drug regimens, as well as stay alert

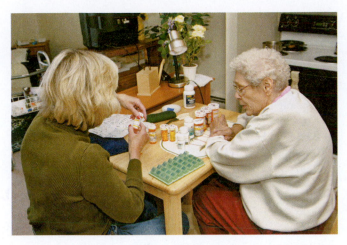

FIGURE 37-10 Keeping track of daily medications often requires the help of family members.
Source: Dennis MacDonald/PhotoEdit Inc.

to possible interactions and duplications in their patients' medications.

Some of these conditions affect the patient's mental abilities, but even the most alert patients can become confused about how and when to take their various medications. With each new medication, the possibility of drug–drug and drug–disease interactions increases; this includes OTC drugs and products. This is especially true among older patients, who constitute only 12% to 17% of the population buying OTC drugs, but consume about 30% of all OTC medications. In fact, older patients are projected to consume more than 50% of all OTC medications by the year 2012. Often patients take OTC medications without the physician's knowledge. In addition, geriatric patients may purchase medications from more than one pharmacy and see more than one prescribing doctor. When a patient is getting prescriptions from a cardiologist, a rheumatologist, an internist, and an ophthalmologist, for example, polypharmacy is almost inevitable. Coordinating these various medications and prescriptions is critically important—and far from easy.

To help solve the problem of polypharmacy and avoid complications and adverse drug interactions, pharmacists and pharmacy technicians must record *every* medication their patients are taking and keep a current patient profile. One good way to do this is the *brown bag method*. The patient is asked to bring *all* his medications to the pharmacy where he meets with the pharmacist so that the pharmacist can record each one. This ensures that no medication is forgotten and creates a complete profile for the pharmacy. Patients should be sure to include any herbal, diet, or vitamin supplements, topical preparations, and OTC products, as well as prescription medications. Encourage the patient to bring this *bag* in once a year for review. Emphasize the importance of notifying the pharmacy and physician of any new drugs as soon as they are added.

PROFILE IN PRACTICE

Mrs. Landon is an older patient who comes to your pharmacy with her daughter. The daughter states that her mother takes 15 medications and was recently diagnosed with and hospitalized for diabetes. The nurse in the hospital told Mrs. Landon and her daughter about certain types of infections being prominent in diabetic patients. The daughter wants to know what preventive measures she can take to help her mother, and what kind of diabetes monitoring machine she should buy.

▸ *As a technician, what can you do to help this patient choose a diabetes monitoring system?*
▸ *What information about infection prevention can you provide to these clients?*

❝ **Workplace Wisdom** **The Baby Boomers Are Aging**
In the United States, there are currently 77 million *baby boomers* of middle adult age, and the fastest-growing age group is 85 and older. By the year 2050, the population of older people will increase to approximately 72 million. ❞

Medicare Part D

The Medicare Prescription Drug, Improvement, and Modernization Act of 2003, which became effective on January 1, 2006, extends prescription coverage to all patients who are eligible for Medicare benefits. It is a voluntary insurance program to provide some drug coverage for those who experience hardships or have high-cost medications. The patient must sign up within three months of becoming eligible for Medicare (three months before reaching age 65 or three months after), or possibly face a penalty. Patients in the program are given a variety of drug coverage plans to choose from, each of which includes a yearly deductible (between $0 and $265) and a monthly premium. Each plan has its own formulary (list of drugs) and specific costs. For patients on high-cost medications, the pharmacist may provide and charge for medication management therapy (MMT). This therapy may take the form of an in-depth annual review of the patient's medications through a program such as the *brown bag*, for instance. Medication management by a pharmacist provides a safety feature and ensures a complete profile for the pharmacy record.

Pharmacy technicians can play an important role in gathering information for the pharmacist who is providing MMT as well as participating in billing and online adjudication. A current profile that includes all of a patient's OTC medications, as well as the physicians that the patient sees, is necessary to ensure safe medication therapy. A technician is often the first person the older customer sees at the counter. Asking questions about these matters, finding about any allergies, and noting any changes in insurance coverage are all great ways to keep the patient's history current for the pharmacist to review.

Cognitive Impairment

Cognition is an umbrella concept referring to an individual's mental ability and process to acquire knowledge and understanding through thought, experience, and the senses. Cognition consists of attention, decision making, language, memory, mental imagery, pattern recognition, problem solving, reading, reasoning, sensory perception, storing and retrieving information, and writing. Mild cognitive impairment (MCI) is considered a normal part of the aging process, as research shows that 17% to 34% of elders exhibit MCI. Evidence of MCI includes forgetfulness and what we refer to as *senior moments*.

Significant cognitive impairment, which includes delirium and dementia, is less common. Delirium is often reversible and is associated with a number of common conditions, such as chronic obstructive pulmonary disease (COPD), congestive heart failure (CHF), dehydration, diabetes, medication, pneumonia, upper respiratory infections, urinary tract infections, and surgery. On the other hand, dementia, which includes diseases such as Alzheimer's, is quite different from delirium (see Table 37-3). Alzheimer's disease accounts for up to 70% of dementia cases in older people.

Cognitive impairment can also be drug-induced. According to Beers Criteria for Potentially Inappropriate Medication

Use in Older Adults, the following drugs are associated with cognitive changes in older people:

- Acyclovir
- Antchloinergics
- Anticonvulsants
- Asparaginase
- Atropine
- Baclofen
- Barbituates
- Benzodiazepines
- Beta-blockers
- Buspirone
- Caffeine
- Chlorambucil
- Chloroquine
- Clonidine
- Clozapine
- Cytarabine
- Digitalis glycosides
- Disulfiram
- Dronabinol
- Ganciclovir
- H-2 antagonists
- Ifostamide
- Interleukin-2
- Ketamine
- Levodopa
- Maprotiline
- Mefloquine
- Methyldopa
- Methylphenidate
- Metriazamide
- Metronidazole
- Pergolide
- Phenylpropanolamine
- Pilocarpine
- Propafenone
- Quinidine
- Salicylates
- Seligiline
- Sulfonamides
- Trazadone
- Tricyclic antidepressants

Elder Abuse

According to the World Health Organization, elder abuse is defined as "a single, or repeated act, or lack of appropriate action, occurring within any relationship where there is an expectation of trust which causes harm or distress to an older person." Elder abuse is more common than you might expect. According to the National Elder Mistreatment Study, 10% of community-dwelling adults aged 60 or older reported some form of abuse, excluding financial, in recent years. Elder abuse takes place in many forms—physical, sexual, psychological, financial, neglect, and self-neglect. Although a federal standard does not exist, most states have laws requiring mandatory reporting requirements for elder abuse. While some states apply such laws to *any person*, other states provide a list of responsible individuals such as law enforcement officials, social service providers, and health care professionals. As a pharmacy technician, you need to be familiar with your state regulations and be prepared to report any evidence of elder abuse.

TABLE 37-3 Delirium Versus Dementia

Feature	Delirium	Dementia
Onset	Acute and abrupt	Subtle and gradual
Symptoms	Fluctuate	Consistent
Duration	Hours or weeks	Continuous and progressive
Short-term memory	Severely impaired	Declines slowly

info

National Center on Elder Abuse

The National Center on Elder Abuse (NCEA), which is directed by the U.S. Administration on Aging, provides assistance, services, and resources related to elder care, adult protective services, and elder abuse. For information on state reporting numbers, government agencies, state laws, and resources, the NCEA can be contacted at 1-800-677-1116 or by visiting **www.ncea.aoa.gov**

Summary

Pediatric patients are physiologically different, and thus present special medication considerations and challenges. Respiratory diseases such as asthma, infectious diseases such as colds, and heart diseases such as rheumatic fever are just a few of the special challenges that face pediatric patients.

Dosage calculations often involve small quantities and require special formulations using manufacturers' guidelines. Lack of organ development, as well as verbal communication ability, also ensures many unique challenges when medicating this patient population. A technician should always take special precautions when calculating doses and reconfirm orders often to prevent medication errors. The health care team must provide education for the patient's family, as well as participating in a tracking and quality assurance system to ensure that mistakes are reviewed and learned from. These are just a few of the ways to ensure correct pediatric medication dispensing.

The aging process causes pharmacokinetic changes in geriatric patients, such as slower metabolism and excretion. Organ size, blood flow, and cardiac output all generally decrease with age. These factors decrease drug absorption and can delay the onset of drug action. These same factors often require a reduction in medication dosage because of the greater pharmacological effects that occur with slower metabolism and increased drug retention. Other considerations and complications, such as multiple medication therapy (polypharmacy), the presence of several diseases, and noncompliance, are significant in proper treatment of geriatric patients. Special aids, such as easy-open lids, medication organizers, complete patient profiles, and alternate dosage forms, are just a few of the ways to improve compliance and prevent drug interactions.

It is estimated that by the year 2050, geriatric persons will constitute 20.4% of the population. The great strides being made in the medical field not only increase both life expectancy and quality of life but also increase the challenges of pharmacy, with a significantly higher number of prescriptions and demand for trained personnel to accomplish the tasks of good pharmacy practice. Education is the key to quality geriatric medication therapy. Quality therapy will take a dedicated team of health care workers, and the pharmacy technician will play an even greater role on this team in the future.

Chapter Review Questions

1. Pediatric patients aged one month to two years are considered _____.
   a. neonates
   b. infants
   c. children
   d. adolescents

2. Geriatric patients experience a/an _____ in body fat as they age.
   a. increase
   b. delay
   c. decrease
   d. hardening

3. After a medication gains access to the bloodstream, it is then _____ to the organs and tissues.
   a. metabolized
   b. distributed
   c. excreted
   d. absorbed

4. Geriatric patients metabolize certain drugs, such as pain medications, _____ younger adults.
   a. slower than
   b. faster than
   c. the same as
   d. none of the above

5. Geriatric patients generally require a/an _____ in medication dosages due to the _____ rate of elimination.
   a. decrease; slower
   b. increase; faster
   c. decrease; faster
   d. increase; slower

6. One way of calculating dosages for pediatric medication, based only on a child's age, is known as _____.
   a. Young's rule
   b. Clark's rule
   c. mg/kg/day
   d. alligations

7. Polypharmacy is best described as _____.
   a. getting prescriptions from several pharmacies
   b. taking multiple medications
   c. getting prescriptions from several physicians
   d. all of the above

8. The most common physiological cause of otitis media in pediatric patients is _____.
   a. foreign objects placed in the ear
   b. a middle-ear tube that is shorter than in adults
   c. fluid buildup in the nasal cavity
   d. bacterial drug resistance

9. By the year 2050, geriatric persons are expected to constitute what percentage of the population?
   a. 4.1
   b. 8.1
   c. 12.8
   d. 20.4

10. As much as _____ of all over-the-counter drugs sold today are consumed by older patients.
    a. 50%
    b. 30%
    c. 59%
    d. 55%

Critical Thinking Questions

1. Explain why slow metabolism rates in pediatric patients can lead to toxic drug levels.

2. What pediatric dosage calculation method do you think is the best? Explain why.

3. Explain why slow metabolism rates in geriatric patients can lead to toxic drug levels.

4. What factors contribute to noncompliance in the geriatric population, and how can a pharmacy technician help prevent them?

Web Challenge

1. Look up a website for medication management, and search for information about the role that pharmacy technicians will play in the future. Discuss how you as a pharmacy technician can help educate patients about better ways to manage their many medications and diseases. Give three examples of medication devices currently available for patients who may be experiencing polypharmacy situations.

2. Look up Alzheimer's disease, and discuss the symptoms, treatments, and current medications being used in the treatment of this disease. Name a medication being used today, and describe how it works. Are any others being researched?

References and Resources

Davidson, M.W., M.L. London, and P.W. Ladewig. *Olds' Maternal-Newborn Nursing & Women's Health Across the Lifespan*. 9th ed. Upper Saddle River, NJ: Pearson, 2011. Print.

Fick D.W., J.W. Cooper, W.E. Wade, et al. "Updating the Beers Criteria for Potentially Inappropriate Medication Use in Older Adults; Results of a US Consensus Panel of Experts." *Archives of Internal Medicine*. 163 (2003): 2716–2724.

Fusco, J.A. "Elder Abuse." In: Richardson M., Chant C., Chessman K.H., Finsk S.W., Hemstreet B.A., Hume A.L., et al., eds. *Pharmacotherapy Self-Assessment Program*. 7th ed. *Geriatrics*. Lenexa, KS: American College of Clinical Pharmacy, 2011. Print.

Haase, M.R. "Poisoning and Envenomation." In: Richardson M., Chant C., Chessman K.H., Finsk S.W., Hemstreet B.A., Hume A.L., et al., eds. *Pharmacotherapy Self-Assessment Program*. 7th ed. *Pediatrics*. Lenexa, KS: American College of Clinical Pharmacy, 2010. Print.

Hilas, O. and C.E. Danielle. "Immunizations in the Elderly." In: Richardson M., Chant C., Chessman K.H., Finsk S.W., Hemstreet B.A., Hume A.L., et al., eds. *Pharmacotherapy Self-Assessment Program.* 7th ed. *Geriatrics.* Lenexa, KS: American College of Clinical Pharmacy, 2011. Print.

Hitner, H. and B. Nagle. *Pharmacology: An Introduction.* 6th ed. New York, NY: McGraw-Hill, 2011. Print.

Holland, L.N. and M. Adams. *Core Concepts in Pharmacology.* 3rd ed. Upper Saddle River, NJ: Pearson, 2010. Print.

Johnston, M. *The Pharmacy Technician: Foundations and Practices.* 1st ed. Upper Saddle, River, NJ: Pearson. 2009. Print.

Soriano, R., Fernandez, H., Cassel, C., Leipzig. *Fundamentals of Geriatric Medicine: A Case-Based Approach.* New York, NY: Springer, 2007. Print.

Wick, J.Y. *Pharmacy Practice in an Aging Society.* Binghamton, NY: Pharmaceutical Products Press, 2006. Print.

"World Population Ageing 2009." *United Nations.* United Nations. December 2009. Web. 27 May 2012.

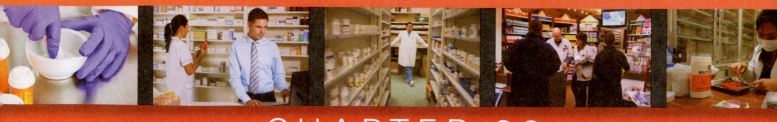

CHAPTER 38

Biopharmaceuticals

LEARNING OBJECTIVES

After completing this chapter, you should be able to:

- Name at least two drugs developed by using recombinant DNA technology, and outline their uses.

- Discuss the four steps in the genetic engineering process.

- Explain briefly how a company gets approval for a biopharmaceutical drug from the FDA.

- Discuss why biopharmaceuticals, genetic engineering, and stem cell research are important in the future of pharmacy and the practice of medicine.

KEY TERMS

allergenics, p. 651

biologics, p. 651

biopharmaceuticals, p. 650

biopharmacology, p. 650

biotechnology, p. 651

Gaucher's disease, p. 651

genetically modified organism (GMO), p. 652

neutropenia, p. 651

rheumatoid arthritis, p. 651

transform, p. 652

vector, p. 652

INTRODUCTION

Biopharmacology is a growing field of research similar to pharmacokinetics (see chapter 23). It is the branch of pharmacology that studies the use of biologically engineered drugs. Biopharmaceuticals are substances created using biotechnology. They can be proteins like antibodies, or even consist of DNA and RNA. Research is being conducted in this area to find new therapeutic medications to treat such life-threatening diseases as AIDS, various cancers, and Parkinson's disease.

The majority of **biopharmaceuticals** are derived from life forms existing in nature, such as plants and animals, although the medications are produced by means other than direct extraction from a biological source. Genetic engineering is another way to create new drugs, and stem cell research offers tantalizing

---

biopharmacology the branch of pharmacology that studies the use of biologically engineered drugs.

biopharmaceuticals substances created using biotechnology.

opportunities for new therapeutic treatments and is making significant strides in the development of new medications used today. This chapter discusses these three forms of biopharmacology, their impact on the pharmaceutical industry, and their role in the future of pharmacology.

What Are Biopharmaceuticals?

The terms biologic, biopharmaceutical, products of pharmaceutical biotechnology, and biotechnology medicines are often used interchangeably; however, they can mean different things to different people. **Biologics** refer to medicinal products derived from blood, as well as vaccines, toxins, and allergen products. Biopharmaceuticals, a term originated in the 1980s, describes a class of therapeutic protein produced by biotechnological techniques such as genetic engineering. Biological medicine, or products of pharmaceutical biotechnology, has the broadest definition, referring to the use of biological systems, such as cells or tissues, or biological molecules, such as enzymes or antibodies, in the manufacturing of commercial products. This classification includes a wide variety of medicinal products, such as vaccines, blood products, **allergenics**, and proteins (including antibodies). Biopharmaceuticals may be composed of sugars, proteins, and even living tissue or cells. Louis Pasteur's work in 1857 could be considered the first use of biotechnology, because he converted a food source into another form.

Recombinant therapeutic proteins (RTPs), which are also produced by **biotechnology**, are at the forefront of biomedical technology. RTPs are artificial forms of recombinant DNA that have been created by combining or inserting one or more DNA strands into a single molecule (see Figure 38-1). One of the first biotechnological substances to be approved by the Food and Drug Administration (FDA) was Humulin insulin, or recombinant human insulin (rHI), manufactured by the Eli Lilly Company beginning in 1982. RTPs can also be made and used to treat a variety of medical conditions for which no other treatments are available. Some of the biopharmaceutical drugs currently being used include Cerezyme for

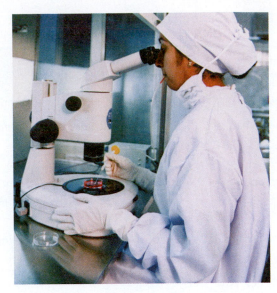

FIGURE 38-1 Scientist performing research in DNA technology.
Source: AP Photo/Jayanta Saha

Gaucher's disease, Leukine for **neutropenia**, and Synvisc and Hyalgan for **rheumatoid arthritis**.

Recombinant DNA technology has had four primary positive impacts on the production of pharmaceutically important proteins: (1) It resolves the problem of source availability; (2) It addresses the problems of product safety; (3) It provides an alternative to direct extraction from inappropriate or dangerous source materials; (4) It aids the generation of engineered therapeutic proteins offering advantages over the native protein products.

❝ Workplace Wisdom Storing Biological Drugs

The FDA imposes special requirements on biological drugs. These drugs are often still in the research or clinical trial stage and require extensive documentation for FDA review. Pharmacy technicians should always be aware of any special precautions, storage requirements, labeling instructions, or ordering and inventory information regarding these drugs. The FDA website contains all necessary information pertaining to biologicals.

Table 38-1 lists some of the biologics made with recombinant DNA technology that are currently on the market and the diseases they are used to treat. ❞

Process of FDA Approval

When a company develops a new biopharmaceutical drug, the company must apply for a *patent*, which gives it the sole and exclusive rights to manufacture and sell that drug. It takes approximately 12 years to move a drug from the experimental stage to the pharmacy.

During the first, *preclinical* phase, the new drug is tested against a targeted disease through laboratory and animal studies. This process also evaluates the acute toxicity of the drug to discover if it is reasonably safe to use in humans. This entire process can take from three to five years.

---

biologics a group of varied medicinal products, such as vaccines, blood products, allergenics, and proteins.

allergenic a substance that can cause an allergic reaction.

biotechnology the use of biological substances or microorganisms to perform specific functions, such as the production of drugs, hormones, or food products.

Gaucher's disease a disease in which fatty materials collect in the liver, spleen, kidneys, lungs, and brain and cause the person to be susceptible to infections.

neutropenia a disease in which there is an abnormal number of the white blood cells that are responsible for fighting infections.

rheumatoid arthritis an autoimmune disease that causes chronic inflammation of the joints.

TABLE 38-1 Biologics Made with Recombinant DNA Technology

Generic Name	Trade Name	Condition Used for
abatacept	Orencia	Rheumatoid arthritis
adalimumab	Humira	Rheumatoid arthritis
alefacept	Amevive	Chronic plaque psoriasis
erythropoietin	Epogen	Anemia from cancer Therapy, chronic renal failure
etanercept	Enbrel	Rheumatoid arthritis, psoriasis
infliximab	Remicade	Crohn's disease
trastuzumab	Herceptin	Breast cancer
ustekinumab	Stelara	Psoriasis

After the preclinical phase, the company files an Investigational New Drug (IND) application with the FDA. The IND shows the results of the animal pharmacology and toxicology studies that have already been done, along with detailed information and protocols for future clinical studies that will help determine if initial-phase drug trials will be safe enough to involve human subjects. The IND must also include the chemical structure of the compound and the company's plans for its manufacture. This helps the FDA assess whether the company can produce and supply consistent batches of the drug.

vector an organism that does not itself cause disease, but spreads disease by distributing or carrying pathogens from one host to another.

transform alter an organism or a cell itself in the genetic engineering process.

genetically modified organism (GMO) an organism whose genetic material has been altered using the genetic engineering techniques known as recombinant DNA technology.

The IND becomes effective if the FDA does not disapprove it within 30 days. The next three steps are clinical trials, which are conducted with volunteers in clinics and hospitals, under the care of a physician. These trials, which take several years (see Figure 38-2), use varying groups of volunteers; a study may involve as few as 20 patients or as many as 3,000.

Following the successful completion of all three IND phases, the company can then file a new drug application (NDA) with the FDA; approval of an NDA can take as long as 30 months. Once the FDA gives its approval, the drug becomes available for physicians to prescribe. However, the FDA often requires some additional annual reporting to evaluate long-term effects.

Since 1978, the number of patents on drugs has risen significantly. For example, in 1978, only 30 patents were issued for FDA-approved drugs; by 2001, more than 34,000 patents had been granted. Several countries, including Argentina, China, and Egypt, are involved in research to develop new drugs, and their respective governments are funding these endeavors with huge financial grants each year. Approval can cost a company as much as $400 million. Even after a patent is granted and the drug is released to the market, it is still monitored for several more years to ensure safety and performance.

Genetic Engineering

Genetic engineering, which is the direct manipulation of an organism's genes, is another way to produce new medications. The first genetically engineered drug was approved by the FDA for therapeutic use in 1982. It was rHi, also known as Humulin insulin. In 1986, the FDA approved a genetically engineered vaccine for hepatitis B and since then many new products have

info

New Drug Applications (NDAs)

Did you know? An NDA runs 10,000 or more pages. Only about one in five drugs on which the clinical testing is done makes it through the FDA trials and approval process.

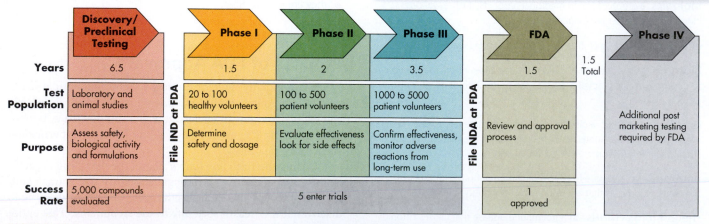

FIGURE 38-2 The FDA approval process for a new biopharmaceutical.

been approved, such as Pulmozyme for cystic fibrosis and Alferon N for genital warts.

The genetic engineering process has four basic steps. The first step is to isolate the desirable gene, such as resistance to a particular disease. Next, that gene is inserted into a **vector**, which is any organism that does not itself cause disease but spreads it by distributing pathogens from one host to another. Bacteria containing plasmids or extrachromosomal DNA molecules that can replicate themselves make good vectors.

During the third step, scientists use the vector to **transform**, or genetically alter, the cells of another organism. Finally, the new **genetically modified organism (GMO)** is isolated from cells that did not take up the vector. The GMO is packaged with resistant genes and then placed in a culture with penicillin to ensure that only cells that have incorporated the vector survive.

Examples of GMOs are synthetic human insulin (approved by the FDA in 1982) and a hepatitis vaccine (approved in 1987). With synthetic human insulin, the human gene that directs the production of insulin was inserted into a harmless bacterial cell. This enabled the large-scale production of insulin under controlled conditions. Genetically modified (GM) viruses have been used to treat severe immune deficiency and some genetic diseases such as sickle cell anemia, muscular dystrophy, and cystic fibrosis. When the DNA of a virus is removed through the genetic engineering process (as described above), the virus is no longer able to inject its DNA into healthy cells. This limits the spread of disease and enables creation of a safe vaccine. Finally, GM foods, such as vegetables, have been created: some resist certain bacterial infections, some were made resistant to pests, and some were modified to stay fresh longer.

Stem Cell Research

Stem cell research also plays a significant role in the discovery of new pharmaceutical products and medical treatments (see Figure 38-3). Scientists are interested in the potential use of embryonic stem cells to treat disease for three reasons. First, stem cells have a special ability to renew themselves many times through cell division in a process called *proliferation*. Second, unlike nerve or muscle cells, which perform specific functions in the body, stem cells are unspecialized (undifferentiated). Third, under certain conditions, stem cells can transform into specialized cells, such as heart muscle, through a process called *differentiation*.

Only since 1998, scientists have been able to isolate stem cells from human embryos, so discovering the full potential of stem cells in the treatment of a disease is an ongoing process. One way they may eventually be useful is in the widespread testing of experimental medications, before the new medications are used in human clinical drug trials. Cancer research, as well as treatments for other life-threatening diseases, such as Parkinson's disease, is already benefiting from the discoveries made in this area. For example, cancer cell lines are currently being used to screen for potential antitumor drugs. Stem cells could also offer a renewable source of replacement cells and tissue for treatment of diseases such as Parkinson's, diabetes, and Alzheimer's (see Figure 38-4). In Parkinson's disease, the brain cells that release dopamine die, causing a chemical imbalance in the brain. Characteristics of this chemical deficiency are tremors and a shuffling gait. Human genes that correct this imbalance were packaged in a virus and then injected into the brain cells of 59-year-old Nathan Klein, who had suffered from Parkinson's disease for more than four years.

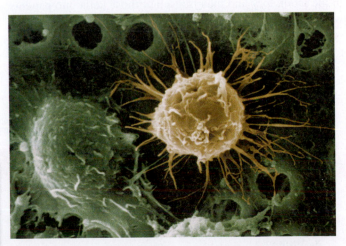

FIGURE 38-3 Color-enhanced scanning electron micrograph (SEM) of a stem cell collected from human bone marrow.
Source: Andrew Paul Leonard/Science Source

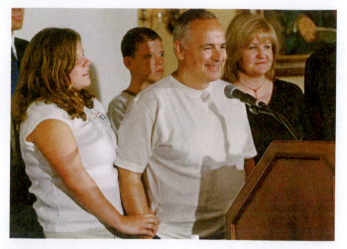

FIGURE 38-4 Nathan Klein, the first person to have gene therapy for Parkinson's disease.
Source: AP Photo/Frank Franklin II

About six months after treatment, he reported feeling better. Although the effects of the gene therapy started wearing off in 2010, he is now having to take only six pills a day, compared to 30 at one point.

The Political Climate

The field of biotechnology is politically charged and highly contentious. Despite the medical breakthroughs that have been accomplished through biopharmacy, genetic engineering, and stem cell research, some groups argue that biotechnology is morally wrong: First, because only God creates life, not scientists; second, because currently human embryos—potential human life—must be used as the source of stem cells. Furthermore, although some scientists argue that this research is necessary to combat both existing and future diseases, develop better medical treatments, and improve crop yields in a hungry world, others are concerned about the health consequences of consuming genetically engineered plants and animals.

Significant strides have been made in the treatment of many diseases such as diabetes with Humulin and rheumatoid arthritis with Epogen. Companies in countries across the globe are spending millions of dollars every day on research in a race to find new biopharmaceutical products. Imaging of the basic cellular structure has now become an integral part of clinical trials in the hopes that one day such information will be used to develop new, better, and more effective products. The availability and use of stem cells has increased; however, the field remains politically divisive.

Summary

Biopharmaceutical research is a growing field of pharmaceutics, and there is a growing need for the drugs that are the end products of this research. Biopharmaceuticals are used today to treat cancers, diabetes, hepatitis, multiple sclerosis and other life-threatening conditions. Genetic engineering and stem cell research play a very important role in the discovery of new products and the treatment of disease. For example, using stem cells, it may become possible to grow healthy heart muscle cells in the laboratory and then transplant those cells into patients with chronic heart disease. Genetic engineering could be used someday to repair damaged genes or replace missing genes in people who have genetic disorders such as cystic fibrosis.

Even though the FDA process for approval of a new drug is long and very expensive, the discovery of new drugs and the development of new technologies are crucial to our health. Biotechnology holds many opportunities for the future, especially as new diseases develop and old ones reemerge. The pharmaceutical industry will need to develop new vaccines and antibiotics for prevention and cure of diseases, to accelerate the drug discovery process, and to determine more accurate medication dosages. With today's extended life expectancy and the number of prescriptions on the rise, improved pharmacy service is even more important. As members of the pharmacy health care team, pharmacy technicians need to better understand diseases and find new and better ways to provide treatment so that we can provide the best possible patient care.

Chapter Review Questions

1. _____ specifically refers to medicinal products derived from blood, as well as vaccines, toxins, and allergen products.
   a. Biologics
   b. Biopharmaceuticals
   c. Biological medicines
   d. Products of pharmaceutical biotechnology

2. Artificial forms of DNA produced by biotechnology are known as _____.
   a. vectors
   b. GMOs
   c. recombinant therapeutic proteins
   d. none of the above

3. Enbrel is a biologic drug made with recombinant technology and is used to treat _____.
   a. breast cancer
   b. rheumatoid arthritis
   c. tumors
   d. Crohn's disease

4. Ustekinumab is a biologic drug made with recombinant technology and is used to treat _____.
   a. rheumatoid arthritis
   b. Crohn's disease
   c. breast cancer
   d. psoriasis

5. All of the following statements about biopharmaceuticals are true *except* _____.
   a. they are products derived from live plants and animals
   b. they can be used for diagnostic purposes
   c. they are not patentable
   d. they are produced by biotechnology

6. The first genetically engineered substance approved by the FDA for therapeutic use was _____.
   a. Enbrel
   b. Humira
   c. Humalog
   d. Humulin

7. In the process of genetic engineering, _____ is the actual alteration of the cell.
   a. isolation
   b. transformation
   c. vectoring
   d. extraction

8. Genetic engineering is the process of _____.
   a. direct manipulation of an organism's genes
   b. making products using biotechnology
   c. direct extraction from a native biological source
   d. making cells and tissues for medical therapies

9. It takes approximately _____ years from the time a new drug is introduced until a physician can prescribe it.
   a. 11
   b. 12
   c. 5
   d. 3

10. Required by the FDA, the _____ typically consists of 10,000 pages of information.
    a. IND
    b. GMO
    c. rHI
    d. NDA

Critical Thinking Questions

1. Explain why some people consider stem cell research to be wrong.

2. What challenges will arise for pharmacy in the future because of the number of people living longer and requiring more medication? How can biopharmaceuticals help meet these challenges?

3. List three advantages and three disadvantages of the development of biopharmaceuticals.

Web Challenge

1. Visit the FDA's website and search for current regulations on biopharmaceutical products.

2. Using the FDA website as a source, list at least 10 biopharmaceuticals that are currently on the market, and name their therapeutic uses.

References and Resources

"Access Excellence." The National Health Museum. Web. 27 May 2012.

"BioSpace." BioSpace. Web. 27 May 2012.

Johnston, M. The Pharmacy Technician: Foundations and Practices. 1st ed. Upper Saddle, River, NJ: Pearson. 2009. Print.

"Stem Cell Basics." National Institute of Health. 2008. Web. 27 May 2012.

Walsh, G.. Biopharmaceuticals: Biochemistry and Biotechnology. 2nd ed. Chichester, West Sussex: Wiley, 2003. Print.

Appendix A:
Common Over-the-Counter Products

Category	Trade Name(s)	Form	Active Ingredients
Analgesics/ antipyretics— acetaminophen, adult	Tylenol	Tablet	Acetaminophen 325 mg
	Tylenol Arthritis	Tablet	Acetaminophen 650 mg
	Tylenol Rapid Release	Gelcap	Acetaminophen 500 mg
	Tylenol Extra Strength	Tablet	Acetaminophen 500 mg
	Tylenol Rapid Blast	Liquid	Acetaminophen 500 mg/5 mL
	Alka-Seltzer Plus Cold, Sinus, Non-Drowsy Effervescent	Tablet	Acetaminophen 250 mg/phenylephrine 5 mg/aspirin 325 mg
	Anacin Advanced Headache Formula	Tablet	Acetaminophen 250 mg/aspirin 250 mg/ caffeine 65 mg
	Excederin Tension Headache	Geltab	Acetaminophen 500 mg/caffeine 65 mg
	Percogesic Original Strength Pain Reliever	Tablet	Acetaminophen 325 mg/diphenhydramine 12.5 mg
Analgesics/ antipyretics— acetaminophen, pediatric	Children's Tylenol Meltaways	Tablet	Acetaminophen 80 mg
	FeverAll Infant	Suppository	Acetaminophen 80 mg
	FeverAll Children's	Suppository	Acetaminophen 160 mg
	Feverall Junior Strength	Tablet	Acetaminophen 325 mg
	Children's Tylenol	Liquid	Acetaminophen 160 mg/5 mL
	Infant's Tylenol Drops	Drops	Acetaminophen 80 mg/0.8 mL
Analgesics/ antipyretics— aspirin, adult	Bayer Low-Dose, St. Joseph's, Ecotrin	Chewable tablet	Acetaminophen 81 mg
	Genuine Bayer	Tablet	Acetaminophen 325 mg
	Extra-Strength Bayer	Tablet	Acetaminophen 500 mg
Analgesics/ antipyretics— NSAID, adult	Advil, Advil Migraine, Motrin IB	Caplet, capsule, gelcap, tablet	Ibuprofen 200 mg
	Aleve, Midol Extended Relief	Caplet, gelcap, tablet	Naproxen sodium 220 mg
	Doan's Extra Strength, Percogesic Maximum	Caplet, capsule	Magnesium salicylate 580 mg
Antipyretics— NSAID, pediatric	Children's Advil, Children's Motrin	Liquid	Ibuprofen 100 mg/5 mL
	Infant's Motrin Concentrated Drops	Drops	Ibuprofen 50 mg/1.25 mL
	Jr. Strength Motrin	Chewable tablet	Ibuprofen 100 mg

Category	Trade Name(s)	Form	Active Ingredients
Antihistamines, adult	Claritin, Alavert	Chewable tablet, liquid, tablet	Loratadine 10 mg, 5 mg/5 mL
	Zyrtec	Capsule, liquid, tablet	Cetirizine 10 mg, 5 mg/5 mL
	Allegra 12 hr	Tablet	Fexofenadine 60 mg
	Allegra 24 hr	Tablet	Fexofenadine 180 mg
	Benadryl	Capsule, liquid	Diphenhydramine 25 mg, 12.5 mg/5 mL
Antitussives	Coricidin HBP Cough and Cold	Tablet	Dextromethrophan 30 mg/ Chlorpheniramine 4 mg
	Dimetapp Children's Long Acting Cough Plus Cold	Liquid	Dextromethrophan 7.5 mg/ chlorpheniramine 1 mg/5 mL
	Scot-Tussin DM Maximum Strength	Liquid	Dextromethrophan 15 mg/ chlorpheniramine 2 mg/5 mL
	Safetussin CD		Dextromethrophan 15 mg/Phenylephrine 2.5 mg/5 mL
Decongestants	Contact Cold and Flu	Tablets	Acetaminophen 500 mg/phenylephrine 5 mg
	Sudafed 12 hr	Capsule, liquid	Pseudoephedrine 120 mg; 30 mg/5 mL
	Sudafed Maximum	Tablet	Pseudoephedrine 30 mg
	Sudafed Children's	Liquid	Pseudoephedrine 15 mg/5 mL
	Sudafed Children's Cough and Cold	Liquid	Pseudoephedrine 15 mg/ dextromethrophan 7.5 mg/5 mL
	Advil Cold and Sinus	Tablet	Pseudoephedrine 30 mg/ibuprofen 200 mg
	PediaCare Relief Cough and Cold	Liquid	Pseudoephedrine 15 mg/ dextromethrophan 7.5 mg/5 mL
	Sudafed PE	Tablet	Phenylephrine 10 mg
	Sudafed PE Congestion	Tablet	Phenylephrine 10 mg/ dextromethrophan 15 mg
	Sudafed PE Children's, PediaCare Children's	Liquid	phenylephrine 2.5 mg/5mL
Expectorants	Mucinex	Tablet	Guaifenesin 600mh
	Mucinex Kids	Liquid	Guaifenesin 100 mg/5 mL
	Mucinex Kids Mini Melts	Meltables	Guaifenesin 50 mg/packet
	Robitussin, Vicks Chest Congestion	Liquid	Guaifenesin 100 mg/5 mL; 200 mg/5 mL
	Humabid Maximum Strength ER	Capsule	Guaifenesin 1,200 mg
	Coricidin HBP Chest Congestion and Cough	Tablet	Guaifenesin 200 mg/dextromethropan 10 mg
Antacids, adult	Tums	Chewable tablet	Calcium carbonate 500 mg
	Tums EX		Calcium carbonate 750 mg

Category	Trade Name(s)	Form	Active Ingredients
	Rolaids	Chewable tablet	Calcium carbonate/magnesium hydroxide 110 mg
	Alka-Seltzer Heartburn Relief	Effervescent tablet	Sodium bicarbonate 194 mg/citric acid 1,000 mg
	Gaviscon	Liquid	Aluminum hydroxide 95 mg/ magnesium carbonate 358 mg
	Mylanta Ultimate Strength	Chewable tablet	Calcium carbonate 750 mg/magnesium hydroxide 300 mg
Antacids, pediatric	Maalox Children's Relief, Children's Pepto	Chewable tablet	Calcium carbonate 400 mg
Antacids, H2 receptor antagonists	Tagamet HB	Tablet	Cimetidine 300 mg
	Axid AR	Tablet	Nizatidine 75 mg
	Pepcid AC	Tablet	Famotidine 10 mg
	Zantac	Tablet	Ranitidine 75 mg or 150 mg
Antacids, PPIs	Prilosec OTC	Capsule	Omeprazole 20 mg
	Zegrid	Capsule	Omeprazole 20 mg/sodium bicarbonate 1,100 mg
	Prevacid 24 hr	Capsule	Lansoprazole 15 mg
Antidiarrheals	Imodium A-D	Caplets, chewable tablet, liquid	Loperamide 2 mg; 1 mg/7.5 mL
	Imodium Advanced	Caplet, chewable tablet	Loperamide 2 mg/simethacone 12.5 mg
	Kaopectate, Maalox, Pepto-Bismol	Caplet, liquid	Bismuth subsalicylate 262 mg; 262 mg/15 mL
	Kaopectate Extra, Pepto-Bismol Extra	Liquid	Bismuth subsalicylate 525 mg/15 mL
Antiemetics	Bioband, Sea-Bond	Wristband	Acupressure wrist band(s)
	Marezine	Chewable tablet	Cyclizine 50 mg
	Bonine Kids	Chewable tablet	Cyclizine 25 mg
	Dramamine Orange	Chewable tablet	Dimenhydrinate 50 mg
	Bonine, Dramamine Less Drowsy	Chewable tablet	Meclizine 25 mg
	Emetrol	Liquid	Phosphorus acid 21 mg/dextrose 1.87 gm/ fructose 1.87 gm/5 mL
Antiflatulents	Gas X	Chewable tablet	Simethacone 80 mg
	Gas X Extra Strength, Mylanta	Chewable tablet	Simethacone 125 mg
	Gas X Ultra Strength	Chewable tablet	Simethacone 180 mg
	Mylicon Infant Drops	Drops	Simethacone 40 mg/0.6 mL
	Activated Charcoal	Capsules, tablets	Activated charcoal 260 mg
	Beano	Drops, tablets	Alpha-galactosidase 150 U; 150 U/5 drops
	Lactaid Original Strength	Capsule	Lactase enzyme 3,000 U

Category	Trade Name(s)	Form	Active Ingredients
Antihemorrhoidals	Americaine	Ointment	Benzocaine 20%
	TUCKS	Ointment	Pamoxine 1%, zinc oxide 12.5%, mineral oil 46.6%
	Preparation H	Gel, suppositories	Witch hazel 50%, phenylephrine 0.25%, cocoa butter 85.39%, shark liver oil 3%
Laxatives	Citrucel	Powder	Methylcellulose 2 gm
	Fibercon	Caplets	Calcium polycarbophil 625 mg
	Metamucil	Powder	Psyllium fiber 3 gm
	Colace	Capsules	Docusate sodium 50 mg
	Fleet Mineral Oil Enema	Liquid	Mineral oil 100%
	Kondremul Emulsion	Liquid	Mineral oil 55%
	Magnesium Citrate	Liquid	Magnesium citrate 1.745 gm/30 mL
	Milk of Magnesia	Liquid	Magnesium hydroxide 400 mg/5 mL
	Fleet Enema	Liquid	Monobasic sodium phosphate 19 gm/118mL; dibasic sodium phosphate 7 gm/118 mL
	Fleet Glycerin Suppository	Suppository	Glycerin 2 gm
	MiraLax	Powder	Polyethylene glycol 3350 17 gm/capful
	Ducolax	Tablet	Bisacodyl 5 mg
	Senokot	Tablet	Sennosides 8.6 mg
	Senokot-S	Tablet	Sennosides 8.6 mg/docusate sodium 50 mg
Acne treatments	Clean & Clear, Oxy	Gel	Benzyl peroxide 5%, 10%
	Neutrogena Rapid Defense	Gel	Salicylic acid 2%
	Gly Derm, Total Skin Care	Gel	Glycolic acid
	DDF Sulfur Therapeutic Mask	Mask	Sulfur 10%
	Clearasil Stay Clear	Cream	Resorcinol 2%/sulfur 8%
Alopecia treatments	Rogaine, Rogaine Women's	Topical solution	Minoxidil 2%
	Rogaine Extra Strength, Rogaine Topical Foam	Topical solution, foam	Minoxidil 5%
Anti-infectives	Betadine First Aid Anitbiotics + Moisturize	Ointment	Polymyxin b sulfate 10,000 U/gm, bacitracin zinc 500 U/gm
	Neosporin	Ointment	Polymyxin b sulfate 5,000 U/g, bacitracin zinc 400 U/g, neomycin base 3.5 mg/gm
	Neosporin Plus Pain Relief	Cream, ointment	Bacitracin zinc 500 U/gm, polymyxin b sulfate 10,000 U/gm, neomycin base 3.5 mg/gm, pramoxine HCL 10 mg
	Polysporin	Ointment, powder	Polymyxin b sulfate 10,000 U/gm, bacitracin zinc 500 U/gm

Category	Trade Name(s)	Form	Active Ingredients
Corns and callus treatments	Curad Mediplast, Dr. Scholl's Gel Corn & Callus Remover Disk, Freezone One Step	Liquid	Salicylic acid 40%
	Dr. Scholl's Corn/Callus Remover	Liquid	Salicylic acid 12/6%
Wart removers	Compound W	Liquid	Salicylic acid 17%
	Duo Film	Liquid	Salicylic acid 40%
Dandruff treatments	Head and Shoulders	Shampoo	Pyrithione zine 1%
	Denorex, DHS Zinc	Shampoo	Pyrithione zine 2%
	Selsun Blue	Shampoo	Selenium sulfide 1%
	Head and Shoulders Intensive	Topical solution	Selenium sulfide 1%
	DHS Tar	Shampoo	Coal tar 0.5%
Dermatitis treatments	Aquaphor	Ointment	Petrolatum 41%
	Aveeno Daily Moisturizing Lotion	Lotion	Dimethasone 1.25%, cetyl alcohol, oat kernel flour, glycerin
	Aveeno Soothing Bath Formula	Bath solution	Colloidal oatmeal 100%
	Carmol 10	Lotion	Urea 10%
	Carmol 20	Lotion	Urea 20%
	Cetaphil	Liquid	Cetyl alcohol, stearl alcohol, PEG
	Eucerin	Ointment	Petrolatum, mineral oil, mineral wax
Head lice treatments	A-200	Shampoo	Pyrethins 0.33%, piperonyl butoxide 4%
	Pronto Lice Killing Shampoo	Shampoo	Permethrin 1%
	RID Max Strength	Shampoo, foam	Pyrethrins 0.33%, piperonyl butoxide 4%
Sunburn treatments	Solarcaine	Gel, spray	Lidocaine 0.5%
	Dermoplast	Spray	Benzocaine 20%, menthol 0.5%
	Xylocaine	Ointment	Lidocaine 2.5%
	Zinc Oxide Desitin	Ointment	Zinc oxide 20%
	Americaine	Spray	Benzocaine 20%
	Lanacane Maximum Strength	Cream	Benzocaine 20%, Benzethonium chloride 1%
Ophthalmic antihistamines	Alaway, Claritin Eye, Zaditor, Zyrtec Itchy Eyes	Drops	Ketotifen 0.025%
	Vasacon A	Drops	Antazoline phosphate 0.5%/naphazoline 0.05%
	Visine A	Drops	Pheniramine maleate 0.3%/naphazoline 0.025%
Ophthalmic decongestants	All Clear	Drops	Naphazoline 0.012%

Category	Trade Name(s)	Form	Active Ingredients
	Murine Tears Plus	Drops	Tetrahydrozoline 0.05%
	Visine LR	Drops	Oxymetazoline 0.025%
	Relief	Drops	Phenylephrine HCl
	Clear Eyes ACR	Drops	Naphazoline 0.012%/zinc sulfate 0.25%, glycerin 0.2%
	Visine Allergic Relief, Zincfrin	Drops	Tetrahydrozoline 0.05%, zinc sulfate 0.25%, BAK 0.01%
	Opcon-A	Drops	Pheniramine maleate 0.315%, naphazoline 0.002675%
	Vasacon-A	Drops	Antazoline phosphate 0.5%, Naphazoline 0.05%
Otic agents	Auro Ear Drops, Debrox	Drops, solution	Carbamide peroxide 6.5%/anhydrous glycerin
	Auro-Dri, Swim Ear	Drops, oil	Isopropyl alcohol 95%, anhydrous glycerin
Oral pain treatments	Anbesol, Zilactin B	Gel, liquid	Benzocaine 10%
	Anbesol Maximum Strength, Orabase	Liquid, ointment	Benzocaine 20%
	Campho-Phenique	Gel, liquid	Petrolatum 59.14%
	Abreva	Cream	Docosanol 10%

Appendix B:
Top 200 Drugs

Please note, duplicates indicate different manufacturers.
Data provided by IMS Health for 2012.

Rank	Based on Total Dollars	Based on Prescription Count
1	Nexium	HYCD/APAP
2	Abilify	Levothyroxine Sodium
3	Crestor	HYCD/APAP
4	Advair Diskus	Lisinopril
5	Cymbalta	HYCD/APAP
6	Humira	Simvastatin
7	Enbrel	Azithromycin
8	Remicade	Proair HFA
9	Copaxone	Crestor
10	Neulasta	Levothyroxine Sodium
11	Singulair	Synthroid
12	Rituxan	Nexium
13	Plavix	Atorvastatin Ca
14	Atripla	Ibuprofen (Rx)
15	Spiriva Handihaler	Trazodone HCl
16	Oxycontin	Metoprolol Tartrate
17	Januvia	Azithromycin
18	Avastin	Warfarin Sodium
19	Lantus	Cymbalta
20	Truvada	Fluticasone Propionate
21	Lantus Solostar	Singulair
22	Epogen	Hydrochlorothiazide
23	Diovan	Ventolin HFA
24	Lyrica	Advair Diskus
25	Lipitor	Pravastatin Sodium
26	Celebrex	Amoxicillin
27	Herceptin	Amlodipine Besylate
28	Gleevec	Omeprazole (Rx)
29	Namenda	Omeprazole (Rx)

Rank	Based on Total Dollars	Based on Prescription Count
30	Actos	Amoxicillin
31	Avonex	Lisinopril/HCTZ
32	Lucentis	Metoprolol
33	Vyvanse	Hydrochlorothiazide
34	Suboxone	Amlodipine Besylate
35	Seroquel	Diovan
36	Zetia	Alprazolam
37	Methylphenidate ER	Metformin HCl
38	Androgel	Metformin HCl
39	Incivek	Simvastatin
40	Diovan HCT	Fluconazole
41	Lidoderm	Oxycodone/APAP
42	Atorvastatin Calcium	Omeprazole (Rx)
43	Symbicort	Omeprazole (Rx)
44	Rebif	SMX/TMP
45	Novolog	Lorazepam
46	Seroquel XR	Meloxicam
47	Tricor	Prednisone
48	Alimta	Clonazepam
49	Eloxatin	Tramadol HCl
50	Levemir	Furosemide
51	Combivent	Sertraline HCl
52	Viagra	Plavix
53	Proair HFA	Gabapentin
54	Procrit	Fluoxetine HCl
55	Niaspan	Simvastatin
56	Nasonex	Vitamin D
57	Novolog Flexpen	Lisinopril
58	Lovaza	Atorvastatin
59	Humalog	Calcium
60	Flovent HFA	Fluticasone
61	Neupogen	Propionate
62	Reyataz	Simvastatin
63	Vytorin	Citalopram HBR
64	Isentress	Lantus

Rank	Based on Total Dollars	Based on Prescription Count
65	Budesonide	Ibuprofen (Rx)
66	Janumet	Amoxicillin/Clavulanate Potassium
67	Aranesp	Vyvanse
68	Cialis	Metoprolol
69	Aciphex	Ciprofloxacin HCl
70	Adderall XR	Lipitor
71	Restasis	Escitalopram
72	Pradaxa	Metformin HCl
73	Gilenya	Spiriva Handihaler
74	Prezista	Alprazolam
75	Betaseron	Celebrex
76	Orencia	Zolpidem Tartrate
77	Varivax	Alprazolam
78	Vesicare	Sertraline HCl
79	Victoza 3-Pak	Lyrica
80	Dexilant	Citalopram HBR
81	Lexapro	Atenolol
82	Synagis	Tramadol HCl
83	Benicar	Nasonex
84	Lunesta	Simvastatin
85	Evista	Carvedilol
86	Prevnar 13	Cephalexin
87	Enoxaparin Sodium	Tramadol HCl
88	Synthroid	Warfarin Sodium
89	Renvela	Venlafaxine HCl ER
90	Atorvastatin Calcium	Cyclobenzaprine
91	Xeloda	Abilify
92	Zyvox	Lisinopril
93	Ventolin HFA	Furosemide
94	Velcade	Zolpidem
95	Xolair	Januvia
96	Sensipar	Metformin HCl
97	Erbitux	Lisinopril
98	Humalog Kwikpen	Lisinopril
99	Stelara	Naproxen

Rank	Based on Total Dollars	Based on Prescription Count
100	Xgeva	Methylphenidate ER
101	Benicar HCT	Cyclobenzaprine
102	Sandostatin LAR	Diovan HCT
103	Mirena	Prednisone
104	Zostavax	Cyclobenzaprin
105	Focalin XR	Viagra
106	Tarceva	Metoprolol Succinate
107	Cubicin	Lantus Solostar
108	Detrol LA	Potassium Cl
109	Zometa	Zetia
110	Treanda	Furosemide
111	Colcrys	Suboxone
112	Solodyn	Namenda
113	Escitalopram Oxalate	Clonazepam
114	Gardasil	Zolpidem
115	Pristiq	Lorazepam
116	Pegasys Convenience Pack	Amoxicillin
117	Invega Sustenna	Cialis
118	Strattera	Prednisone
119	Trilipix	Amphetamine Salts
120	Revlimid	Methylprednisolone
121	Asacol	Pantoprazole Sodium
122	Bystolic	Diazepam
123	Viread	Allopurinol
124	Enoxaparin Sodium	Furosemide
125	Loestrin 24 Fe	Amoxicillin Trihydrate/ Clavulanate Potassium
126	Yervoy	Lorazepam
127	Avodart	Gabapentin
128	Lexiscan	Escitalopram Oxalate
129	Lovenox	Ranitidine HCl
130	Epzicom	Atenolol
131	Exelon	Omeprazole
132	Amphetamin Salt ER	Digoxin
133	Gamunex-C	Bystolic
134	Nuvaring	Amitriptyline

Rank	Based on Total Dollars	Based on Prescription Count
135	Amphetamin Salt Er	Flovent HFA
136	Escitalopram Oxal	Pravastatin
137	Provigil	Loestrin 24 Fe
138	Norvir	Risperidone
139	Epipen 2-Pak	Oxycontin
140	Forteo	Simvastatin
141	Risperdal Consta	Simvastatin
142	Premarin	Carvedilol
143	Zytiga	Paroxetine HCl
144	Welchol	Triamterene/HCTZ
145	Metoprolol Succinate	Potassium Cl
146	Onglyza	Doxycycline Hyclate
147	Xifaxan	Bupropion
148	Byetta	Doxycycline Hyclate
149	Aggrenox	Lovastatin
150	Opana Er	APAP/Codeine
151	Aloxi	Ciprofloxacin
152	Privigen	Klor-Con M20
153	Lumigan	Lexapro
154	Intuniv	Tricor
155	Travatan Z	Temazepam
156	Pulmozyme	Albuterol
157	Pneumovax 23	Gabapentin
158	Zyprexa	Cyclobenzaprin HCl
159	HYCD/APAP	Famotidine
160	Angiomax	Triamcinolone Acetonide
161	Lialda	Alprazolam
162	Cimzia	Alendronate Sodium
163	Geodon	Oxycodone HCl
164	Actonel	Amoxicillin
165	Prograf	Triamterene/HCTZ
166	Fentanyl	Atorvastatin Calcium
167	Ortho-Tri-cyclen Lo 28	Alprazolam
168	Novolog Flxpen Mix	Clindamycin
169	Ranexa	Tamsulosin HCl

Rank	Based on Total Dollars	Based on Prescription Count
170	Qvar	Levothyroxine Sodium
171	Afinitor	Atenolol
172	Invega	Lisinopril
173	Tysabri	Ranitidine HCl
174	Temodar	Benicar
175	Nuvigil	Symbicort
176	Sprycel	Mupirocin
177	Tasigna	Niaspan
178	Adacel	Lovaza
179	Valcyte	Prednisone
180	Exforge	Premarin
181	Nutropin AQ	Nuvaring
182	Zosyn	Dexilant
183	Amphetamine Salts	Metoprolol
184	Effient	Cheratussin AC
185	Claravis	Hydrochlorothiazide
186	Advair HFA	Metoprolol Tartrate
187	Chantix	Levoxyl
188	Reclast	Penicillin VK
189	Vidaza	Metronidazole
190	Abraxane	Amlodipine Besylate
191	Gammagard Liquid	HYCD/APAP
192	Tamiflu	Azithromycin
193	Complera	Naproxen
194	Maxalt	Allopurinol
195	Ciprodex	Actos
196	Activase	Diazepam
197	Vimpat	Bupropion HCl XL
198	Simponi	Losartan Potassium
199	Synvisc-One	Lidoderm
200	Sutent	Gabapentin

Appendix C:
Advanced Career Path Options

There are numerous advanced career path opportunities for properly trained pharmacy technicians. Although the vast majority of positions available fall within standard community and health-system pharmacy settings, pharmacy technicians should consider all career opportunities available.

The following provides a brief introduction to just a few of the advanced career options for pharmacy technicians. The National Pharmacy Technician Association (NPTA) has developed a two-disc audio program, entitled *Exploring Your Career Paths in Pharmacy*, which provides insight on how to explore and evaluate 50 career path options for pharmacy technicians. For more information on this resource, visit www.pharmacytechnician.org or call 1-888-247-8700.

Clinical Pharmacy Technician

The role of *clinical pharmacy technician* is an emerging trend within certain health-system pharmacies. Rather than working within the central or satellite pharmacy, clinical pharmacy technicians are assigned to a specific unit, working with a clinical pharmacist.

Clinical pharmacy technicians have been used to manage the delivery of initial dosages, locate missing medications, review floor stock inventory levels, and assist in collecting patient-specific data for analysis by the clinical pharmacist.

Specific areas of utilization for clinical pharmacy technicians include the following:

- Congestive heart failure (CHF) clinics
- Coumadin therapy
- Diabetes management
- Intensive care unit (ICU) lab profiles
- Lipid clinics

Federal Pharmacy

Federal pharmacy refers to the practice of pharmacy within the federal government, such as the military, the Public Health Service, federal correctional facilities, or the Department of Veterans Affairs. Federal pharmacy is unique in that it is not regulated by a state board of pharmacy and therefore need not meet certain requirements such as state-specified pharmacist-to-technician ratios.

Military

Military pharmacy services, which are overseen by the Department of Defense, provide pharmaceutical care for active-duty military personnel and their families. Each branch of the military (the U.S. Army, the U.S. Navy, the U.S. Air Force, the U.S. Marine Corps, and the U.S. Coast Guard) maintains its own facilities and pharmacy personnel.

Military pharmacy technicians can be either civilian or enlisted (military) personnel. Civilian pharmacy technicians are not required to complete military basic training. Enlisted pharmacy technicians, who are required to complete basic training, are classified as noncommissioned officers; they are eligible for rank advancements within the military.

Public Health Service

The *Public Health Service (PHS)*, which is part of the Department of Health and Human Services (DHHS), provides pharmaceutical care to specific populations or communities. Pharmacy technicians work in numerous divisions of PHS, including:

- Agency for Health Care Policy and Research
- Agency for Toxic Substances and Disease Registry
- Centers for Disease Control and Prevention (CDC)
- Food and Drug Administration (FDA)
- Health Resources and Services Administration
- Indian Health Service (IHS)
- National Institutes of Health (NIH)
- Substance Abuse and Mental Health Services Administration

Federal Correctional Facilities

Federal correctional facilities, also known as *federal prisons*, are responsible for providing medical and pharmaceutical care to their inmates. Pharmacists and pharmacy technicians work securely onsite at these facilities, with little to no interaction with the inmates themselves.

Department of Veterans Affairs

Through the Veterans Health Administration (VHA), the Department of Veterans Affairs (VA) provides pharmaceutical care to those who previously served in the U.S. military. There are hundreds of VA medical facilities located across the United States, including VA hospitals, and most of them employ pharmacy technicians. In addition, pharmacy technicians can work at VA mail-order facilities.

Home Infusion Pharmacy

Home infusion pharmacies prepare intravenous (IV) solutions to be administered at the patient's home. In addition to IV solutions, home infusion pharmacies prepare enteral nutrition therapy and other injectable solutions.

Home infusion pharmacies focus solely on preparation of sterile products; therefore, the pharmacists and pharmacy technicians must be properly trained in aseptic technique. After the infusion therapies have been prepared at the pharmacy, they are delivered to the patient for administration.

The most common home infusion therapies are the following:

- Anti-infectives, including for HIV/AIDS
- Biotechnology
- Chemotherapy
- Chronic pain management
- Hydration
- Nutrition (TPN and enteral nutrition)

Mail-Order Pharmacy

Mail-order pharmacies are facilities that dispense maintenance medications to patients via the mail (U.S. Postal Service and other carriers). Unlike community pharmacies, mail-order pharmacies are not designed to provide medications for acute needs.

Major mail-order pharmacies, such as CVS/Caremark and Medco, operate numerous facilities strategically located across the United States to provide faster deliveries to their patients. These pharmacies are considered extremely high volume, with some facilities processing and dispensing more than 30,000 prescriptions per day.

Because of the high volume of prescriptions, mail-order pharmacies employ vast numbers of pharmacists and pharmacy technicians and generally operate 24 hours a day. Pharmacy technicians typically work in the call center or translate and input new prescription orders.

Mail-order pharmacies are completely automated, using robotics to pull, count, and label prescription orders. Each order is then verified by a staff pharmacist, who compares the prepared order with an electronic image of the original prescription and electronic images of what the medication being dispensed should look like.

Nuclear Pharmacy

Nuclear pharmacies, or *radiopharmacies*, prepare and dispense radioactive drugs, known as *radiopharmaceuticals*, which are used to diagnose and treat diseases. There are two types of nuclear pharmacies: institutional and centralized.

Institutional nuclear pharmacies operate within a large health system's nuclear medicine department. Centralized nuclear pharmacies operate in an offsite facility and prepare radiopharmaceuticals for various facilities that outsource this service.

The two main types of radiopharmaceuticals are positron emission tomography (PET) drugs and radioactive blood elements. PET drugs are used in diagnostic imaging, and because they have a very short half-life, they are prepared only in institutional nuclear pharmacies. Radioactive blood elements include red blood cells, white blood cells, and even platelets that are combined with radionuclides to be used in diagnosis.

Because they must handle advanced issues and have potential exposure to radioactive elements, pharmacy technicians must complete extensive training to work in a nuclear pharmacy. These training programs are administered by employers such as Syncor.

Appendix D:
Practice Certification Exams

Practice Certification Exam I

This practice test has been designed to simulate the certification exam, both in the number/style of questions, as well as the content. You should complete this exam within 110 minutes.

1. The failure of one or more drugs to be mixed in the same solution due to a physical or chemical interaction is called _____.
   a. precipitation
   b. incompatibility
   c. intolerance
   d. injunction

2. A preparation of finely divided undissolved drugs dispersed in a liquid vehicle is known as _____.
   a. elixir
   b. solution
   c. syrup
   d. suspension

3. A system in which the item is deducted from inventory as it is sold or dispensed is known as _____.
   a. turnover
   b. scantron
   c. Baker cell
   d. POS system

4. An inert substance added to the active drug ingredient to increase the bulk and make the tablet a practical size for compression is called a_____.
   a. diluent
   b. binder
   c. facilitator
   d. emulsifying agent

5. Effective communication in pharmacy practice can be hindered by which one of the following?
   a. visual impairment
   b. auditory loss
   c. speech impairment
   d. all of the above

6. "OBRA 90" is an acronym for _____.
   a. Omnibus Budget Recommendation Act of 1990
   b. Omnibus Budget Reconciliation Act of 1990
   c. Omni Bus Reconciliation Act of 1990
   d. Omni Bus Recognition Act of 1990

7. A substance or a mixture of substances added to a tablet to facilitate its break up or disintegration after administration is called _____.
   a. terminator
   b. disintegrator

   c. binder
   d. diluent

8. A solid dosage form in which the drug substance is enclosed in either a hard or soft soluble container or shell of a suitable form of gelatin is called a_____.
   a. capsule
   b. pill
   c. tablet
   d. suppository

9. Softening of the cornea due to vitamin A deficiency is called _____.
   a. conjunctivitis
   b. glaucoma
   c. pellagra
   d. keratomalacia

10. The only drug approved to treat high blood pressure during pregnancy is _____.
    a. lidocaine
    b. clonidine
    c. metoprolol
    d. methyldopa

11. The only antihypertensive drug available as a transdermal delivery system is _____.
    a. nicotine
    b. clonidine
    c. nitroglycerin
    d. lidocaine

12. From the following formula, calculate the amount in grams of cetyl ester wax needed to make 1 lb of cold cream.

Cetyl ester wax	12.5 parts
White wax	12.0 parts
Mineral oil	56.0 parts
Sodium borate	0.5 parts
Water	9.0 parts

   a. 56.75
   b. 12.5
   c. 60
   d. 0.125

13. An imbalance between oxygen supply and oxygen demand in cardiac muscle may produce a condition known as _____.
    a. congestive heart failure
    b. heartburn

  c. myocardial infarction
  d. angina pectoris

14. From the following formula, calculate in kilograms the quantity of Miconazole needed to prepare 12 kg of powder.

Zinc oxide	1 part
Calamine	2 parts
Miconazole	1.5 parts
Bismuth subgalate	3 parts
Talc	8 parts

  a. 15.5
  b. 0.097
  c. 1.16
  d. 1.5

15. Frequently patients on thiazide diuretics are told to take supplements of, or eat, foods high in which element?
  a. calcium
  b. sodium
  c. chlorine
  d. potassium

16. Renal tubules produce urine through all the following *except* _____.
  a. adsorption
  b. filtration
  c. reabsorption
  d. secretion

17. The structural and functional unit of the kidney is the _____.
  a. loop of Henle
  b. glomerulus
  c. nephron
  d. cortex

18. An antihistamine nasal spray is _____.
  a. Nasacort
  b. Nasonex
  c. Astelin
  d. Afrin

19. What anesthetizes the stretch receptors in the airway, lungs, and pleura but does not affect the respiratory center?
  a. benzonatate
  b. guaifenesin
  c. codeine
  d. dextromethoraphan

20. A cycle of inflammation of the nasal mucosa caused by repeated application of nasal decongestants is called _____.
  a. allergic rhinitis
  b. rhinorrhea
  c. rhinitis medicomentosa
  d. nasal congestion

21. In pharmacies, controlled substances may be stored in which one of the following manner?
  a. Controlled substances may be stored in an unlocked cabinet.
  b. Controlled substances may be stored in a securely locked substantially constructed cabinet.
  c. Controlled substances (CIII through CV) may be dispersed on the pharmacy shelves among noncontrolled substances in a manner to deter theft.
  d. b and c

22. Drug agent extracted from cattle lung is _____.
  a. Proventil HFA
  b. Survanta
  c. Bonine
  d. Serevent

23. Patients taking which one of the following medication should always be warned to avoid any consumption of alcohol?
  a. Metronidazole
  b. Tetracycline
  c. Albuterol
  d. Prednisone

24. Legislation that was a direct result of the thalidomide disaster and made manufacturers more accountable for their products was the _____.
  a. Comprehensive Drug Abuse Prevention and Control Act
  b. Medical Device Amendment
  c. Durham–Humphrey Amendment
  d. Kefauver–Harris Amendment

25. Patients should be advised not to drink milk or eat dairy products while taking which one of the following medications?
  a. calcium carbonate
  b. tetracycline
  c. penicillin
  d. calciferol

26. Patients should be advised to drink plenty of water and to avoid the sun while taking which one of the following medications?
  a. TMP-SMZ
  b. cephalexin
  c. propranolol
  d. warfarin

27. A class of pharmaceutical agents that kill or inhibit the growth of infection-causing microorganisms is _____.
  a. anesthetics
  b. antilipidemics
  c. antibiotics
  d. antihistamines

28. Which one of the following is a hospital-acquired infection?
  a. nosocomial infection
  b. institutional infection

c. HA infection
d. viral infection

29. The substance/agent capable of killing bacteria is called _____.
   a. bacteriostatic
   b. antiviral
   c. antifungal
   d. bactericidal

30. The agency that oversees the Controlled Substances Act is the _____.
   a. Central Intelligence Agency
   b. Armed Forces
   c. Food and Drug Administration
   d. Drug Enforcement Agency

31. The substance/agent capable of inhibiting growth or multiplication of bacteria is called _____.
   a. bacteriostatic
   b. anti-inflammatory
   c. antifungal
   d. bactericidal

32. All of the following are true statements *except* _____.
   a. all controlled substances must be inventoried on the day the pharmacy first dispenses controlled substances.
   b. the inventory of CII medications requires an exact count or measure while other schedules may be estimated
   c. prescriptions are the primary records of acquisition by a pharmacy
   d. the beginning inventory plus all acquisitions minus dispensing by prescriptions or to other practitioners should equal the current inventory count

33. Substances active against both gram-positive and gram-negative bacteria are called _____.
   a. neg-gram
   b. bacteriostatic
   c. broad spectrum
   d. narrow spectrum

34. A patient weighs 165 lb. How many kilograms does the patient weigh?
   a. 165,000
   b. 75
   c. 363
   d. 330

35. Testing process to identify bacteria and to determine the drugs that may combat the infection is called _____.
   a. culture and sensitivity
   b. cross sensitivity
   c. cultivation
   d. Bacto test

36. The types of ulcers include all of the following *except* _____.
   a. stress
   b. gastric

c. duodenal
d. colon

37. Estrogen is contraindicated with _____.
   a. migraines
   b. smokers
   c. thrombosis history
   d. all of the above

38. A substance with a high potential for abuse, that has no currently accepted medical use in the United States, and for which there is a lack of accepted safety for use would be classified as _____.
   a. CI
   b. CII
   c. CIII
   d. CIV

39. The thyroid hormones T3 and T4 are both stored as _____.
   a. serotonin
   b. thyroglobulin
   c. acetylcholine
   d. norepinephrine

40. The feedback mechanism that controls the thyroid is the _____.
   a. adrenocorticotrophic hormone autoregulator
   b. hypothalmic–pituitary axis
   c. homeostasis
   d. hirsutism

41. Legislation that requires that most prescription drugs be dispensed in a childproof container is the _____.
   a. Poison Prevention Act
   b. Safe Medical Devices Act
   c. Prescription Drug Marketing Act
   d. Medical Device Amendment

42. Which drug should be taken with 8 oz. of water before the first food of the day, and the patient must avoid lying down for at least 30 minutes after taking?
   a. Miacalcin
   b. Didronel
   c. Fosamax
   d. Hydrocortisone

43. Glial cells surrounding the capillaries in the CNS that present a barrier to many water-soluble components are referred to as _____.
   a. central glial cells
   b. blood–brain barrier
   c. glial barrier
   d. aqua barrier

44. Legislation that placed all hormones that promote muscle growth or are similar to testosterone under the Controlled Substances Act was the _____.
   a. Comprehensive Drug Abuse Prevention and Control Act
   b. Medical Device Amendment

c. Anabolic Steroid control Act

d. Poison Prevention Act

45. A chemical mediator that produces intense uterine contraction, reduces blood pressure, increases heart rate and cardiac output, and inhibits gastrointestinal secretions is called _____.
    a. epinephrine
    b. serotonin
    c. dopamine
    d. prostaglandin

46. Joint action of drugs in which their combined effect is more intense or longer in duration than the sum of their individual effects is called _____.
    a. opportunistic
    b. pharmakon
    c. synergism
    d. contraindications

47. Legislation that prohibits the sale of drug samples, reimportation of prescriptions, and established fair pricing guidelines is the _____.
    a. Orphan Drug Act
    b. Prescription Drug Marketing Act
    c. Durham–Humphrey Amendment
    d. Kefauver–Harris Amendment

48. Decrease in susceptibility to a drug's effects from continued use is called _____.
    a. addition
    b. synergism
    c. sensitivity
    d. tolerance

49. Which of the following DEA numbers is valid?
    a. Dr. Russ   AR123456879
    b. Dr. Black AB56897
    c. Dr. Jones AJ1234563
    d. Dr. Smith CS2468217

50. The traditional agent of choice for accidental poisonings in the home and which is commonly sold in pharmacies is _____.
    a. activated charcoal
    b. demulcent
    c. syrup of ipecac
    d. diphenhydramine elixir

51. Microorganism utilized in the production of Novo Nordisk's Novolin is _____.
    a. baker's yeast
    b. Escherichia coli
    c. Salmonella
    d. Pseudomonas

52. The rate at which inventory is used is known as _____.
    a. sales journal
    b. sales volume
    c. turnover
    d. net profit

53. Low blood glucose is called _____.
    a. glucosuria
    b. hypoglycemia
    c. polyuria
    d. hyperglycemia

54. Certain controlled substances do not bear the federal caution legend and may be sold without a prescription. These products have small quantities of controlled substances included in them and may be sold if certain requirements are met and the proper records kept. The restrictions on the sale include the following *except* _____.
    a. the sale must be made by the pharmacist or a certified pharmacy technician
    b. the purchaser must be at least 18 and must either be known to the pharmacist or have substantial identification
    c. not more than 8 oz. or more than 48 dosage units of any substance containing opium in any 48-hour period may be furnished to the purchaser. Not more than 4 oz. or 24 dosage units of any other controlled substance in any 48-hour period may be sold.
    d. pharmacists must maintain a record in a bound book regarding the sale

55. Sources of insulin include all of the following *except* _____.
    a. cow
    b. horse
    c. pig
    d. human

56. The human skin comprises approximately what percent of the body weight of the average adult?
    a. 10   **c.** 15
    b. 12.5   **d.** 20

57. Legislation that was directed toward recipients of Medicare and Medicaid. Pharmacists must offer consultation under this regulation.
    a. Durham–Humphrey Amendment
    b. Omnibus Budget Reconciliation Act
    c. Prescription Drug Marketing Act
    d. Orphan Drug Act

58. Therapies that in a certain concentration redden the skin to produce a feeling of warmth, but do not cause inflammation are _____.
    a. crepitus
    b. thermotherapy
    c. cryotherapy
    d. rubefacients

59. The National Drug Code number provides specific information about the product. Which of the following statements is true?
    a. The NDC contains 10 digits.
    b. NDC numbers indicate the date the product was produced.

c. NDC numbers are divided in two sections with the first section indicating the manufacturer and the second section indication the specific product.

d. NDC numbers are divided into three sections with the first five digits indicating the manufacturer, the next four digits indicating the product name, strength, and dosage form, and the last two digits indicating the package size.

60. A rare, acute, life-threatening condition that occurs primarily in children or teenagers in the course of, or while recovering from, a mild respiratory tract infection, flu, chicken pox, or other viral illness and sometimes linked to salicylate use is _____.
    a. Reye's syndrome
    b. Legionnaires disease
    c. Viral meningitis
    d. Herpes simplex

61. A device that produces a nonheated mist to increase humidity is _____.
    a. humidifier
    b. peak flow meter
    c. vaporizer
    d. HEPA filter

62. A document that contains the goals, policies, and procedures relevant to the employee and the job the employee is assuming is known as _____.
    a. employee handbook
    b. corporate prospectus
    c. planogram
    d. administration handbook

63. What is used to record the balances that private patients, government agencies, insurance companies, managed care contractors, and insurers owe the pharmacy?
    a. balance sheet
    b. accounts receivable ledger
    c. cash disbursements journal
    d. sales journal

64. Control of the amount, type, and quality of health care provided to patients within a benefit program is referred to as _____.
    a. health insurance
    b. managed care
    c. benefit plans
    d. pharmaceutical care

65. Three systems of measurement are used in pharmacy. Which of the following is correct?
    a. metric system
       weight
       volume
       length
       apothecary system
       weight
       volume
       avoirdupois system
       weight
    b. metric system
       weight
       volume
       length
       apothecary system
       volume
       avoirdupois system
       weight
    c. metric system
       weight
       volume
       length
       apothecary system
       weight
       volume
       avoirdupois system
       volume
    d. metric system
       weight
       volume
       length
       height
       apothecary system
       weight
       volume
       avoirdupois system
       weight

66. The principle that states that patients have the right to full disclosure of all relevant aspects of care and must give explicit consent to treatment before treatment is initiated is called _____.
    a. confidentiality
    b. fidelity
    c. informed consent
    d. moral reasoning

67. The provision of drug therapy intended to achieve outcomes that improve the patient's quality of life as it is related to the cure or prevention of a disease, elimination or reduction of a patient's symptoms, or arresting or slowing of a disease process is called _____.
    a. pharmaceutical care
    b. managed care
    c. socialized medicine
    d. pharmacy practice

68. The FDA recall of a product that will cause serious or fatal consequences is classified as _____.
    a. class I
    b. class II
    c. class III
    d. class IV

69. Devices _____.
    a. do not have any restrictions
    b. are defined as instruments, apparatuses, implements, machines, etc.

c. may be restricted to sale only upon the written or oral order of a practitioner licensed to administer such a device

d. b and c

70. A company that buys from the manufacturer and sells to hospitals, pharmacies, and other pharmaceutical dispensers is known as _____.
   a. Food and Drug Administration
   b. wholesaler
   c. retailer
   d. mass merchandiser

71. Drugs that are not intended to be sold, but are intended to promote the sale of the drug are called _____.
   a. legend drugs
   b. sample drugs
   c. investigational drugs
   d. over-the-counter drugs

72. Legislation that created the legend class of drugs was the _____.
   a. Comprehensive Drug Abuse Prevention and Control Act
   b. Medical Device Amendment
   c. Durham–Humphrey Amendment
   d. Kefauver–Harris Amendment

73. Mixing ingredients in order to provide a prescription for a specific patient or a small group of patients is known as _____.
   a. manufacturing
   b. compressing
   c. compounding
   d. adjudication

74. A prescription is written for 1 lb. of 3% salicylic acid in white petrolatum. How many milligrams of salicylic acid are needed?
   a. 13,620
   b. 13.62
   c. 1,362
   d. 48

75. The portion of the cost of prescriptions that patients with third-party insurance must pay is called _____.
   a. co-pay
   b. deductible
   c. U&C
   d. MAC

76. All of the following defines the term drug *except* _____.
   a. articles intended for use in the diagnosis, cure, mitigation, treatment, or prevention of disease in man or other animals
   b. articles recognized in the USP, NF, and the Homeopathic Pharmacopoeia of the United States
   c. devices that are utilized for life-sustaining or life-supporting functions
   d. articles (other than food) intended to affect the structure or any function of the body

77. All of the following methods for filing prescriptions are allowed *except* _____.
   a. a system using three separate prescription file drawers
      prescriptions for CII substances
      prescriptions for CIII, CIV, and CV
      all other prescriptions
   b. a system using two prescription file drawers
      prescriptions for scheduled II–V substances, provided all CIII–CV have a letter AC no less than one inch high stamped in red ink on the lower right corner
      all other prescriptions
   c. a system using five prescription file drawers
      schedule II prescriptions only
      schedule III prescriptions only
      schedule IV prescriptions only
      schedule V prescriptions only
      all other prescriptions
   d. a system using two prescription file drawers
      schedule II prescriptions only
      all other prescriptions, including CIII–CV provided the controlled prescriptions bear the red letter AC as described above

78. Each of the following is a characteristic desired in an intravenous solution *except* _____.
   a. pH of 6
   b. sterility
   c. clarity
   d. isotonic

79. A prescription calls for a sliding scale dosage of prednisone. How many 5-mg tablets would it take to fill the following?

   20 mg/day $\times$ 2 days

   15 mg/day $\times$ 2 days

   5 mg bid $\times$ 2days

   2.5 mg bid $\times$ 2 days

   2.5 mg/day $\times$ 2 days
   a. 20 tablets
   b. 21 tablets
   c. 22 tablets
   d. 15 tablets

80. Calculate the flow rate for an IV of 1,000 mL to run in over eight hours with a set calibrated at 20 gtts/mL.
   a. 41.6 gtts/minute
   b. 17.36 gtts/minute
   c. 125.1 gtts/minute
   d. 50 gtts/minute

81. A pharmacist may manufacture without registering as a manufacturer an aqueous or oleaginous solution or solid dosage form containing a narcotic-controlled substance not exceeding _____ of the complete solution or mixture.
   a. 25%
   b. 20%
   c. 30%
   d. 50%

82. A set amount that must be paid by the patient for each benefit period before the insurer will cover additional expenses is called _____
    a. co-pay
    b. deductible
    c. garnishment
    d. MAC

83. An IV of 150 cc is to infuse at a rate of 80 mL/hour. What is the infusion time?
    a. 10 hours
    b. 1.8 hours
    c. 6.6 hours
    d. 47 minutes

84. A device designed to reduce the risk of airborne contamination during the preparation of an IV admixture by providing an ultraclean environment is called _____.
    a. laminar flow hood
    b. HEPA
    c. autoclave
    d. automix

85. Carrying out a procedure under controlled conditions in a manner that minimize the chance of contamination caused by the introduction of microorganisms is called _____.
    a. pharmaceutical care
    b. aseptic technique
    c. sterilization
    d. autoclaving

86. Maximum and minimum inventory levels for each drug are called _____.
    a. reorder points
    b. M&M inventory
    c. POS points
    d. Maxim system

87. When a drug is substantially degraded or destroyed by the liver's enzymes before it reached the circulatory system, this is called _____.
    a. enzyme induction
    b. tolerance
    c. first pass effect
    d. metabolism

88. Legislation that classified drugs according to their potential for abuse was the _____.
    a. Comprehensive Drug Abuse Prevention and Control Act
    b. Medical Device Amendment
    c. Durham–Humphrey Amendment
    d. Anabolic Steroid Control Act

89. The time at which the minimum effective concentration is reached and the drug response occurs is called _____.
    a. onset of action
    b. peak concentration
    c. minimum inhibitory concentration
    d. site of action

90. The cellular material at the site of action that interacts with the drug is called _____.
    a. dock
    b. receptor
    c. channel
    d. gap junction

Practice Certification Exam II

This practice test has been designed to simulate the certification exam, both in the number/style of questions, as well as the content. You should complete this exam within 110 minutes.

1. Which route of medication administration is used to inject drugs into the top skin layers?
   a. subcutaneous
   b. hypodermic
   c. intradermal
   d. intra-arterial

2. A connection between two or more computer systems that allows for the transfer of data is a(n) _____.
   a. interface
   b. terminal
   c. bar code
   d. window

3. Certification is _____.
   a. the process of granting recognition or vouching for conformance with a standard
   b. the process by which a nongovernmental agency or association grants recognition to an individual who has net certain predetermined qualifications specified by that agency or association
   c. the general process of formally recognizing professional or technical competence
   d. the process of making a list or being enrolled in an existing list

4. An ongoing systematic process for monitoring, evaluating, and improving the quality of pharmacy services is _____.
   a. peer review
   b. quality assurance
   c. process validation
   d. none of the above

5. Sterile products should be prepared at least _____ inches inside the laminar airflow hood.
   a. 6
   b. 10
   c. 2
   d. 3

6. The main concern of pharmacy practice today is the _____.
   a. provision of optimal drug therapy for all patients
   b. preparation and compounding of medications for patients
   c. bulk preparation and distribution of drug products
   d. safe ordering, procurement, and storage of medications

7. A policy and procedure manual may provide guidance in each of the following areas *except* _____.
   a. personal orientation, training, and evaluation
   b. correct aseptic (sterile) technique
   c. activities of technicians outside the workplace
   d. position or job descriptions

8. All of the following are requirements for a prescription label *except* _____.
   a. name and address of the pharmacy
   b. name of the prescriber
   c. serial number of the prescription
   d. telephone number of the patient

9. A prescription can usually be refilled _____.
   a. only once
   b. as many times as the pharmacist deems necessary
   c. as many times as the prescriber indicates on the prescription within a specified time period
   d. only at the location where it was originally filled

10. Which of the following best describes controlled substances in schedule I (one)?
    a. drugs with no accepted medical use in the United States
    b. drugs with a low to moderate potential for physical dependence
    c. drugs with no potential for abuse
    d. drugs that are available without a prescription

11. A 500 mL quantity of D10W contains how many grams of dextrose?
    a. 100
    b. 10
    c. 50
    d. 20

12. What is the seventh digit of the following DEA number, AB369145_?
    a. 3
    b. 8
    c. 4
    d. 0

13. The Poison Prevention Packaging Act of 1970 mandated all of the following *except* _____.
    a. prescription drugs may be exempt if the prescriber or consumer requests noncompliant packaging
    b. household cleaners must be packaged in childproof containers
    c. a limited number of prescription drugs is exempt (e.g., sublingual nitroglycerin)
    d. the special packaging requirements are extended to nonprescription drugs

14. Sublingual tablets are _____.
    a. placed under the tongue
    b. dissolved in a liquid and release bubbles
    c. placed inside the cheek
    d. chewed before swallowing

15. Which of the following terms refers to the acidic or basic nature of a solution?
    a. osmolarity
    b. osmolality
    c. isotonicity
    d. pH

16. The Omnibus Budget Reconciliation Act of 1990 (OBRA 90) required pharmacists to perform which of the following functions for patients receiving Medicaid?
    a. drug therapy review
    b. counseling
    c. financial consultation
    d. a and b

17. A patient presents a prescription for hydrochlorothiazide (HCTZ). Other items related to his prescription that he might purchase include all of the following *except* _____.
    a. home blood pressure monitoring device
    b. potassium-containing salt substitute
    c. pseudoephedrine-containing decongestant
    d. sunscreen

18. Which statement concerning Synthroid is correct?
    a. The generic name is levothyroxine.
    b. The usual dose is 50–100 gm/day.
    c. It is usually given three times a day.
    d. It is used to treat diabetes.

19. Nonprescription drugs are also known as _____.
    a. legend drugs
    b. new drugs
    c. over-the-counter drugs
    d. investigational drugs

20. All of the following are true concerning patient participation in an investigational drug study *except* _____.
    a. the patient must sign an informed consent
    b. participation is voluntary.
    c. the patient may withdraw from the study at any time
    d. the patient must be paid

21. You receive a prescription for Ceclor suspension 125 mg/5 mL, 1.5 tsp tid x 10 days. The appropriate quantity to dispense would be _____.
    a. 125 mL
    b. 150 mL with one refill
    c. 200 mL
    d. 225 mL

22. When filling a prescription for Tylenol with Codeine 30 mg, a technician should do all the following *except* _____.
    a. file the prescription as a schedule III controlled substance
    b. affix an auxiliary label cautioning against performing tasks requiring alertness or driving
    c. verify that the patient is not allergic to Tylenol or codeine
    d. inform the patient that this medication is a potent anti-inflammatory agent

23. When a prescription is received for Cortisporin drops, use as directed, the technician should _____.
    a. have the pharmacist ascertain whether an ophthalmic or otic product is to be dispensed
    b. tell the patient to take the prescription back to the physician to be corrected
    c. affix a "For the eye" auxiliary label
    d. wash hands before dispensing so that the drops will remain sterile

24. Which of the following drug pairs is most likely to be associated with a medication error?
    a. digoxin and captopril
    b. prednisone and dexamethasone
    c. quinidine and quinine
    d. fluoxetine and fluorouracil

25. For a hospital inpatient order for ceftriaxone 1 gm qd IV piggyback, the technician should do all the following *except* _____.
    a. prepare the dose in the laminar airflow hood using sterile technique
    b. inform the pharmacist if the patient has a penicillin allergy recorded
    c. convert the dosage from grams to grains, so the nurse will know how much to give
    d. confirm that he/she has the right drug—many other drugs sound similar (ceftaxime, ceftizoxime)

26. The following term(s) may be used to describe a prepackaged unit _____.
    a. unit dose
    b. closed system
    c. blister pack
    d. a and c

27. All of the following are true about cimetidine *except* _____.
    a. an over-the-counter preparation is available
    b. it reduces the acidity of the stomach
    c. using samples of this product is a good way to save money in the hospital
    d. it interacts with many other drugs

28. The computer insurance error message "patient not found" or "invalid ID number" indicates _____.
    a. the customer is not a legitimate patient
    b. the patient does not appear to be enrolled in the insurance program; check for errors such as misspelling of the patient's name
    c. the patient does not have any condition that requires treatment
    d. the patient cannot find his/her prescription

29. As a technician, you are asked to prepare an IV solution with insulin.
    a. You should use only regular insulin. The other insulins cannot be given IV.
    b. You do not need to bother making the IV in the laminar airflow hood since insulin is an antibiotic.

    c. Because the dose is in units, you cannot measure the volume in milliliters.
    d. You must sign out the dose on the narcotic log.

30. The portion of prescription costs that the patient must pay in a given time period before the third-party insurer will begin paying is the _____.
    a. fee-for-service
    b. co-payment
    c. deductible
    d. none of the above

31. If a pediatric patient is to receive oral ampicillin as a suspension, which of the following is not necessary?
    a. Ensure that the patient's allergies are recorded in the computer.
    b. Affix an expiration date to the label after preparing the suspension.
    c. Affix an auxiliary label stating, "shake well before using."
    d. Prepare the medication in the laminar airflow hood.

32. A resource that may be used to determine if a parenteral medication must be filtered is _____.
    a. the packaging insert
    b. *Handbook on Injectable Drugs*
    c. the manufacturer
    d. all of the above

33. The offer to counsel under OBRA 90 may be made _____.
    a. in writing
    b. orally
    c. by a technician
    d. all of the above

34. When filling an inpatient's medication drawer, the technician notices that the fill list contains both enalapril and lisinopril. The technician should _____.
    a. fill only one drug; they are both the same kind of drug
    b. notify the pharmacist that the patient has orders for two drugs of the same class
    c. call the doctor to see which drug to use
    d. tell the nurse that there is a dangerous interaction between these drugs

35. If you believe someone has presented a fraudulent prescription at your pharmacy, the appropriate action would be to _____.
    a. call 911 immediately
    b. call the physician whose name appears on the prescription
    c. discreetly notify the pharmacist so that the appropriate action may be taken
    d. ask the customer how he/she got the prescription

36. You receive an order for etoposide. In preparing this drug, you should _____.
    a. wear gloves only of you are allergic to etoposide
    b. flush the extra contents of the vial down the sink drain
    c. prepare it in a biological safety cabinet (BSC)
    d. not add any extra labels—they are too confusing to the nurse

37. While a mother is waiting for an antibiotic preparation for her 6-year-old, she asks the technician what to give the child for fever. The technician should _____.
    a. suggest aspirin; it is the least expensive antipyretic
    b. inform the pharmacist that the mother would like help choosing a nonprescription product
    c. offer to sell the mother some drug samples
    d. suggest over-the-counter diphenhydramine

38. You receive the following prescription:

    Vanceril (beclomethasone) inhaler; Dispense #1; Sig: ii puffs inhaled bid. In filling the prescription, the technician should _____.
    a. inform the patient that this drug is a corticosteroid that has many serious side effects
    b. include the following specific directions on the label: "Inhale 2 puffs into each nostril three times a day."
    c. provide the patient with the "For the Patient" instructions included with the inhaler
    d. tell the patient to use this inhaler only when he/she really needs it

39. When accepting a prescription for warfarin from a patient the technician should _____.
    a. notify the pharmacist if the patient is also buying aspirin. There is an interaction with these medications
    b. give the lower dose just to be safe if the strength is unclear (10 mg vs. 1.0 mg)
    c. tell this patient to take an iron supplement, because this drug thins the blood
    d. tell the patient that he/she should eat foods high in vitamin K

40. When selling an over-the-counter nasal decongestant spray (phenylephrine), which question can the technician answer without referring the customer to the pharmacist?
    a. Can I take this drug with my blood pressure medicine?
    b. I keep using this spray, but my nose seems to get stuffier. Should I use it more often?
    c. Is there a less expensive generic of this nose spray available?
    d. I have had this cold for four weeks. Do you think I should see the doctor?

41. The pharmacist asks you to prepare the following prescription:

    Amoxicillin suspension 5 mL po tid × 10 days

    You notice that the prescriber did not indicate the concentration of the suspension on the prescription. You should _____.
    a. dispense the capsules instead
    b. alert the pharmacist to the problem
    c. ask the patient which concentration he/she prefers
    d. prepare the prescription with the 250 mg/mL concentration because it is most frequently ordered.

42. Which of the following could contribute to a medication error?
    a. failure to rotate stock appropriately
    b. preparing one prescription at a time
    c. reading the drug product label carefully
    d. none of the above

43. The risk of a decimal point error is reduced by writing "seven milligrams" as _____.:
    a. 0.7 gm
    b. 7 mg
    c. 7.0 mg
    d. 0.70 gm

44. Pharmaceutical compounding may involve which of the following ingredient(s)?
    a. Aquaphor
    b. simple syrup
    c. coal tar
    d. all of the above

45. A patient calls the pharmacy asking why his heart medication is white instead of the usual yellow color. Upon investigation, you learn that the prescription was filled with 0.25 mg of digoxin instead of the 0.125 mg strength. Which of the following is the most appropriate action to take?
    a. Tell the patient to cut the tablets in half and take one-half tablet daily.
    b. Ask the patient to bring the prescription back to the pharmacy so that you can secretly exchange it for the correct dose.
    c. Explain the situation to the pharmacist, correct the error, and document the error per procedures.
    d. Prepare a new prescription with the 0.125 mg strength, and inform the patient that pharmacists are solely responsible for the accuracy of prescriptions.

46. Position or job descriptions _____.
    a. are the same for technicians from hospital to hospital
    b. are written descriptions outlining employee responsibilities
    c. are the same for pharmacists and technicians
    d. apply only to upper hospital managers

47. Which of the following reasons corresponds to why it is important to follow established policies and procedures at your institution/company to prevent medication errors?
    a. Policies and procedures formally establish a system to prevent the occurrence of medication errors.
    b. It is important to follow policies and procedures for good performance in your position.
    c. Policies and procedures are a good resource when confronted with an unusual request by a patient.
    d. Patients usually ask the technicians if policies and procedures are followed in the institution/company.

48. A technician reading a medication order for a patient notices an abbreviation with which he or she is not familiar. Which of the following are acceptable ways to clarify the meaning of the abbreviation?
    a. Call the prescriber and ask the meaning of the abbreviation.
    b. Ask the pharmacist the meaning of the abbreviation.
    c. Refer to the lists of approved abbreviations in the policy and procedure manual.
    d. b and c

49. A physician calls the pharmacy asking about the maximum dose of a new medication. The technician answering the phone remembers hearing the pharmacist answer this question earlier that same day. How should the technician handle this call?
    a. Inform the physician that the maximum dose is 500 mg twice daily, since that was the dose the pharmacist gave earlier that day.
    b. Ask another technician and relay the information to the physician.
    c. Look up the answer to the question in *Facts and Comparisons* and inform the physician.
    d. Refer the question to the pharmacist.

50. A prescription with the directions to be given a.d. should be administered to _____.
    a. both eyes
    b. left eye
    c. right ear
    d. left ear

51. The usual dose of milk of magnesia is 30 cc. This is equivalent to _____.
    a. 3 Tbsp
    b. 3 tsp
    c. 1 tsp
    d. 2 Tbsp

52. Which vaccine has to be stored frozen before use?
    a. oral polio
    b. injectable polio
    c. influenza
    d. pneumococcal

53. If a product labeled to expire August 2015 what is the last date it should be used by?
    a. 8/01/15   c. 7/31/15
    b. 9/01/15   d. 8/31/15

54. The only type of insulin that may be added to an IV solution is _____.
    a. isophane insulin
    b. regular insulin
    c. NPH insulin
    d. extended insulin zinc

55. Which agent is not used for the treatment of tuberculosis?
    a. pyrazinamide
    b. rifampin

56. Refill limitations for a schedule III controlled substance prescription are _____.
    a. maximum of five refills and not more than six months after date of issuance
    b. maximum of five refills and not more than one year after date of issuance
    c. maximum of 10 refills and not more than six months after date of issuance
    d. maximum of 10 refills and not more than one year after date of issuance

57. Which cytotoxic drug does not require refrigeration?
    a. vinblastine
    b. cyclophosphamide
    c. asparaginase
    d. carmustine

58. The set of procedures for preparation of sterile products that is designed to prevent contamination is called _____.
    a. eutectic mixing
    b. filtration
    c. trituration
    d. aseptic technique

59. An example of a drug used as an anticonvulsant is _____.
    a. aspirin
    b. levothyroxine
    c. phenobarbital
    d. lithium

60. Which of the following statements is true regarding quality?
    a. Quality control is a process of checks and balances.
    b. Quality is defined by what our customers perceive.
    c. Quality improvement is an important part of meeting regulatory agency (e.g., JCAHO) requirements.
    d. All the above statements are true.

61. Triazolam would most likely be ordered as _____.
    a. tid prn
    b. bid
    c. qam
    d. qhs prn

62. Cortisporin is ordered "a.u." Which of the following medications should be dispensed?
    a. otic suspension
    b. ophthalmic solution
    c. topical ointment
    d. ophthalmic ointment

63. Reason(s) why a technician should always refer patients with medication or health-related questions to a pharmacist include _____.
    a. possibility of drug–drug interaction
    b. possibility of drug–disease state interaction

c. need for physician referral
d. all of the above

64. A type of reimbursement whereby a pharmacy receives a predetermined amount of money for a defined group of patients regardless of the number of prescriptions filled is _____.
a. fee-for-service
b. co-payment
c. capitation
d. no payment

65. Typical data collected from the patient at the prescription take-in window include _____.
a. weight for children and infants
b. allergies
c. emergency phone numbers
d. all the above

66. If a patient is noted to have experienced an allergic reaction to a medication, the technician should _____.
a. tell the patient that the doctor made a mistake, and refuse to fill the prescription.
b. tell the patient to take the medication anyway since it is a doctor's order.
c. ask the patient the type of allergic reaction experienced, note the patient's response, and alert the pharmacist.
d. none of the above

67. If a prescription is written generically and is marked "may not substitute." This means _____.
a. a generic drug can usually be dispensed (state law may vary)
b. the specific brand name drug must be dispensed, because it is marked "may not substitute."
c. send the patient back to the physician's office for clarification
d. none of the above

68. Endocarditis is an infection involving which part of the body?
a. bone
b. heart
c. joint
d. skin

69. Three fluid ounces is equal to _____ mL.
a. 120
b. 90
c. 100
d. 150

70. Fentanyl has a concentration of 0.05 mg/mL. How many milliliters do you need for a 950 mcg dose?
a. 190
b. 0.19
c. 19
d. 1.9

71. According to most insurance coverage, if a prescription is written for a brand name product and "may substitute" is marked, this means that _____.
a. the brand name drug must be dispensed
b. the generic drug must be dispensed
c. the generic drug can be dispensed if the patient and the pharmacist agree
d. the prescription is written incorrectly

72. The last step in the prescription-processing function is _____.
a. computer data entry
b. prescription filling
c. dispensing
d. compounding

73. During prescription computer entry, the technician is responsible for all the following *except* _____.
a. entering accurate patient demographic information
b. entering any allergies the patient reports
c. handling insurance claims messaging
d. handling drug interaction messaging

74. The computer error message "refill too soon" indicates _____.
a. the patient is attempting to get the prescription earlier than the "day supply" indicated
b. the pharmacy should not refill the prescription under any circumstances
c. a and b
d. none of the above

75. You receive an order for amoxicillin suspension (125 mg/5 mL) with a dose of 250 mg tid for 10 days. How many milliliters do you need to dispense?
a. 300
b. 150
c. 100
d. 120

76. When receiving a drug–drug, drug–disease state, or drug–allergy interaction computer message, the technician should _____.
a. inform the patient that the prescription cannot be filled.
b. call and alert the doctor of the mistake.
c. ignore the message if you have seen the interaction before.
d. alert the pharmacist to the problem.

77. All of the drugs listed below are antidotes *except* _____.
a. activated charcoal
b. Digibind
c. cefazolin
d. naloxone

78. Which of the following is not required on a prescription label?
a. the prescription number
b. directions on how to take the medication
c. the prescribing physician's name
d. the physician's DEA number

79. The sterile parts of a syringe that may never be touched are the _____.
    a. plunger and barrel
    b. tip and plunger
    c. barrel and hub
    d. tip and hub

80. The advantage of using a vertical laminar airflow hood in preparing chemotherapy medication is _____.
    a. there is no advantage
    b. contaminated air is not blown at the operator
    c. the vertical airflow hood provides a better sterile environment than horizontal airflow hoods
    d. horizontal airflow hoods are to be used in preparing chemotherapy medications

81. Which of the following medications must be protected from light?
    a. amphotericin B
    b. heparin
    c. tobramycin
    d. lanoxin

82. All of the following medications must be stored in the refrigerator, but not frozen, *except* _____.
    a. tetanus toxoid
    b. insulin
    c. tobramycin
    d. nitroglycerin

83. Which of the following is not a common disease treated in the home care environment?
    a. sepsis
    b. osteomyelitis
    c. chronic pain
    d. malnutrition

84. All of the following medications must be prepared in a vertical laminar airflow hood *except* _____.
    a. cisplatin
    b. cyclophosphamide
    c. cefotaxime
    d. etoposide

85. All of the drugs listed below are laxatives *except* _____.
    a. bisacodyl tablets
    b. Citrucel powder
    c. FiberCon tablets
    d. Pancrease capsules

86. Examples of quality control measures utilized when preparing an IVPB include _____.
    a. pulling the drug from the shelf and double checking to ensure the vial is correct
    b. calculating the correct dose and volume to withdraw from the vial to ensure the vial is correct
    c. checking the IVPB for particulate matter after injecting the medication
    d. all the above

87. All of the drugs listed below are scheduled narcotics *except* _____.
    a. Vicodin tablets
    b. Seconol capsules
    c. Duragesic patches
    d. Toradol tablets

88. The concentration of tobramycin is 80 mg/2 mL. An order is written for 130 mg of tobramycin in 100 mL NS. How many milliliters of tobramycin do you inject into the IVPB bag?
    a. 0.325
    b. 3.25
    c. 1.625
    d. 16.25

89. A 1,000-mL bag of Ringer's lactate is to infuse over eight hours. What is the flow rate of the infusion?
    a. 62.5 mL/hour
    b. 12.5 mL/hour
    c. 6.25 mL/hour
    d. 125 mL/hour

90. Schedule II narcotic prescriptions may be refilled how many times?
    a. 6
    b. 1
    c. 0
    d. 12

Practice Certification Exam III

This practice test has been designed to simulate the certification exam, both in the number/style of questions, as well as the content. You should complete this exam within 110 minutes.

1. A patient in the hospital needs KCl 8 mEq IV stat. The pharmacy stocks KCl 20 mEq/mL in a 10 mL multidose vial. What will the correct volume of the stat dose be?
    a. 2.5 mL
    b. 4 mL
    c. 0.4 mL
    d. 0.04 mL

2. What document is used as proof-of-receipt of a controlled substance according to the DEA?
    a. packing slip
    b. invoice
    c. purchase order
    d. DEA222C form

3. The pharmacy has a 10% strength and a 2% strength of a certain ointment. A patient turns in a prescription for 4 oz of this ointment but in a 5% strength. Using correct calculations, which of the following would be needed to compound the ointment for the patient?
    a. 45 gm of 2% ointment
    b. 120 gm of 10% ointment
    c. 75 gm of 2% ointment
    d. 75 gm of 10% ointment

4. What is the correct temperature for storing an item in the refrigerator?
   a. 2°–8° C
   b. <36° F
   c. 15°–30° C
   d. 59°–86° F

5. In an inpatient setting, the pharmacy must receive a direct copy of a physician's order before filling an initial dose. Which of these choices listed is not considered a direct copy?
   a. fax
   b. photocopy
   c. computer-generated transfer
   d. phone call acknowledging the verbal order

6. 125 mL of a Cipro 5% suspension contains how many grams of active ingredient?
   a. 0.625
   b. 6.25
   c. 62.5
   d. 60.25

7. Which of the following professional concepts most specifically refers to the protection of the identity and health information of patients?
   a. motility
   b. confidentiality
   c. mortality
   d. compatibility

8. According to federal law, what is the maximum number of refills permitted for a schedule III controlled substance?
   a. six refills within one year
   b. three refills within 90 days
   c. five refills within six months
   d. no refills are allowed

9. In the following NDC number, 69907-3110-01, what do the numbers 3110 identify?
   a. manufacturer
   b. drug product
   c. package size
   d. number of tablets in the bottle

10. The trade name for glipizide is _____.
    a. Diabinese
    b. Micronase
    c. Glucophage
    d. Glucotrol

11. What is the total volume of fluid needed if D5W is to run at 50 mL/hour for 24 hours?
    a. 1,200 mL
    b. 2,083 mL
    c. 480 mL
    d. 2,000 mL

12. Gentamicin injection is normally given to a patient at 5 mg/kg/day in three divided doses. If a patient weighs 164 lbs, what is the approximate strength per dose that the patient should receive?
    a. 25 mg
    b. 75 mg
    c. 124 mg
    d. 142 mg

13. Which of the following drugs is classed as an H2 antagonist medication?
    a. clonidine
    b. ranitidine
    c. loratadine
    d. clemastine

14. KCl supplements are most often used in combination with _____.
    a. labetalol
    b. lisinopril
    c. naproxen
    d. furosemide

15. If a patient called in for refills on Prinivil and Diabeta, which of the following combinations of medications would need to be filled for the patient?
    a. lisinopril and glipizide
    b. enalapril and glyburide
    c. enalapril and glipizide
    d. lisinopril and glyburide

16. How much neomycin powder must be added to fluocinolone cream to dispense an order for 60 gm of fluocinolone cream with 0.5% neomycin?
    a. 120 mg
    b. 240 mg
    c. 300 mg
    d. 600 mg

17. Which of the sig codes given refers to the following directions: Take two tablets by mouth every four to six hours as needed?
    a. 2 tablets q4–6h prn
    b. 2 tablets po q4–6h prn
    c. 2 tablets po q4–6h
    d. none of the above

18. The pharmacy receives an order for 10% ointment. Only the 15% and 5% strengths of the particular ointment are kept in stock. In what ratio would the two stock ointments need to be mixed in order to correctly compound the prescription order?
    a. 1:1
    b. 1:2
    c. 2:1
    d. 1:3

19. Which of these drugs listed is most likely to cause photosensitivity?
    a. nifedipine
    b. naproxen
    c. tetracycline
    d. glyburide

20. How many 250 mg doses of Claforan could be withdrawn from a 2-gm vial of the injection?
    a. 8
    b. 6
    c. 4
    d. 2

21. A medication that should be protected from exposure to light is _____.
    a. promethazine
    b. tetracycline
    c. erythromycin
    d. nitroglycerin

22. The blower on the Laminar Flow Workbench should remain on at all times. If it is turned off for any reason, it should remain on at least _____ before being used to prepare IV admixtures and other products.
    a. 15 minutes
    b. 1 hour
    c. 30 minutes
    d. 45 minutes

23. Which of the following needle sizes has the largest bore?
    a. 23 gauge
    b. 18 gauge
    c. 27 gauge
    d. 29 gauge

24. When metronidazole is dispensed for a patient, which auxiliary label should be affixed to the dispensing container?
    a. no alcohol
    b. no dairy products
    c. take with food or milk
    d. may cause drowsiness

25. If 500 mL of a 15% solution is diluted to 1,500 mL, how would you label the final strength of the solution?
    a. 20%
    b. 5%
    c. 0.05%
    d. 0.20%

26. A prescription reading "iii gtts as tid prn pain" should have which set of directions printed on the dispensing label?
    a. Instill three drops in the left eye three times daily as needed for pain.
    b. Instill three drops in the left ear three times daily as needed for pain.
    c. Instill three drops in the right ear two times daily as needed for pain.
    d. Instill three drops in the right eye three times daily as needed for pain.

27. A patient with a penicillin allergy is most likely to exhibit a sensitivity to _____.
    a. tetracycline
    b. erythromycin
    c. cephalexin
    d. gentamicin

28. A Tylenol#3 tablet contains 30 mg of codeine. The amount of codeine is also equivalent to _____.
    a. 1/4 grain
    b. 1/2 grain
    c. 1 grain
    d. 2 grains

29. An IV infusion order is written for 1 L of D5W/0.45% NS to run over 12 hours. The set that will be used delivers 15 gtts/mL. What should the flow rate be in drops per minute?
    a. 7
    b. 21
    c. 25
    d. 8

30. To ensure that it is working properly, the Laminar Flow Workbench should be inspected by qualified personnel at least _____.
    a. every six months
    b. every year
    c. every three years
    d. every five years

31. Zovirax and Epivir are both classed as _____ agents.
    a. antimalarial
    b. tuberculosis
    c. antiviral
    d. antifungal

32. A physician writes an order for a patient to receive KCl 40 mEq/1 L NS. The fluid is to be infused at 80 mL/hour. What amount of KCl will the patient receive per hour?
    a. 6.8 mEq
    b. 3.2 mEq
    c. 2.3 mEq
    d. 8.6 mEq

33. Na is the chemical symbol for which of the following elements?
    a. nitrogen
    b. nickel
    c. copper
    d. sodium

34. When withdrawing medication from an ampule, what size filter needle will be sufficient to filter out any tiny glass fragments that may have fallen into the solution?
    a. 0.2 micron
    b. 0.5 micron
    c. 2 micron
    d. 5 micron

35. Which of the following conditions is the drug rifampin used to treat?
    a. influenza
    b. tuberculosis
    c. nail fungus
    d. urinary tract infection

36. When measuring liquid in a graduated cylinder, where is the volume of liquid read?
    a. top surface of the liquid
    b. top of the meniscus
    c. center of the meniscus
    d. bottom of the meniscus

37. How many grams of 2% silver nitrate ointment will deliver 1 gm of the active ingredient?
    a. 25
    b. 4
    c. 50
    d. 20

38. The federal law enacted in 1970 that requires the use of child-resistant safety caps on all dispensing containers unless otherwise desired by the patient is known as the _____.
    a. Controlled Substance Act of 1970
    b. Poison Prevention Act of 1970
    c. Bueller-Ferris Act of 1970
    d. Harrison Narcotic Act of 1970

39. Into what size bottle will a prescription for 180 mL of cough syrup will best fit?
    a. 2 oz
    b. 4 oz
    c. 6 oz
    d. 8 oz

40. If a patient should receive a medication at 15 mg/kg/day in three equally divided doses, what will be the approximate dose if the patient weighs 142 lb?
    a. 968 mg
    b. 323 mg
    c. 2,904 mg
    d. 284 mg

41. If one of your pharmacy's patients has had an adverse drug reaction, the _____ form should be used to report it.
    a. HCFA form
    b. Medwatch form
    c. DEA222C
    d. Universal Claim Form

42. Of the following choices, which pair of drugs are H2 antagonists?
    a. Zantac and Prevacid
    b. Prinivil and Tagamet
    c. Pepcid and Zantac
    d. Vasotec and Motrin

43. A pharmacy wants to make a 30% profit on an item that costs $4.50. What would the retail selling price have to be in order to make such a profit?
    a. $6.23
    b. $7.10
    c. $5.85
    d. $6.40

44. Which statement is true concerning the drug tetracycline?
    a. It should be given with food or milk for best absorption.
    b. It should not be given with milk products or antacids for best absorption.
    c. It should be given with milk because it is upsetting to the stomach.
    d. Exposure to sunlight will not affect a patient taking this medication.

45. What schedule of controlled substances does the drug Darvocet N 100 fall under?
    a. II
    b. III
    c. IV
    d. V

46. When storing an item at room temperature, the correct temperature of the room should range from _____.
    a. 2°–8° C
    b. 36°–46° F
    c. >30° C
    d. 15°–30° C

47. A list of medications that a physician may prescribe from within a given setting is called _____.
    a. an MSDS Sheet
    b. a formulary
    c. a closed panel of drugs
    d. an open system

48. Which of the following sig codes refers to these directions: Take one tablespoonful after meals as needed for indigestion.
    a. 1 Tbsp pc for indigestion
    b. 1 Tbsp pc prn for indigestion
    c. 1 tsp ac prn for indigestion
    d. 1 tsp pc prn for indigestion

49. If while preparing IV admixtures, a vial slips from your hand and breaks onto the floor or other surface, a spill kit should be used to clean the area if the vial contained which of the following medications?
    a. vinblastine
    b. adenosin
    c. amphotericin b
    d. methylprednisolone

50. During cleaning of the Laminar Flow Workbench in preparation to make IV admixtures, which of the following statements is true?
    a. The work surface should be cleaned first using a continuous side-to-side motion.
    b. 70% isopropyl alcohol should be sprayed onto the HEPA filter to ensure its cleanliness.
    c. The sides should be cleaned from top to bottom working outward from the filter.
    d. None of the above

51. What volume of 5% aluminum acetate solution will be needed if 120 mL of 0.05% solution are extemporaneously compounded for patient use?
    a. 12 mL
    b. 1.2 mL
    c. 8.3 mL
    d. 0.83 mL

52. Ampicillin powder for injection should be reconstituted with and diluted in _____ for best stability.
    a. D5W
    b. normal saline
    c. Lactated Ringers
    d. none of the above

53. How many 1-L bags will be needed if D5W is to run at 60 mL/hour for 16 hours?
    a. 1
    b. 2
    c. 3
    d. 4 or more

54. Which of the drugs listed is classified as an antidiarrheal medication?
    a. labetalol
    b. loperamide
    c. cimetidine
    d. nalbuprofen

55. A pharmacy has 20 mL of a 1:200 solution in stock. If the pharmacist has asked the technician to dilute the solution to 500 mL, how should the final strength of the solution be labeled?
    a. 2%
    b. 2.5%
    c. 25%
    d. 0.02%

56. When an antibiotic injection is given in a small volume of solution that is connected to the main line of IV fluids the patient receives, it is commonly known as getting _____.
    a. IV bag
    b. IV injection
    c. IV piggyback
    d. IV push

57. Of the drugs listed, which one could not be phoned in or filled with refills added?
    a. hydrocodone
    b. acetaminophen
    c. codeine
    d. gabapentin

58. The largest gelatin capsule use for extemporaneous compounding is _____.
    a. 000
    b. 0
    c. 10
    d. 5

59. All manipulations in the Laminar Flow Workbench should take place at least _____ inches within the hood.
    a. 4
    b. 6
    c. 8
    d. 10

60. Which of these medications listed should always be dispensed in a glass container?
    a. aminophylline
    b. dopamine
    c. potassium
    d. nitroglycerine

61. How many teaspoons are in one tablespoon?
    a. 2
    b. 3
    c. 4
    d. 5

62. When using a torsion prescription balance, the first thing you should do after placing it on a level surface is _____.
    a. place the weights in the left pan and the substance to be weighed in the right pan
    b. place the weights in the right pan and the substance to be weighed in the left pan
    c. place the substance to be weighed onto the scale
    d. unlock the balance and level it to zero

63. An air vent on a vented administration set should be a _____ micron filter vent to be considered a sterilizing filter.
    a. 0.2
    b. 0.5
    c. 5
    d. none of the above

64. How many tablets will a patient need if he/she is to take 1 tablet po bid for 10 days?
    a. 10
    b. 20
    c. 30
    d. 40

65. Of the following tasks involved in pharmacy practice, which is allowed by law for technicians to perform?
    a. giving or receiving a verbal copy
    b. counseling a patient on the use of their medication
    c. receiving a verbal order from a physician
    d. filling a unit dose cart

66. Which organization requires that oral products be stored separate from inhaled products and topical preparations be separated from injectables and so on?
    a. American Society of Health System Pharmacists
    b. Pharmacy Technician Certification Board
    c. American Pharmacists Association
    d. Joint Commission

67. An automatic stop order is most likely to be issued with which of the following medicines?
   a. clonidine 0.3-mg tablets
   b. acetaminophen/codeine 325-mg/60-mg tablets
   c. amlodipine 5-mg tablets
   d. furosemide 40-mg tablets

68. Which of the choices listed would not be equal to one pound?
   a. 454 gm
   b. 1 lb
   c. 16 oz
   d. 240 gm

69. Amphotericin B should only be mixed in _____ for compatibility.
   a. 0.9% sodium chloride
   b. Lactated Ringers
   c. 0.45% sodium chloride
   d. dextrose

70. There are several different types of automated dispensing systems. Which of the following is not an automated dispensing system?
   a. Kirby-Lester
   b. Omnicell
   c. Pyxis
   d. Baker

71. Personal protective equipment should be used properly when handling hazardous medications. This would consist of _____.
   a. gloves
   b. gown
   c. mask
   d. all of the above

72. After preparation of IV admixtures are completed, how should the used needles be disposed of?
   a. Needles should be recapped and discarded in a trashcan.
   b. Needles should be bent, so they cannot possibly be reused.
   c. Needles should be disposed in a sharps container without recapping.
   d. None of the above

73. The retail price of a prescription is $18.23. The patient pays with a $20 bill. How should the patient receive change from the money given?
   a. one dollar bill, three quarters, one nickel, and two pennies
   b. one dollar bill, two quarters, three dimes, and seven pennies
   c. one dollar bill, three quarters, and two pennies
   d. one dollar bill, two quarters, one nickel, and two pennies

74. Which of the following items is not necessary to be present on a valid prescription?
   a. dispensing pharmacist's initials
   b. name of medication
   c. prescriber's signature
   d. patient's name

75. Which of the drugs listed would not likely be found stored in an emergency crash cart?
   a. epinephrine injection
   b. cimetidine injection
   c. lidocaine injection
   d. dopamine injection

76. To be considered a generic substitute for a trade named drug product, the substitute must be _____.
   a. bioequivalent
   b. the same color
   c. made by the same manufacturer
   d. none of the above

77. On the following perpetual inventory for a schedule II controlled substance, in what line is the error made?

Line#	Patient's Name	Quantity Dispensed	Quantity Received	Current Balance
1	Received from wholesaler		100	100
2	Barbara Jones	42		58
3	Nancy Smith	36		32
4	Thomas Watkins	24		8

   a. 1
   b. 2
   c. 3
   d. 4

78. When a pharmacy is audited by a third-party payer such as Medicaid, what shows proof that the medications filled by the pharmacy were, in fact, picked up by the patient or a representative of that patient?
   a. the prescription number
   b. a recorded signature of the patient or patient's representative
   c. the computer profile of the patient
   d. none of the above

79. What is the best defense against the spread of bacteria and infection?
   a. spraying with Lysol
   b. hand washing
   c. mopping with chlorine bleach
   d. wearing gloves

80. An injection that is given in the spinal column is known as _____.
   a. a peritoneal injection
   b. an interspinal injection

c. an intrathecal injection

d. an intravenous injection

81. A hard copy of the original prescription should remain on file in a retail pharmacy for at least _____ years.
    a. 2
    b. 3
    c. 4
    d. 5

82. Which of the following medications is indicated for the induction of labor contractions?
    a. ritodrine
    b. oxytocin
    c. medroxyprogesterone
    d. estrogen

83. When dispensing _____, a patient information package insert should be included with the medication.
    a. oral contraceptives
    b. diet pills
    c. insulin
    d. nasal drops

84. An instrument used to determine a patient's blood pressure is known as a _____.
    a. glucometer
    b. sphygmomanometer
    c. tempanometer
    d. electrocardiogram

85. Which of the following classes of antibiotics are not recommended for young children and adolescents?
    a. penicillins
    b. erythromycins
    c. flouroquinolones
    d. cephalosporins

86. If an accident should occur involving a hazardous substance that is stored in the pharmacy, what document would give instructions on actions that need to be taken?
    a. policy and procedure manual
    b. MSDS sheet
    c. employee handbook
    d. OSHA "*Right to Know*" pamphlet

87. When preparing a TPN solution containing calcium, phosphate, and other ingredients, which of the following statements would be true?

a. The calcium and phosphate should be mixed together in the same syringe before being injected into the TPN solution.

b. The phosphate should be added first to avoid precipitation of the calcium additive.

c. The calcium should be added after all other ingredients have been added.

d. The phosphate should be added last after the addition of calcium and other ingredients, which will allow for dilution of the calcium to prevent precipitation.

88. The pharmacist has asked the technician to dilute 50 mL of a 50% solution to 3% and repackage the diluted solution into 2 oz bottles. How many bottles will the technician be able to fill?
    a. 5
    b. 6
    c. 13
    d. 14

89. A patient is being provided with hyperalimentation. The following order has been sent to the pharmacy for preparation. If the pharmacy stocks magnesium sulfate 10% (0.8 mEq/mL) in a 10-mL vial, what is the volume of injection to be added during preparation of this TPN solution?

2L over 24hrs
Dextrose 25%
Phosphorus 20mEq/2L
$MgSO_4$ 24mEq/2L
Calcium Gluconate 26mEq
KCl 40mEq/L
Na 80mEq/2L

a. 0.3 mL

b. 0.8 mL

c. 2.15 mL

d. 30 mL

90. What is the maximum volume that can be injected subcutaneously in a single dose?
    a. 0.5 mL
    b. 1 mL
    c. 2 mL
    d. 3 mL

Glossary

absorption the process by which a drug is moved from the site of administration into the bloodstream.

acceptable macronutrient distribution range (AMDR) the range of intake levels that provide adequate amount of a nutrient and are associated with a reduced risk of disease.

acidosis excessive acid in the body fluids.

acne infection accompanied by an overproduction of sebum.

addiction a pattern of compulsive substance abuse characterized by a continued psychological and physiological craving or need for the substance and its effects.

adipose fat.

adjudication the process of transmitting a prescription electronically to the proper insurance company or third-party biller for approval and billing.

adjuvant helping or assisting.

adulterated altered and causing an undesirable effect.

adverse effects undesirable and potentially harmful drug effects.

aerobic requires oxygen for life.

afferent sending an impulse toward the CNS.

agonist a type of drug that activates the receptor to produce a predicted action.

allegation a principle relating to the solution of questions concerning the compounding or mixing of different ingredients.

allergen a substance capable of causing a hypersensitivity reaction.

allergy the result of the immune system's reaction to a foreign substance.

alopecia hair loss.

ambulatory pharmacy community-based pharmacy; includes chain retail drugstores, grocery store pharmacies, home health care, mail-order facilities, and other pharmacies from which patients can obtain medications without living onsite.

anaerobic does not require oxygen for life.

analgesic a drug that is used to help reduce pain.

anhydrous without water.

antacid a drug that reduces stomach acid.

antagonist a type of drug that prevents receptor activation.

antibodies proteins that specifically seek and bind to the surface of pathogens or antigens.

antidiarrheal a drug that is used to help eliminate diarrhea.

antiemetic a drug used to subside or reduce nausea and vomiting.

antiflatulent a drug used to rid the intestinal tract and stomach of excess gas or air.

antigens specific molecules that trigger an immune response.

antihemorrhoidal a drug used to help reduce or eliminate hemorrhoids.

antihistamine a drug that blocks histamine and leukotriene receptors and relieves common allergy symptoms.

antineoplastics agents, such as medications, that prevent the growth of malignant cells.

antioxidant a molecule that slows or prevents the oxidation of other molecules.

antipyretic a drug that is used to help reduce or eliminate fever.

antitussive a drug that suppresses unproductive coughs.

anxiety a mental state characterized by apprehension and uneasiness stemming from the anticipation of danger.

anxiolytic a drug used in the treatment of anxiety.

apothecary Latin term for pharmacist; also used as a general term to refer to the early pharmacy practice.

apothecary system an old English system of measurement of weight, based on the grain.

applications software programs designed to perform specific functions such as creating databases, spreadsheets, e-mail, or graphics, or performing word processing.

aqueous containing water; water-soluble.

aromatic having a strong or fragrant smell (aroma).

arterioles the smallest arteries.

aseptic technique the process of performing a procedure under controlled conditions in a manner that minimizes the chance of contamination of the preparation.

association a group of individuals who voluntarily form an organization to accomplish a common purpose.

asthma a respiratory disease characterized by wheezing, shortness of breath, and bronchoconstriction.

asymptomatic showing no evidence of disease or disordered condition.

atrioventricular valves include the tricuspid and mitral valves of the heart.

attire clothing.

attitude a way of acting, thinking, or believing.

autonomy the condition or quality of being independent.

avoirdupois system the current American system of measurement of weight, based on 1 lb being equivalent to 16 oz.

bactericidal kills microorganisms.

bacteriostatic inhibits the growth and/or reproduction of microorganisms.

bench (countertop) model a horizontal laminar flow hood that sits on top of a counter; the space underneath it can be used for storage.

beneficence the quality of being kind or charitable.

bevel the sharp, pointed, diagonally cut end of a needle.

bilirubin a substance produced by the breakdown of hemoglobin.

bioavailability the degree to which a drug becomes available to body tissue(s) after administration.

biological safety cabinet a vertical laminar flow hood used to provide protection for the worker, the work environment, and the drug.

biologics a group of varied medicinal products such as vaccines, blood products, allergenics, and proteins.

biometrics a technology that measures and analyzes human body characteristics such as fingerprints, for authentication purposes.

biopharmaceuticals substances created using biotechnology.

biopharmacology a branch of pharmacology that studies the use of biologically engineered drugs.

biotechnology the use of biological substances or microorganisms to perform specific functions such as the production or modification of drugs, hormones, or food products.

blepharitis inflammation of the eyelid margins accompanied by redness.

blister packs unit-dose packages.

bone marrow the spongy type of tissue found inside most bones; responsible for the manufacture of red blood cells, some white blood cells, and platelets. Also acts as storage area for fat.

bones specialized form of dense connective tissue consisting of calcified intercellular substance that provides the shape and support for the body. Bones are made of calcium and phosphate. Injuries can result in fractures.

buffer capacity the ability of a solution to resist a change in pH when either an acidic or an alkaline substance is added to the solution.

capsule a solid dosage form in which the active ingredient and any excipients are enclosed in a soluble gelatin shell that will dissolve in the stomach.

carcinoma malignant tumor.

carrier/insurer/provider the insurance company.

cartilage soft tissues that line every joint and give shape to the ears and nose. Injuries can result in tears or degeneration of the cartilage and arthritis.

cassette systems drug containers that can hold hundreds or thousands of tablets and are affixed to a counting machine.

cataract an ocular opacity or obscurity in the lens of the eye.

cellulitis inflammation of the connective tissue of the skin.

Celsius (centigrade) an international unit of measurement for temperature.

central nervous system (CNS) the part of the nervous system made up of the brain and spinal cord.

central processing unit (CPU) the brain of a computer system; it interprets commands, connects the various hardware components, runs software applications, and controls speed and use of memory space.

centralized pharmacy system a system in which all pharmacy-related activities are performed from one location and medications are delivered to various patient care units throughout the facility.

cerebrospinal fluid (CSF) the fluid surrounding the brain and spinal cord.

certification the recognition granted by a nongovernmental agency attesting that an individual has met the required levels of competency.

certified nursing assistant (CNA) an individual who is certified to assist RNs and LPNs in providing patient care but is not permitted to administer medication.

certified pharmacy technician (CPhT) an individual who is certified to assist pharmacists in providing pharmaceutical care but is not permitted to dispense medication or counsel patients; certification is achieved by passing a national certification exam.

chain pharmacy a retail, or ambulatory, pharmacy that is owned by a corporation operating multiple pharmacy facilities at various locations.

channel a gesture, action, sound, written or spoken word, or visual image used in transmitting information.

chemotherapy the drug therapy used to treat cancer and other diseases.

chronic obstructive pulmonary disease (COPD) a condition resulting from continual blockage of oxygen exchange in the lungs; an umbrella term for emphysema and chronic bronchitis.

chyme the liquid that food turns into before it passes into the small intestine.

cilia the tiny hair-like organelles found in the nose and bronchial passageways.

civil law any law dealing with the rights of private citizens.

claim a request for reimbursement, for products or services rendered, from a health care provider to an insurance provider.

Clark's rule formula for solving pediatric dosage calculations based on the patient's weight in pounds.

class 100 environment the classification of an airflow unit capable of producing an environment containing no more than 100 airborne particles of a size 0.5 micron or larger, per cubic foot of air.

clearance the time it takes a drug to be eliminated from the body.

combining form a root word with an added vowel.

comminuting the process of reducing the particle size of a substance by grinding; also known as trituration.

common fractions fractions written with a numerator that is separated by a fraction line and positioned above a denominator.

community pharmacy name commonly used for an ambulatory or retail pharmacy.

compassion a deep awareness of and sympathy for another's suffering.

complement a large group of proteins that are activated in sequence when cells are exposed to a foreign substance; activation eventually results in the death or destruction of the substance. In general, complements amplify or enhance the effects of antibodies and inflammation.

complex fraction a fraction in which both the numerator and the denominator are themselves common fractions.

compounding the practice of extemporaneously preparing medications to meet the unique need of an individual patient according to the specific order of a prescriber; producing, mixing, or preparing a drug by combining two or more ingredients.

concentration term for the strength of active pharmaceutical ingredient in a medication.

conjunctivitis an acute or chronic inflammation of the eye conjunctiva.

consequentialism the theory that the value of an action derives solely from the value of its consequences.

console model a horizontal laminar flow hood that sits on the floor.

context the setting, or circumstances, in which communication occurs.

contraception birth control.

contractility the ability to contract; also, the degree of contraction.

contracts written agreements.

co-pay a portion of the cost of a service or product that a patient pays out of pocket each time it is provided.

correctional facilities more commonly referred to as prisons; places in which individuals are physically confined and usually deprived of a range of personal freedoms.

corticosteroid steroidal hormones produced in the adrenal cortex.

counseling the process of providing patients and customers with pharmaceutical and general health-related advice; provided only by registered pharmacists or doctors of pharmacy.

counting machines electronic devices that automatically and precisely count capsules and tablets, based on weight.

criminal law any law dealing with crime or punishment.

cross-multiplication a principle used in solving pharmacy calculations; you set up two ratios or fractions in relationship to each other as a proportion and solve for the unknown variable.

cycloplegic causing relaxation and paralysis of the intraocular muscles.

cytotoxic poisonous or destructive to cells.

databases lists of information ordered in specific ways.

DAW instructions from the prescriber to "dispense as written," without generic substitution.

days supply the expected duration for a prescription being dispensed; how long the amount of medication dispensed will last if taken as directed.

decentralized pharmacy system the pharmacy service system consisting of a central, or inpatient, pharmacy and multiple satellite pharmacies, as well as an outpatient pharmacy.

decimal fractions fractions written as a whole number with a zero and a decimal point in front of the value.

decongestant a drug that aides in reducing sinus and mucosal buildup.

deductible a set amount that a client pays up front before insurance coverage applies.

deep venous thrombosis (DVT) a blood clot in one of the veins of the legs or other deep veins.

defendant the party against which a legal action is brought.

defense mechanisms unconscious mental processes used to protect one's ego.

denial a defense mechanism characterized by refusal to acknowledge painful realities, thoughts, or feelings.

denominator the bottom value of a fraction; placed beneath the fraction line.

dependency the state of being dependent.

depression a mental state characterized by lack of energy, feelings of despair, guilt, and misery, and changes in sleep pattern and eating habits.

dermatitis a condition that results in dry, flaky, or itchy skin.

dialysis a medical procedure that removes waste from the blood of patients with renal failure.

diction the clarity and distinctness of pronunciation in speech.

Dietary Reference Intakes (DRI) nutritional guidelines that include both recommended intakes and tolerable upper intake levels.

diluent a substance used to dilute another substance.

"dispense as written" (DAW) a notation by the prescriber instructing the pharmacy to use the exact drug written (usually brand).

dispensing quantity the total amount of medication to be dispensed.

displacement a defense mechanism in which there is an unconscious shift of emotions, affect, or desires from the original object to a more acceptable or immediate substitute.

distribution the process by which an absorbed drug is moved from the bloodstream to body tissues or receptors.

DNA deoxyribonucleic acid; a nucleic acid that carries genetic information and is capable of self-replication and synthesis of RNA.

doctor of medicine (MD) a licensed individual, trained to examine patients, diagnose illnesses, and prescribe and administer medication.

doctor of osteopathy (DO) a licensed individual, trained to examine patients, diagnose illnesses, and prescribe and administer treatments using manipulative techniques on the musculoskeletal system in conjunction with conventional treatments.

doctor of pharmacy (PharmD) an individual who has completed a doctoral degree in pharmacy and is licensed to practice pharmacy in a specific state.

dosage calculations pharmacy calculations pertaining to the number of doses, dispensing quantities, and/or ingredient quantities.

dosage form the actual form of the drug (tablet, capsule, suppository, solution, etc.); also called dosage formulation.

dose the amount of medication prescribed to be taken at one time.

drop factor an abbreviated form referring to a specific drip rate.

drops per minute (gtts/minute) the volume of medication to be administered each minute.

drug drug interaction an interaction between two or more drugs administered to a patient, resulting in either an increase or a decrease in the therapeutic effects of one or more of the drugs, or an adverse effect.

drug of choice (DOC) the drug preferred for the treatment of a particular condition or disease.

drug per hour (mg/hour) the dosage, or amount of medication in milligrams, that will be administered per hour of infusion.

dyscrasia an abnormal condition of the body, especially a blood imbalance.

eczema an inflammatory skin condition characterized by itching, redness, blistering, and oozing.

edema swelling.

efferent sending impulses away from the CNS.

electroencephalogram (EEG) a graphic record of the electrical activity of the brain.

emergency medication order a specific type of STAT order for a medication that is required for a physician to be able to respond to a medical emergency.

emollient softening and soothing to the skin.

empathy a feeling of concern and understanding for another's situation or feelings.

emulsion a suspension that consists of two immiscible liquids and an emulsifying agent to hold them together; liquid mixture of water and oil.

endometrium the lining of the uterus.

epiglottis the small, leaf-shaped cartilage attached to the tongue that prevents substances other than air from entering the trachea.

epitope a region on the surface of an antigen that is capable of producing an immune response.

ethics a system of principles and duties; often associated with a profession.

excipient any substance added to a prescription to confer a suitable consistency or form to the drug.

excretion the process by which drugs are eliminated from the body; usually occurs through urine, feces, or the respiratory system.

exogenous from outside the organism.

expectorant a drug that loosens and thins mucus and phlegm buildup in the chest.

expired drugs drugs that have not been dispensed as of the manufacturer's printed expiration date.

Fahrenheit American unit of measurement for temperature.

feedback the return of information, or a message, in the communication process.

felony a serious crime such as rape or murder.

fidelity faithfulness to obligations and duties.

floor stock a distribution system in which medications are kept on each floor for distribution to patients.

flow rate duration the length of time for which an IV will be administered, or how long an IV bag will last before it must be changed.

flow rates a term used to describe a number of common pharmacy calculations used in the preparation of IV infusions.

formulary a listing of drugs approved for specific uses or for reimbursement.

fortified with an added nutrient for enrichment.

fraction line a symbol representing the division of two values; placed between the numerator and the denominator of a fraction.

franchise pharmacy a retail, or ambulatory, pharmacy that consists of facilities at multiple locations, although each pharmacy may be separately owned.

Fried's rule formula for solving pediatric dosage calculations based on the patient's age in months.

front end the over-the-counter (OTC) section of a retail pharmacy.

Gaucher's disease a disease in which fatty materials collect in the liver, spleen, kidneys, lungs, and brain and cause the person to be susceptible to infections.

genetically modified organism (GMO) an organism whose genetic material has been altered using the genetic engineering techniques known as recombinant DNA technology.

geometric dilution a technique of starting with the ingredient of the smallest amount and doubling the portion by adding the other ingredients, in order of quantity, until fully mixed.

geriatric refers to persons over the age of 65.

glaucoma a group of eye diseases characterized by an increase in intraocular pressure.

gonads testes and ovaries.

grain the primary unit of weight in the apothecary system.

gram metric system's primary unit of weight.

gray matter a major component of the nervous system, composed of nonmyelinated nerve tissue with a gray-brown color.

gross profit how much above cost the pharmacy is paid for a given product, or the selling price minus the cost.

group purchasing system a purchasing system in which a pharmacy joins a group purchasing organization (GPO), which contracts with pharmaceutical manufacturers collectively for all members of that GPO.

half-life the time required for serum concentration levels of an absorbed and distributed drug to decrease by one-half.

hard drive the main storage device of a computer; can be either external or internal.

hardware the mechanical and electrical components that make up a computer system.

health maintenance organization (HMO) a type of health care/insurance plan.

health-system pharmacy classification of pharmacy setting in which patients reside onsite at the facility where the pharmacy is located (such as hospitals, nursing homes, and long-term care facilities).

hematopoiesis the formation and development of blood cells.

hematopoietic blood-forming.

hematuria blood in the urine.

HEPA a high-efficiency particulate air filter; used in flow hoods.

high-density lipoprotein (HDL) good cholesterol.

homeostasis a stable and constant environment.

homogenous having all the same qualities within a group.

hordeolum an infection of one (or more) of the sebaceous glands of the eye.

hormone a chemical substance, produced by an organ or gland, that travels through the bloodstream to regulate certain bodily functions and/or the activity of other organs and glands.

hospice provides palliative care (care designed to help ease suffering) and supportive services to individuals at the end of their lives.

hospital pharmacy the most common type of health-system pharmacy; a pharmacy located within a hospital facility serving patients who have been admitted or are being discharged.

household system the measurement system commonly used by Americans for general measuring and cooking.

humor a body fluid.

hydrophobic repels water.

hyperlipidemia high concentrations of lipids in the blood.

hypermetabolic metabolizing at an increased rate.

hyperplasia the reproduction of cells within an organ at an increased rate.

hypersensitivity allergy.

hypertension high blood pressure.

hypertonic solutions solutions that have greater osmotic pressure than cell contents. Hypertonic solutions cause cells to dehydrate and shrink.

hypotension abnormally low blood pressure.

hypotonic solutions solutions that have a lower osmotic pressure than cell contents. Hypotonic solutions cause cells to take on water and expand.

improper fraction a fraction in which the value of the numerator is larger than the value of the denominator.

independent purchasing system a purchasing system in which the pharmacy establishes contracts directly with each pharmaceutical manufacturer.

infant child between the ages of one month and two years.

infection an invasion of pathogens into the body; an infection occurs when a pathogenic microbe is able to multiply in the tissues (colonize).

inflection alteration in pitch or tone of the voice.

infusion a relatively large volume of solution given at a constant rate.

inpatient pharmacy (IP) portion of a facility that is responsible for medication packaging, centralized inventory, sterile product preparation, and the preparation and delivery of medication carts. It provides pharmaceutical services to patients admitted to a facility.

input devices hardware that allows information, or data, to be entered into a computer system.

institutional pharmacy a pharmacy found in places such as hospitals, long-term care facilities, extended living facilities, and retirement homes, which require patients to reside onsite.

intellectualization a defense mechanism used to protect oneself from the emotional stress and anxiety associated with confronting painful personal fears or problems; characterized by excessive reasoning.

International Units (IU) measurement of a drug in terms of its action, not its physical weight.

intradermal parenteral injection in the dermis of the skin.

intramuscular (IM) within or into a muscle; parenteral injection in the muscle.

intraocular within the eye.

intrathecal parenteral injection in the spine.

intravenous parenteral injection in the vein.

investigational medication order an order for medication used in facilities that participate in research programs.

iridotomy an incision made in the iris of the eye to enlarge the pupil.

isotonic containing the same tonicity concentration as red blood cells.

isotonic solutions solutions that have an osmotic pressure equal to that of cell contents.

IV admixture a mixture of a solution and drug(s) prepared aseptically to be administered via a vein.

IV infusion a compounded solution that provides fluids, specific medications, nutrients, electrolytes, and minerals to a patient.

joint the location or position where bones are connected to each other. A joint contains synovial fluid and cartilage.

justice the principle of moral rightness and equity.

Kegel exercises pelvic muscle training and toning exercises.

ketone a by-product of fat metabolism.

keyboard the primary input device of a computer system, used to enter information (both alphabetic and numeric) into the computer.

kilocalories (kcal) a unit of measurement for food energy.

laminar flow hood a device containing a HEPA filter; used for preparing sterile products.

larynx the voicebox.

laxative a drug used to reduce or eliminate constipation.

leukocyte white blood cell.

licensed nursing assistant (LNA) an individual who is licensed to assist RNs and LPNs in providing patient care but is not permitted to administer medication.

licensed practical nurse (LPN) an individual who is licensed to provide basic care, such as administering medication, under the supervision of a registered nurse.

licensing permission granted by a government entity for an individual to perform an activity.

ligaments strong fibrous bands of connective tissue that hold bones together. Injuries can result in sprains.

lipid fat.

lipid-soluble dissolvable in fats; describes drugs that pass readily into cell membranes composed mostly of fatty substances such as the brain.

liter metric system's primary unit of volume.

long-term care (LTC) facility facility that provides rehabilitative, restorative, or ongoing skilled nursing care to individuals who need assistance with activities of daily living.

low-density lipoprotein (LDL) bad cholesterol.

lozenge a solid dosage form administered orally to be dissolved in the mouth.

lumen the hollow space inside a needle.

lymphocyte type of white blood cell.

lysis the destruction of cells.

macrophage white blood cell, found primarily in connective tissue and the bloodstream.

malabsorption an abnormality in digestion that causes nutrients to be absorbed poorly or not at all.

markup the difference between the selling price and the cost, stated in dollars and cents.

mastication chewing.

Medicaid the health insurance program for individuals and families with low incomes or disabilities.

medical device any instrument or apparatus used in the diagnosis, prevention, monitoring, treatment, or alleviation of disease.

medical ethics principles and moral values of proper medical care.

medical malpractice the negligent treatment of a patient by a health care professional.

Medicare the health insurance program for individuals aged 65 or older, younger people with disabilities, and people with end-stage renal disease.

medication order term for a patient prescription in a health system.

message the substance, or information, being transferred in communication.

metabolism the chemical alteration of drugs, food, or foreign compounds in and by the body; the process of transforming drugs in the body; also known as biotransformation.

metabolite any substance produced by the metabolic process.

meter metric system's primary unit of length.

metric system the international and scientific standard system of measurement; based on the meter, the gram, and the liter.

mg/kg/day formula for solving dosage calculations based on the patient's weight in kilograms.

microdrip the most commonly used drip rate; 60 gtts/mL.

milliequivalent (mEq) unit of measurement based on the number of grams of a drug in 1 mL of a normal solution.

misbranded drug a drug that has been misleadingly or fraudulently labeled.

misdemeanor an offense or infraction less serious than a felony.

mitigate to lessen or decrease severity.

modem a hardware device used for connecting computer systems that are remotely located, via a telephone line or cable; can be installed either internally or externally.

monitor the visual display screen of the computer system.

monocyte a type of white blood cell.

monograph a detailed document pertaining to a specific drug.

monosaccharide the simplest form of carbohydrate (e.g., glucose, fructose).

mouse a device that rolls on a hard, flat surface and controls the movement of the cursor, or pointer, on the screen.

mucopurulent containing or composed of mucus and pus.

multiple sclerosis (MS) a chronic, inflammatory disease of the white matter areas of the brain and spinal cord in the central nervous system. In later stages of the disease, some level of permanent disability affects the patient.

muscle a specialized tissue that contracts when stimulated.

mydriatic causing dilation of the pupil of the eye.

myocyte a muscle cell.

narcolepsy a condition characterized by frequent and uncontrolled periods of deep sleep.

National Drug Code (NDC) number a unique identifying number assigned to each drug by the manufacturer.

negative feedback the process by which the body is able to return to homeostasis.

neighborhood pharmacy an independent pharmacy that is privately owned, small in size, and usually fills an average of 100 to 300 prescriptions per day.

neonate child from birth to one month of age.

net profit the money left over after you have paid invoice cost (cost of goods sold) and overhead.

neutropenia a disease in which there is an abnormal number of the white blood cells that are responsible for fighting infections.

nomenclature set of names; way of naming.

noncompliance when a patient does not follow a prescribed drug regimen.

nonconsequentialism the theory that certain actions, in and of themselves, are wrong.

nonverbal communication the imparting or interchanging of thoughts, opinions, or information without the use of spoken words.

numerator the top value of a fraction; placed above the fraction line.

nurse practitioner (NP) an individual who is licensed to work closely with a physician in providing patient care and typically may prescribe medications under the supervision of a physician.

nursing home facility that provides skilled and custodial care to older Americans who do not need the intensive, acute care of a hospital but who can no longer manage independent living.

occlusive closing or blocking; refers to a substance that closes or covers a wound and keeps the air from reaching the wound.

ointment a semisolid topical preparation that is applied to the skin or mucous membranes.

oleaginous containing oil; having oil-like properties.

oocyte an immature egg.

operating system the primary software program used to connect the various hardware components of a computer and allow them to perform their essential functions.

ophthalmic pertaining to the eye.

otic for or of the ear.

otitis media infection and inflammation of the middle ear.

outpatient pharmacy a pharmacy that is available to patients who are being discharged from the hospital or who are being treated by a physician without requiring overnight admission.

output devices hardware devices that produce and release data in a visual or tangible, printed form.

ovaries the female reproductive organs that produce eggs.

over-the-counter (OTC) products medications and devices that do not require a prescription for purchase and use.

ovulation the process in which the ovarian follicle ruptures and releases the egg.

ovum a mature egg.

palliative reducing the severity of symptoms.

parasite an organism that lives on or inside another organism.

parenteral nutrition complex admixtures used to provide nutritional support to patients who are unable to take in adequate nutrients through the gastrointestinal tract.

pathogen a disease-causing microorganism.

patient prescription stock system a system in which medication orders are reviewed, prepared, and verified, and then the medications are taken to the floor and dispensed to the patient.

patient profile an electronic record, stored in the pharmacy computer system, that details the patient's personal and billing information, prescription records, and medical conditions.

pepsin a digestive enzyme needed to break down food proteins.

pepsinogen precursor to pepsin.

percent strength representation of the number of grams of active ingredient contained in 100 mL.

% Volume/Volume (%v/v) percent strength concentration of a liquid active ingredient contained within a liquid base.

% Weight/Volume (%w/v) percent strength concentration of a solid active ingredient contained within a liquid base.

% Weight/Weight (%w/w) percent strength concentration of a solid active ingredient contained within a solid base.

peripheral nervous system (PNS) all parts of the nervous system excluding the brain and spinal cord.

personal digital assistant (PDA) a handheld electronic device that is battery powered and operates like a computer.

pH the measure of acidity or alkalinity of a solution or substance; 7 is the neutral point on this scale (less than 7 is acidic and greater than 7 is alkaline).

phagocyte a specialized cell that engulfs and ingests other cells.

pharmacist an educated, skilled individual licensed to practice pharmacy and dispense medication.

pharmacist in charge (PIC) an individual designated on the records of the State Board of Pharmacy as the primary, onsite pharmacist.

pharmacodynamics the study of the biochemical and physiologic effects of drugs and their mechanisms of action.

pharmacogenomics the study of individual genetic differences in response to drug therapy.

pharmacokinetics the study of the processes of absorption, distribution, metabolism, and excretion of drugs; the study of the time course of a drug and its metabolites in the body following drug administration.

pharmacology the study of drugs.

pharmacopoeia a compilation or listing of pharmaceutical products that also contains their formulas and methods of preparation.

pharmacy the profession of preparing and dispensing medications, as well as supplying drug-related information to patients and consumers.

pharmacy clerk/cashier a noncertified/unlicensed individual who is authorized to do only nonpharmacy-related tasks such as operating the cash register.

pharmacy manager an individual, almost always a pharmacist, who is appointed to supervise all aspects of the daily pharmacy operations.

pharmacy technician an educated, skilled individual trained to work in a pharmacy, under the supervision of a pharmacist.

pharynx the part of the throat from the back of the nasal cavity to the larynx.

physician assistant (PA) a licensed individual who is trained to coordinate patient care under the supervision of a medical or osteopathic doctor.

piggyback bags minibags that hold 50 mL or 100 mL of solution and are used to administer drugs intermittently.

pigmentation color.

pitch the property of sound that is determined by the frequency of sound wave vibrations reaching the ear.

plaintiff the party that initiates a legal action.

plaque a fatty deposit that is high in cholesterol.

POE system a point-of-entry computer system, networked within the health system to allow prescribers and nurses to enter medication orders directly for the pharmacy;

sometimes referred to as a computerized physician order entry (CPOE) system.

polydipsia the ingestion of abnormally large amounts of fluids.

polyphagia excessive hunger or eating.

polypharmacy the administration of more medications than clinically indicated.

polyuria excessive urination.

powder a solid dosage form made from blended active ingredients and excipients.

precipitate a solid that forms within a solution.

prefix a part of a word attached to the beginning of the root word that gives a specific meaning to the root.

prescription an order, by an authorized individual, for the preparation or dispensing of a medication.

priapism a painful, extended-duration erection.

printer the primary output device of a computer system, used to produce paper documents.

PRN order a medication order used when a patient is to receive a medication only as necessary, as with pain medication.

processing components hardware devices used to organize, manage, and store data.

processor a company hired by the insurer to process claims.

profession an occupation that requires advanced education and training.

profit the difference between the selling price and the costs associated with a product. There are two types of profit calculated by businesses—gross profit and net profit.

projection a defense mechanism whereby one's own attitudes, feelings, or suppositions are attributed to others.

pronunciation the manner in which someone utters a word.

proper fraction a fraction in which the value of the numerator is smaller than the value of the denominator.

proportion two, or more, equivalent ratios or fractions that both represent the same value.

protease an enzyme that begins protein breakdown.

psoriasis a noncontagious, chronic skin disease characterized by rapid skin cell turnover resulting in thick, red, and scaly skin.

psychotic a mental state characterized by a loss of orientation to reality.

pulmonary edema fluid collection in the pulmonary vessels or lungs.

purchasing system an organization's strategy or procedure for obtaining medications, devices, and products.

quality assurance (QA) a program of activities used to ensure that the procedures used in the preparation of compounded products meet specific standards.

random-access memory (RAM) temporary memory used while information is being input into the computer.

rash a skin condition characterized by redness and inflammation.

ratio the expression of a relationship of two numbers, separated by a colon (:).

rationalization a defense mechanism whereby one's true motivation is concealed by explaining one's actions and feelings in a way that is not threatening.

reaction formation a defense mechanism characterized by action at the opposite extreme of one's true feelings, as overcompensation for unacceptable impulses.

read-only memory (ROM) permanent memory used for essential operating instructions for the computer system.

recall the process in which a drug manufacturer or the FDA requires that specific drugs or devices be returned to the manufacturer because of a specific concern about the recalled product.

receiver the person to whom a communication message is sent.

receptor a molecular structure located on the surface of the cell that binds with a particular chemical or chemicals. When a chemical binds with a receptor, the receptor is stimulated to either produce or inhibit a specific action.

registered nurse (RN) an individual who is registered to assist physicians with specific procedures, administer medications, and provide patient care.

registered pharmacist (RPh) an individual who has completed a bachelor's degree in pharmacy and is licensed to practice pharmacy in a specific state.

registration the process of listing, or being named to a list.

regression a defense mechanism characterized by reverting to an earlier or less mature pattern of feeling or behavior.

repression a defense mechanism characterized by the exclusion of painful impulses, desires, or fears from the conscious mind.

retinopathy a noninflammatory disease in which the retina of the eye is damaged.

rheumatoid arthritis an autoimmune disease that causes chronic inflammation of the joints.

rhinitis inflammation of the nasal passages.

rhinorrhea runny nose.

RNA ribonucleic acid; a nucleic acid needed for the metabolic processes of protein synthesis. In viruses, RNA may carry the genetic information of the virus.

Roman numerals letters and symbols used to represent numbers.

root words words or parts of a word that identify the major meaning of a term.

rosacea a facial skin disorder accompanied by chronic redness and inflammation, and/or acne.

route of administration how a drug is introduced into or on the body.

Rx abbreviation for prescription.

sarcomere one of the segments into which a fibril of striated muscle is divided.

satellite pharmacies subunits of a central pharmacy, located near specific patient care areas in a facility, such as cardiology, operating rooms, and chemotherapy treatment centers.

scanner a hardware device used to input a photographic image into the computer system.

sebum an oily substance produced by the sebaceous glands in the skin.

seizure a disturbance of brain activity characterized by changes in consciousness, activity, and sensation.

semilunar valves include the aortic and pulmonary valves of the heart.

semisynthetic a naturally occurring compound that has been chemically altered.

sender the person who originates or imparts a communication message.

sexually transmitted disease (STD) a disease caused by a pathogen (virus, bacterium, parasite, or fungus) that is spread from person to person through sexual contact.

sexually transmitted infection (STI) a sexually transmitted disease.

side effects drug effects other than the intended one; usually undesirable but not harmful.

SIG specific directions provided on a prescription for the patient to follow, such as dosages, schedule and frequency of administration, and additional instructions.

simple fraction a proper fraction, with both the numerator and denominator reduced to lowest terms.

site of action the location where a drug will exert its effect.

social contract an understood agreement between individual members of a society.

software the programs and applications that control the functioning of computer hardware and direct the operation of the computer.

specific gravity a measure of the density of a substance as compared to water; the specific gravity of water is 1.

standing order a medication order used when a patient is to receive a specific medication at specific intervals throughout the day; also called a scheduled order.

STAT order a medication order used when a patient requires a medication immediately; this is an urgent order and thus takes priority over other orders and requests.

statute a law, decree, or edict.

sterile free from bacteria and other microorganisms.

store manager an individual appointed to supervise all aspects of the daily store operations, including the pharmacy department.

stye an infection of one (or more) of the sebaceous glands of the eye.

subcutaneous parenteral injection in the skin.

sublimation a defense mechanism in which unacceptable instinctual drives and wishes are modified to take more personally and socially acceptable forms.

sublingually under the tongue; preparations may be administered by placing them under the tongue and allowing them to dissolve.

suffix a part of a word attached to the end of the root word that gives a specific meaning to the root.

suppository a solid dosage form used to administer medication by way of the rectum, vagina, or urethral tract.

suspension a liquid containing ingredients that are not soluble in the vehicle.

synovial fluid a liquid that fills the space between the cartilage of each bone; provides smooth movement by lubricating the cartilage.

synthesized produced in a laboratory to imitate a naturally occurring compound.

synthetic drugs that are not naturally occurring; produced in a laboratory.

tablet a solid dosage form that may be administered orally, sublingually, vaginally, or under the skin.

target cell general term referring to a large number of cells, all of which are similar, on which a particular drug is intended to act.

telepharmacy the practice of using advanced telecommunications technology to provide pharmaceutical care to patients in rural and medically underserved areas from a distance.

tendons cords of connective tissue that attach muscle to bone. Injuries can result in strains, ruptures, or inflammation.

teratogenic causing congenital malformations (birth defects).

testes the male reproductive organs that produce sperm.

thrombi blood clots (singular, thrombus).

thrombophlebitis inflammation of a vein with a thrombus.

tinnitus ringing or buzzing in the ear that is not caused by an external source; may be caused by infection or a reaction to a drug.

tolerance when a person requires (psychologically or physiologically) larger doses of a drug to achieve the same effect.

tonicity a state of normal tension of the tissues by virtue of which the parts are kept in shape, alert, and able to function properly.

total parenteral nutrition (TPN) a solution made to supply many of the body's basic nutritional needs via parenteral administration.

toxicity drug poisoning; can be life-threatening or extremely harmful.

trachea the windpipe.

transdermal gel a gel that penetrates the skin and allows the active ingredient to be easily absorbed into the body; also known as a PLO gel.

transfer a situation in which the patient would like to have the prescription refilled at a pharmacy other than where it was originally delivered or filled.

transform alter an organism or a cell itself in the genetic engineering process.

trituration the process of reducing the particle size of a substance by grinding; also known as comminuting.

troche interchangeable term for lozenge, but sometimes prepared in soft form.

type 1 diabetes mellitus a metabolic disorder formerly called insulin-dependent diabetes mellitus (IDDM).

type 2 diabetes mellitus a metabolic disorder formerly called noninsulin-dependent diabetes mellitus (NIDDM).

unit-dose a distribution system in which each medication order is filled in the pharmacy in a way that provides each dose in a package ready to administer to the patient. Usually, not more than a 24-hour supply is dispensed at one time.

urobilinogen a substance produced by the breakdown of bilirubin.

vector an organism that does not itself cause disease, but spreads disease by distributing or carrying pathogens from one host to another.

venules the smallest veins.

veracity truthfulness; the quality of conforming with the truth.

verbal communication the imparting or interchanging of thoughts, opinions, or information through the use of spoken words.

viscous thick; almost jelly-like.

void empty the bladder.

volatile evaporates rapidly.

volume the loudness of a communication.

volume per hour (mL/hour) the amount of fluid, or solution, that will be administered to the patient intravenously per hour.

water-soluble dissolvable in water; describes drugs that are composed mostly of water and can be excreted by the kidneys.

white matter a major component of the CNS, composed of myelinated nerve tissue that is white in color.

written communication the imparting or interchanging of thoughts, opinions, or information through the use of written words.

Young's rule formula for solving pediatric dosage calculations based on the patient's age in years.

Index

Page references followed by "f" indicate figure; and those followed by "t" indicate table.